Pharmacology and Pharmacotherapeutics

Pharmacology and Pharmacotherapeutics

TWENTY-SEVENTH EDITION

R.S. SATOSKAR
M.B.B.S., B.Sc. (Med.), Ph.D. (Sheffield)
Formerly, Professor and Head, Department of Pharmacology, Seth G.S. Medical College; T.N. Medical College; L.T.M. Medical College and Associate in Clinical Medicine, K.E.M. Hospital, Mumbai

NIRMALA N. REGE
M.D. & Ph.D. (Pharmacology), D.N.B. (Clin. Pharmacology)
Professor Emeritus, Department of Pharmacology and Therapeutics Seth G.S. Medical College and K.E.M. Hospital, Mumbai
and
Professor, Department of Pharmacology Era's Lucknow Medical College, Lucknow

RAAKHI K. TRIPATHI
M.D. (Pharmacology)
Associate Professor, Department of Pharmacology and Therapeutics Seth G.S. Medical College and K.E.M. Hospital, Mumbai

SANDHYA K. KAMAT
M.D. (Pharmacology)
Professor and Head, Department of Pharmacology and Therapeutics Seth G.S. Medical College and K.E.M. Hospital, Mumbai

ELSEVIER

Co-published with

Popular Prakashan
www.popularprakashan.com

ELSEVIER

RELX India Pvt. Ltd.
Registered Office: 818, Indraprakash Building, 8th Floor, 21, Barakhamba Road, New Delhi 110001
Corporate Office: 14th Floor, Building No. 10B, DLF Cyber City, Phase II, Gurgaon-122002, Haryana, India

Popular Prakashan Pvt. Ltd.
Registered Office: 301, Mahalaxmi Chambers, 22, Bhulabhai Desai Road, Mumbai-400026

Pharmacology and Pharmacotherapeutics, 27e, R.S. Satoskar, Nirmala N. Rege, Raakhi K. Tripathi and Sandhya K. Kamat

First Edition, 1969; Russian Edition, 1985; Twentieth Edition, 2007; Reprinted 2007, 2008, July 2008; **Twenty-first Edition, 2009;** Reprinted May 2010, December 2010; **Twenty-second Edition, 2011;** Reprinted July 2012; **Twenty-third Edition, 2013;** Reprinted September 2014; **Twenty-fourth Edition 2015; Twenty-fifth Edition 2017; Twenty-sixth Edition 2021, Twenty-seventh Edition 2024**

ISBN: 978-81-312-6794-3

This Twenty-seventh edition of ***Pharmacology and Pharmacotherapeutics*** by R.S. Satoskar, Nirmala N. Rege, Raakhi K. Tripathi and Sandhya K. Kamat is co-published by arrangement with RELX India Pvt. Ltd. and Popular Prakashan Pvt. Ltd.

First Printed in India 2024, Reprinted 2025

Content Strategist: Arvind Koul
Content Project Manager: Subodh Kumar
Sr Production Executive: Dhan Singh
Cover Design: PealiDezine

Printed in India by Multivista Global Pvt Ltd.

Preface to the Twenty-Seventh Edition

Pharmacology is a vast and ever-evolving discipline, with continuous additions of new drugs and combinations each year. While it is essential to stay updated with the latest advancements, we firmly believe that understanding the fundamental principles and their applications in practice is the key to prescribe rationally. Prescribing is an art and science and has become more intricate than ever before. As future physicians, one must possess the skills to make informed and evidence-based decisions during clinical practice, wherein one treats not the disease but the patient. How the drug is used is far more important than what is used. Sir William Osler said, "*The good physician treats the disease; the great physician treats the patient who has the disease.*" Since its first edition in 1969, this book has laid emphasis on a comprehensive and integrated approach to pharmacology so that the readers can understand how to use the drugs in real-life medical scenarios.

The current competency-based curriculum of National Medical Commission (NMC), India fortunately echoes these thoughts. It has included prescribing competency as one of the essential competencies that students should possess at the time of graduation. Prescribing competency includes a sound knowledge about drugs and apt skills for prescribing drugs while using your professional judgement and experience. The present curriculum also lays stress on clinical skills, communication, professionalism, life-long learning and leadership. The new curriculum has also brought in alterations in the student assessment. The emphasis is on task-oriented questions that assess ability to integrate, analyse and reason rather than recall based questions. Introduction of case scenario based MCQs demands not just application of knowledge learned in the subject but its integration with other disciplines. Such approach requires clinically oriented integrated learning, which has been followed in this book since its first edition.

Since pharmacology is not an isolated discipline but an interconnected web that weaves together relevant elements from other disciplines such as physiology, biochemistry, pathology, microbiology and medicine, the content in the book is presented in a similar fashion. Both the drug information as well as therapeutics have been given equal weightage. Various therapeutic approaches and options have been discussed for clinical conditions based on symptom profiling of patients and variations in disease stages. The importance of counselling has also been highlighted while discussing the management of disease. Ethics related to drug development, writing prescriptions, and managing clinical conditions have been discussed. The approach of this book is patient-oriented and not examination-oriented. It is neither possible nor necessary to remember all the information in this book. We have always believed that pharmacology is not merely memorization; it is a means to an end – the end being optimal patient care. "*The young physician starts life with 20 drugs for each disease, & the old physician ends life with one drug for 20 diseases*" – Sir William Osler.

This book is not only for the second year undergraduate medical students but it continues to remain a companion of graduating students throughout their medical education and beyond. It is updated every 2-3 years so that it can serve as an authentic, reliable and practical source of information for physicians who wish to revisit it during their clinical practice.

Maintaining the tradition, the current edition has undergone extensive revision, with additional coloured figures, boxes and tables to engage the students with the text. All the positive features of earlier edition such as learning objectives, key terms, flow charts, background colour highlights to focus on key points in pharmacology and therapeutics have been retained. At the end of the book case scenario based MCQs have been added, which can challenge the readers to think critically and self- assess their learning. Attention has been paid to keep the text simple and student friendly.

We miss Dr. SD Bhandarkar, who contributed to this book for many years by bringing in clinical relevance and strengthening the integration of basic pharmacology with clinical medicine. He will always remain in our hearts and keep inspiring us while we work on this book. Lastly we wish our readers a fruitful and fulfilling learning through this book. Any feedback and suggestions to strengthen this book are always welcome.

R.S. Satoskar
Nirmala N. Rege
Raakhi K. Tripathi
Sandhya K. Kamat

Mumbai
October 2023

Preface to the First Edition

Pharmacology has undergone phenomenal growth during the last twenty years and drug therapy now forms a major aspect of therapeutics. So far, pharmacology was traditionally associated with the study of drugs in dogs, cats and rats, while therapeutics or clinical application was regarded as an entirely independent and a mystical skill. Now it is generally agreed that the major object of teaching pharmacology to the medical students is to provide a rational basis for choosing and using drugs skilfully to relieve patients' ailments. This is becoming more and more important as the practising doctor is now confronted with so called "newer drugs" at such a great pace that even a full-time pharmacologist sometimes finds it difficult to keep abreast of their merits and demerits. It is highly desirable, therefore, that students of pharmacology should be educated to develop a critical outlook towards various drugs, as they are introduced. This means that book on pharmacology meant for medical students should not only give detailed account of various pharmacological actions but should also furnish a critical appraisal of their present day use in therapeutics. We have attempted in this book to combine these two important aspects. In addition, an outline of experimental evaluation of drugs in animals and man is also provided. While doing this, it was thought essential to give the relevant information from other disciplines like physiology, pathology and clinical medicine. This, though a repetition to a certain extent, is no doubt useful to understand the basis of rational therapeutics. After all, pharmacology is in some respects a bridge between basic medical sciences on one hand and clinical medicine on the other. Most of the presently available text books, except a few classics written by many authors, fail to achieve this goal. It is a common experience of those who teach pharmacology in this country to find it difficult to recommend one single book to the undergraduate medical students. Many books which give excellent information about pharmacological actions treat the therapeutics very cursorily while others that give delightful therapeutics probably assume that students know most of the basic pharmacology. It is not practicable to recommend routinely the classical multi-author books to undergraduate students, as they have many other subjects to go through, which are equally important and advanced. This book is written to fill up this gap between a big book and a concise, less informative work, so that students will get all the necessary information by reading one book. While doing this, obviously we have to restrict the size of the book, lest it would be unwieldy and defeat the very purpose for which it is written. In order to achieve this, history and chemistry are reduced considerably while diagrams are included strictly to facilitate the understanding of the subject. The coverage is given according to the importance of the subject in therapeutics. Wherever multiple drugs of similar type are available, only the important prototype is discussed in detail, while others have received only a brief mention.

Although the book is written mainly for undergraduate medical students, it will also prove useful to postgraduates and practising doctors. The therapeutics part includes many details so that the book would continue to be useful even after passing pharmacology and is expected to serve as a pharmacotherapeutic reference work. The big multi-author books on this subject are no doubt excellent and authoritative but are not easily accessible to practising doctors in an emergency. In such circumstances this book should find its use.

The book is not written 'with an eye on examination' but it is the hope of the authors that by reading this book students would develop an attitude of thinking towards newer drugs which are many times made to appear like "therapeutic marvels". It is not expected that undergraduate students should 'cram' this book and try to remember everything that is given. It is neither possible nor necessary. They are expected to learn the basic pharmacology of the drugs in common clinical use and their rational application in therapeutics. However, the authors will feel rewarded, if students can grasp the ideology and spirit behind presentation of this book.

Drug therapy related to tropical problems is emphasized; this topic is often dismissed summarily in other works of this size. Proprietary names are included wherever necessary so that their pharmacological identity is recognised by the reader. No detailed reference list is given as this would have added many more pages. Instead, the books, reviews, symposia and monographs referred to are enlisted at the end of the book. The enthusiastic reader may refer to these for a more extensive reference list. Preparations included in the Indian Pharmacopoeia are marked as I.P. and those included in British Pharmacopoeia are listed in a separate list at the end.

It is not possible to present a book of such a size without generous help of others and the authors are deeply grateful to their many colleagues at Seth G.S. Medical College and Lokmanya Tilak Municipal Medical College, Bombay. Particularly, the help rendered by Drs. B.S. Kulkarni, S.M. Chittal, S.V. Gokhale, M.G. Wagh, C.H. Kewalramani, Mr. N.K. Dadkar, Mr. V.S. Jathar, Dr. S.M. Karandikar and Miss P. Mirwankar is gratefully acknowledged. We also would like to express our grateful thanks to many authors and publishers who promptly conceded our requests and granted permission to reproduce certain tables and diagrams, as indicated in the text. We are greatly indebted to Dr. A.F. Golwalla, Hon. Professor of Medicine, Seth G.S. Medical College and K.E.M. Hospital, Bombay for his encouragement and permission to reproduce E.C.G. records. Finally, our thanks are due to Popular Prakashan and Popular Press (Bom.) Pvt. Ltd., who as publishers and printers respectively are responsible for delivering this book in your hand expeditiously.

R.S. Satoskar
A.K. Kale
S.D. Bhandarkar

Bombay,
November, 1968

Acknowledgements

We thank our residents Dr. Ajinkya Parhe, Dr. Sujit Bhilwade, Dr. Pooja Redkar, Dr. Soham Sinha, Dr. Abhilash Saravanan, Dr. Jay Maradia, Dr. Ajay Gattani, Dr. Vinoodh Kumar Kumaresan and Dr. Rhea Monterio for their help in drawing additional figures, conducting literature search, participating in discussions while reworking on this edition and reading the proofs.

We sincerely thank Mr. Harsha Bhatkal, Publisher, Popular Prakashan Pvt. Ltd., Ms. Asmita Mohite, and Ms. Armaity Motafram for converting our manuscript into an attractive book and excellent co-operation. We thank Mr. Ram Das, the manuscript designer for his painstaking efforts. We appreciate the creativity of PealiDezine for the cover design. We acknowledge the support of Elsevier India and its staff for the help rendered.

Table of Contents

SECTION 1
General Pharmacology

SECTION 2
Drugs Acting on the Central Nervous System

SECTION 3
Local Anaesthetics

SECTION 4
Autonomic Nervous System

SECTION 5
Other Biogenic Amines and Polypeptides

SECTION 6
Drugs Used in Respiratory Disorders

SECTION 7
Cardiovascular Drugs

SECTION 8
Drugs Acting on Blood and Blood Forming Organs

SECTION 9
Drugs Affecting Renal Functions

SECTION 10
Drugs Used in Disorders of the Gastrointestinal Tract

SECTION 11
Oxytocics and Uterine Relaxants

SECTION 12
Chemotherapy

Dosage Note

Pharmacology and drug therapy, like medicine, is an everchanging science. As new information accumulates, changes in drug therapy are inevitable. The authors and publishers of this book have taken special care to provide drug information and dosage schedules, that are generally in accord with the accepted standards at the time of publication. However, it may be noted that in view of the possibility of human error or advances in medicinal sciences, such therapeutic approaches are liable to change. Neither the authors nor the publishers nor any other party who has been involved in the publication of this work warrants that the information contained herein is in every respect accurate and complete. We urge the readers to confirm the information with other sources and refer to the manufacturers' recommendation for all dosages, especially for the new drugs and for those used infrequently in clinical practice.

Competency Code	Competency	Core (Y/N)	Chapter No.
PH1.1	Define and describe the principles of pharmacology and pharmacotherapeutics*	Y	1, 2, 3, 5
PH1.2	Describe the basis of Evidence based medicine and Therapeutic drug monitoring	Y	1, 3, 4
PH1.3	Enumerate and identify drug formulations and drug delivery systems	Y	1, 69
PH1.4	Describe absorption, distribution, metabolism & excretion of drugs	Y	1
PH1.5	Describe general principles of mechanism of drug action	Y	2, 5
PH1.6	Describe principles of Pharmacovigilance & ADR reporting systems	Y	4
PH1.7	Define, identify and describe the management of adverse drug reactions (ADR)	Y	2, 23, 52
PH1.8	Identify and describe the management of drug interactions	Y	3
PH1.9	Describe nomenclature of drugs i.e. generic, branded drugs	Y	3, 4
PH1.10	Describe parts of a correct, complete and legible generic prescription. Identify errors in prescription and correct appropriately	Y	3
PH1.11	Describe various routes of drug administration, eg., oral, SC, IV, IM, SL	Y	1, 20, 70
PH1.12	Calculate the dosage of drugs using appropriate formulae for an individual patient, including children, elderly and patient with renal dysfunction.	Y	1, 3
PH1.13	Describe mechanism of action, types, doses, side effects, indications and contraindications of adrenergic and anti-adrenergic drugs	Y	17, 18, 70
PH1.14	Describe mechanism of action, types, doses, side effects, indications and contraindications of cholinergic and anticholinergic drugs	Y	17, 19, 20, 70
PH1.15	Describe mechanism/s of action, types, doses, side effects, indications and contraindications of skeletal muscle relaxants	Y	22
PH1.16	Describe mechanism/s of action, types, doses, side effects, indications and contraindications of the drugs which act by modulating autacoids, including: anti-histaminics, 5-HT modulating drugs, NSAIDs, drugs for gout, anti-rheumatic drugs, drugs for migraine	Y	11, 23, 24, 25, 70, 73
PH1.17	Describe the mechanism/s of action, types, doses, side effects, indications and contraindications of local anesthetics	Y	16, 70
PH1.18	Describe the mechanism/s of action, types, doses, side effects, indications and contraindications of general anaesthetics, and pre- anesthetic medications	Y	7
PH1.19	Describe the mechanism/s of action, types, doses, side effects, indications and contraindications of the drugs which act on CNS, (including anxiolytics, sedatives & hypnotics, anti-psychotic, anti- depressant drugs, anti-maniacs, opioid agonists and antagonists, drugs used for neurodegenerative disorders, anti-epileptics drugs)	Y	8, 9, 10, 13, 14, 15
PH1.20	Describe the effects of acute and chronic ethanol intake	Y	6
PH1.21	Describe the symptoms and management of methanol and ethanol poisonings	Y	6
PH1.22	Describe drugs of abuse (dependence, addiction, stimulants, depressants, psychedelics, drugs used for criminal offences)	Y	3, 7, 8, 10, 12, 13, 18, 21
PH1.23	Describe the process and mechanism of drug deaddiction	Y	3, 8, 10, 18, 21
PH1.24	Describe the mechanism/s of action, types, doses, side effects, indications and contraindications of the drugs affecting renal systems including diuretics, antidiuretics- vasopressin and analogues	Y	30, 31, 37

*Disease-specific therapeutic principles run across the book, available in multiple chapters, viz. (Chapters 8, 9, 11, 13, 14, 15, 19, 23, 24, 27, 29, 30, 31, 32, 37, 38, 40, 41, 50, 51, 52, 59, 62, 64, 68, 69, 70, 71).

(Continued)

Competency Code	Competency	Core (Y/N)	Chapter No.
PH1.25	Describe the mechanism/s of action, types, doses, side effects, indications and contraindications of the drugs acting on blood, like anticoagulants, antiplatelets, fibrinolytics, plasma expanders	Y	32, 33
PH1.26	Describe mechanisms of action, types, doses, side effects, indications and contraindications of the drugs modulating the renin- angiotensin and aldosterone system	Y	30, 31
PH1.27	Describe the mechanisms of action, types, doses, side effects, indications and contraindications of antihypertensive drugs and drugs used in shock	Y	23, 30, 32
PH1.28	Describe the mechanisms of action, types, doses, side effects, indications and contraindications of the drugs used in ischemic heart disease (stable, unstable angina and myocardial infarction), peripheral vascular disease	Y	29
PH1.29	Describe the mechanisms of action, types, doses, side effects, indications and contraindications of the drugs used in congestive heart failure	Y	31
PH1.30	Describe the mechanisms of action, types, doses, side effects, indications and contraindications of the antiarrhythmics	N	28
PH1.31	Describe the mechanisms of action, types, doses, side effects, indications and contraindications of the drugs used in the management of dyslipidemias	Y	38
PH1.32	Describe the mechanism/s of action, types, doses, side effects, indications and contraindications of drugs used in bronchial asthma and COPD	Y	27
PH1.33	Describe the mechanism of action, types, doses, side effects, indications and contraindications of the drugs used in cough (antitussives, expectorants/ mucolytics)	Y	26
PH1.34	Describe the mechanism/s of action, types, doses, side effects, indications and contraindications of the drugs used as below: 1. Acid-peptic disease and GERD 2. Antiemetics and prokinetics 3. Antidiarrhoeals 4. Laxatives 5. Inflammatory Bowel Disease 6. Irritable Bowel Disorders, biliary and pancreatic diseases	Y	38, 39, 40, 41
PH1.35	Describe the mechanism/s of action, types, doses, side effects, indications and contraindications of drugs used in hematological disorders like: 1. Drugs used in anemias 2. Colony Stimulating factors	Y	34, 35, 36
PH1.36	Describe the mechanism of action, types, doses, side effects, indications and contraindications of drugs used in endocrine disorders (diabetes mellitus, thyroid disorders and osteoporosis)	Y	62, 63, 68
PH1.37	Describe the mechanisms of action, types, doses, side effects, indications and contraindications of the drugs used as sex hormones, their analogues and anterior Pituitary hormones	Y	61, 62, 64, 65, 66, 67
PH1.38	Describe the mechanism of action, types, doses, side effects, indications and contraindications of corticosteroids	Y	64, 70
PH1.39	Describe mechanism of action, types, doses, side effects, indications and contraindications the drugs used for contraception	Y	66
PH1.40	Describe mechanism of action, types, doses, side effects, indications and contraindications of 1. Drugs used in the treatment of infertility, and 2. Drugs used in erectile dysfunction	Y	66, 67
PH1.41	Describe the mechanisms of action, types, doses, side effects, indications and contraindications of uterine relaxants and stimulants	Y	42
PH1.42	Describe general principles of chemotherapy	Y	43, 49
PH1.43	Describe and discuss the rational use of antimicrobials including antibiotic stewardship program	Y	49

Competency Code	Competency	Core (Y/N)	Chapter No.
PH1.44	Describe the first line antitubercular dugs, their mechanisms of action, side effects and doses.	Y	52
PH1.45	Describe the dugs used in MDR and XDR Tuberculosis	Y	52
PH1.46	Describe the mechanisms of action, types, doses, side effects, indications and contraindications of antileprotic drugs	Y	53
PH1.47	Describe the mechanisms of action, types, doses, side effects, indications and contraindications of the drugs used in malaria, KALA-AZAR, amebiasis and intestinal helminthiasis	Y	54, 55, 56, 58
PH1.48	Describe the mechanisms of action, types, doses, side effects, indications and contraindications of the drugs used in UTI/ STD and viral diseases including HIV	Y	50, 51, 56, 57
PH1.49	Describe mechanism of action, classes, side effects, indications and contraindications of anticancer drugs	Y	59
PH1.50	Describe mechanisms of action, types, doses, side effects, indications and contraindications of immunomodulators and management of organ transplant rejection	Y	70, 72
PH1.51	Describe occupational and environmental pesticides, food adulterants, pollutants and insect repellents	Y	19, 60, 74, 75
PH1.52	Describe management of common poisoning, insecticides, common sting and bites	Y	2,19, 23, 71
PH1.53	Describe heavy metal poisoning and chelating agents	N	74
PH1.54	Describe vaccines and their uses	Y	52, 71
PH1.55	Describe and discuss the following National Health Programmes including Immunisation, Tuberculosis, Leprosy, Malaria, HIV, Filaria, Kala Azar, Diarrhoeal diseases, Anaemia & nutritional disorders, Blindness, Non-communicable diseases, cancer and Iodine deficiency	Y	51, 52, 53, 54, 58, 62, 71, 77
PH1.56	Describe basic aspects of Geriatric and Pediatric pharmacology	Y	3
PH1.57	Describe drugs used in skin disorders	Y	69
PH1.58	Describe drugs used in Ocular disorders	Y	70
PH1.59	Describe and discuss the following: Essential medicines, Fixed dose combinations, Over the counter drugs, Herbal medicines	Y	3
PH1.60	Describe and discuss Pharmacogenomics and Pharmacoeconomics	N	1
PH1.61	Describe and discuss dietary supplements and nutraceuticals	N	38, 77
PH1.62	Describe and discuss antiseptics and disinfectants	Y	60
PH1.63	Describe Drug Regulations, acts and other legal aspects	Y	4, Practical
PH1.64	Describe overview of drug development, Phases of clinical trials and Good Clinical Practice	Y	4
PH2.1	Demonstrate understanding of the use of various dosage forms (oral/local/ parenteral; solid/liquid)	Y	Practical
PH2.2	Prepare oral rehydration solution from ORS packet and explain its use	Y	39
PH2.3	Demonstrate the appropriate setting up of an intravenous drip in a simulated environment	Y	Practical
PH2.4	Demonstrate the correct method of calculation of drug dosage in patients including those used in special situations	Y	1, 3
PH3.1	Write a rational, correct and legible generic prescription for a given condition and communicate the same to the patient	Y	3
PH3.2	Perform and interpret a critical appraisal (audit) of a given prescription	Y	Practical
PH3.3	Perform a critical evaluation of the drug promotional literature	Y	Practical

(Continued)

Competency Code	Competency	Core (Y/N)	Chapter No.
PH3.4	To recognise and report an adverse drug reaction	Y	2, 40
PH3.5	To prepare and explain a list of P-drugs for a given case/condition	Y	3
PH3.6	Demonstrate how to optimize interaction with pharmaceutical representative to get authentic information on drugs	N	Practical
PH3.7	Prepare a list of essential medicines for a healthcare facility	Y	3
PH3.8	Communicate effectively with a patient on the proper use of prescribed medication	Y	3
PH4.1	Administer drugs through various routes in a simulated environment using mannequins	Y	Practical
PH4.2	Demonstrate the effects of drugs on blood pressure (vasopressor and vaso-depressors with appropriate blockers) using computer aided learning	Y	2, 18, 19
PH5.1	Communicate with the patient with empathy and ethics on all aspects of drug use	Y	Communication skill
PH5.2	Communicate with the patient regarding optimal use of a) drug therapy, b) devices and c) storage of medicines	Y	Communication skill
PH5.3	Motivate patients with chronic diseases to adhere to the prescribed management by the health care provider	Y	Communication skill
PH5.4	Explain to the patient the relationship between cost of treatment and patient compliance	Y	Communication skill
PH5.5	Demonstrate an understanding of the caution in prescribing drugs likely to produce dependence and recommend the line of management	Y	Communication skill
PH5.6	Demonstrate ability to educate public & patients about various aspects of drug use including drug dependence and OTC drugs	Y	Communication skill
PH5.7	Demonstrate an understanding of the legal and ethical aspects of prescribing drugs	Y	Communication skill
PY3.5	Discuss the action of neuro-muscular blocking agents	Y	22
MI1.6	Describe the mechanisms of drug resistance, methods of antimicrobial susceptibility testing and monitoring of antimicrobial therapy.	Y	49
MI3.6	Describe the etio-pathogenesis of Acid Peptic Disease (APD) and the clinical course. Discuss the diagnosis and management of the causative agent of APD	Y	41
CM19.1	Define and describe the concept of Essential Medicine List (EML)	Y	3
CM19.2	Describe roles of essential medicine in primary health care	Y	3
CM19.3	Describe counterfeit medicine and its prevention	Y	3
FM4.25	Clinical research & Ethics: Discuss human experimentation including clinical trials	N	4
FM8.2	Define the terms Toxicology, Toxicology and poison	Y	1
FM8.6	Describe the general symptoms, principles of diagnosis and management of common poisons encountered in India	Y	2
FM8.8	Describe basic methodologies in treatment of poisoning: decontamination, supportive therapy, antidote therapy, procedures of enhanced elimination	Y	2
FM9.1	Describe General Principles and basic methodologies in treatment of poisoning: decontamination, supportive therapy, antidote therapy, procedures of enhanced elimination with regard to Caustics Inorganic – sulphuric, nitric, and hydrochloric acid Organic- Carboloic Acid (phenol), Oxalic and acetylsalicylic acids.	Y	11, 60
FM9.2	Describe General Principles and basic methodologies in treatment of poisoning: decontamination, supportive therapy, antidote therapy, procedures of enhanced elimination with regard to Phosphorus, Iodine, Barium	Y	2

Competency Code	Competency	Core (Y/N)	Chapter No.
FM9.3	Describe General Principles and basic methodologies in treatment of poisoning: decontamination, supportive therapy, antidote therapy, procedures of enhanced elimination with regard to Arsenic, lead, mercury, copper, iron, cadmium and thallium	Y	34, 74
FM9.4	Describe General Principles and basic methodologies in treatment of poisoning: decontamination, supportive therapy, antidote therapy, procedures of enhanced elimination with regard to Ethanol, methanol, ethylene glycol	Y	6
FM9.5	Describe General Principles and basic methodologies in treatment of poisoning: decontamination, supportive therapy, antidote therapy, procedures of enhanced elimination with regard to Organophosphates, Carbamates, Organochlorines, Pyrethroids, Paraquat, Aluminium and Zinc phosphide	Y	19, 60
FM9.6	Describe General Principles and basic methodologies in treatment of poisoning: decontamination, supportive therapy, antidote therapy, procedures of enhanced elimination with regard to Ammonia, carbon monoxide, hydrogen cyanide & derivatives, methyl isocyanate, tear (riot control) gases	Y	75
FM10.1	Describe General Principles and basic methodologies in treatment of poisoning: decontamination, supportive therapy, antidote therapy, procedures of enhanced elimination with regard to: i. Antipyretics – Paracetamol, Salicylates ii. A nti-Infectives (Common antibiotics – an overview) iii. N europsychotoxicology Barbiturates, benzodiazepines, phenytoin, lithium, haloperidol, neuroleptics, tricyclics iv. N arcotic Analgesics, Anaesthetics, and Muscle Relaxants v. Cardiovascular Toxicology Cardiotoxic plants – oleander, odollam, aconite, digitalis vi. Gastro-Intestinal and Endocrinal Drugs – Insulin	Y	6, 8, 9, 10 11, 12, 13, 14, 19, 20, 22, 31
DR5.3	Enumerate and describe the pharmacology, administration and adverse reaction of pharmacotherapies for scabies	Y	69
DR7.3	Describe the pharmacology and action of antifungal (systemic and topical). agents Enumerate side effects of antifungal therapy	Y	48
DR8.7	Enumerate the indications and describe the pharmacology, administration and adverse reaction of pharmacotherapies for common viral illnesses of the skin	Y	51, 69
DR9.4	Enumerate, describe and identify lepra reactions and supportive measures and therapy of lepra reactions	Y	53
DR9.5	Enumerate the indications and describe the pharmacology, administration and adverse reaction of pharmacotherapies for various classes of leprosy based on National Guidelines	Y	53
DR9.6	Describe the treatment of Leprosy based on WHO guidelines	Y	53
DR10.3	Enumerate the indications and describe the pharmacology, administration and adverse reaction of pharmacotherapies for syphilis	Y	51
DR10.8	Enumerate the indications and describe the pharmacology, indications and adverse reactions of drugs used in the non- syphilitic sexually transmitted diseases (chancroid, donovanosis and LGV)	Y	51
DR11.3	Enumerate the indications and describe the pharmacology, administration and adverse reaction of pharmacotherapies for dermatologic lesions in HIV	Y	51
DR14.5	Enumerate the indications and describe the pharmacology indications and adverse reactions of drugs used in the urticaria and angioedema	Y	23
DR15.3	Enumerate the indications and describe the pharmacology indications and adverse reactions of topical and systemic drugs used in treatment of pyoderma	Y	69
AS4.1	Describe and discuss the pharmacology of drugs used in induction and maintenance of general anaesthesia (including intravenous and inhalation induction agents, opiate and non-opiate analgesics, depolarising and non-depolarising muscle relaxants, anticholinesterases	Y	7, 19, 22
AS4.3	Observe and describe the principles and the practical aspects of induction and maintenance of anesthesia	Y	7

(Continued)

Competency Code	Competency	Core (Y/N)	Chapter No.
AS5.4	Observe and describe the pharmacology and correct use of commonly used drugs and adjuvant agents in regional anesthesia	Y	16
AS8.3	Describe the pharmacology and use of drugs in the management of pain	Y	11
AS8.4	Describe the principles of pain management in palliative care	Y	11, 59
AS8.5	Describe the principles of pain management in the terminally ill	Y	11, 59
PS4.4	Describe the treatment of alcohol and substance abuse disorders including behavioural and pharmacologic therapy	Y	6
PS4.6	Enumerate and describe the pharmacologic basis and side effects of drugs used in alcohol and substance abuse	Y	6
PS5.3	Describe the treatment of schizophrenia including behavioural and pharmacologic therapy	Y	13
PS5.5	Enumerate and describe the pharmacologic basis and side effects of drugs used in schizophrenia	Y	13
PS6.4	Describe the treatment of depression including behavioural and pharmacologic therapy	Y	14
PS6.6	Enumerate and describe the pharmacologic basis and side effects of drugs used in depression	Y	14
PS7.4	Describe the treatment of bipolar disorders including behavioural and pharmacologic therapy	Y	14
PS7.6	Enumerate and describe the pharmacologic basis and side effects of drugs used in bipolar disorders	Y	14
PS8.4	Describe the treatment of anxiety disorders including behavioural and pharmacologic therapy	Y	14
PS8.6	Enumerate and describe the pharmacologic basis and side effects of drugs used in anxiety disorders	Y	14
PS18.1	Enumerate the indications and describe the pharmacology, dose and side effects of commonly use drugs in psychiatric disorders	Y	13, 14
IM1.24	Describe and discuss the pharmacology of drugs including indications & contraindications in the management of heart failure including diuretics, ACE inhibitors, Beta blockers, aldosterone antagonists and cardiac glycosides	Y	31
IM1.27	Describe and discuss the role of penicillin prophylaxis in the prevention of rheumatic heart disease	Y	44
IM2.15	Discuss and describe the medications used in patients with an acute coronary syndrome based on the clinical presentation	Y	29, 33
IM2.18	Discuss and describe the indications, formulations, doses, side effects and monitoring for drugs used in the management of dyslipidemia	Y	38
IM2.20	Discuss and describe the assessment and relief of pain in acute coronary syndromes	Y	29
IM2.23	Describe and discuss the indications for nitrates, anti platelet agents, gpIIb - IIIa inhibitors, beta blockers, ACE inhibitors etc in the management of coronary syndromes	Y	29, 33
IM3.12	Select, describe and prescribe based on the most likely aetiology, an appropriate empirical antimicrobial based on the pharmacology and antimicrobial spectrum	Y	43, 44, 47, 49
IM3.13	Select, describe and prescribe based on culture and sensitivity appropriate empaling antimicrobial based on the pharmacology and antimicrobial spectrum.	Y	44, 47, 49
IM4.22	Describe and discuss the pharmacology, indications, adverse reactions, interactions of antimalarial drugs and basis of resistance	Y	54
IM4.23	Prescribe drugs for malaria based on the species identified, prevalence of drug resistance and National Programs	Y	54

Competency Code	Competency	Core (Y/N)	Chapter No.
IM4.26	Counsel the patient on malarial prevention	Y	54
IM5.7	Enumerate and describe the causes and pathophysiology of drug induced liver injury	Y	2
IM5.16	Describe and discuss the management of hepatitis, cirrhosis, portal hypertension, ascites spontaneous, bacterial peritonitis and hepatic encephalopathy	Y	37, 40, 45
IM6.13	Describe and enumerate the indications and side effects of drugs for bacterial, viral and other types of diarrhea	Y	39
IM6.17	Discuss and describe the principles of HAART, the classes of antiretrovirals used, adverse reactions and interactions	Y	51
IM6.18	Discuss and describe the principles and regimens used in post exposure prophylaxis	Y	51
IM7.20	Select, prescribe and communicate appropriate medications for relief of joint pain	Y	73
IM7.21	Select, prescribe and communicate preventive therapy for crystalline arthropathies	Y	73
IM7.22	Select, prescribe and communicate treatment option for systemic rheumatologic conditions	Y	73
IM7.23	Describe the basis for biologic and disease modifying therapy in rheumatologic diseases	Y	73
IM8.14	Develop an appropriate treatment plan for essential hypertension	Y	30
IM8.15	Recognise, prioritise and manage hypertensive emergencies	Y	30
IM9.14	Prescribe replacement therapy with iron, B12, folate	Y	34
IM10.25	Identify and describe the priorities in the management of ARF including diet, volume management, alteration in doses of drugs, monitoring and indications for dialysis	Y	37
IM11.16	Discuss and describe the pharmacologic therapies for diabetes their indications, contraindications, adverse reactions and interactions	Y	63
IM11.18	Describe and discuss the pharmacology, indications, adverse reactions and interactions of drugs used in the prevention and treatment of target organ damage and complications of Type II Diabetes including neuropathy, nephropathy, retinopathy, hypertension, dyslipidemia and cardiovascular disease	Y	30, 38, 63
IM12.13	Describe the pharmacology, indications, adverse reaction, interactions of thyroxine and antithyroid drugs	Y	62
IM12.14	Write and communicate to the patient appropriately a prescription for thyroxine based on age, sex, and clinical and biochemical status	Y	62
IM12.15	Describe and discuss the indications of thionamide therapy, radio iodine therapy and General Surgery in the management of thyrotoxicosis	Y	62
IM14.13	Describe and enumerate the indications, pharmacology and side effects of pharmacotherapy for obesity	Y	38
IM15.14	Describe and enumerate the indications, pharmacology and side effects of pharmacotherapy of pressors used in the treatment of Upper GI bleed	Y	33
IM15.15	Describe and enumerate the indications, pharmacology and side effects of pharmacotherapy of acid peptic disease including Helicobacter pylori	Y	41
IM16.13	Describe and enumerate the indications, pharmacology and side effects of pharmacotherapy for parasitic causes of diarrhea	Y	39
IM16.14	Describe and enumerate the indications, pharmacology and side effects of pharmacotherapy for bacterial and viral diarrhea	Y	39
IM16.16	Describe and enumerate the indications, pharmacology and side effects of pharmacotherapy including immunotherapy	Y	39
IM17.11	Describe the indications, pharmacology, dose, side effects of abortive therapy in migraine	Y	24

(Continued)

Competency Code	Competency	Core (Y/N)	Chapter No.
IM17.12	Describe the indications, pharmacology, dose, side effects of prophylactic therapy in migraine	Y	24
IM17.13	Describe the pharmacology, dose, adverse reactions and regimens of drugs used in the treatment of bacterial, tubercular and viral meningitis	Y	46, 52
IM19.8	Discuss and describe the pharmacology, dose, side effects and interactions used in the drug therapy of Parkinson's syndrome	Y	15
IM19.9	Enumerate the indications for use of surgery and botulinum toxin in the treatment of movement disorders	Y	22
IM20.7	Enumerate the indications and describe the pharmacology, dose, adverse reactions, hypersensitivity reactions of anti-snake venom	Y	71
IM20.8	Describe the diagnosis, initial approach, stabilisation and therapy of scorpion envenomation	N	71
IM20.9	Describe the diagnosis, initial approach, stabilisation and therapy of bee sting allergy	N	23
IM21.1	Describe the initial approach to the stabilisation of the patient who presents with poisoning	Y	2
IM21.2	Enumerate the common plant poisons seen in your area and describe their toxicology, clinical features, prognosis and specific approach to detoxification	Y	10, 20, 31
IM22.3	Describe the approach to the management of hypercalcemia	N	68
PE13.5	Propose a management plan for Fe Deficiency Anaemia	Y	34
PE14.1	Discuss the risk factors, clinical features, diagnosis and management of Lead Poisoning	N	74
PE14.3	Discuss the risk factors, clinical features, diagnosis and management of Organo phosphorous poisoning	N	19
PE14.4	Discuss the risk factors, clinical features, diagnosis and management of paracetamol Poisoning	N	11
PE24.5	Discuss the role of antibiotics, antispasmodics, anti-secretory drugs, probiotics, anti- emetics in acute diarrheal diseases	Y	39
PE24.8	Discuss the causes, clinical presentation and management of dysentery in children	Y	39
PE34.3	Discuss the various regimens for management of Tuberculosis as per National Guidelines	Y	52
PE34.4	Discuss the preventive strategies adopted and the objectives and outcome of the National Tuberculosis Control Program	Y	52
SU13.2	Discuss the Principles of immunosuppressive therapy. Enumerate indications, describe surgical principles, management of organ transplantation	Y	72
PM3.5	Enumerate the indications and describe the therapies for spasticity including medications, serial casts, nerve blocks, botulinum toxin injections	Y	16, 22
PM7.6	Enumerate the indications and describe the pharmacology and side effects of commonly used drugs in neuropathic bladder	Y	20
CT1.14	Describe and discuss the pharmacology of various antituberculous agents, their indications, contraindications, interactions and adverse reactions	Y	52
CT1.15	Prescribe an appropriate antituberculosis regimen based on the location of disease, smear positivity and negativity and co- morbidities based on current national guidelines including directly observed tuberculosis therapy (DOTS)	Y	52
CT2.16	Discuss and describe therapies for OAD including bronchodilators, leukotriene inhibitors, mast cell stabilisers, theophylline, inhaled and systemic steroids, oxygen and immunotherapy	Y	27, 55, 75

Competency Code	Competency	Core (Y/N)	Chapter No.
OR3.1	Describe and discuss the aetiopathogenesis, clinical features, Investigations and principles of management of Bone and Joint infections a) Acute osteomyelitis b) Subacute osteomyelitis c) Acute suppurative arthritis d) Septic arthritis and HIV infection e) Spirochaetal infection f) Skeletal tuberculosis	Y	52, 73

Some Abbreviations Used in the Text

ACE: Angiotensin converting enzyme
ACh: Acetyl choline
AChE: Acetylcholinesterase
ACTH: Adrenocorticotropic hormone
AD: Alcohol dehydrogenase
ADHD: Attention deficit hyperactivity disorder
ADP: Adenosine diphoshate
ADR: Adverse drug reaction
AMPA: Aminomethylphosphonic acid
ANC: Acid neutralizing capacity
ANF/P: Atrial natriuretic factor/peptide
APD: Action potential duration
APP: Acute phase proteins
ARDS: Adult respiratory distress syndrome
ATA: Atmosphere absolute
ATP: Adenosine triphosphate
ATS; Antitetanus serum
AUC: Area under curve
AVP: Arginine vasopressin
BBB: Blood–brain barrier
BCG: Bacillus Calmette–Guérin
BDZ: Benzodiazepines
BMD: Bone mineral density
BMI: Body mass index
BMR: Basal metabolic rate
BNP: (human) Brain-type natriuretic peptide
BPH: Benign prostatic hypertrophy
CCB: Calcium channel blocker
CDK: Cyclin-dependent kinases
CFS: Chronic fatigue syndrome
cGMP: Cyclic guanosine monophosphate
CHF: Chronic heart failure
CL: Corpus luteum
CLDII: Continuous, low dose, insulin infusion
CMI: Cell-mediated immunity
CMRNG: Chromosomally mediated resistant *N. gonorrhoeae*
COC: Combined oral contraceptives
COMT: Catechol-O-methyltransferase
COPD: Chronic obstructive pulmonary disease
COX: Cyclooxygenase
CPDA: Citrate-phosphate-dextrose-adenine
CPK: Creatine phosphokinase
CPPD: Calcium pyrophosphate dihydrate
CSF: Cerebrospinal fluid
CTZ: Chemoreceptor trigger zone
CVP: Central venous pressure
CYP: Cytochromes P450
DA: Dopamine
DDT: Dichlorodiphenyltrichloroethane
DES: Daytime excessive sleepiness
DIC: Disseminated intravascular coagulation
DM: Diabetes mellitus
DOPA: Dihydroxyphenylalanine
DPI : Dry powder inhalers
DTP: Diptheria, tetanus toxoid, pertusis
DUB: Dysfunctional uterine bleeding
DVT: Deep-vein thrombosis
DVT: Deep vein thrombosis
EAA: Excitatory amino acids
ECF: Extracellular fluid
ECT: Electroconvulsive therapy
EDRF: Endothelium-derived relaxing factor
EGFR: Epidermal growth factor receptor
ENL: Erythema nodosum leprosum
EPR: Extrapyramidal reaction
ERP: Effective refractory period
ET: Endothelin
FAD: Flavin adenine dinucleotide
FADH2: Reduced flavine adenine dinucleotide
FDC: Fixed-dose combination
FFA: Free fatty acids
FMN: Flavin mononucleotide
FSH: Follicle-stimulating hormone
GABA: Gamma-aminobutyric acid
GBH: Gamma benzene hexachloride
GERD: Gastroesophageal reflux disease
GFR: Glomerular filtration rate
GLUT: Glucose transporter
GM-CSF: Granulocyte/macrophage colony stimulating factor
GnRH: Gonadotropin-releasing hormone
GPCR: G-protein-coupled receptors
GRA: Glucocorticoid-remediable aldosteronism
HACEK: *Haemophilus* species, *Aggregatibacter* species, *Cardiobacterium*, *Eikenella*, *Kingella kingae*
hCG: Human chorionic gonadotropin
HDCV: Human diploid cell inactivated vaccine
HDL: High-density lipoprotein

HF: Heart failure
HPV: Human papilloma virus vaccine
HRT: Hormone replacement therapy
HVA: Homovanillic acid
IBD: Inflammatory bowel disease
IBS: Irritable bowel syndrome
IGF: Insulin-like growth factor
IHD: Ischaemic heart disease
IL: Interleukin
ILA: Insulin-like activity
INH: Isoniazid
IOP/IOT: Intraocular pressure/intraocular tension
IRI: Immunoreactive insulin
IRMA: Immunoradiometric acid
IRS: Insulin receptor substrate
LABA: Long acting beta-2 agonist
LDL: Low-density lipoprotein
LES: Lower esophageal sphincter
LH-RH: Luteinizing hormone-releasing hormone
LMWH: Low-molecular-weight heparins
LSD: Lysergic acid diethylamide
LT: Leukotriene
LTH: Luteotropic hormone
LTP: Long-term potentiation
LVEF: Left ventricular ejection fraction
LVF: Left ventricular failure
MAC: Minimum alveolar concentration
MAC: Mycobacterial avium complex
MAP: Muscle action potential
MDI: Metered dose inhaler
MDR: Multi-drug resistant
MHPG: 3 methoxy-4-hydroxy phenol glycol
MI: Myocardial infarction
MIC: Minimum inhibitory concentration
MMR vaccine: Measles, mumps and rubella vaccine
MND: Motor neurone disease
MRP: Multidrug-resistant associated protein
MRSA: Methicillin-resistant *Staphylococcus aureus*
NAD: Nicotnamide adenine dinucleotide
NADH: Reduced nicotinamide adenine dinucleotide
NADP: Nicotinamide adenine dinucleotide phosphate
NADPH: Reduced nicotinamide adenine dinucleotide phosphate
NANC: Non-adrenergic, non-cholinergic
NAP: Nerve action potential
NARES: Non-allergic, non-infectious rhinitis with eosinophilia
NE/NA: Norepinephrine/noradrenaline
NEP: Neutral endopeptidase
NGU: Non-gonococcal urethritis
NK: Natural killer
NK: Neurokinins
NMDA: N-methyl-D-aspartate
NSAID: Nonsteroidal anti-inflammatory drug
NT: Neurotransmitter
OPV: Oral poliomyelitis vaccine;
ORS/ORT: Oral rehydration solution/therapy
OTC: Over-the-counter
PVRV: Purified Vero-cell vaccine
PAOP: Pulmonary artery occlusive pressure
PAS: Paraaminosalicylic acid
PAT: Paroxysmal atrial tachycardia
PCECV: Purified chick embryo cell vaccine
PCOS: Polycystic ovarian syndrome
PCR: Polymerase chain reaction
PDE: Phospodiasterase
PEP: Postexposure prophylaxis
PG: Prostaglandin
PKPD: Pharmacokinetics–pharmacodynamics
PMTCT: Preventing mother-to-child transmission
POMC: Pro-opio-melanocortin
PPD: Purified protein derivative
PPNG: Penicillinase-producing *N. gonorrhoeae*
PRA: Plasma renin activity
PrEP: Pre-exposure prophylaxis
PUFA: Polyunsaturated fatty acids
PVT: Paroxysmal ventricular tachycardia
RA: Rheumatoid arthritis
RAAS: Renin–angiotensin-aldosterone system
RE: Reticuloendothelial
REM: Rapid eye movement
RIMA: Reversible inhibitor of MAO
RPCFT: Reiter protein complement fixation test
SABA: Short-acting beta-2 agonists
SAM: s-Adenosyl methionine
SLC: Solute carrier
SLE: Systemic lupus erythematosus
SNpc: Substatia nigra pars compacta
SNRI: Serotonin norepinephrine reuptake inhibitor
SR: Sarcoplasmic reticulum
SSKI: Saturated solution of potassium iodide
SSRI: Selective serotonin reuptake inhibitors
STD: Sexually transmitted disease
TDM: Therapeutic drug monitoring
TI: Therapeutic index
TNF: Tumor necrosis factor
t-PA: Tissue-type plasminogen activator
TSS: Toxic shock syndrome
TSST-1: Toxic shock syndrome toxin-1
UDPG: Uridine diphospho-glucose
URTI: Upper respiratory tract infection
UTI: Urinary tract infection
UVA/B: Ultraviolet A/B
VMA: Vanilylmandelic acid
VMAT: Vesicular monoamine transporter
VMR: Vasomotor rhinitis
VREF: Vancomycin-resistant *Enterococcus faecium*
VTE: Venous thromboembolism
WPW: Wolff-Parkinson-White
XDR-TB: Extensively drug-resistant TB

Good health is not just the absence of disease. It is the positive dynamic energy state in which internal organs work in perfect harmony and concord, and external behaviour is smooth and relaxed.

— Swami Vivekananda

1
SECTION

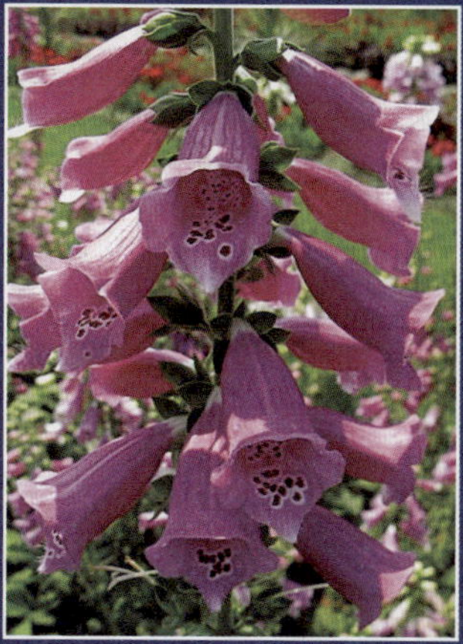

Digitalis purpurea

General Pharmacology

Section Outline

This section consists of the following chapters:

CHAPTER 1

General Considerations and Pharmacokinetics

Learning Objectives

This chapter will enable the reader:

1. To enumerate the sources of drugs.
2. To state the different sources of drug information.
3. To discuss the advantages and disadvantages of routes of drug administration and dosage forms.
4. To enlist the important dosage forms to be administered by a specified route.
5. To enlist the drug delivery systems.
6. To define the term bioavailability and state its significance.
7. To explain the mechanisms involved in the absorption, and distribution of a drug.
8. To explain the processes of biotransformation and drug elimination.
9. To describe the strategies for prolongation of drug action.
10. To state the indications for therapeutic drug monitoring (TDM).
11. To describe the clinical implications of TDM.

KEY TERMS

pharmacokinetics, p. 4
gene-based therapy, p. 7
stem cell therapy, p. 7
local application, p. 8
oral or enteral route, p. 10
parental route, p. 11
drug delivery systems, 14
drug absorption, p. 16
bioavailability, p. 17
drug distribution, p. 20
fate of a drug, p. 23
plasma half-life, p. 27
therapeutic drug monitoring, p. 30

Illness has been man's heritage from the beginning of his existence, and the search for remedies to combat it is perhaps equally old. The world's oldest known therapeutic writings come from India and China. The earliest Indian records are the *Vedas. Rigveda* (3000 BC), the earliest *Veda* mentions diseases and medicinal plants. *Ayurveda*, the Indian system of Traditional Medicine, mentions various medicinal preparations of herbal and mineral origin. These are presented in ancient treatise *Charaka Samhita, Sushruta Samhita* and *Vagbhata*. Babylonian clay tablets (700 BC) have been found to mention about 300 drugs. The Chinese materia medica *Pan Tsao* was probably written in 2735 BC and contains many plant and metallic preparations and some animal products. The ancient Egyptian medical papyri (1900 BC) contain remedies to treat symptoms of various illnesses. PH 1.1

DEFINITIONS

The word **pharmacology** is derived from two Greek words **pharmacon** (an active principle) and *logos* (a discourse or treatise). **It is the science that deals with drugs.** Pharmacology consists of detailed study of drugs, particularly their actions on living animals, organs and tissues. The actions may be beneficial or harmful.

The objective of pharmacology is mainly to provide such scientific data, using which one can choose a drug treatment of proven efficacy and safety from the various options available, to suit the patient. Over a period of time, it has evolved into the following branches (Fig. 1.1):

Pharmacognosy is the science of identification of drugs from natural sources.

Pharmacy is the science of identification, selection, preservation, standardisation, compounding and dispensing of medicinal substances.

Clinical pharmacy is the science of drug formulations, their stability, shelf life, handling and also education of the patient about compliance and

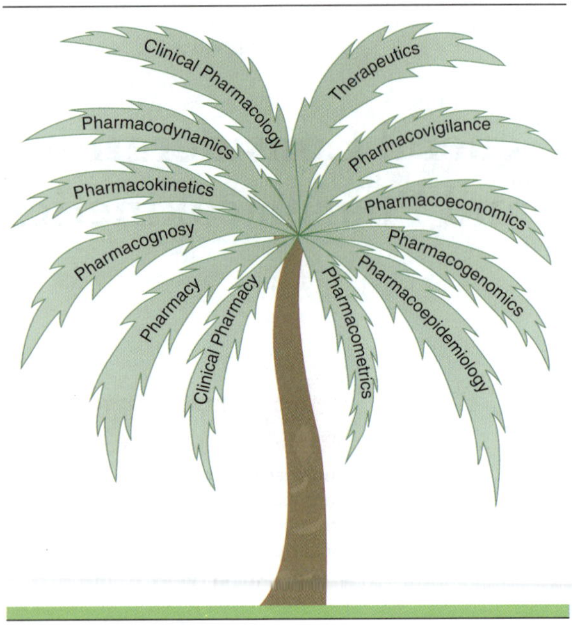

FIG. 1.1 Branches of Pharmacology.

counselling him on how to take the medication. It also includes monitoring for errors in drug therapy. The clinical pharmacist optimises the patient care with the help of the physician.

PH 1.1

Pharmacokinetics (PK) is a study of absorption, distribution, metabolism and excretion of drugs, and their relationship to pharmacologic response (**what the body does to a drug**).

Pharmacodynamics (PD) is the quantitative study of the effects of drugs (**what the drug does to the body**) (Fig. 1.2). Studies on pharmacodynamics elucidate the site and mechanism of drug action.

Therapeutics is a branch of medicine concerned with prevention and cure of disease or relief of symptoms with drug therapy (pharmacotherapeutics) and non-drug measures. The word means *to care for, to tend to or to nurse.* It involves not only scientific knowledge and judgement (obtained from the books) but also skills, wisdom and the sense of responsibility. FM 8.2

Toxicology is the science of poisons, which are harmful, dangerous or fatal to human. It includes detection and knowledge about the nature and effects of poisons as well as treatment of poisoning. Many drugs in large doses act as poisons.

Chemotherapy is concerned with the effect of drugs upon microorganisms and parasites, living and multiplying in a living organism. It now includes the drug treatment of cancer as well.

Pharmacoepidemiology is the study of the use and effects of drugs in large number of people. It helps to gain further insight into the efficacy and safety of new drugs after they are released for community use. PH 1.6

Pharmacoeconomics is the analysis of the cost of drug therapy and its benefits to the health care system and the society. It examines the quantitative relations between the cost and the benefit (*cost–benefit analysis*).

Pharmacovigilance is the science and activities related to the detection, assessment, understanding and prevention of adverse effects or any other drug-related problem (WHO). It involves the surveillance of drugs once they are released for use in the community and relies on voluntary reporting, prescription monitoring, medical records and statistical studies in the population.

Pharmacogenetics is the study of genetic basis for variations in drug metabolism and response in humans. It deals with identifying inherited variations mediated through single gene.

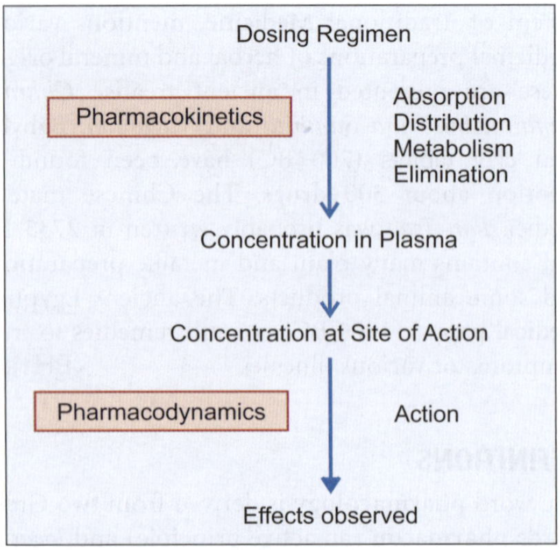

FIG. 1.2 Pharmacokinetics and pharmacodynamics.

PH 1.60

Pharmacogenomics is the science that examines genomic variability to assess its effects on the drug response of humans (see later in this chapter), microbes (antimicrobials) and tumours (anticancer drugs) and explores the ways these variations can be used to predict the patient's response, either good or poor, to the drug. This may help in the development of target-specific personalised and safer drugs.

Pharmacometrics is a science that deals with evolving a quantitative relationship between exposure to the drug (PK) and its response (PD), derived by constructing mathematical models based on few observations (PKPD modelling). Such models are used to predict the response or the dose, e.g. deriving dose for patient with renal dysfunction or predicting undesirable effect to a given dose.

The word *drug* is derived from the French word *drogue*, a dry herb. **A drug is defined as any substance used for the purpose of diagnosis, prevention, relief or cure of a disease in man or animals.** According to WHO, 'A drug is any substance or product that is used or intended to be used to modify or explore physiological systems or pathological states for the benefit of the recipient'. PH 1.9

Drug nomenclature is based on the following nomenclature systems:

- Chemical/Molecular/Scientific name
- Generic / Non-Proprietary / Approved / Official name
- Brand / Trade / Proprietary name

1. **Chemical name:** It depicts the chemical/molecular structure of the drug accompanied by its diagram e.g. chemical name of paracetamol is as acetyl-p-amino-phenol. Chemical names are cumbersome and not suitable for use in drug prescribing.
2. **Generic name:** This is the abbreviated (from the chemical name) and approved name of the drug. It is the official medical name assigned by the manufacturer (innovator) in collaboration with the drug regulatory authority (Licensing) of the given country. Sometimes during drug development, a manufacturer assigns a code name for convenience and simplicity before an approved name is coined. For example, an agent with the code name, RO 151788 was later named as flumazenil. The generic name removes the confusion of giving several names by different manufacturing companies to the same drug. All member countries of the WHO agree to use the Recommended International Nonproprietary Name (rINN) to maintain uniformity in name across the countries.
3. **Proprietary name:** These are the names given to a drug by the manufacturing/ marketing company. They are copyrighted terms selected by a manufacturer to designate a particular product. Copyright laws prevent any other company from using the same name, while other laws prevent use of this name for any other chemically identical products. A single drug may have many brand names e.g. paracetamol has several proprietary names e.g. Crocin, Tylenol, Paramol, Panadol, Calpol etc.

THE NATURE AND SOURCES OF DRUGS

The various sources of drugs are as follows:

1. **Minerals,** e.g. liquid paraffin, magnesium sulphate, kaolin and aluminium trisilicate.
2. **Animals,** e.g. heparin, gonadotropins and antitoxic sera.
3. **Plants,** e.g. morphine, atropine, aspirin, artemisin and taxane. Plants contain several chemical constituents such as alkaloids, glycosides, resins, oleoresins, tannins, oils etc. These vary from plant to plant. Some of them are responsible for pharmacological effects (*active principles*), e.g. the alkaloids like morphine in opium and atropine in *Atropa belladonna*, respectively; the glycoside digoxin in *Digitalis purpurea*; and phytoestrogens like genistein or daidzein in soy preparations. Several drugs used in modern medicine have been derived from plants.
4. **Microorganisms,** e.g. bacteria and fungi, isolated from soil, are important sources of antibacterial substances, e.g. penicillin.
5. **Synthetic,** e.g. nonsteroidal anti-inflammatory drugs (NSAIDs), hypnotics, anticancer drugs and ACE inhibitors. Majority of the drugs currently used in therapeutics are synthetic.

6. **Genetic engineering** (DNA recombinant technology), e.g. insulin and hepatitis B vaccine.

The drugs developed from the above-mentioned sources (1 to 6) are called as 'Pharmaceuticals'.

7. **Biologicals,** e.g. growth factors, monoclonal antibodies, cytokines. In the last decade many biological agents have also become available for therapeutic purposes. This is a heterogeneous group and includes complex protein molecules that interact with cytokines or cell surface markers. PH 1.59

Herbal medicines/remedies: These include a plant derived material or preparation with therapeutic or other human health benefits which contains either raw or processed ingredients from one or more plants. They are available in the market as **traditional medicines**. These cannot be prescribed by practitioners of Modern Medicine who do not have any training or expertise in prescribing these drugs. One should check whether their efficacy and safety is proved by adequate scientific evidence and they are approved by the regulatory authorities – Drug Controller of India (DCI).

The following points have to be remembered by the treating physician while recommending herbal medicines:

- The regulations by DCI, applicable to the modern drugs, are not applicable to them.
- Standardized herbal medicines may not be available as they are difficult to standardize.
- If not processed properly, herbal or herbo-mineral formulations (*bhasmas*) can lead to toxicity.
- Herbal medicines may not be safe. Those previously thought to be innocuous have been found to be potentially toxic. The best example of this are the Chinese herbal teas, which have been reported as hepatotoxic.
- Their safety during pregnancy is unknown.
- The herbal combinations and their recommended doses are many a times not supported by any scientific data. Tall claims are sometimes made about their efficacy without adequate scientific data.
- It is almost impossible to test for the presence of the ingredients mentioned in the package insert/container label.
- They are not always as cheap as claimed.

Some of the so called 'herbal medicines' have been found to be adulterated with modern drugs such as glucocorticoids, diclofenac, benzodiazepines, phenytoin, statins and sildenafil. Caution should be taken before recommending such herbal medicines.

Recently new entity **phytopharmaceutical drug** has been emerged which may overcome some of the above mentioned issues with herbal medicines. Phytopharmaceutical drug is defined as a purified and standardized fraction with defined minimum four bio-active or phytochemical compounds (qualitatively and quantitatively assessed) of an extract of a medicinal plant or its part, for internal or external use of human beings or animals for diagnosis, treatment, mitigation, or prevention of any disease or disorder but does not include administration by parenteral route. These drugs can be marketed with approval from DCI, which is given based on the scientific and credible data. These can then be prescribed by practitioners of Modern Medicine.

The prescriber can offer the following therapies as an adjuvant or substitute for drug therapy:

PH 1.61

I. **Dietary supplements/ health supplements:** They may be used to supplement the normal diet and include concentrated source of one or more nutrients. These nutrients may include amino acids, enzymes, minerals, proteins, vitamins, other dietary substances, plants or botanicals, prebiotics, probiotics and substances from animal origin or other similar substances with known and established nutritional or beneficial physiological effect. They are offered alone or in combination. The quantity of nutrients added to the food articles does not exceed the recommended daily allowance.

PH 1.61

II. **Nutraceutical:** The term combines the two words, "nutrient," which is a nourishing food component, and "pharmaceutical," which is a medical drug. A nutraceutical is a food or food related component that provides extra health or medical benefits, encompassing improvement of health, prevention and treatment of disease, in addition to the basic nutritional value. The Food Safety and Standards Authority of India (FSSAI) has issued regulations for approval of nutraceuticals in the Indian market. Nutraceuticals are usually expensive and do not necessarily substitute cheap balanced diet.

III. **Gene-based therapy:** The developments in biotechnology have made it possible to synthesise short nucleotide sequences (genes). These are responsible for the *in vivo* synthesis of proteins critical in certain metabolic pathways. They can be introduced into human beings for therapeutic purposes. The gene therapy aims to introduce functional genetic material into cells to replace or supplement the activity of defective genes.

A variety of diseases are due to inherited deficiencies of single genes; e.g. thalassaemia, phenylketonuria and cystic fibrosis. In these conditions, serious metabolic disturbances result because of either deficiency or faulty protein product of the abnormal gene; or accumulation of precursors which cannot be metabolised further because of the enzyme deficiency. This metabolic abnormality can be corrected if the synthetic gene is delivered to the target tissue(s). In contrast, in acquired diseases such as cancer gene therapy adds new molecular function(s) capable of altering the course of the disease, or to block an existing function.

Gene-based therapy is in its infancy and many technological and ethical problems remain to be solved.

IV. **Stem cell therapy:** Recently stem cells (either embryonic or adult pleuripotent cells) have been used as a therapeutic approach for regeneration and proliferation of functional cells in the body, e.g. in myocardial infarction, osteoarthritis and diabetes mellitus. This approach has great potential in therapeutics but much remains to be done.

SOURCES OF DRUG INFORMATION

It is essential to select drugs for treating a disease in rational manner – based on logical thinking supported by comprehensive and objective information. The sources that provide information about the drug are of three types:

1. *Primary information sources* include original research publications in the journals and reports of clinical drug trials. They serve as basic foundation to provide factual data.
2. *Secondary information* sources are derived from the primary and include review articles, meta-analyses, systematic reviews and compilations of published articles or their parts done by bibliographic, abstracting, or indexing services like Medline, Current Contents, International Pharmaceutical Abstracts, Index Medicus, Excerpta Medica.
3. *Tertiary information sources* are documents written by individuals or groups and are often peer reviewed. These include formularies, standard treatment guidelines, textbooks, general reference books, drug bulletins, the National List of Essential Medicines (NLEM) and drug compendia.

Digital (Electronic) sources

The above-mentioned drug information sources apart from being available as print version are now also available on the internet. It is important for the prescriber to have up-to-date medical information, which may be easily done by resorting to internet sources. Furthermore, majority of educated patients feel that their health care provider should be competent in directing them to appropriate sources of drug information on the internet. Due to the unregulated nature of the internet, it is of utmost importance to identify unbiased, authentic and scientific drug information.

An authentic and credible website delineates the following:

- Information regarding who runs the site and who is responsible for the content. This should be clearly visible on the home page or in the "About Us" section.
- The source of funding for the given website. If it is a company or organization that stands to profit from the content, bias may be suspected and reader must critically review the information displayed on the site. The source of funding may be apparent in the suffix of the web site address (e.g. addresses

ending in ".gov" are government-sponsored; ".edu" are sponsored by educational institutions; ".org" represent non-commercial organizations).

- The source of the content and appropriate references.
- Provision of the date of last update. This ensures that the information is current.
- Display of the credibility check of the information using various tools like the Medication Website Assessment Tool (MWAT), Health On the Net (HON) Foundation Code of Conduct, and the Healthcare Website Assessment Tool (HWAT 3.0).

The websites preferred as sources of health information are university/academia–based websites, consumer websites sponsored by medical journals or publications, and government agency websites while pharmaceutical manufacturer or media driven websites are the least preferred. Examples of such credible websites include www.nlm.nih.gov, www.cochrane.org.

Pharmacopoeia is an official code containing a selected list of the established drugs and medicinal preparations with descriptions of their physical properties and tests for their identity, purity and potency. Pharmacopoeia defines the standards which these preparations must meet, and may mention their average doses for an adult. Examples are the *Indian Pharmacopoeia* (IP), the *British Pharmacopoeia* (BP), the *United States Pharmacopoeia* (USP) and the *European Pharmacopoeia*. They have legal standing from the point of view of drug regulatory authority.

A **formulary** is not a regulatory document but provides information about the available drugs, based on original and reputed drug information sources as well as experts' recommendations. It provides up-to-date guidance to prescribers and aids rational prescribing and dispensing drugs, e.g. the National Formulary of India (NF), *WHO Model Formulary*, and the *British National Formulary* (BNF).

Martindale: The Complete Drug Reference is a compendium, which provides unbiased information about drugs and medicines used throughout the world, including their trade names and manufacturers' contact information. The drug information is backed by references, systematic reviews and metaanalyses or evidence-based guidelines. Thus, it serves as an excellent source of drug information.

*Different brands of same medicine are marketed by different manufacturers. Information about the brands, their formulations, strengths, cost, dose, precautions, adverse effects and contraindications is available in publications such as the Physician's Desk Reference (**PDR**), the Indian Drug Review (**IDR**), the Monthly Index of Medical Specialities (**MIMS**) or the Current Index of Medical Specialities (**CIMS**) India website. Various therapeutic guidelines are also available in form of country-specific Standard Treatment Guidelines (STGs).* PH 1.3. 1.11

ROUTES OF DRUG ADMINISTRATION AND DOSAGE FORMS

Drugs may be applied locally, or may be administered orally and or parenterally. The forms in which the drugs are administered are termed as **dosage form**. In the dosage form, a drug exists with different substances such as diluents, binders, stabilizers etc. These substances are termed as **excipients**. This final medicinal product in the dosage form is developed through various pharmaceutical processes (termed as **drug formulation**) based on physical, chemical and mechanical properties of the drug and need for type/s of excipients. Sometimes for certain dosage forms special drug delivery systems are required. Various routes of administration, dosage forms and examples of drugs are presented in Table 1.1.

Local Application

Dusting powder, cream, lotion, gel, ointment or spray exert action at the site of application (*topical action*). The other topical forms include **bougie** for urethra, **pessary** for vagina, **inhalers** for bronchi and **suppository** for the vagina and rectum.

Drugs used for local effects on mucous membranes are likely to be absorbed and may produce adverse systemic effects. During irrigation or spraying of the nose, a compound may find its way into the middle ear through the Eustachian tube. Lipoid pneumonia following aspiration of an oily solution into the respiratory tract has been reported.

Table 1.1 Routes of Drug Administration and Dosage Forms with Examples PH 1.11, PH 1.3

Route	Dosage Forms	Drugs
A. Local application		
• Skin	Creams	Clobetasol
	Ointments	Povidine iodine
	Lotions	Calamine
	Gels	Lignocaine
	Sprays	Diclofenac
	Dusting powder	Clotrimazole
• Urethral	Bougie	Alprostadil
• Vaginal	Suppository	Clotrimazole
	Cream	Estrogen
	Pessary	Nystatin
• Rectal	Suppository	Bisacodyl
	Enema	Soap water
• Ear	Drops	Ciprofloxacin
• Eye	Drops	Timolol maleate
	Ointment	Gentamicin
• Nose	Sprays	Xylometazoline
• Inhalation	Metered dose inhaler	Salbutamol
	Dry powder inhaler	Tiotropium bromide
	Nebulisers	Ipratropium bromide
B. Oral/enteral		
	Tablets	Paracetamol
	Capsules	Tramadol
	Syrups	Lactulose
	Solutions	Cetrizine
	Suspensions	Ibuprofen
	Elixirs	Promethazine
C. Parenteral		
Inhalational	Gases	Isoflurane
Intradermal	Solution	BCG vaccine
Subcutaneous	Solution	Insulin
Intramuscular	Solution	Hepatitis B vaccine
Intravenous	Solution	Aminophylline
Intra-arterial	Solution	5-fluorouracil
Intraperitoneal	Solution	Dialysis fluid
Intraosseous	Solution	Dopamine
Intra-articular	Solution	Hydrocortisone
Intrathecal	Solution	Lignocaine
Epidural	Solution	Morphine
Intracavernosal	Solution	Papaverine
D. Transcutaneous		
Transdermal	Patch	Fentanyl
Inunction	Ointment	Nitroglycerin
Jet injection	Solution	Insulin
Iontophoresis	Gel	Diclofenac
E. Transmucosal		
Sublingual	Tablet	Isosorbide dinitrite
Buccal	Tablet	Lorazepam

Table 1.1 Routes of Drug Administration and Dosage Forms with Examples—cont'd

Route	Dosage Forms	Drugs
F. Transrectal	Suppository	Diazepam
	Enema (evacuation)	Soap water
	Enema (retention)	Prednisolone
G. Transnasal		
Nasal spray	Solution	Nafarelin

Administration of a medicament in a liquid form into the rectum is called *enema*. Enemata are of the following two types:

1. **Evacuant enema** (e.g. soap water enema): The aim is to remove the faecal matter and the flatus. The water stimulates the rectum by distension while soap acts as a lubricant/softener. The quantity of fluid administered is about 600 mL. It is useful in treating selected cases of constipation. It is also administered before surgical operations, delivery and radiological investigation of the gastrointestinal (GI) tract.
2. **Retention enema:** The fluid containing the drug is retained in the rectum for local action as with prednisolone enema for ulcerative colitis; or it may act systemically after absorption through the mucous membrane. The quantity of fluid administered is usually 100–120 mL.

For systemic absorption by transrectal route, see later.

Oral or Enteral Route

This is the most commonly employed route for drug administration:

Advantages

- Convenient and safe.
- Economical.
- Complications of parenteral therapy are avoided.

Disadvantages

- The onset of drug action is tardy.
- Irritant and unpalatable drugs cannot be administered.
- The absorption of certain drugs can be irregular or negligible, e.g. aminoglycosides.
- Not useful in the presence of vomiting and diarrhoea.
- Cannot be employed in an unconscious or uncooperative patient nor in an emergency.
- Not for drugs destroyed in GIT, e.g. insulin and enzymes for systemic action. Furthermore, some drugs like testosterone, though absorbed, get inactivated in the intestinal wall and the liver (first-pass metabolism) and only a small portion reaches the systemic circulation.

Oral dosage forms such as tablets or capsules are often made more acceptable by various types of coatings, colouring agents and flavouring agents.

Precautions

- Capsules and tablets should be washed down with a glass of water with the patient in upright posture, either sitting or standing, as this enhances the passage into the stomach and permits rapid dissolution.
- Avoid oral administration to a recumbent patient, especially in the case of drugs which can damage the oesophageal mucosa, e.g. tetracyclines, iron salts, slow-release potassium preparations and alendronate.

Enteric-Coated Tablets. Sometimes, tablets are coated with cellulose acetate phthalate, gluten and anionic copolymers of methacrylic acid and its esters. These substances resist the acid juice of the stomach but permit disintegration in the intestinal alkaline juices. Enteric coating is done to:

- Prevent gastric irritation and destruction of the drug in the stomach.
- Achieve the desired concentration of the drug in the small intestine.
- Retard the absorption of the drug.

However, if the coating is very hard, a tablet may pass out without being dissolved in the GI (Fig. 1.3A and B).

Parenteral Routes

Routes of administration other than the alimentary tract (the *enteron*) are called *parenteral.*

Advantages

- Can be employed in an unconscious or an uncooperative patient.
- Can be employed in cases of vomiting and diarrhoea and in patients unable to swallow.
- Irritant drugs or those drugs which are not absorbed orally can be administered.
- No modification occurs as seen on oral route.
- Rapid action and accuracy of dose are ensured.

Disadvantages

- Inconvenient for use or for self-medication.
- Less safe, and liable to cause infection if proper aseptic care is not exercised.
- Likely to injure important structures such as nerves and arteries.
- More expensive.

The parenteral routes include the following methods:

1. **Inhalation:** Drugs may be administered by this route, using the following dosage forms:
    - Pressurised, metered dose aerosols, e.g. salbutamol and beclomethasone
    - Dry powders from inhalers activated by patient's inhalation, e.g. salbutamol
    - Oxygen or compressed air driven nebulised solutions, e.g. salbutamol
    - Gases, e.g. general anaesthetics, vapours of volatile oils

    Drugs given by inhalation produce rapid effects. Thus, nicotine, morphine and tetrahydrocanabinol are rapidly absorbed following the inhalation of tobacco, opium or marijuana smoke, respectively. Drugs go directly to the left side of the heart through the pulmonary veins and may produce cardiac toxicity. Local irritation may cause bronchospasm and increase the respiratory tract secretion.

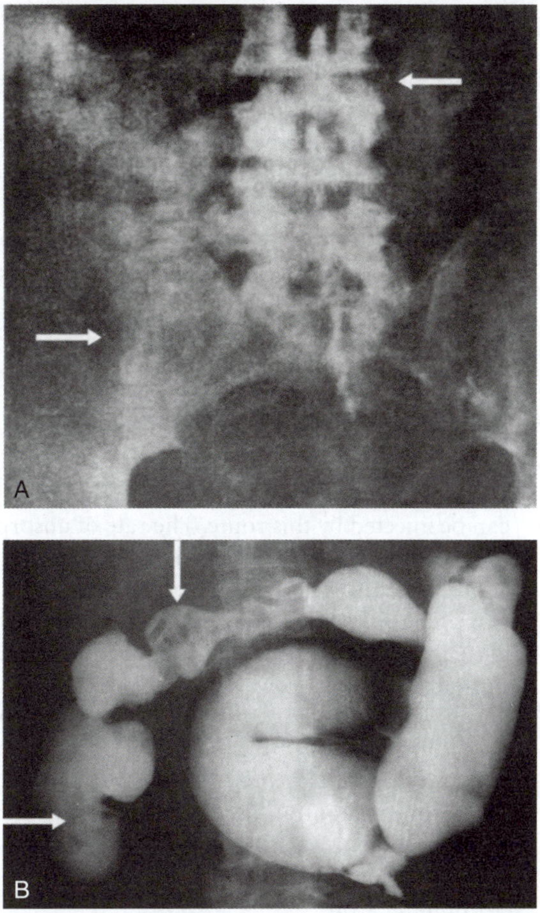

FIG. 1.3 Radiographs (A and B) showing intact tablets in the GI tract. Arrows indicate presence of tablets which are not dissolved.

2. **Injectable parenteral** routes wherein the *drugs are injected* using strict aseptic technique:
    Intradermal (ID): This is given into the layers of the skin, e.g. BCG vaccine. Only a small quantity can be administered by this route and the injection may be painful. It is also employed for testing drug sensitivity.
    Subcutaneous (SC): Only nonirritant substances can be injected by this route. The commonest drug used by this route is insulin. The drug absorption is slower than with intramuscular (IM) route. However, the action is sustained and uniform. Absorption by this route is unreliable in shock. SC drug implants can act as 'depot' therapy, e.g. testosterone implants.
    Hypodermoclysis is a technique, of administration

of large quantities of fluids (usually saline; at a rate of 1 ml/min with approx. 3 L per day from two sites in 24 hrs) subcutaneously. The common sites of infusion are arm, back, abdomen or thighs. Drug absorption from the SC area can be enhanced by the addition of the enzyme hyaluronidase (Chapter 76). *It is a suitable way of fluid administration for mild to moderate dehydration, especially in the elderly, and in those under palliative care when oral intake or intravenous infusion is not possible.* The adverse effects are usually local and mild e.g. subcutaneous edema may occur, which can be treated by local massage or systemic diuretics.

Intramuscular (IM): In addition to soluble substances, mild irritants, suspensions and colloids can be injected by this route. The rate of absorption is reasonably uniform and the onset of action is rapid. The rate of absorption is faster from deltoid and vastus lateralis than from gluteus maximus. The volume of injection should not exceed 10 mL. *However, IM absorption is not always faster than oral absorption, e.g. diazepam, hydrocortisone, digoxin and phenytoin are absorbed more slowly intramuscularly than orally.*

Drugs injected intramuscularly, especially irritants, may:

- Cause local pain and even necrosis, e.g. quinine, iron.
- Damage the nerve causing severe pain and even paresis of the muscles supplied by it.

IM injections should not be administered in the buttock until the child starts to walk, as the gluteus maximus muscle mass is less till the child starts to walk; the lateral aspect of the thigh should be used.

Intravenous (IV): Drugs given directly into a vein produce very rapid action, and the desired blood concentration can be achieved rapidly with a smaller dose. Titration of the dose is possible. A drug may be injected intravenously:

a. *As a bolus*, e.g. furosemide
b. *Over 5–10 min*, diluted in 10–20 mL of isotonic glucose or saline, e.g. aminophylline
c. *In an infusion* in 50–100 mL or larger in volume

An infusion is employed to:

a. **Slow the administration of the drug** to avoid toxicity, e.g. morphine.
b. **Maintain a constant plasma level** of the drug, e.g. insulin or dopamine.
c. **Administer large volumes** either rapidly or over prolonged periods of time, e.g. fluids in shock or dehydration.

The **disadvantages** of this route are as follows:

- Once the drug is administered by this route, its action cannot be halted.
- Local irritation can lead to phlebitis.
- Self-medication is difficult.
- Extravasation of certain substances may cause irritation and even sloughing (Box 1.1).

Precautions during IV therapy:

a. Before injecting, ensure that the needle and the syringe are air-free, and that the needle is in the vein. Irritating solutions should be administered by piggybacking into a running IV drip or through a central line. If they are administered through a peripheral vein, the IV site should be rotated at regular intervals. If extravasation occurs, attempts to aspirate the extravasated substance through the cannula should be made before removing the cannula.
b. The injection should be given slowly in case of certain drugs such as iron and aminophylline, as a sudden high blood concentration may be dangerous.
c. Only the minimum quantity required to elicit a particular effect should be injected.

Intra-arterial drug administration produces a sudden high concentration in arterial blood and hence, may be harmful locally or damaging to tissues supplied by the artery. This route is used in diagnostic studies, such as angiograms, and in embolisation therapy. Certain antimalignancy compounds are administered by regional intra-

Box 1.1 Drugs causing tissue damage on extravasation

- Acidic, alkaline or hypertonic solutions
- Potassium and calcium solutions
- Noradrenaline and other vasopressors
- Aminophylline
- Iron
- Cancer chemotherapy agents
- Quinine, thiopental, phenytoin, diazepam, nitroglycerine, ethyl alcohol, radiocontrast media

arterial infusion in localised malignancies.

Intrathecal administration involves introduction of drugs such as spinal anaesthetics into the subarachnoid space. The drugs act directly on the CNS. This route also is convenient for producing high local concentrations in the subarachnoid space, e.g. certain antibiotics and antimalignancy drugs.

Lignocaine is used extradurally to produce anaesthesia for pelvic surgery. The epidural use of morphine for analgesia is described in Chapter 10.

Intraperitoneal: This route is sometimes used in infants for giving fluids like glucose saline, as the peritoneum offers a large surface for absorption. It is also used for peritoneal dialysis.

Intraosseous (intramedullary) cannulation: Drugs injected into the bone marrow of the iliac crest or the tibia (using a special gadget) are rapidly absorbed into the circulation. Adrenaline injected in this manner may be of great help in adults in severe shock, and those with sudden cardiac arrest, and no immediate access to a vein. In infants and children, drugs such as adrenaline and dopamine have been used in this manner for resuscitation in acute, life-threatening situations when standard venous access methods have failed.

Intra-articular and intralesional: Certain drugs are administered directly into a joint for the treatment of local conditions. This ensures a high local concentration of the drug, e.g. hydrocortisone acetate in the treatment of rheumatoid arthritis. Repeated injections may damage the joint. Glucocorticoids and local anaesthetics have been administered intralesionally into painful and tender lesions.

Intracavernosal and transurethral: See Chapter 67.

Ocular: Subconjunctival, retrobulbar, intracameral and intravitreal. See Chapter 70.

3. **Transcutaneous/transdermal:**

Iontophoresis: In this procedure, a galvanic current allows the penetration of drugs applied to the skin into the deeper tissues. Salicylates have been used by this method.

Inunction: Certain drugs when rubbed into the skin (inunction) can get absorbed and produce systemic effects, e.g. nitroglycerin ointment in angina pectoris and NSAIDs for sprain. Certain potent glucocorticoids when applied to skin lesions for local effects may get absorbed and cause systemic adverse effects.

Jet injection (dermojet): This needleless method involves the transcutaneous introduction of a drug by means of a high velocity jet produced through a microfine orifice. It is used for giving insulin or mass vaccination.

Transdermal delivery system: See under' Drug delivery systems'.

It must be emphasised that percutaneous absorption of topically applied drugs is greater in infants and children, particularly in prematures and if the skin is burnt or excoriated. This can enhance drug toxicity.

4. **Transmucosal:**

Sublingual: A tablet containing a medicament is placed under the tongue and is allowed to dissolve in the mouth. The active agent thus gets absorbed through the buccal mucous membrane directly into the systemic circulation. Drugs commonly administered by sublingual route are nitroglycerin in angina pectoris and buprenorphine as an analgesic. Some other drugs which may be administered sublingually are nifedipine, diazepam, lorazepam, domperidone, ondansetron and ergotamine. Advantages of this route are shown in Box 1.2.

Transnasal: DAVP, a synthetic analogue of vasopressin, GnRH agonist (nafarelin) and calcitonin are the *drugs administered by this route. A toxic substance should not be administered by this route, as it may directly reach the brain along with lymphatic channels.* Also see status epilepticus in Chapter 9.

Transrectal: The rectum has rich blood and lymph supply, and drugs can cross the rectal mucosa like the other lipid membranes; thus, unionised and lipid-soluble substances are readily absorbed. The portion absorbed from

Box 1.2 Advantages of Sublingual Route

- Can be employed in patients who are vomiting,
- Rapid onset of action,
- Quick termination of the drug effect on spitting the tablet,
- Avoidance of degradation of the drug in the stomach and
- Bypassing its rapid inactivation in the intestinal wall and the liver (first pass).

the upper rectal mucosa is carried by the superior haemorrhoidal vein into the portal circulation whereas that absorbed from the lower rectum enters directly into the systemic circulation via the middle and inferior haemorrhoidal veins. Thus approximately 50% of drug absorbed by the rectum bypasses the liver. In addition, CYP3A4 is absent in the lower intestine. Hence, chances of first pass metabolism are lower than after the oral dose. Examples of drugs that can be given rectally are paracetamol for fever and diazepam for status epilepticus.

The **advantages** of this route are as follows:

- Gastric irritation is avoided.
- Duration of action can be controlled, if suitable solvent is used.
- Avoids first pass metabolism.
- Convenient route for long-term care of geriatric and terminally ill patients.
- Administration of a rectal suppository or a capsule is a simple procedure which can be undertaken by unskilled persons and by the patient himself.

The **disadvantages** include the following:

- Incomplete and erratic absorption
- Irritation of rectal mucosa by drugs

Endotracheal route: In patients who have an indwelling endotracheal tube, certain drugs (e.g. adrenaline, atropine, diazepam, naloxone lignocaine) can be administered by this route for an immediate effect. The drug is diluted in 5–10 mL of isotonic saline before administration.

A drug may exert different effects when given by different routes. Thus, oral magnesium sulphate acts as saline laxative. When *injected*, it is a depressant of the CNS and acts as an anticonvulsant. On the other hand, hypertonic magnesium sulphate, given as a *retention enema*, can be used to reduce cerebral oedema. PH 1.3

DRUG DELIVERY SYSTEMS

The conventional (or immediate release) dosage forms serve only the purpose of introducing specific amounts of drug into the body. They do little to maintain uniform body drug concentration. In order to produce a therapeutic concentration at the site of action, much larger quantities of the drug are needed to be administered, which can cause adverse reactions. Additional disadvantages include the need for frequent dosing, problems related to concomitant food intake for orally administered drugs and long-term patient compliance.

Various drug delivery systems, which incorporate drugs in a dosage form that releases the medication in different ways over a longer period are called as modified release (MR) dosage forms. Various suffixes are used to denote the type of delivery of drug such as ER/XR (extended release), TR (time release), DR (delayed release), SR (Sustained release), XL(extra long, extra large) and CR (Controlled release). Sometimes the term extended release formulations is used as an umbrella term to include the rest under it. These dosage forms release drugs over along time so that frequency of intake of medication is reduced, thereby increasing compliance. They also reduce the peak related adverse effects and fluctuations in concentrations during the day. Some novel formulations release the drug at a predetermined rate (CR formulations) or at a predetermined site (Targeted delivery), over an extended period of time from a single application. CR formulations need a therapeutic system including drug reservoir and mechanism for predictable release of drug. This helps in maintaining constant level of the drug in body. Some of the modified release formulations are as follows:

1. For drugs administered orally

- *Extended release/XR/XL preparations:* release the drug over an extended period of time and generally once daily dosing is required e.g. divalproex is ER, venalaflaxine is XR and metformin is XL.
- *Time-release preparations* (timsules, spansules) Such preparations have the particles of drug covered with coatings which dissolve at different time intervals. The coating which dissolves early releases an amount of the drug which establishes its action quickly; the coating which dissolves more slowly ensures a slow release of the remainder of the drug, thus providing uniform drug concentration over a prolonged period.
- *Sustained release:* Using pharmaceutical tech-

niques like barrier coating, complexing with macromolecules or using vehicle with low solubility the release of the drug from the dosage form is slowed down to last for longer time e.g. alprazolam.

- *Delayed release preparations:* These release drug after a lag period after administration. This prevents disintegration of dosage form too early before reaching site of action or to lessen potential ADRs due to breakage in oesophagus. The example is sulfasalazine DR which is used for ulcerative colitis.
  Enteric coated tablets are also examples of DR preparations.
- *Controlled-release preparation:* Prazosin is available as osmotic controlled- release oral system (OROS).

The **disadvantages of the above oral preparations**, particularly ER, is that their size may be too large to swallow. These preparations should not be cut, crushed or chewed. In patients with irritable bowel syndrome having tendency for "*intestinal hurry*", the dosage form reaches quickly to colon, where the absorption is poor and erratic. They are more expensive than their IR counterparts.

2. For drugs administered topically

- *Ocusert*, when placed under the eyelid, delivers a steady flow of pilocarpine round the clock for seven days without causing any discomfort, and avoiding the need for repeated eye drops.
- *Intrauterine device*, e.g. mirena containing levonorgestrel, when placed in the uterine cavity produces contraceptive effect for 5 years.
- *Transdermal therapeutuic system:* It is available as an adhesive unit to deliver drugs slowly through skin producing prolonged systemic effect, e.g. scopolamine for prevention of motion sickness, nitroglycerine for angina prophylaxis and fentanyl for cancer pain.
- *Drug eluting stents(DES)* consist of a metallic stent backbone covered with a polymer, containing a drug (sirolimus or paclitaxel). The drug is gradually released over the next 14–30 days and modifies the local healing response within the stented artery. Used during coronary angioplasty and stenting, they help to reduce the incidence of restenosis.
- *Metered dose inhalers or rotainhalers (See chapter 27).*

3. For drugs administered intravenously

For optimal drug effect, computerised, miniature, syringe pumps are now available for:

- Continuous administration of insulin and nitroglycerine.
- Intermittent, pulsed administration of GnRH.

4. Targeted delivery systems

- *Liposomes are* concentric, spherical shells of phospholipids in a watery medium, into which drugs are incorporated. They are administered by the IV route. Drugs which have been administered via liposomes are anticancer drugs (daunorubicin and doxorubicin), antifungal drug (amphotericin B) and the antibiotic gentamicin.
- *Nanomedicines:* These are synthesised using nanotechnology. The nanomedicines have size and shape in the nanoscale range (1–100 nm). They have very high surface/volume ratio. Their outer surface or their core can be loaded with chemicals (either a metal or an organic substance); and can be administered either intralesionally (paclitaxel, doxorubicin for cancer) or intravenously (for therapeutic purpose or as contrast agent for diagnostic imaging).
- *Others:* Monoclonal antibodies against cancer cell antigens is one of the innovations to deliver anticancer drugs to cancer cells. These antibodies *home in* on the cancer cells and release lethal concentrations of the drug selectively to the cancer tissue. A device for rapid nasal delivery of anticonvulsant lorazepam to the CNS has been developed (Chapter 9).

Box 1.3 Factors to be Considered while Selecting Route of Drug Administration and Dosage Form.

- Indended target site where drug is to be delivered
- Desired effect on the target
- Desired time to onset of action
- Condition of the patient
- Nature of the disease
- Available drug formulation: Chemical and physical properties of the drug
- Bioavailability of the drug by selected route
- Dose required

Box 1.3 lists the factors responsible for the selection of an appropriate route of drug administration and dosage forms.

PHARMACOKINETICS

The passage of a drug from the site of administration to the site of action is under the influence of four pharmacokinetic processes *viz.*, absorption, distribution, metabolism and excretion (ADME). These are important determinants of the drug concentration in systemic circulation, which in turn determine its concentration at the site of action (target concentration). Pharmacological effects of a drug are proportional to the target concentration. Based on ADME, dosage form of the drug, dose, its frequency of administration, onset of effect and how to maintain the target concentration to get the desired effect can be decided. Hence to prescribe rationally, a prescriber should be aware of pharmacokinetics of a drug. Moreover, it is possible to modulate the ADME processes to sustain the adequate concentration at the target site. PH 1.4

ABSORPTION AND BIOAVAILABILITY

Absorption is the process by which drugs enter the systemic circulation. Absorption of a drug from various sites, its movement among various body compartments and its distribution within the cell are all determined by the properties of the drug and those of biological membranes in the body.

For understanding the drug absorption, drugs can be divided into three groups:

1. Those that do not ionise are nonpolar and lipid soluble and, hence, are easily diffusible.
2. Those that always get ionised are water-soluble polar (lipid insoluble) and almost nondiffusible (strongly acidic/basic drugs).
3. Those that are partly ionised and partly nonionised and, hence partly water soluble and partly lipid soluble (weakly acidic/basic drugs).

Weakly acidic drugs remain unionised at acidic pH hence are diffusible at acidic pH, whereas weakly basic drugs remain unionised at alkaline pH, hence are diffusible at alkaline pH.

Molecules, including drug molecules, cross a biological membrane by the following methods:

1. **Simple or passive diffusion** is the commonest means by which a drug gets absorbed and distributed in the tissues. In this process, the drug molecules move across the cell membrane, in proportion to their concentration, from higher to lower concentration. *Cellular energy is not required and the system does not become saturated.* Passive diffusion may be either *lipid diffusion* (or *aqueous diffusion*. Thus, lipid-soluble drugs undergo lipid diffusion whereas water-soluble substances of small molecular weight (<700 Da) such as urea and alcohol undergo aqueous diffusion.
2. **Transport using transmembrane transporters:** Transporters are proteins located across the mucosal cells of the intestine (enterocytes), hepatocytes, renal tubules and in the capillary endothelium of vital organs. They pick up an endogenous substance or a drug at one border of the cell and release it at another. They are of two types:
   a. **Solute carriers (SLCs)** which are either *facilitatory* transporters for nonionic solutes, e.g. glucose transporter (GLUT) for glucose or *ion-coupled secondary active* transporters for neurotransmitter reuptake, e.g. VMAT for norepinephrine (NE) (Chapter 17)
   b. **ATP-binding cassettes (ABC) family** includes ubiquitous membrane proteins involved in active ATP-dependent movement of a range

of substrates, including ions, lipids, peptides, steroids, e.g. p-glycoprotein (ABCB1). It facilitates the efflux of anticancer drugs from cancer cells.

Membrane transporters are functionally of two types:

1. **Uptake transporters** which allow the transport of organic anions and cations *into the cells.*
2. **Efflux transporters** which allow the transport of agents only *out of the cells*, even against high concentration gradient, e.g. p-glycoprotein family. p-Glycoprotein is expressed on both, the enterocytes and hepatocytes, where they serve as an efflux pump. It is also present at the BBB.

Transmembrane transport occurs:

- **By facilitated diffusion** in which an SLC moves molecules *down the chemical/concentration gradient* or moves ions *down the electrical gradient*). Examples are transport of glucose and amino acids into cells.
- **By active transport,** which requires input of energy:
  a. Where a *carrier protein* moves molecules uphill *against the chemical or electrical gradient*, e.g. iodide transport into the thyroid follicular cells against concentration gradient. Other examples are folic acid antagonists and hormonal analogues.
  b. *Via ion channels* in the cell membrane (Chapter 2). Examples are inorganic ions such as Na^+, K^+, Ca^{++} and Cl^- and the ionised fraction of ionisable drugs.
  c. **By endocytosis,** comprising
     i. *Receptor mediated endocytosis*, e.g. insulin.
     ii. *Pinocytosis (cell drinking)* e.g. large, highly charged drug molecules such as lipid droplets.

Majority of the drugs, being lipid soluble, are absorbed by passive diffusion, a few by other modes. As a rule, drugs which are neither lipid soluble nor water soluble, e.g. barium sulphate, are not absorbed from the gut.

Information regarding the rate of absorption of a drug is necessary:

- To determine the frequency of its administration
- To ascertain the duration of effective action
- To predict the onset of desired or undesired effects of the drug

The time between the administration of a drug and the development of response is known as the **biological lag**. The route of administration determines the biological lag, which is minimum for IV route.

Oral absorption mostly occurs in the upper GI tract. Drugs given orally may be inactive systemically because of:

- *Enzymatic degradation* of polypeptides within the lumen of the GI tract, e.g. insulin, adrenocorticotropic hormone (ACTH).
- *Poor absorption* from the GI tract, e.g. aminoglycoside antibiotics.
- Inactivation by first pass metabolism.

These can be partly overcome by using Prodrugs.

Prodrug

Prodrug is an inactive chemical compound that, after administration, undergoes biotransformation to the pharmacologically active drug. Such prodrugs may overcome the barriers limiting the usefulness of a drug. For example, dopamine does not cross the BBB, and hence its prodrug 1-DOPA is used to treat Parkinson's disease, which increases the availability of dopamine in the CNS. Altering the polarity of ampicillin by esterifying ampicillin to form talampicillin improves its absorption. Prodrugs may also be used to achieve longer duration of action, e.g. esters of antipsychotic phenothiazines like fluphenazine. Another important use of prodrugs is to provide site-specific delivery of drugs. Thus, methenamine is a prodrug for formaldehyde; it is converted to formaldehyde and ammonia at the acidic urinary pH and acts as a urinary tract antiseptic.

Bioavailability of a Drug

It is defined as the amount or percentage of an active drug that is absorbed from a given dosage form

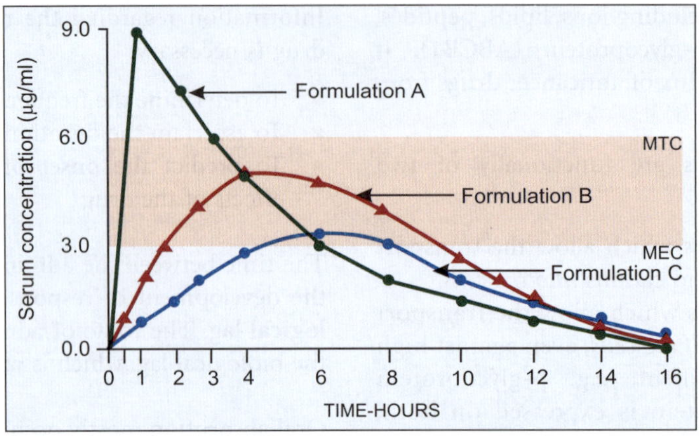

FIG. 1.4 ***The plasma drug level curves following oral administration of three formulations of the same basic drug.*** **MTC, minimum toxic concentration; MEC, minimum effective concentration. The pink area indicates the therapeutic range. For formulation A and B, the areas under the curves are identical. However, formulation A would produce quick onset and short duration of action compared to formulation B whose effect would last much longer. Formulation C gives in-adequate plasma levels and is, therefore, likely to be therapeutically ineffective.**

following its nonvascular administration, and reaches systemic circulation, to be available at the desired site of action. When the drug is given intravenously, the bioavailability is 100%.

Single dose bioavailability test involves an analysis of plasma or serum concentration of the drug at various time intervals after its oral administration and plotting a serum concentration versus time curve (Fig. 1.4). It provides information about the following:

1. Maximum concentration achieved after absorption (**Cmax**)
2. Time taken to achieve Cmax (**Tmax**)
3. Area under the curve (**AUC**) which gives idea about extent of absorption
4. Shape of the AUC which gives idea about rate of absorption

The bioavailability *F* is determined by comparing the AUC after oral administration of a drug with the AUC after IV administration of the same dose of the drug.

$$F = \frac{\text{AUC after oral dose}}{\text{AUC after IV dose}} \times 100$$

Drug formulations are considered to be **pharmaceutically equivalent** if they contain the same active ingredients and are identical in strength, concentration and dosage forms. The pharmaceutically equivalent drug formulations are considered to be **bioequivalent** when the rates and extent of bioavailability of the active ingredients in the two formulations do not differ significantly when tested by standard procedures. Such substances are likely to be **therapeutically equivalent**.

Factors affecting drug absorption and its bioavailability are listed in Box 1.4.

1. **Physical properties**
   Physical state: Liquids are absorbed better than solids and crystalloids are absorbed better than colloids.
   Lipid or water solubility: At the cell surface, the lipid-soluble drugs penetrate into the cell more rapidly than the water-soluble drugs. Bile salts emulsify the fat-soluble vitamins A and D in the small intestine and assist their absorption.

2. **Dosage forms**
   Particle size: Small particle size is important for absorption of corticosteroids, antibiotics like chloramphenicol and griseofulvin, certain oral anticoagulants and spironolactone. By reducing the particle size, the dosage of the active drug can be reduced without lowering its efficacy. On the other hand, for an antihelminthic such as

Box 1.4 Factors Affecting Oral Drug Absorption and Its Bioavailability

Drug related
- Physical properties of the drug
- Nature of the dosage form

Patient related
- Physiological factors
- Pharmacogenetic factors
- Disease states

bephenium hydroxynaphthoate, the particle size should be large enough to reduce its absorption. Particle size is of no consequence in the case of freely water-soluble drugs.

Disintegration time and dissolution rate: The effect of the physical factors is commonly evaluated by determining:

a. **The disintegration time** which measures the rate of breakup of the tablet or the capsule into the drug granules.
b. **The dissolution rate** which is the rate at which the drug goes into solution.

The dissolution rate is perhaps, a better parameter than the disintegration rate. This is because, in addition to disintegration time and particle size, other factors such as crystalline form (polymorphism), saturation solubility and solvation can modify the bioavailability.

Formulation: *The method of formulation can markedly influence the drug absorption and thus determine its bioavailability.* Usually, substances like lactose, sucrose, starch and calcium phosphate or lactate are used as inert diluents in formulating powders or tablets. Such fillers may not be totally inert but may affect the absorption as well as stability of the medicament. Thus, calcium and magnesium ions reduce the absorption of tetracyclines and bisphosphonates, while calcium phosphate used as a diluent for calciferol has caused calcium toxicity, when given in large doses. Replacement of calcium phosphate by lactose made a marked difference in the efficacy of a reformulated phenytoin preparation. *A faulty formulation can render a useful drug therapeutically useless.* The study of the influence of formulation on the therapeutic activity of drugs is known as **biopharmaceutics**.

3. **Physiological factors**

Ionisation: At the body pH, most drugs exist in two forms: (1) an unionised component, predominantly lipid soluble and (2) an ionised, water-soluble component. The unionised fraction can cross the cell membrane rapidly by passive diffusion. The amount of the drug which crosses the gut wall is determined by the gradient of its concentration between the lumen of the gut and the portal venous blood. If the absorbed unionised form gets rapidly decreased by binding with plasma proteins, then its low levels in portal venous blood facilitates its own absorption from the gut lumen.

pH of the GI fluid and the blood: Weakly acidic drugs are rapidly absorbed from the stomach as they exist in the acidic medium of the stomach in an unionised form. e.g. salicylates and barbiturates. However, major portion of these weakly acidic drugs is absorbed from the duodenum because of their solubility in the alkaline medium and availability of larger absorbing surface area. **Weakly basic drugs** are not absorbed until they reach the alkaline environment of the small intestine., in which these drugs exist in an unionised form facilitating their absorption. Their actions are delayed when administered orally, e.g. morphine.

GI transit time: The presence of food, and the volume, viscosity and tonicity of the gastric contents can influence drug absorption by altering the gastric emptying time. Rapid absorption occurs if the drug is given on an empty stomach. Box 1.5 shows the effect of food on the GI absorption of drugs.

Increased peristaltic activity, as in diarrhoea, reduces the drug absorption. Anticholinergic drugs, which prolong gastric emptying time, also

Box 1.5 The Effect of Food on Drug Absorption

Food aids the absorption of
Chloroquine, carbamazepine, griseofulvin, lithium, nitrofurantoin, riboflavin, spironolactone

Food interferes with the absorption of
Ampicillin, aspirin, captopril, digoxin, isoniazid, levodopa, penicillin G, rifampicin, tetracycline

impair absorption of concomitantly administered drugs such as l-DOPA.

Enterohepatic cycling: involves excretion of drug or its metabolite into the intestine. Such drug may undergo reabsorption. The conjugated metabolite may undergo enzymatic deconjugation by intestinal bacteria, which will liberate the parent drug to get reabsorbed. This increases the bioavailability of a drug, e.g. oral contraceptives, morphine.

Area of the absorbing surface and local circulation: As majority of the drugs are better absorbed from the small intestine because of its larger surface area, any major GI resection reduces the drug absorption. Increased vascularity can increase absorption.

First-pass elimination: The bioavailability of certain drugs is reduced by rapid metabolic degradation during the first passage through the gut wall (isoprenaline) or the liver (propranolol). The other examples are opioids, beta-adrenergic blockers, progesterone, isosorbide dinitrate, etc.

Presence of other agents: Vitamin C enhances the absorption of oral iron, while phytates retard it. The absorption of fat-soluble vitamins is reduced in the presence of liquid paraffin. Calcium, present in milk and in antacids, forms insoluble complexes with the fluoroquinolones and reduces absorption.

4. **Pharmacogenetic factors:** Chapter 3.
5. **Disease states:** Structural changes in the GI mucous membrane result in malabsorption syndrome. GI mucosal oedema significantly depresses the absorption of drugs such as hydrochlorothiazide in patients with congestive heart failure. Absorption and first pass metabolism may be affected in conditions like thyrotoxicosis, achlorhydria, cirrhosis of the liver and biliary obstruction.

The only valid tests of bioavailability of a drug preparation are as follows:

- The levels of the drug in biological fluids such as plasma, urine and saliva
- An objectively measurable variable of its therapeutic efficacy, e.g. heart rate and BP

Therapeutically, bioavailability is more important in the case of drugs with a narrow therapeutic index, e.g. digoxin and aminophylline.

PH 1.4

DISTRIBUTION OF A DRUG

After absorption, a drug enters or passes through the several body fluid compartments depending upon its physicochemical properties (Table 1.2). They are as follows:

- Plasma
- Interstitial fluid compartment
- Transcellular fluid compartment, e.g. fluids in the GI tract, bronchi, CSF
- Intracellular fluid compartment

Apparent Volume of Distribution (V_d)

It is defined as the volume into which the total amount of a drug in the body appears to be uniformly distributed. It is calculated as the total amount of drug in the body divided by the concentration of the drug in the plasma at zero time. For many drugs, V_d is constant over a wide dosage range.

$$V_d(\text{L}) = \frac{\text{Total amount administered}}{\text{Plasma concentration}}$$

Table 1.2 Distribution of Drugs in Different Body Compartments

Body Compartment	Types of Drugs
Total body water (60%)	Small, water-soluble molecules such as alcohol and antipyrine
Extracellular space (20%)	Large water-soluble molecules such as mannitol
Intravascular space (5%)	Very large, strongly protein-bound molecules such as heparin
Body fat (2%–5% in men; 10%–13% in women)	Highly lipid-soluble molecules such as DDT and thiopentone
Bones (12%–15%)	Fluoride and lead

Some drugs pass into the cells whereas others are distributed extracellularly. *However, a drug can penetrate into and exist in more than one compartment.* The rate of passage of a drug through a membrane is dependent upon the pH of the body compartment and the **dissociation constant (pK$_a$)** of the drug. *pK$_a$ is the pH at which the nonionised and ionised drug concentrations are equal.*

Nonionised, lipid-soluble drugs (the vast majority) readily cross membranes and are distributed throughout the body; they have large volumes of distribution. On the other hand, drugs which are highly protein bound (e.g. warfarin) or ionised (gentamicin) remain largely within the vascular compartment and have very low volumes of distribution. A drug like amoxicillin with V_d = 15 L is likely to be distributed in extracellular fluid (ECF), which includes plasma and interstitial fluid. Where the V_d exceeds the total volume of body water (42 L), there is a possibility of a drug accumulating in a tissue, e.g. V_d for digoxin is 420 L as it accumulates in the skeletal muscles. Chloroquine exhibits V_d of 13,000 L as it is concentrated in the liver. *Such drugs cannot be easily removed by dialysis.*

Protein Binding

After absorption, the drug circulates in the blood either in the free form or bound to plasma proteins either albumin or alpha-acid glycoprotein. These proteins are termed as **acceptors**. *Albumin is the main binding protein for many endogenous substances and drugs.* The fraction bound to protein usually falls as the total concentration of the drug increases and the binding sites get saturated.

Box 1.6 lists the effects of protein binding on drugs. Diffusion across the intestinal wall continues as long as the concentration within the gut exceeds that of the unbound fraction in the portal capillaries.

Box 1.6 Effects of Protein Binding on Drugs

- Assists enteral absorption of a drug,
- Acts as a temporary store for it and thereby prolongs its action,
- Causes prolonged, low levels of free drug,
- Delays its metabolic degradation,
- Delays its excretion
- Diminishes its penetration into the CNS

Protein binding:

- *Assists absorption of orally administered drugs*
- *Acts as a temporary 'store' of a drug* and tends to prevent large fluctuations in concentration of unbound drug in the body fluids.
- *Reduces diffusion of the drug into the cells and thereby delays its metabolic degradation*, e.g. 90% of long-acting sulphonamides and 98% of warfarin circulate in bound form whereas protein binding is negligible with ethosuximide and amoxycillin.
- *Reduces the amount of drug available for filtration* at the glomeruli and hence delays its excretion.
- *Reduces the drug clearance.*
- *Reduces concentrations of free drug to be available for desirable effect*, e.g. highly protein bound drug may have too low concentration in interstitial fluid, CSF and tissue cells to combat dangerous infections, e.g. sulphadoxine.

The extent of drug binding depends on the binding protein concentration in the plasma. Thus, in pregnancy, the protein bound fraction of thyroxine increases due to a rise in the concentration of the specific binding protein in the plasma. Conversely, in hypoproteinaemia, there is a rise in the free fraction due to low plasma albumin levels; the therapeutic dose required may thus be smaller.

Administration of concomitant drugs which get bound to the same binding sites on plasma proteins may result in a sudden increase in the free concentration of one of them, possibly to a dangerous level (Chapter 3). Thus, if a patient stabilised on the anticoagulant warfarin takes glibenclamide in addition, a sudden increase in free concentration of warfarin may occur due to its displacement from the binding sites by glibenclamide and may result in haemorrhage.

Drug Storage

The concentration of a drug in certain tissues such as fat and liver after a single dose may persist even when its plasma concentration has decreased to low or undetectable levels, e.g. on IV administration, 70% thiopentone is taken up by the body fat from which it is released slowly. Iodine is similarly concentrated in the thyroid tissue. Membrane transporters are involved in drug targeting to a specific tissue, e.g. metformin concentrates in the liver with the help of SLC type influx transporters.

Because of such storage, repeated exposure to certain drugs (e.g. chloroquine)/ chemicals (e.g. DDT), even in small doses, may lead to chronic toxicity. Arsenic gets incorporated in the hair follicles on prolonged administration. This phenomenon is used for detection of arsenic poisoning.

Drugs showing such preferential accumulation are listed in Box 1.7.

Termination of drug effects mainly occurs due to biotransformation and excretion and to a lesser extent by redistribution of the drug from its site of action into other tissues or sites (e.g. Thiopentone see Chapter 7).

Placental Transfer

The passage of drugs through the placenta into the fetal circulation is determined by the properties of the drug, the properties of the placenta and the altered maternal blood levels due to changing pharmacokinetics in pregnancy. There are a number of influx transporters in placenta making the placental barrier imperfect. The effect on the fetus is determined by its gestational age (Chapter 78).

Box 1.7 Preferential Accumulation of Drugs

Site	Drugs
Thyroid	Iodine
Kidney	Mercury
Liver	Chloroquine
Eye	Chloroquine
Bones & teeth	Lead, Tetracycline
Adipose tissue	Thiopental, DDT
Skeletal muscles	Digoxin, Statins

Blood-Brain Barrier (BBB)

A specialised system i.e. Blood Brain Barrier (BBB) not only maintains the special composition of CSF in the face of fluctuating composition of the plasma, but also protects the brain from toxic substances.

BBB allows free passage of lipid-soluble drugs such as diazepam. Ionisable organic molecules (which many drugs are) are largely denied such passage from blood into the brain. However, substances can pass freely between CSF in the subarachnoid space and the ECF in the brain; hence, drugs such as antibiotics introduced into the CSF can enter the brain ECF in adequate concentration. Drugs may penetrate into the brain using **uptake transporters** for endogenous substances and nutrients.

Apart from the anatomical features, *functional BBB and blood–CSF barrier involve membrane transporters such as p-glycoproteins (MDR1) and organic anion transporting polypeptides (OATPs) which extrude a large number of structurally diverse drugs and protect the brain from their adverse effects.* Membrane transporters in the choroid plexus actively secrete drugs from the CSF into the blood. Drugs and endogenous metabolites, irrespective of their molecular size and lipid solubility, exit with bulk flow of the CSF through the subarachnoid villi into the venous sinuses in the brain.

The classical BBB, however, is absent in certain areas of the brain such as the pineal gland and the area postrema of the fourth ventricle (**Chemoreceptor trigger zone- CTZ**). These areas act as brain sensors for changes in the composition of the plasma.

The BBB becomes less efficient in the presence of inflammatory diseases such as meningitis and encephalitis. Parenterally administered antibiotics can then reach therapeutic concentrations in the brain ECF. When the infection is controlled and the inflammation subsides, the BBB tends to be restored. *As that may happen while viable microorganisms persist in the CSF, drug dosage should not be reduced till the CSF is sterilised.*

FATE OF A DRUG

PH 1.4

Human body treats drugs as foreign chemical substances (xenobiotics). Alteration of a drug within a living organism is known as **biotransformation.**

After absorption, drugs could undergo three possible fates:

1. **Biotransformation by enzymes:** which may be microsomal, cytosolic or mitochondrial. The biotransformation of drugs usually:
   a. Inactivates an active drug (metabolism) to make it more polar and water soluble (i.e. metabolite), so that it can be excreted by the kidneys.
   b. Activates an inactive drug (prodrug).
   c. Generates active metabolite(s) of an active drug (Table 1.3).
2. **Spontaneous change into other substances** without the intervention of enzymes, e.g. the anticancer drug mechlorethamine (a prodrug) changes spontaneously into the active ethyleniminium cations at the slightly alkaline pH of the plasma or similar inactivation of the muscle relaxant atracurium (Hofmann reaction).
3. **Excreted unchanged:** A highly polar and water-soluble drug is not metabolised and gets excreted as such, e.g. aminoglycosides.

Table 1.3 Effects of Biotransformation on Drugs

Effect of Biotransformation	Examples
Inactivation of an active drug	Chloramphenicol by conjugation
Activation of an inactive drug to an active product	*Therapeutically useful:* L-DOPA to dopamine and enalapril to enalaprilat *Toxic:* parathion to paraxone
Generation of active metabolites of an active drug	*More active:* diazepam to oxazepam *Having a different activity:* pethidine, a CNS depressant, to norpethidine, CNS stimulant

There are many tissues which can metabolise drugs, but by far the most active tissue per unit weight is the liver. The enzymes which metabolise drugs (namely microsomal and non microsomal enzymes) are distinct from those which function in the intermediary metabolism.

Hepatic microsomal enzymes: These enzymes are located in the **liver microsomes** which form a part of the smooth membrane of the endoplasmic reticulum of the hepatic cells. These enzymes catalyse a variety of oxidative and reductive reactions, e.g. superfamilies of enzymes-cytochrome P450 (*CYP*), flavin-containing monooxygenases (*FMOs*) and epoxide hydroxylases (*EHs*) as well as some phase II enzymes like esterases, amidases, glucuronyl transferases.

- **CYPs** are involved in the metabolism of many dietary and xenobiotic compounds (Chapter 3) and in synthesis of endogenous agents (e.g. steroids, bile acids from cholesterol). A drug bound to CYP may be either oxidised or reduced. There are many isozymes of the enzyme CYP, each of which is encoded by a separate gene. *Variations in their gene structure explain the differences in the drug metabolism among different individuals and ethnic groups.* CYP3A4 is involved in the metabolism of several drugs, followed by CYP2D6. The other important isoenzymes are CYP2C9, CYP2C19 and CYP1A2.
- **FMOs** are minor contributors to drug metabolism. H_2 receptor antagonists, clozapine, itopride are metabolised by them. The metabolites cause no drug–drug interaction.
- **EH** deactivates potentially toxic metabolites produced by CYPs, e.g. carbamazepine 10,11-epoxide, an active metabolite of the carbamazepine is inactivated by microsomal EH.

Nonmicrosomal enzymes: Drugs are also metabolised by nonmicrosomal enzymes, present in liver, plasma and tissues including placenta and even by those present in the intestinal microorganisms (**microfloral enzymes**), e.g. monoamine oxidase (MAO), alcohol dehydrogenase, xanthine oxidase.

The xenobiotic enzyme reactions involved in metabolic transformations are as follows:

Phase I (Nonsynthetic)

- Oxidation
- Reduction
- Hydrolysis

Phase II (Synthetic)

- Synthesis (conjugation or transfer reactions).

Phase I Reactions

Oxidation, reduction and hydrolysis introduce polar groups such as hydroxyl, amino, sulphhydryl and carboxy into drugs, which convert them to water soluble and pharmacologically less active metabolites. Thus, metabolism of drugs is essentially a detoxification process. However, during the initial stages of metabolism of certain drugs, active and even toxic compounds may be produced, e.g. imipramine, an antidepressant drug is biotransformed into an active compound desipramine; cyclophosphamide, sulindac and enalapril are activated by oxidation.

Oxidation: A drug may be oxidised by more than one mechanism and for the same drug this may differ in different species of animals. The reactions include the following:

- **Microsomal oxidation** which involves
  a. ***Hydroxylation***, wherein hydroxyl group is introduced into the drug molecule, e.g. conversion of salicylic acid to gentisic acid.
  b. ***Dealkylation***, wherein an alkyl group is removed, e.g. conversion of phenacetin to the active compound *p*-acetaminophenol.
  c. ***Deamination***, wherein an amino group is removed, e.g. conversion of amphetamine to benzyl–methyl-ketone.
  - **Nonmicrosomal oxidation**, e.g. ethyl alcohol is oxidised to carbon dioxide and water. Methyl alcohol is oxidised to toxic formic acid and formaldehyde.
  - **Mitochondrial oxidation:** A mitochondrial enzyme MAO causes oxidative deamination of substances like adrenaline, 5-HT and tyramine.

Reduction: Many halogenated compounds and nitrated aromatic compounds are reduced by the microsomal enzymes, e.g. halothane and chloramphenicol; drugs like chloral hydrate, disulfiram and nitrites are reduced by nonmicrosomal enzymes.

Hydrolysis: This is usually carried out by enzymes 'carboxy esterases' that hydrolyse (split with addition of water) the esters and amide containing compounds. These enzymes are microsomal, nonmicrosomal and microfloral in origin. They are usually of low specificity and exhibit considerable species variation. Drugs like atropine, neostigmine and phenytoin, are hydrolysed by esterases. Digitalis glycosides are rendered inactive by hydrolysis.

Methanamine mandelate, a urinary antiseptic, is hydrolysed in the urinary tract, at an acid pH, to formaldehyde and ammonia.

Phase II Reactions

Conjugation or transfer reaction: This is a synthetic process by which a drug or its metabolite is combined with an endogenous substance, resulting in various conjugates such as glucuronides, ethereal sulphates, methylated compounds and amino acid conjugates. Conjugation invariably results in inactivation of the compound. After such inactivation, large molecules are eliminated in the bile whereas smaller molecules are excreted in the urine.

Glucuronides are produced by the combination of a hydroxyl, carboxyl or amino group of drug molecule with glucuronic acid. Compounds like morphine, paraamino benzoic acid (PABA), stilboesterol and salicylic acid are excreted mainly in the form of glucuronides. Ethereal sulphates are produced by the combination of sulphate and hydroxyl or amino group. A classical example of amino acid conjugation is the combination of benzoic acid with glycine to form hippuric acid.

A drug may be metabolised and inactivated by more than one successive reaction, e.g. progesterone is first reduced to pregnanediol which is then conjugated; chloramphenicol is similarly reduced and then conjugated.

> *In practice, patients may differ in their response to a standard dose of a drug. This is largely due to variations in the rate of drug metabolism among individuals. Factors affecting drug metabolism are listed in Box 1.8. The major factors are: genetic, environmental and disease related.*

Box 1.8 Factors Affecting Drug Metabolism

- Animal species and strain
- Age and sex
- Genetic determinants
- Nutritional status
- Hypothermia
- Route and duration of administration
- Environmental determinants such as air pollution
- Simultaneous administration of other drugs (enzyme induction and inhibition)
- Presence of disease, hepatic/renal damage

The ability of the microsomal enzymes to metabolise drugs is poor in premature infants and neonates as compared to adults. Hence, the liver of a premature infant is unable to conjugate chloramphenicol to the same extent as in adults, resulting in very high serum concentration of chloramphenicol causing cyanosis of infants (**grey baby syndrome**). Undernutrition depresses the functional capacity of these enzyme systems, and this should be borne in mind particularly in countries where undernutrition is common.

The diseased liver has poor ability to metabolise drugs. Morphine and methadone which are metabolised in the liver may thus have an unusually prolonged action in hepatic cirrhosis. Reduc-tion in hepatic blood flow in shock and congestive heart failure can cause marked reduction in the metabolic degradation of lignocaine.

Certain agents, such as ethanol, barbiturates, on repeated administration, stimulate the synthesis of microsomal enzyme system. This is called **enzyme induction**. It takes 2–3 weeks to induce enzymes. Once the enzymes are induced, they metabolise drugs, which are their substrates, more rapidly. Thus, exposure to the insecticide DDT accelerates the biotransformation of drugs, leading to their faster elimination. Enzyme induction also occurs to a limited extent in the kidney, lung, skin and gut. For **enzyme inhibition**, see Chapter 3. PH 1.4

DRUG EXCRETION

The important routes of excretion are:

- Renal
- Extrarenal (GIT, lungs, skin etc.)

Renal

The processes which determine the elimination of a drug by kidneys are as follows:

1. Passive Glomerular Filtration. Only the unbound fraction of unionised drugs is filtered at the glomerulus; but they are reabsorbed by diffusion back from the tubular lumen into the cells lining the tubules. Thus, ultimately a very small amount of the drug appears in the urine.

Ionised drugs which are poorly absorbed are excreted almost entirely by glomerular filtration and are not reabsorbed.

2. Active Tubular Secretion. Many weak acids (anionic substances) and weak bases (cationic substances) are actively secreted by proximal tubules by carrier-mediated systems involving transporters such as **p-glycoprotein** and the **multidrug-resistance-associated protein type 2** (MRP2). These transporters are also responsible for excretion of conjugated metabolites of drugs (Box 1.9).

Tubular secretion of weak organic acids such as penicillin can be blocked by probenecid, and their half-lives can be prolonged. Secretion of weak

Box 1.9 Some Drugs Secreted by Proximal Tubule into Urine

Cationic (weakly acidic)	Anionic (weakly basic)
Atropine	Acetazolamide
Cimetidine	Antibiotics (penicillin, cephalosporins)
Ethambutol	Ciprofloxacin
Metformin	Diuretics (loop diuretics, thiazides)
Procainamide	Probenecid
Pseudoephedrine	Salicylate
Quinine	Sulphonamides
Trimethoprim	Sulphonylureas

bases by renal tubules can also be blocked but the blocking agents are too toxic for any therapeutic utility.

3. Passive Renal Tubular Reabsorption. Passive diffusion is a bidirectional process and drugs may diffuse across the tubules in either direction depending upon the drug concentration, lipid solubility and the pH, e.g. salicylates.

The pH of the urine influences the excretion of certain weak acids and weak bases. Thus, *weak acids are quickly eliminated in an alkaline urine as they undergo ionization minimizing their tubular reabsorption, e.g. barbiturates and salicylates; while weak bases are rapidly excreted in an acidic urine, e.g. pethidine and amphetamine.* On the other hand, the action of these substances in the body can be prolonged if the urinary pH is not favourable for their excretion. Elimination of weak acids and weak bases can thus be accelerated by

- Maintaining a high rate of urine flow by the use of diuretics.
- Adjusting the urinary pH. PH 1.12, PH 2.4

In the presence of renal damage, the ability of the kidney to excrete drugs is impaired. This might result in unacceptable high blood levels and prolonged drug action with normal doses. *Great care must, therefore, be exercised when drugs like aminoglycosides or coumarin anticoagulants are used in the presence of kidney damage.* Similarly, potassium salts may produce dangerous hyperkalaemia if the kidney function is impaired. Some other drugs, the dose of which must be adjusted in renal failure are as follows:

1. **Only in severe renal failure:** Cotrimoxazole, carbenicillin, cefotaxime, metronidazole and fluoroquinolones
2. **Even in mild renal failure:** Cephalexin, ethambutol, amphotericin B, acyclovir and flucytosine.

In patients with impaired renal function, the dose of drugs, which are eliminated almost completely (90%) by kidney needs to be reduced. This can be calculated based on creatinine clearance.

Creatinine clearance *in adults* can be estimated from serum creatinine by the **Cockroft and Gault formula:**

Creatinine clearance (mL/min) in males

$$= \frac{(140 - \text{Age in years}) \times \text{Weight (kg)}}{72 \times \text{serum creatinine (mg/dL)}}$$

Creatinine clearance (mL/min) in females

$$= 0.85 \times \frac{(140 - \text{Age in years}) \times \text{Weight (kg)}}{72 \times \text{serum creatinine (mg/dL)}}$$

Thus, if the serum creatinine is 2.5 mg/dL in a 50-year-old male who weighs 60 kg and has height 158 cm, then his calculated creatinine clearance is 30 mL/ min. *This Creatinine clearance refers to an adult with 1.73 square metre body surface area (BSA).* Thus it should be corrected to the BSA of the patient.

Hence, based on the weight and height of the patient, the calculated BSA is 1.6 *square metre*. Using this corrected creatinine clearance is calculated, which is 27.7 mL/min.

The dose of the drugs then equals:

$$\frac{\text{Corrected creatinine clearance} \times \text{the usual daily dose.}}{100}$$

If the adult dose is 5 mg, then the dose to be administered in the above patient will be:

$$\frac{27.7 \times 5}{100} = 1.38\text{mg}$$

However, the first dose in such patients should be the same as the initial dose used in a patient with normal renal function (**loading dose**).

In clinical practice the dosages are not calculated manually. The automated calculators use CKD EPI creatinine equation (2021) to estimate glomerular filtration rate (eGFR). One requires serum creatinine levels, age of the patient and ethnicity as black or non black.

It is beyond the scope of this book to give detailed instructions about dose adjustment for each drug in renal impairment. The manufacturer's instructions should be consulted for this purpose.

Protein binding reduces the amount of the drug available for glomerular filtration but protein bound drugs may still be available for secretion by the proximal renal tubules, e.g. salicylic acid. This is because the bound form of the drug is released from its combination with plasma proteins when the peritubular fluid concentration of the free form of the drug is lowered.

Since drugs, metabolites and toxins are concentrated in the kidneys during their excretion, this organ is frequently the site of drug-induced renal toxicity.

EXTRARENAL ROUTES

Lungs

Volatile general anaesthetics and alcohol are partially excreted by the lungs. Their presence can be recognised by the odour they impart to the breath.

Bile

Transport systems similar to those in the kidneys are present in the hepatocytes which actively secrete drugs and their metabolites into the bile. Drugs such as phenolphthalein, doxycycline and cefoperazone appear in high concentrations in the bile. Such drugs may get repeatedly reabsorbed from the intestine and re-excreted in bile, thereby exerting a prolonged action (**enterohepatic circulation**).

Intestines

Drugs and their metabolites can be:

- Actively secreted from the systemic circulation into the intestinal lumen using transporters.
- Passively diffuse from the blood into the intestinal lumen, depending on their pK and the luminal pH. Laxatives like cascara and senna, which act on the large bowel, are partly excreted into that area from the blood stream, after their absorption from the small intestine. Heavy metals are also excreted through the intestine and can produce intestinal ulceration.

Skin

Arsenic and heavy metals like mercury are excreted in small quantities through the skin.

Saliva and Milk

Certain drugs like iodides and metallic salts are excreted in the saliva. Lead compounds deposited as lead sulphide produce a blue line on the gums. Secretion of drugs in milk is discussed in Chapter 78.

PH 1.1

PLASMA HALF-LIFE AND ITS SIGNIFICANCE

Information about the time course of drug absorption, distribution and elimination (Pharmacokinetics) can be expressed in mathematical terms. As mentioned earlier, pharmacokinetic parameters aid in the selection and adjustment of drug dose schedules. *However, they are not a substitute for, but rather a supplement to, clinical monitoring and judgement.* These parameters include bioavailability, V_d, half-life (t½) and clearance. Significance of bioavailability and V_d is discussed earlier. Clearance and dose determine the magnitude of the steady state (SS).

Drugs are eliminated from the body by

- **First-order kinetics or**
- **Zero-order kinetics.**

Elimination of most drugs occurs exponentially (**first-order kinetics**) i.e. a constant fraction of the drug in the body disappears in each equal interval of time. Thus, following a single IV dose, the plasma concentration of the drug falls exponentially (Fig. 1.5A). *That is, the drug is removed from the body not at a constant rate but at a rate proportional to its plasma concentration.* In the case of an exponentially eliminated drug, a plot of the log of concentration against time gives almost a straight line. The rate of an exponential process may be expressed either:

1. in terms of its rate constant (K) which expresses the fractional change per unit of time, or
2. in terms of its half-life (t½), the time required for 50% completion of the process (**elimination half-life, plasma half-life**). Half-life of a drug can be computed using following formula:

$$t\frac{1}{2} = \frac{0.693}{K}$$

For drugs following first order kinetics, the elimination half-life is independent of the dose, the route of administration and the plasma concentration(C). It depends on V_d as well as on the clearance from the body i.e. metabolism and the renal excretion ($t½ = 0.693 \times V_d/CL$). However, the actual quantity of the drug removed per unit time is smaller at lower plasma concentrations and larger at higher plasma concentrations. Furthermore, it should be noted that t½ during long-term oral administration of a drug may be different from that after a single IV dose. Reduced clearance of the drug due to disease is expected to prolong biological half-life and the drug effect. *This reciprocal relationship is valid only as long as the V_d of the drug does not change.*

Simple calculation shows that **when a single dose of the drug is administered, nearly 93.75% of the drug is eliminated in four half-lives**. Since 4–5 half-lives are required for complete exponential elimination, repeated dosing intervals shorter than this leads to drug accumulation. Thus, a drug administered in equal doses, intermittently, at constant time intervals (equal to half-life), will *accumulate exponentially* to a plateau (**steady state;** *SS*) plasma level. The concentration at SS = dose rate/clearance.

After the steady state is reached, drug elimination equals drug absorption during the dose interval (Fig. 1.5B). The time taken to attain the SS depends only upon on *its half-life* (t½). **It takes five elimination half-lives for the drug to reach the plateau level in the plasma.** Thus, in practice, dobutamine with t½ of 2 min, given by infusion, reaches a SS in 10 min, whereas it takes 7.5 days for oral diazepam (t½ 36 h).

The drug concentration maintained during the SS is directly proportional to both elimination t½ and the quantity of the drug given per unit time (as dose/dosage interval).

With certain drugs such as phenytoin, alcohol, dicoumarol, probenecid, oral propranolol and large doses of salicylates, the elimination is exponential with lower dosage levels, but *when the dose exceeds a certain critical level, the eliminating mechanisms get saturated and then a fixed quantity of the drug is eliminated per unit time.* This is called **dose-dependent elimination** or **saturation kinetics** or **zero-order kinetics.** With such drugs, an increase in the dose can cause a disproportionate increase in the plasma level as only a fixed amount is getting excreted. This can result in drug toxicity (Fig. 1.6).

Dose of a drug: It is the specific amount of medication to be taken at a given time. The average daily amount of a drug that is actually prescribed is termed as **prescribed daily dose** (PDD). It is based on the pharmacokinetic considerations and also varies with

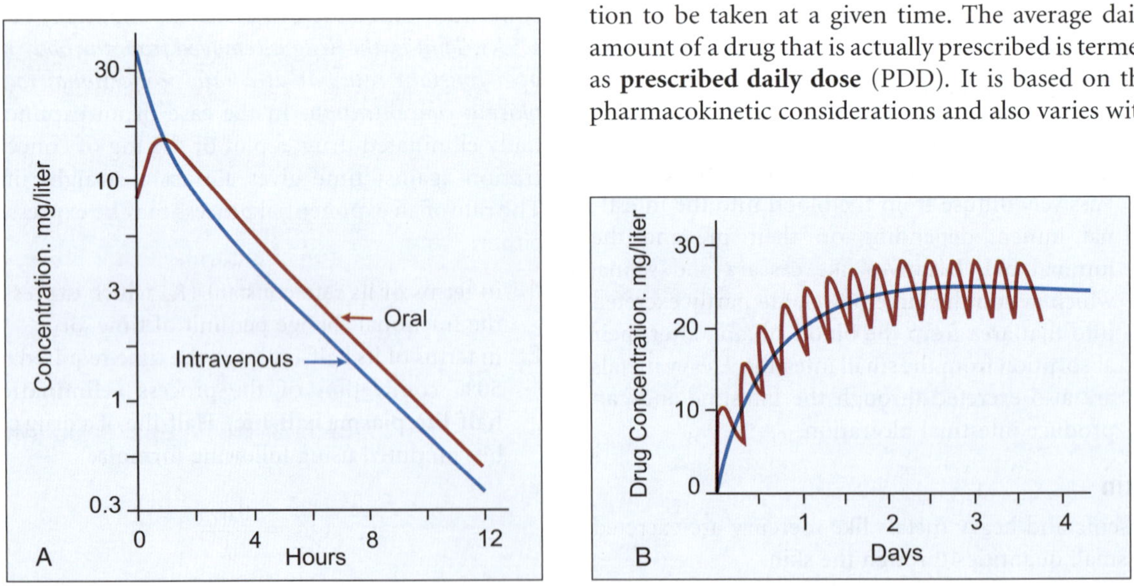

FIG. 1.5 **(A)** ***Exponential curves of plasma concentration of a drug following oral and IV administration.*** **The slope is independent of the route of administration (first-order kinetics). (B)** ***Rise of drug concentration to a plateau (steady-state) level during repeated oral administration of a constant dose.*** **Peaks are the high points of the fluctuations whereas troughs are the low points of the fluctuations.**

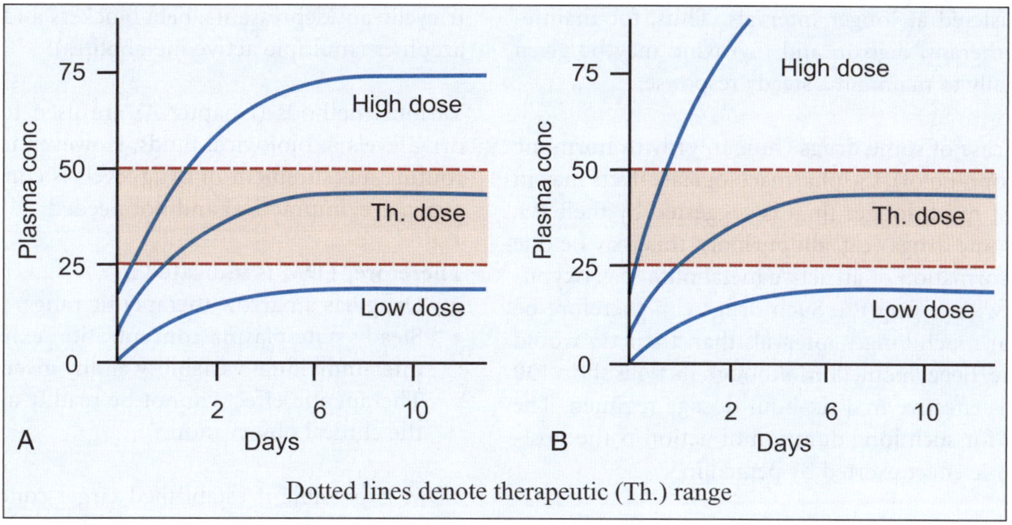

FIG. 1.6 Comparison of nonsaturation and saturation kinetics for drugs, given orally, 12 hourly.
Fig. 1.6 A shows plasma concentration curves of a drug that follows nonsaturation kinetics (first order). Note that, the steady-state plasma concentration is directly proportional to the dose. Fig. 1.6 B shows curves for a drug that follows saturation kinetics (zero order), e.g. phenytoin. Note that, no SS is reached with high doses and that even a small increase in the dose results in a disproportionately large (perhaps toxic) plasma concentration.

patient characteristics and severity of the disease (Chapter 3). PH 1.12

To compare drug use across different countries or different health care facilities in a given country, a measurement unit has been introduced by WHO, which is termed as **defined daily dose** (DDD). DDD is an assumed average maintenance dose per day of a drug used for its main indication in adults. This standard is used in pharmacoepidemiological studies to measure drug consumption in a given population. It does not necessarily reflect the recommended dose or PDD.

Dose determination: Sometimes, for achieving the therapeutic drug concentration, a **loading dose** of the drug is administered, followed by **maintenance doses**. The loading dose is defined as the one or series of doses given initially that are higher than the subsequent doses. It is administered for achieving the desired plasma concentration rapidly. *A loading dose is a product of V_d and desired plasma concentration.* Its disadvantage is the possible toxic effect caused by large initial drug concentration particularly in sensitive individuals.

The subsequent doses are required for maintaining a steady-state plasma drug concentration in the therapeutic range. In a patient with impaired hepatic, renal or cardiovascular function, the maintenance dose must be reduced in order to prevent unduly high plasma drug levels. This may be achieved either by reducing each individual dose or by lengthening the dosage interval in proportion to the increase in the biological half-life.

Dosing frequency: When a drug with rapid absorption or **short biological half-life** is administered repeatedly in the same dose at fixed, long intervals of time, marked fluctuations in the plasma concentration (during plateau state) may occur between the doses. These fluctuations can be reduced by giving the drug at shorter intervals, say by giving half doses at half intervals. Thus, during levodopa therapy, steady plasma levels and a steady clinical response can be maintained only by giving the drug in at least four divided doses per day. Insulin with a very short t½ of a few minutes is best administered by a continuous, IV infusion for maximum efficacy in diabetic coma. On the other hand, in **drugs with long t½**, such fluctuations in the plasma concentration at plateau are less marked, and hence, these drugs may be administered at longer intervals. Thus, for maintenance therapy, digoxin and thyroxine may be given once daily to maintain a steady response.

In the case of some drugs (human growth hormone and propranolol), the pharmacological effects may in fact last much longer than is suggested by their t½. With some drugs (e.g. allopurinol), this may be due to the formation of an active metabolite (e.g. oxypurinol) with a long t½. Such drugs can therefore be given at much longer intervals than their t½ would indicate. Benzylpenicillin, although its t½ is short (30 min), is effective in a six-hour dosage regimen. The reason for such long duration of action is the post-antibiotic effect exerted by penicillin.

The concentrations of many drugs at their site(s) of action are in equilibrium with their plasma concentration. Hence, the therapeutic response to such drugs correlates better with plateau plasma levels than with dosages.

Variations in plasma levels following similar doses (on weight basis) observed in different subjects are due to variations in the rates of pharmacokinetic processes either due to disease condition or Genetic differences. With drugs such as theophylline and phenytoin, there may be as much as 3–5-fold variation in the plasma concentration achieved in different individuals given similar doses. Furthermore, drug concentration in certain tissues may persist even when the plasma drug concentration is low or undetectable after stopping the drug, thus giving a prolonged effect, e.g. digoxin in the ventricular muscle. PH 1.2

Therapeutic Drug Monitoring (TDM): Monitoring of concentrations of drugs in body fluids, usually in plasma but also in serum and blood is done to enhance the efficacy of a drug and minimize toxicity. It allows a prescriber to individualize the drug dosage so that plasma drug concentrations remain within a targeted therapeutic range or window. However, TDM is not required for drugs whose dose can be correlated with clearly measurable indices such as BP, blood sugar, urine volume or blood coagulation parameters. Similarly, it is of no value when the plasma drug concentration correlates poorly or not at all with the drug effect as with anticancer drugs, tricyclic antidepressants, beta blockers and benzodiazepines (multiple active metabolites).

Various methods (Chapter 4) are used to estimate drug levels in biological fluids. However, in practice, routine measurement of drug levels is cumbersome, expensive, impractical and not needed.

Therefore, TDM is indicated if:

- Drug has a narrow therapeutic range.
- Steady state plasma concentration exhibits large inter-individual variability at any given dose.
- Therapeutic effect cannot be readily assessed by the clinical observation.

TDM is possible if established target concentration range (Box 1.10) and cost-effective drug assay techniques are available.

The plasma samples are collected only when the drug reaches SS (i.e. 4–5 t½ after starting therapy) because at SS, plasma concentration of a drug is usually proportional to the target site concentration. During the dosing interval, the drug concentration keeps on changing, especially in the distribution phase. Less variations are observed during the elimination phase;

Box 1.10 Some Drugs Suitable for TDM and their Therapeutic Range

Drug	Therapeutic Range
Phenytoin	10-20 mg/L
Sodium Valproate	50-100 mg/L
Carbamazepine	5-12 mg/L
Lamotrigine	1.5–3 mg/L
Gentamicin	Peak 7–10mg/L; Trough 1-2 mg/L
Amikacin	Peak 4–12 mg/L; Trough 4 mg/L
Vancomycin	Trough 10–20 mg/L
Cyclosporin	50-200 mcg/L (serum or plasma) 150–400 microgram/L (whole blood)
Sirolimus	5–15 microgram/L (whole blood)
Tacrolimus	5–20 microgram/L (whole blood)
Amiodarone	1–2.5 mg/L for ventricular arrhythmia 0.5–1.5 mg/L for atrial arrhythmia
Theophylline	5-20 mg/L
Lithium	
- Acute Mania	0.8-1.2 mmol/L
- Maintenance	0.4-1.0 mmol/L
Digoxin	0.8-2 mcg/L

the least variable point being just prior to the next dose (trough or pre-dose concentration). Near peak concentrations are measured to detect toxicity for the drugs that show specific symptoms related to peak concentrations (e.g. carbamazepine and lithium) or to calculate AUC for antibiotics. For the latter, both peak and trough concentrations are needed.

It is important to note that TDM involves not only **measuring drug concentrations**, but also the **clinical interpretation** of the result. It requires knowledge of pharmacokinetics, sampling time, details of drug intake and patient's clinical condition. On the basis of all this information, TDM:

- Supports prescribing decisions following a change in dosage regimen or when there is sudden change in clinical state of a patient.
- Prevents/confirms the drug toxicity and helps to treat it.
- Finds out reasons for non-responsiveness: whether the concentrations are subtherapeutic or the patient is under-treated or is non-compliant.
- Helps when manifestations of drug toxicity and clinical symptoms of disease state overlap.
- Detects potential drug interaction in patient receiving multiple drug therapy.
- Guides withdrawal of therapy.

METHODS OF PROLONGING THE DURATION OF ACTION OF A DRUG

The drug action can be prolonged by using the following methods:

1. **Retarding drug absorption:** Oral absorption of a drug can be retarded by administering it on full stomach or by giving it in various coated formulations, e.g. *sustained release preparations* of nitroglycerine. Such formulation, however, does not always prolong the action of a drug.
   Absorption of a drug after **parenteral administration** can be retarded by:
   i. **Reduction in the vascularity of the absorbing surface:** This can be achieved by administration of a vasoconstrictor along with the drug, e.g. adrenaline with lignocaine.
   ii. **Reduction in the solubility of the drug:** This can be achieved by combining the drug with a compound having poor water solubility or giving the drug in a suspension form. Thus, penicillin is combined with procaine, a compound with poor water solubility.
   iii. **Administration of the drug in oily solution** testoterone injections
   iv. **Combination of the drug with a protein** from which it is released slowly, e.g. protamine zinc insulin.
   v. **Esterification:** Steroidal sex hormones such as testosterone and estrogens, when esterified with carboxylic acids, give compounds such as benzoate, propionate, enanthate and cypionate which are absorbed slowly.
   vi. **Pegylation**, i.e. combination with polyethylene glycol (PEG), e.g. interferons.
   vii. **Depot preparations** (e.g. DOCA in Addison disease) or *of steroid filled silastic capsules* (e.g. progestogens for contraception).
   viii. Transdermal patches of nitroglycerine, estradiol, scopolamine and fentanyl when applied on the skin, the drug is slowly absorbed at constant rate into the systemic circulation.
2. **Retarding drug metabolism:** The hepatic microsomal enzyme systems concerned with metabolism may be inhibited by certain drugs, such as MAO inhibitors leading to prolonged drug action. The action of levodopa can be extended by combining it with a DOPA decarboxylase inhibitor which inhibits its metabolism in the blood.
3. **Retarding renal excretion of the drug:** The tubular secretion of certain drugs can be blocked by using compounds which share the same tubular secretory pathway. Thus, probenecid is used to reduce the penicillin excretion (Chapter 44).
4. **Increased protein binding of the drug in the plasma:** Long-acting sulphonamide sulphamethoxypyridazine is bound to plasma proteins more extensively than short-acting sulphadiazine. Suramin, used in the treatment of trypanosomiasis, is extensively bound to the plasma proteins. Such drugs have prolonged action.

Drugs that are sequestered in the adipose tissue (such as quinestrol, a derivative of estradiol) have a prolonged action.

CHAPTER 2

PH 1.1

Pharmacodynamics – Drug Receptor Interactions; Adverse Drug Reactions

Learning Objectives

This chapter will enable the reader:

1. To explain different mechanisms (receptor and nonreceptor) of drug action with suitable examples.
2. To classify various drug receptors, illustrating drug receptor interactions.
3. To interpret drug response relationship from drug response curves.
4. To differentiate between various types of antagonisms giving examples.
5. To explain the terms therapeutic index and therapeutic window and their application while using a drug.
6. To discuss the factors that modify drug action and drug effects.
7. To define the term 'adverse drug reaction (ADR)'.
8. To classify ADRs giving suitable examples.
9. To explain various allergic and idiosyncratic reactions giving examples.
10. To discuss how to prevent or treat ADR.
11. To discuss management of acute poisoning.

KEY TERMS

Pharmacological and biochemical effects of a drug occur when it reaches the site of action in the body. These effects may be desirable or undesirable and sometimes toxic. *The site of drug action or where a drug acts, and the mechanism of its action or how a drug acts, are the two fundamental and complex elements in pharmacodynamics.* Understanding pharmacodynamics is essential as it provides the basis not only for rational selection of drugs but also for their judicious use to produce the maximum benefit with minimum risk to the patient.

SITE OF DRUG ACTION

- **Locally**, i.e. at the point of application, e.g. glucocorticoid ointment for skin lesion; counterirritants such as methyl salicylate; gastric antacids.
- **Systemically**, i.e. after absorption into systemic circulation
  a. During passage through the body, e.g. osmotic diuretics.
  b. By reaching an effective concentration in a *particular tissue* (general anaesthetics in the brain or diuretics in the kidneys) or *in a cell type* (e.g. anticancer drugs within the cancer cells or antibiotics within microbes).

STRUCTURE ACTIVITY RELATIONSHIP (SAR)

The activity of a drug is intimately related to its chemical structure. Knowledge about the chemical structure of a drug is useful as seen from the following examples:

1. **Synthesis of new compounds:**
   New compounds or drug substitutes may be designed for the following purposes:
   a. **To increase or decrease the duration of action of the original drug or to get a more potent compound:**
   i. Procaine, a local anaesthetic, gets rapidly hydrolysed in the plasma. Hence reduction of cardiac

rate and excitability is too transient with it. A structurally similar compound, procainamide, is resistant to hydrolysis, has a longer duration of action and is used to treat cardiac arrhythmias.

ii. Atropine, when instilled into the eye, produces mydriasis and cycloplegia (Chapter 20). These effects persist for about a week. Structurally similar homatropine reduces their duration to 24 h.

b. **To restrict the drug action to a particular system of the body:** Atropine is a nonselective muscarinic receptor blocker which acts on cardiovascular system, GIT, glands and smooth muscles such as bronchi. Hence it causes multiple effects which are not desirable when used therapeutically. Ipratropium bromide is an atropine derivative which has selective action on bronchial smooth muscles.

c. **To reduce the adverse reactions, and/or enhance the kinetic or dynamic properties of the drugs:** Benzyl penicillin, given orally, is inactivated by gastric acid. Penicillins have been synthesised which are gastric acid resistant and hence can be given orally, e.g. phenoxymethyl penicillin. Staphylococci develop resistance to benzyl penicillin fairly fast. Hence, penicillinase resistant penicillin, cloxacillin, was synthesised.

2. **Synthesis of competitive antagonists:**
   a. The respiratory depression by morphine is antagonised by the structurally similar nalorphine (Chapter 10).

3. **Understanding the mechanism of drug action:** Adrenaline stimulates both the alpha and the beta-adrenergic receptors. A related compound, isoprenaline, selectively stimulates the beta-adrenergic receptors, whereas a very closely similar compound propranolol, blocks the beta-adrenergic receptors. The difference in mechanism of action is due to its chemical structure.

Chirality: Many commonly used drugs (atenolol, ibuprofen, warfarin) exist as racemates, i.e. 50:50 mixtures of mirror image stereoisomers (**enantiomers**). The two types of molecules may have either the same pharmacological action with different intensities on account of pharmacokinetic differences, e.g. verapamil; or entirely different actions, e.g. thalidomide in which the l-thalidomide is a potent hypnotic whereas the d-thalidomide is a potent teratogen. This fact, unknown then, accounted for the thalidomide disaster in pregnant women in the 1960s. Drugs have now been developed as single enantiomer to have selective pharmacological action and reduced risk of adverse reactions; e.g. l-atenolol, *s*-omeprazole, *s*-zopiclone, and l-salbutamol. PH 1.5

MECHANISM OF DRUG ACTION

The terms **drug action** and **drug effects** are often used as synonyms. However, the drug action always precedes the drug effects. Drug action is the initial interaction of a drug with cells at the site of action; the resultant physiological and biochemical consequences are the drug effects.

The drug action and drug effects depend upon the drug concentration achieved at the site of action, which in turn is determined by:

- ADME (absorption, distriibution, metabolism and excretion) of the drug
  - First pass metabolism
  - Tissue affinity, e.g. ultra short-acting barbiturate like thiopental is mainly concentrated in the central nervous system.
- Condition of the body or the *milieu interior*, e.g. iron is absorbed more rapidly in individuals with iron deficiency anaemia.

A drug may act by virtue of its:

1. **Physical properties:**
   Colour: Dyes such as sunset yellow when added to liquid medications may exert a psychological effect, e.g. tincture of cardamom. Ferric oxide in calamine lotion imparts it a pink colour that matches with the skin colour and the applied medication is not noticed easily. This makes it cosmetically acceptable and psychologically relieves anxiety of the consumer.
   Physical mass: Agar and psyllium seeds are used as laxatives as they absorb water, swell and initiate peristalsis.
   Smell: Peppermint oil is used in mixtures to mask the unpleasant smell of drugs.
   Taste: Compounds with a bitter taste are used to

improve the appetite as they reflexly increase the flow of hydrochloric acid.

Osmolality: Magnesium sulphate is used as a laxative due to its osmotic property.

Adsorption: Activated charcoal adsorb toxins and is used in the treatment of nonspecific diarrhoeas and poisoning.

Soothing demulcents: Syrups as pharyngeal demulcents are used for cough (Chapter 26); calamine lotion is used for eczema (Chapter 69).

Reduction in surface tension: By virtue of this property, cationic surfactants like cetrimide exert a cleansing effect and serve as antiseptics.

Electrical charge: Heparin, a strongly acidic compound, exerts its anticoagulant effect due to its negative charge (Chapter 33).

Radioactivity: ^{131}I is used in the treatment of hyperthyroidism (Chapter 62).

Radio-opacity: Barium sulphate as 'barium meal' and organic iodine compounds are used for the visualisation of the biliary and urinary tracts, respectively.

2. **Chemical properties:**

   Acidity or alkalinity: Antacids like magnesium hydroxide and aluminium hydroxide are used in the treatment of peptic ulcer to neutralise gastric acid (Chapter 41).

   Chelation: Dimercaprol is used in arsenic poisoning and forms stable ionised ring complexes with it which get easily excreted (Chapter 74).

3. **Ability to modulate**

   Neurotransmitters (NTs), hormones, growth factors: Drugs may resemble these body function regulators, bind to the specialised constituents of cells and mimic or oppose their actions. They may replace the endogenous substances when the production of endogenous substances decreases. **Replacement** finds an important application in the treatment of hormone deficiencies, e.g. exogenous insulin in diabetes mellitus, thyroxine in hypothyroidism, and hydrocortisone in Addison disease.

Drugs may target:

1. Enzymes: Drugs may act by either increasing the rate of enzymatic reactions in the body (**enzyme stimulation**) or decreasing such rate (**enzyme inhibition**).

Enzyme stimulation by drugs, which are foreign substances, is unusual; it occurs commonly with endogenous substances such as hormones, e.g. adrenaline stimulates adenylyl cyclase.

Enzyme inhibition with drugs is either nonspecific, e.g. denaturing by alcohol when used as an antiseptic or specific, e.g. inhibition of cholinesterase by physostigmine, inhibition of carbonic anhydrase by acetazolamide and that of angiotensin converting enzyme (ACE) by enalapril.

2. Transport processes: Various transport processes such as Na^+–K^+ ATPase pump, voltage gated Ca^{++} and K^+ channels regulate the ionic concentrations of the cells and control the cell functions. Drugs may bind to the proteins subserving these transport processes and alter the activity of cells. For example, digoxin binds to and inhibits Na^+–K^+ ATPase pump; verapamil blocks the calcium channel; while minoxidil opens the K^+ channel.

Drugs may interfere with NT uptake, e.g. Serotonin reuptake transporter (SERT) is a target for the antidepressant fluoxetine which inhibits serotonin reuptake and increases its concentration in the synapse. Noradrenaline is taken up by neurons by NET(Norepinephrine transporter). This can be a target for indirectly acting sympathomimmetics as well as tricyclic antidepressants.

3. Structural proteins: Drugs may also bind to structural proteins of the body. For example, colchicine used to treat gout binds to tubulin of inflammatory cells and prevents their chemotaxis. Cyclosporine, an immunosuppressant binds to immunophillins.

4. Other cell constituents such as cell wall and DNA: Many antiviral and anticancer drugs are structural analogues of nucleic acids and compete with them to get incorporated in cellular RNA or DNA, interfering with cellular division, e.g. folic acid antagonist-methotrexate. Penicillin interferes with cell wall synthesis by binding to PBP (penicillin binding proteins).

5. Receptors: For details, see Drug receptor section.

TYPES OF DRUG EFFECTS: *A drug produces only a quantitative and not a qualitative change in the function of the target organ.* Drugs may produce their effects by:

Stimulation: Increase in the activity of specialised cells is called stimulation. Excessive stimulation may ultimately lead to depression. A drug may specifically stimulate certain portions of a particular system but depress others, e.g. morphine stimulates the vagus and the oculomotor nuclei and the CTZ but depresses the respiratory and the cough centres.

Depression: Decrease in the activity of specialised cells is called depression. Quinidine depresses the myocardium, whereas barbiturates depress the central nervous system.

Irritation: The term irritation indicates that a drug produces adverse effects on the growth, nutrition and morphology of living tissues. Irritation is a nonspecific phenomenon that can occur in all the tissues. It produces changes in the cellular structure and can produce inflammation, corrosion and necrosis. Heavy metals like mercury and silver are irritants. Mild irritation may have therapeutic utility, e.g. senna and cascara stimulate the mucosal cells of the gut and act as laxatives. The cellular changes produced are:

1. **Astringent effect** (precipitation of proteins): This may sometimes be beneficial. The irritant, however, may dissolve the precipitated proteins resulting in deeper penetration of the irritant and causing more extensive tissue damage. This effect is called as **corrosive effect.** Many strong acids and alkalis exert a corrosive effect.
2. **Dehydration**
3. **Cytotoxic action** (damage to the cell wall or the nucleus), e.g. anticancer drugs

When an irritant agent is applied locally to the skin to relieve deep seated pain, it is referred to as **counterirritant.** Volatile oils like turpentine oil are often used in this fashion. The counterirritant is applied to the skin situated over the organ responsible for pain. The basis for pain relief is that:

- It stimulates the sensory nerve endings in the skin and the afferent impulses are relayed in the cerebrospinal axis to efferent vasomotor fibres supplying the internal organ. Thus, the increased circulation to the skin has its counterpart in the deep integumental structures and viscera innervated from the same segmental level of the central nervous system (CNS).
- In addition, the sensory impulses emanating from the skin may interfere with the transmission of pain impulses coming from the viscera and may even produce their partial or complete exclusion by occupying the final common sensory pathway (**Gate control theory**). The vasodilatation and blockade of pain impulses may explain the relief of deep seated pain.

Antimicrobial effects: Drugs are used for prevention, arrest and eradication of infections; they act specifically on the causative organisms, e.g. antibiotics (Chapter 43).

Modification of immune status: Vaccines, sera and certain other agents (levamisole and corticosteroids) act by modulating the immune status (Chapters 71 and 72).

DRUG RECEPTORS

The receptors are **specific protein macromolecules** in the *cell membrane, the cytosol or the nucleus.* Numerous receptors for hormones, neurotransmitters and drugs have been identified, purified, cloned and their structure has been determined. Many drugs (*ligands*) bind to:

1. Receptors for the endogenous substances
2. Enzymes
3. Other constituents, which serve as receptors for the drugs.

Such ligand binding alters enzyme activity, changes permeability to ions, leads to conformational change or introduces genetic material in the nucleus.

The receptor serves a dual function:

- **It acts as a recognition molecule for specific ligand/s** (molecules which bind to it) from among numerous molecular species present in the fluid that bathes the cell.
- **It initiates biochemical reactions which transmit the signal from the ligand to proteins in the cell membrane and within the cell (post-**

receptor events); such events amplify the original signal by a cascade effect and regulate the function of the cell. The receptor, its cellular target and the intermediary molecules (transporters) if any, are designated as **receptor-effector system** (signal transduction system).

Biologically, the receptor is generally inactive till a ligand binds to it; only then it gets 'activated' and triggers the post-receptor events. An exception occurs when the receptor in a target endocrine gland undergoes **constitutive activation** due to a genetic mutation (Chapter 61). In such a case, the target gland overproduces its hormone, and a disease state sets in, e.g. an overfunctioning, solitary, thyroid nodule ultimately becomes a toxic nodule (Plummer disease).

The principal elements which characterise the interaction between a ligand and a receptor are **selectivity** and **affinity.**

Selectivity of binding of drugs to receptors depends on their physicochemical structure.

Affinity is a measure of the 'strength' of binding between the drug and its receptor and is defined by a constant in the binding relationship between the drug and the receptor.

The ability of the drug to elicit a response after its interaction with the receptor is termed as the **intrinsic activity** or the **efficacy** of the drug. The biological response to a drug is also regulated by alteration in the receptor number and affinity.

An **agonist** is a drug which initiates pharmacological action after binding to the receptors (same site or other allosteric site). It is a drug with high affinity for the receptor and also high intrinsic activity.

An **antagonist** is a drug which after binding to the receptors does not elicit a pharmacological action but causes receptor blockade. An antagonist, therefore, has the same affinity for the receptor as the agonist but its intrinsic activity is poor.

Partial agonist is a drug with affinity equal to or less than that of the agonist but less intrinsic activity. Such a drug, no matter how high its concentration, will not produce the full response which the tissue is capable of. Further, a partial agonist, because of its ability to occupy receptors, diminishes the action of an agonist when the two are used simultaneously.

In the case of opioids (Chapter 10), which act on several types of receptors, some act as agonists or partial agonists on one type of receptor but as antagonists on another type of receptor, e.g. pentazocine and nalbuphine act as agonists on k receptors but as antagonists on μ receptors. Such drugs are called **mixed agonist-antagonists.**

Inverse agonist is a drug which after combination with certain receptors produces actions opposite to those produced by a pure agonist (*affinity but negative efficacy*). Thus, beta carbolines through interaction with benzodiazepine binding sites on $GABA_A$ receptors produce anxiety, arousal and increase in muscle tone, actions opposite to those produced by diazepam.

A receptor exists in two conformational states, active (R_a), and inactive (R_i) which are in equilibrium (**two state-receptor model theory**). The *relative affinity* of a drug for any of these two conformations shifts the equilibrium towards either R_a state or R_i state. Thus a drug having higher affinity for the R_a activates the receptor and is termed as a **full agonist**. The one having moderate affinity for the R_a displays intermediate intensity of effects and is a **partial agonist.** A drug that binds with equal affinity to both the conformations, R_a and R_i, does not alter the equilibrium and acts as a **competitive antagonist**, whereas the one with selective preferential affinity for R_i produces an effect opposite to that of a full agonist and is an **inverse agonist**.

Multiple receptor 'types' and 'subtypes' for a ligand are common. A neurotransmitter may activate several receptor types, e.g. dopamine and adrenaline have five receptors each, histamine has four, whereas acetylcholine has seven.

Increasing concentrations of an agonist evoke a progressively increasing tissue response until the maximum response is reached. If another drug that acts on the same receptor system produces quantitatively different maximum response, then its **efficacy** (intrinsic activity) must differ. Hence, difference in maximum responses can form the basis for comparing intrinsic activities of drugs. In practice, this means that drug 'X' produces a therapeutic effect larger than the maximum effect produced by drug 'Y'(Fig. 2.1B). e.g. as a diuretic furosemide is more efficacious than hydrochlorothiazide.

The term **potency** of the drug, on the other hand, means that weight for weight, drug 'X' has a greater concentration than drug 'Y' i.e. drug X is less potent then drug Y as higher concentration is required to get the same effect; the maximum effect obtainable is, however, similar (Fig. 2.1A) for example prednisolone is more 'potent' than hydrocortisone.

Some agents are so potent that only a few molecules have to interact with their receptors to induce a massive response. This obviously needs **an amplifier system.** The simplest amplifier unit is an enzyme molecule that is activated by a drug molecule which then converts several substrate molecules into product molecules. If such units are coupled, the product molecules in their turn activate a second enzyme, and so on. Most hormones and neurotransmitters exert their effects without entering the cell. They interact with specific receptors which are coupled to various effector or amplifier systems responsible for generating internal signals or **second messengers**, which initiate a further sequence of enzyme reactions. In such *amplifier system model*, the active agent needs to activate only a fraction of its receptors to obtain maximal response from the effector system. Thus, there is a *spare capacity* for the specific receptors.

Spare receptors are qualitatively similar to the occupied receptors and are available for action. Thus, adrenaline can elicit the maximum cardiac inotropic response even when 90% of the cardiac β_1 adrenergic receptors are occupied by relatively irreversible antagonists. This indicates that the cardiac tissue possesses a large number of spare β_1-receptors.

Continued exposure to the drug/hormone, blunts receptor-mediated responses to drugs and hormones with time. This phenomenon is termed **desensitisation, refractoriness or tolerance**. Thus, repeated administration of ephedrine and adrenergic agonists in bronchial asthma causes a reduction in therapeutic response. Desensitisation is usually reversible.

The density of receptors on cells, their occupancy and their capacity to respond (efficacy) can change in response to the agonist or antagonist. The cell can increase or decrease the number of receptors in response to a given signalling molecule. Cells do this to maintain the overall homeostasis. When they increase the number of receptors, it is called **upregulation**, whereas when they decrease the number of receptors to become less responsive to certain ligands, it is designated as **downregulation**. Such balancing act between upregulation and downregulation is the characteristic of physiological homeostatic patterns.

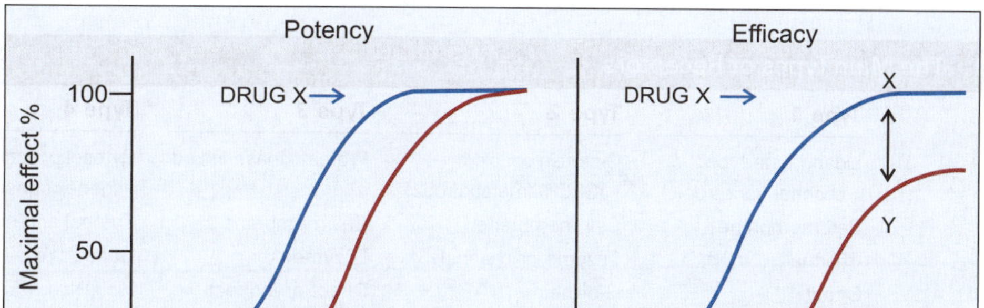

FIG. 2.1 Relative potency and relative efficacy of two agonist drugs X and Y (see text).

Downregulation occurs more slowly than desensitisation and is less rapidly reversible. It involves net degradation of the cell receptors.

Continous exposure to β_2 agonist causes downregulation of β_2 receptors. Thus if salbutamol is used repeatedly in patients with asthma, then its effect decreases with time, ultimately resulting in complete loss of effect. Hence salbutamol is preferred only as a reliever for bronchospasm and not for maintenance therapy for asthma.

In contrast, the continued occupation of cell receptors by antagonists may increase the number of cell receptors (**upregulation**). Such receptors become accessible to the endogenous agonist. When the antagonist is stopped suddenly, the stimulation of increased number of receptors causes an exaggerated response to agonist.

Thus, chronic administration of beta-adrenergic blocker, propranolol, is accompanied by increase in the number of beta-adrenergic receptors. Its sudden withdrawal in a patient with ischemic heart disease makes him more susceptible to the effects of endogenous noradrenaline and may precipitate angina.

Types of Receptors (Table 2.1 and Fig. 2.2):

- **Type 1:** Ligand gated ion channel (Ionotropic)
- **Type 2:** G-protein coupled (GPCR) (Metabotropic)
- **Type 3:** Receptors linked to enzymes
- **Type 4:** Receptors that regulate DNA (gene) transcription

Ligand gated ion channel receptors are cell-membrane spanning proteins. Agents binding with them open a transmembrane channel and permit ions to cross the membrane phospholipid bilayer. Thus, opening of the nicotinic receptor channel permits sodium ions to cross the membrane into the cell and cause depolarisation of the membrane. On the other hand, the gamma-aminobutyric acid (GABA) receptor channel allows chloride ions to permeate into the cell, and hyperpolarises the cell membrane. Opening of the potassium channels allows potassium ions to leak out of the cell and thus hyperpolarises the cell membrane, e.g. sulphonylurea receptor. Many drugs (benzodiazepines and $5HT_3$ antagonists) act by modifying the function of receptor channels.

G protein-coupled receptors (GPCR) are receptors which are coupled to a specific class of proteins, G proteins or guanine nucleotide binding proteins and mediate their effects through secondary messengers. GPCR are found on all cell types and are abundant in the brain and the gut. They are either **stimulatory (Gs) or inhibitory (Gi)** in action. The G in the name refers to guanosine diphosphate or triphosphate. A ligand binding to GPCR promotes binding of GTP to G-proteins. The activated G-proteins in turn activate effector systems such as enzymes (adenylyl cyclase and phospholipase) and ion channels (Ca^{++} and K^+). The second messengers for such actions are:

1. Intracytoplasmic calcium ion
2. Cyclic AMP

Table 2.1 The Main Types of Receptors

	Type 1	Type 2	Type 3	Type 4
Class	Ligand gated ion channel (ionotropic)	G-protein coupled (GPCR) (metabotropic)	Protein kinase linked	Cytosolic, acting on DNA (gene) transcription
Location	Cell membrane	Cell membrane	Cell membrane	Cytosol and nucleus
Effector	Channel	Enzyme or channel	Enzyme	Gene
Coupling	Direct	G-protein	Direct or indirect	Via DNA
Examples of receptors	nACh, $GABA_A$, glycine	mACh, beta adrenergic, TSH, H_2	Insulin, growth factor, cytokine, ANF	Steroid/thyroid hormone
Second messenger	None	cAMP, cGMP, Ca^{++}	None	None
Lag period for effect	Millisecond	Seconds	Hours	Hours

Notes: ANF, atrial natriuretic factor; cAMP, cyclic AMP; cGMP, cyclic GMP; n, nicotinic; m, muscarinic; H, histaminic; Ach, acetylcholine.

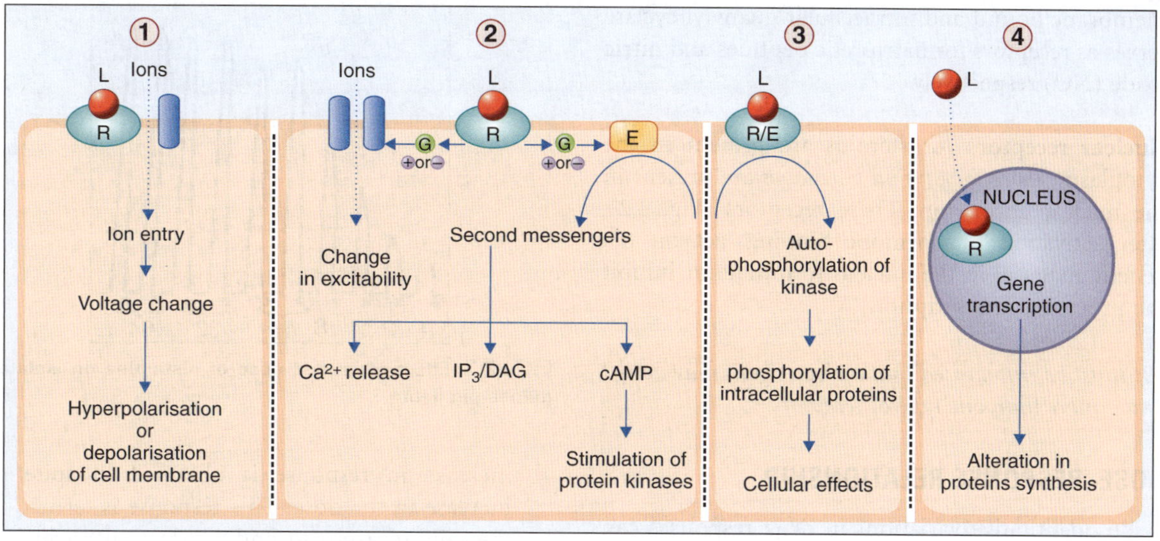

FIG. 2.2 **Types of receptor-effector linkage. 1, ligand-gated ion channel (ionotropic receptors); 2, G-protein coupled receptor (Metabotropic); 3, kinase-linked receptors; 4, nuclear receptors; R, receptor; G, G-proteins; E, enzyme; L, ligand. Modified from *Pharmacology* by Rang H.P. et al., 5th edition, Churchill Livingstone, 2003.**

Types of drug receptors.

3. Inositol 1,3,5-triphosphate (IP_3) and diacylglycerol (DAG) released from the phospholipid in the cell membrane.

In some instances, these three are interlinked.

The classic examples of GPCR (Fig. 2.2) are the adrenergic β_1 and α_2 receptors and dopamine receptors. Thus:

1. The extracellular ligand binds to a cell-surface GPCR, which in turn,
2. Activates G-protein located on the cytoplasmic face of the plasma membrane.
3. The activated G-protein alters the activity of the effector element such as the adenylyl cyclase enzyme (or an ion channel).
4. Adenylyl cyclase converts intracellular ATP to cyclic AMP, the second messenger.

ACh and GABA can activate ligand gated ion channels as well as GPCR.

Many drugs such as opiates act on GPCR either as agonists or as antagonists. **Nearly 65% of the drugs act via GPCRs.**

Receptors linked to enzymes (Fig. 2.2), the third family of cell surface receptors, are linked to enzymes like **tyrosine kinases**. They serve as receptors for insulin and epidermal growth factor. Tyrosine kinases undergo auto-phosphorylation after the hormone binds to them and then phosphorylates intracellular proteins on the tyrosine residues. Certain receptors do not have tyrosine kinase in built in their structure but after ligand binding they undergo dimerisation to bind to intracellular tyrosine kinase termed as **Janus kinase (JAK)**. Subsequently, JAK phosphorylates other proteins termed as **signal transducers and activators of transcription (STAT)** which translocate to nucleus and regulate transcription, e.g. gamma interferon, growth hormone receptors. This entire pathway is called **JAK-STAT pathway**.

Similarly receptors expressed on haemopoetic cells are called **Toll-like receptors (TIRs)**. Ligands like cytokines, lipids, peptidoglycans, viruses, etc., use these receptors and lead to series of complex reactions, using intracellular factors and enzymes, which ultimately phosphorylates NF-kB transcription factors and finally translocate them to the nucleus resulting in transcriptional activation of inflammatory genes.

Membrane bound and intracellular guanylyl cyclase serves as receptors for natriuretic peptides and nitric oxide (NO) respectively.

Nuclear receptors for steroids are present in the cytoplasm; *those for thyroid hormones* are present in the nuclear chromatin. These receptors (Fig. 2.2), after activation by hormone binding, act on the genetic material in the nucleus to initiate or inhibit the process of transcription.

It must be emphasised that a given agent may activate more than one type of receptors.

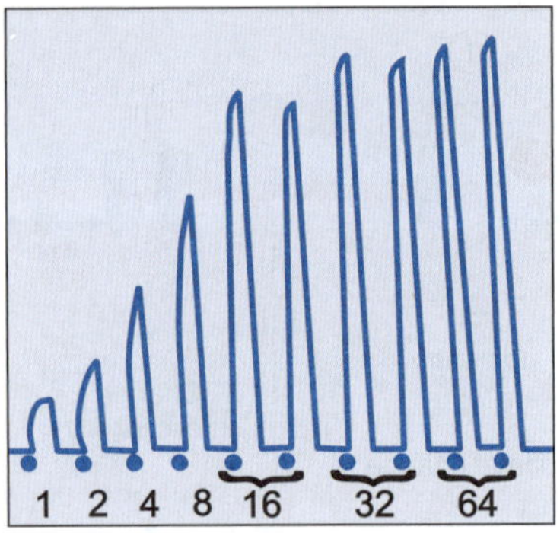

FIG. 2.3 Effect of graded dose of histamine on isolated guinea-pig ileum.

DOSE–RESPONSE RELATIONSHIP

Wide quantitative variations in drug responses can occur between different species and within the same species under different conditions. Methods have, therefore, been devised to study the phenomenon of variation in pharmacological drug response and to minimise the errors of prediction in therapeutic use of drugs.

Each drug has a characteristic dose–response curve for a specified set of conditions. In general, the log dose–response curve conforms to the S-shaped (sigmoid type) curve or to segments of the sigmoid. The magnitude of the drug effect is a function of the dose administered. Two basic types of dose effect relationship have been observed:

1. **Graded or quantitative dose–response relationship:** This type of relationship relates the magnitude of the response in a single biological unit to the dose of the drug. As the dose administered to a single individual or discrete organ or tissue is increased, the pharmacological response also increases in graded fashion provided the dose has exceeded some critical level called the **threshold dose** (Fig. 2.3). The graded dose–response relation is partially a reflection of the extent of occupancy of the receptors by the drug. Since an entire dose–response relationship is determined from one animal, the curve does not tell us about the degree of biological variation inherent in a population.
   The responses increase with increasing doses of a drug till a stage, beyond which no further increase in response is obtained in spite of increase in the dose. This response is termed as the **ceiling response**, and the dose with which it is obtained is the **ceiling dose**. If the dose exceeds the ceiling dose, there is no further increase in the therapeutic effect. In fact, such a dose may provoke undesirable responses. The ceiling dose allows us to compare the **therapeutic efficacy** of various compounds.
   Fig. 2.4A shows a 'dose versus response' curve, whereas Fig. 2.4B shows the same data in the form of a 'log-dose versus response' curve. The latter is particularly useful for the comparison of various compounds.

2. **Quantal or all or none dose–response relationship:** In contrast to graded responses, the quantal responses are all or none. The quantal curve shows the frequency with which any dose of a drug evokes a stated, fixed (all or none) pharmacological response in a given population. It is, therefore, essentially a frequency distribution of the responders (actual numbers or percentage of the total number of individuals) to different doses of the drug. Each individual is categorised as responder or nonresponder, according to a pre-decided criterion for the response. While studying an antiepileptic drug in animals, each animal is classified as a responder (seizure-free) or not responder at a specified time after the drug treatment. Obviously, sensitive animals will respond to smaller doses while some will be resistant and need very large doses. Usually, the sensitivity of animals to

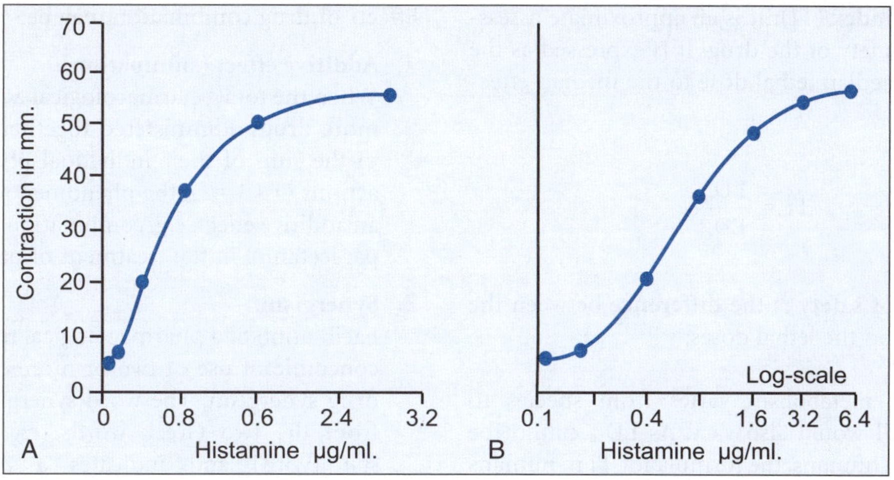

FIG. 2.4 **(A) Dose–response relationship curve from the data in Fig. 2.3. (B) Same dose–response relationship plotted on logarithmic-scale.**

different doses is distributed normally with respect to the logarithm of the dose. Thus, for a given drug, if log dose is plotted on the horizontal axis and the % responding to the various dose levels is plotted on the vertical axis, a **normal (Gaussian) distribution curve** is obtained (Fig. 2.5). The curve represents the distribution of sensitivity of a group of animals to the given drug. In this figure about 10% of the animals in a given group remain seizure-free at a dose level of log dose '0', whereas another 10% do not respond until the dose is increased to log dose '2'. Majority of the animals, however, respond at doses between '0.5' and '1.5' on the log-scale. The same data, plotted as the cumulative number of animals that responded against

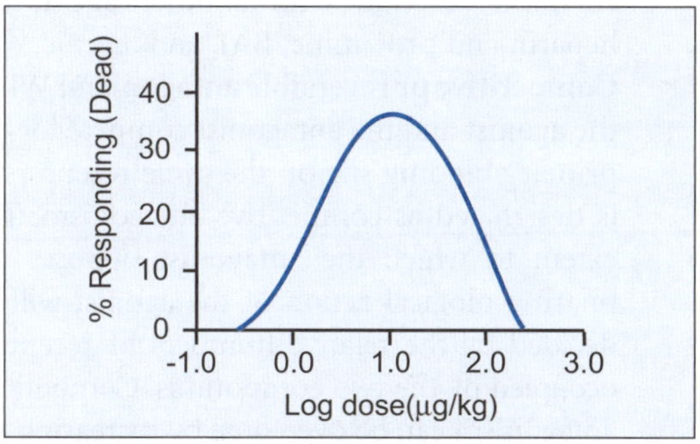

FIG. 2.5 **Quantal dose–response curve.**

log dose, would give an S shaped cumulative frequency curve. *For a given dose of a drug, a cumulative frequency curve gives the per cent of animals responding to that dose and to lower doses.*

The quantal dose–response curve, however, is not always exactly symmetrical or bell-shaped but may show 'skewing' or 'truncation'. This shows that besides polygenic random variation, nonrandom but inter-coupled events like other actions of the drug and experimental limitations influence the quantal dose–response curve. Further, there are drugs that undergo biotransformation controlled by a single gene. Variant of such gene may segregate the animals into distinct groups as slow or fast metabolizers. A bimodal quantal log-dose–response curve may be obtained in such cases.

The median lethal dose or LD_{50}: This is the dose (mg/kg) which would be expected to kill one-half of an unlimited population of the same species and strain.

The median effective dose or ED_{50}: This is the dose (mg/kg) which produces a desired response in 50 per cent of the test population. ED_{50} can be obtained from either quantal or graded dose–response curves.

Therapeutic index (TI): It is an approximate assessment of the safety of the drug. It is expressed as the ratio of the median lethal dose to the median effective dose:

$$TI = \frac{LD_{50}}{ED_{50}}$$

The margin of safety is the **difference** between the therapeutic and the lethal doses.

As the drug metabolism varies from species to species, the TI would also vary. As LD_{50} cannot be worked out in humans, the formula for TI in humans can be restated as:

$$TI = \frac{\text{Dose which produces a defined } \textit{unwanted effect} \text{ (e.g. tachycardia due to salbutamol) in 50\% of the test subjects}}{\text{Dose producing } \textit{therapeutic effect} \text{ (specified reduction in airway resistance) in 50\% of the test subjects}}$$

The larger the TI, the safer is the drug. For safe therapeutic application of a compound, its TI must be more than one. *Such drugs have very little dose-related toxicity.* Thus, penicillin has a very high TI, whereas it is much smaller for digoxin, aminophylline and lignocaine.

In practice, no drug produces only a single effect but has a spectrum of effects. Further, a drug may be selective in one respect but nonselective in another. Thus, although antihistaminics selectively block histamine actions, most of them cause significant sedation. For therapeutic purposes, selectivity of a drug effect is an important property. Thus depending upon its effect, a drug may have many therapeutic indices. The margin of safety of aspirin when used for headache is far greater than its margin of safety for the relief of arthritic pain or in rheumatic fever. This is because the latter use requires much larger doses.

RESPONSE TO DRUG COMBINATIONS

In clinical practice, there is often a need to use two or more drugs concurrently. The resultant effect may vary depending on the combination used.

Effects of drug combination may be:

1. **Additive effect (summation):**
   When the total pharmacological action of two or more drugs administered together is equivalent to the sum of their individual pharmacological actions (1+1=2), the phenomenon is termed as an additive effect, e.g. combination of aspirin and paracetamol in the treatment of pain and fever.

2. **Synergism:**
   Facilitation of a pharmacological response by the concomitant use of two or more drugs is called drug synergism. The word synergism is derived from the two Greek words, *ergo* (work) and *syn* (with) and indicates a pharmacologic co-operation. This co-operation usually results in a total effect greater than the sum of their independent actions (1+1>2), e.g. codeine and aspirin for pain; hydrochlorothiazide and amlodipine for hypertension.
   If the synergism results in prolongation of action of one of the drugs, it is termed *time synergism*, e.g. lignocaine and adrenaline combination increases the duration of action of lignocaine. The term **potentiation** is often loosely employed for synergism and should be avoided, as the word 'potentiate' means 'to endow with power', which no drug is really capable of achieving.

3. **Antagonism:**
   The phenomenon of opposing actions of two drugs on the same physiological system is termed as drug antagonism. Antagonism can be:
   - **Chemical antagonism:** The biological activity of a drug can be reduced or abolished by a chemical reaction with another agent, e.g. heparin and protamine, BAL and arsenic.
   - **Competitive or reversible antagonism:** When the agonist and the antagonist compete for the primary binding site on the same receptors, it is designated as competitive antagonism. The extent to which the antagonist opposes the pharmacological action of the agonist will be decided by the relative numbers of receptors occupied by the two compounds. Competitive antagonism can be overcome by increasing the concentration of the agonist at the receptor

site, e.g. acetylcholine and atropine antagonism at muscarinic receptors. If the concentration of acetylcholine at the receptor level is increased by the administration of an anticholinesterase, the blockade produced by atropine can be reversed (**reversible antagonism**). Similar is the case between noradrenaline and prazosin, an alpha-adrenergic blocking agent.

A competitive antagonist shifts the dose–response curve to the right. The maximal response to agonist is, however, not impaired (Fig. 2.6A).

- **Noncompetitive antagonism:** In this type of antagonism, an antagonist inactivates the receptor (R) so that an effective complex with the agonist cannot be formed, irrespective of the concentration of the agonist. This may happen in various ways:
  - i. The antagonist might combine with R at the same site, but the combination is so firm that even higher agonist concentration cannot displace it (**irreversible**).
  - ii. The antagonist binds to an allosteric site so as to prevent the expected characteristic biologic response to the agonist; or
  - iii. The antagonist might itself induce a certain change in R so that the reactivity of the binding site where agonist should interact is reduced or abolished, e.g. noradrenaline and phenoxybenzamine on vascular smooth muscle; acetylcholine and decamethonium at the neuromuscular junction.

  Although the agonist curve shifts to the right, the slope is reduced and the maximum response diminishes. The extent of inhibition produced depends on the characteristics of the antagonist; the agonist has no influence upon the degree of antagonism or its reversibility (Fig. 2.6B).
- **Physiological antagonism:** This term is sometimes used where a drug reverses the effects of another drug by acting on different receptors, e.g. adrenaline given in anaphylactic reaction to counteract effects of histamine. Sometimes the term 'functional antagonism' is used to represent the interaction of two agonists that act independently of each other but cause opposite effects, e.g. acetylcholine and adrenaline.

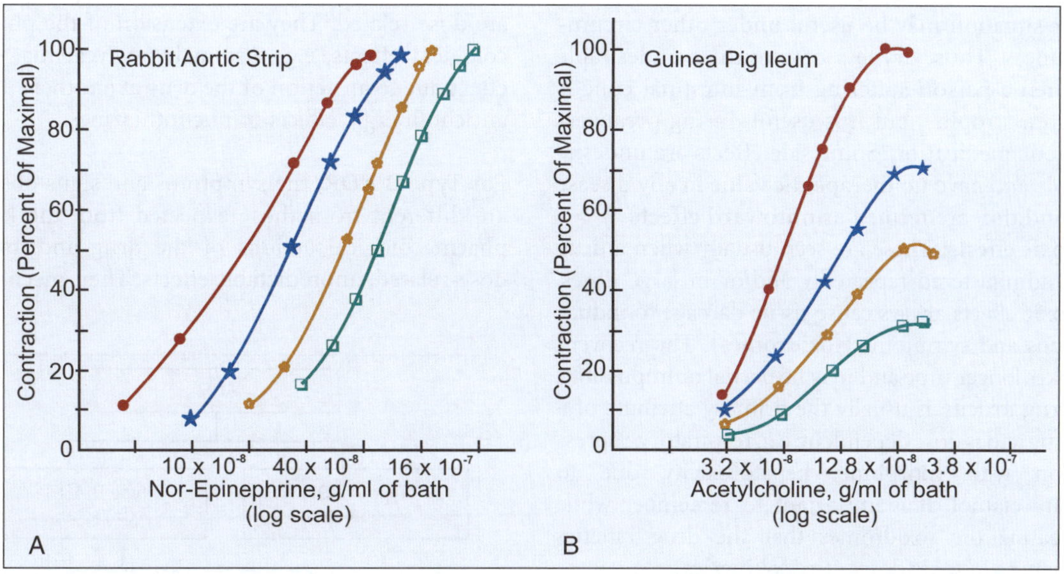

FIG. 2.6 **(A) Characteristic of competitive antagonism between noradrenaline and an antagonist. Black dots denote the control curve. Subsequent curves are drawn with increasing concentrations of the antagonist. Note that the curves are almost parallel and maximum response could be obtained with noradrenaline on each occasion. (B) Characteristic of non-competitive antagonism. Note the decrease in maximum response to acetylcholine following the increase in antagonist concentration.**

Importance of drug antagonism:

- **To correct adverse effects of drug**, e.g. chlorpromazine induced extrapyramidal reactions which are due to cholinergic activation can be countered by benzhexol (Chapter 13).
- **To treat drug poisoning**, e.g. morphine with naloxone, organophosphorus compounds with atropine.
- **To predict whether newly prescribed drug for a patient, who is already receiving another drug may result in reduced efficacy,** e.g. if the patient is on beta blocker for angina pectoris and develops anaphylactic shock, then the usual dose of adrenaline is not effective.

ADVERSE DRUGS REACTIONS (ADR) PH 1.7

The administration of a drug may result in the development of:

- **Side effects:** Side effects are in fact *pharmacological effects produced with therapeutic dose of the drug*, e.g. dryness of mouth with atropine. These effects are not harmful and recovery is quick on stopping the drug or reducing the dose. Side effects which might be troublesome in a particular situation may be useful under other circumstances. Thus, dryness of mouth is undesirable when a person suffering from intestinal colic is given atropine, but it is useful during preanaesthetic medication. Some side effects are undesirable and have no therapeutic value in any disease condition are termed as **untoward effects**.
- **Toxic effects:** These are seen usually when a drug is administered repeatedly and/or in large doses. Toxic effects always cause tissue damage to induce signs and symptoms (**toxidromes**). The recovery takes longer time and may be partial or impossible. Drug toxicity is usually the primary attribute of a drug and is dose dependent, e.g. respiratory depression with morphine; hepatotoxicity due to paracetamol. It is important to remember while treating the toxidromes that the drug kinetics changes in toxic doses (**toxicokinetics**).

According to WHO, **adverse drug reaction** (**ADR**) is defined as 'any response to a drug that is noxious and unintended and that occurs at doses used in man for the prophylaxis, diagnosis or therapy of disease or for modification of physiological function'. It includes both, side effects and untoward effects and excludes adverse reactions due to drug overdose (poisoning), drug abuse and therapeutic errors.

ADR could be either local (irritation, necrosis or thrombophlebitis) or systemic. The basic cause of an ADR may be discernible (pharmaceutical, pharmacokinetic or pharmacodynamic) or may be unknown.

ADRs are generally classified into **Type A** (Augmented); **Type B** (Bizarre) (Fig. 2.7); **Type C** (Chronic) **Type D** (Delayed), **Type E** (End of dose) and **Type F** (Unexpected failure of therapy). The differences between Type A and Type B ADRs are listed in Table 2.2. Type C ADRs are both time and dose-related (e.g. analgesic nephropathy) whereas Type D ADRs are only time-related (e.g. carcinogenesis). Type E ADR is seen after sudden stoppage of drug (e.g. beta blockers or clonidine). Type F ADR often occur due to drug interactions (e.g. failure of oral contraceptives when given concurrently with rifampicin).

Type A ADR, is largely predictable on the basis of the known pharmacological actions of a drug and usually are dose related. They are extension of the pharmacological effects, e.g. insulin hypoglycaemia, or an effect due to an action of the drug at another site, e.g. anticholinergic effects of phenothiazines.

For **Type B ADR,** the symptoms and signs observed are different from those expected from the known pharmacological actions of the drug and are not dose-related, unpredictable effects. Their mechanism

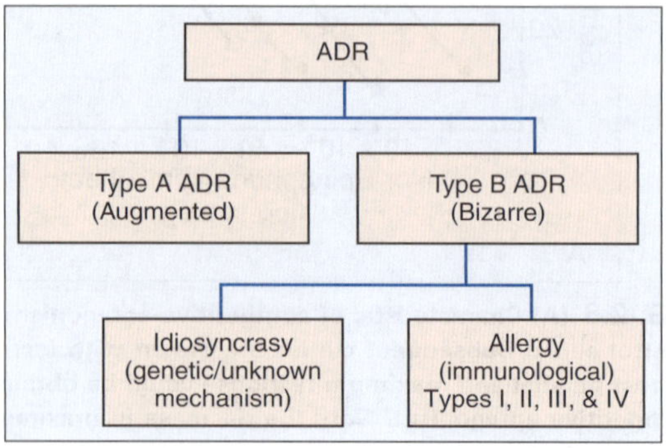

FIG. 2.7 Classification of ADR.

Table 2.2 Comparison between Type A and Type B ADR

	Type A	Type B
Nature of ADR	Augmented/ Quantitative Normal response	Totally abnormal/ Qualitative Bizarre response
Mechanism	Hyper-response	Genetic, immuno-logical/unknown
Pharmacologically predictable	Largely yes	No
Dose dependent	Yes	No
Incidence and morbidity[a]	High	Low
Mortality[a]	Low	High
Treatment	Adjust dose	Stop the drug

[a]In the community.

is sometimes known (genetic or immunological) but may often be unknown (Fig. 2.7).

Idiosyncrasy is a Type B ADR wherein the abnormal response to a drug is either due to a genetic or unknown mechanism. Thus, sometimes genetically determined absence or reduced activity of certain enzyme(s) in an individual is responsible for the ADR. Drugs like primaquine, salicylates and sulphonamides cause haemolysis in individuals whose RBC lack the enzyme G6PD. In many cases, however, the cause of the idiosyncrasy is unknown, e.g. chloramphenicol-induced aplastic anaemia.

In general, all unusual, idiosyncratic reactions should be considered genetically determined until proved otherwise. As against idiosyncrasy, allergy always has immunological basis.

DRUG ALLERGY (HYPERSENSITIVITY)

The word *allergy* is derived from Greek words 'allos' meaning altered and 'ergos' meaning energy. Most of the drugs/sera used in therapeutics are capable of causing allergic reactions, which are type B ADR. They may be mild or very severe like anaphylaxis and have immunological basis. They occur in individuals who have been sensitised following the prior administration of the same drug or structurally similar drug.

To understand how drugs cause immunologically mediated reactions, it is necessary to know some basic immunological concepts. These are described in Chapter 71.

Generally, proteins with molecular weight of over 5000 Da administered intramuscularly/intravenously, readily stimulate the production of antibodies. Peptides of molecular weight less than 5000 Da are less immunogenic. Nonprotein compounds such as drugs can become immunogenic after chemical coupling to a carrier protein in the body and produce antibodies that can react with the drug which thus behaves as a **hapten**. *A hapten is a substance which is antigenic in the sense that it reacts with an antibody but itself is incapable of stimulating antibody production unless combined with a carrier protein.*

Prior exposure to the drug may cause sensitisation and on subsequent exposure results in clinical manifestations such as rash, fever, eosinophilia and blood dyscrasias can occur. The manifestations are dose independent.

The patient must be informed about the drugs he is allergic to, in order to prevent such reactions in the future.

The immune reactions underlying allergy are as follows:

1. **Type I reactions (Immediate Hypersensitivity):** These are **IgE mediated,** where in the antigen reacts with a specific class of antibody, **reaginic antibodies (IgE)**, bound to the surface of mast cells and basophils. This interaction causes degranulation of mast cells and basophils with massive liberation of histamine and other mediators of immediate hyperresponse, leading to anaphylaxis. Mediators released are as follows:
   - *Those that increase vascular permeability and contract smooth muscles*, e.g. histamine, PAF, SRS-A, bradykinin.
   - *Those that are chemotactic for or activate other proinflammatory cells*, e.g. leukotriene B4, eosinophil and neutrophil chemotactic factors.

- *Those that modulate the release of other mediators*, e.g. bradykinin, PAF, prostaglandins.
- *Those which cause termination of the inflammatory response.*

Mast cell triggering forms a vital part of the acute inflammatory defence reaction. This may either result in **(a) systemic i.e. anaphylaxis** or **(b) local allergic reactions (atopic allergy)**.

Death due to anaphylaxis is usually due to laryngeal oedema, a feature unique to man, bronchospasm leading to asphyxia, or vasodilatation with circulatory collapse.

Such systemic reactions are known to occur in a sensitised human subject following a repeat injection of a drug like penicillin or antitoxic serum. This is the phenomenon of *anaphylaxis.*

As compared to systemic anaphylaxis, **atopic allergy** to extrinsic antigens (allergens) such as pollen, animal danders, mites in house dust, and absorbed foodstuffs occur more frequently in man. Combination of the allergen with cell bound IgE antibody in the bronchial tree, the nasal mucosa or the skin releases mediators of anaphylaxis giving rise to localised reactions such as, asthma, rhinitis (Chapter 27), eczema (Chapter 69) or urticaria (Chapter 23). The offending antigen can be identified by intradermal prick test. There is a strong familial tendency. The symptoms of atopic allergy are to a certain extent controllable with antihistaminic drugs and other mediator antagonists (Chapter 23). Courses of antigen injection may desensitise by forming blocking IgG or IgA antibodies, or by turning off IgE production. Fig. 2.8 summarises the therapeutic approaches to atopic allergy.

Anaphylactoid (pseudo-allergic) reactions mimicking anaphylactic shock sometimes occur after oral administration of aspirin (Chapter 11) and after IV administration of iodine containing diagnostic contrasts (Chapter 62). *They are not immunological in nature.*

2. **Type II reaction (cytotoxic):** In this case, the IgG and IgM antibodies formed bind to an antigen present on the cell surface and promote their destruction by lysis/phagocytosis by polymorphs and macrophages or by nonadherent lymphoid killer cells through an extracellular mechanism. Transfusion reactions, anti-D antibodies in Rhesus incompatibility and antibodies to kidney glomerular basement membrane are examples of this type of reaction. *Methyldopa-induced haemolysis is a Type II reaction.*

3. **Type III reaction (immune complex mediated):** The union of soluble antigen with IgG antibody *in vivo* forms immune complexes which may ultimately cause histamine release, activation of kinin system and aggregation of platelets resulting in microthrombi, small vessel damage and further release of vasoactive amines. The attracted polymorphs release tissue-damaging enzymes on contact with the complex. In case of high levels of circulating antibodies, the antigen is precipitated near the site of its entry into the body. The reaction in the skin is characterised by erythema, oedema and cellular infiltration, maximal at 3–8 h (**Arthus reaction**). When the antigen is relatively in excess, soluble complexes formed circulate in the body and are deposited at preferred sites such as the skin, the joints, the renal glomeruli and the choroid plexus. This type of reaction is manifested as **serum sickness** following the injection of large

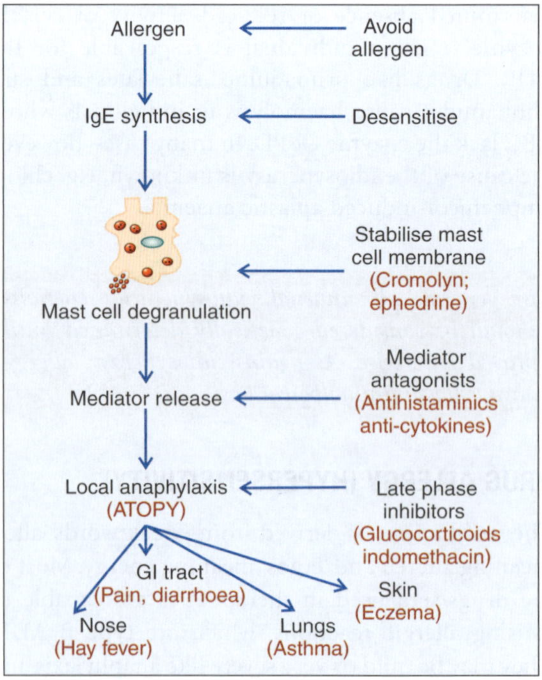

FIG. 2.8 **Atopic allergy and targets for therapy.**

quantities of foreign protein, e.g. horse serum; skin reactions of *SLE (systemic lupus erythematosus) induced with isoniazid or hydrallazine and vasculitis with sulphonamides.*

Chemotherapy may cause an abrupt release of microbial antigens, producing dramatic immune complex mediated reactions such as erythema nodosum leprosum in lepromatous leprosy treated with dapsone and the Jarisch–Herxheimer reaction in syphilitics treated with penicillin.

4. **Type IV reaction (cell-mediated or delayed hypersensitivity):** In this case, T-lymphocytes carrying a specific receptor on their surface are activated by the antigen to release certain active factors. This phenomenon is observed in contact dermatitis and in diseases caused by chemicals, dusts, mycobacteria, chlamydia, fungi and helminths and in the rejection of transplants. *Inflammatory reactions initiated by mononuclear lymphocytes and not by antibody alone are called delayed hypersensitivity reactions.* The word delayed indicates the secondary cellular response appearing at 48–72 h after the antigen (drug) exposure. In contrast, the **immediate hypersensitivity response** seen within 12 h of the antigen (drug) challenge is initiated by basophil mediated reactions (Type I) and by preformed antibodies (Types II and III). A typical delayed hypersensitivity response is observed in the Mantoux reaction following the intradermal tuberculin injection, wherein an indurated and erythematous reaction occurs within 48 h. **Delayed types of reactions** *are often observed:*
   a. With drugs that are capable of binding to body constituents and forming new antigens, e.g. *sulphonamides* and *penicillin.*
   b. Following insect bites.
   c. Following contact with certain plants or food in sensitised individuals.

Desensitisation:

In therapeutic practice, a course of graded injections of an antigen (drug) is given to a hypersensitive patient in order to render him less allergic to the antigen. This process is termed as desensitization and is believed to be due to formation of blocking antibodies (see Chapter 71).

MANIFESTATIONS OF ADR

PH 1.7, PH 3.4

Drugs can cause ADR-related to almost all tissues and organs. Some important ADR are as follows:

1. **Gastrointestinal:** Several drugs cause anorexia, nausea, vomiting (e.g. metronidazole, chloroquine), diarrhoea/constipation (e.g. iron salts, morphine). Aspirin and other NSAIDs can cause gastric ulceration and even bleeding.
2. **Haemopoietic:** It ranges from anaemia to blood dyscrasias like leucopenia, agranulocytosis, aplastic anaemia and thrombocytopenia (Chapter 36). The reduction in clotting factors may lead to haemorrhages. IM 5.7
3. **Hepatocellular:** Drugs can damage the liver:
   - *By direct action,* (Type A), either themselves or more commonly through their metabolites (e.g. paracetamol and tetracycline). Other organs such as the kidney may also be affected.

Table 2.3 Drug induced Idiosyncratic Hepatotoxicity

Idiosyncratic hepatotoxic Reactions	Causative Drugs
Nonspecific hepatitis	Isoniazid, pyrazinamide, cotrimoxazole, phenytoin, halothane
Bridging hepatic necrosis	Methyldopa
Cholestasis with hyperbilirubinemia	Certain anabolic steroids
Cholestatic hepatitis	Chlorpromazine, amoxicillin-clavulanic acid, oxacillin, erythromycin estolate, oral contraceptives
Sclerosing cholangitis	Floxuridine
Vanishing bile duct syndrome (destruction of intrahepatic biliary ductules)	Carbamazepine, chlorpromazine, haloperidol, amitriptyline, azathioprine
Steatohepatitis (due to mitochondrial hepatotoxicity)	Zidovudine, protease inhibitors
Hepatic venoocclusive disease	Cyclophosphamide, melphalan, busulfan

- *Due to idiosyncratic reaction* (Type B; Table 2.3). Sometimes extrahepatic general allergic manifestations may be present such as rash, arthralgias, fever, leukocytosis, and eosinophilia.

  Patients with genetic absence of CYP2D6 also experience hepatotoxicity with desipramine, propranolol, and quinidine.

In case of some drugs such as methyldopa, sodium valproate, and isoniazid both, direct and idiosyncratic mechanisms can operate.

The hepatic effects of potentially hepatotoxic drugs are generally monitored by periodic measurement of SGPT. However, mild, transient, nonprogressive increase in SGPT can be seen with isoniazid, valproate, phenytoin, and statins.

4. **Cardiac:** Drugs can cause cardiotoxicity directly. Thus, they may precipitate arrhythmias or even cardiac arrest (e.g. digoxin, quinine, aminophylline, flecainide). Fenfluramine is known to cause valvular fibrosis (Chapter 38).
5. **Renal:** Drugs can cause albuminuria, haematuria and even tubular necrosis. Nephrotoxicity is either direct or immunologically mediated (Chapter 37).
6. **Abnormalities of taste and smell:** Drugs are known to produce abnormalities of taste and smell sensations: **hypogeusia** is a decrease in taste acuity; **ageusia** is total loss of ability to recognise taste; **dysgeusia** is distortion of taste sensation; Hyposmia, anosmia and dysosmia represent the corresponding abnormalities of the sense of smell. Some drugs associated with the above abnormalities are d-penicillamine, pyrazinamide, ACE inhibitors, methimazole, biguanides, l-DOPA and bromocriptine.
7. **Ocular:** See Chapter 70.
8. **Otological:** Some topical preparations and certain drugs (aminoglycosides) can cause ototoxicity and impair hearing (Box 2.1).
9. **Dermal:** The skin is a common target organ for various allergic and photosensitivity reactions. Anticancer drugs can cause hair loss. Heavy metals like mercury, arsenic are secreted in the sweat and can produce exfoliative skin rashes (Chapter 69).
10. **Electrolyte disturbances:** Diuretics like thiazides and furosemide may produce hyponatremia or hypokalaemia. NSAIDs may cause sodium retention and oedema.

Box 2.1 Drugs Causing Ototoxicity

- Salicylates
- Aminoglycosides, macrolides
- Loop diuretics (furosemide)
- Antimalarials (quinine, chloroquine)
- Anticancer drugs (cisplatin, bleomycin)
- Chelating agent (desferrioxamine)
- Ear drops (chloramphenicol, polymyxin, propylene glycol, acetic acid 2%)

11. **Endocrine disturbances:** Chlorpromazine may produce menstrual irregularities, galactorrhoea and amenorrhoea. Combination oral contraceptives may arrest lactation in nursing mothers. Glucocorticoids depress the synthesis of ACTH and endogenous cortisol. Abrupt withdrawal of these compounds may, therefore, precipitate acute hypocorticism (Addisonian crisis) whereas vigorous therapy may cause Cushing syndrome.
12. **Infertility and sexual impotence:** Chapters 66 and 67.
13. **Behavioural and neurological:** Amphetamine may cause disorientation, confusion and inability to concentrate; glucocorticoids may produce euphoria, restlessness and psychosis; and benzodiazepines may cause anterograde amnesia (Chapter 8). For behavioural teratogenicity, see Chapter 78. Ethambutol can cause optic neuritis, whereas dystonic reactions can occur following phenothiazines.
14. **Carcinogenesis:** Estrogens exacerbate mammary carcinoma in females. Increased risk of developing endometrial cancer has been reported in women receiving prolonged estrogen therapy without concomitant progestin.
15. **Teratogenicity:** A teratogen is an agent which can cause a **fetal physical malformation** and **behavioural effects** when maternal administration results in significant exposure during organogenesis (18th to 60th days of fetal life). After that period, during the remainder of pregnancy, exposure to fetotoxic drugs may cause functional disability or an alteration in growth of the organs/fetus but no physical defects. The word teratogenicity is derived from the Greek word *teratos* which means monster.

The sedative '**thalidomide**', prescribed to pregnant women with morning sickness, was found to produce various types of developmental anomalies in the newborns. The commonest anomalies were 'amelia' or total absence of limbs, and 'phocomelia' or absence of one or more limbs (Fig. 2.9).

16. **Unmasking and exacerbation of disease:** Drugs can exacerbate an already existing disease or unmask a latent condition, e.g. glucocorticoids unmask latent diabetes and may exacerbate an existing peptic ulcer. Isoniazid may unmask latent epilepsy.
17. **Production of a disease (Iatrogenic disease):** Sometimes, drugs themselves may produce certain pathological syndromes. The diseases produced as a result of therapeutic measures are known as iatrogenic diseases, the Greek word *iatros* meaning 'physician'. Thus, glucocorticoid therapy can precipitate hypertension, congestive heart failure and Cushing syndrome. Glucocorticoids, aspirin and indomethacin may precipitate perforation of duodenal ulcer. Repeated doses of NSAIDs can cause renal damage.
18. **Immunosuppression:** Chapter 72.
19. **ADR due to drug interaction:** This can occur when two or more drugs are administered concurrently (Chapter 3).
20. **Adverse reactions precipitated by abrupt drug withdrawal:** Abrupt cessation of administration of drugs after prolonged use can cause either of the following:
    - **Resurgence/rebound of underlying disease**
    - **A typical 'withdrawal syndrome' in case of drug dependence.**
    - **Symptoms as a result** of physiological adaptation, e.g. pituitary suppression by glucocorticoids.

The withdrawal syndromes after abrupt stoppage of drugs such as CNS depressants, antiepileptics, clonidine and nitrates are described in the respective chapters. Such drugs must be withdrawn gradually with small decrements and under close medical supervision. Sometimes, substituting a drug with a longer half-life (e.g. methadone in patients taking morphine) is helpful.

MANAGEMENT OF ADR

PH 1.7, PH 3.4

ADR will never completely be eliminated but every attempt should be made to minimize their occurrence by working to prevent them. When a patient presents with new or worsening symptoms, a physician should think of an ADR and review the prescribed drug/s. Reporting of suspected ADR to the pharmacovigilance centre (either institutional or National) is valuable as that can lead to further regulatory actions e.g. making changes in prescribing inserts or drug labels, restricting its use or banning the drug.

Not all the ADR need treatment. Some may settle with time even with continuation of drug due to development of tolerance (Chapter 3). In case of type A ADR, reduction in dose may suffice, but type B ADR may need discontinuation of the drug. These decisions are based on the severity of ADR, chances of developing permanent damage, risk involved in withdrawal of suspected drug, availability of suitable alternative. If the patient is receiving multiple drugs, one should withdraw the least necessary and most likely drug first. If the reaction is mild, then one can

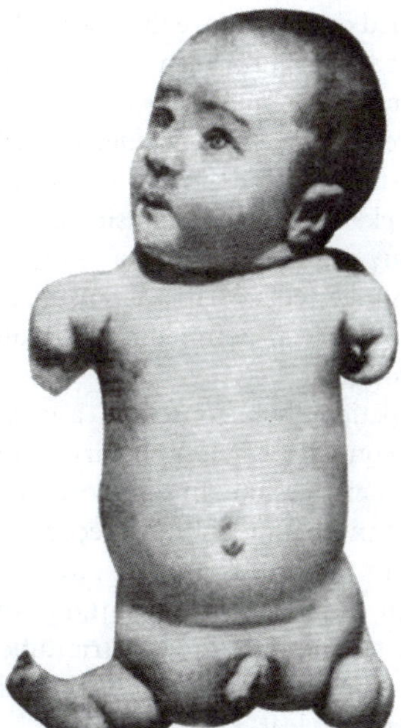

FIG. 2.9 Limb abnormalities (Seal limbs) following thalidomide administration in the mother. With courtesy of Dr. R. A. Pfeiffer from the Univ – Kinderkilinic, Munster. Direktor: Prof. Dr. H. Mai.

identify the causative drug by withdrawing them one by one. But if the reaction is severe, all the drugs have to be stopped. When an ADR is not a prime effect of the drug, it can be managed symptomatically by using a second drug e.g. anti-emetics given to prevent chemotherapy induced nausea-vomiting. **These basic principles of management are elaborated wherever relevant in subsequent chapters on systemic pharmacology of drugs.**

PH 1.52, FM 8.6, FM 8.8, IM 21.1

TREATMENT OF ACUTE DRUG POISONING

Drug poisoning could be accidental, homicidal or suicidal. Box 2.2 outlines the principles of treatment of acute poisoning.

1. **Removal of the poison:** If the patient is conscious and visits a doctor within 4 h of poison ingestion, then vomiting can be induced by tickling the back of the pharynx. Ipecac syrup 15–30 mL (adult dose) followed by 200 mL of water is useful in inducing vomiting in many cases including infants. Ipecac may be repeated after 20 min, if needed. If there is no emesis, gastric lavage should be carried out to remove the ipecac. Though concentrated salt solution can induce vomiting it may cause hypernatremia.

   Induction of emesis is contraindicated if the patient:

   a. Is stuporous, delirious or comatose; is in shock; is getting convulsions; has an inadequate gag reflex.
   b. Has ingested a corrosive poison, a CNS stimulant, or a petroleum distillate such as kerosene.

   If the patient is unconscious, aspiration of the gastric contents is helpful if carried out within 4 h of poison ingestion. In comatose patients, endotracheal intubation should precede gastric intubation to prevent aspiration. After withdrawing stomach contents, 10–15 mL/kg of saline is administered via the nasogastric tube and withdrawn. The process is continued until the lavage fluid returns clear.

   Absorption of a poison from the GI tract can be reduced in certain cases by using **activated charcoal** in the dose of 50 g (25 g in children). Activated charcoal adsorbs most of the drugs and poisons except alkalies, arsenic, lithium carbonate, cyanide, mineral acids and ferrous sulphate. *Charcoal should not be administered concurrently with ipecac or a specific antidote as it may adsorb them and render them ineffective.* As most poisons do not dissociate from activated charcoal if it is present in excess, there is no need to remove the charcoal from the GI tract. If activated charcoal is not available **Universal Antidote** may be substituted. It consists of two parts of powdered charcoal with one part of tannic acid and one part of magnesium oxide. Activated charcoal is particularly useful for reducing the absorption of alkaloids from the gut. A homemade substitute for the universal antidote is two parts of burnt toast, one part of strong tea and one part of milk of magnesia.

   Repeated oral doses of activated charcoal (50 g initially, followed by 25 g every 4 h, in adults) enhance the elimination of some drugs which are excreted back into the GI tract after they are absorbed; e.g. aspirin, carbamazepine, barbiturates, phenytoin and theophylline. Oral administration of polyethylene glycol (PEG) may be used for total bowel clearance in case of poisoning (Chapter 40). PEG is administered at a rate 25–40 mL/kg/h until the rectal effluent is clear.

2. **Enhancement of elimination of the poison:**

   a. **By increasing the urine output with diuretics like mannitol, furosemide:** Mannitol, an osmotic diuretic, is given intravenously, initially in the dose of 100–120 mL of 25% solution. Subsequently, a sustained infusion of 5% mannitol alternately in a litre of normal

Box 2.2 Principles of Treatment of Acute Poisoning FM 8.6

- Supporting measures: attention to 'Airway, Breathing, Circulation, Disability, Exposure' (ABCDE), maintain hydration and nutrition
- Removal of the poison by emesis/gastric lavage
- Use of activated charcoal
- Accelerated elimination of the poison by diuresis, dialysis, haemoperfusion
- Identification of the poison
- Specific antidote, if available
- Patients with altered mental status should receive oxygen, i.v. glucose and i.v. thiamine (100 mg)
- Follow-up and psychiatric counselling in case of suicidal poisoning

saline and a litre of 5% dextrose is administered at the rate of 500 mL/h for next 3 h. The infusion is thereafter adjusted depending upon urine output and the state of hydration. Potassium chloride (10–20 mEq) is added to each litre according to serum chemistry, and alkalinisation with sodium bicarbonate may be conveniently carried out through the drip. An average urine volume of 10–12 L in 24 h (a flow rate of 8–10 mL/min) is considered as satisfactory diuresis. The dose of mannitol should not be more than 20 g/h. Diuresis is terminated on awakening.

Alternatively, **furosemide** is used in the dose of 20 mg along with 500 mL of 1.2% sodium bicarbonate and 1 L of 5% dextrose intravenously in the first hour. The urine flow should be above 5 mL/min at the end of the hour. If it is not, furosemide should be given intravenously in large doses (up to 500 mg per 24 h); *it is essential to monitor the serum chemistry, central venous pressure and urine output.*

Such **forced diuresis** is useful in poisoning due to drugs which are less protein bound are more ionised at the achievable urine pH. *Shock, cardiac failure and renal impairment are absolute contraindications to forced diuresis.* It must be noted that forced diuresis is a potentially dangerous procedure and should only be considered for those patients who have taken the poison in such doses that they are unlikely to survive with supportive therapy alone. It is not a substitute for the intensive supportive therapy as outlined below as most of the deaths are because of failure to maintain adequate tissue oxygenation.

b. **By adjusting the pH of urine:** Weakly acidic drugs such as phenobarbitone (Chapter 6), salicylates (Chapter 11), chlorpropamide, methotrexate and chlorphenoxy herbicides are excreted faster in an alkaline urine. Alkalinisation of the urine is achieved by administration of Sodium bicarbonate 3.75 g (45 mEq) as 50 mL of a 7.5% solution, which is added to every litre of fluid intended for i.v. administration. The urinary pH should be maintained between 7.5 and 8.5. *Prior to alkalinisation hypokalemia must be treated since it will hamper efforts to alkalinise the urine due to H^+–K^+ exchange in the kidney. Urine alkalinisation is contraindicated in renal failure, pulmonary oedema and congestive cardiac failure.*

c. **By extracorporeal drug removal techniques** including **haemodialysis** or **charcoal haemoperfusion.** For haemodialysis to be effective, the drug must have low molecular weight, low volume of distribution (<1 L/kg), high water solubility and minimal protein binding. Haemodialysis is attempted for overdoses of salicylate, methanol, ethylene glycol, lithium, carbamazepine and valproic acid. Drugs with high protein binding can be removed by charcoal haemoperfusion wherein the poison will be adsorbed on charcoal and then cleared by haemodialysis. Peritoneal dialysis is the least effective method for the removal of the drugs.

In general, dialysis is more suitable than forced diuresis in patients who have severe cardiac and renal impairment. Extracorporeal drug removal techniques are usually used when patient fails to respond to supportive treatment, drug elimination routes are impaired, extremes of age and high serum levels of poison.

3. **Administration of specific antidote** (Table 2.4 and other chapters).
4. **Supportive treatment** includes:
   a. **Adequate tissue oxygenation:** Maintenance of a patent airway and ventilation is important. Oxygen can be given by a nasal catheter. Endotracheal intubation is performed when spontaneous respiration is inadequate and also to remove secretions. If assisted ventilation is required for more than 24 h, tracheostomy is usually performed. Frequent monitoring of blood gases and blood pH is helpful. Respiratory physiotherapy minimises lung complications.
   b. **Maintenance of BP by fluids and vasopressor agents:** Intravenous fluids must be given as an adjuvant to forced diuresis to prevent dehydration and for maintaining the blood volume.

Table 2.4 Antidotes for Emergency Treatment of Certain Poisonings FM 8.8

Poison	Antidote
Paracetamol	*N*-Acetylcysteine
Theophylline	Propranolol
Mercury, arsenic and copper	BAL
Atropine and other antimuscarinics	Physostigmine
Carbon monoxide	Oxygen
Cyanide	Dicobalt edetate; amyl nitrite followed by sodium nitrite, then sodium thiosulphate
Methyl alcohol and ethylene glycol	Ethyl alcohol; Fomepizole
Lead	Calcium disodium edetate; dimercaptosuccinic acid
Nitrites	Methylene blue
Opioids	Naloxone
Benzodiazepines	Flumazenil
Organophosphate compounds	Atropine; pralidoxime
Warfarin	Vitamin K_1
Beta-adrenergic stimulants	Propranolol
Beta blockers	Glucagon
CCB	Calcium gluconate
Iron	Desferrioxamine
Methotrexate	Leucovorin
INH	Pyridoxine

For management of shock see Chapter 32. Overloading of the circulation should be avoided.

c. **Prevention of secondary infection:** Prophylactic antibiotics should not be used routinely but may be necessary in patients requiring tracheostomy or catheterisation.

Self-medication is often an important cause of drug poisoning. This is particularly true of commonly used and 'available over the counter' drugs like fever and pain remedies (paracetamol) and vitamin D preparations. The other common agents to cause self-poisoning are ingestion of adulterated alcohol (methyl alcohol) and insecticides.

CHAPTER 3

PH 1.1

Principles of Drug Prescribing; Factors Modifying the Effects of a Drug; and Drug Interactions

Learning Objectives

This chapter will enable the reader:

1. To discuss the principles involved in prescribing a drug.
2. To be aware of factors that determine drug dose.
3. To define the terms p-drug, essential drugs and orphan drugs.
4. To state the importance of standard treatment guidelines/essential drug list in rational use of medicine.
5. To classify various factors that modify drug effects.
6. To differentiate between drug tolerance and drug dependence.
7. To explain the consequences of use of drug combinations.
8. To classify drug interactions giving suitable examples.

KEY TERMS

PH 1.2

Modern therapeutics is not just an art but is more of a science. It is now more and more dominated by **evidence-based medicine (EBM)** that is defined by Dr. David Sackett as the 'the conscientious, explicit and judicious use of current, best evidence in making decisions about the care of individual patients'. Thus, it is essential for the physician, before prescribing any therapy, to examine objectively all the available evidence for patient care resulting from systematic research, and to integrate the same with individual clinical expertise.

In practice, the treatment of a sick person includes many aspects, and administration of drugs is one of them. In certain patients, drugs are of the greatest importance, while in others, they have a less important role to play.

In all situations, the *doctor–patient* communication (verbal as well as non-verbal) is of prime importance. 'Words have the potential to "heal" or to "sicken". Words that bring expectations are interventions on their own. Words may not "cure" but they can affect attitudes and emotions, and ultimately body sensations; the right words can lead a patient to optimism, whereas the wrong words can produce despair.'

DRUG PRESCRIBING

PH 1.1

A practitioner who prescribes drugs must know the:

- Natural course of the disease he/she is treating
- Pharmacological actions and adverse effects of a drug he / she is prescribing
- Reasons for choosing a particular drug
- Methods of assessing drug efficacy and safety
- Possible interactions when several drugs are administered concurrently

Drugs should be prescribed only when:

- There is a clear indication for their use
- The benefit of their use outweighs the possible harms

PH 1.9

Drugs should be prescribed by their **generic** names rather than by **brand** names. PH 1.2

Practitioners, should have a critical approach towards

newly marketed drugs. New drugs are often marketed with excessive claims regarding their properties and superiority over the established drugs. Moreover, these new entrants to the drug market are invariably costly. Surprisingly, such drugs are often prescribed to patients even though there is poor evidence of their efficacy and safety. Hence, physicians should have skills to critically appraise drug promotional literature and assess new drugs objectively so that they are able to distinguish marketing claims from true ef-fectiveness, advantages and make reliable prescribing decisions.

It should also be remembered that, many costly preparations sold in the market are neither new nor necessarily better than older, established and inexpensive preparations. In fact, these 'me too' drugs are often introduced in the market under various brand names, either alone or as fixed dose combinations and are sold at a fancy price, purely with effective advertisement, promotional literature and other modern sales promotion techniques. Real wonder drugs are rarely born and do not require much advertisement; an important principle of marketing and sales promotion is *to create a demand where real need does not exist.*

How you use a drug is often more important than which drug you prescribe: Rational use requires familiarity with both therapeutic and adverse effects of drugs. This is difficult if one switches from one drug to another frequently. Usually, it is beneficial to be slow while adopting any new agent (be neither the first nor the last to start a new drug). In practice, the initial choice of the drug and the dose regimen depends upon the:

- Correct diagnosis,
- Severity of the disease,
- Presence of complications/co-morbidities
- Risk/benefit of using the drug
- Cost/efficacy ratios (affordability) of the drugs.

It is unfortunate that doctors often overprescribe drugs for trivial complaints. Although this has some relation to increased demand by patients for drugs, the major fault lies with the medical profession. Many busy practitioners find it difficult to keep in touch with the current literature and are easily persuaded by the promotional techniques used by the pharmaceutical industry. Others probably would like to impress their patients by their 'most up-to-date' knowledge about 'the latest drugs', while some may not even bother about what preparation they prescribe and what drug the branded product contains. Majority of them are neither aware of nor do they bother to find out the cost of the preparation.

It cannot be emphasized enough that while selecting a drug, its **cost-effectiveness** (getting the maximum benefit at the minimal cost) and **cost–benefit ratio** should be taken into consideration. While trying to prolong the patient's life, ensuring that his/her quality of life is also enhanced is equally important. Hence, while selecting a drug it is the doctor's duty to keep in mind its real need, cost and affordability to the patient. How many practitioners know that the cost of the same drug promoted under different brand names may vary as much as 5–10 times? Dermal preparations containing the newer potent steroids are far more expensive than equally effective, well established older preparations.

Cost being a major consideration in long-term treatment (e.g. hypertension), only cost-effective drugs should be prescribed; *this often means prescribing drugs by their generic names.* Pharmacoeconomic studies compare various drugs/treatments for a given disease from cost perspective (Chapter 1).

Dosing during therapy: *As experience accumulates, physicians find that smaller doses work equally well and are safer, and more economical.* It is well known that individuals vary in their response to drugs. The importance of phar-macogenomics is also being increasingly recognised. New drugs are often introduced at a dose that will be effective in about 90% of the target population, because this is known to help market penetration. Doses are also partly determined by an irrational preference for round numbers. A sizeable minority (30%) are likely to require smaller doses than those recommended during early marketing period of a new drug and hence may be subjected to adverse effects due to overdosage. This should be borne in mind while prescribing a drug, especially a recently marketed one. Dose searching is continued even after a drug is marketed.e.g. Ethinyl estradiol was initially used in the dose of 50 mcg, in a combined oral contraceptive pill. Subsequently the dose was reduced to 20 mcg as it was found to be equally effective, and more safer.

Various formulae used earlier to calculate the dose give only gross estimation. They are based on the average body weight of 70 kg. In many countries, average body weight is less than 70 kg. Furthermore, *it is now established that quantitative response to drug differs in different population,* e.g. Asians need smaller doses of psychotropic and antihypertensive drugs than Caucasians.

The drug regimen should be as simple as it can be kept: as few drugs as possible and once or twice a day administration, if permissible. A wise general policy is 'start low, go slow', particularly in children and the elderly, except perhaps during an emergency. It is important to note that elderly (> 65 years) may suffer from dementia; they may forget to take the drugs or swallow more amount. This makes it mandatory to monitor compliance, to the prescribed drug regimen. PH 1.59

Fixed-dose combinations (FDCs): A FDC drug includes two or more active pharmaceutical ingredients combined in a single dosage form, wherein the individual ingredients are in fixed doses (ratio) e.g. combination of l- DOPA + Carbidopa is a single tablet containing 100 mg l-DOPA and 25 mg carbidopa and thus the content ratio is 4:1. Use of rational FDCs is helpful. They:

- *Are convenient to use and improve compliance*
- *Enhance the efficacy of therapy*, e.g. antituberculosis therapy, which is more effective and prevents drug resistance; and combined estrogen–progesterone contraceptive pills which demonstrate synergy
- *Reduce drug toxicity*, e.g. levodopa–carbidopa combination
- Are cheap due to cost saving in post-manufacturing processes (packaging to distribution)

However, using FDCs:

a. may expose the patient to additional toxicity (e.g,. ornidazole + ofloxacin)
b. may reduce the effectiveness of therapy
c. makes dosage adjustment of the individual drug difficult (e.g., alprazolam + sertraline),
d. may be expensive and may not have a complementary mechanism of action (e.g., famotidine + domperidone).

Often, such combinations:

1. Contain inadequate dose of the main ingredient, e.g. ampicillin and cloxacillin (250 mg of each)
2. Contain a second agent of doubtful efficacy, e.g. serratiopeptidase added to paracetamol or an NSAID
3. Have ingredients that may exert only additive effects, e.g. ibuprofen and paracetamol
4. Have ingredients which exhibit pharmacokinetic mismatch
5. Are not supported by scientific evidence and may even be irrational (trypsin and chymotrypsin)

Hence, a FDCs should be prescribed unless there is reason to consider that the patient needs all the drugs in the formulation and that the doses are appropriate and will need no individual dose adjustment.
PH 1.10, PH 3.8

It is not only important to know what drugs to prescribe but also how to write a prescription properly without any errors. A prescription is a written order by the prescriber to a pharmacist for compounding and/or dispensing the prescribed medicines along with instructions for the patient. It has the following parts: 1. **Superscription** (prescriber and patient's details, date of prescription and the sign Rx, take thou); 2. **Inscription** (medicines/ingredients prescribed with oral medicines first, followed by injections and then topical and their quantities); 3. **Subscription** (instruction to the pharmacist about how to prepare the medicine from the ingredients or the amount of medicine to be dispensed) and 4. **Transcription** (instructions for the patient about how to take the medicines, which are to be transferred by the pharmacist on the label pasted on the dispensed medicines. It also includes signature and name of the prescriber).

However, now a days many prescriptions include only marketed medicines. Hence there is no need to instruct the pharmacist about how to prepare the medicine but the amount to be dispensed by the pharmacist and instructions to the patient are written on the

PH 3.1, PH 3.8

Box 3.1 Principles of Prescription Writing

'Prescribe right drug to right patient in right dose by right route at right time intervals.'

- Write the prescription on your letterhead which has your name, qualification, registration number and contact number.
- Write legibly and indelibly.
- Write the patient's name, age, sex and address.
- Write the medicine's name in capital and as generic name. Do not abbreviate names of drugs/preparations(s) or instructions about taking the medicines. Write 'Units' not 'u'. Write mcg not µg. When decimals are unavoidable, write, say, 50 mcg, not 0.05 mg, Write clearly dose (so many tablets/capsules/puffs), dosing interval (so many hours), time of the day, relation to meals and duration of therapy. Also mention when to follow up and if any investigations to be done before that so that those reports can be brought on follow up day .
- When prescribing a drug 'as required', write the minimum dosing interval and the maximum number of doses per day.
- In case of scheduled drugs, write the quantity of drug to be supplied at a time and how many times the prescribed drugs may be supplied without revalidation.
- Advise the parents/patients that: no medicine should be added to the infant's feeding bottle; tablets/capsules should be taken in sitting position and washed down with plenty of water; ointments should be used as supplied and not diluted before use; residual ointment after use by one patient should be discarded and not stored for future use; medicines should be stored beyond the reach of children.
- Sign the prescription. If prescription is on the hospital case paper, write your name.
- Write date and your registration number.
- Avoid painful IM injections in children whenever possible. Liquid preparations are more suitable for children and old persons.

Some abbreviations used in prescription orders are o.d., once a day; /d, per day; b.i.d., twice a day; t.i.d., thrice a day; q.i.d., four times a day; q as in q4h, 4 hourly; HS, at night; sos, as required, e.g. a sleeping pill (Chapter 8); prn (pro re nata), an extra dose as required, in addition to the basal orders, e.g. an analgesic (Chapter 11).

prescription itself, which is handed over to the patient. Hence it is more important to remember the principles of prescription writing as outlined in Box 3.1 rather than the parts of the prescription.

A good prescription is one which has minimum number of effective, better tolerated and affordable drugs, prescribed with specific objectives in mind giving clear instructions to patients/relatives. Prescribing 'fancy and expensive tonics' to patients who can hardly afford two meals a day is also unethical.

It is mandatory to explain to the patient in a simple language, the reason for prescribing the drug(s) and what to expect when treatment is taken; what is prescribed and how to take it (regimen); possible common and serious ADRs; any specific instructions or warnings and when to come for follow up. Adherence to the prescribed therapy is better if the physician clarifies doubts of the patient, makes him/her recite the important points told earlier and provides optimal reassurance. For the patients who are mentally challenged, incapable of understanding or remembering instructions or unable to take care of themselves, care givers (parents in case of a child) should be instructed.

Patient compliance: Once the drugs are dispensed, it is the patient's responsibility to take the prescribed medicines except when hospitalized. However, patients often do not follow the prescribed course of treatment. This is known as non-compliance to medication and there are several reasons for noncompliance:

- Complexity of the regimen (several drugs to be taken several times a day)
- Cost of treatment
- Adverse reactions
- Poor motivation
- Length of therapy
- Natural disinclination to take injectable preparations

The patient's compliance may be improved by personal contact and constant reminders that '*drugs do not work unless you take them*'. A sympathetic discussion about the difficulties of drugs prescribed and about the possible adverse effects is likely to have a beneficial effect on compliance. On the other hand, mere distribution of printed leaflets about drugs prescribed, diet, etc., may educate the patient but is less effective in improving patient compliance. Moreover, they are useless in an illiterate population. Occasionally, it is necessary to take into confidence the patient's care-givers, particularly with old or mentally disturbed patients. A surprise check on urine or plasma level of the drug or its metabolite also helps to detect defaulters, but it not practical.

It is not enough simply to note the failure of drug therapy and the adverse reactions produced. If one has to make any purposeful decision about the future use of the drug, it is necessary to know more about it. What is the cause of the failure? How useful is the drug usually? Is it commonly used? For what condition is it usually given? What good does it do? Is the risk in its use worth the benefits expected? Can therapy be improved? This constitutes a *therapeutic audit* and would help the doctor in using drugs in future cases more rationally and effectively.

Drug 'generations': Newer drugs belonging to an existing group are often promoted as second and third 'generation' drugs, implying that they are universally superior to the older members of the group. Often, 'first generation' means that these drugs have been available for many years while second generation drugs are made available later. The differences may be minor and mostly in pharmacokinetics ('me too' drugs). Moreover, long-term safety of the newer generation of drugs is not known, e.g. gatifloxacin, a second generation fluoroquinolone was withdrawn due to ADR after it was marketed but the first generation fluoroquinolones are still being used. One must remember that the 'first-generation' drugs may also be the drugs of choice in selected indications e.g. cephalosporins of the first generations are still the preferred drugs in Gram positive infections.

Drugs expiry date: Do the drugs become useless after the expiry date mentioned by the manufacturers? No. Drug companies, because of certain legal compulsions and liability concerns, will not advocate such use after the expiry date mentioned on the package. Shelf-life of a drug is the time where a given product, stored under reasonable conditions, is expected to remain stable ('90% of potency). Most of the drugs remain stable for a long time beyond their expiry dates. According to Medical Letter (Volume 44, 93, 2002), 'There are virtually no reports of toxicity from degradation products of outdated drugs (except tetracycline). How much of their potency they retain varies with the drug and the storage conditions, especially humidity, but many *drugs stored under reasonable conditions* retain 90% of their potency for at least 5 years after the expiration date on the label, and sometimes much longer.' However, one has to be more careful in case of biological agents (Chapter 72).

CM 19.3

Poor quality drugs are the substandard spurious/falsely-labelled/falsified/counterfeit (**SSFFC**) drugs that pose serious health problem to consumers. World Health Organization (WHO) defines SSFFC medicines as 'medicines which are deliberately and fraudulently mislabelled with respect to identity and/or source, and also which may include products with correct ingredients or with the wrong ingredients, without active ingredients, with insufficient or too much active ingredient, or with fake packaging'. Globally, counterfeit medicines may constitute 10% of the available products. For detection of counterfeit drugs, one needs a good infrastructure for vigilance and for strict enforcement of drug regulations.

PH 1.1, PH 3.5

P-DRUGS (PERSONAL DRUGS)

In practice, the physician usually needs 50–60 drugs routinely to treat common ailments. P-drugs are the drugs one chooses for prescribing regularly and with which one becomes familiar. Such a list would spare the physician repeated search for a better drug from among the many available. Guidelines for choosing P-drugs are outlined in Box 3.2.

Sometimes, a drug may be very efficacious, but it may not be suitable in a given patient because of other patient-related factors such as renal/hepatic damage, diabetes mellitus, pregnancy, lactation or drug allergy. The cost of treatment and, especially, the cost/benefit ratio of a drug or a dosage form is also a major selection criterion. Many patients may have to be treated with a less-than-ideal drug which has to be accepted because of the unaffordable cost or nonavailability of the ideal drug.

*Personal treatment **(P-treatment)** and P-drugs are not identical.* Not every P-treatment includes a P-drug,

Box 3.2 Steps for Selecting P-Drugs

- Define the diagnosis (pathophysiology)
- Specify the therapeutic objective(s)
- Make an inventory of the effective drug groups
- Choose a group and select the individual drug from the group according to efficacy, safety, suitability and cost
- Prescribe treatment for a standard duration

Adapted from: *Guide to Good Prescribing*, WHO Action Programme on Essential Drugs, 1999 e.g. life style modifications in obesity. As with P-drugs, the choice of P-treatment is guided by the therapeutic objectives in a given patient, and depends upon efficacy, safety, suitability and cost of the treatment.

With the availability of increasing number of drugs and formulations, and the flood of promotional material, it is desirable to prepare one's own pocket P-drug formulary. It should contain not only names of P-drugs but also dosage form, dosage, frequency and duration of administration of the drugs; patient-teaching material about the drugs; and patient monitoring information for doctor's own use. *Of course, one has to keep oneself well informed about the merits and demerits of new drugs, and revise one's P-drug list from time to time.* PH 3.7, PH 1.59, CM 19.1

ESSENTIAL DRUGS

As per WHO definition: 'Essential drugs are those drugs that satisfy the healthcare needs of the majority of the population. They should, therefore, be available at all times in adequate amounts and in appropriate dosage forms, at a price the individual and the community can afford.'

The list of such drugs is presented at *two levels.*

1. The **core list** which indicates the minimum drug needs of a basic health care system, listing the most cost-effective drugs for priority conditions.
2. The **complementary list** which consists of drugs for priority diseases that are cost-effective but not necessarily affordable, or may need specialised health care facilities. This list also includes essential drugs for less frequent diseases. The section on reserve anti-infective agents could thus be integrated into the complementary list.

This concept, advocated for use in hospitals, has many **advantages:**

- It improves the practitioner's knowledge of the drugs he is prescribing and hence the quality of prescribing
- It reduces the cost of patient care CM 19.2

The drugs from such selected lists should be made available at all times, even at the remotest places in the country. Obviously, the list will differ according to factors such as local disease pattern, disease incidence, available infrastructure and the financial resources at disposal. Genetic, environmental and demographic factors have also to be taken into account. Hence, drug utilisation studies are necessary both, from urban and rural areas to understand the above-mentioned factors and deficiencies in the healthcare systems.

Only those drugs which are of proven value, relatively safe and cost-effective are included. Such lists are revised from time to time. *Fixed-dose combinations* are acceptable only when the dosage of each ingredient meets the requirements of a defined population group, and the combination has advantage over a single compound in therapeutic effects, safety and compliance, e.g. antituberculosis drugs. Many countries have now prepared essential drug lists based on their priorities.

Of course, it is not correct to say that drugs not included in such lists are all 'nonessential' and hence not required. Some of them are indeed useful for special indications under specific circumstances, e.g. anticancer drugs.

ORPHAN DRUGS

Orphan drugs are drugs meant for the diagnosis, prevention or treatment of rare diseases. According to Indian Regulatory Authority, rare disease is the one that affects not more than 5 lakh persons. They are not easily available because their manufacture is not commercially viable for various reasons which include:

- Their limited demand
- Enormous cost of production
- Nonpatentability of the drug
- The complex and costly procedure for establishing the efficacy and safety of the drug, and for the governmental approval process

Some examples of orphan drugs are certain anticancer and antiviral drugs; certain antiparasitic drugs (pentamidine) and drugs used in the treatment of rare genetic enzyme deficiencies. Furthermore, one should also remember that some of the older drugs, which had been proven useful for many years and have high cost-effectiveness for routine use, have now become 'orphan drugs' because their commercial production is no longer profitable, e.g. cyanocobalamine. Drugs such as chlorpropamide, reserpine and diloxanide furoate are not easily available. They have become 'the victims of myth (that newer drugs are necessarily superior), master-marketing and fashionable prescribing'.

FACTORS MODIFYING THE EFFECTS OF A DRUG

Individuals differ both in the degree and the character of the response that a drug may elicit. The doses of official preparation of drugs are, therefore, always expressed in the form of a range which gives the therapeutic effect in majority of subjects. The important factors which influence the effect of a drug are as follows:

1. **Body weight:** The average dose is mentioned either in terms of mg per kg body weight or as the total single dose for an adult weighing 50–100 kg. The smaller dose should be used in Indians whose average weight is about 50 kg. However, dose expressed in this fashion may not apply in cases of excessively obese individuals or those suffering from oedema, dehydration or emaciation. Nutritional factors can sometimes alter drug metabolising capacity and this should be kept in mind in undernourished patients. PH 1.56

2. **Age and gender:** Children may not react to all drugs in the same manner as young adults. The pharmacokinetics changes with age. Thus, gastric emptying is prolonged and gastric pH fluctuates in neonates and infants. Their liver capacity to metabolise drugs is low, renal function is less well-developed and proportion of body water is higher in the infants. The metabolic clearance of drugs such as chloramphenicol, barbiturates, pethidine, salicylates, sulphonamides, diazepam and aminoglycosides is less in infants than in adults.

   The *pharmacodynamics* of drugs in children may differ from that in adults as well. Drugs may show unique effects in children, not seen in adults. Thus, some substances may disturb the patterns of growth and development that occur only during particular periods of life, e.g. tetracyclines and glucocorticoids in children. Metoclopramide and other dopamine antagonists produce acute dystonic reactions more often in children and adolescents than in adults. With few exceptions, drugs are more active and more toxic in the newborn than in adults. The doses of antidiphtheria serum and antitetanus serum, however, are not modified by age. PH 1.12, PH 2.4

   The **paediatric doses** are expressed in terms of body weight (mg/kg per dose or per day) or in terms of body surface area (mg/m^2/dose or per day). Following formulae can be used to calculate doses in child:

   1. **Young's formula**
      Adult Dose × [Age ÷ (Age+12)] = Child's Dose
   2. **Clark's formula**
      Adult Dose × (Weight in lbs ÷ 150) = Child's Dose (1 kg = 2.2 ls)

   These formulae do not take into account all the potential sources of pharmacokinetic differences in children (Chapter 78). Moreover, those who need long term treatment will need dose adjustments as they grow. It is also important to remember that these calculated doses may not be optimum for some children due to high interindividual variability and dose adjustments may be required according to the clinical response. Obese children can be dosed using ideal body weight. If actual weight is used to calculate the dose, then there is a risk of administration of high dose of the drugs that do not distribute into fat e.g. paracetamol.

   It is always better to verify the calculated dose with recommended dose mentioned by the manufacturer on the drug label. One may use handy worked-out table for paediatric doses, if available (Table 3.1). More precision in doses will come when we have algorithm based on modelling and simulation tools or data emerged from drug trials in children. PH 1.12

   Elderly also present problems in dosage adjustment and this may vary widely with different people. While prescribing the drugs for elderly (particularly after 60 years), it is important to remember that in the elderly the body fat may increase while total water and lean body mass decrease. Furthermore, plasma albumin concentration may be lower. *As age advances, liver and kidney mass and blood flow decreases so that the metabolic inactivation and renal excretion of drugs slows down.* In the elderly, the serum creatinine level may be within normal range even though *the creatinine clearance is markedly reduced*. These

Table 3.1 Determination of Children's Doses from Adult Doses on the Basis of Body Surface Area[a]

Weight (kg)	Approx. Surface Area in Square Meters	Approx. Percentage of Adult Dose[b]
2	0.15	9
4	0.25	14
6	0.33	19
8	0.40	23
10	0.46	27
15	0.63	36
20	0.80	46
25	0.95	55
30	1.08	62
35	1.20	70
40	1.30	75
45	1.40	81
50	1.51	87
55	1.58	91

Source: A.M.A. Drug Evaluation 1973 (2nd edition).
[a]Based on Done, A.K.: *Drugs for Children* in Modell, W. (Ed) Drugs of Choice 1972–73. St. Louis: The C.V. Mosby Co., 1972.
[b]Based on average adult surface area of 1.73 sqm. A.M.A. Drug Evaluation 1973 (2nd ed.)

changes demand modification of dosage regimen. Pharmacodynamically, the elderly are more sensitive to CNS drugs such as neuroleptics, hypnotics, sedatives and respiration depressants. The response to drug acting on β adrenergic receptors is attenuated while possibility of postural hypotension with antihypertensive is increased due to reduced sensitivity of baroreceptors. It is known that *incidence of ADR rises with age*. Hence, it is important to select appropriate (less toxic) drugs, dose regimen and formulation while prescribing for the elderly. *Often, elderly suffer from senile dementia which makes it necessary to monitor compliance. In addition, remember that in the elderly, 'stopping a drug is equally important as starting it'.*

Some drugs which need to be prescribed with caution in the elderly are listed in Box 3.3. Central depressants such as hypnotics and antipsychotics may produce confusional states or falls in the elderly.

In general, in elderly patients detailed, previous, drug history should be elicited before prescribing drugs and their mental status should be assessed. They should be prescribed as few drugs as possible, preferably those with less serious ADR, for short periods.

Gastric metabolism of alcohol is lower in women than in men, which is responsible for gender-related differences in blood alcohol levels.

3. **Pregnancy and lactation:** Special care should be exercised when drugs are prescribed during pregnancy and lactation (Chapter 78).
   Drugs which may stimulate the uterine smooth muscle are contraindicated during pregnancy. Furthermore, many drugs administered to the mother are capable of delaying the onset of labour or of crossing the placenta and affecting the fetus.
4. **Diet, tobacco, alcohol and environment:** Medicines are usually taken after a meal to reduce the risk of gastric irritation, nausea and vomiting. Food, however, can have significant effect on the pharmacokinetics of drugs (Box 1.5). Generally, food depresses the rate and the extent of drug absorption. However, some drugs are better absorbed when administered with food, e.g. vitamin D, griseofulvin and saquinavir. Drugs may be given on empty stomach (i) to prevent mixing with the foodstuffs, e.g. the anthelmintics, (ii) to get an immediate action, e.g. drugs used for motion sickness and (iii) to prevent drug inactivation in the stomach, e.g. penicillin V. Tetracyclines form insoluble chelates with aluminium, calcium and magnesium salts, which reduces their absorption. Captopril, digoxin, thyroxine sodium and rifampicin are examples of drugs better absorbed on empty stomach.

Box 3.3 Some Drugs to be Used with Caution in the Elderly

- NSAID
- CNS depressants
- Neuroleptics
- Antihypertensives and other drugs causing postural hypotension
- Diuretics
- Anticholinergics and drugs with anticholinergic adverse effects
- Digoxin
- Drugs causing bone marrow depression
- Nephrotoxic drugs

The dose of a hypnotic required to produce sleep during daytime is higher than that required to produce sleep at night. High altitude with low barometric pressure diminishes the capacity of the body to oxidise drugs and this may precipitate drug toxicity.

Polycyclic hydrocarbons present in cigarette smoke and hydrocarbon pesticides such as DDT induce hepatic microsomal CYP enzymes. This accelerates the biodegradation of several drugs.

Alcohol modifies the response to many drugs. It also induces hepatic enzymes and causes rapid metabolism of certain drugs. On the other hand, hepatic injury due to alcohol can enhance response to drugs (Chapter 6).

5. **Route of administration:** Intravenous doses of the drugs are usually smaller than oral doses, particularly in case of drugs which are incompletely absorbed orally, e.g. digoxin. The onset of drug action is quicker with the IV route; this might enhance the chances of drug toxicity.

6. **Psychological factors:** The personality of the physician may influence the drug effect considerably, particularly if the drug is intended for use in a psychosomatic disorder. Inert dosage forms called placebos are known to produce therapeutic benefit in psychosomatic conditions (Chapter 4). The personality of the patient and the physician may also modify the drug effect. The dose of chlorpromazine required to produce calming effect in an otherwise normal individual is 50–100 mg/day. However, the same drug may have to be administered in the dose of 500–1000 mg/day to achieve the quietening effect in highly agitated schizophrenic patients.

7. **Genetic factors:** Variations in the human genome determine the genetically mediated differences in drug metabolism and response (**pharmacogenomics**). The latter are usually due to defective/deficient enzyme systems responsible for inactivating the drug. Often, this results in drug accumulation and toxicity. *Patients with hereditary disorders of intermediary metabolism such as diabetes mellitus rarely show a disturbance in the metabolism of drugs and other foreign compounds.* This is because the microsomal enzyme system, involved in the metabolism of drugs, does not participate to a significant extent in the intermediary metabolism. Some examples of genetic variations:

Acetylation and hydroxylation of drugs: The rate of acetylation of INH, dapsone, hydralazine and some sulphonamides is controlled by an autosomal recessive gene and the dosage of these drugs depends upon the acetylator status of individuals. Similarly, slow hydroxylators are liable to exaggerated responses (excessive beta blockade with metoprolol) and to drug toxicity (lactic acidosis with phenformin).

Plasma cholinesterase (pseudo-cholinesterase): Some persons inherit a modified type of esterase (atypical pseudocholinesterase) that is less efficient than the normal enzyme in hydrolysing the drug succinylcholine. Such people may develop prolonged respiratory paralysis even with a therapeutic dose of succinylcholine.

Phenytoin hydroxylation: Certain epileptic patients are unable to *p*-hydroxylate diphenylhydantoin and develop marked toxicity.

Hepatic CYP2D6 enzyme variation: Tricyclic antidepressants (TCA) are mostly metabolised by CYP2D6. Patients with mental depression exhibiting slow metabolism need much smaller doses of TCA than the fast metabolisers. On the other hand, failure to respond to TCA is common in ultra-fast metabolisers.

Erythrocyte diaphorase: The enzyme erythrocyte NAD-diaphorase protects the erythrocytes by reducing methemoglobin to haemoglobin. Individuals with a hereditary deficiency of this enzyme are likely to develop methemoglobinemia after administration of drugs such as sulphonamides and nitrites.

Glucose-6-phosphate dehydrogenase (G6PD): Primaquine and certain other drugs cause haemolysis in individuals with a deficiency of G6PD (Chapter 36).

Miscellaneous: These include inherited abnormal drug response such as:

a. Resistance to coumarin anticoagulants
b. Response to lower doses of propranolol by Chinese as compared to the Caucasians although the metabolism of propranolol is significantly faster in the Chinese
c. Slow metabolism of alcohol in about 90% of Whites as compared to the rate observed in

90% Orientals is due to the presence of a variant of alcohol dehydrogenase enzyme in their liver. In 50% of Asians, inactive form of aldehyde dehydrogenase is observed due to mutation; as a result they have higher levels of acetaldehyde following alcohol ingestion, which causes facial flush and other intense responses

d. Precipitation of an acute attack of porphyria by barbiturates in susceptible individuals is due to enhanced activity of the hepatic enzyme, delta-aminolevulinic acid synthetase, which leads to a marked rise in the rate of porphobilinogen synthesis
e. Precipitation of severe hyperpyrexia, muscle rigidity, hyperkalemic cardiac arrest and death (malignant hyperthermia, an autosomal dominant condition) by anaesthetics such as halothane, methoxyflurane and cyclopropane

8. **Metabolic disturbances:** Changes in water-electrolyte and acid–base balance, body temperature and other physiological parameters may modify the effects of drugs, e.g.
   a. Aspirin reduces body temperature only in the presence of pyrexia
   b. The vasoconstrictor effect of noradrenaline is reduced in the presence of metabolic acidosis
   c. The absorption of iron from the gut is maximum if the individual has an iron deficiency anaemia. Hypokalaemia can enhance digoxin cardiotoxicity

9. **Presence of disease (comorbidity):** Drugs like morphine and chlorpromazine may produce unusually prolonged effect in cirrhotic patients. Antibiotics like streptomycin and kanamycin, excreted mainly by the kidneys may prove toxic if the kidney function is impaired. In myxoedema, morphine acts for a much longer time because of the low rate of oxidation. In congestive heart failure, the clearance of lignocaine may diminish by 50%. Pulmonary and GI disease may also alter pharmacokinetics.

10. **Cumulation:** If a drug is excreted slowly, its repeated administration may build up a sufficiently high concentration in the body to produce toxicity, e.g. digoxin, emetine and heavy metals. Sometimes, a cumulative effect is desired, e.g. with phenytoin in the treatment of epilepsy. Most often, however, it is undesirable. Substances like lead can remain deposited in bones without producing toxic effects. This is called *passive cumulation*; toxic manifestations occur as soon as it is released into the blood.
    To avoid cumulation:
    a. One must know if the drug is eliminated slowly or rapidly
    b. Stop the drug administration at the appearance of the first warning symptom
    c. Select carefully the form in which the drug is to be administered
    d. Check liver and kidney function before and during drug administration, as even an otherwise noncumulative drug would produce cumulation in the presence of hepatic and renal damage

11. **Other drugs and chemicals:** Previous or concurrent therapy with certain drugs may result in stimulation or inhibition of the metabolism of other drugs. Both tobacco smoke and alcohol consumption induce CYP450 liver enzymes. They accelerate the metabolism of a number of drugs, leading to a reduction in their therapeutic effects.
12. **Additive effect** (summation): See Chapter 2.
13. **Synergism:** See Chapter 2.
14. **Antagonism:** See Chapter 2.
15. **Drug tolerance:** When a large dose of a drug is required to elicit an effect ordinarily produced by its normal therapeutic dose, the phenomenon is termed as drug tolerance. **Drug tolerance** is of two types:
    a. **True tolerance:** This is seen on both oral and parenteral administration of a drug and can be: (i) natural or (ii) acquired.
    i. **Natural tolerance:** This is seen in various animal species and also among the various human races. It includes:
    - **Species tolerance:** Certain animal species can tolerate certain drugs in quantities lethal to man, e.g. some rabbits can tolerate large quantities of belladonna. This is attributed to the enzyme atropine esterase in their liver and plasma, which rapidly detoxifies belladonna.
    - **Racial tolerance:** A solution of ephedrine

instilled into the conjunctival sac of the Caucasians produces prompt dilatation of the pupil but in Negroes it may not produce any dilatation.

ii. **Acquired tolerance** results only on repeated administration of a drug and may take weeks or months to develop, e.g. opiates, barbiturates, nitrates and xanthines. Tolerance is sometimes desirable, e.g. barbiturates, when used in the treatment of epilepsy, produce tolerance for their soporific but not for their antiepileptic effect. Generally however, tolerance is undesirable.

- **Tissue tolerance:** In this type, the development of tolerance is confined to certain effects or to certain systems, e.g. morphine produces tolerance for its euphoriant effect, but the pupils and the GI tract do not become tolerant. Thus, the same dose of morphine invariably produces pinpoint pupils and constipation but may fail to produce euphoria.
- **Cross tolerance:** If an individual initially develops tolerance to a drug belonging to a particular group, he also shows tolerance to other drugs from the same group. This phenomenon is known as cross tolerance, e.g. that between alcohol and the general anaesthetics like ether.

b. **Apparent or pseudotolerance:** The feudal kings, much worried about poisons, were often in the habit of taking small doses of arsenic by mouth. This apparently rendered them immune to oral arsenic but poisoning could occur if any other route was chosen. This tolerance is probably due to the *local changes developed by the GI tract which prevent the poison from getting absorbed from the gut.*

PH 4.2

Mechanism of development of tolerance:

a. **Pharmacokinetic (dispositional) tolerance** is due to changes in drug pharmacokinetics leading to decreased intensity and duration of contact between a given drug and the target tissue. Thus, the barbiturates after repeated administration enhance their own degradation by inducing hepatic microsomal enzyme systems. In many tumours, *p*-Glycoprotein transporters pump out the administered anticancer drugs and make them resistant to therapy.

b. **Pharmacodynamic (functional) tolerance** is probably due to changes in the properties and functions of the target tissue, that make them **less sensitive** to a given drug concentration. Thus, it is associated with some cellular changes. With some drugs, this may be related to a decrease in drug receptors (**downregulation**). With compounds like morphine, alcohol and barbiturates, it has been demonstrated that the cells of the CNS, which usually develop tolerance to these drugs, become capable of normal physiological functions in the presence of high concentrations of these drugs. The adaptive mechanisms involved are not clearly understood.

Tachyphylaxis: Tolerance to drugs as described above usually takes some time to develop. However, with certain drugs like ephedrine, tyramine, amphetamine and 5-hydroxytryptamine, tolerance may appear within a few minutes in isolated preparations as well as in the intact animals. Thus, if any of these drugs is administered repeatedly, at very short intervals, the pharmacological response elicited decreases progressively. This phenomenon is known as *tachyphylaxis* or **acute tolerance** (Fig. 3.1). Repeated doses of ephedrine at short intervals, in the treatment of bronchial asthma, may produce diminishing response.

Various mechanisms are responsible for the appearance of tachyphylaxis. With tyramine, it is due to depletion of the noradrenaline stores from the sympathetic nerves. However, with sympathomimetics like ephedrine and amphetamine, tachyphylaxis can occur without appreciable depletion of the noradrenaline stores. Tachyphylaxis probably can occur if the drug dissociates slowly from its binding to the receptor, thus continuing receptor blockade while losing its intrinsic activity and hence its pharmacological effect. Tachyphylaxis with isoprenaline is accompanied by a decline in beta receptor number while receptor affinity for the agonist remains unaltered. With other

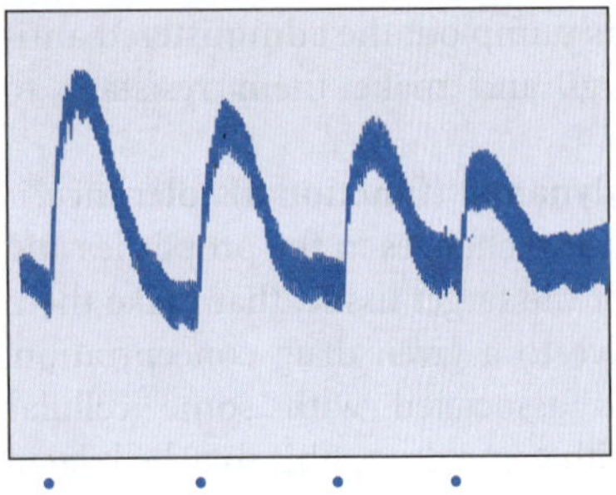

FIG. 3.1 **Effect of repeated doses of tyramine on BP in anaesthetised dog. Black dots denote administration of the same dose. Note the decreasing response.**

drugs, however, tachyphylaxis is probably due to some unidentified 'adaptive response' of the tissue concerned.

PH 1.22

10. **Drug dependence:** Man has long sought ways of enhancing his pleasure and of easing his discomfort. Various agents are consumed to achieve this goal. However, repeated administration of certain agents may induce dependence. Commonly used beverages like tea and coffee stimulate the CNS and are capable of producing dependence but are usually harmless. Tobacco (nicotine), on the other hand, is a dependence-producing agent capable of causing physical harm but it produces relatively little stimulation of the CNS.

Types of Drug Dependence (Box 3.4):

a. Psychological
b. Physical
c. Combined

A condition in which a drug produces 'a feeling of satisfaction and a psychic drive that requires periodic or continuous administration of the drug to produce pleasure or to avoid discomfort', is called **psychic dependence**. In case of **physical dependence**, the body 'achieves' an adaptive state that manifests itself by intense physical symptoms when the drug is withdrawn (**withdrawal syndrome**). The drugs that cause physical dependence (e.g. opioids, benzodiazepines and nicotine) are termed as **hard drugs** while those which cause only psychic dependence are called as **soft drugs** (cannabis, lysergic acid diethylamide [LSD]).

If the agent causing dependence is not made available to the individual, he develops withdrawal symptoms characterised by psychic/physical disturbances (see later). WHO has defined drug dependence as 'a state, psychic and sometimes also physical, resulting from the interaction between a living organism and a drug, characterised by behavioural and other responses that always include a compulsion to take the drug on a continuous or periodic basis in order to experience its psychic effects and sometimes to avoid the discomfort of its absence'. Tolerance may or may not be present. A person may be dependent on more than one drug. **Compulsive drug use is commonly but not necessarily associated with the development of tolerance and physical dependence.** There are some drugs where tolerance and physical dependence develop after chronic use; but they are not self-administered nor used compulsively.

Mechanism of drug dependence: The exact mechanism is not known. Alteration of the cellular

Box 3.4 Important Drugs Known to Cause Dependence PH 1.22

I. ***Drugs that cause severe psychic as well as physical dependence:***
   i. **Opiate or morphine type:**
      Morphine and its congeners like codeine, dihydromorphinone, heroin
      Synthetic morphine substitutes such as meperidine (pethidine) and its congeners, methadone and its congeners, morphinan compounds, pentazocine, diphenoxylate
   ii. **Alcohol-barbiturate type:**
      Ethyl alcohol, barbiturates, paraldehyde, chloral hydrate, meprobamate, benzodiazepines, methaqualone
   iii. **Nicotine** (tobacco)

II. ***Drugs that cause definite psychic but mild or questionable physical dependence:***
   i. **Opiate antagonist type:**
      Morphine antagonists like nalorphine; morphinan antagonists like levallorphan
   ii. **Amphetamine type:**
      Amphetamine, methamphetamine and phenmetrazine. Piperidines like methylphenidate and pipradol

III. ***Drugs that cause only psychic dependence:***
   Cocaine, LSD, psilocybin, mescaline, cannabis (marihuana, hashish), caffeine (coffee, tea)

IV. ***Volatile substances:*** Glue, nail varnish, petrol, paint solvents, hair spray, etc.

metabolism of the **CNS is a prime factor in the development of dependence** (Chapter 6). It appears that these drugs affect the glutaminergic and dopaminergic transmission in the amygdala and ventral striatum of the forebrain. *Other systems may become tolerant to the drug but only the CNS is capable of developing physical dependence*. Withdrawal of the drug produces distorted homeostasis leading to the development of a **withdrawal syndrome or an abstinence syndrome**. The withdrawal syndrome may vary from a mild-to-severe one, sometimes resulting in fatality. The symptoms of the withdrawal syndrome are usually characterised by rebound effects in the same physiological systems that were initially modified by the drugs. Thus, general CNS depressants, on withdrawal, cause hyperexcitation, while withdrawal of the central stimulant amphetamine produces fatigue, lethargy, drowsiness and depression. Withdrawal symptoms due to drugs with long half-lives, e.g. phenobarbitone are usually less severe but more protracted.

The term '**addiction**' denotes the phenomenon involving both psychic and physical dependence and is currently designated as **drug abuse**. Its characteristics include:

- An overpowering desire (compulsion/craving) to continue taking the drug in spite of knowing its harmful effects
- A tendency to increase the dose
- A high tendency to develop withdrawal symptoms

Addiction is now considered as a **chronic complex brain disease** affecting both, its structure and function. It can produce devastating effects on the individual, families and the society in general. Most of the drugs used by the addicts have CNS effects which can be physical, emotional and behavioural. Drugs such as opiates, barbiturates, alcohol and cocaine all produce a sense of well-being in the user. This is termed as **euphoria** (pleasurable feeling or high). They act on specific reward sites in the brain and drug induced increase in dopamine in the Nucleus Accumbensis now considered responsible for the feeling of euphoria (see Chapter 6). However, when exposed to these drugs under similar environmental influences, all the recipients do not develop dependence. It is not clear why some individuals stop after initial experimentation. Others continue drug use but do not become dependent and still others become compulsive drug users or addicts. **Addiction has both, genetic and environmental components** ('seed' and 'soil') and is often triggered by traumatic life events, chronic stress or repeated use of mood altering drugs, in susceptible subjects.

A potential addict may start and continue taking a dependence inducing drug:

- Following its medicinal use
- To achieve a sense of relief from stresses and tension of life
- To satisfy curiosity about drug effects
- To achieve a sense of belonging, to be 'accepted' by others in the group
- To express hostility or independence
- To have pleasurable (euphoric), new, thrilling or even dangerous experiences
- To gain an improved understanding or creativity
- To escape from reality and to have a dreamy state

Drugs of abuse are usually taken orally, and sometimes intravenously or by inhalation. The latter routes give much higher plasma concentrations, which are associated with a feeling of 'kick' or 'flash' resembling an orgasm. Drugs may be abused continuously, e.g. heroin, or intermittently to produce short-term euphoric effects during rave parties, e.g. cocaine, cannabis or methamphetamine.

The experience achieved by the individual under the influence of the drug is so impressive that he develops a craving for it. The drugs of abuse are **powerful reinforcers** and the individual finds it difficult to give it up. Such drugs affect the normal functioning of an individual by causing psychic and physical dependence, e.g. cocaine and heroin. Factors which appear to facilitate the initiation of drug abuse are given in Box 3.5.

PH 1.23

Addiction, once developed, can be treated but cannot be cured. *To achieve any success, complete co-operation and life-long commitment of the individual to abstain from the drug is vital.*

Box 3.5 Factors which Facilitate Initiation of Drug Abuse

- Ready availability of drugs as in case of doctors and medical students
- General public acceptance of the use of mood modifiers such as alcohol
- Increasing mobility particularly of youth
- Peer group pressure
- An abundance of information about drug effects and sources
- Lack of adequate publicity given to harmful effects of these agents
- Unstable or broken homes, sociocultural pressures and social ills

Box 3.6 Principles of Treatment of Drug Addiction PH 1.23

- Hospitalisation of the patient
- Gradual or sudden withdrawal of the drug
- Substitution therapy
- Psychotherapy and occupational therapy
- Specific drug therapy, e.g. disulfiram in alcohol addiction
- Correction of nutritional deficiencies
- Community treatment and rehabilitation

Box 3.6 summarises the principles of treatment of addiction (Deaddiction therapy). The details are described in the respective chapters.

It is highly desirable that drugs which are likely to be administered over a prolonged period should be screened for their dependence liability in animals. PH 1.8

DRUG INTERACTIONS

Drug interactions may result from the use of two or more drugs. This may lead to enhanced or diminished effect that may be useful or harmful. The **useful drug interactions** are illustrated by synergistic combinations of drugs such as antibiotics, antihypertensives or antidiabetics. **Harmful drug interactions** are, unfortunately, more numerous and are discussed below.

A new symptom appearing during treatment with a drug may be due to the disease or the drug. This can be perplexing enough. But, if the patient is receiving several drugs and two or more drugs are capable of causing the same new symptom as the underlying disease, or if two drugs in concert elicit symptoms that would not otherwise appear, the physician is in a quandary. In this situation, he may attribute the new symptom wrongly to the disease itself or to idiosyncrasy to one of the drugs, *instead of recognising it as a drug interaction. The incidence of ADR rises with the number of drugs used.* A physician who uses multiple drugs must, therefore, be constantly alert to the possibility of drug interaction. Furthermore, he must be aware of both, 'drugs posing high risk to the patients' (Box 3.7) and 'conditions which increase the susceptibility of patients to ADR and drug interactions' (Box 3.8) in this respect. Although it is relatively easy to detect cardiovascular, renal or hepatotoxic effects, there is a possibility to miss psychological effects (anxiety, depression, insomnia, amnesia or cognitive disorders). Several drugs used in routine practice can cross BBB, and therefore one has to be aware of such possibility. Physician should rely on his/her own observations rather than wait for warnings issued by the drug regulatory authorities.

It is absolutely essential that when a patient's clinical condition changes, particularly if he is severely ill or elderly, all drug treatment should be carefully reviewed.

Box 3.7 High-Risk Drugs

- ***Affecting a vital process in the body,*** e.g. warfarin, chlorpromazine, morphine
- ***Having a steep dose–response curve,*** e.g. verapamil, levodopa, chlorpropamide
- ***Having saturable kinetics,*** e.g. phenytoin, theophylline, salicylates
- ***Demonstrating dose-dependent toxicity,*** e.g. digoxin, lithium, aminoglycosides, methotrexate
- ***Leading to a breakthrough of disease,*** due to loss of effect, e.g. quinidine, glucocorticoids, antiepileptics

Box 3.8 Patients with High Susceptibility to ADR and Drug Interactions

- Elderly patients receiving many drugs
- Patients with liver/kidney damage
- Patients with unstable disease, e.g. epileptics, brittle diabetics, demented patients and those with cardiac disease
- Patients dependent upon drug treatment for survival, e.g. transplant recipients and patients with Addison's disease
- Patients who have more than one prescribing doctor

Drug interactions may occur either outside the body or in the body.

1. **Drug interactions outside the body:**
   The most glaring examples of this are seen when several drugs are mixed in an IV infusion. One or more of the drugs may get inactivated or even precipitated. This is often attributable to changes in the pH of the solutions. The following are some of the examples:
   a. **Use of wrong vehicle for infusion:** No drug should ever be added to blood, plasma, amino acid solutions, fat emulsions (which tend to crack), sodium bicarbonate solution, mannitol solution (from which mannitol tends to crystallise) and to heparin infusion. An infusion set should be discarded after administration of blood and not used for other infusion fluids.
      Highly acidic solutions (pH may be as low as 3.5) such as dextrose or fructose are unsuitable as vehicles for sodium or potassium salts of weakly acidic drugs such as phenytoin, barbiturates, methicillin and novobiocin, as the latter tend to get precipitated at this pH. Drugs such as benzyl penicillin, ampicillin, heparin and aminophylline are unstable at the pH of these solutions. Dextrose solution is, however, eminently suitable for infusing noradrenaline which is stable at the acidic pH. Isotonic saline is slightly acidic or neutral and is a suitable vehicle for most drugs with the exception of noradrenaline. If noradrenaline has to be infused in isotonic saline, vitamin C should be added to the infusion.
      Most antibiotics become unstable and deteriorate in large volumes of fluid. Erythromycin lactobionate is unstable in electrolyte solutions but may be diluted with 5% dextrose solution. Amphotericin B should be diluted with 5% dextrose of a pH recommended by the manufacturer, but not with saline.
   b. **Addition of drugs to an infusion:** Drugs should be added to infusion containers only when constant plasma concentrations are needed or when the administration of a more concentrated solution would be harmful.
      No more than one drug should be added to any infusion container and the components should be compatible. Solutions should be mixed thoroughly and checked for absence of particulate matter before use. The container should be labelled with the patient's name and the quantity of the additive and with the date and time of the addition. Infusion should be examined from time to time for cloudiness, crystallisation or change of colour; if any sign of deterioration is observed, discontinue the infusion. Phenytoin, phenothiazines, vitamin B complex (±vitamin C), amphotericin, sulphadiazine and furosemide should not be mixed with any other drug in solution.
      Beta-lactam antibiotics should not be mixed with any proteinaceous material for fear of forming immunogenic and allergenic conjugates. Some drugs lose their effects when added to large volume infusions, e.g. ampicillin in glucose or lactate containing infusions; mustine hydrochloride in isotonic saline; gentamicin-carbenicillin added to the same infusion.
      Also see Chapter 1 for IV infusions.

2. **Drug interactions in the body can be:**
   a. **Pharmacokinetic**, one drug affecting the absorption, distribution, transport, metabolism or excretion of another drug
   b. **Pharmacodynamic**, one drug altering the pharmacological action of another drug

Drug absorption:

- Drugs given orally can interact in the gut to form complexes which may not be absorbed. Thus, calcium, magnesium, aluminium and iron salts interfere with absorption of tetracycline and of prednisolone. Sucralfate reduces the bioavailability of phenytoin. Such interactions can be avoided by separating the administration of the two drugs by at least 2 h.
- A drug altering the gastric pH can alter the solubility of another agent and thus may influence its absorption, e.g. sodium bicarbonate reduces the absorption of tetracycline. Drugs can also affect the absorption by modifying the gut motility and gastric emptying. Antimuscarinic drugs and opioids can slow down the absorption of other drugs by delaying gastric emptying.

- Sorbitol accelerates the gastrointestinal absorption of paracetamol.
- A few women taking low dose, combination oral contraceptives may be put to risk of pregnancy by the concurrent administration of a broad spectrum antibiotic (ampicillin or tetracycline). By reducing the bacterial flora in the intestines, these antibiotics disrupt the deconjugation and hence reabsorption of the steroids secreted into the intestine.

Drug distribution: Some drugs are bound strongly to plasma proteins and remain pharmacologically inactive. Certain groups of drugs seem to share a limited number of protein binding sites and can be displaced from them by each other. This results in an increase in the unbound and pharmacologically active form of one of the drugs leading to toxicity. However, this type of drug interaction is clinically significant only with drugs which are extensively (>90%) protein bound, have a small apparent volume of distribution (Vd) and have effects proportional to their concentration, e.g.

- Gemfibrozil can displace warfarin sodium from the binding sites, leading to a bleeding tendency.
- Salicylates can displace glibenclamide from the binding sites, leading to hypoglycaemia.

Drug transport: Guanethidine and the related adrenergic neurone blocking drugs are actively transported into adrenergic neuron by the same transport system that is responsible for noradrenaline uptake into the neuron. This system is inhibited by the antidepressant imipramine, which interferes with the antihypertensive activity of guanethidine.

Drug metabolism:

- **Stimulation:** The synthesis of the drug-metabolising microsomal enzymes is enhanced (**enzyme induction**) by a number of commonly used drugs, insecticides and polycyclic hydrocarbons (Table 3.2). This reduces the efficacy and increases the therapeutic dose of the drugs metabolised by the microsomal enzymes. It should be noted that different inducers are relatively selective for certain families of CYP450 enzymes.
- **Inhibition:** Inhibition of the metabolism of one drug by another may lead to toxicity of the former (see Table 3.3).

Table 3.2 Drug-Induced Acceleration of Metabolism of Drugs

Inducer	Drugs Whose Metabolism is Accelerated (Victim Drugs)
Barbiturates	Barbiturates, oral anticoagulants, steroids (oral contraceptives, testosterone and glucocorticoids), vitamins (D and K), thyroxine, phenylbutazone, phenytoin, griseofulvin, chloramphenicol, theophylline
Phenytoin	Glucocorticoids, vitamin D, theophylline
Griseofulvin	Warfarin
Rifampicin	Oral contraceptives, glucocorticoids, metoprolol, propranolol
Carbamazepine	Vitamin D

Note: *Dicophane* and *gamma benzene hexachloride* are powerful inducers of drug-metabolising microsomal enzymes. Hence, research on drug metabolism could be misleading if the animal quarters are sprayed with either of these insecticides. *Nicotine* is also a powerful enzyme inducer.

Table 3.3 Drug-Induced Inhibition of Metabolism of Drugs

Inhibitor	Drugs Whose Metabolism Is Inhibited (Victim Drugs)
Allopurinol	Tolbutamide, methotrexate, probenecid
Disulfiram	Alcohol, tolbutamide, warfarin, phenytoin
Isoniazid	Glucocorticoids, oral contraceptives, carbamazepine, phenytoin
Chloramphenicol	Tolbutamide, probenecid, phenytoin
Cimetidine	Warfarin and diazepam
Fluoxetine	Warfarin, phenytoin, some benzodiazepines
Erythromycin	Amiodarone, digoxin, antipsychotics, warfarin, theophylline
Ketoconazole	Cyclosporin, astemizole, terfenadine
Phenylbutazone	Phenytoin, tolbutamide
Ethanol	Methanol (beneficial effect)
Valproate	Lamotrigine
Grape fruit juice[a]	Cyclosporin, terfenadine and most calcium channel blockers

Note: Many drugs inhibit the *p*-hydroxylation of phenytoin, increasing the chance of phenytoin toxicity. They include dicoumarol, isoniazid, disulfiram, chloramphenicol and methylphenidate.
[a]Contains psoralen.

Table 3.4 Enzymes of CYP Family with Examples of Substrates and Inhibitors

Isoenzyme	Substrate	Inhibitor	Results of Interaction
CYP3A4	Terfenadine, astemizole, cisapride	Antifungal azoles, macrolide antibiotics (except azithromycin), Cimetidine	Potassium channel blockade with QT prolongation
	Felodipine	Grapefruit juice	Hypotension
CYP2D6	Codeine, TCA	Quinidine, antipsychotics, SSRI, TCA	No pain relief with codeine adverse effects of TCA increased
CYP2C9	NSAIDs, warfarin	Fluconazole	Variable warfarin levels, effects
CYP2C19[a]	Anticonvulsants, diazepam, TCA, omeprazole	Ketoconazole, INH, omeprazole	More ADR of substrate
CYP1A2[b]	Theophylline, imipramine propranolol, clozapine	Fluroquinolones	More ADR of substrate

[a]Absent in 20%–30% Asians, who require low dose of substrate drugs.
[b]Induced by tobacco smoking.

Clinically significant drug interactions involving CYP family are shown in Table 3.4.

Drug excretion: This can be facilitated or interfered with by certain drug combinations. Thus, the excretion of weakly acidic drugs like sulphonamides, salicylates and barbiturates can be enhanced by making the urine alkaline. Probenecid inhibits the tubular secretion of penicillin, indomethacin and riboflavine. Quinidine, verapamil and amiodarone can double the plasma digoxin concentration.

Receptor site (pharmacodynamic interaction): In this case, drugs acting on the same receptor site or at different active receptors may enhance or decrease the response, e.g. tubocurarine and aminoglycoside antibiotics may accentuate the block at the neuromuscular junction; marked CNS depression is caused by concurrent administration of morphine and barbiturates. Several examples of pharmacodynamic drug interactions are described in respective chapters.

Changes in electrolyte and fluid balance: Drugs that cause potassium depletion may potentiate the effects of digitalis and nondepolarising muscle relaxants, but antagonise the antiarrhythmic action of lignocaine, quinidine and procainamide.

Interactions among chemotherapeutic agents: Injudicious combinations of chemo-therapeutic agents may prove harmful in therapeutics (Chapter 49).

Drug interactions are not always predictable. Hence, the physician should always be wary of including too many drugs in the prescription so as to minimise this danger. *Furthermore, the physician should always enquire about alcohol and tobacco consumption by the patient. Numerous drug interactions between alcohol and other drugs have been reported* (Chapter 6). *One should be careful in distinguishing between drug interactions which are clinically significant and those which are not.*

Lastly, one must remember that in practice apart from prescribing drugs, advice about diet, exercise, counseling (sometimes for patient's relatives) are often useful in the recovery process and in improving the quality of life, particularly in chronic diseases. In some patients such advice is perhaps more important than the use of drugs.

Management of drug interactions: Many drug interactions listed in the literature are theoretical or clinically not important. But there are a few, which have serious or life-threatening consequences. Luckily, they are usually predictable based on pharmacodynamic-

Box 3. 9 Management of drug interactions: Prevention and Management Strategies PH 1.8

Strategies to minimize drug interactions

- Minimize the number of prescribed drugs
- Do not prescribe for patients receiving five or more medications
- Review prescribed therapy time to time
- Consider non-pharmacologic options
- Check the risk factors in patients (Age > 65 years, bradycardia, underlying heart, kidney or renal disease, electrolyte imbalance) before prescribing
- Educate the patient regarding possible drug interaction when a potential warning symptom can be anticipated

Strategies to Manage drug interactions

- Early detection of drug interaction: Monitor for therapeutic effects, ADR or laboratory data
- Adjust dosages of medications (reduce warfarin dose by 30-50% upon initiation of amiodarone)
- Limit duration of therapy (antipsyhotics and hypnotics)
- Adjust administration times (l-dopa and anticholinergic drugs)
- Modify drug combinations:
  - a. Prescribe an alternative, non-interacting drug
  - b. Stop the interacting drug temporarily

pharmacokinetic properties of the drug and patient related factors. The best strategy is to avoid them, if possible. For this, a doctor should be aware of the most common and clinically relevant drug interactions. Strategies to avoid/minimize drug interactions and to manage them are presented in Box 3. 9.

CHAPTER 4

Drug Invention, New Drug Development, and Drug Assay

Learning Objectives

This chapter will enable the reader:

1. To describe briefly the process of new drug development.
2. To state objectives of preclinical animal studies.
3. To describe animal toxicity studies mandatory for preclinical testing.
4. To comment on the predictive values of animal studies.
5. To enumerate various phases of clinical drug development stating their objectives, requirements, type and number of participants, study design and duration.
6. To differentiate between generic and branded drugs.
7. To discuss the role of placebo in clinical trial and clinical practice.
8. To list various drug assay methods

KEY TERMS

new drug, p. 71
drug invention, p. 71
animal toxicity study, p. 71
phases of clinical drug development, p. 74
placebo, p. 78
generic drugs, p. 77
repurposing of drugs, p. 77
drug assay, types, p. 79

A new drug is defined as a new substance of chemical, biological or biotechnological origin for which adequate data need to be generated and submitted to the regulatory authority in order to judge its efficacy and safety for the proposed claim. In India the new drug applications are reviewed and approved by the Drugs Controller General of India (DCGI) office under Central Drugs Standard Control Organization (CDSCO). Even marketed drugs are considered new if there is change in their dose, route of administration, indication or if they are combined with other drugs as a fixed-dose combination.

Advances in cell biology and receptor technology have helped in developing automated screening systems for new drugs. One of the popular techniques today is high content screening (HCS), in which *in vitro* or cell-based assays are used to screen large numbers of compounds for their effects on cellular or subcellular targets. With the help of computer-aided drug design (CADD), HTS and HCS, 'hits and leads' are invented. *A **Hit** is a molecule with confirmed structure, confirmed activity in primary throughput screening and a good profile in secondary assay; whereas a **Lead** is a hit series with proven structure activity relationship both in vitro and in vivo.* The leads are then tested by the pharmacological methods to determine their efficacy and safety initially in animals and later on in humans by clinical pharmacological studies. **Ethics Committee Approval** is mandatory before conducting such studies in animals and humans. Regulatory approval is required before conducting clinical trials with new drugs.

Prior to any clinical evaluation, the investigator should obtain reasonably clear answers to the important questions:

- Are the data from animal studies adequate?
- What is the probable risk involved in giving the drug to humans? Is it worth the risk?
- Is there any need for a new drug for the disease under consideration?
- Does the new drug seem promising?

The objectives of animal studies are outlined in Box 4.1. PH 1.63, PH 1.64

ANIMAL TOXICITY STUDIES

In order to assess the safety of a drug, various toxicity studies are carried out in animals such as mice, rats,

Box 4.1 Objectives of Animal Studies

To evaluate:
- Efficacy
- Toxicity
- Receptor selectivity
- Mechanism of action
- Pharmacokinetics

guinea pigs, dogs and monkeys, under varying conditions of drug administration. The important tests include the following:

1. **Systemic toxicity studies:**
   a. ***Single-dose toxicity studies:*** The main objective of a single-dose study is to determine minimum lethal dose (MLD), maximum tolerated dose (MTD) and if possible, the target organ of toxicity.
   In these studies a drug is tested for the effects of a single dose. Graded doses are given in two rodent species (mice and rats of both sexes), using the same route as that intended for humans. One additional route is used in one of the species to ensure systemic absorption of the drug. Animals are observed for mortality for up to 14 days (72 h if the administration is parenteral). Detailed observations are made of the effects of the drug on important physiological functions and body weight. Microscopic examination of grossly affected organ is carried out.
   b. ***Repeated-dose toxicity studies:*** These studies are also carried out in at least two species, of which one should be nonrodent. After the initial dose-ranging studies for MTD, the final systemic toxicity study (FSTS) is carried out. Three doses are selected: (1) **the highest dose** having observable toxicity; (2) **mid-dose** causing some symptoms but no gross toxicity or death; and (3) **the lowest dose** free of toxicity and comparable to the intended therapeutic dose or its multiple. A control group treated with vehicle is a must for comparison. Selected doses are administered depending on the duration of intended use in humans and the phase of the proposed clinical trial. The route of drug administration should be the same as that proposed for human use.
   Variables for safety include cage side observations for eye changes, loss of fur, behavioural and physiological observations, body weight changes, food/water intake, blood chemistry, haematology and examination of organs. The sites of injections are inspected for gross and microscopic changes. ECG and fundoscopy are done in nonrodent species. Sometimes, '**high-dose reversal study**' is included wherein animals are studied after stopping the treatment or after recovery from signs of toxicity.
2. **Local toxicity studies**: The drug is applied to an appropriate site, e.g. skin, vagina or cornea to determine local effects in suitable species (guinea pigs or rabbits). If the drug gets absorbed from such site, appropriate systemic toxicity studies will also be required.
3. **Specialised toxicity studies:**
   a. ***Male fertility studies*** detect effects of a drug on structure and functions of male reproductive organs.
   b. ***Female reproduction and fetal developmental toxicity studies*** include observations on the mating behaviour, progress of gestation, parturition, health during pregnancy and in postpartum period. Ability of the drug to induce fetal malformations and/or death *in utero* (i.e. **teratogenicity**) when given throughout organogenesis is looked for. **Perinatal toxicity study** is undertaken if the drug is to be given to pregnant or nursing mothers for long periods or where possibility of adverse effects on fetal development is high; the drug is administered throughout the last trimester. These studies are carried out in one rodent species (preferably rat) and one nonrodent species (rabbit).
   c. ***Allergenicity/hypersensitivity*** tests are carried out in guinea pigs to determine the minimum irritant dose and the effect of a challenge after sensitisation.
   d. ***Genotoxicity tests:*** Certain drugs are known to produce genetic abnormalities. Which

may produce various types of overt and covert anomalies in the subsequent generations. These are *in vivo* and *in vitro* tests conducted to detect genetic damage, if any.

e. ***Carcinogenicity studies*** detect the ability of a drug to induce malignancy. They are performed for all drugs that are expected to be used clinically for more than 6 months, as well as for those which are intended to be used frequently in an intermittent manner.

Generation of pharmacokinetic data during the toxicity studies (**toxicokinetic data**) helps to relate doses and systemic exposures achieved with toxicological findings.

A new drug with a completely novel structure and with novel pharmacological action is rarely born. It is often discovered by chance observation (serendipity) as in the case of penicillin, antidiabetic sulphonylureas and thiazide diuretics. Most of the new drugs synthesised are related to, or are very similar to, already known drugs. Obviously, the benefit offered by such imitative, **me-too** agents to the patient is generally small; and sometimes the new drug may even be worse than the well-tried parent compound. The clinical studies with such imitative drugs are justifiable only if the other established drugs are far from ideal and if animal studies indicate distinct advantages over the parent compound in clearly defined terms. *Effectiveness of the drug in very small doses, in itself, is not a justification for human studies, as the toxic effects are known to run parallel with 'higher potency'.* Such a preparation would be difficult to dispense and difficulties in regulating its dosage may be enormous. A clinical trial is justified if the new drug is shown to be more efficacious or at least potentially less toxic without significant reduction in its therapeutic efficacy.

A drug with a completely new structure and/or a new mode of action, if found reasonably safe in animal studies, certainly deserves to be studied clinically. Human pharmacological studies with such a compound with particular reference to its mode of action and its actions on various systems of the body may eventually lead to formulation of a new potentially useful structure. A new compound with different chemical structure is likely to produce more novel actions than a closely related imitative compound and hence, it certainly deserves clinical studies.

Interpretation of Animal Data

No tests on animals, however meticulous and prolonged, can ever prove with absolute certainty the *efficacy or safety* of a new drug in man. Animal pharmacological studies would only indicate the probable beneficial and toxic effects that may be expected during human trials; one must weigh the probable benefits against possible harm that could occur. Almost every drug with biological activity will produce some adverse effects. Drugs that are claimed to be absolutely harmless are also likely to be therapeutically useless.

Although animal studies can eliminate obvious toxicity, certain serious adverse reactions such as allergy, neuropsychological toxicity and blood dyscrasias are difficult to detect in animals. It is known that pharmacokinetics and pharmacodynamics of a drug differ both qualitatively and quantitatively in different species. *A drug found highly effective in animals may be totally ineffective in humans because of differences in genomic profiles.* Thus, penicillin, a potent and reasonably safe antibiotic used in humans, can produce fatal toxicity in guinea pigs even in small doses. Further, the animals used in toxicity studies are not necessarily suffering from the disease for which the drug would be used in humans. Hence, such studies should be carried out in many species and, if possible, in both healthy and diseased animals. In toxicological experiments, high doses of the drug are used to bring out the possible toxic effects, and subacute and chronic toxicity studies in animals must always precede the chronic administration of the drug in man. Such studies in animals help the physician to understand and treat the effects of over-dosage of drugs in man.

Subjective responses like nausea, headache, tinnitus, weakness and loss of libido due to a new drug are difficult to discover by animal studies. Such effects, if severe, could considerably reduce the therapeutic utility of the drug.

The relative usefulness of animal studies would be decided by the relevance of animal tests to the human condition, where the drug would be used. Thus, the animal studies regarding a potential diuretic or hypotensive or an antibacterial drug will provide more useful information than those regarding drugs supposed to be effective in human mental diseases, since similar conditions cannot be produced experimentally in animals.

While deciding the dose to be administered for the first time in humans, it should be remembered that dose in smaller animals tends to be larger (on mg/kg basis) than that in larger animals, and dosage schedule based on weight basis in animals, should never be applied to human studies. If possible, the pharmacological actions of a new drug in humans should be controlled by measuring blood levels guided by similar estimations done in different species of animals. It has been suggested that during the first cautious trial in humans, about one-tenth to one-fifth of the predicted effective dose should be administered and then increased gradually.

CLINICAL EVALUATION

A clinical investigator who has an adequate background in interpreting animal studies and who studies drugs cautiously and critically in humans, with continuing analysis of the result achieved is called a clinical pharmacologist. **Clinical pharmacology** involves the study of various aspects of pharmacodynamics and pharmacokinetics in humans, both in health and in disease; and, therefore, is a discipline which is a part of medicine as a whole. It helps in defining guidelines for rational drug prescribing, and includes studies on pharmacoeconomics, pharmacovigilance and pharmacoepidemiology.

The Clinical Pharmacologist should be a combination of a pharmacologist and a clinician. Clinical pharmacologists can be clinicians working in the disciplines of medicine, therapeutics, cardiology, anaesthesiology or surgery, and having interest in pharmacology. Obviously, one should restrict such work to the field of one's specialisation where one has the requisite experience and full knowledge of the ever increasing advances in the subject. *This is essential because the safety and effectiveness of new drugs solely depend on his strict, unbiased and uncompromising adherence to the highest scientific standards.* More than the equipment and finances, it is the honesty, commitment and calibre of the investigator involved that matters the most.

It is essential to have information about the chemical and pharmaceutical properties (such as solubility and stability) of a new drug before it is evaluated in clinical trials. PH 1.63, FM 4.25

In India, the clinical development of drugs is carried out as per New Drugs and Clinical Trials Rules, 2019. Good Clinical practices (GCP) guidelines should be followed throughout the clinical evaluation. GCP provides standards for design, conduct, monitoring, auditing, recording and reporting of clinical trials. Adherence to them provides assurance that the generated data and reported results are credible and accurate and the rights, safety and well-being of the participants in the studies are protected.

All clinical trials need to be approved by the institutional **Ethics Committee** and regulatory authority. Further, prior **informed consent** of both, volunteers and patients is mandatory. Healthy subjects with **risk factors** for an ADR, e.g. age less than 18 years, old age, reproductive age in women, history/family history of drug allergy, organ dysfunction, and so on, are *generally* excluded from the drug trials. 'A risk factor is a personal attribute (age and gender), an aspect of behaviour or lifestyle, environmental exposure, or inborn/inherited characteristic. On the basis of *epidemiologic evidence*, it is known to be associated with a health-related condition considered important to prevent.' PH 1.64, FM 4.25

Phases of New Drug Development

Phase 1 clinical trials (human pharmacology): These are carried out at a few selected centres. The main aim is to obtain precise information about safety and tolerability of the drug from the smallest number of **healthy volunteers** in the minimum possible time. Both subjective and objective evaluation is done along with relevant laboratory studies, to evaluate safety of the drug.

Once the safety is proved in volunteer studies, further studies are carried out in pathological states which the new drug is expected to modify in other phases of drug development. The prime requisites for such an evaluation are:

- Uniformity of subjects with respect to age, sex, nutritional status, and so on
- Precise diagnosis in the case of patients
- A clear index of response relevant to the therapeutic objective

The clinical investigator must decide how far it is ethical to withhold a known treatment for the sake of trial with a new drug and whether any additional ancillary therapy is needed. If other known drugs are also to be administered simultaneously for some reasons, it is necessary to watch for drug interactions.

In certain fields like endocrinology or infectious diseases, where the aetiopathology is precisely known, the clinicopharmacological studies with the new compound could be precise, quantitative and predictable, e.g. penicillin in pneumonia and thyroxine in hypothyroidism. But such information about the disease is often not available and the natural history of the disease is such that the correct assessment of a new drug becomes difficult as in atherosclerosis, psychiatric disorders and rheumatoid arthritis. Clinical assessment is also difficult in case of drugs expected to produce subjective relief of symptoms such as pain, anorexia and sleeplessness. Hence, controlled clinical trials are absolutely necessary to prove or disprove the therapeutic usefulness of the drug and for comparing it with the previously established drug. These evaluations are carried out in Phase 2 and Phase 3 studies.

Phase 2 clinical trials (therapeutic exploration): In this phase, clinical evaluation is carried out in patients to explore efficacy, and to determine dose regimen (dose finding) for the next phase. Mostly these trials are placebo controlled.

Phase 3 clinical trials (therapeutic confirmation): These studies include *controlled clinical trials.* A controlled trial may be defined as one where a new drug is compared with (a) the previously established drug (active control) or (b) placebo control, under standardised conditions. It is designed to ensure that the comparisons made are precise, informative and as convincing as possible. Such studies are mainly conducted in two ways:

- Where the test drug is given to one group and results are compared with those administered the established drug/placebo in the other group (parallel design)
- Where the test drug is alternated with either a placebo or with the previously established drug, in the same patient (crossover design)

In the first method, patients are allocated to various groups. In order to balance the groups and to avoid any bias, allocation should be carried out by **randomisation** by a person who is completely unaware of the therapy allotted to an individual group. One of the groups gets the new treatment while the other receives established therapy in a similar form and in similar way as the drug under evaluation.

When both the evaluating clinician and the subject are unaware of the nature of the drug being administered, the procedure is called a **double-blind controlled trial**. It effectively reduces the influence of extratherapeutic factors. In case any laboratory investigations are involved, the specimens should be submitted to the laboratory under a code number. The treatments are decoded only after the trial is over.

In the second method, the patient acts as his own control. This reduces the chances of erroneous results due to individual variation amongst the patients. Allocation of the patient to either the new therapy or the established treatment first is decided by *randomisation* and the evaluating clinician should not know the sequence of drug administration before completion of the trial. As in the first method such a study can be made a double-blind controlled trial.

Finally, the results of such controlled trials at a few centres are confirmed by broad **multicentric clinical trials** at many centres before the drug is marketed.

PH 1.6

Phase 4 clinical trials (postmarketing surveillance): Since ADRs continue to occur even after a new drug is released for use in the community, careful **pharmacovigilance** (Chapter 1) must continue to avoid tragedies like that which occurred following the use of thalidomide. After marketing new drugs, the pharmaceutical companies collect all the safety data (ADR occurring in clinical practice) for 4 years through post marketing surveillance studies and report the same to the regulatory authority. It is during this phase, that astute observation by practising doctors leads not only to early detection of ADR but also sometimes recognition of additional benefits which helps in identifying new indications for drugs, e.g. beta blockers for glaucoma and minoxidil for baldness.

The ADR of marketed drug are later captured under the PVPI program of India. For this, ADR monitoring centres have been established in various parts of the country. Any ADR observed in the clinical practice is reported to these centres by the physician. The details of this programme are available at https://cdsco.gov.in/PVPI.

Table 4.1 Characteristics of Clinical Trials Conducted in Various Phases of Drug Development PH 1.64

Characteristic	Phase 1 First in Human	Phase 2 First in Patient	Phase 3 Multicentre Trial	Phase 4 Postmarketing Surveillance
Study types	Human pharmacology studies	Therapeutic exploratory studies	Therapeutic confirmatory studies	Therapeutic use (variety of studies)
Participant number	10–100	50–500	A few hundred to a few thousand	Thousands
Type of participants	Usually healthy volunteers; occasionally patients according to class of drugs	Patients	Patients	Patients prescribed approved drug
Study design	Open label	Randomised and controlled (usually placebo as comparator); may be blinded	Randomised and controlled (placebo or standard drug as comparator); blinded	Open label
Primary objective	Determine safety and tolerability	To study: • Efficacy • Dose–response relationship • Dose and regimen for next phase	Confirm efficacy in larger population for use in the intended indication	Optimise drug's use: Relatively rare and unpredicted ADR, compliance, drug–drug interactions, pharmacosurveillance, pharmacoeconomics, comparison with other drugs.
Other objectives	Characterisation of pharmacokinetics Assessment of pharmacodynamics when drug activity is readily measurable	Safety and tolerability in patients Evaluation of potential study endpoints, therapeutic regimens (including concomitant medications) and target populations (e.g. mild versus severe disease)	Safety and tolerability Further exploration of the dose–response relationship, or use in wider populations, in different stages of disease, or in combination with another drug	New therapeutic applications during wider use in the community
Study duration	Months to 1 year	1–2 years	3–5 years	No fixed duration
Success rate	50%	30%	25%–50%	–

The characteristics of clinical trials conducted in various phases of drug development are summarised in Table 4.1.

Phase 0 studies, recently recommended by regulatory authority of the USA (US FDA) for some drugs, are exploratory, first-in-human studies. A very small number of patients (10–15) are given subtherapeutic microdoses of the drug for approximately one week. Such doses are less likely to be toxic but are pharmacologically active to exhibit effects on molecular target in an assay system. Sometimes they are used to study the suitability of pharmacokinetic properties. Such early data help to make suitable modifications or to select only those candidates, which are capable of producing the effect as observed in the preclinical studies. This approach is cost-saving as early weeding out of ineffective agents is possible. It also increases efficiency of drug development programme by allowing effective drugs to enter further clinical studies. *The drugs to be tested in Phase 0 should have wider therapeutic index, a known target and validated biomarker with assay system.* PH 1.9

Generic versus branded drugs

Developing a new drug is a costly affair! After the discovery of a new drug at least 10 years are spent to fulfil all the regulatory requirements for its marketing. Besides, there is always a risk of failure in the later stage of development and after marketing its commercial success cannot be guaranteed. Hence, for every new drug, exclusive marketing authority is given by the regulatory authority, to the pharmaceutical company (innovator) developing the drug. This exclusivity lasts for 20 years from the date of filing the patent by the innovator. It serves as the incentive to the innovator company to allow recovery of its research expenditure expenses. The new drug is marketed under the brand name given by the company. No other company can manufacture or market the same drug without a license from the innovator company. e.g., Rimegepant for migraine by the innovator 'Biohaven Pharmaceuticals' having the brand name NURTEC.

After the expiry of patent, the same drug can be marketed by many other pharmaceutical companies under the generic name or international non-proprietary name (INPN) and is termed as a generic drug e.g., paracetamol, diazepam etc. This generic drug contains the same active drug that was originally protected but may vary in excipients. Its dosage form, strength, route of administration, efficacy and safety, quality and intended use is same as that of innovator and is bioe-quivalent (WHO). The generic drug cost around 40 to 60 percent less than the innovator and are affordable. Sometimes these off patented generic drugs are given brand names by the manufacturing companies e.g., Crocin to paracetamol, Alergin to cetrizine. Such drugs are termed as 'branded generic' drugs. They are more expensive than their unbranded generic counterparts.

Prescribing unbranded generics to patients across India is increasing slowly. However, many a times physicians are not aware of concept of generics or they may not have confidence in their quality especially as there are incidences of poor quality generics in the Indian market. In addition, there is a competitive promotion of branded generics. The Indian Government is trying overcome these hurdles. e.g. since 2017 bioequivalence testing has been made mandatory for the manufacture of a generic medicine in India. In '*Pradhan Mantri Bhartiya Janaushadhi Pariyojana (PMBJP)*' un-branded generics are used and efforts are being made to increase their numbers and control their prices. Rational prescribing includes prescribing affordable and quality drugs and prescribing unbranded generic medicines to the patients is one step towards it.

Repurposing of Drugs

Due to the substantial costs and slow pace of new drug development, pharmaceutical companies identify drugs, already available in the market or in the later stages of development, for the treatment of conditions different from the indication for which they are being developed or are marketed. As these drugs have already been proven sufficiently safe in animal and early human studies, their evaluation for the new indications require substantially less cost and time. This approach is termed as repurposing or repositioning of a drug and is increasingly becoming an attractive proposition.

Some examples of repurposed drugs are as follows: Thalidomide, a teratogenic drug was serendipitously found to be effective for erythema nodosum leprosum (ENL) and decades later for multiple myeloma. Minoxidil, an antihypertensive agent, has been found to cause hair growth as an adverse effect and has been repurposed for treatment of baldness. Sildenafil originally developed as an antihypertensive has been repurposed for erectile dysfunction based on clinical data analysis. Systematic screening using cellular or animal model systems can result in the identification of a new use for an old drug. For example, disulfiram, a drug used for alcohol abuse was found to be a selective antineoplastic agent for prostate cancer in cell based assays. Using a model of tobacco dependence in zebrafish, topiramate, an antiepileptic drug has been repurposed as smoking cessation remedy. During COVID-19 pandemic many clinical studies were conducted to repurpose the available drugs (e.g. hydroxychloroquine, ivermectin, dexamethasone, remdesivir) for the treatment of COVID-19.

Role of Placebo

Placebo is a Latin term which means, 'I may please you'. The placebo effect is an effect attributable to the patients' participation in a therapeutic encounter, and is not due to any specific pharmacodynamic property of the substance for the condition being treated. Placebo effect may be defined as 'how the patient's perception of treatment influences his/her response'. *Placebo effects are not just effects of an 'inert' substance but involve complex neurobiological mechanisms involving neurotransmitters and activation of 'specific quantifiable and relevant areas' of the brain.* Thus these effects are genuine biopsychosocial phenomena and not just spontaneous reactions. Therapeutically placebo mainly relieves subjective and self-appraised symptoms. They do not alter the pathophysiology of the disease process. Placebos are used:

- During clinical trials as a part of drug development, to eliminate the possibility that the benefit of the drug is solely due to chance
- As therapeutic agents that work psychologically

The placebo helps to: (i) Differentiate the drug effects from natural fluctuations in a disease like asthma; and (ii) Sort out the real drug-related ADR from those simply due to the procedure.

During clinical trials, an inert substance like starch or lactose is used as a placebo to eliminate the effect of bias of the physician and the patient, particularly in evaluating a drug claimed to be effective in conditions such as bronchial asthma, angina pectoris, pain and psychiatric disorders. In such cases the placebo should be indistinguishable from the active medicament in physical properties like colour, smell, taste and dosage form.

Placebos can often produce relief of subjective symptoms observed in psychosomatic conditions. This includes relief from anxiety, headache, pain, insomnia and breathlessness. Hence, placebos are often employed in the treatment of certain diseases where the psychic element is suspected to be responsible for subjective symptoms. Objective responses such as increase or decrease in neutrophils and eosinophils may sometimes be seen with placebos.

When administered for its therapeutic effects, the placebo preparation:

- Must appear to be relevant to the illness
- Must be harmless
- Should preferably conform to the patient's expectations

To be effective, the 'potency' of the preparation must be shown by some signs such as strong taste, a colourful capsule or a tablet of odd shape and sometimes even by obvious but harmless side effect like coloured urine.

Placebo effect may be modified by:

1. **Personality of the physician:** Reassurance and optimistic outlook often achieve a better effect. 'The doctor himself must inspire confidence. It is difficult to define this quality. Some doctors have it and some do not. In this respect, the hospital specialist is in a better position than the GP because he is backed by a temple of healing, which is clearly nearer the seat of power than a wayside shrine. Since few doctors are good enough actors to simulate the confidence they do not have, it often happens that one who is kind and credulous is a better healer than another who is informed and critical. Placebo reactions go faster when both the parties have faith and in this respect knowledge is an inhibitor.'
2. **Personality of the patient:** Some individuals are amenable to suggestions. Such people are termed

placebo reactors, and since a placebo acts by suggestion, they derive benefit from the use of placebos. Neurotics are great placebo reactors, whereas depressed or psychotic subjects are usually resistant. Individuals who are of conservative, suspicious, or sceptical nature are not likely to benefit from placebos and may become worse as per their 'own expectations'. Such patients may complain of drowsiness, headache, dryness of mouth, fatigue, insomnia, constipation, impotence, difficulty in concentrating and a 'drugged feeling'. These anticipatory or perceived adverse effects are known as '**Nocebo effects**'.

3. **Form of administration:** It is not surprising that the greatest placebo effect (as high as 81%) is achieved with injections. This may perhaps explain the preference for the use of injections by the practitioners! Colour, taste, presence or absence of stress are other factors which modify placebo effect.

Even when an active drug is used, its placebo effect often comforts the patient long before the drug is effective. It is well known that patients often get some immediate relief as soon as the doctor's medicine is administered, because of their faith in the doctor that things will go well in his hands and these effects are the essence of what makes medicine a healing profession. PH 1.2

Interpretation of Clinical Data

After the completion of the clinical trial, the results are subjected to statistical analysis. If the difference between the two groups of treatment is so large that the probability of its occurrence simply by chance is less than 5 times in 100 ($p < 0.05$), then the new drug is said to have produced a significant effect. It is necessary, however, to rule out all other possible explanations for such difference, before the verdict is accepted.

Various statistical designs have been suggested to ensure that the results obtained are as precise as possible without interference by other biological factors and individual bias; and there is no doubt that such statistical safeguards are essential. *However, elaborate statistics cannot validate a poorly designed and executed clinical trial.* Further, in a given study it is more important to know whether a new drug is significantly better than the older one or placebo in terms of its 'clinical effect' and not merely statistically. In fact, an effect whose reality is revealed only after elaborate statistics is hardly likely to be clinically important. **Statistical significance** and **Therapeutic significance** of results are not necessarily equivalent. Often statistics would show 'a statistically significant difference', but it cannot tell whether such difference really matters in therapeutics. Thus, a drug may lower the plasma cholesterol concentration statistically but may not prevent myocardial infarction.

Most of the new drugs are not 'wonder drugs' and need proper clinical assessment. As pointed out by the Lancet, there is no doubt that a prior design of the trial is important but 'It is clearly not worth devoting such energy to trial design if the trained observer is not both trained and observing. After all, the controlled trial requires as much in 'clinical observation' as it does in design. No one should play at clinical trials.'

Meta-analysis

For various reasons, the results of multiple clinical trials of a drug may vary. Many times, such trials are conducted in a limited number of patients, with different study designs. This poses difficulty in drawing clear cut (**evidence-based**) conclusions regarding the merits of the drug. Hence, in a systematic review, the results from such trials conducted with the same objective are pooled and analysed collectively, using elaborate statistical methods. Such analysis is called meta-analysis. Although the procedure is not full proof, in practice, it does help in judging the merits/demerits of a drug and thus in therapeutic decision-making.

DRUG ASSAY

Assay is the estimation of the amount or the activity of an active principle in a unit quantity of the preparation. It can be:

- Chemical
- Biological
- Immunological

1. **Chemical assay:** In this assay, the mass concentration of the active principle is estimated by means of a chemical method, e.g. the salicylates, sulphonamides and many others. It is the most commonly used procedure. The useful techniques are spectrophotometry, fluorometry, gas chromatography, mass spectrometry, high pressure liquid chromatography and liquid chromatography–mass spectrometry (LC–MS).

2. **Bioassay:** Bioassay is a measure of the concentration of the specific active ingredient in a sample of biological material and is performed by determining the amount of the unknown sample required to produce a defined effect on a suitable test animal or organ under standard conditions. Thus, bioassays can be performed on whole animals either singly or in groups and on isolated tissues or even cells.
   To be useful, the bioassay procedures must satisfy the following requirements:
   a. **High sensitivity.**
   b. **Specificity**, e.g. the ileum of the guinea pig contracts with both acetylcholine and histamine. The tissue, therefore, has to be atropinised for the bioassay of histamine.
   c. **Reproducibility:** The pharmacological response with the same dose should remain the same under identical conditions.
   d. **Accuracy.**
   e. **Stability:** The animal or the tissue should remain 'bioassay fit' for a sufficiently long time.
   f. **Easy availability of the animals**

3. **Immunoassay:** Unlike the bioassay *in vivo* or *in vitro*, the radioimmunoassay (RIA) is a physicochemical assay and depends upon the reaction between an antigen (say hormonal) and its specific antibody in the test tube. The antibodies used are generally obtained from the sera of animals, such as rabbits, which have been previously immunised by repeated injections of the hormone (antigen). Such antibodies raised in animals are polyclonal. Monoclonal antibodies prepared by the hybridoma technique give superior immunoassays.

Immunologic methods measure all the immunologically active components, some of which may be less active biologically, e.g. insulin (Chapter 63) or LH (Chapter 65). Further, the reliability of the results depends largely on the specificity of the antiserum (antibody).

When the results of such an assay differ from those obtained by the biological assay, the latter should not be ignored.

Radioreceptor assays embodying the principles of both bioassay and RIA are more sensitive and more specific than the RIAs.

Labelled antibody (instead of labelled antigen) is used in **immunoradiometric assays** (IRMA). They are more specific and more sensitive than RIAs. Such assays are commonly used to measure protein hormones, e.g. TSH.

Enzyme-linked immunosorbent assays (ELISA), in which enzymes such as alkaline phosphatase and penicillinase are used in place of radioactive iodine to label the ligands, are widely used to assay hormones, e.g. hCG.

More sensitive and specific methods of measuring drug in the biological materials such as **Enzyme – Multiplied Immunoassay Technique (EMIT), Fluorescence Polarization Immunoassays (FPIA)**, and **chemiluminescence** assay are also now available.

2

SECTION

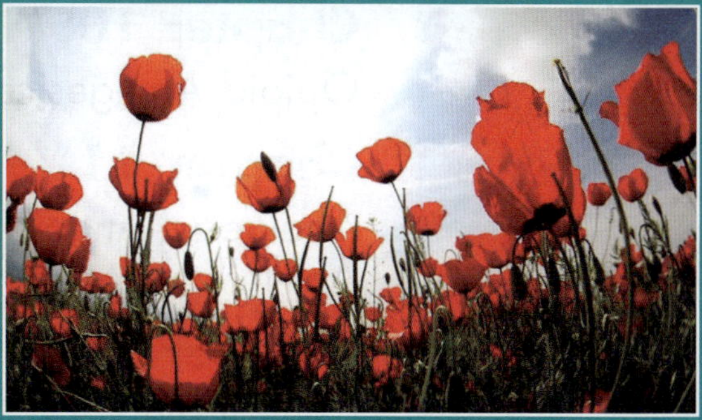

Papaver somniferum

Drugs Acting on the Central Nervous System

Section Outline

This section consists of the following chapters:

SECTION 2

Drugs Acting on the Central Nervous System

CHAPTER 5

General Considerations

Learning Objectives

This chapter will enable the reader:

1. To state functions of various parts of the central nervous system (CNS).
2. To describe different types of effects that a drug may show on interacting with the CNS.
3. To appreciate that drug effects are secondary to modulation of neurotransmission.
4. To describe distribution, effects and receptors of neurotransmitters of the CNS.
5. To state target sites for action of CNS drugs at the synaptic level with suitable examples.
6. To enumerate various methods to investigate a drug acting on the CNS.

KEY TERMS

Anatomically, the nervous system can be divided into the central nervous system (CNS) and the peripheral nervous system consisting of somatic and autonomic nerve fibres (Chapter 17).

The CNS and peripheral nervous system process information received from both internal and external sources and send out instructions to various tissues to produce appropriate responses such as:

- **Psychic**, as manifested by change in emotions, thought and attitude
- **Somatic**, as demonstrated by various types of body movements
- **Autonomic**, as indicated by changes in respiration, circulation and visceral functions

Functions of various parts of the CNS are described in Table 5.1

DRUGS AND CNS

Drugs exert their effects on the CNS by:

- **Directly** acting on the neurons and modifying their functions,
- **Reflexly** sending afferent impulses to the CNS via the chemoreceptors, baroreceptors and peripheral nerves, thereby eliciting psychic, somatic or visceral responses, OR
- **Affecting the nutrition and oxygen supply of the CNS** by altering its blood supply or affecting its metabolism, e.g. hypoglycaemia or ammonia intoxication.

To reach the CNS, a drug must have a high lipid solubility (high oil/water partition coefficient) or a specialised transport mechanism. Ionised drugs normally cannot cross BBB.

The condition of the meninges to a certain extent alters the penetrability of drugs into the CNS, e.g. aminoglycosides which are polar drugs cross the BBB only in the presence of meningeal inflammation (meningitis) (Chapter 1).

Types of Drug Effects

Drugs may either (i) stimulate or (ii) depress the CNS. In therapeutic doses, the stimulant action is usually

Table 5.1 Functions of Various Parts of Central Nervous System

Part of CNS	Functions Attributed
Cerebral cortex	Higher functions like judgement, memory, fine voluntary movements, and special senses. It is a prime coordinator to control lower centres.
Frontal lobes	Thinking and integration of emotional behaviour.
Limbic system	Integrates emotional state with motor and visceral activities.
Basal ganglia	Extrapyramidal control of skeletal muscle tone and coordination of posture.
Thalamus	Relay centre for sensory pathways to cortex. Conscious appreciation of pain, temperature and crude touch sensations. Exerts regulatory control over visceral functions.
Hypothalamus	Control of the autonomic nervous system, control of pituitary gland functions. Important centre for integration of eating, drinking, sexual behaviour, tem-perature regulation, sleep, circadian rhythms and other vegetative functions.
Cerebellum	Control of vestibular function and body posture.
Reticular formation	Sleep–wakefulness cycle, control of blood pressure, respiration, swallowing, vomiting; transmission of crude pain, voluntary muscle tone and posture; control of upper motor neurons.
Spinal cord	Reflex movements, control the upper and the lower motor neurons and muscle tone.

selective (confined to specific areas of the CNS), whereas toxic doses may cause convulsions. Excessive CNS stimulation is followed by its depression.

Suppression of inhibitory areas in the CNS may result in an **apparent stimulation**. Thus, ethyl alcohol eliminates the inhibitory control exerted by the higher cortical centres and leads to garrulousness and hilarity.

Depression or inhibition of the CNS may be achieved through more than one mechanism. The CNS contains a number of inhibitory and excitatory chemical transmitters. In presynaptic inhibition there is reduced quantity of the excitatory transmitter released in the synaptic cleft reducing the impulses from the post synaptic neuron, whereas in postsynaptic inhibition there is active release of an inhibitory transmitter that causes hyperpolarization of postsynaptic neuron. An example of postsynaptic inhibition is that exerted by the inhibitory interneurons, Renshaw cells of the spinal cord, on the α-motor neurons by releasing glycine.

Depression can be generalised or localised. Thus, depressants like general anaesthetics and barbiturates have a more generalised action, whereas drugs like phenytoin sodium and chlorpromazine depress only certain areas in the cortex.

The action of a CNS depressant may be modified by the internal environment; the amount of a general anaesthetic required to anaesthetise a highly excited subject is more than that required in a normal person. Similarly, barbiturates may induce anxiety and apprehension when used in the presence of pain.

Although receptor selectivity for action may be remarkable, a drug can affect several CNS functions to varying degrees, which could cause ADR.

A specific depressant may produce unusual excitation under certain circumstances, e.g. benzodiazepines cause paradoxical excitation in children and elderly patients instead of sedation.

NEUROCHEMICAL TRANSMISSION IN CNS

There are three processes occurring in connection with impulse transmission within the nervous system as described below.

Neurotransmission is a fundamental property of all neurons, by which an impulse is transmitted across a synapse between two neurons. **Neurotransmitters (NTs)** are released into the synaptic cleft and either stimulate or inhibit the postsynaptic neuron. (Fig. 5.1)

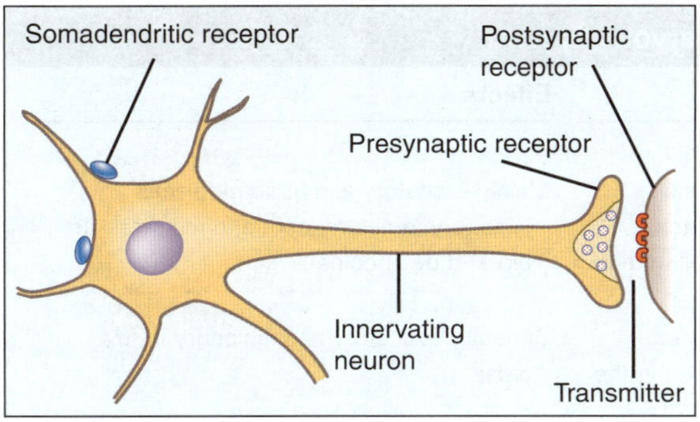

FIG. 5.1 **Pre- and postsynaptic receptors.**

A substance must satisfy certain criteria in order to be accepted as a NT:

- It must be present in the neurons and presynaptic nerve endings and should have a discrete rather than a uniform pattern of distribution.
- It must be released from the presynaptic nerve terminals on stimulation of the neuron, to produce clearly demonstrable effects.
- Enzymatic mechanisms capable of synthesising and degrading the substance should be present within the neurons
- Local concentration of the substance should correlate with the integrity of neuronal structure and function.
- Fluctuations in its concentration should take place in response to the functional changes in the neuron.
- Clearly demonstrable effects should be obtained by increasing or decreasing the local concentration of such substance in the CNS.
- When applied to the postsynaptic neuron, the substance or its agonists should mimic the action of the synaptically released chemical transmitter. Known antagonists of this substance should block its effects.

Regulation of NT Release

NT are stored in the vesicles in the presynaptic neurons. They are rapidly released in the synaptic cleft following neuronal depolarization that causes the, influx of Ca^{++} ions in the neuron.

Released NT may also act at the **presynaptic receptors** (Fig. 5.1), and inhibit or enhance further release of NT. These presynaptic receptors are also called as **autoreceptors**.

Presynaptic receptors are of several types, including members of both **G protein linked** (*metabotropic*) and **multiunit ion channel** (*ionotropic*) types. Activation of both types regulate NT release in different situations. Activation of the G protein linked receptors usually leads to a reduction in evoked NT release, thereby closing a negative feedback loop. Activation of the ionotropic receptors enhances the release of NT as a result of their ability to raise the calcium concentration in the terminals directly. Many NTs use several of these mechanisms.

The presynaptic terminals may also have receptors responding to NTs released from other neurons e.g. noradrenaline presynaptic neuron bears serotonin receptors and *vice versa*. Activation of these receptors, **heteroreceptors**, can also influence the NT release. Presynaptic receptors are thus important from the neurophysiological point of view and as potential targets for therapeutic agents.

Neuromediation implies the elicitation of the postsynaptic responses to the released NTs through second messengers (neuromediators) such as cAMP, cGMP and inositol phosphate (Chapter 2).

Neuromodulation is a less clearly defined process. It is thought to occur at pre- and postsynaptic levels to regulate the release of NTs, modulate the postsynaptic excitability or induce long-term changes by affecting gene transcription. Neuromodulators arise from neurons as well as from the nonneuronal cells. They are not stored or released like the NTs. They act with a longer latency of action, and have a longer duration of action. Examples are adenosine, prostaglandins and nitric oxide.

Some neurons release a chemical into the blood circulation from the nerve terminals, which is called as **neurohormone**, e.g. hypothalamic hormones released into the hypothalamo-pituitary portal circulation.

Neurotrophic factors: These neuropeptides, produced by neurons, astrocytes, microglia and inflammatory/immune cells, assist in repairing tissue damage.

CNS NEUROTRANSMITTERS

The CNS has both *excitatory* and *inhibitory* chemical

Table 5.2 Some Neurotransmitters Found in the Nervous System

Name	Distribution	Effects
	Amines	
Acetylcholine (ACh)	Widely distributed in almost all regions in CNS, predominantly in cerebral cortex, ascending reticular system, cerebellum and spinal cord	Mainly excitatory and at some places inhibitory in nature; central effects can be blocked by atropine
Noradrenaline (NA)	High concentration in the hypothalamus, limbic system and reticular formation in the brainstem	Generally excitatory and inhibitory in few areas
Dopamine (DA)	Mainly in the basal ganglia, to some extent in the median eminence of hypothalamus, adenohypophysis and frontal cortex	Predominantly inhibitory action and in some areas excitatory; deficiency causes extrapyramidal disturbances
5-Hydroxytryptamine (5-HT, serotonin)	Extends into the cerebral cortex, raphe nucleus in pons and medulla, hippocampal areas	Both excitatory and inhibitory effects
Histamine (H)	Distribution similar to NA and 5-HT but irregular	Mainly inhibitory effects; functions uncertain
	Amino acids	
l-Glutamic acid and aspartic acid (EAA)	Widely distributed in CNS and spinal cord	Excitatory effects
Gamma-aminobutyric acid (GABA), glycine	GABA in CNS; glycine mainly in the spinal cord and brainstem	Inhibitory effects in the brain and spinal cord
	Peptides	
Substance P	Hypothalamus, thalamus, basal ganglia; the dorsal column and dorsal roots of the spinal cord; enteric nervous system (ENS)	Excitatory
Cholecystokinin	Brain (cortex, hippocampus, limbic system and hypothalamus), pancreas	Inhibits eating and stimulates oxytocin release

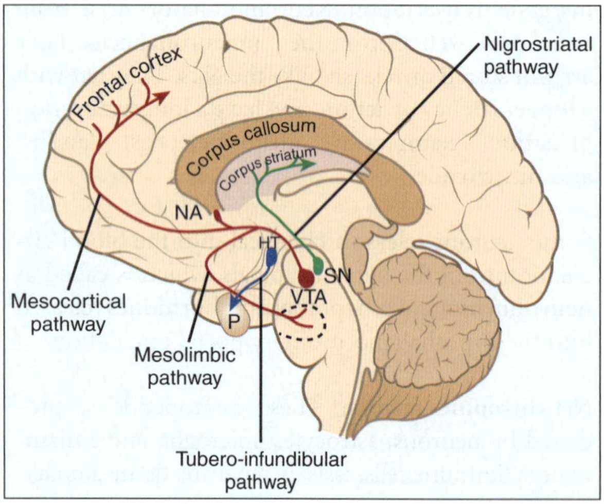

FIG. 5.2 Sagittal section of the brain showing dopaminergic pathways. VTA, ventral tegmental area; SN, substantia nigra; HT, hypothalamus; P, pituitary; NA, nucleus accumbens.

transmitters which may be amines, amino acids or peptides (Table 5.2).

Many drugs which modify the functions of the CNS affect the concentration of one or more of NTs in the central as well as the peripheral nervous system. For details, see Chapters 17 and 24. The details of noradrenaline and acetylcholine as NT is depicted in Chapter 17.

Dopamine, an important NT of the brain has three main pathways (Fig. 5.2):

1. **Mesolimbic/mesocortical pathways:** Dopamine is secreted by the neurons in the ventral tegmental area (VTA) which projects into the limbic system especially into the hippocampus, amygdala, anterior caudate nucleus and part of the prefrontal cortex. Dopamine has been

Table 5.3 Distribution and Properties of D_1 and D_2 Receptors

Location	Type of D Receptors	Functions
Limbic system	D_1 and D_2	Mood and emotional stability; stereotypy
Corpus striatum	D_1 and D_2	Motor control
Hypothalamus	Mainly D_1	Autonomic control
Pituitary	Mainly D_2	Inhibition of prolactin secretion
Blood vessels	Mainly D_1	Dilatation
Heart: muscle	Mainly D_2	Stimulation of inotropic function (Chapter 31)
Heart: sympathetic fibres	Mainly D_2	Inhibition of NA release

Note: Mechanism of action: D_1 increases cAMP synthesis; D_2 decreases cAMP synthesis.

implicated as a possible cause of schizophrenia and D_2 receptor blockers are used to treat it (Chapter 13).

2. **Nigrostriatal pathway:** Dopamine deficiency due to degeneration of SN is major cause of symptoms and signs of Parkinson's disease (Chapter 15).
3. **Tuberoinfundibular pathway:** Dopamine acts as prolactin-inhibiting factor (PIF) in this pathway and its inhibition causes release of prolactin.

Table 5.3 lists the distribution and properties of D_1 and D_2 Receptors.

GABA: This is a major inhibitory amino acid NT in the brain; its synthesis from glutamate is catalysed by the enzyme glutamic acid decarboxylase. It binds to either $GABA_A$ or $GABA_B$ receptor following its release from the presynaptic vesicles. $GABA_A$ receptor is part of a complex that surrounds and regulates a chloride ion channel (**ionotropic receptor**). Most GABA receptors are composed of α, β and γ subunits. Receptors composed of α and β subunits produce functional $GABA_A$ receptors that respond to barbiturates but not to benzodiazepines. Coassembly with γ subunits is necessary for assembly of benzodiazepine receptors. $GABA_B$ receptor is a **metabotropic receptor**; its activation by the drug baclofen causes muscle relaxation.

Glutamate and aspartate (excitatory amino acids, EAA): These amino acids, present in various parts of the brain, play an important role as excitatory NTs. Glutamate released from the presynaptic terminals binds to glutamate receptor subtypes; their activation increases the conductance of Na^+ and Ca^{++} through ligand gated ion channels into the cells, leading to depolarisation (**ionotropic glutamate receptors**); or it stimulates phosphatidyl inositol turnover (**metabotropic G protein–coupled glutamate receptors**). The three ionotropic glutamate receptors are as follows:

a. *N*-Methyl-d-aspartate (NMDA) receptors
b. AMPA (α-amino-3 hydroxy-5-methyl-4-isoxazole propionic acid,) receptors
c. Kainate receptors

NMDA and AMPA receptors are usually colocalized and are found in cortex, basal ganglia and sensory pathways. Kainate distribution, on the other hand, is limited.

AMPA and in some regions of brain kainate receptors mediate the fast excitatory neurotrans-mission associated with excitatory postsynaptic potentials at glutamatergic synapses.The activation of NMDA receptors promotes Ca^{++} entry and long-term potentiation (LTP), causing a prolonged increase in the size of a postsynaptic response to a presynaptic stimulus.

EAA are involved in synaptic plasticity and excitotoxicity. The former deals with long term adaptive changes in synaptic connections, which underlie the brain functions such as learning, memory and thinking; pathological changes in synaptic plasticity have been observed in epilepsy, chronic pain or drug dependence. Very high concentrations of extracellular glutamate however has negative impact on synaptic plasticity and permits entry of excess Ca^{++} in cells causing neuronal cell death. This excitotoxicity plays a role in acute brain injury due to ischaemic stroke, trauma and status epilepticus. Chronic excitotoxicity with mitochondrial dysfunction has been implicated in many neurodegenerative diseases like Alzheimer's disease, Parkinson's disease, multiple sclerosis and Huntington chorea.

Metabotropic glutamate receptors (mGlu) are present on neurons and glia. The postsynaptic ones allow intracellular Ca^{++} release and alter the responses through ionotropic receptors. They too play a role in glutamate-mediated synaptic plasticity and excitotoxicity. The presynaptic mGlu serve as autoreceptors for glutamate or heteroreceptors for other NTs (e.g. GABA) and inhibit their release. Thus they decrease synaptic transmission and neuronal excitability.

Several endogenous peptides have been discovered in the brain, e.g. angiotensin, endorphins, vasopressin, endocrine peptides, gut peptides and orexin. They regulate neuronal function by themselves or in concert with other NTs.

Basis of Drug Action PH 1.1, PH 1.5

Excess of NT or its deficiency may cause a disorder which may or may not be treatable. When used in the treatment, the drugs may:

- **Modify the synthesis, storage, release, reuptake or metabolism, of the inhibitory or excitatory NTs,** e.g. Tricyclic antidepressants and SSRI inhibit the reuptake of NA or 5HT and act as antidepressants.
- **Modify the ionic fluxes across the cell membrane**, e.g. phenytoin sodium.
- **Antagonise NT** by acting at postsynaptic receptors, directly (e.g. chlorpromazine blocks dopamine receptors) or by antagonising the effects of endogenous NTs, e.g. central anticholinergics given for Parkinson's disease.
- **Act as neuromodulators.**
- **Modify the energy supply of the CNS**. This may be achieved by inhibition of action of certain enzymes involved in cellular respiration and energy processes or by altering the availability of the substrate for energy production.

Under certain circumstances, the central and the peripheral effects of a drug may be antagonistic. Atropine in small doses stimulates the central vagal nucleus and induces bradycardia, whereas the therapeutic doses usually induce tachycardia by peripheral cholinergic blockade.

We know more about what the brain does than how it does!

CHAPTER 6

The Alcohols and Barbiturates

Learning Objectives

This chapter will enable the reader:

1. To describe pharmacological actions of alcohol.
2. To discuss various metabolic pathways for alcohol stating their clinical relevance.
3. To correlate blood alcohol levels with behavioural changes.
4. To state indications for ethyl alcohol.
5. To outline pharmacotherapy of acute alcohol intoxication.
6. To describe management of alcohol withdrawal syndrome.
7. To outline the management of alcohol dependence/addiction.
8. To describe the pharmacological basis for the use of anticraving drugs in the treatment of alcohol dependence.
9. To give examples of clinically relevant interactions of ethyl alcohol with other drugs.
10. To state toxic effects of methanol poisoning and discuss its treatment.
11. To describe pharmacotherapy of ethylene glycol poisoning.
12. To correlate pharmacokinetic features of various barbiturates with their clinical uses.
13. To state the role of barbiturates in clinical practice with reasons.
14. To outline the management of acute barbiturate poisoning.

KEY TERMS

Both, alcohol and barbiturates are CNS depressants. Consumption of alcohol in one form or another is increasing all over the world, sometimes for its medical use but often for its pleasurable, stress relieving and blissful effects on the mind/mood. In doing so, alcohol has become the **major drug of abuse.** Barbiturates, a group of sedative-hypnotic drugs, are not preferred now due to availability of safer agents like benzodiazepines. Adverse reactions to the barbiturates was the prime concern in clinical practice and cases of overdosing and poisoning were common. However, some of the barbiturates have few specific indications, e.g. thiopental as a general anaesthetic agent (Chapter 7) and phenobarbitone as an antiepileptic drug (Chapter 9). Their use is also on the decline.

ALCOHOL

Aliphatic alcohols are hydroxy (OH) derivatives of the aliphatic hydrocarbons. They contain one, two or more OH groups and are designated as follows:

- **Monohydroxy,** e.g. ethyl, methyl and propyl alcohols
- **Dihydroxy**, also called glycols due to the sweet taste, e.g. ethylene glycol and propylene glycol
- **Trihydroxy**, e.g. glycerol or glycerine
- **Polyhydroxy,** e.g. mannitol and sorbitol

Of these, ethyl alcohol is the main constituent of alcoholic beverages.

ETHYL ALCOHOL (Ethanol): It is obtained by fermentation of sugars by yeast. The alcohol is separated by simple distillation. It is a colourless, volatile and inflammable liquid. Neutral spirit contains 90%–95% alcohol by volume. Wines containing more than 16% of alcohol are prepared by fortification with neutral spirit. The alcohol content of various beverages varies from 4% to 55% by volume. Whisky (40%) and vodka (35%–50%) are more concentrated beverages, whereas beer contains 4%–6% (v/v) of alcohol.

Pharmacological actions

Topical: Applied to the skin,

(a) It evaporates quickly. It has a cooling and refreshing effect and is used for reducing the temperature in fevers. *Eau-de-cologne* and aftershave lotion are other examples of cosmetic preparations used for *their* cooling effect.
(b) In concentrations of 40%–50%, it has a rubefacient and mild irritant action.
(c) Higher concentrations denature proteins by partial precipitation and dehydration and act as astringents and germicidals. In the concentration of 70% it acts as an antiseptic (Chapter 60).

PH 1.20

Central nervous system: Ethanol has widespread actions on many NTs and receptors. It is a CNS depressant and acts by enhancing the inhibitory $GABA_A$ receptor activity and inhibiting the excitatory NMDA receptors. It also affects the functioning of the other receptors such as dopamine, $5\text{-}HT_3$, NA, endorphin and adenosine.

The **euphoric** (pleasurable) **effects** are mediated by a dopaminergic pathway that projects from the ventral tegmental area to the hypothalamic nucleus accumbens. Other pleasure-giving activities such as eating, sex and consumption of other substances of abuse (e.g. opium and cannabis) also act through this *central dopamine reward system.*

The desire to drink alcohol can be due to **craving** that has been linked to dopaminergic, 5-HTergic and opioid systems that cause reinforcement or to prevent withdrawal, which is mediated through GABAergic, glutamatergic and noradrenergic systems.

Long-term exposure to alcohol brings about adaptive changes in the neuronal systems including downregulation of the inhibitory neuronal GABA receptors and upregulation of the excitatory glutamatergic receptors leading to tolerance to many effects of alcohol.

The initial CNS effect is due to depression of the reticular activating system. The cortex is thus released from the inhibitory control required for purposeful activity.

Alcohol:

1. Removes inhibitions and thus diminishes such processes as hesitation, caution and self-criticism, which are required to live a disciplined life as desired by the society. The pattern of behaviour depends on the environment and the basic personality of the individual. The initial euphoria, during which the individual may do silly and harmless antics, is commonly followed by mood swings and uncontrolled emotional outbursts, and a person may become violent and antisocial.
2. *Reduces visual acuity and interferes with muscular coordination, even in small doses.* It impairs the ability of the brain to coordinate motor activity such as typing, standing and hand steadiness. It lengthens the reaction time for both, visual and auditory stimuli. In a mildly intoxicated person, the reaction time may be lengthened by 10%–15%. *Hence, even moderate drinking is considered dangerous to public and individual safety.*
3. *Causes difficulty in speech, unsteadiness of gait and finally complete loss of self-control, if consumed in excess amount.*
4. *Can cause unconsciousness* when consumed in large quantities. Respiration becomes slow, noisy and laboured; the face becomes pale and cyanotic; and the BP falls. Death occurs due to medullary depression, mainly the respiratory centre. Some of the CNS effects of alcoholic beverages are probably due to the presence of adulterants such as ethyl acetate, isoamyl alcohol and butanol. In epileptics, alcohol may precipitate convulsions. *Chronic alcohol abuse causes shrinking of the brain by its neurotoxic action.*

Alcohol alters the patient's reaction to pain from one of concern to one of relative detachment. It reduces both, REM and deep sleep. However, it is neither used as an analgesic, nor as a hypnotic.

Sudden withdrawal of alcohol causes excitation and hyperactivity of the CNS.

Gastrointestinal tract: Taken orally, it gives a local feeling of warmth and increases the salivary secretion probably by reflex action. It has an irritant action on the gastric mucosa and enjoys reputation as an appetizer; 50 mL of 7%–10% alcohol increases the gastric secretion, by releasing histamine and gastrin from the gastric antrum, in addition to its psychic and local irritant effects. Concentrations higher than 15% inhibit both, gastric motility and secretion and this effect may persist for many hours. It has a direct toxic effect on gastric mucosa. It may cause gastritis and gastric erosions, giving rise to pain, nausea, vomiting and even bleeding. Many chronic alcoholics suffer from gastritis and achlorhydria. *The irritant effect of alcohol on the gastric mucosa is accentuated by aspirin and other NSAIDs* (Chapter 11) *which inhibit the local synthesis of prostaglandins (PG).* Alcohol is frequently the cause of gastro-esophageal reflux disease (GERD) and esophageal cancer.

Liver: Ethanol causes dose-related hepatotoxicity. The common effects are fatty infiltration and hepatomegaly. This results in the following:

- **Impaired gluconeogenesis**
- **Glycogen depletion**
- **Reduced synthesis of albumin and transferrin**
- **Diminished fatty acid oxidation**
- **Increased synthesis of VLDL, with consequent hypertriglyceridaemia**

Hypoglycaemia and hepatomegaly are the two important manifestations in chronic alcoholics. The hepatomegaly may be (a) simple hepatomegaly with normal hepatic architecture or (b) due to fatty degeneration.

Alcohol has a direct toxic effect on the liver. Elevated serum level of gamma glutamyl transpeptidase (γ-GTP) is the most sensitive index of alcoholic liver disease; the spectrum includes alcoholic hepatitis, cirrhosis or hepatoma.

Acute alcohol ingestion inhibits the hepatic microsomal CYP450 enzyme systems, whereas chronic ingestion induces them with the resultant increase in the rate of metabolism of drugs such as phenobarbitone, warfarin and steroids. However, alcohol itself is metabolically degraded by alcohol-inducible CYP450 system to a minimal extent.

Cardiovascular system: Alcohol in moderate amounts dilates skin vessels by depressing the vasomotor centre, resulting in flushing and feeling of warmth. This effect prevents normal cutaneous vasoconstriction on exposure to cold. Hence, it may be harmful to take alcohol for warming up in cold weather as the body would lose more heat. Taken in concentrated form (brandy 15–20 mL), alcohol probably stimulates the vital medullary centres reflexly by irritating the pharyngeal mucosa, resulting in a slight rise in BP, tachycardia and an increase in the cardiac output. Hence, it is sometimes used as a household remedy for fainting attacks.

The epidemiological evidence that regular drinking in small amount reduces the risk of ischaemic heart disease (IHD) is controversial. Alcohol may relieve angina, but that is more likely due to its central action. The false sense of well-being induced by alcohol may prompt the patient to ignore the warning given by the chest pain. *In fact, regular consumption of alcohol is often associated with hypertension. Even small amounts of alcohol depress the myocardial function in patients with preexisting heart disease.* Alcohol affects the conduction system of the heart and may precipitate arrhythmias. Further, alcoholism is an important causative factor in cardiomyopathy and stroke. *Hence it is not justifiable to advise/encourage alcohol consumption as a protective measure against the development of ischaemic heart disease (IHD).*

Kidney: Alcohol inhibits ADH release and causes diuresis due to decreased tubular reabsorption of water. It increases the excretion of magnesium and calcium.

Skeletal muscle: Ethanol may cause damage to muscle tissue (alcoholic myopathy).

Reproductive system: Alcohol has an erroneous reputation as a sexual stimulant (aphrodisiac). The feeling of false confidence produced by the loss of inhibitory control is probably responsible for that. But as Shake-speare correctly noted in *Macbeth*, 'Lechery, Sir, it provoketh and unprovoketh; it provoketh the desire, but it taketh away the performance'. In fact, it depresses the sexual responsiveness. In men, chronic alcohol ingestion causes a reduction in plasma testosterone, impotence, sterility, gynaecomastia, prostatic congestion and acute urinary retention.

In women, repeated drinking can cause amenorrhoea and infertility.

Teratogenic effects: Drinking during early pregnancy can cause fetal damage. The fetus has been described to have 'characteristic facial appearance, microcephaly, growth retardation, mental deficiency and an increase in the frequency of other major abnormalities' (the **fetal alcohol syndrome**). *Even moderate alcohol consumption during pregnancy increases the risk of spontaneous abortion and low birth weight.*

Miscellaneous: Chronic alcohol use is associated with various types of anaemia, *macrocytic anaemia being common due to folate deficiency.* It may also cause leucopenia, decrease in T cells, mutagenesis and decrease in IgG production. *Chronic alcoholics may also suffer from lower bone density, hyperlipidaemia, hyperuricaemia, hypomagnesaemia and pancreatitis.*

Absorption, fate and excretion: Ethyl alcohol, being highly lipid soluble and diffusible, is absorbed very rapidly from the stomach, duodenum and small intestine, 50% within 15 min and 100% within 1–2 h. The absorption is delayed by the presence of food in the stomach, whereas it is accelerated following rapid gastric emptying. It is largely (90%) metabolised by gastric and hepatic alcohol dehydrogenase enzyme. *Aspirin inhibits this enzyme in the stomach, and increases the bioavailability of alcohol*. Alcohol is distributed throughout the body water and is stored in all tissues; it diffuses back into the blood when its blood level falls.

In the lungs, alcohol passes from blood to breath, which smells of alcohol. *The ratio of concentrations of alcohol in blood and alveolar air is constant and is about 2100:1*. Because of this high ratio, it is difficult to wash out blood alcohol by artificial ventilation.

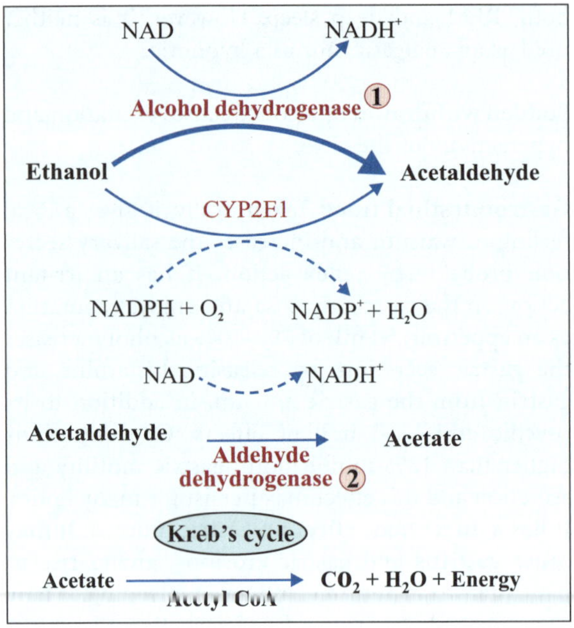

FIG. 6.1 Metabolism of alcohol. NAD, nicotinamide adenine dinucleotide; NADPH, nicotinamide adenine dinucleotide phosphate; 1: Inhibition by fomepizole; 2: Inhibition by disulfiram.

It is primarily metabolised by cytosolic and mitochondrial oxidative enzymes in the liver.

Alcohol dehydrogenase oxidises alcohol to acetaldehyde, which is converted to acetate by *aldehyde dehydrogenase*. The acetate is oxidised to carbon dioxide and water by liver and other tissues such as the stomach and brain (Fig. 6.1).

At very low concentrations, alcohol is metabolised by *first-order kinetics* (Chapter 1). At higher plasma concentrations (>10 mg/dL), it is metabolised at a constant rate which is independent of blood alcohol concentration (**zero-order kinetics**). As NAD is consumed during the degradation of alcohol, the availability of hepatic NAD serves as the rate controller for alcohol metabolism and determines change from first order kinetics to zero order kinetics.

Increased production of toxic metabolites such as acetaldehyde, NADH and Acetyl CoA can cause organ damage in chronic alcoholics. Fomepizole inhibits alcohol dehydrogenase (Fig. 6.1), whereas certain drugs such as disulfiram, metronidazole, trimethoprim and cefotetan inhibit aldehyde dehydrogenase.

Is alcohol a food? One gram of alcohol gives 7.1 calories in the form of acetate. *Although it can spare carbohydrates, alcohol is not a food, because it has no protein, vitamin or any other nutrients ('empty calories').* Despite this alcohol is widely used at various personal or social occasions under the pretext of enjoyment, celebration, socialization, relaxation and relief from stress or grief. Its effects vary from person to person and are harmful to users or to those around them depending upon quantity ingested, frequency, age, health status, use of other drugs and family history. **Consumption of alcohol before driving is hazardous.** Table 6.1 lists certain groups of people who should avoid alcohol drinking.

Indications for ethyl alcohol: It is a solvent for various active ingredients. It is sometimes used:

- **In the symptomatic treatment of fever** because of its topical cooling effect on the skin.
- **In the prevention of bed sores** as it hardens the skin.
- **As an antiseptic** (70%).
- **As an appetiser** (10%).
- **In methyl alcohol poisoning** (see section on Methyl alcohol).
- **To wash out phenol** in cases of accidental skin contamination.
- **By local injection to destroy a nerve** as in trigeminal neuralgia. PH 1.21

ACUTE ALCOHOL INTOXICATION

Chemical analysis of blood is useful to decide the degree of intoxication in an individual who has ingested alcohol (Table 6.2). *However, it is difficult to associate a particular blood alcohol concentration with a specific degree of impairment.* Blood alcohol estimation gives accurate results only if done within 6 h of alcohol consumption.

Approximately 600 mL of pure alcohol can produce a fatal effect in an individual of 70 kg body weight. Coma after an acute alcoholic bout may be due to

Table 6.1 Who should avoid alcohol drinking and why?

Alcohol Drinking Should be Avoided By	Why
■ Individuals involved in driving or operating machinery	Affects skill, coordination, and alertness
■ Patients taking medicines like	
■ First generation antihistaminics for cold/ cough, sedatives	Increased risk of sedation and CNS depression
■ Antiinflammatory drugs , anticoagulants	Increased risk of GI bleeding
■ Sulfonylreas	Increased risk of hypoglycemia
■ Antiepileptics like phenytoin, levetiracetam	Increased risk of seizures
■ Statins, anti-TB drugs	Increased risk of liver damage
■ MAOI	Increased risk of hypertensive crises due to interaction with tyramine in alcoholic beverages (beer and wine)
■ Antihypertensives	Increased risk of arrhythmia and hypotension
■ Patients with concomitant medical conditions e.g. liver failure, epilepsy	Worsens the conditions (hepatotoxic effect of alcohol, lowers seizure threshold)
■ Addicts who are recovering from alcohol use disorder or are unable to control the amount that they drink	Promotes dependence
■ Individuals < 21 years of age	Liability for abuse
■ Pregnant women or those who wish to plan pregnancy	Teratogenicity

Table 6.2 Correlation of Blood Alcohol Levels with Behavioural Changes

Blood Concentration (mg/100 mL)	Behavioural Changes	Interpretation
<50	Not significant	Not under the influence of alcohol but may affect the reaction time
50–100	Feeling of exaltation, talkativeness	Possibly under the influence
100–200	Emotionally unstable, motor incoordination, nystagmus	Probably under the influence
200–300	Staggering, loss of self-control	Definitely under the influence
300–400	Stupor-dead drunk	Grossly intoxicated
400–500	Coma, anaesthetic effect	
>500	Respiratory arrest and death	

CNS depression, head injury or severe hypoglycaemia which especially occurs in fasting individuals. Hypomagnesaemia is common. Some individuals may develop severe acute hepatitis. Death due to acute alcohol poisoning is, however, uncommon. After death, the degradation of alcohol ceases but levels of alcohol in the brain and blood remain constant for some time. Hence, postmortem samples of blood can give reliable estimates about the degree of intoxication at the time of death. FM 9.4

The **treatment** consists of the following:

- **General nursing care**
- **Maintenance of vital functions**
- **Thiamine** 100 mg (bolus) IV
- **Glucose** 50%, 50 mL IV, for hypoglycaemia
- **Magnesium sulphate** 2–4 g IV over 1–2 h

If the acutely intoxicated patient is not comatose but only rowdy, careful use of a sedative such as a benzodiazepine is indicated. PH 1.20

CHRONIC ALCOHOLISM

'At risk' (heavy) drinking is defined by National Institute on Alcohol Abuse and Alcoholism (NIAAA, USA) as consuming greater than 14 drinks per week or more than 4 drinks on any day for men, and greater than 7 drinks per week or more than 3 drinks on any day for women. A 'drink' is that amount of any alcoholic beverage which contains 14 g of alcohol.

Chronic alcoholics are liable to suffer from:

- **Neuropsychiatric syndromes** such as cognitive problems like dementia, Korsakoff psychosis, hallucinosis, suicidal tendencies and Wernicke encephalopathy.
- **Nutritional deficiencies** such as polyneuritis due to thiamine deficiency and anaemia. Organ damage leading to hepatic cirrhosis, chronic pancreatitis, cardiomyopathy, peripheral neuropathy and optic nerve degeneration.

Withdrawal Syndrome

Sudden withdrawal of alcohol in alcoholics leads to *withdrawal syndrome* (Box 6.1). **Delirium tremens,** though rare, is the most severe component of the abstinence syndrome which develops some days after sudden withdrawal of alcohol in chronic alcoholics. The symptoms consist of restlessness, insomnia, tremors and hallucinations generally involving great fear, delirium, autonomic instability and even convulsions.

Box 6.1 Alcohol Withdrawal Syndrome

8 h: Tremulousness, anxiety, irritability, nausea and vomiting (Tremulous syndrome)
24 h: Hyperexcitability, insomnia, disordered perception and convulsions (Seizure syndrome)
2–5 days: Tremor, hallucinations, disorientation and ANS overactivity (Delirium tremens)

The treatment of withdrawal syndrome is outlined in Box 6.2.

Box 6.2 Symptomatic Treatment of Alcohol Withdrawal Syndrome

- Maintenance of nutrition and electrolyte balance
- Thiamine IV (100 mg)
- Glucose IV *for* hypoglycaemia
- Diazepam IV *to treat* seizures and delirium
- Alpha-adrenergic agonist clonidine 0.1–0.4 mg q.i.d., or beta-blocker atenolol (orally) 50–100 mg daily, *to combat* autonomic hyperactivity; haloperidol for agitation
- Carbamazepine *to prevent* seizures
- Watch for arrhythmia

ALCOHOL TOLERANCE

Repeated ingestion causes alcohol tolerance which can be:

1. ***Pharmacokinetic or metabolic tolerance*** that develops within 2–3 weeks and is due to increased metabolism of alcohol (30%).
2. ***Pharmacodynamic or cellular tolerance*** wherein physiological functions remain near normal in spite of alcohol concentration.
3. ***Behavioural tolerance*** wherein subject learns to control his/her behaviour even on excess alcohol consumption.

ALCOHOL DEPENDENCE (ADDICTION)

Although all those who drink alcohol are not addicts, repeated ingestion can lead to dependence. Alcoholism is a polygenic disorder with both genetic and environmental determinants, in which the subject continues drinking in spite of adverse medical or social consequences. The intensity of craving is such that the 'desire to drink' remains uncontrollable and is the major interest in life. This leads to **alcohol use disorder,** which creates many social and occupational problems. Nearly 50% of Asians have abnormal inactive enzyme aldehyde dehydrogenase, which causes higher levels of acetaldehyde following alcohol intake, thus resulting in severe nausea and vomiting. This may decrease the risk of excessive drinking.

Though precise mechanism for alcohol dependence is not known, upregulation of NMDA receptors and voltage sensitive Ca^{++} channels occurs. This is associated with downregulation of $GABA_A$ mediated responses. PH 1.23, PS 4.4 & PS 4.6

Treatment of alcohol dependence (Deaddiction) is as follows:

1. **Detoxification** which aims at providing safe withdrawal to make the patient alcohol-free
2. **Support therapy** to prevent relapses and to assist the patient in maintaining abstinence
3. **Rehabilitation** which includes (a) psychotherapy and (b) institutional therapy

The major part of the treatment includes education, counselling and cognitive-behavioural therapy; drugs form only a small part.

Detoxification

Following a thorough physical examination for existing complications (such as liver failure, GI bleeding and nutritional deficiencies) in an alcoholic who wishes to stop alcohol drinking, alcohol is withdrawn. Adequate nutrition and oral multiple B vitamins, including 50–100 mg of thiamine daily is instituted. However, IV fluids are not necessary unless dehydration signs or history of recent bleeding, vomiting, or diarrhoea are present. Glucose is administered intravenously if there is hypoglycaemia.

Benzodiazepines (BZD), particularly the long acting ones, such as diazepam (10 mg) or chlordiazepoxide (25–50 mg), considered as the substituting drugs for alcohol, are the treatment of choice. They are given orally every 4–6 h on the first day, with tapering of doses over the next 5 days. Abatement of symptoms such as anxiety and agitation occurs within 3–5 days of therapy, but regaining normal sleep pattern may take several months. Lorazepam and oxazepam are preferred in the elderly and those with liver failure. Every 4 hourly dosing of these drugs is needed to avoid plasma level fluctuation that may precipitate seizures.

Carbamazepine, an antiepileptic drug (Chapter 9), is an effective alternative to benzodiazepines in treating mild to moderate withdrawal symptoms. It prevents seizures and does not cause respiratory depression nor impairs memory. It is relatively safe.

BZD in high doses are effective in decreasing agitation and preventing seizures in delirium tremens, but they do not change confusion state. **Clonidine** 0.1–0.4 mg q.i.d., or **Atenolol** 50–100 mg daily may be used to control autonomic hyperactivity.

Support Therapy

Anticraving drugs help in preventing relapses and support complete abstinence during rehabilitation. They are as follows:

1. **Opioid antagonists**, e.g. naltrexone, nalmefene
2. **NMDA receptor antagonist:** e.g. acamprosate
3. **Aversion drugs,** e.g. disulfiram,
4. **Dopaminergic antagonists,** e.g. tiapride (experimental)
5. **Supporting drugs**, e.g. lithium, carbamazepine, topiramate

The pharmacological basis for use of these drugs lies in the neurobiology of dependence. Brain **dopamine** is probably the body's natural 'Happy chemical'. It is involved in bringing pleasure and promoting reward-motivating behaviour. During alcohol dependence, there is excessive activation of *dopamine-rich ventral tegmental reward system,* which gives the feeling of pleasure or reward by stimulating nucleus accumbens (NAc) and the prefrontal cortex. In addition, other neurotransmitters, inhibitory GABA and excitatory glutamate are also involved in alcohol dependence. The interplay between them is complex and varies with stages of alcohol dependence.

The drugs used in alcohol dependence with their mechanisms of action are listed in Table 6.3.

NALTREXONE: Naltrexone, 50–100 mg once daily, has to be given for 12–16 weeks or more after detoxification. Once-a-month injection of naltrexone is available. The most common side effect of naltrexone is nausea. It may cause dose-dependent hepatotoxicity. Disulfiram and naltrexone should not be combined as both are hepatotoxic.

Nalmefene, an analogue of naloxone with a greater bioavailability, has a longer duration of action. It does not cause dose-dependent hepatotoxicity.

ACAMPROSATE: This analogue of GABA is as effective as naltrexone and can be combined with it. It is largely excreted by the kidneys. Adverse effects are usually mild and include diarrhoea, rash and headache. The usual dose is two enteric coated tablets (333 mg each) thrice daily.

DISULFIRAM (tetraethylthiuram disulphide): After ensuring that alcohol has not been consumed for at least 12 h, disulfiram treatment is initiated with 500

Table 6.3 Drugs Used in the Treatment of Alcohol Dependence (Deaddiction) PS 4.6

Drug Name	Mechanism of Action	Effects
Naltrexone and other mu opioid antagonists	1. Blocks opioid mu receptors involved in the pleasant sensations associated with drinking which removes the inhibition on GABA release 2. Blocks dopamine release in the NAc	Reduces craving and urge to drink alcohol and thus maintains the abstinence
Acamprosate	1. Acts as an agonist at the GABA receptors 2. Weak antagonist at the NMDA receptors, hence reduces glutamate-induced hyperexcitability associated with alcohol withdrawal	Reduces voluntary alcohol consumption and craving that occur in alcohol withdrawal and early abstinence
Disulfiram	1. Inhibits aldehyde dehydrogenase and blocks the oxidation of acetaldehyde 2. Inhibits dopamine beta oxidase and thus interferes with the synthesis of NA	Raises the blood level of toxic acetaldehyde, which directly causes unpleasant symptoms such as nausea, vomiting, dizziness, headache, chest pain, hypotension, perspiration flushing of the skin (antabuse reaction)

mg as a single daily dose for 1–2 weeks, followed by 125–250 mg o.d. as the maintenance dose.

After a week's therapy, even a small amount of alcohol produces **antabuse reaction** (Table 6.3). The patient realises that, while on this drug, he/she cannot tolerate even small amounts of alcohol and abstains from drinking. *Severe violent reactions can occur even with the first dose, and hence this treatment should be carried out in a hospital. However, the drug hardly improves the success rate of continued abstinence nor does it delay the resumption of drinking.*

Adverse reactions: It can cause drowsiness, nausea, headache, cramps, fatiguability, a metallic taste in the mouth and acidosis. It can also cause depression, psychosis and peripheral neuropathy. It is hepatotoxic.

It is **contraindicated** in

- **Hepatic and circulatory diseases**
- **Uncontrolled diabetes mellitus**
- **Obvious personality changes in alcoholics**

***Drug interactions:** Disulfiram inhibits metabolic degradation of warfarin, theophylline, benzodiazepines, carbamazepine, tricyclic antidepressants and phenytoin. The first and the last interactions can be hazardous.*

LITHIUM: Oral lithium carbonate acts as a mood stabiliser and reduces alcohol consumption. It may be used as an adjunct to treat alcohol withdrawal (Chapter 14).

An antiemetic **ondansetron,** a $5HT_3$ receptor antagonist, is effective in early-onset alcoholics by reducing the desire to drink but has no effect on its pharmacokinetics. **Topiramate,** an antiepileptic, is also claimed to have anticraving effect.

Among the various drugs for the treatment of alcohol dependence, the evidence for efficacy is strongest for naltrexone and acamprosate. A combination of two or more treatment modalities is useful rather than using a single drug.

Psychotherapy by a sympathetic doctor can often give rewarding results during early stages. Dependence is reversible if the addict realises that his/her drinking has become a problem to him. Complete cooperation by the patient is very essential, and he/she should be explained that indulgence in even small quantities of alcohol again would lead to a relapse.

Rehabilitation

In all alcoholics, the possibility of an underlying psychiatric disorder such as schizophrenia, anxiety disorder, panic disorder or depression must be considered.

- **Institutional therapy:** Psychotherapy and drug therapy can be reinforced by institutional therapy (**Alcoholics Anonymous**, *AA*) where the patient sees for himself/herself the ex-alcoholics who have become abstainers and are living a happy life. This helps to boost the patient's morale. A religious and spiritual approach is also helpful.

Certain abnormalities of personality develop in very chronic cases which make the treatment far more difficult. Thus, in Korsakoff psychosis, there is a marked impairment of memory, disorientation in space, impaired physical capacity and diminution of will power. In such cases, the results of aversion therapy with drugs are generally disappointing.

Drug interactions: Numerous drug interactions between alcohol and other drugs have been described (Box 6.3). This should be borne in mind while prescribing these drugs to alcoholics.

METHYL ALCOHOL (methanol): This is used as a solvent and is added in a 5% concentration to denature ethyl alcohol. It is not used therapeutically but often misused for adulteration of ethyl alcohol. Its absorption and distribution are similar to those of ethyl alcohol; the rate of metabolism, however, is very slow. It is mainly oxidised to formaldehyde and subsequently to formic acid, which is toxic. The latter reaction is folate dependent and causes folate depletion. PH 1.21

Pharmacological actions: Following its ingestion, initial symptoms resemble those of ethyl alcohol ingestion. The later symptoms are due to the following:

Box 6.3 Interactions of Ethyl Alcohol with Other Drugs

- CNS depressants such as opioids, hypnotics, tranquillizers, antihistaminics, reserpine, methyldopa and clonidine can cause *severe CNS depression* in the presence of alcohol.
- Vasodilators (hydralazine and nitroglycerine) can cause additive *orthostatic hypotension.* On the other hand, heavy consumption of alcohol is known to cause transient *hypertension.*
- Alcohol *potentiates* the adverse effects of aspirin and other NSAID (GI bleeding), sulphonylureas (hypoglycaemia) and oral anticoagulants (bleeding).
- Isoniazid can cause *hepatic toxicity* in chronic alcoholics because of increased conversion to a toxic metabolite.
- Chlorpropamide, metronidazole and its analogues, griseofulvin, tolbutamide, cephalosporins and phenylbutazone, can cause a mild *disulfiram-like reaction* in alcohol users.

Box 6.4 Treatment of Methanol Poisoning PH 1.21

- Hospitalisation, nursing care
- Gastric lavage, activated charcoal
- Treatment of acidosis/hypoglycaemia
- Inhibition of methanol metabolism
  - (a) Ethyl alcohol 10% IV; 0.6 g/kg loading dose, followed by 10 g/h infusion, in adults
  - (b) Fomepizole: 100 mg, diluted with 250 mL of isotonic saline and infused slowly over 45 min.
- Promote metabolic degradation of formate:
  Folinic acid 1 mg/kg (Max. 50 mg) IV, together with folic acid 1 mg/kg IV, 4 hourly for six doses.
  - Diuretics, urine alkalinisation
  - Haemodialysis in severe case
  - Maintenance of nutrition

- **CNS depression**
- **Acidosis** following the production of formic and other organic acids.
- **Toxic effects of formaldehyde and formic acid on the retinal cells.**

The symptoms may be delayed, particularly if ethanol is also consumed simultaneously. Usually, headache, vertigo, nausea, vomiting severe abdominal pain, dyspnoea and motor restlessness occur. Bradycardia has a bad prognostic significance. Coma can develop very rapidly, followed by death. Death is usually preceded by blindness. *However, total blindness could occur with as little as 15 mL of methyl alcohol, while ingestion of 30 mL is fatal.* Several deaths have been reported following the ingestion of methyl alcohol or alcoholic brew adulterated with methyl alcohol for its ethyl alcohol-like effects. FM 9.4

Treatment of toxicity: This is summarised in Box 6.4. It is directed mainly at supporting respiration and rapid correction of acidosis by IV sodium bicarbonate. The development of blindness is enhanced by acidosis. Hypokalaemia, if present, needs correction, so also the maintenance of adequate nutrition and water and electrolyte balance. The patient's eyes should be protected from strong light.

Specific therapy aims at suppression of metabolism of methanol by alcohol dehydrogenase and enhancement of its removal by haemodialysis.

The IV infusion or oral/ nasogastric administration (600 mg/kg) of ethyl alcohol has been recommended on the basis that it has higher affinity for alcohol dehydrogenase than methanol. Hence, it slows down the oxidation of methyl alcohol by competing for the same metabolic pathway. Ethanol administration can be life saving if, for some reasons, alkali therapy is delayed. Folic acid can accelerate metabolism of formate to CO_2 and H_2O.

FOMEPIZOLE: This 4-methyl pyrazole is useful in the treatment of poisoning with methyl alcohol and ethylene glycol (see below). It inhibits alcohol dehydrogenase rapidly, and the effect remains prolonged. It is well tolerated. Headache, nausea, dizziness and, sometimes, minor allergic reactions may occur. Its use appears to be more effective and safe than ethyl alcohol, but fomepizole is expensive.

Methyl alcohol is oxidised slowly, and hence acidosis can recur even after adequate initial alkali administration. It is necessary, therefore, to observe the patient closely for several days.

ETHYLENE GLYCOL (EG): This compound is used as an antifreeze in automobile radiators and as an industrial solvent. The therapeutic misuse of industrial glycerol contaminated with EG causes fatal nephrotoxicity. The initial transient excitation is followed by CNS depression. The acid metabolites and NADH-induced lactic acidosis (Fig. 6.2) cause metabolic acidosis, while oxalate and other intermediates which are nephrotoxic can cause tubular necrosis and acute renal failure. Ingestion of about 100 mL of EG, if untreated, can be fatal. FM 9.4

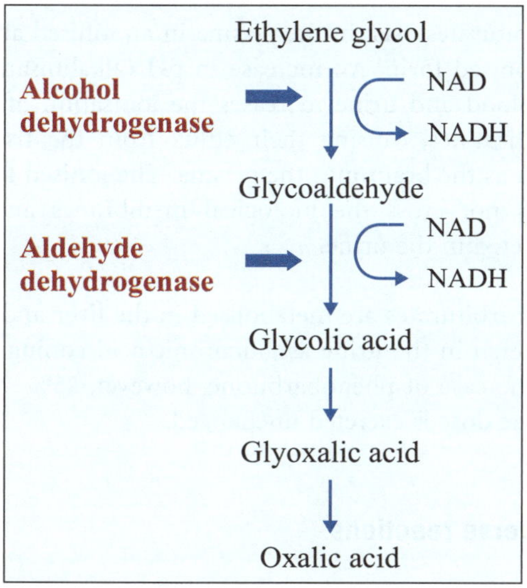

FIG. 6.2 Hepatic metabolism of ethylene glycol.

Treatment of EG poisoning: It is similar to that of methanol poisoning (Box 6.4). In addition, pyridoxine should be administered intravenously in the dose of 100 mg daily to promote the conversion of glyoxalic acid to glycine. Methyl alcohol and EG are rapidly cleared by the kidneys if the renal function is normal. Diuretics, urinary alkalinisation and early haemodialysis (which removes EG from the blood) may be helpful.

BARBITURATES

These are the derivatives of barbituric acid (Fig. 6.3).

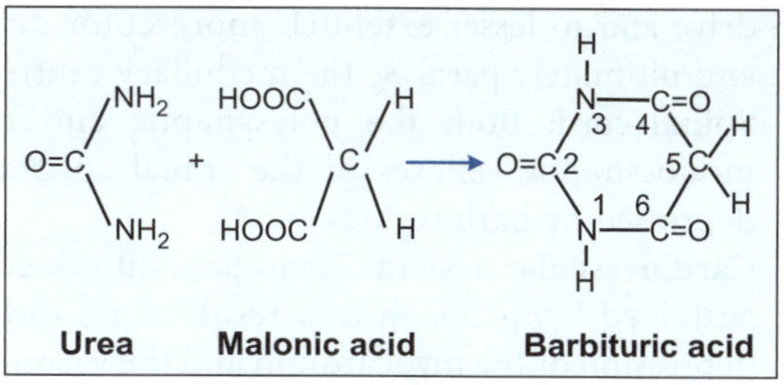

FIG. 6.3 Synthesis of barbituric acid.

Classification of barbiturates

1. Long acting (8 h or more), e.g. phenobarbitone
2. Intermediate acting (4–8 h), e.g. pentobarbitone
3. Short acting (less than 4 h), e.g. secobarbitone
4. Ultra short acting (in minutes), e.g. thiopentone/thiopental

Mechanism of action: Barbiturates cause reversible depression of all excitable tissues, the CNS being exquisitely sensitive. They bind to the beta subunit of the inhibitory $GABA_A$ receptor, *a site distinct from the site at which benzodiazepines (BZDs) bind* (Chapter 8; Fig 8.3). At lower doses, they enhance the action of GABA, whereas, in therapeutic doses, they open the chloride channels directly. They also inhibit the excitatory AMPA-glutamate receptors.

Pharmacological actions: Barbiturates are **less selective than BZDs and act at multiple sites in the CNS:**

Central nervous system: Barbiturates depress the CNS in a dose-dependent manner.

- **Sedation and hypnosis:** (Chapter 8). *In elderly and children, barbiturates occasionally produce dysphoria or excitement and a state of confusion.*
- **Anaesthetic effect:** Thiopentone IV produces general anaesthesia (Chapter 7).
- **Anticonvulsant and antiepileptic effect:** Barbiturates administered in anaesthetic doses inhibit or abolish drug-induced convulsions and those due to epilepsy and tetanus. **Phenobarbitone has a selective antiepileptic action** (Chapter 9).
- **Respiration:** Barbiturates cause dose-dependent depression of the respiratory centre. High doses suppress the neurogenic and hypoxic

drive and to lesser extent chemoreceptor drive and ultimately paralyse the medullary centre.

- **Spinal cord:** Both the polysynaptic and the monosynaptic reflexes of the spinal cord are depressed by barbiturates.
- **Cardiovascular system:** Toxic doses produce a sustained hypotension as a result of (i) direct depression of the myocardium and the vasomotor centre and (ii) hypoxia.
- **Kidney:** Barbiturate anaesthesia results in a reduction of urinary output as a result of the decrease in the GFR, and stimulation of secretion of ADH. Acute barbiturate poisoning is often associated with oliguria largely due to severe hypotension.
- **Liver:** Barbiturates exert various actions on certain liver enzymes.
  - *On acute administration*, barbiturates competitively inhibit CYP450 enzymes and therefore the metabolism of drugs and endogenous steroids.
  - *Chronic administration causes* **induction of hepatic microsomal enzymes** (Chapters 1 and 3), leading to an increased inactivation of certain drugs, including barbiturates themselves. This may explain the phenomenon of tolerance to barbiturates.
  - *They induce delta-amino-levulinic acid (ALA) synthetase, a mitochondrial enzyme, and aldehyde dehydrogenase, a cytoplasmic enzyme.* An increase in ALA synthetase results in an increase in ALA and porphobilinogen synthesis. *In patients suffering from acute intermittent porphyria, barbiturates may precipitate a severe attack resulting in paralysis and even death.*
  - *Phenobarbitone increases the hepatic glucuronyl transferase and the bilirubin-binding Y-protein and stimulates the metabolism of bilirubin.* Hence it was previously used to treat neonatal jaundice. Phototherapy and in severe cases, exchange transfusion are preferred now.

Absorption, fate and excretion: Barbiturates are weak acids and undergo absorption mainly from the stomach. Absorption also occurs from the intestine and the rectum. The barbiturates are well distributed in the body. They readily cross the placental barrier and small amounts may be secreted in milk. The factors which affect the distribution and fate of various barbiturates are their:

- **Lipid solubility**
- **Degree of protein binding**
- **Extent of ionisation**

The short-acting barbiturates are highly lipid soluble and hence, have a rapid onset of action. They are more rapidly metabolised, but at the same time tend to get completely reabsorbed by the kidney tubules.

Barbiturates exist in the plasma in an ionised and a unionised form. An increase in pH (alkalinisation) of blood and urine increases the ionisation of the barbiturates, causing their efflux from the tissues such as the brain into the plasma. The ionised form does not cross the biological membranes and is excreted in the urine.

All barbiturates are metabolised in the liver and are excreted in the urine as glucuronic acid conjugates. In the case of phenobarbitone, however, 25%–30% of the dose is excreted unchanged.

Adverse reactions:

- **Intolerance:** They may cause excitement (with hypnotic doses) headache, nausea, vomiting, diarrhoea and lassitude. Occasionally, barbiturates themselves may produce paroxysmal pain.
- **Allergic reactions** include urticaria, angioedema, other skin reactions, agranulocytosis and thrombocytopenic purpura.
- **Anaemia:** Prolonged phenobarbitone therapy may produce megaloblastic anaemia which responds to folic acid (Chapter 35).
- **Depression of fetal respiration:** Barbiturates, if administered to a woman during labour, may depress the foetal respiration.
- **Porphyria:** Barbiturate administration may precipitate an attack of acute intermittent hepatic porphyria.
- **Drug automatism:** When a barbiturate is employed as a hypnotic, because of confusion and amnesia, a patient may repeatedly take the

barbiturate at night and poison himself. This phe-nomenon is known as drug automatism.

- **Tolerance:** Repeated administration of barbiturates causes tolerance to their sedative and hypnotic actions. It can be attributed to: (a) Increased hepatic inactivation and (b) adaptation of the neuronal tissue to the drug. Barbiturate addicts often show cross-tolerance to other general CNS depressants such as general anaesthetics. *However, tolerance to the hypnotic effect of barbiturates fails to modify their lethal dose significantly.* Acquired barbiturate tolerance usually disappears completely within 1–2 weeks of abstinence.

PH 1.22, PH 1.23

- **Drug dependence:** Repeated ingestion of barbiturates causes drug dependence. The manifestations of chronic barbiturate intoxication are thick slurred speech, ataxia, impaired reflexes, hypotonia, nystagmus and difficulty in accommodation. The nutrition is usually unimpaired.

  The treatment of barbiturate dependence is purely symptomatic. Generally, the withdrawal should be gradual, over 10 days to 3 weeks, depending on the severity of the dependence. If desired, replacement could be made with a hypnotic such as chlordiazepoxide 50 mg, or diazepam 10 mg.

Drug interactions: See Box 6.5.

Indications:

- **As anticonvulsants:** See Chapter 9.
- **General anaesthesia:** See Chapter 7.
- **Psychiatric uses:** Amylobarbitone, pentobarbitone and thiopentone given by IV route produce a state of deep sedation in which the cortical inhibitions are abolished. This may bring forth the suppressed psychic disturbances; the patient becomes more communicative and amenable to suggestions. This procedure of *narcoanalysis* or amylobarbitone interview is useful in interrogation or lie detection.

  Barbiturates are no longer used as sedatives or hypnotics. FM 10.1

Box 6.5 Important Drug Interactions of Barbiturates

Severe CNS depression: Other CNS depressants (alcohol, benzodiazepines and antihistaminics) and monoamine oxidase inhibitors
Hepatic microsomal enzyme induction with diminished efficacy of other drugs: see Chapter 3

Acute barbiturate poisoning: Acute barbiturate poisoning causes marked CNS depression, particularly the respiratory failure, and a peripheral circulatory collapse. The frequent and often fatal complications are atelectasis, pulmonary oedema and bronchopneumonia or acute renal shutdown.

Treatment of acute barbiturate poisoning: The severity of barbiturate poisoning is assessed by clinical signs before treatment and correlates well with plasma levels of barbiturate. The presence of reflexes, response to painful stimuli and maintenance of BP and of respiration without external assistance indicate better prognosis, whereas cases showing deep coma with absent reflexes, respiratory depression and cardiovascular collapse have a high mortality.

Box 6.6 summarises the principles of management of acute barbiturate poisoning. The treatment is similar to that of any drug overdose (for details, see Chapter 2) and includes supportive care, GI decontamination, and enhancement of elimination.

Box 6.6 Principles of Management of Acute Barbiturate Poisoning

- Hospitalisation
- Attention to *airway, breathing and circulation* (ABC)
- Gastric lavage with 50 g activated charcoal
- Forced alkaline diuresis; adequate IV fluids; electrolyte balance
- Peritoneal dialysis, haemodialysis, haemoperfusion
- Nursing care, nutrition
- Prophylactic antibiotics

Haemodialysis is about 40 times more effective than forced diuresis in promoting elimination of long acting barbiturates. Charcoal haemoperfusion is now considered superior to haemodialysis for the same purpose.

CHAPTER 7

PH 1.18

General Anaesthetics

Learning Objectives

This chapter will enable the reader:

1. To classify general anaesthetic agents.
2. To describe various mechanisms of action of general anaesthetics.
3. To state the factors that influence kinetics of inhalational anaesthetic agents.
4. To describe salient features of various general anaesthetic agents used in practice.
5. To state advantages of neuroleptanalgesia, giving examples of drugs that produce it.
6. To describe factors that help in rational selection of an anaesthetic agent and technique(s) for its administration.
7. To discuss reasons for the use of preanaesthetic medications.
8. To state the drugs/drug groups used during the perianaesthetic period, giving a pharmacological basis for their use.

KEY TERMS

minimum alveolar concentration, p. 103
stages of anaesthesia, p. 103
balanced anaesthesia, p. 104
volatile liquid anaesthetics, p. 104
gaseous anaesthetics, p. 106
diffusion hypoxia, p. 107
nonvolatile general anaesthetics, p. 107
second gas effect, p. 107
dissociative anaesthesia, p. 110
neuroleptanalgesia, p. 111
anaesthetic agents, rational use, p. 112
preanaesthetic medication, p. 112

General anaesthetics are the agents which bring about a loss of all modalities of sensation, particularly pain (analgesia), inhibition of autonomic reflexes, relaxation of skeletal muscle, amnesia and a reversible loss of consciousness. Nitrous oxide was discovered by Priestley in 1776, but it was used for the first time in 1844 by Horace Wells, a dentist in Hartford, USA, for a painless tooth extraction. William Morton, a second year medical student, in 1846 successfully showed the use of ether as a general anaesthetic in the first classic demonstration held in the operating room of the Massachusetts General Hospital, Boston, USA. Since then, anaesthesiology has progressed considerably, and many safer agents are now available for use. AS 4.1. PH 1.18

Classification of General Anaesthetics

I. Inhalational general anaesthetics

- **Volatile liquids:** Diethyl ether; ethyl chloride; trichloroethylene; halothane; enflurane; isoflurane, desflurane, sevoflurane
- **Gases:** Nitrous oxide

II. Intravenous general anaesthetics

- **Ultra short-acting barbiturates:** Thiopental sodium; methohexital
- **Propofol**
- **Benzodiazepines:** Midazolam, diazepam
- **Phencyclidine derivative:** Ketamine
- **Opioid analgesics:** Morphine, fentanyl, sufentanil
- **Miscellaneous:** Etomidate, dexmedetomidine

PH 1.18

Mechanisms of action:

Molecular targets for anaesthetic agents are primarily proteins of the neuronal ligand gated ion channels.

1. Almost all the anaesthetic agents **potentiate the effect of inhibitory NT**, GABA at $GABA_A$ receptors. Their site of interaction at $GABA_A$ receptor subunits may vary.
2. They also act on other major channels associated with nicotinic receptors, $5\text{-}HT_3$, and glycine.
3. Volatile and gaseous anaesthetic agents activate the two-pore domain K^+ channels, which are

background K+ channels and **reduce neuronal excitability**. These are not affected by IV anaesthetics.

4. Nitrous oxide and ketamine **inhibit excitatory synaptic transmission** by binding to NMDA receptors. *The inhalational anaesthetics may also act on NMDA receptors.*
5. Some may inhibit presynaptic Na^+ channels and agents **inhibit the release of the presynaptic excitatory neurotransmitters.**

Thus the specific receptors vary from anaesthetic to anaesthetic (e.g. nicotinic receptors and NMDA for nitrous oxide; $GABA_A$ for most IV anaesthetics; and NMDA for ketamine). A single agent may have multiple mechanisms of action. Specific behavioural effects of an anaesthetic agent are attributable to the selectivity of the ion channel it acts on.

Although the general anaesthetics are capable of depressing all the functional elements of the CNS including the spinal cord, their clinical effects vary, depending on their chemical structure, and their ability to localise within CNS and interact with target sites. Specific cortical areas exhibit different sensitivities to inhalational and IV anaesthetics.

In general, the neurophysiological changes in midbrain reticular formation, thalamic sensory relay nuclei and part of cortex contribute to unconsciousness and analgesia. Loss of reflex responses to painful stimuli occur due to inhibition at spinal cord level. Short term amnesia is due to hippocampal inhibition. With increasing concentration, the motor, autonomic and respiratory controls are gradually lost. The margin between anaesthetic concentration required for surgical anaesthesia (see under 'Stages of anasthesia') and respiratory and cardiovascular depression is very narrow. Hence to maintain appropriate level of anaesthesia requires a skilled personnel.

INHALATIONAL GENERAL ANAESTHETICS

The factors which control the transfer of an inhalation anaesthetic agent from the alveoli to the blood, and from there into the brain, are as follows:

- **Its solubility in blood**
- **Its density:** The lighter the gas, the faster does it diffuse into and out of the tissues
- **Its partial pressure** in the anaesthetic mixture (solubility in blood is inversely proportional to the partial pressure), in the arterial and mixed venous blood, and in the tissues.
- **The rate of blood flow through the lungs and the tissues**

The lower the solubility of an anaesthetic agent in blood, the more rapid is the rise in partial pressure in arterial blood, e.g. nitrous oxide, desflurane, sevoflurane have low blood solubility, but they rapidly reach high arterial tensions. This leads to rapid equilibrium with the brain producing rapid induction. The highly soluble anaesthetic agents with high blood/gas partition coefficient, such as diethyl ether, show slow induction, slow recovery and a slow change in the depth of anaesthesia.

The higher the concentration of an anaesthetic agent in the inspired gas mixture, the greater will be the rise in partial pressure in the blood. Moderately soluble agents such as halothane enflurane and isoflurane can be used at a higher concentration to achieve rapid induction of anaesthesia, which can then be maintained with a lower concentration.

In addition, with a higher rate and depth of ventilation, the rise in partial pressure of anaesthetic agents with moderate to high blood solubility is high. Ventilation changes, however, do not influence the speed of induction of low-solubility agents.

The general anaesthetics have a low margin of safety, and the therapeutic indices vary from 2 to 4. It is also difficult to estimate the dose accurately. The anaesthesiologists describe the measure of potency of inhalation anaesthetic agents in terms of **minimum alveolar concentration** (MAC) of the anaesthetic, at 1 atm pressure, that produces ablation of movement in response to the surgical incision. Usually, 0.5–2 MAC is required for adequate anaesthesia. The MACs required for halothane and enflurane are 0.75 and 1.68, respectively, while the MAC for nitrous oxide is 105. Thus, nitrous oxide is a poor anaesthetic, when used alone.

Stages of anaesthesia: Guedel, in 1920, referring mainly to the anaesthetic ether, outlined the four stages of general anaesthesia as follows (Fig. 7.1):

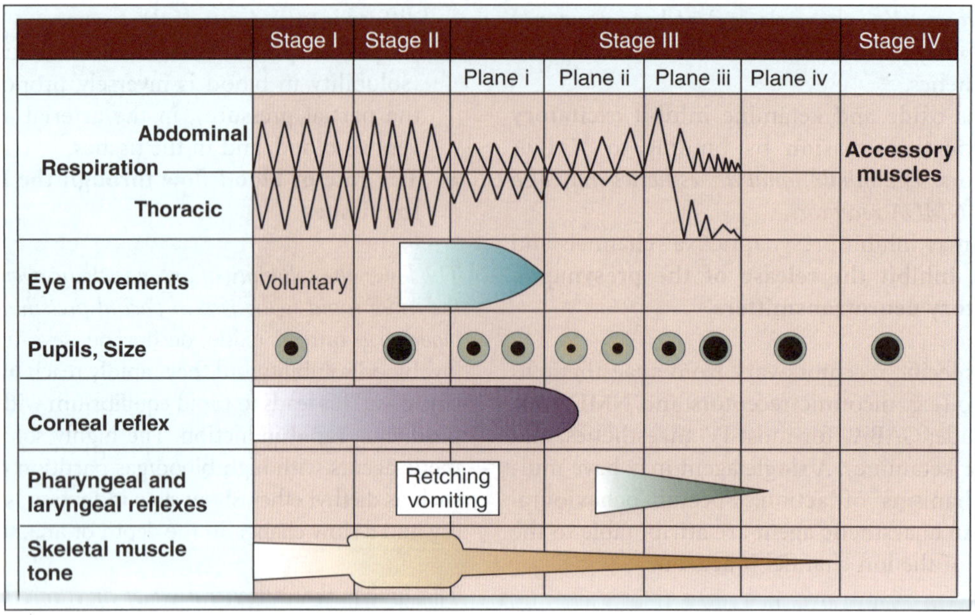

FIG. 7.1 The signs and stages of ether anaesthesia.

1. **Stage of analgesia**
2. **Stage of delirium or excitement**
3. **Stage of surgical anaesthesia:**
   This stage is further divided into 4 planes (i-iv) based on pupilary dilatation, muscle relaxation, BP and the pulse rate, and the loss of laryngeal reflex, pupillary light reflex and corneal reflex.
4. **Stage of respiratory paralysis**

In modern anaesthetic practice, the stages are never discerned separately because a combination of agents (balanced anaesthesia) is used. Usually a rapid and smooth induction is achieved with the help of an intravenous agent such as thiopental or propofol; the anaesthesia is maintained with inhalational drugs such as halothane or nitrous oxide– oxygen plus a volatile anaesthetic such as isoflurane. Such combinations are termed as **balanced anaesthesia** techniques, which utilise optimally favourable properties of anaesthetic agents, minimising their adverse effects.

Inadequate anaesthesia is indicated by the following:

- **Signs of ANS overactivity**, such as tachycardia, rise of BP, sweating and lacrimation
- **Grimacing**
- **Other muscle activity**

Surgical anaesthesia is indicated by the following:

- **Loss of eyelash (lid) reflex**
- **Development of rhythmic respiration**

Deep anaesthesia is suggested by the following:

- **Depression of respiration**
- **Hypotension**
- **Asystole**

Associated blood loss and hypoxia can aggravate the situation. They must be avoided.

Computer-assisted, EEG-based indices are now used to monitor cerebral functions and to decide anaesthetic requirements.

PH 1.18

VOLATILE LIQUID ANAESTHETICS

The volatile general anaesthetics which are liquid at room temperature are all extremely potent but relatively more soluble in blood, cell water and fat; hence, both induction and recovery with these agents are slower than that with the gaseous general anaesthetics.

DIETHYL ETHER: Ether (Fig. 7.2) is a colourless, volatile liquid with a pungent odour. Anaesthetic ether contains 96%–98% diethyl ether. Ether, when exposed to air, moisture or light may form ether peroxides or acetic aldehyde, which are irritant. To avoid this conversion, ether is marketed in sealed containers or amber-coloured bottles covered with a black paper.

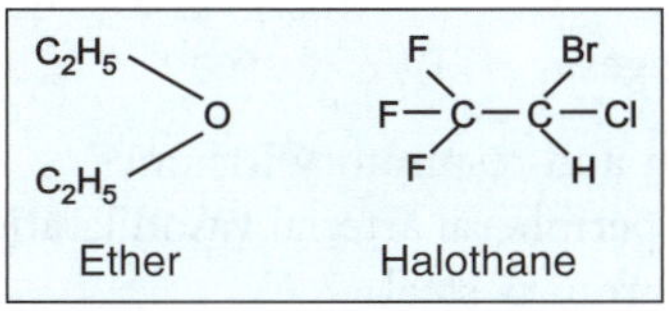

FIG. 7.2 **Chemical structures of ether and halothane.**

A concentration of 10%–15% of ether in the inspired air is usually required for induction, while a concentration of 4%–5% ensures a satisfactory maintenance of anaesthesia in plane iii (Fig. 7.1); with a concentration of more than 7%, respiratory failure may develop.

Absorption, fate and excretion: Only a minor portion of ether is oxidised within the body; 85%–90% is eliminated through the lungs and the remainder through the skin, urine, milk and sweat. Ether crosses the placental barrier and reaches comparable concentrations in the foetal blood.

Advantages:

- Can be administered without complicated apparatus and air can be used as a diluent and source of oxygen
- Can be used during an emergency without pre-anaesthetic medication
- Has a wide margin of safety
- Excellent analgesic
- Curarimimetic and hence causes satisfactory muscle relaxation
- Reflex stimulant of respiration and bronchodilator
- Less likely to precipitate cardiac arrhythmias
- Little hepato-/nephrotoxicity
- Can be used during delivery
- Cheap

Disadvantages:

- Inflammable and explosive, and therefore potentially hazardous; cautery cannot be used
- Induction is slow and may be stormy; and recovery slow
- Irritant and may cause nausea/vomiting. Increase in salivary and bronchial secretion may cause cough/laryngeal spasm
- May rarely cause cardiac arrest
- May cause convulsion, especially in children
- Exhibits cross-tolerance with ethyl alcohol

HALOTHANE: It is a fluorinated volatile anaesthetic with structural similarity to chloroform (Fig. 7.2). It is a heavy, colourless liquid with a characteristic sweet, fruity odour.

Halothane readily attacks most of the metals including stainless steel, brass and copper and may also affect the rubber elements of the anaesthetic equipment.

Halothane produces the loss of consciousness in a concentration of 2%–3% in oxygen vapour, and the anaesthesia can be maintained by using 1%–2% of halothane vapour with oxygen and nitrous oxide.

Absorption, fate and excretion: About 60%–80% of halothane is eliminated unchanged through the lungs in the first 24 h. About 20% appears to be retained in the body and is probably metabolised.

Advantages:

- Noninflammable and nonirritant to the respiratory tract; hence not unpleasant for induction. It has a fruity odour
- Potent anaesthetic with speedy induction and recovery
- Inhibits pharyngeal and laryngeal reflexes, making tracheal intubation easy. It does not cause laryngospasm, bronchospasm or coughing but in fact causes bronchodilatation
- Postoperative vomiting infrequent
- Can induce controlled hypotension and a bloodless field; to be used only by experts for this purpose

Disadvantages:

- Special apparatus is required
- Inadequate muscular relaxation for abdominal surgery; slow postoperative recovery
- Poor analgesic
- Depresses respiration

- Can raise intracranial tension due to cerebral vasodilatation
- Causes hypotension by direct depression of the myocardium, and sensitizes the heart to catecholamines, causing cardiac arrhythmias; a major drawback
- Postoperative recovery of mental function slow; shivering during recovery common
- Induces hepatocellular microsomal enzyme; rarely, may cause delayed allergic hepatic necrosis due to the toxic metabolite and trifluoroacetyl chloride
- Can cause malignant hyperthermia in susceptible individuals.

ENFLURANE: This halogenated volatile liquid anaesthetic is chemically 2-chloro 1, 1, 2-trifluoroethyl difluoromethyl ether. It is noninflammable, with mild, sweet odour and boils at 57°C. Chemically, it is very stable. About 80% of enflurane is excreted unchanged by the lungs and only 2%−5% is metabolised by the liver.

Anaesthesia produced by enflurane resembles that produced by halothane, except that the muscular relaxation is better and tachypnoea is uncommon. It causes hypotension, and it potentiates the activity of nondepolarising muscle relaxants. Further, it depresses the myocardial contraction force and sensitises the heart to the actions of catecholamines. Hence, it **can cause cardiac arrhythmias**. Like halothane, it causes bronchodilatation.

The compound could produce seizures and involuntary motor activity during deep anaesthesia. Hence, it is relatively contraindicated in patients with epilepsy and brain lesions. Compared to halothane, liver damage is rare.

ISOFLURANE: This volatile liquid with pungent odour is related to enflurane. Its pharmacological properties are similar to those of halothane, but it is less liable to cause hypotension. The drug is metabolised only to the extent of 0.2%.

Advantages:

- Physically stable and noninflammable
- Rapid induction and recovery of anaesthesia
- Bronchodilator
- Good muscle relaxant
- Potent coronary vasodilator; does not affect renal blood flow
- Less likely to sensitise the myocardium to adrenaline
- Hepatotoxicity rare
- Considered by many as the 'near ideal' anaesthetic; the preferred agent in neurosurgery

Disadvantages:

- Pungent and respiratory irritant
- Causes peripheral arterial vasodilatation and can cause coronary steal
- Does not protect against local ischemia

Desflurane has properties similar to those of isoflurane. It is extremely volatile, with pungent odour. It has a rapid onset of action and rapid recovery. It may cause cough, salivation and bronchospasm. Hence, it is not preferred for induction of anaesthesia. **Sevoflurane** is nonirritating to the respiratory tract and can be used for induction of anaesthesia in children as it is pleasant to inhale.

GASEOUS ANAESTHETICS

NITROUS OXIDE: Nitrous oxide is a colourless, inorganic gas with a sweet taste. It does not undergo significant decomposition in the body.

Nitrous oxide, if administered along with air, produces a stage of excitement and delirium and also produces amnesia. Hence the name 'laughing gas'. It is commonly used together with oxygen and other agents such as isoflurane.

Nitrous oxide produces analgesia when inhaled in the concentration of 35%–40% with air. Loss of consciousness occurs with the concentration of 65%–70%, and plane i of surgical anaesthesia can be reached with an 80:20 mixture of nitrous oxide and oxygen. A further increase in the concentration of the anaesthetic agent produces hypoxia.

Nitrous oxide has no serious, deleterious effects on circulation, respiration, the liver and the kidneys, and it is probably the safest anaesthetic agent.

Absorption, fate and excretion: Nitrous oxide is not altered within the body and is carried in the form of a physical solution in the blood. It is rapidly eliminated through the lungs within 2–5 min after its withdrawal.

Advantages:

- Noninflammable and nonirritant
- Rapid induction and recovery
- Analgesic in subanaesthetic concentration
- Nausea and vomiting are uncommon

Disadvantages:

- Not a potent anaesthetic agent by itself; must be supplemented with another pre anaesthetic agent or a muscle relaxant
- Excitement may be violent
- CO_2 accumulation and hypoxia may develop during prolonged use
- Diffusion hypoxia develops at the time of discontinuation of nitrous oxide and is dangerous in patients with a low cardiopulmonary reserve, which can be prevented by the administration of 100% oxygen while discontinuing nitrous oxide
- A special apparatus is required
- *An increase in spontaneous abortions has been reported in the wives of male dentists and in female chairside, dentists' assistants*
- Any closed gas-filled space tends to expand during the administration of nitrous oxide; therefore, contraindicated in patients with collections of air in the pleural, pericardial or peritoneal cavities; intestinal obstruction; occlusion of the middle ear; chronic obstructive airway disease; or emphysema; also contraindicated in patients who have recently undergone pneumoencephalography
- May cause hallucinations; female patients might allege sexual misbehaviour by the doctor; also seen after propofol anaesthesia

Indications: It may be used for tooth extraction, obstetric analgesia and during painful procedures such as changing dressings in burns patients, cleaning and debridement of wounds and cauterisation.

When nitrous oxide is given in a high concentration (70%–80%) with another potent inhalational anaesthetic such as halothane, it facilitates delivery of the latter to blood at a higher rate and helps in achieving faster induction. This effect is termed as **second gas effect**.

On the other hand, when nitrous oxide is discontinued, a large amount of nitrous oxide rapidly diffuses into the alveoli from the blood owing to its low blood solubility. This dilutes the alveolar air causing a drop in the partial pressure of oxygen in the alveoli. The gas also dilutes the alveolar carbon dioxide, causing a decreased drive for ventilation. During this time, breathing room air results in hypoxia, which is termed as **diffusion hypoxia**. This hypoxia can be prevented by the administration of 100% oxygen 5–10 min after discontinuing nitrous oxide.

Other Indication: Measurement of coronary/cerebral blood flow by the Fick principle.

Xenon: It is a rapidly acting potent inhalational anaesthetic agent, which is very expensive. It is a noncompetitive antagonist of NMDA receptors and agonist of TREK channels (two-pore K^+ channels). It is well tolerated even by elderly.

As modern surgery makes increasing use of electronic devices, inflammable and/or explosive anaesthetics such as ether are now considered obsolete in many advanced countries. *Open ether, however, is still being used in many developing countries and is considered as a relatively safe anaesthetic despite its inflammable and explosive nature, particularly when a qualified anaesthetist and anaesthetic equipment are not available.*

NONVOLATILE GENERAL ANAESTHETICS

Ultra short-acting barbiturates: These have very high lipid solubility compared to other barbiturates (Chapter 6). Their chemical structure (*viz.* presence of sulphur at C2 instead of oxygen) is responsible for it. Because of high lipid solubility, they have rapid onset and short duration of action. Hence they are used intravenously to produce general anaesthesia. The agents employed most commonly are **thiopental** and **methohexitone**. Methohexitone is twice as potent as thiopental and shorter acting.

THIOPENTAL: Thiopental sodium is readily soluble in water, but the solution deteriorates on keeping. The clinically used solution is intensely alkaline (pH 10.5 -11) and can cause local irritation and venous thrombosis. Given intravenously, it rapidly induces hypnosis and anaesthesia – without analgesia.

Anaesthetic action: The induction is very quick and pleasant. Consciousness is lost first, then the reflex activity and muscle tone, and lastly, the vital medullary centres are depressed. Pupils react to light and remain contracted in light hypnosis. The corneal reflex remains active until deep anaesthesia is achieved. *Cerebral blood flow and cerebral metabolic rate are reduced, and there is a marked reduction of intracranial tension. It also reduces cerebral metabolism. It is, therefore, a choice for patients with cerebral swelling.*

A fairly reliable sign of an adequate induction by thiopental is the absence of the eyelid reflex. The presence of swallowing, phonation and reflex movements of eyes during anaesthesia indicates a need for further injection.

Although the reflexes return in 10–30 min, after stoppage the patient remains disoriented for several hours, and hence must not be left alone (see below).

Absorption, fate and excretion: Thiopental being highly lipophilic, distributes very rapidly to highly perfused tissues like brain. The rapid accumulation in brain results in induction of anesthesia within minutes after its IV administration. However, thiopental also leaves the brain tissue rapidly to get distributed throughout the body into the moderately or poorly perfused tissues such as the muscle and fat. This **redistribution phenomenon** is responsible for its short duration of action and rapid recovery from anesthesia.

The rapid metabolism of the drug by the liver may also contribute to its short duration of action. With successive doses, body fat depots get saturated with the drug. Slow release of the stored drug back into the plasma is responsible for the prolonged recovery and continuation of drowsiness observed after the cessation of anaesthesia. Large doses or IV infusion progressively increases accumulation of drug, and also the steady state blood concentration. This results in saturation of its metabolism. The resultant zero order kinetics elimination decreases the safety margin. *Hence it is used only for induction and not for maintenance of anaesthesia.*

Thiopental readily crosses the placental barrier and appears in breast milk.

Advantages:

- Nonexplosive and nonirritant; easy to administer
- Very rapid and smooth induction, and rapid recovery after small doses
- Quiet respiration; no cardiac arrhythmias.
- Nausea, vomiting, excitement and postoperative complications are infrequent

Disadvantages:

- Poor analgesic and muscle relaxant
- Conducting anaesthesia and judging its depth are difficult as the usual stages of anaesthesia are not discernible
- Pharyngeal and laryngeal reflexes persist, permitting occurrence of coughing, apnoea, laryngospasm and bronchospasm; hence, *equipment for controlled ventilation must be available*
- Depression of the respiratory centre
- Depresses the myocardium and vasomotor centre and produces hypotension; *must never be given to a patient who is sitting,* for example, in a dental chair
- Highly irritant if extravasated; nerve palsy and limb gangrene reported
- Relaxes gastroesophageal sphincter, causing silent regurgitation
- *Can precipitate acute attack in patients with acute intermittent porphyria*

Barbiturate anaesthesia is to be used with great caution in the presence of hepatic and/or renal damage, in shock, in airway obstruction, in individuals with a past history of bronchial asthma or severe cardiovascular disease.

Preparations and dosages:

i. Thiopental sodium, 0.5–1.0 g powder; used as a freshly prepared, 2.5%–5% solution for IV anaesthesia. It is administered at a dose of 100–150 mg for induction of anesthesia via IV route. This dose should be repeated every 30–60 sec but not exceeding 500 mg.

ii. Methohexitone: twice as potent as thiopental and shorter acting; used as a 1% solution. The IV induction dose is 50–120 mg at rate of 10 mg every 5 seconds and maintenance dose is 20–40 mg every 4–7 minutes. Alternatively, it can be given as continuous infusion using a 0.2% solution at 3 mL/min.

Indications:

- **For induction** of general anaesthesia
- **As anaesthetic agent for operations of short durations**, e.g. fracture reduction, dilatation and curettage, laryngoscopy and bronchoscopy; methohexitone preferred during electroconvulsive therapy (ECT) as it increases ictal activity
- **As an anaesthetic** in patients with a history of malignant hyperthermia, head injury and brain tumour to lower intracranial pressure.
- **As anticonvulsant** in the emergency treatment of intractable seizures

PROPOFOL: This IV anaesthetic causes rapid induction and rapid recovery with a small hangover effect. It is generally used for sedation, induction and maintenance of general anaesthesia and for brief ambulatory procedures. It causes dose-dependent cortical depression and is an anticonvulsant. It is largely (88%) metabolised by the liver and partly cleared by the other mechanisms.

Advantages:

- Has a specific antiemetic action and is less likely to cause bronchospasm
- Has no effect on the hypoxic, pulmonary vascular reflexes
- Because of quick and pleasant recovery from anaesthesia, is now preferred to thiopental for intubation, endoscopy and day-care surgery
- Is safe during pregnancy
- May be combined with an ultra-short-acting opioid such as remifentanil

Disadvantages:

- Narrow therapeutic window
- Excess dose can cause greater sedation, myocardial and respiratory depressant effects than other IV agents
- Prolonged IV infusion can lead to cumulation with sedation and acidosis; results in **propofol infusion syndrome** seen in patients with a head injury.
- The emulsion formulations painful; pretreatment/mixing with lignocaine can reduce the pain.

Preparations and dosage:

Propofol emulsion, 1% (10mg/ml) and 2% (20mg/ml) for injection or infusion. Approximate dose is 40 mg every 10 secs, which is titrated against the patient's response until clinical signs show the onset of anesthesia.

Fospropofol, a water-soluble prodrug, is claimed to cause less pain on IV injection. It is hydrolysed by endothelial alkaline phosphatase to propofol.

MIDAZOLAM: This short-acting benzodiazepine (BZD; Chapter 8) is used either intramuscularly or intravenously for sedation and anaesthesia. It is also used as pre-medication or as anaesthetic adjuvant due to its sedative, anxiolytic and amnestic properties. Its onset of action is rapid, and t½ is 2−4 h.

Indications: For induction, an initial IV dose of 0.3 to 0.35 mg/kg is administered over 20 to 30 seconds. The effect is observed after 2 min. For complete induction, increments of approximately 25% of the patient's initial dose may be used or induction may instead be completed with inhalational anesthetics. If the patient has received opioid pre-medication, the recommended doses should be reduced to 0.15 to 0.35 mg/kg.

For sedation/anxiolysis/amnesia, 0.07 to 0.08 mg/kg IM (approximately 5 mg IM) is administered upto 1 hour before surgery.

With the IV administration of midazolam, the same precautions are required as with IV diazepam. It is water soluble and less irritant to the veins than diazepam (Chapter 8). It has also been used by SC infusion (by a syringe pump) as an anticonvulsant. It is a relatively safe drug.

Remimazolam is an ultra-short-acting IV BZD (Chapter 8) for sedation and general anaesthesia. For induction of anesthesia, a short infusion of 6 or 12 mg/kg/h and for maintenance, continuous infusion of 1–2 mg/kg/h is employed. It has faster onset of action and short duration (30 min) than midazolam. This is because of its metabolism by carboxylesterase 1 (CSE1).

Both the BZD have low liability for respiratory and cardiovascular depression; they cause minimal pain on injection and they have reversal agent flumazenil (Chapter 8).

BZD do not produce true general anaesthesia, as the awareness about the surrounding remains, so also the mobility; hence, surgical procedures are difficult to carry out under BZD anaesthesia given alone. Hence they are co-administered with opioid analgesic like fentanyl/ remifentanil and neuromuscular blocker like rocuronium. PH 1.22

KETAMINE: This agent is chemically related to phencyclidine and acts as an antagonist at NMDA receptors. It probably acts on the cerebral cortex, particularly the limbic system. It has the analgesic property in subnarcotic doses, and light anaesthesia usually does not cause depression of the protective pharyngeal and laryngeal reflexes. It is a potent bronchodilator.

Given intravenously, it is quick acting, although the onset of action is slower than that of thiopental. Following a single dose, it induces a state of **dissociative anaesthesia** characterised by complete analgesia combined with amnesia and catatonia, with or without the loss of consciousness. The patient can open his eyes and can obey instructions. Respiratory support is not needed. Analgesia lasts for about 40 min, whereas anaesthesia lasts for about 15 min due to rapid redistribution.

Anaesthesia can be induced by both IM (5−10 mg/kg) and IV (1−2 mg/kg) routes. A low dose 0.2 to 0.5 mg/kg IV or 0.06−0.12 mg/kg/h infusion produces adequate *analgesia* and is an alternative to opioids to minimise respiratory depression.

The drug increases the BP, heart rate and cardiac output by activating central sympathetic system and preventing peripheral reuptake of NA. It can be used in patients in shock. **However, it should be avoided in patients with an ischemic heart disease.**

Disadvantages

- Sometimes causes nystagmus, involuntary movements and hypertonus.
- May cause delirium, hallucinations and colourful dreams during induction and recovery, especially in adults; diazepam, midazolam or propofol given prior to ketamine can prevent these disturbances
- Rarely, laryngospasm may occur; salivation may be troublesome
- Muscular relaxation inadequate
- Increases intraocular and intracranial pressures
- *Is a drug of abuse* **(date rape drug)**

Indications: It can be used as an inducing agent, but its use in low dose, in combination with other anaesthetic agents such as propofol, is preferred. It is of choice in poor-risk elderly, children and patients with asthma. It is used for short-lasting diagnostic procedures such as cardiac catheterisation and bronchoscopy, dressing of burns, forceps delivery, breech extraction, manual removal of the placenta and dental work.

It is not used:

- In patients suffering from hypertension, cardiac decompensation or a cerebrovascular accident.
- For surgery of the pharynx, larynx or bronchi.
- In abdominal surgery, as it relieves visceral pain poorly.
- In thyrotoxic patients, in whom it may cause rise in blood pressure.
- In pregnant women at term, because of its oxytocic activity. *However, it may be used during caesarian section as it causes less fetal and neonatal depression.*
- During operations on the eye, as it causes a rise in the intra-ocular pressure.
- In the presence of psychiatric disorders such as acute psychosis and schizophrenia.

Barbiturates and diazepam are chemically incompatible with ketamine. They should never be administered from the same syringe or via the same infusion set.

ETOMIDATE: This drug, a carboxylated imidazole, has potent hypnotic and anaesthetic properties. A single IV dose of 0.3 mg/kg produces the loss of consciousness within 10 s and a state of anaesthesia, followed by sleep. Recovery is rapid and complete due to redistribution. In fact, cardiovascular stability during and after induction is considered to be a major advantage of etomidate; hence, it is preferred in elderly patients prone to hemodynamic instability and those with a poor cardiovascular reserve. The drug, however, commonly causes pain on injection, myoclonus and postoperative nausea and vomiting.

Indication: It is primarily used for induction, along with opioid analgesics, as etomidate has no analgesic effect. Opioids help during endotracheal intubation and reduce involuntary muscle movements.

NEUROLEPTANALGESIA

Neuroleptics (antipsychotics) are a group of drugs which induce a state of apathy and mental detachment in which the patient is mildly sedated and uncaring about his or her surroundings. These compounds are used in the treatment of major psychoses and are discussed in detail in Chapter 13. **Neuroleptanalgesia** is a method of IV anaesthesia which combines the use of a **neuroleptic drug with an opioid analgesic drug**. Such a combination produces a state which differs from the classical general anaesthesia in that the subject is conscious and is able to cooperate during the operative procedure. The most favoured combination in clinical practice is that of the neuroleptic droperidol and the analgesic fentanyl.

DROPERIDOL: This is a butyrophenone derivative like haloperidol. Its pharmacological actions are similar to those of chlorpromazine (Chapter 13), but it is short acting (2−3 h) and more potent than haloperidol. Apart from typical behavioural effect of calming, droperidol also has antiemetic and alpha-adrenergic blocking (adrenolytic) actions. Like all neuroleptic drugs, it can produce extrapyramidal reactions.

FENTANYL: This drug belongs to the group of 4-acylanilino piperidines. It is a morphine-like opioid analgesic (Chapter 10) that is used exclusively as a supplementary analgesic in inducing general anaesthesia. Like morphine, it suppresses the respiratory and cough centres and causes nausea, vomiting and miosis. It is 80-100 times more potent than morphine. However, its action is of shorter duration. These actions can be antagonised by naloxone.

Droperidol 2.5 mg and **fentanyl citrate** 50 mcg in 1 mL, given intravenously, causes complete analgesia and amnesia sufficient for surgical procedures without marked hypnosis. The onset of anaesthesia is slow.

Major **advantages** of this procedure are as follows:

- Smooth onset and rapid postanaesthetic recovery
- Less danger of hypotension and other circulatory disturbances
- Suppression of vomiting and coughing
- Continued analgesia in the postoperative period
- Availability of patient's cooperation during the operative procedures such as eye, oral and orthopaedic surgery, angiocardiography, myelography and bronchoscopy

Because the combination does not disturb the cardiovascular dynamics, it is claimed to be very useful in old people and in 'poor risk' cases. Furthermore, the combination can be used to induce anaesthesia which can then be continued with other general anaesthetic agents such as nitrous oxide−oxygen mixture and muscle relaxants.

Adverse reactions: They are due to toxicity of individual drugs. They include hallucinations, mental depression, extrapyramidal disturbances due to droperidol and respiratory depression due to fentanyl. The latter may be marked and assisted, and controlled ventilation is necessary. Post-operative drowsiness and cardiac dysrhythmias may precipitate due to the combination.

As compared to droperidol, fentanyl has a shorter duration of analgesic action (30 min) and supplementary doses of fentanyl (1 mcg/kg) may be needed after 20 min.

Fentanyl, alfentanil sufentanil and **remifentanil** are sometimes used as IV analgesics in short operations because of their brief duration of action. They can be used as coinducing agents.

A high dose of morphine can be used with benzodiazepines to achieve anaesthesia in patients for cardiac surgery when the circulatory reserve is limited.

AS 4.3

RATIONAL USE OF ANAESTHETIC AGENTS

Selection of appropriate general anaesthetic agent depends on **drug-related factors** and the **host-related factors**. The former include characteristics of the drug, its pharmacokinetic features, effects on the homeostasis and ADR. Host-related factors include the procedure the patient is undergoing, the time required for the same, patient's characteristics such as age, comorbid conditions and concomitant medications.

Careful attention needs to be paid to minimise adverse effects of the drugs, maintain homeostasis and facilitate smooth postanaesthetic recovery. Minor surgical and diagnostic procedures can be performed safely under judicious use of sedation-based techniques without using general anaesthesia.

Many protocols are available to achieve analgesia and deep sedation using various agents in combination. For example, in **monitored anaesthesia care technique,** midazolam IV is used as pre-medication followed by propofol infusion for deep sedation and opioid analgesic/ketamine for analgesia.

Conscious anaesthesia technique employs use of small doses of IV anaesthetics such as propofol and midazolam along with opioid analgesics to produce pain and an anxiety-free altered level of consciousness. *In this state, no respiratory support is needed and the patient can respond to commands.* This technique can also be used in ICU for patients under stress and on mechanical ventilators by using additional agents such as muscle relaxants and dexmedetomidine.

Deep sedation technique produces a state like light GA from which the patient cannot be aroused easily. The protective reflexes are lost, and surgical stimuli do not elicit any verbal responses. Thiopental, midazolam, propofol, ketamine and potent opioid analgesics given intravenously can be used for this purpose.

PH 1.18. AS 4.1

PH 1.18. AS 4.1

PREANAESTHETIC MEDICATION

Preanaesthetic medication is the term applied to drugs used before the administration of an anaesthetic agent, with the object of making anaesthesia safer and more agreeable to the patient. The reasons for such medication are as follows:

- *For sedation, to reduce anxiety and apprehension* without producing much drowsiness
- *To obtain an additive or synergistic effect, so that induction could be smooth and rapid* and the dose of the general anaesthetic could be reduced
- *To counteract certain adverse effects of the anaesthetic drug used* such as salivation, bradycardia and vomiting
- *To relieve pre- and postoperative pain*
- *To suppress respiratory secretions and to reduce reflex excitability*

There is no single drug which can achieve all these objectives, and hence usually a combination of drugs is used. It must be emphasised, however, that factors other than drugs can favourably affect preoperative psychological preparation, and a preoperative visit by the anaesthesiologist and a sympathetic discussion with the patient about the events of the next day have a high therapeutic value.

The drugs commonly used for preanaesthetic medication are as follows:

1. **Opioid analgesics** such as morphine (10−15 mg IM), pethidine (50−100 mg IM) and buprenorphine (300 mcg IM) are generally employed for their sedative and analgesic properties before major surgery. Epidural and intrathecal routes allow a low dose to produce analgesia with less systemic side effects. Buprenorphine has a longer duration of action than morphine and pethidine (Chapter 10). They also reduce the amount of general anaesthetic required.
   Disadvantages:
   - They may depress respiration and may cause respiratory arrest. Furthermore, drugs like morphine increase the tone of smooth muscles such as bronchial muscles. In emphysema or in kyphoscoliosis where the pulmo-

nary reserve is already low, the use of opioids may precipitate pulmonary insufficiency.

- They may cause vasomotor depression and may decrease the ability of circulation to respond to stress. They often delay the awakening as their clinical effect lasts for 4−6 h.
- Morphine may induce vomiting and cause antidiuresis.
- Pethidine by its vagolytic action may produce tachycardia.
- Both these drugs are histamine liberators. Fentanyl and its congeners are used to overcome some of these effects (See earlier). Fentanyl is administered as 50 to 100 mcg intramuscularly 30 to 60 minutes prior to surgery or intravenously immediately before surgery.

2. **Sedatives:** Benzodiazepines (midazolam diazepam, lorazepam) are preferred because of their safety, muscle relaxant property and less respiratory depression (Chapter 8). They also provide amnesia. Diazepam in dose of 5 to 20 mg has been most widely used. It is active orally and can also be given parenterally, although its action is less predictable by the latter route. Other sedatives used belong to the phenothiazine class. Phenothiazines possess sedative, antiarrhythmic, antiemetic and antihistaminic properties. Phenothiazines commonly employed are promethazine and trimeprazine. They can be given orally as well as parenterally (Chapter 13).
   Phenothiazines and benzodiazepines should not be combined with opioids particularly in patients with respiratory insufficiency.
   Dexmedetomidine: This imidazole derivative causes analgesia and sedation with very little respiratory depression by its central and peripheral α_2 adrenergic receptor agonist action. Its main adverse effects are hypotension and bradycardia. It is used intravenously for short-term sedation of critically ill adults and as an anaesthetic adjunct.
3. **Antimuscarinic drugs:** Atropine (600 mcg IM) is generally combined with morphine to block the vagal actions, so as to reduce salivary and respiratory secretions and to prevent parasympathetically induced reflex hypotension and bradycardia. It may thus lessen the possibility of cardiac arrhythmias during the induction stage. Because of the blockade of cardiac vagal action, atropine may produce tachycardia.
   However, with newer anaesthetics, atropine is less commonly used. Instead, a synthetic long-acting quaternary amine, such as **glycopyrrolate,** is now the preferred antimuscarinic agent because of its less central actions and less tendency to cause excessive tachycardia (Chapter 20).
4. **Antiemetics:** The commonly used phenothiazines such as **promethazine** and **trimeprazine** have antiemetic properties and may thus help to prevent the postoperative nausea and vomiting. This advantage should, however, be weighed against the possible hypotension following these drugs. 5-HT_3 antagonist, ondansetron, is also used. Other drugs used are **cyclizine**, 50 mg, **trimethobenzamide** 200 mg and **benzquinamide** 25−50 mg.
5. **Other drugs:** In addition to the use of above mentioned drugs, proper pre-evaluation and specific pre-medication are needed in patients with special problems such as a chronic lung disease, emphysema, ischemic heart disease, diabetes mellitus, hypertension, undernutrition and in debilitated and old people. Antibiotic prophylaxis may be needed (Chapter 49).

The risk of stopping long-term medication before surgery is often greater than the risk of continuing it during surgery. This applies particularly to glucocorticoids, analgesics, antiparkinsonian drugs, antiglaucoma drugs, and thyroid or antithyroid drugs. On the other hand, it is advisable to discontinue combined oral contraceptive pills 4 weeks before major surgery; monoamine-oxidase inhibitors 2 weeks before surgery; warfarin 3−5 days before surgery; aspirin 7 days before surgery; and lithium 2 days before surgery.

DRUGS ADMINISTERED DURING ANAESTHESIA

AS 4.1

- **Skeletal muscle relaxants** such as succinyl choline and curarimimetics to achieve good muscle relaxation (Chapter 22).
- **A very short-acting ganglion blocking agent** such as trimethaphan camphor sulphonate or sodium nitroprusside to produce controlled hypotension (Chapter 30).

- **Drugs administered to counter the anaesthetic complications,** for example, vasopressor agents (such as methoxamine or phenylephrine) to correct hypotension, antiarrhythmics to correct cardiac arrhythmias and anticonvulsants. FM 10.1

The prophylactic administration of supplementary glucocorticoids to patients receiving steroid therapy or those with a history of such therapy within 2 years before surgery is necessary to avoid serious hypotension and shock during surgery. Antibiotics such as streptomycin and neomycin (aminoglycosides) have a neuromuscular blocking action and hence can produce skeletal muscle paralysis when instilled into pleural or peritoneal cavity during anaesthesia; these drugs can also potentiate the actions of curarimimetic, skeletal muscle relaxants (Chapter 45). Patients on beta-adrenergic blockers tend to develop hypotension more often following certain anaesthetic agents. FM 10.1

Malignant hyperthermia is a serious but rare complication of general anaesthesia (see Chapter 22).

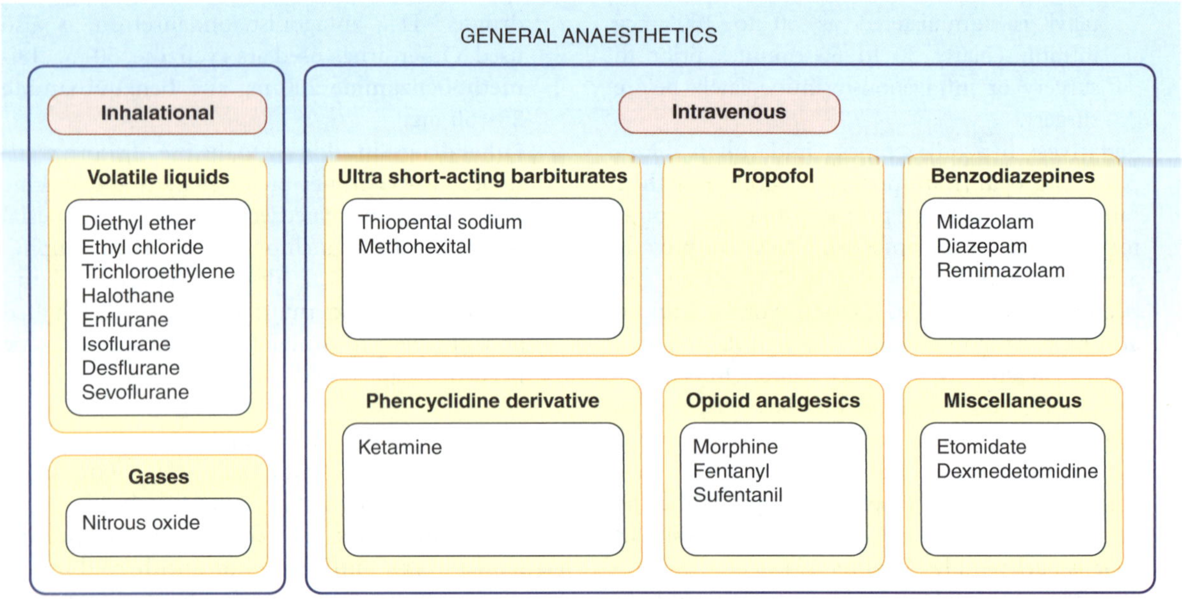

CHAPTER 8

Sedatives, Hypnotics and Pharmacotherapy of Sleep Disorders

Learning Objectives

This chapter will enable the reader:

1. To be aware of components of sleep cycle with EEG changes.
2. To classify hypnotics.
3. To describe the mechanism of action, pharmacological effects, ADR, salient pharmacokinetic features and indications for benzodiazepines.
4. To compare benzodiazepines with nonbenzodiazepines, selective melatonin receptor agonists, orexin receptor antagonists, low doses of antidepressants and sedative antihistaminics with respect to hypnotic effects, adverse effects and use in therapy.
5. To explain the pharmacological basis for the use of flumazenil in benzodiazepine overdosage.
6. To state limitations of barbiturates as a hypnotic agent.
7. To discuss the management of insomnia based on its types.
8. To enlist the drugs causing insomnia.
9. To mention the drugs used to treat other sleep disorders, giving the rationale.

KEY TERMS

Good refreshing sleep is necessary for a healthy life. Physiologically, sleep is regarded as the absence of wakefulness where the responses to environmental stimuli are greatly reduced. But, in fact, it is an active state, related to definite anatomic structures as well to several neurotransmitters and biogenic amines. Yet, its exact mechanism is not known.

The determinants of natural sleep are many, but the most important regulator is probably a 'central pacemaker' (or the biological clock) in the ventrolateral preoptic (VLPO) hypothalamus. Clock genes determine the circadian rhythm that maintains the normal daily sleep–awake cycle. REM sleep, modulated by the circadian system, is associated with increased melatonin secretion by the pineal gland.

Melatonin acts mainly on two receptors MT1 and MT2 which are found in hypothalamus, hippocampus, cerebellum and other parts of the brain. It is involved in the sleep–wake cycle, lowering of the body core temperature (thermal regulator) and an increased plasma concentration of cortisol. Physiologically, nocturnal high plasma concentration of melatonin correlates with an increased sleep propensity. It plays an important role in the circadian timings system (*chronobiotic actions*).

On the basis of electrophysiological studies (EEG, electromyogram and electro-oculogram), sleep has been classified as (a) **nonrapid eye movement sleep** (NREM) and (b) **rapid eye movement sleep** (REM).

While falling asleep, one passes sequentially through stages N1, N2, and N3 of NREM sleep. After about 75–90 min of NREM sleep, REM sleep occurs, lasting for 10–30 min. The NREM–REM cycle repeats four to five times during the night, with progressive lengthening of the REM bouts and shortening of N3 until one awakens from REM (not NREM) sleep in the morning. Both, NREM and REM stages are important for sleep efficiency and quality.

In general, NREM stages N1 and N2 constitute 50%–60%, NREM stage N3 (slow wave) 15%–25%, whereas REM 20%–25% of the total sleep in young adults. Slow wave sleep is prominent in children and decreases with the age, so that it may even be absent in healthy old people.

Table 8.1 Sleep Characteristics of NREM and REM Sleep

NREM	REM
No Rapid Eyeball Movements	Rapid Eyeball Movements
Peaceful and sound sleep	Not so restful
Predominance of parasympathetic activity	Predominance of sympathetic activity
Decrease in the heart rate, cardiac output, peripheral vascular resistance, respiratory and metabolic rate, slowing of eye movements	Marked increase in the heart rate, BP, cardiac output, peripheral vascular resistance, small airway resistance and metabolic rate. Breathing becomes fast and shallow with short periods of central apnoea
Secretion of adrenal steroids is at their lowest and of growth hormone is at its highest	
Progressive diminution of muscle tone (except those muscles which hold the chin up and keep the middle respiratory passages open)	All voluntary muscles, especially arm and leg muscles remain flaccid (except extraocular muscles)
Sleep deepens progressively during its 3 stages and to awaken a person becomes increasingly difficult	Easy to awaken a person.
Brain activity is low	Brain is highly active with an increased oxygen consumption
Dreams infrequent and are rarely recalled	75% of the dreams in REM sleep; vivid, bizarre and often sexual, with erections occurring in the males.
EEG shows slow waves (Delta waves) in N3 stage	EEG resembles that of an awake and alert person. It shows a beta rhythm,
Incidences of ischaemic cerebrovascular strokes due to relative hypotension during N3 stage	Incidences of obstructive sleep apnoea due to excessive muscle hypotonia and hypertensive–hypoxic cardiovascular events due to catecholamine secretion

The differences between NREM and REM sleep are depicted in Table 8.1

A normal person spends about one-third of his life in sleep. In practice, many individuals complain of disturbed or lack of sleep, **insomnia**.

A **hypnotic** drug is one which produces sleep that resembles natural sleep. A **sedative**, on the other hand, is a drug that reduces excitement, calms the patient, and is commonly used as an **anxiolytic**. Hypnotics and sedatives both depress the CNS, the difference being quantitative. PH 1.19

Classification of Hypnotics

All hypnotics act on different subunits of GABA receptors (Chapters 5 and 9). They are classified as follows:

I. **Selective, benzodiazepine, $GABA_A$ receptor agonists:**
   a. **Benzodiazepines**, e.g. diazepam, oxazepam and lorazepam
   b. **Nonbenzodiazepines**, e.g. zopiclone, zolpidem, zaleplon (Z drugs)

II. **Melatonin receptor agonist:** Ramelteon

III. **Orexin receptor antagonist:** Suvorexant

IV. **Miscellaneous:**
   a. **Sedative antihistaminics**, e.g. diphenhydramine and promethazine
   b. **Tricyclic antidepressants**, e.g. doxepin, amitriptyline

Before the advent of BZD, barbiturate class of drugs were available as sedative-hypnotics. However their use is currently restricted to antiepileptic (Chapter 9) and anaesthetic agents (Chapter 7). Drugs such as morphine and pethidine, besides acting as opioid analgesics, also possess hypnotic property. Hence, they are grouped as **Anodyne hypnotics**. However, they should not be used as hypnotics in the absence of severe pain (Chapter 10).

BENZODIAZEPINES

These compounds such as **diazepam, lorazepam, oxazepam** etc (Fig. 8.1) have largely replaced the barbiturates as hypnotics (Chapter 6).

Mechanism of action: GABA, the most potent inhibitory transmitter in the CNS controls the state of neuronal excitability. It acts by binding to the neuronal $GABA_A$ receptor (Fig. 8.2) and opens the chloride channels. BZDs bind selectively to subunits of the $GABA_A$ receptors, a site distinct from that of GABA or the barbiturates-binding site and is designated as *benzodiazepine-binding site*. They increase the frequency of chloride channel opening and the chloride ion concentration in the neuron. This causes hyperpolarisation of the neuronal membrane, making it more difficult for the excitatory neurotransmitters to depolarise the cell. *They enhance the effectiveness of GABA by increasing its affinity for the $GABA_A$ receptors and thus lowering the concentration of GABA required for opening the chloride channels.*

Although all the BZDs have similar pharmacological properties, they differ in their selectivity and vary in their clinical usefulness owing to the existence of multiple subtypes of BZD-binding sites in the CNS. Thus, the **antispasticity effect** appears to involve the $GABA_A$ receptors in the brain stem and the spinal cord, whereas the **sedative and anxiolytic actions** are localised to the limbic system.

Pharmacological actions: Benzodiazepines act as:

- **Anxiolytics** (see Chapter 14)
- **Sedative hypnotics**
- **Anticonvulsants**
- **Muscle relaxants**
- **Anaesthetics**

Sedative–hypnotic action: In small doses, BZDs produce relief from anxiety and in larger doses, they induce sleep. All benzodiazepines are qualitatively similar in their effects on the important sleep parameters. Thus, they decrease the time to onset of sleep, prolong stage 2 of sleep, and significantly shorten stages 3 and 4 and REM sleep. The total sleep time is increased with diminished awakenings.

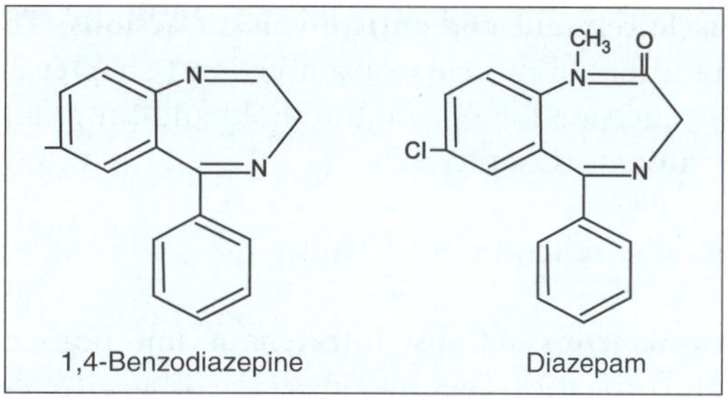

FIG. 8.1 **Chemical structures of l,4- benzodiazepine nucleus and diazepam.**

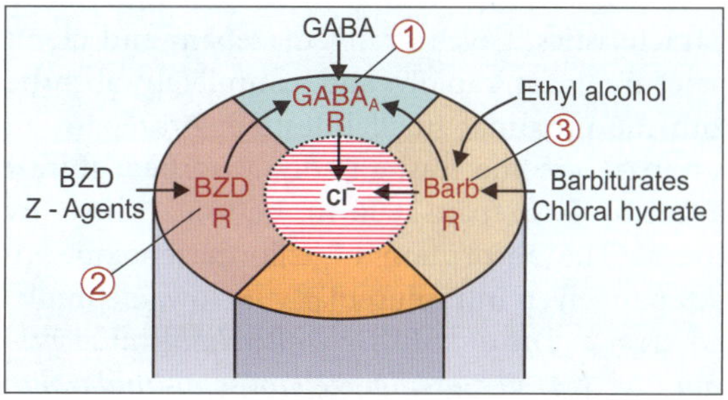

FIG. 8.2 **$GABA_A$–BZD–barbiturate binding sites on the GABAA receptor. R, binding site; Z-agents, Zolpidem, etc. Note: Selective BZD–$GABA_A$ receptor agonist acts through $GABA_A$ receptor. Barbiturates in therapeutic doses directly open the chloride channel.**

Clinically, BZDs are preferred as hypnotics because they

- *Induce sleep which is more refreshing and with fewer hangover symptoms* such as drowsiness, dysphoria, and mental or motor depression.
- *Preserve near-normal sleep, remain effective as hypnotics for longer periods of time, and cause less rebound of REM sleep* after withdrawal.
- *Can induce sleep even in the presence of pain and do not cause hyperalgesia.*
- *Do not exert a significant action on respiration and CVS even in large doses. Hence its use in patients having asthma is not contraindicated.*
- *Have a higher therapeutic index.*
- *Cause fewer drug interactions and have less potential for drug abuse.*

However, all can induce **anterograde amnesia**, where there is impairment of memory for events following the drug administration.

Muscle relaxant and anticonvulsant actions: They have a central muscle relaxant action (Chapter 22). They increase the seizure threshold and act as anticonvulsants (Chapter 9).

Anaesthetic action: See Chapter 7.

Miscellaneous actions: Intravenous injections can dilate coronaries. They may lower the BP and decrease the respiratory rate.

Absorption, fate and excretion: The various BZDs differ from one another in their pharmacokinetic characteristics. Given orally, diazepam and clorazepate are most rapidly and completely absorbed from the proximal small intestine; prazepam and oxazepam are the least rapidly absorbed; flurazepam and lorazepam fall in between these two groups. The absorption of chlordiazepoxide and diazepam given intramuscularly is slow, incomplete and erratic. *The only BZDs with reliable absorption from the IM site are lorazepam and midazolam.* Rectal and nasal route for diazepam, as well as nasal route for midazolam is generally used in the convulsing patient, preferably in children.

The duration of action following a single dose depends on the rate and extent of drug distri-bution and of metabolic degradation. BZDs are metabolised by hepatic microsomal CYP3A4 and 2C19 enzymes (except lorazepam, oxazepam and temazepam), and hepatic damage prolongs their action. *The t½ is prolonged in subjects over 60 years of age and in infants due to reduced hepatic clearance; hence, dosage should be reduced in such individuals.* **Remimazolam**, an ultra-short-acting IV BZD, gets metabolised by tissue carboxylesterase 1(CSE1) to form an inactive metabolite, resulting in a very short duration of action of 30 min (Chapter 7). Depending on their elimination t½, they can be grouped as shown in Table 8.2.

Some of the BZDs are biotransformed to clinically active metabolites, some of them with a longer

Table 8.2 Benzodiazepine Derivatives and Oral Doses

Name	Bedtime Hypnotic Single Dose (mg[a])	Total[b] Daily Anxiolytic Dose (mg)
I. Effective half-life more than 24 h[c]		
Chlordiazepoxide	–	30–100
Diazepam[d]	5	5–30
Flurazepam	15–30	15–30
Clorazepate (prodrug with active metabolite, nordazepam)	3.75–20	15–60
II. Effective half-life 5–24 h		
Nitrazepam	5–10	–
Lorazepam	1–2	1–4
Oxazepam	15–30	45–60
Temazepam	7.5–30	–
Alprazolam	0.75–3	0.75–4
Estazolam	1–2	–
III. Effective half-life less than 5 h		
Triazolam	0.125–0.25	–
Midazolam	7.5–15	–
IV. Effective half-life less than 1h		
Remimazolam	–	–

[a]Use half the dose in old people.
[b]In divided doses.
[c]These compounds are metabolised to clinically important active metabolites with elimination half-life values ranging between 36 and 200 h.
[d]For IV use, inject 5 mg directly and slowly.

half-life than the parent compound. Thus, desmethyldiazepam (t½ 36−200 h), a major metabolite, plays an important role in the clinical effects of chlordiazepoxide, diazepam, prazepam and clorazepate. Clorazepate and prazepam are in fact pro-drugs and reach the systemic circulation only as desmethyldiazepam. Flurazepam is converted to the active metabolite desalkylflurazepam. *Multiple-dose therapy with such drugs leads to accumulation of the long half-life, active metabolites, resulting in prolongation of the effect, and may cause unwanted daytime sedation.* However, it should be noted that the clinical drug effects do not necessarily increase in direct proportion to plasma concentration because of the development of tolerance.

Because of a long half-life, clinically significant amounts of chlordiazepoxide, diazepam or desmethyl-diazepam may persist in the blood and in the body for many days/weeks after the termination of prolonged therapy. This could be beneficial in anxiety state as it prevents the rapid return of anxiety and delays the development of withdrawal symptoms.

Lorazepam and **oxazepam** lack active metabolites and are preferred in the elderly and in lactating women.

Preparations and doses: See Table 8.2.

Adverse reactions: Benzodiazepines in general are well tolerated.

a. The common side effects are due to dose-related depression of CNS: drowsiness, lethargy and ataxia. They also cause impairment of visual–motor coordination, behavioural changes, daytime sedation, and anterograde amnesia.
b. Occasionally they produce personality changes and may cause a paradoxical increase in hostility, irritability and anxiety, especially in the elderly. They should be used cautiously in the presence of respiratory, liver and cardiac diseases.
c. Miscellaneous: Rarely, BZDs cause leucopenia, allergy, photosensitisation, vertigo, headache, impaired sexual function and menstrual irregularities.

PH 1.22, PH 1.23

Patients develop **tolerance** to the sedative (but not to the anxiolytic) action, as well as physical and **psychic dependence.** Withdrawal syndrome includes insomnia, agitation and rarely convulsions. The **withdrawal symptoms are more intense** following the discontinuation of shorter acting BZD than of longer acting BZD. The treatment is similar to that of barbiturate dependence (see the section, Barbiturates).

Use of BZD in early pregnancy can increase the risk of spontaneous abortions and fetal malformations. Administration of BZD to the mother before delivery can cause apnoeic spells, reluctance to feed, hypotonia and hypothermia in the newborn (**floppy baby syndrome**).

Drug interactions: They enhance the effects of CNS depressants such as alcohol, barbiturates and amitriptyline. Microsomal enzyme inhibitors such as clarithromycin, isoniazid and cimetidine retard their elimination, whereas inducers (rifampin) can decrease their effectiveness. However, serious drug interactions are rare. Alcohol is an inhibitor of CSE 1, the enzyme metabolizing remimazolam and can prolong its effects.

Indications:

- **As hypnotics** (see the section, Pharmacotherapy of insomnia)
    - For procedural sedation: Remimazolam is used for induction (5 mg) and maintenance (with additional top-up of 2.5 mg as required) of sedation in adults undergoing short surgical procedures like upper GI endoscopy, colonoscopy, bronchoscopy. Its pharmacokinetic profile allows these procedures to be conducted faster with low liability for deep and/or prolonged sedation.
- **In anxiety states** (Chapter 14)
- **During withdrawal of alcohol** (Chapter 6)
- **As skeletal muscle relaxants** (Chapter 22)
- **As anticonvulsants** (Chapter 9)
- **As preanaesthetic and anaesthetic medication:** midazolam and remimazolam are used as IV anaesthetic agents (Chapter 7).

FM 10.1

Benzodiazepine Receptor Antagonist

FLUMAZENIL, an imidazo-benzodiazepine, binds competitively to BZD-binding sites and acts as an antagonist of BZD. It does not block the pharmacologic effects of GABA or all GABA-mimetics. Given alone, it has minimal effect on the CNS. The drug can cause withdrawal syndrome in patients dependent on BZD. Clinically, it rapidly reverses the effects of BZD and facilitates the return of consciousness within 5–15 min in patients with BZD poisoning.

Given orally, it is rapidly absorbed and has a high hepatic clearance. It is metabolised in the liver, and little is excreted unchanged. It is given intravenously initially in the dose of 0.2 mg over 30 s, and followed by 0.3 mg every minute to a total of 3 mg. It can also be given by IV infusion. The duration of action of a single dose is 30–60 min.

Indications:

- **In BZD poisoning**
- **For reversal of sedative effect of a BZD** administered during general anaesthesia, a diagnostic or therapeutic procedure

It is **contraindicated** in patient with seizure disorders, a raised intracranial pressure as after a severe head injury, and those on tricyclic antidepressants.

NONBENZODIAZEPINE, BENZODIAZEPINE-RECEPTOR AGONISTS

Nonbenzodiazepines such as **zolpidem, zaleplon, zopiclone** and **eszopiclone (Z agents)** are the newer sedative hypnotic agents which have varied chemical structures (Table 8.3). They bind selectively to a subset of BZD-binding sites and enhance the effect of GABA. Their characteristic features are as follows:

- *As sedative hypnotics, they are as effective as BZD* and provide normal architecture of sleep.
- *They are rapid in onset and have short duration of action.* Zaleplon is perhaps the best (even with middle-of-night use) because of its ultra-short t½.
- Their ADR profile is similar to BZD. *They have adverse effects on memory and cognitive function.* They often cause headache, and impair the next morning driving performance. Hallucinations have been reported.
- *They are metabolised in the liver by CYP3A4.* Zopiclone has active metabolites.
- *They lack anixiolytic, anticonvulsant and muscle relaxant properties.*
- *Their effects can be antagonised by flumazenil.*
- *Dependence, drug abuse and withdrawal symptoms have been reported.*

Hence they should be used in low doses than recommended, e.g. 5 mg of zolpidem instead of 10 mg.

Table 8.3 Comparison of Eszopiclone, Zolpidem and Zaleplon

Property	Eszopiclone	Zolpidem	Zaleplon
Structure	Cyclopyrrolone	Imidazopyridine	Pyrazolopyrimidine
Elimination half-life (h)	6	1.5–2.4	1–1.5
Bioavailability	80%	70%	30%
Sleep duration (h)	8	8	
Memory effects	+	+	+/–
Cognitive effects	+	+	+/–
Negative effects on memory and cognition next day	+	+	+/–
Common adverse effect	Metallic after-taste	Headache	Headache
Abuse potential	+	++	++

Note: ±, very mild effect; +, mild effect.

Zaleplon is effective in reducing sleep latency and therefore used in insomnia with difficulty in falling asleep. But it does not decrease premature awakening or increase the total sleep time. Zopiclone, with a longer t½, can be used for initiating and maintaining sleep. Zolpidem also decreases nocturnal arousal; its low dose sublingual formulation may be used for treating midnight awakenings.

Eszopiclone is the S-isomer of zopiclone and has similar actions. Its plasma t½ is 6 h.

In general, they do not appear to be superior to the short-acting BZD.

MELATONIN RECEPTOR AGONISTS

MELATONIN: The sleep regulating hormone, melatonin, has been used to prevent jet lag and to induce post-travel sleep in air travellers. Jet lag causes daytime drowsiness, insomnia, frequent awakenings, anxiety and GI upset (**circadian rhythm disorder**). Melatonin reduces these symptoms and aids the person sleeping post-travel. The doses prescribed are 0.5−5 mg on the evening of departure and one−three nights after arrival at the new destination.

Given orally as 0.3–5 mg at night 3−5 h before the desired time of sleep, it may help to improve onset, duration and quality of sleep. It is not so effective when taken at bedtime. It increases REM sleep. It is generally well tolerated. It may cause day time drowsiness, fatigue, dizziness, headache and irritability. As it has an inhibitory action on the pituitary LH and testicular aromatase enzymes, *it should not be used in pregnancy*. It is also avoided in nursing mothers because it inhibits prolactin release. It has no abuse potential.

It is also used in benzodiazepine withdrawal syndrome as a 2 mg controlled release tablet. For nicotine withdrawal syndrome, 0.3 mg is administered 3 h after smoking the last cigarette.

Ramelteon and **tasimelteon** are the newer analogues of melatonin. Ramelteon is used in transient as well as chronic insomnia, especially for sleep onset problems. It has an active metabolite. It does not cause rebound insomnia. Adverse reactions are similar to those of melatonin. It is contraindicated in liver failure and in those taking inhibitors of CYP2C9 and CYP1A2.

OREXIN RECEPTOR ANTAGONISTS

Orexin A and B (hypocretins 1 and 2) are neuropeptides that are released by the hypothalamic neurons, which project their axons widely throughout the CNS. They act on G protein coupled receptors, OX1 and OX2, to stimulate orexin, monoaminergic and cholinergic neurons in the hypothalamus/brainstem regions and promote wakefulness. This effect is long lasting. Inhibition of orexin neurons decreases wakefulness and increases non-REM sleep time. Loss of orexin signalling causes narcolepsy. The orexin system is also believed to be involved in autonomic functions, energy balance and reward system.

SUVOREXANT: This drug promotes sleep by preventing orexin neuropeptides from binding to their receptors. It is indicated for the treatment of insomnia, characterized by difficulties with sleep onset and/or sleep maintenance. Given orally, it has a long half-life and high protein binding. Next-day somnolence is common, and cataplexy-like symptoms can occur. It is a substrate for CYP3A4.

MISCELLANEOUS

In addition to the drugs described earlier, which have a primary hypnotic action, various other drugs have hypnotic action as their prominent side effect. These are listed in Box 8.1.

H_1 receptor antagonists, **diphenhydramine** and **promethazine,** are sometimes preferred as hypnotics in paediatric practice. They can cause anticholinergic side effects.

Antidepressants: **Amitriptyline** (5−25 mg), **doxepin** (3−6 mg) and **trazodone,** are used as hypnotics, often

Box 8.1 Drugs with Sedation as a Prominent Side Effect

- **Antipsychotics** : chlorpromazine
- **Antidepressants** : amitriptyline, doxepin
- **Antihistaminics** : diphenhydramine, promethazine
- **Anticholinergics** : scopolamine
- **Antiepileptics** : primidone

as alternatives to BZD receptor agonists. They have affinity for central H_1 receptors and antagonize them. They are effective in low doses and lack abuse potential. Trazodone (25–75 mg) has a short t½ and much less anticholinergic activity that may be advantageous in elderly. They are well tolerated and reasonably safe (Chapter 14). Quetiapine, an antipsychotic drug with H_1 antagonistic properties is also used to treat insomnia (Chapter 13).

Some drugs used as hypnotics (phenothiazine antihistaminics and chlorpromazine) may cause insomnia as an idiosyncratic reaction.

Barbiturates such as phenobarbitone given in small doses acts as a daytime sedative. Larger doses produce sleep. The sleep resembles natural sleep.

However, they:

a. cause more reduction in duration of REM sleep and number of cycles than BZDs.
b. exhibit hangover (residual sedation and headache on waking) more than with BZDs.
c. cannot induce sleep in the presence of pain, whereas BZDs can.
d. cause rebound increase in REM sleep on sudden withdrawal; this can lead to increased dreaming and nightmares during the withdrawal period, especially in addicts.
e. produce motor incoordination, ataxia even at hypnotic doses.
f. have a narrow therapeutic index, liability for abuse and overdose toxicity, the main safety concerns with their use (Chapter 6).

Barbiturates are no more recommended as hypnotics.

Dexmedetomidine: See Chapter 7.

Chlormethiazole: This thiazole derivative with sedative, hypnotic and anticonvulsant actions was used earlier in the treatment of delirium tremens induced by alcohol withdrawal and also for short term management of insomnia or restlessness. It is no longer preferred because of its toxicity and availability of much safer BZD.

PHARMACOTHERAPY OF INSOMNIA AND OTHER SLEEP DISORDERS

Ability to go to sleep is a very personal attribute and people are either 'good sleepers' or 'poor sleepers'. The latter, on the whole, take longer to fall asleep, sleep less, awaken more often have less REM and stage 4 NREM sleep, and have higher physiological arousal (heart rate, body temperature) than good sleepers. At the extreme end of the spectrum of poor sleepers is the person who sleeps through the whole night in several cat naps instead of sleeping continuously. A reduced total sleep time without any subjective or objective consequences suggests that the subject may be a physiologically short sleeper. As with all other things in life, most people learn to live with their own sleeping pattern.

Length of total daily sleep in normal individuals varies between 4 and 10 h (average 7 h). Its duration decreases in the elderly (average < 6 h).

Clinically, sleep disorders manifest as described in the following section.

Insomnia

Insomnia is defined as 'a repeated difficulty with sleep initiation, duration, consolidation or quality that occurs despite adequate time and opportunity for sleep and results in some form of day time impairment and lasting for at least one month' (American Academy of Sleep Medicine, 2005). In practice, insomnia is said to be present when an individual complains of inability to fall or stay asleep, of reduction in the total sleep period, of sleep disturbed by nightmares or of sleep that does not refresh.

Insomnia can be acute or chronic.

1. **Acute insomnia**, which may be *transient* (<3 nights) or *short-term* (*acute*) *insomnia* (<3 weeks). It may occur in the absence of disease and is then due to stress caused by reactions to life changes, environmental factors, grief, job demands, travelling through time zones, etc. Other than this, acute insomnia may be due to physical discomfort such as pain, dyspnoea, cough, fever or psychiatric

causes such as anxiety. It may occasionally be induced by drugs, such as adrenergic agonists and aminophylline.

2. **Chronic insomnia** by definition lasts for at least 3 weeks and needs detailed evaluation. It can be primary or secondary. A 2 week sleep diary and an interview with the sleep partner may be useful. It is a complex process and rarely benefits from hypnotics alone.

Insomnia secondary to pain, fever, dyspnoea or myalgia, usually responds to appropriate treatment of the cause. If organic disease is responsible for insomnia (such as COPD, GERD and hyperthyroidism), it should be treated. *Sudden fearful awakening with palpitation and sweating should arouse the suspicion of an associated major disorder such as* IHD, *hypoglycaemia or severe anxiety state.*

About 30%–60% of the patients with chronic insomnia have a recognisable psychiatric illness such as chronic anxiety, depression or psychosis. These should be looked for and treated. Difficulty in staying asleep is a frequent complaint of depressed patients. It is not benefitted by hypnotics, and treatment of depression is of prime importance (Chapter 14).

Rational therapy of insomnia depends on the accurate diagnosis, and its precipitating and perpetuating factors. These can be easily identified in subjects with acute insomnia.

Nonpharmacological therapy: In patients with 'primary' insomnia, a definite cause cannot be ascertained. In almost 30% of such cases, simple, *nonpharmacological* measures (Box 8.2) may help the subjects to establish good sleep habits. Other measures are (a) **cognitive therapy** given by a specialist and (b) **behavioural therapy** which could be advised by the practitioners.

Behavioural strategies include bedtime restrictions, stimulus control therapy and relaxation and education about sleep hygiene. **Bedtime restriction** involves a reduction in the time spent in bed closely to match the actual time spent asleep. This simple procedure is useful for the people who spent lots of time in bed but are not sleeping. **Stimulus control** involves instructions related to reassociate bed and bedroom with sleep and re-establish a regular sleep pattern. *In chronic primary insomnia, drugs are prescribed only as a last resort because although they may provide a short time improvement, such benefits are not persistent.*

Box 8.2 Nonpharmacological (Sleep Hygiene) Measures for Treating Insomnia

The patient is advised to

- Avoid daytime naps
- Take moderate exercise in the morning or afternoon; it has been shown to increase stage 4 NREM sleep
- Avoid the consumption of alcohol, tobacco and caffeinated beverages close to bedtime
- Establish a regular bedtime hour and condition oneself to go to bed only when feeling sleepy; one should not remain in bed if one cannot sleep soon
- Use the bed for sleeping not for eating, reading or watching television
- Avoid all complex mental activity prior to bedtime

Further

- One may need a change in the mattress
- The elderly should restrict fluids in the evening to decrease nocturia
- Some fill up for the stomach such as a glass of warm milk is useful; milk contains tryptophan, and d-tryptophan is known to reduce the time to onset of sleep in volunteers
- Training in relaxation, and meditation can be helpfu

Drug therapy: It is empirical and gives only symptomatic relief. Pharmacologically, it is impossible to clearly separate sedative, antianxiety and hypnotic drugs. It would appear that with most drugs belonging to these classes, the desired effect can be produced by an appropriately adjusted dose.

In therapeutic doses, most 'hypnotic' drugs have similar actions. They

- **Decrease the latent period of sleep.**
- **Increase the total sleep time.**
- **Decrease the awake time and the awakenings.**
- **Reduce the period of REM sleep.**

There are more similarities than differences among the various hypnotic drugs. The differences are, however, of practical importance. They are as follows:

1. Rapidity of action

Box 8.3 Principles of Drug Therapy of Insomnia PH 1.1

I. ***Transient insomnia***
- Use the lowest dose of hypnotic with a short duration of action for 2–3 nights

II. ***Short-term insomnia***
- Counselling
- Use lowest effective dose of hypnotic, 30 min before retiring to bed.
- After getting 1–2 nights' acceptable sleep, skip a dose.
- Use it intermittently (2–4 times a week) for a short time, not more than 3 weeks at a time and then discontinue gradually.
- Be alert to rebound insomnia after stopping

III. ***Chronic insomnia***
- Psychotherapy and behavioural therapy
- Chronotherapy
- Treatment of associated depression or psychosis
- Use hypnotics as adjuvants every third night and discontinue gradually after 3–6 months.

2. Duration of action
3. Differences in the degree of suppression of REM sleep
4. Adverse reactions, especially liability to produce hangover, respiratory depression, dependence and impairment of cognitive function

The principles of drug therapy of insomnia are outlined in Box 8.3. Transient insomnia can be helped by a short course for 2–3 nights.

BZD receptor agonists, *because of their flexible pharmacokinetics, efficacy, tolerability and safety, are to be preferred.* If an elderly person has difficulty in falling asleep (sleep onset insomnia), a drug that is rapidly effective such as a short-acting BZD like oxazepam should be administered 20–30 min before the usual bedtime. For persons with difficulty in maintenance of sleep, longer acting drugs such as nitrazepam, lorazepam or temazepam may be preferred. Long half-life BZDs such as diazepam and flurazepam are preferred when daytime sedation is also desired. *Newer Z agents are not superior to BZDs and offer only a marginal advantage.*

Doxepin can be substituted for BZD. It has an advantage that it does not cause dependence and drug abuse, but may have other side effects such as anticholinergic effects.

Whichever hypnotic is chosen, it should be used initially in a small dose and should be increased only if absolutely necessary. Once a good night's sleep is obtained, attempts should be made to omit the drug for a few nights. The drug should be used to condition the patient to sleep better and should not be allowed to make a slave out of him/her. He/she should be explained that he/she can now sleep well without the drug and that an occasional night of imperfect sleep will do no harm.

Rebound insomnia can occur following sudden withdrawal of hypnotic drugs used for a longer time. Hence they should be tapered off slowly. *As far as possible, hypnotics should be used for a short duration and intermittently.*

Limitations of hypnotics: The major drawbacks of all hypnotics is the 'hangover' and dependence liability. All of them impair performance the next day. Even smaller amounts used as daytime sedative can impair social judgement and performance. Patients should be warned not only about the possible interactions of hypnotics with alcohol and other drugs, but also about the possibility of impaired performance such as car driving the next day. However, the newer benzodiazepines with a short t½ such as lorazepam and the nonbenzodiazepines are relatively safer.

Rarely, these drugs can cause (a) severe hypersensitivity reactions including anaphylaxis and/or angioedema and (b) hazardous sleep-related activities such as sleep driving, telephoning while asleep, and preparing and eating food while asleep.

Sedatives and hypnotics are indicated in various situations in children, but they should not be employed as a substitute for other important measures such as discussion/counselling with the parents about their children's behavioural problems and the importance of change in parental attitudes. A routine use of hypnotics for conditions such as tics, nightmares, breath-holding attacks, masturbation, aggressiveness, fears and school phobias, and head banging is not considered justifiable.

Insomnia in the elderly: The commonest causes of insomnia in this population are age-related changes in the sleep cycle and daytime napping. *One should always look for causes such as medical illnesses, loneliness, depression, anxiety, dementia and loss of family support.* The patient should understand that improvement rather than total relief of insomnia is an achievable goal. Because of reduced body water, renal and hepatic function and increase in body fat, the pharmacological profile of hypnotics may be altered in the elderly, with prolongation of their half-life (Chapter 1). The following points are important while treating insomnia in this age group:

1. Restriction of fluids in the evening.
2. Smaller than usual doses of short-acting BZD, e.g. oxazepam, which are the hypnotics of choice.
3. If BZDs are not tolerated, use zolpidem and zaleplon.
4. Avoid sedative antihistaminics as they are liable to cause delirium and antimuscarinic side effects.
5. Think about possible psychiatric problems particularly depression and treat if present.
6. Help to resolve socioeconomic problems. *Often a change in behaviour of the other family members towards the patient can produce remarkable effects.*

Points to remember

- *Detailed history must be taken* to rule out causes such as severe anxiety or depression; and consumption of drugs (Box 8.4), excessive tea, coffee and colas.
- *Periodic loss of sleep in itself is not harmful* and, therefore, does not require treatment with drugs.

Box 8.4 Drug-Induced Insomnia

Adrenergic agonists: Salbutamol, ephedrine, amphetamine, nasal decongestants
Central stimulants: Methylphenidate, caffeine, aminophylline, nicotine
Bupropion
Antidepressants: MAO inhibitors, SSRI
Levodopa
Amantadine
Antimicrobials: Chloroquine, metronidazole, fluoroquinolones
Diuretics
Systemic glucocorticoids

Professionals such as doctors, nurses and seamen who also lose sleep on and off remain resilient and healthy.

- *The clinician should not have a negative approach* to what lies behind the presented symptom of sleeplessness, and hypnotics must not be prescribed readily 'on demand'.
- *One should be critical in repeating the 'sleeping pill' prescription* and try to avoid its continuation.
- *No hypnotic is safe*, all can cause harm and none is effective in helping patients with problems underlying their insomnia. Special caution is necessary in patients with respiratory diseases, suicidal tendencies and history of drug dependence. *The risk of falls and fractures increases especially in the elderly patients using hypnotics and other psycho-therapeutic agents.*
- *Moreover some of these drugs lose their effectiveness on repeated administration.*
- *The difficulties of stopping the hypnotic in chronic users could be enormous.* They should be tapered off slowly.
- *Effectiveness and safety are still the main considerations in choosing a hypnotic drug.*
- *Chronic insomnia usually needs a long-term strategy for its management,* mainly with cognitive, behavioural therapy and cautious use of drugs to a limited extent.
- *Hypnotics should not be used in patients with sleep apnoea.*

Hypersomnia

Its treatment is discussed in Chapter 14.

Parasomnia

Sleepwalking, night terrors and nightmares are designated as *parasomnias.*

Sleepwalking and night terrors are the mild and severe manifestations of parasomnia, occurring about 1–3 h after the onset of sleep, when stages N3 is more prevalent. The disorders are idiopathic when they begin in childhood and benefit from (a) safety precautions and (b) the use of drugs such as diazepam and flurazepam which suppress stages N3 of sleep.

An organic cause such as a brain tumour must be ruled out in adult patients.

Nightmares, commonly known as bad dreams, occur during REM sleep. They may occur in normal children and in children with fever. Other environmental causes should be looked for. The best way to handle them is to avoid terrifying stories, movies and frightening television programmes. *When they occur for the first time in adult life, depression is an important cause, and such depressed patients may be at increased risk for suicide. They are treated with REM suppressants such as tricyclic antidepressants* (Chapter 14).

Miscellaneous

This involves (a) circadian rhythm disorders (disturbed sleep schedule) and (b) restless leg syndrome.

The cause of restless leg syndrome (RLS) is not known. Clinically, it responds to some extent to gabapentin (Chapter 9) and dopamine agonists, pramipexole and ropinirole (Chapter 15).

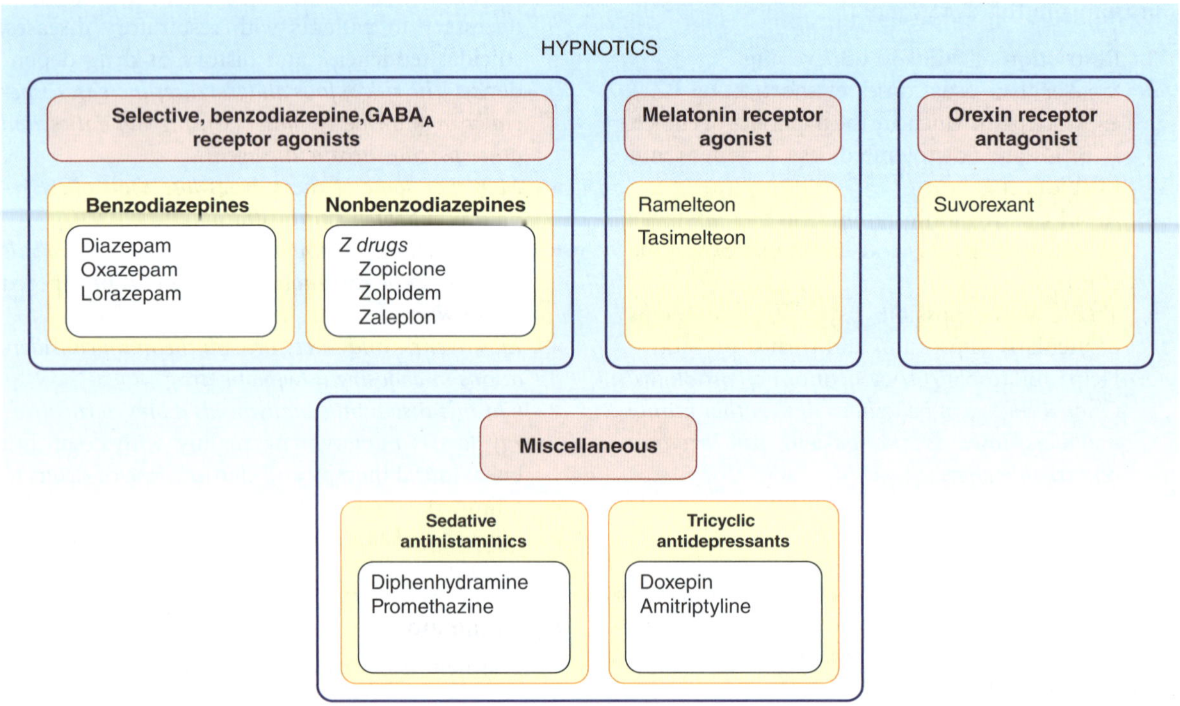

CHAPTER 9

Drugs Effective in Seizure Disorders

Learning Objectives

This chapter will enable the reader:

1. To be aware of different types of epileptic seizures and their clinical manifestations.
2. To explain neurophysiological mechanisms responsible for seizures.
3. To classify antiepileptic drugs based on the mechanism of action.
4. To describe the mechanism of action, pharmacological effects, ADR, salient pharmacokinetic features and indications for phenytoin, phenobarbitone, carbamazepine, ethosuximide, sodium valproate, vigabatrin, tiagabin, gabapentin, benzodiazepines, lamotrigine, topiramate, levetiracetam, zonisamide, lacosamide and perampanel.
5. To discuss the principles of management of epilepsy.
6. To state precautions to be taken during pregnancy of a patient having epilepsy.
7. To state antiepileptic drug(s) of choice and alternatives for various types of epilepsy.
8. To outline the management of status epilepticus.
9. To enlist the drugs causing seizures.
10. To enumerate nonepileptic uses of antiepileptic drugs.

KEY TERMS

Seizure is a sudden and transient episode (signs and/or symptoms) due to abnormal excessive electrical discharges from a group of CNS neurons. The rapid, rhythmic, and synchronous firing may occur due to epilepsy or due to a systemic disorder such as hypoglycaemia or hypocalcaemia, or an intracranial/severe systemic infection. Some drugs used for other indications can also induce seizures (see Box 9.1).

Epilepsy is a collective term for a group of chronic disorders characterised by recurrent seizures associated with the disturbance of consciousness and/or a characteristic body movement (**convulsion**), and sometimes autonomic hyperactivity.

In cases of other seizures, generally there is no environmental or physiological trigger such as emotions, exercise, flashing lights or loud music immediately preceding the seizure. They are self-limited and are called **nonepileptic seizures** (**NES**). Their main treatment comprises that of the cause.

Box 9.1 Drug-Induced Seizures

1. **Sympathomimetics and central stimulants:** Ephedrine, amphetamine, terbutaline, aminophylline, cocaine
2. **Some tricyclic antidepressants**
3. **Phenothiazines** (antipsychotics and antihistaminics) and **haloperidol**
4. **Bupropion, lithium, flumazenil**
5. **Withdrawal of alcohol, short acting BDZ/barbiturates**
6. **Anaesthetic agents** such as ether, halothane, ketamine, lignocaine
7. **Analgesics:** Tramadol, pethidine
8. **Antimicrobial and antiviral:** Penicillin, cephalosporins, imipenem, quinolones, INH, acyclovir, ganciclovir
9. **Immunomodulators:** Methotrexate, cyclosporine, tacrolimus

Drugs used in the treatment of seizure disorders can be divided into the following:

1. **Anticonvulsants:** Drugs which are used to abolish seizures (antiseizure).
2. **Antiepileptics:** Drugs which are administered prophylactically to prevent seizures. PH 1.19

Classification of Antiseizure Drugs

- **Centrally acting,** e.g. general anaesthetics, diazepam, paraldehyde, barbiturates (Chapters 7 and 8) and specific antiepileptics
- **Acting mainly on the spinal cord,** e.g. Mephenesin (Chapter 21)
- **Peripheral skeletal muscle relaxants,** e.g. d-Tubocurarine, Pancuronium and Succinylcholine (Chapter 22)

Box 9.2 Types of Seizures

I. **Generalised onset seizures**
Absence seizures (petit mal): Typical, atypical, myoclonic, eyelid myoclonia
Tonic–clonic seizures (grand mal)
Tonic seizures
Atonic seizures
Myoclonic seizures
Epileptic spasms

II. **Focal onset seizures**

III. **Unknown onset (focal, generalised) seizures**

TYPES OF EPILEPSY

The drug treatment of epilepsy is guided by the nature of seizures. The currently used classification of seizures is based on history, clinical findings, EEG recording and imaging studies. Thus, the seizures can be divided into (a) **Generalized onset seizures**, (b) **Focal onset seizures** and (c) **unknown onset seizures** (Box 9.2).

The drugs used for all focal seizures are generally the same, whereas in the case of the generalised seizures, they depend on the type of seizure in the different subgroups.

1. **Generalised seizures.** They can be non-motor type (absence seizures) or motor type (tonic-clonic, tonic, clonic, atonic, myoclonic, epileptic spasms).
   a. **Absence seizure (petit mal):** It consists of sudden impairment of consciousness *without convulsive movement* and *without loss of postural control.* The patient appears to go blank for less than 30 s, and there may be accompanying fluttering of eyelids or small chewing movements. Awareness of the surroundings is regained quickly at the end of an attack, and the patient may not even know that one has occurred. The EEG is diagnostic with diffuse, bilaterally synchronous 3 per second wave and spike discharges. Absence seizures almost always begin in childhood. The child may outgrow these seizures.
   b. **Tonic–clonic seizures:** These are accompanied by a generalised abnormality in the EEG (**grand m***al or major epilepsy). They are characterised* by a sudden loss of consciousness *without any warning (aura)*, followed by generalised stiffening (tonic), and finally jerking (clonic) convulsions lasting for 1–2 min. This is followed by a period of headache, drowsiness and sleep. The attack may be accompanied by tongue biting, frothing and urinary incontinence.
   c. **Tonic seizure:** As above but without a clonic phase.
   d. **Atonic seizure** (drop attack): Such a seizure consists of a sudden loss of postural tone, without accompanying tonic or clonic movements. The head may drop for a few seconds or the child may drop to the floor without any apparent cause.
   e. **Myoclonic seizure:** This is a sudden, brief, repetitive muscle contraction involving a body part or the whole body. In the latter case, there is a violent fall without a loss of consciousness. Myoclonic seizures may occur by themselves or coexist with other seizures. The EEG changes are characteristic.
   f. **Epileptic spasms:** They are focal or generalized, with or without alteration of awareness. Generalized epileptic spasm presents as brief seizures with sudden flexion at the trunk and flexion or extension of the limbs. They commonly occur in clusters. Although they can occur at any age, they are most often seen during infancy **(infantile spasms)** and may be due to immature CNS. The EEG shows diffuse, giant slow waves with a background of irregular, multifocal spikes and sharp waves.
2. **Focal seizures** originate in a localised area of the brain (usually a medial temporal lobe or inferior frontal lobe) *with a localised focus of EEG abnormality*, and may or may not become generalised. The manifestations depend on the brain region or regions involved. The interictal EEG is either normal or shows epileptiform spikes, but EEG during seizure is nonlocalising.

a. **Focal aware seizures:** Focal seizures can cause motor, sensory, autonomic or psychic symptoms without impairment of cognition. *The patient is conscious and is aware of the event which lasts for a few seconds to a few minutes.* These seizures can be of (i) focal motor onset or (ii) focal non-motor onset. The former begins with recurrent contractions of a particular muscle group and has epileptic focus in motor cortex. The patients with focal non-motor onset experience either numbness, paraesthesia, flushing, sweating, olfactory, auditory, gustatory or psychic symptoms as the focal epileptic discharges spread into limbic system.
b. **Focal impaired awareness seizures:** These can be of motor and non-motor type. Usually these consist of an aura (unusual smell, sudden intense emotional feelings), *followed by impaired consciousness (for 30 s to 1 h)*. The ictal phase begins with repetitive motor activity such as lip smacking, swallowing or aimless wandering or unconscious performance of highly skilled activities such as car driving *(automatisms)* or motionless stare. There is amnesia for the entire period of the seizure or a postictal aphasia. Only 70%–80% of the seizures arise from the temporal lobe. *Hence, although the terms psychomotor, temporal and limbic have been used synonymously, all such seizures are not the same.* Focal slowing or sharp wave activity or both, on the EEG, provides confirmation.
c. **Focal to bilateral tonic–clonic seizures:** These start as focal seizures and develop into one of the generalised seizures by spreading to cerebral hemispheres (secondarily generalized). *Distinguishing between primarily generalised seizure and focal changing to generalised seizure is important as the choice of drugs differs for both.*

Status epilepticus (SE): Prolonged seizures (more than 5–10 min) or repetitive seizures (of any variety) without recovery of consciousness between attacks comprise SE. When tonic–clonic seizures go into SE, the situation can be life-threatening and *is a medical emergency* (see section, Drug therapy of epilepsy).

The above description applies to a classification of the 'seizures'. The classification of 'epilepsies', on the other hand, must also take into account seizure types, aetiology, age of onset, genetic factors, EEG findings, associated neurologic defects, imaging results, response to treatment and prognosis. *Defining a specific epilepsy syndrome is more helpful in judging the prognosis and in selecting the drug treatment rather than taking into consideration only the seizure characteristics.*

In about 10% of persons with true seizures, multiple EEG studies reveal no abnormalities. *Therefore, a normal EEG does not rule out a seizure disorder in a person with a diagnostic clinical picture.*

Neurophysiology: Depending on the neurotransmitter released, the brain neurons are grouped as *excitatory* and *inhibitory. The primary inhibitory transmitter in the brain is GABA, whereas the excitatory transmitter is mostly the amino acid glutamate.* GABA acts on the GABA receptors, and glutamate acts through the N-methyl-D aspartate (NMDA) and non-NMDA receptors (Chapter 5). Activation of these receptors modifies various voltage-gated Na^+, K^+, Ca^{++} and Cl^- ion channels and excites or inhibits the neuron. Normally, the neurons fire action potentials singly or in short runs, and the excitability is kept under control by powerful inhibitory influences.

Pathophysiology: It involves two, importantly related events:

1. **Hyperexcitability** is the abnormal responsiveness of the neurons to an excitatory input, leading to multiple discharges. Chronic hyperexcitability can result from a number of mechanisms.
2. **Hypersynchrony** refers to the recruitment of a large number of nearby neurons to an abnormal firing mode. Thus, *epilepsy is a network phenomenon involving the participation of many neurons firing simultaneously.*

The characteristic pathophysiologic event in a seizure is believed to be a **paroxysmal depolarisation shift (PDS)** of the neuronal membrane potential and associated burst discharge. *Excitatory neurotransmitters are probably involved in the initiation and spread of the seizure discharge, and the inhibitory transmitter GABA is responsible for its termination.*

The normal brain contains billions of neurons which 'fire' asynchronously (i.e. at different times). Inhibitory feedback loops in the normal brain regulate the frequency of firing of individual neurons and prevent synchronisation. When such inhibitory feedback is defective, a large number of cells in a given area of the brain fire at the same time (i.e. they synchronise) and produce a self-regenerating electrical impulse. Such an area constitutes an **epileptic focus.** Such foci may be cortical or subcortical. They may discharge intermittently, only to be shown up on the gross surface EEG, but may not cause symptoms.

The clinical type of seizure is determined by the site of the abnormal focus and is independent of the brain pathology. The response to treatment correlates best with the site of the focus.

PH 1.19

ANTIEPILEPTIC DRUGS

Antiepileptic drugs (AEDs) act by preventing the generation and/or spread of the seizure. Drugs for focal seizure inhibit mainly the voltage-activated Na^+ channels, whereas antipetit mal seizure drugs inhibit voltage-activated Ca^{++} channels. The agents modulating GABA transmission are effective against focal and tonic–clonic seizures.

Classification of AEDs (According to their mechanism of action)

1. **Decrease in the neuronal excitability by delaying the recovery of inactivated Na^+ channels:** Phenytoin, carbamazepine, lamotrigine, topiramate
2. **Decrease in the low threshold calcium currents (T-current) in the thalamic neurons:** Ethosuximide
3. **Action similar to both phenytoin and ethosuximide as mentioned earlier:** Sodium valproate, zonisamide
4. **Enhancement of inhibition through GABA:**
   a. Acting through GABA-related receptors: Barbiturates and benzodiazepines
   b. By releasing GABA from neuronal endings: Gabapentin
   c. By inhibiting GABA transaminase: Sodium valproate and vigabatrin
   d. By inhibiting neuronal reuptake of GABA: Tiagabine
5. **Decrease release of excitatory neurotransmitter glutamate:** Lamotrigine
6. **Miscellaneous:** Levetiracetam and acetazolamide

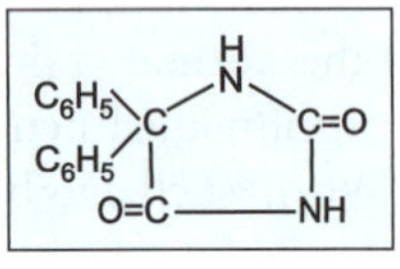

FIG. 9.1 Diphenylhydantoin.

An antiepileptic drug may act through multiple mechanisms

1. **AEDs delaying the recovery of inactivated Na^+ channels:** Phenytoin carbamazepine, lamotrigine, topiramate
   I. **DIPHENYLHYDANTOIN** (phenytoin sodium): This drug is still an important drug in the treatment of epilepsy with the exception of petit mal and myoclonic seizures (Fig 9.1).

Mechanism of action: The drug slows the recovery of voltage-dependent Na^+ channels, resulting in a decreased permeability to sodium ions (**stabilising effect**) of all neuronal membranes, including the peripheral nerves as well as other nonexcitable and excitable membranes.

Reduction in the neuronal Na^+ concentration causes the following:

a. Reduction in PDS.
b. Decreases post-tetanic potentiation (PTP) which is responsible for the spread of the seizure activity.
c. Inhibits the spread of seizure discharge and shortens the duration of after discharge.

In patients in whom it is effective, the generalised abnormality in EEG disappears, but the *abnormal focal electrical activity persists.*

High concentrations of phenytoin also augment the brain level of GABA, 5-HT and homovanillic acid. This may contribute to its toxicity.

Pharmacological actions:

CNS actions: It exerts a selective antiepileptic action without causing drowsiness. The onset of action is slow even on IV injection, but the action persists for a considerable time after the cessation of therapy.

Cardiovascular actions: It has a cell membrane-stabilising effect on the myocardium (Chapter 28).

Absorption, fate and excretion: Its absorption is

slow and variable, with the plasma peak level at 3–12 h after ingestion. In plasma, it is 70%–95% albumin bound and is metabolised mainly by parahydroxylation in the liver. The drug is concentrated in bile and is reabsorbed from the intestine as parahydroxyphenol. Individuals with deficient liver parahydroxylase can develop toxicity even with small doses.

At plasma concentration less than 10 mcg/mL (subtherapeutic), elimination is exponential, and the plasma t½ is about 24 h. As it approaches the therapeutic concentration of 20 mcg/mL, its metabolism becomes saturated; it then exhibits dose-dependent (zero order) elimination, and the plasma concentration rises disproportionately to the dose increment; the elimination t½ increases. *Hence, the dose increments must be smaller with increasing dosage.* About 94% of a single dose is excreted in urine within 48 h. *It induces hepatic microsomal enzymes.* Hence on chronic medication, the drug disappears from the plasma within 3 days after stopping.

FM 10.1

Adverse reactions: Within the therapeutic range of plasma phenytoin level (10–20 mcg/mL), the drug is usually well tolerated.

With higher plasma levels (>20 mcg/mL), the half-life increases to 35 h or longer. When this happens, even a slight increase in the dose can cause increased toxicity. However, the toxicity disappears equally quickly on reducing the daily dose. Death due to phenytoin is rare.

- **Intolerance:** Urticarial, scarlatiniform and measles-like skin rashes may occur. They may be accompanied by lymphadenopathy, hepatomegaly and jaundice.
- **Central nervous system:** Mild toxicity consists of drowsiness, fatigue, headache and confusion. Larger doses can cause a **vestibulocerebellar syndrome** characterised by vertigo, ataxia, nystagmus and dysarthria. Ocular pain with blurring of vision, delusions, hallucinations and other psychotic episodes are sometimes encountered. Rarely, cognitive impairment and behavioural changes may occur. Peripheral neuropathy has been reported particularly in old people. These effects are dose related and are reversible. Ataxia, however, may occasionally persist for long periods.
- **Gastrointestinal tract:** Alkalinity of the drug causes nausea and vomiting which can be prevented by taking the daily dose in divided portions, after meals, with plenty of water.
- **Face and gums:** Hyperplasia and hypertrophy of the gums with oedema and bleeding occur in approximately 15% of patients. It is not related to the dose of phenytoin. Scrupulous dental hygiene can prevent the gingival hyperplasia. In most cases, the gums return to normal within a year after its discontinuation. Long-term phenytoin therapy sometimes causes hypertrophy of the facial subcutaneous tissue, hypertrichosis and coarsening of facial features (**phenytoin facies**).
- **Endocrine effects:** Hypertrichosis is seen especially in children. Less commonly, hyperglycaemia and osteomalacia have been observed.
- **Drug interactions:** Phenytoin is a potent inducer of hepatic microsomal enzymes. It accelerates its own metabolism and that of other drugs such as vitamin D, folate, glucocorticoids, gonadal steroids, thyroxine, OC pills, doxycycline, warfarin and carbamazepine, thereby reducing their therapeutic efficacy. Thus, *it may cause osteomalacia and megaloblastic anaemia* (See Box 9.3).
- **Teratogenicity:** Hydantoins, administered during the first trimester of pregnancy, can cause **fetal hydantoin syndrome**. It comprises midline hypoplasia, ptosis, wide mouth, inner epicanthic folds, short neck, mild webbing of the neck, short phalanges

Box 9.3 Drug Interactions of Phenytoin

- Isoniazid, cimetidine, cotrimoxazole and coumarin anticoagulants *inhibit phenytoin metabolism,* leading to a rise in phenytoin plasma level and toxicity.
- Folic acid, during its chronic administration, *reduces the effectiveness of phenytoin.*
- Phenytoin *competes with drugs* such as sulphonamide, salicylates and vitamin B_{12} *for binding to plasma proteins.*
- Rifampicin and ethanol decrease the plasma phenytoin level because of *hepatic enzyme induction.*

and hypoplastic nails. Some children may develop congenital heart defects, microcephaly and cognitive deficits.

- **Miscellaneous:** Rarely, blood dyscrasias including aplastic anaemia and agranulocytosis may occur. The appearance of LE cells and methaemoglobinaemia can also occur. Rapid IV administration can cause cardiovascular collapse and/or severe CNS depression.

Preparations and dosage: Phenytoin sodium tablets 30, 50 and 100 mg. Capsules of 25, 50, 100 and 300 mg and oral suspension 6 mg/ml are also available. Phenytoin can be given orally at an initial dose of 3–4 mg/kg/day or 150–300 mg daily and the dose can be increased to 200–500 mg daily. The IV preparation 50 mg/mL can be given at a loading dose of 20 mg/kg and at a maintenance dose of 100 mg 6−8 hrly. Intravenous dose should not exceed 25−50 mg/min. *It should not be given intramuscularly because of its poor absorption from this site. Bioavailability of phenytoin may differ with different brands, and the patients should be advised to use the same brand all the time.*

Fosphenytoin sodium, a prodrug of phenytoin, can be given intravenously more rapidly; it causes fewer reactions; it can also be given intramuscularly.

Indications:

- **Grand mal epilepsy:** It abolishes grand mal seizures in nearly 60% of the patients and reduces their frequency in another 15%–20%.
- **Focal seizures:** Phenytoin is preferred to phenobarbitone in this type of seizures. The drug often controls but does not completely abolish the seizure activity. It is also occasionally useful in infantile spasm.
- **Status epilepticus** (see section, Drug therapy of epilepsy).
- **Cardiac arrhythmias:** Chapter 28.
- **Miscellaneous:** It has been used with some success in certain types of neuralgia, e.g. trigeminal neuralgia, in diabetic neuropathy with dysasthesias and in chorea.

II. CARBAMAZEPINE (Fig 9.2)

Pharmacological actions: Its mechanism of action is similar to that of phenytoin, but it is claimed to cause less cognitive impairment.

Carbamazepine is also useful in the treatment of trigeminal neuralgia, a condition characterised by paroxysms of intense stabbing pain within the distribution of trigeminal nerve, without sensory loss. This condition, because of its paroxysmal nature, tendency to relapse and partial response to phenytoin, has been regarded as a type of epilepsy. Carbamazepine is remarkably specific for trigeminal neuralgia and probably for the related syndrome of **glossopharyngeal neuralgia**.

It is also effective in the **deafferentiationpain** in diabetic neuropathy, cancer and multiple sclerosis.

Absorption, fate andexcretion: Oral absorption is slow; overall bioavailability, however, approaches 90%. It is metabolised by the liver (98%). Children metabolise the drug faster than adults. The plasma half-life, initially 24–36 h, falls to around 12 h on chronic dosing because of autoinduction. *It is a potent hepatic microsomal enzyme inducer and accelerates its own me-tabolism as well as that of many other lipid soluble drugs.* Valproate inhibits its metabolism.

Adverse reactions: The drug is usually well tolerated. However, it can cause nausea, anorexia, giddiness, vomiting, ataxia, mental confusion and skin rash. Diplopia and blurred vision may occur, making driving dangerous. The rare but serious toxic effects reported include obstructive jaundice, peripheral neuritis, agranulocytosis, thrombocytopenia and aplastic anaemia. It is a minor teratogen.

Long-term use of carbamazepine may cause fluid retention and insidious development of sluggishness, both mental and physical. The loss of physical and mental drive can be so gradual that the patient and the family may wrongly attribute it to the normal process of ageing.

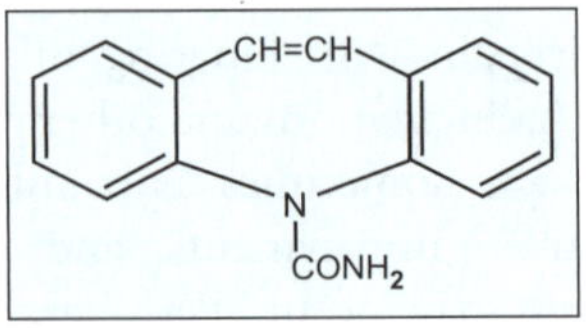

FIG. 9.2 Carbamazepine.

Drug interactions: See Box 9.4.

Box 9.4 Drug Interactions of Carbamazepine

- Induction of hepatic metabolism of oral contraceptives, steroids, vitamin D, theophylline and warfarin
- Inhibition of carbamazepine metabolism by erythromycin, isoniazid, verapamil, cimetidine and sodium valproate

Preparations and dosage: It is available as 100, 200 and 400 mg tablets and as 200, 300 and 400 mg controlled release (CR) tablets. In addition, chewable tablet (as 100 mg), 20 mg/ml oral suspension and rectal suppository (125 and 250 mg) are also available. The initial dose is 100–200 mg once daily or b.i.d., gradually increased to a dose of 0.8–1 g/day in divided doses, not exceeding 1.6–2 g/day in divided doses in focal onset epilepsy and to 400–800 mg in neuralgias.

Indications:

- **Grand mal and focal seizures** where it is used singly or in combination.
- **Trigeminal neuralgia:** see above.
- **Deafferentation pain** in various disorders.
- **Diabetes insipidus of pituitary origin**, where it stimulates ADH release (Chapter 37).
- **As an alternative to lithium** in the management of manic-depressive psychosis and as an adjunct in the treatment of **drug resistant schizophrenia** (Chapter 13).
- **In the treatment of alcohol withdrawal syndrome** (Chapter 6).

Oxcarbazepine, a prodrug, has similar activity and therapeutic uses as carbamazepine, but it is more expensive. Its active metabolite is an s-isomer, **eslicarbazepine**, which is also available as prodrug, **eslicarbazepine** acetate. However, it is used only for focal seizures as an add-on therapy to be given as a single dose. Both oxcarbazepine and **eslicarbazepine** are selective inducers of cytochrome isoenzyme that metabolises estrogens.

III. LAMOTRIGINE:

Mechanism of action: This drug acts like phenytoin on Na+channels. It also inhibits the release of the excitatory amino acid glutamate.

Absorption, fate and excretion: Given orally, it is almost completely absorbed and is eliminated mainly by hepatic metabolism. Its t½ is 24 h.

Adverse reactions: Lamotrigine can cause skin rash, nausea, vomiting, diplopia, ataxia, Stevens-Johnson syndrome and disseminated intravascular coagulation (DIC).

Indications:

- It can be used as monotherapy in primary generalised tonic–clonic, focal and myoclonic seizures.
- It is usually used as an add-on drug in patients with resistant focal and secondarily generalised seizures.
- Due to its membrane-stabilising action, it is also used in the treatment of deafferentation pain.

It is used in the dose of 50 mg b.i.d., increased gradually to 200 mg/day.

Valproic acid inhibits its metabolism, and hence in patients taking valproate, the dose of lamotrigine is reduced to 25 mg on alternate days.

IV. TOPIRAMATE:

Mechanism of action: This drug acts similarly as phenytoin. In addition, it also has some GABA receptor enhancing and weak glutamate receptor inhibiting activity.

Adverse reactions: These are mainly neuropsychological effects, such as dizziness, drowsiness, psychomotor slowing, difficulty in concentrating, confusion, ataxia, depression, acute myopia, glaucoma and raised intracranial tension.

Indications:

- Monotherapy for focal and primary generalised seizures.
- In chronic alcohol addicts as an anticraving drug.
- In obesity as an FDC with pheniramine. It is expensive.

2. AED decreasing the low threshold calcium currents (T-current) in the thalamic neurons

ETHOSUXIMIDE: Its structure is depicted in Fig. 9.3.

Mechanism of action: The drug reduces the low

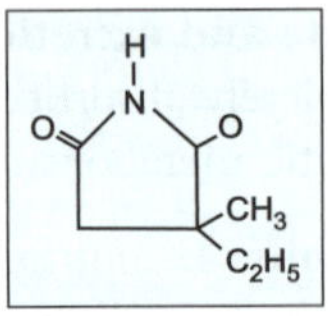

FIG. 9.3 Ethosuximide.

threshold calcium currents (T currents) in the thalamic neurons which are responsible for the generation of the absence seizures.

Pharmacological actions: It is effective only in petit mal epilepsy. It does not induce liver enzymes, and monitoring of blood levels is not required.

Absorption, fate and excretion: It is completely absorbed from the GI tract and is present in the plasma mostly in the free form. About 20% is excreted unchanged in the urine, and the rest is metabolised by the liver.

Adverse reactions: These comprise anorexia, nausea, vomiting, drowsiness, dizziness and occasionally Parkinsonism. Skin rashes, blood dyscrasias, SLE and psychic disturbances may rarely occur. It can unmask grand mal epilepsy.

Preparations and dosage: It is available as 250 mg capsules and as a syrup (250 mg per 5 mL). The usual starting dose is 250 mg/day in children, increased by 250 mg at weekly intervals to usual dose of 500-750 mg twice daily. If necessary, it can be increased upto a maxmimum dose of 1 g twice daily. In adults, it is given initially in a dose of 500 mg daily in 2 divided doses, increased by 250 mg weekly upto a usual dose of 1-1.5 g daily in 2 divided doses, not exceeding 2 g daily.

Indications: It is the drug of choice in petit mal epilepsy. Additional drug(s) may be needed to control associated or unmasked grand mal epilepsy.

3. **AEDs having action similar to both, phenytoin and ethosuximide**

I. **SODIUM VALPROATE:** Chemically sodium valproate is sodium dipropylacetate (Fig. 9.4).

Mechanism of action: It is a **broad-spectrum antiepileptic** which probably acts at multiple sites. Its actions are similar to that of both ethosuximide and phenytoin. Thus, it

a. Inhibits the T type Ca^{++} current.
b. Delays the recovery of the inactivated Na^{+} channels.
c. Inhibits GABA transaminase, thus increasing the GABA activity (Fig. 9.5).

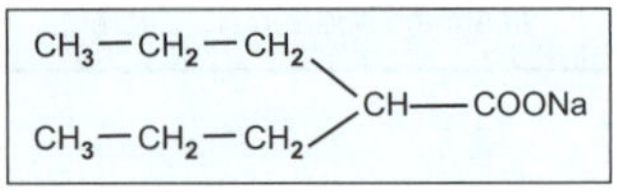

FIG. 9.4 Sodium valproate.

Pharmacological actions: In petit mal, it is as effective as ethosuximide. However, it is more liable to cause GI adverse effects than ethosuximide.

a. *In patients with both petit mal and grand mal seizures, sodium valproate may be the drug of choice as it is able to control both types of seizures.*
b. It is also used in myoclonic seizures with variable success in akinetic seizures and infantile spasms.
c. It is claimed that it does not alter the patient's behaviour, alertness and cognitive function, and therefore does not impair learning ability and performance. *It is well tolerated by the elderly and is the drug of choice in them.*
d. *Sodium valproate does not induce hepatic microsomal enzymes.* In fact it is an inhibitor of these enzymes. Thus it inhibits its own metabolism and that of lamotrigine, phenobarbitone, phenytoin and carbamazepine, and may enhance their toxicity.

Absorption, fate and excretion: Sodium valproate is rapidly and almost completely absorbed after oral administration. Eighty per cent to 95% of plasma valproate is protein bound. More than 90% is metabolised in the liver.

Adverse reactions: The main adverse reactions are nausea and vomiting. It increases appetite and may cause weight gain. Dose related hair loss may occur. Hypoalbuminaemia is common, and **hepatotoxicityis** *its major drawback. Hence it is advisable to do baseline hepatic function studies before starting sodium valproate.*

The other infrequent adverse effects are sedation, ataxia, incoordination, thrombocytopenia and pancreatitis.

It is teratogenic, and spina bifida is associated with its use during pregnancy.

Preparations and dosage:

i. Sodium valproate 100 and 200 mg tablets; 200 and 500 mg modified release/enteric coated tablets; 150 and 300 mg gastro-resistant capsules; 50, 100, 250, 500, 750 and 1 g modified release granules; syrup 200 mg per 5 mL and as 100 mg/ml injection. The therapy is initiated 10 mg/kg/day in two divided doses. This is increased by 5–10 mg/kg/day at weekly intervals up to 20–30 mg/kg/day. Doses as high as 60 mg/kg/day have been used. The IV starting dose is same as oral dose, the total dose is 1–2 g daily to be administered IV over 3–5 minutes.

ii. A combination of sodium valproate with valproic acid in controlled release tablets and valproic acid alone as enteric coated tablets are also available.

iii. **Divalproex sodium** is a stable co-ordination compound comprised of sodium valproate and valproic acid. Divalproex sodium dissociates to the valproate ion in the GIT.

Indications:

It is used as a first line drug in the following:

- **Grand mal seizures**
- **Petit mal seizures**
- **Combined grand mal and petit mal seizures**
- **Myoclonic epilepsy**

It is useful as adjunctive therapy in the following:

- **Focal epilepsy**
- **Manic depressive psychosis** (Chapter 13)
- **As prophylactic in febrile convulsion**

II. **ZONISAMIDE**

This sulphonamide derivative inhibits T type Ca^{++} currents and, like phenytoin, delays the recovery of the inactivated Na^{+} channels. Given orally, it has a long t½ (1–3 days) and is mainly excreted in the urine. The ADR reactions are somnolence, ataxia, anorexia, and fatigue; rarely, renal calculi develop

Indications: As an adjunctive therapy in the treatment of focal seizures in adults.

4. **AEDs that enhance inhibition through GABA:**

a. **Acting through GABA-related receptors**

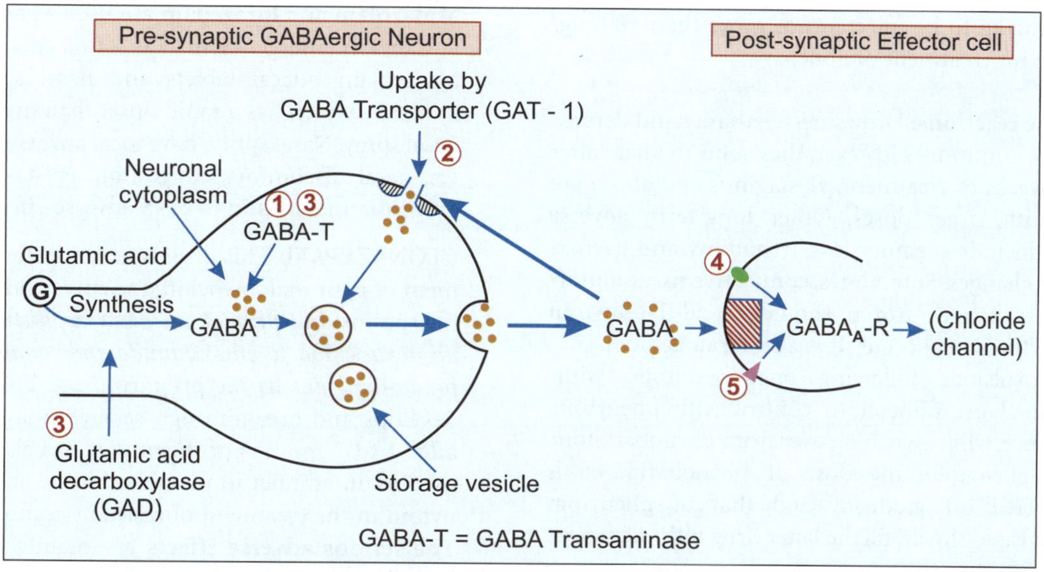

FIG. 9.5 **Antiepileptic drugs acting on GABA metabolism. 1, vigabatrin inhibits GABA-T; 2, tiagabine blocks GABA reuptake; 3, valproate inhibits GABA-T and stimulates GAD; 4, barbiturates activate GABA receptors; 5, benzodiazepines facilitate GABA action.**

PHENOBARBITONE: Phenobarbitone is discussed in Chapter 6. It is concentrated in the epileptic focus. Its antiepileptic activity is similar to that of diphenylhydantoin, but in addition it raises the seizure threshold. However, it has a different mechanism of action (Chapter 6). Hence, it can be combined with phenytoin in the treatment of resistant grand mal, focal cortical seizures and hypsarrhythmia. The daily dose varies from 60 to 180 mg in divided doses or as a single dose at night.

The main advantages of phenobarbitone are as follows:

- *It is well tolerated by most patients.*
- *Its half-life is long, permitting single-dose-a-day therapy, with better compliance.*
- *Therapeutic drug monitoring is usually not necessary.*
- *It is cost-effective.*

Phenobarbitone is of limited value in temporal lobe epilepsy and may aggravate petit mal seizures. It may produce excitement or hyperactivity in children and in old people. Because of its long half-life, it takes 2–3 weeks to reach a steady therapeutic plasma level.

Preparations and dosage:

Phenobarbitone tablets, 15, 30, 60, 100 mg and solution for injection, 3 mg/ml, for IV injection at a dose of 10 mg/kg to be injected not more than 100 mg/minute for treatment of epilepsy

Adverse reactions: Drowsiness, lethargy and depression are common. However, they tend to abate after a few weeks of treatment. Nystagmus and ataxia are seen with larger doses. Other long-term adverse effects include memory loss, irritability and haematologic changes. Sometimes, connective tissue abnormalities such as frozen shoulder and Dupuytren contractures may occur. It is also teratogenic.

Convulsions following phenobarbitone withdrawal are difficult to control with phenytoin. Hence, while switching over from phenobarbitone to phenytoin, the dose of phenobarbitone is tapered off gradually and that of phenytoin increased slowly, till the latter drug fully takes over.

Indications:

- **Grand mal epilepsy** (see the section, Drug therapy of epilepsy).
- **Status epilepticus**

Mephobarbitone and **primidone** are prodrugs and their antiepileptic effect is due to their active metabolite phenobarbitone. Primidone is also used in the treatment of essential tremor resistant to propranolol.

II. BENZODIAZEPINES

Benzodiazepines, in general, are anticonvulsants but not antiepileptics. They increase the effectiveness of the inhibitory neurotransmitter GABA (Chapters 8 and 14).

Benzodiazepines are not a good choice for the long-term treatment of epilepsy because

a. Tolerance can develop and seizures may recur within few months.
b. Drowsiness and ataxia can occur.
c. Status epilepticus on abrupt cessation of these drugs is difficult to treat.

DIAZEPAM: Because of its high lipid solubility and good penetration into the brain, it has a very rapid onset of action. **Given intravenously or rectally, it can be life-saving in status epilepticus and is the treatment of choice in this condition as well as in nonepileptic seizures** (Chapter 8). It is also available as intranasal spray.

Midazolam and **lorazepam** are used as anticonvulsants in emergency such as status epilepticus. Midazolam buccal tablets and nasal spray is available, which has a rapid onset than diazepam nasal spray. Nasal sprays have local adverse effects *viz.* nasal discomfort, congestion, epistaxis and dysgeusia in addition to CNS adverse effects.

CLONAZEPAM: This drug is useful in the treatment of petit mal, myoclonic seizures and infantile spasms. *In petit mal, it is used in patients who do not respond to ethosuximide and sodium valproate and not as the primary drug.* Tolerance develops and breakthrough seizures may occur after 1 to 2 months of therapy. It has also been used as an adjunct to phenobarbitone and phenytoin in the treatment of resistant grand mal.

The serious adverse effects are mainly neurological and comprise drowsiness, ataxia, personality changes, slurred speech, tremor, vertigo and confusion. They are dose related. Skin eruption, anaemia, leucopenia and thrombocytopenia have been reported. It is liable to cause respiratory depression and to increase the salivary and bronchial secretions. The other ADR involve the cardiovascular, the GI and the genitourinary systems. Tolerance is known to occur and psychic and physical dependences have been reported.

Clonazepam is available as 0.5 mg, 1 and 2 mg tablets and oral solution of 100 or 400 mcg/ml and as 1 mg/mL ampoules for IV injection. Therapy is initiated in adults and in children more than 10 years of age with oral administration of 0.5 mg twice a day; the dose is gradually increased to the maximum of 428 mg/day.

CLOBAZAM: It has actions and disadvantages similar to those of diazepam but has less sedative effects. It is used as an adjunct in the treatment of epilepsy. Clobazam is claimed to be useful in short courses in patients in whom seizures occur in clusters.

b. By releasing GABA from neuronal endings

I. GABAPENTIN: This is a GABA molecule bound to a lipophilic cyclohexane ring. However, it does not mimic GABA. Its precise mechanism of action is not known. It binds to the a2d subunit of voltage-gated calcium channels and probably increases the release of GABA.

The drug is well absorbed orally; is not protein bound; does not get metabolised; and is excreted unchanged in the urine. It has a plasma half-life of 5–9 h. Concurrent use of gabapentin does not affect the blood levels of other AEDs.

Adverse reactions: They include mild to moderate somnolence, dizziness, ataxia, fatigue, oedema, blurred vision and vertigo which can interfere with activities such as driving. Tolerance develops to these effects within 2 weeks.

Indications: Gabapentin is used in combination with other drugs, in focal seizures with or without secondary generalisation, resistant to other drug therapy. It is administered in the dose of 100 mg t.i.d., increased gradually to 900–1200 mg/day. **Gabapentin enacarbil** is an extended release formulation.

Pregabalin: This drug, related chemically to gabapentin, has similar mechanism of action, properties, ADR and uses. It is excreted unchanged in the urine. It does not interact with the other AEDs. It is used as an add-on drug in the treatment of focal epilepsy. It is not superior to gabapentin.

Other indications: Both the drugs have also been used in the treatment of migraine, deafferentiation pain such as postherpetic neuralgia and diabetic neuropathy, restless leg syndrome and in bipolar disorders with variable benefits. They are expensive.

c. By inhibiting GABA transaminase

I. Sodium valproate: See earlier.

II. VIGABATRIN (gamma-vinyl GABA): This drug acts as an irreversible GABA transaminase inhibitor (Fig. 9.5), thereby leading to an increased concentration of brain GABA. It is not metabolised but is excreted unchanged in the urine. The adverse effects are weight gain, drowsiness, depression, memory disturbances, diplopia and constriction of visual fields. *Hence, visual field testing is mandatory.* Attacks of acute behavioural changes in some patients is a major disadvantage. Its use is restricted to epilepsy not satisfactorily controlled by other drugs. Vigabatrin is particularly useful in infantile spasm. *It worsens absence seizures and myoclonic seizures.*

d. By inhibiting neuronal reuptake of GABA

TIAGABINE: This drug selectively inhibits the neuronal and astrocytic reuptake of GABA, and thus increases in synaptic GABA concentration. Orally, it is almost completely absorbed. Food de-lays its absorption. The drug is extensively metabolised in the liver and has a half-life of 7 to 9 h. Common adverse reactions include headache, dizziness, somnolence and tremor.

The drug is mainly used as an 'add-on' drug for the treatment of focal seizures, with or without secondary generalisation in adolescents and adults. It is usually administered in a dose of 4 to 12 mg t.i.d.

5. **Decrease release of excitatory neurotransmitter glutamate**
   Lamotrigine: See earlier

6. **Miscellaneous**
   The following drugs have different mechanisms and are mainly used as add-on drugs.

LEVETIRACETAM: This drug binds to synaptic vesicular protein (SV2A) but its precise mechanism of action is not known.

Given orally, it is absorbed rapidly and completely. It can also be given intravenously. It is not bound to plasma proteins and is excreted (70%−80%) unchanged in the urine. Adverse reactions are mild and include drowsiness, asthenia and dizziness. Rare, important side effects are emotional liability, agitation and nervousness. Coordination difficulties and serious skin reactions including Stevens–Johnson syndrome may occur.

Indications: As an add-on drug to treat refractory myoclonic, or focal seizures and uncontrolled generalised tonic–clonic seizures.

Brivaracetam is an analog of levitiracetam with similar actions and ADR.

Lacosamide: This AED, related to amino acid serine, acts by enhancing slow inactivation of Na^+ channels. It is given orally and intravenously. The adverse effects include dose-dependent dizziness, headache, fatigue, ataxia and vomiting. It may also cause sedation, tremor and diplopia.

Indications: Its efficacy for focal onset seizures is similar to other drugs and is used as an add-on drug in resistant cases.

Rufinamide, acts by enhancing slow inactivation of voltage-gated Na^+ channels.

Indications: It is used as an adjunct in the treatment of seizures in children with Lennox−Gastaut syndrome.

Ezogabine: This drug act as a **potassium channel facilitator** and reduces the degree of depolarisation needed to open the K^+ channels in the neurons. As a result, K^+ channels open faster and stay open for a longer time. This slows the repetitive firing of impulses by the neurons.

It is extensively metabolized and excreted by kidneys.

The adverse effects include dizziness, somnolence, fatigue, confusion, vertigo, tremors, disturbances in gait, attention and memory; blurred vision, dysarthria and euphoria. Weight gain, psychotic symptoms, QTc interval prolongation and suicidal tendencies have also been reported. When administered concomitantly with phenytoin/carbamazepine, its serum concentration decreases.

Indications: It may be used as adjunctive therapy for focal seizures.

Perampanel: This is the *first noncompetitive antagonist of AMPA receptors on postsynaptic neurons and inhibits AMPA-dependent calcium entry into the neurons.* It is metabolised by CYP3A4 followed by glucuronidation. The adverse effects include dizziness, somnolence, vertigo, ataxia, aggression, euphoria, blurred vision, weight gain, fatigue and dysarthria. Parampenal can cause serious, life-threatening psychiatric, behavioural adverse effects.

Indications: It is used as adjunct therapy for focal seizures.

Acetazolamide: This diuretic with its carbonic anhydrase inhibitory activity (Chapter 37) is occasionally effective as an adjunct in resistant petit mal and grand mal epilepsies.

AED IN NONEPILEPTIC DISORDERS

These drugs have been used in many nonepileptic disorders with variable results (Table 9.1)

PH 1.1

GENERAL PRINCIPLES OF MANAGEMENT OF EPILEPSY

Seizures are a symptom of an underlying disorder: genetic, traumatic, metabolic, inflammatory, drug induced or due to drug withdrawal. Although treatment of the cause can cure seizures, this may not be possible for all.

Table 9.1 Non-epileptic indications of antiepileptic drugs

Anti epileptic drug	Non-epileptic indications
Carbamazepine	Trigeminal neuralgia and bipolar disorder
Gabapentin	Neuropathic pain syndromes, migraine/tension headache, spasticity, and social phobia
Lamotrigine	Neuropathic pain syndromes
Primidone;	Essential tremor
Topiramate	Migraine/tension headache, essential tremor and binge disorder
Vigabatrin	Spasticity
Sodium valproate	Migraine/tension headache and bipolar disorder
Phenytoin	Digoxin-induced ventricular tachycardia
Phenobarbitone	Neonatal hyperbilirubinaemia

Epilepsy should be considered as an illness and not a social stigma. Occupations involving driving of vehicles and working with machines, near a waterfront or at heights are not suitable for epileptics. Likewise, swimming is a forbidden sport. Within these limits, a well-controlled epileptic may be a good employee if he/she knows his/her limitations.

About 65%−70% of epileptics are found to have an underlying brain lesion (*secondary epilepsy*).

The rational management of epilepsy needs an accurate evaluation of the epileptic syndrome. Currently, there is no drug cure for epilepsy. The main aim is to achieve prolonged seizure-free periods with the lowest risk of drug toxicity, permitting the patient to lead as full a life as his or her capabilities permit. Complete control of symptoms may not always be possible. AEDs are continued even if they prevent the seizures only partly.

Drugs, used regularly, abolish seizures completely in 60%−80% of the patients and reduce their frequency in another 10%−20%. This is usually achieved without producing intolerable adverse effects. Occasionally, these drugs will suppress the abnormal electrical activity and, after therapy for years, may produce complete clinical cure in a few cases. This is especially true in patients with petit mal epilepsy. To achieve best results with drugs, the following must be carefully observed:

- **Proper initial evaluation** is necessary to rule out other neurological events (e.g. syncope) that might be mistaken for seizures.
- A patient who gives history of a single seizure is treated with medication if there is one or more risk factor for recurrence of seizures such as abnormal neurological finding, the presence of structural lesions, abnormal EEG, partial seizures or a family history of seizures; otherwise the patient is only observed and not prescribed drugs. **However, if patient has a history of two or more seizures an AED should be prescribed.** The initial choice of the AED depends on various factors (Box 9.5).
- The drug therapy should be simple and started with a single drug (**monotherapy**) which is effective, least toxic and convenient to take. The AED therapy is initiated in small doses targeting the lower portion of the therapeutic range, and is gradually increased till the maximum benefit is obtained *without an increase in adverse effects.* Commonly used drugs are listed in Table 9.2.
- Mild toxicity can be managed by reducing the dose by 25% – 30% while waiting for tolerance to develop. Most antiepileptics may give rise to skin rash during the first few weeks of therapy. The drug need not be stopped for that reason except for carbamazepine as rash may be the first indication of Steven Johnson Syndrome.
- Changes in therapy should be made after careful weighing of pros and cons and not every time a new drug appears in the market. Adequate trial (for 2–3 months) should be given to an AED before rejecting it in favour of another one.
- Epileptic seizures that initially respond to drug therapy sometimes escape from control. In the

Table 9.2 Drugs Commonly Employed in the Treatment of Epilepsy

Drug	Steady State (days)	Serum Half-Life (h)		Dose[a] (mg/day)	Dose Interval	Therapeutic Plasma Concentration (mcg/mL)
		Adults	Children			
Phenytoin sodium[b]	7–8	24	20	100–400	o.d.	10–20
Carbamazepine[b]	3–4	12	8	200–1500	b.i.d., t.i.d.	4–12
Ethosuximide	7–10	55	30	500–1500	b.i.d., t.i.d.	40–100
Valproate[c]	1–4	15	11	500–2000	b.i.d., t.i.d.	50–100
Lamotrigine	3–6 (5–15 with valproic acid comedication)	15–35 (30–90 with valproic acid comedication)	32	200–500	o.d.	2.5–15
Phenobarbitone[b]	>21	120–140	72–96	60–180	o.d.	10–40

Note: Plasma valproate levels are not a useful index of therapeutic efficacy.
[a]In adults.
[b]Hepatic microsomal enzyme inducers.
[c]Hepatic microsomal enzyme inhibitor.

case of phenobarbitone, primidone, phenytoin and carbamazepine, the *escape may be due to hepatic enzyme induction.*

- Monotherapy with standard drugs results in satisfactory control of seizures, in almost 50% of patients. If adequate control is not achieved by a single drug in maximum tolerated doses and if compliance and absence of precipitating factors (as sleep deprivation, febrile illness and use of concomitant drugs) are confirmed, *another drug is substituted.* If this fails, combined therapy should be considered.
- While changing from one drug to another, the first drug must be tapered off slowly (unless serious ADR demand abrupt stoppage), while the second one is introduced in gradually increasing doses.
- When a drug combination is used, each drug should be prescribed separately and fixed-dose drug combinations should be avoided.
- For phenobarbitone, phenytoin, primidone and ethosuximide, sustained therapeutic plasma levels can be achieved by giving the entire daily dose once a day. Sodium valproate is best prescribed on a twice-a-day basis and carbamazepine 2–3 times a day. Extended release formulations are now available. Young children require frequent doses as they metabolise AED more rapidly than adults.
- When experience shows that, in a given patient, the frequency or likelihood of attacks increases under stressful circumstances, e.g. examination or social events, it is advisable to increase the dose, often to the limit of tolerance, well in advance of the event, and to reduce it gradually afterwards. Trauma, including that of surgery, also increases the drug requirement.
- Clinical monitoring by recording the seizure frequency and ADR is more important than TDM. **TDM is useful** for (a) in adjusting the dose of a drug during the initial days of its use; (b) in detecting noncompliance; and (c) to attribute toxicity to a particular drug and adjust its dose.
- If patients remain seizure free for 2–5 years, an attempt can be made to taper the AEDs slowly over 6–10 weeks. Phenobarbitone, primidone and benzodiazepines should be tapered off over 2–4 months. *However, most patients need treatment for their lifetime, except those with petit mal.*

The risk of recurrence is about 40%–50% in adults and 25% in children. About 80% recurrences occur within 4 months of discontinuation of drugs.

- *Information, instructions and warnings: The patient,*

or in cases of children, the parents, should be counselled regarding the duration of treatment and the need for compliance, to maintain the seizure record in a diary and to attend the follow-up clinic regularly. The patients should be warned not to stop the AED on their own as sudden withdrawal of an AED can precipitate status epilepticus. The patient should be advised to avoid using OTC formulations and drugs from alternative medicine as some of them may contain drugs which lower seizure threshold and precipitate seizures.

Finally, it must be remembered that epilepsy syndromes are often associated with psychiatric, cognitive and social complications, even in cases considered as uncomplicated. Furthermore, age-related brain atrophy leads to increased vulnerability to seizure-induced cognitive defects. In addition, certain AEDs can cause cognitive adverse effects. Phenobarbitone, phenytoin and valproate have negative effects on memory and, motor and cognitive function. On the other hand, carbamazepine and valproate may have positive effects on mood. *Hence it is advisable to screen for psychiatric and cognitive comorbidity in all patients before starting AEDs.*

EPILEPSY AND PREGNANCY

AED should not be stopped abruptly during pregnancy. Their dose should be reduced to a minimum. *Women on AEDs should receive folic acid supplements 5 mg/day starting before the conception, and the drug should be continued throughout the pregnancy.*

Well over 90% of women taking AEDs give birth to healthy babies, and pregnancy need not be terminated in well-controlled epileptics. However, women with epilepsy have almost twice the rate of complications such as toxaemia, intrapartum haemorrhage and premature labour, regardless of the drug used. The major **fetal malformations**, such as cardiac defects, cleft palate, neural tube defects and spina bifida, occur in almost 2% of pregnancies in epileptics; they are probably drug-related. The use of two or more AEDs increases the frequency to 10%. Minor malformations such as nail hypoplasia, low set ears and prominent lips also occur with a higher than normal frequency in infants born of mothers on antiepileptics.

The newborn of mothers who have received an AED during pregnancy should be examined for congenital abnormalities. Most AEDs promote haemorrhagic diathesis in the neonate. Hence, they should receive vitamin K at birth, in order to prevent bleeding due to deficiency of vitamin K–dependent clotting factors. *Furthermore, phytomenadione (not menadione) 20 mg/day should be given to the mother in the last month of pregnancy.*

AED can be used safely during breast feeding. Sometimes, the babies can get sedated. PH 1.19

DRUG THERAPY OF EPILEPSY

Drugs used in the treatment of epilepsy may be clinically classified into the following:

1. **Those that are effective in petit mal:** Ethosuximide, sodium valproate, lamotrigine clonazepam and acetazolamide
2. **Those that are effective in all other varieties:** Diphenylhydantoin, primidone, carbamazepine, lamotrigine, topiramate, valproate, oxcarbazepine and phenobarbitone
3. **Newer add-on drugs:** Lamotrigine, topiramate, levetiracetam, zonisamide and lacosamide are considered as *broad spectrum* as they are useful in both focal and generalised seizures.

Box 9.5 lists the factors which determine the selection of the AED.

Box 9.5 Factors Determining the Selection of the AED

- Type of epilepsy syndrome
- Tolerability and safety of the drug
- Convenience of the drug schedule
- Cost of therapy

PETIT MAL

It is essential to confirm the diagnosis of petit mal by an EEG as the specific drugs are effective only in patients with typical EEG changes. It is also essential to inquire about concomitant grand mal attacks as antipetit mal drugs are liable to aggravate grand mal.

Ethosuximide and **sodium valproate** are equally effective in this condition. Sodium valproate as a single drug is the drug of choice if tonic–clonic seizures also coexist.

Drug treatment of petit mal can be withdrawn 3–4 years after cessation of attacks. It is rare for this variety of epilepsy to recur.

GRAND MAL

Therapy with **sodium valproate** is initiated with 600 mg daily, divided into two doses. It can be increased every third day by 200 mg. The usual maintenance dose is 1–2 g/day.

The other suitable alternative, **carbamazepine,** should be started in the dose of 200 mg twice or thrice a day and the dose should be increased gradually until seizures are controlled or a total daily dose of 1200 mg is reached. If seizures continue, change over to **phenytoin sodium**.

Lamotrigine appears to be effective in epilepsy syndromes with mixed, generalised seizure types and is used as monotherapy as well as adjunctive therapy.

Once seizures are under control, the drug or drug combination must be continued for a least 3–4 years after the last seizure episode.

Epilepsy during drowsiness is a condition where fits occur when the patient is drowsy but not asleep. *Phenobarbitone, which produces drowsiness, increases the frequency of attacks in this condition and must be avoided.*

FOCAL SEIZURES

The drug treatment of this condition is similar to that of grand mal epilepsy. The seizures are often refractory to drug therapy. **Carbamazepine** and **phenytoin** are the preferred drugs in this condition.

MYOCLONIC SEIZURES

Sodium valproate and lamotrigine are the drugs of choice for this condition. Topiramate, levetiracetam and clonazepam serve as the alternatives.

Fig. 9.6 and Table 9.3 summarize the choice of AED for common types of seizures. It also depicts the alternatives that can be used for these seizures.

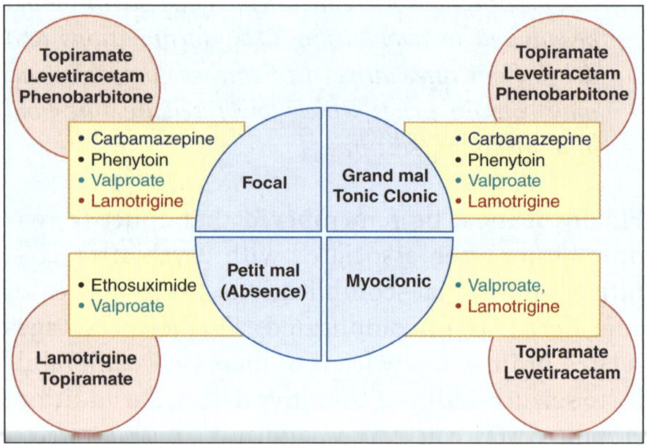

FIG. 9.6 Choice of Antiepileptic drugs for common type of seizures. The drugs listed in yellow boxes are the drugs preferred for the given epilepsy while the drugs listed in the pink circles are the alternative drugs.

POSTTRAUMATIC SEIZURES

Head injury predisposes to the development of seizures. Prophylactic treatment with IV phenytoin should be initiated as soon as possible after injury to decrease the risk of posttraumatic seizures occurring within the first 7 days. Other AED such as carbamazepine, levetiracetam and valproate are also used.

FEBRILE SEIZURES

Febrile convulsions are neither associated with, nor do they cause, mental retardation, affect IQ, poor scholastic performance or behavioural problems; hence, *routine prophylactic administration of AEDs is not warranted.*

Brief febrile seizures need only treatment of the fever (tepid sponging and paracetamol) in an otherwise normal child. If a febrile convulsion lasts longer than 15 min, rectal administration of diazepam in solution (10 mg per 2 mL) in the same dose as in status epilepticus is rapidly effective.

Table 9.3 Choice of Antiepileptic Drugs

Type of Seizure	Drug/s of Choice	Alternative/s – 1	Alternative/s – 2
Petit mal	Ethosuximide Sodium valproate	Lamotrigine Clonazepam	Topiramate
Grand mal (tonic–clonic)	Sodium valproate Carbamazepine Lamotrigine	Topiramate	Phenytoin Phenobarbitone[a]
Petit mal with tonic	Sodium valproate	Lamotrigine	Phenobarbitone + Ethosuximide
Myoclonic	Sodium valproate Lamotrigine	Topiramate Levetiracetam	Clonazepam
Focal	Carbamazepine Lamotrigine Sodium valproate Phenytoin	Topiramate Phenobarbitone Levetiracetam	Newer antiepileptics[b]

[a]In developing countries, because of low cost.
[b]For patients resistant to established drugs.

The risk of developing epilepsy in such children is approximately 10%. When indicated, chronic prophylaxis is initiated with phenobarbitone, or carbamazepine is another alternative. *Phenytoin is not well tolerated by small children, and valproate is more toxic at this age.* The child should be treated for 2 years or for 1 year after the last seizure, whichever is longer.

ECLAMPTIC SEIZURES

Management of eclampsia consists of treatment of seizures, control of blood pressure and ultimately, uneventful delivery of the baby. The drug of choice to treat eclamptic seizures is mag-nesium sulphate. It is administered as a slow intravenous bolus with a loading dose of 4–6 g, followed by a maintenance infusion of 1 to 2 g/ hour. The patient should be monitored for clinical signs of magnesium toxicity, such as loss of patellar reflexes, drowsiness, flushing, slurred speech, muscle weakness and respiratory depression. If toxicity is suspected, then the infusion should be discontinued and if required, IV calcium gluconate should be administered.

The mechanism of action of magnesium sulphate as anticonvulsant is not clear, however it is a potent cerebral vasodilator and reverses cerebral vasoconstriction by blocking calcium influx through the NMDA receptors. Apart from seizure control, maintaining the BP to normal is equally essential and should be achieved by antihypertensive drugs IV hydrallazine or labetalol (Chapter 30). See Chapter 30.

STATUS EPILEPTICUS (Box 9.6)

Status epilepticus (SE) is a life-threatening disorder characterised by an acute, prolonged epileptic crisis without return of full consciousness between seizures.

Box 9.6 Management of Generalised Convulsive SE

- Hospitalise
- Ensure adequate airway
- Prevent aspiration and physical injury
- Initiate cardiorespiratory monitoring
- Obtain appropriate blood samples (glucose, calcium and electrolytes poison screen, if available)
- Establish IV line with normal saline
- Give 50 mL of 50% glucose and 100 mg of thiamine IV, only if hypoglycaemia is documented.
- Give sodium bicarbonate IV if the arterial blood pH is less than 7.2
- Treat fever or hyperthermia
- Give an anticonvulsant, e.g. lorazepam IV followed by an antiepileptic such as phenytoin.
- Institute long-term antiepileptic therapy.

The IV administration of anticonvulsant drugs requires the availability of cardiopulmonary resuscitative support equipment.

There are many different SE syndromes, defined by clinical features, EEG findings and underlying/precipitating factors. SE is an emergency and the patient should be treated in ICU.

SE can be classified as (a) generalised convulsive status epilepticus (**GCSE**), (b) subtle SE (the most severe clinical stage of GCSE with poor prognosis), (c) nonconvulsive SE (e.g. absence and focal onset SE). Among these, GCSE is the most common.

Normally a generalised convulsive seizure resolves spontaneously after 3–5 min. Hence if seizure activity lasts for more than 10 min, it is diagnosed as SE. Such patients need emergency IV medication if death or permanent brain damage, especially hippocampal sclerosis (which can occur in 30–60 min in untreated patients), is to be prevented. Box 9.6 summarises the principles of management of GCSE.

Lorazepam IV is considered as the treatment of choice for controlling seizures. Although diazepam has a longer t½, it has a higher volume of distribution and more lipid solubility. Hence, its therapeutic effects are of a shorter duration than those of lorazepam (2–8 h). The dose of lorazepam is 4–8 mg, given over 1–2 min. It can be repeated if there is no response within 5 min. In patients taking valproate, start IV sodium valproate (25 mg/kg).

Lorazepam has been used by squirting it intranasally, using an atomising pump. It reaches the brain rapidly within minutes. However, this device is not marketed. Instead midazolam nasal spray can be used. Its dose is 5 mg of single spray in one nostril, which can be repeated if no response is seen within 10 min. It is used to treat one episode/3 days (max 5 episodes in a month).

In case lorazepam is not available, IV **diazepam** can be administered. It may be given in the dose of 10 mg IV slowly (more than 5 min) in adults, 5 mg for children more than 7 years of age and 2.5 mg for those between 1 and 7 years of age. The dose may be repeated twice more at 15 min intervals. The dose may be further repeated every 2–4 h, if necessary.

If IV administration is not possible, **diazepam may be given rectally**: 10 mg in adults and children more than 3 years of age, and 5 mg in children 1–3 years of age, and, in elderly patients, it may be repeated, if necessary, after 5 min. **Midazolam** (buccal or IV 10 mg) is an alternative to diazepam.

Propofol or **midazolam or thiopental** is administered in cases of refractory SE in consultation with an anaesthesiologist.

For patients with nonconvulsive status (absence SE) or myoclonic status, sodium valproate IV may be required.

Box 9.7 lists 'The Points to Remember' in the treatment of status epilepticus.

Emergency management of convulsions due to other disorders such as withdrawal of sedatives (including barbiturates), tetanus, eclampsia, cerebral haemorrhage, poisoning from convulsive agents and during the administration of local anaesthetics is similar to that of SE.

Box 9.7 Points to Remember While Treating GCSE

- During prolonged SE, cerebral seizure activity may continue even after convulsions have stopped.
- Do not inject 50% glucose IV routinely; hyperglycaemia can damage cerebral neurons. IV Lorazepam 4–8 mg (2 mg/min) is an anticonvulsant, not an antiepileptic. Do not inject BDZ after convulsions have stopped.
- Phenytoin is incompatible with glucose-containing solutions; is contraindicated in patients having second or third degree heart block; should be injected intravenously at not more than 25 mg/min in elderly patients.
- Phenobarbitone has a rapid and prolonged antiepileptic action. It is indicated when phenytoin is contraindicated or has failed to control convulsions.
- BP normally rises at the onset of SE. Do not allow systolic BP to fall below the high normal level during the course of treatment as otherwise cerebral ischaemic damage may occur.
- Muscle relaxants stop convulsions but do not abolish cerebral seizure activity. Do not use them unless EEG monitoring is available.
- Watch for cardiorespiratory and metabolic derangement.
- Refractory SE is always due to a serious underlying disease.

Diazepam or lorazepam is the drug of choice; paraldehyde IM may also be used. *Phenytoin is not useful.* The same is true of convulsions occurring during the withdrawal of CNS depressant agents in addicts.

Surgical Treatment of Refractory Epilepsy

Surgery can be effective in reducing seizure frequency and providing complete seizure control in patients with refractory epilepsy.

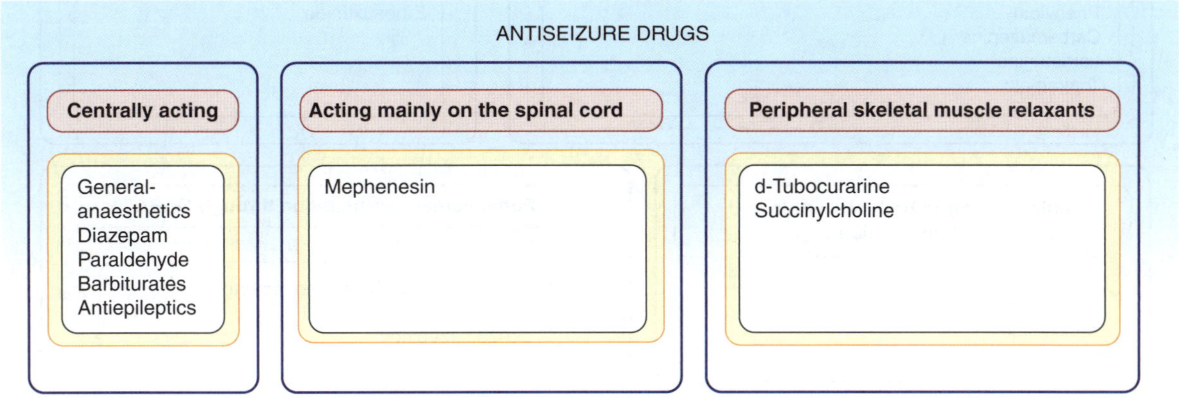

ANTIEPILEPTICS (ACCORDING TO THEIR MECHANISM OF ACTION)

Decrease in the neuronal excitability by delaying the recovery of inactivated Na^+ channels

Phenytoin
Carbamazepine
Lamotrigine
Topiramate

Decrease in the low threshold calcium currents (T-current) in the thalamic neurons

Ethosuximide

Action similar to both phenytoin and ethosuximide

Sodium valproate
zonisamide

Enhancement of inhibition through GABA

Acting through GABA-related receptors:
- Barbiturates
- Benzodiazepines

By releasing GABA from neuronal endings:
- Gabapentin

By inhibiting GABA transaminase:
- Sodium valproate
- Vigabatrin

By inhibiting neuronal reuptake of GABA:
- Tiagabine

Decrease release of excitatory neurotransmitter glutamate

Lamotrigine

Selective enhancer of slow sodium channel inactivation

Lacosamide

Potassium channel opener

Ezogabine

AMPA receptor antagonist

Perampanel

Miscellaneous

Levetiracetam
Acetazolamide

CHAPTER 10

Opioid Analgesics and Antagonists

Learning Objectives

This chapter will enable the reader:

1. To be aware of different types of pain and mechanisms responsible for the same.
2. To define the term 'analgesic' and classify analgesic drugs.
3. To describe endogenous opioid system and its physiological role.
4. To describe pharmacological effects associated with various opioid receptor types.
5. To describe the mechanism of action, pharmacological effects, ADR, salient pharmacokinetic features and indications for morphine.
6. To compare and contrast codeine, pethidine, methadone, pentazocine and buprenorphine with morphine with respect to opioid receptors, pharmacological effects, ADR and indications.
7. To explain pharmacological basis for the use of methadone in the treatment of opioid dependence.
8. To give examples of opioid agonist–antagonists, partial agonists and antagonists and describe their effects in the presence and absence of opioid agonist.
9. To explain the rationale for the use of alvimopan in reducing the risk of opioid-induced bowel dysfunction.

KEY TERMS

Pain is an unpleasant sensory and emotional experience associated with actual or potential tissue damage or described in terms of such damage. It is a subjective experience which cannot be objectively defined or quantified satisfactorily. Pain acts as a warning signal against disturbances in the body and thus has a protective function. However, on many occasions, pain seems pointless, only contributing to the discomfort in the subject. As a symptom, pain demands instant relief, and in practice its dramatic relief highly impresses a layman. Clinically, pain can be considered as follows:

- Somatic pain
- Visceral pain
- Referred pain
- Deafferentation or neuropathic pain
- Psychogenic or functional pain

Somatic pain arises *from the skin and from the deep nonvisceral structures* such as muscles, ligaments, bones and joints. It is usually well defined and is generally caused by an inflammatory reaction in the tissues; it may be accompanied by the contraction of the surrounding skeletal muscles as in patients with rheumatoid arthritis. However, other causes such as direct irritation of a nerve as in trigeminal neuralgia, herpes zoster, increased pulsation of the intracranial arteries as in migraine, or vascular insufficiency as in *thromboangitis obliterans* are also incriminated in the genesis of somatic pain.

Pain arising from the skin and superficial mucous membrane or nerves is felt as pricking, if brief, and stinging, smarting or burning, if prolonged.

Deep nonvisceral (musculoskeletal) pain usually has a dull character, and it may be accompanied by a sickening sensation due to an autonomic response. Sometimes, it spreads to other areas and may even occur as referred pain. BP and pulse, however, are not much affected, unless the pain is acute and severe.

Visceral pain, unlike the somatic pain, is diffuse, less easily localised and often 'referred'. It is dull-aching or colicky in character and is often accompanied by sweating, nausea, fall in BP and even shock. In addition, muscle rigidity and hyperaesthesia are common accompaniments. In practice, visceral pain may be due to spasm (renal or biliary colic), ischemia (myocardial infarction), inflammation (appendicitis and pancreatitis) or stimulation of the sensory nerve endings (peptic ulcer).

Deep pain, whether visceral or somatic in origin, may be misinterpreted as coming from some part of the body other than the actual site of stimulation. This is called **referred pain.** Thus, cardiac pain is commonly referred to the left arm and diaphragmatic pain to the shoulder. Usually, the pain is referred to a cutaneous area which receives its nerve supply from the same spinal segment as the affected viscus.

Various theories have been proposed to explain the pain mechanism, but none can explain all its aspects. The conscious appreciation of pain appears to depend on the widespread activity of the entire cortex, *and individuals differ widely in their reactions to similar painful experiences.*

Deafferentation pain is caused by partial damage to axons and nerve membranes, which become very sensitive to mechanical and chemical stimuli. Such pain may either be of burning, superficial (dysasthetic) type or of stabbing (lancinating) character. It has a peculiarly unpleasant quality about it and may not respond to opioids or to NSAID (see Chapter 11).

Psychogenic or **functional pain** is usually a vague pain which follows no definite anatomical pattern of distribution. Such pain is usually continuous from day to day and involves more than one part of the body. *It, however, does not disturb sleep.* Psychogenic pain is often preceded by a phase of exhaustion, whereas organic pain brings about exhaustion. *However, psychic element is present in all types of pain.*

Nociception

Nociception is a physiological process by which pain is perceived. Pain receptors (nociceptors) are distributed throughout the body. Painful stimuli may primarily be physical stimuli such as pressure or heat, or they may be chemical stimuli from the products of inflammation.

A variety of naturally occurring compounds can elicit pain response in experimental animals, e.g. histamine, acetylcholine, bradykinin, PGs, 5-HT and substance P. These substances are present in venoms and products of inflammation.

It appears that *tactile sensation* is transmitted by a large diameter (L), fast conducting nerve fibres, and *pain* via small diameter (S), slow conducting (C) nerve fibres (**nociceptors**). Activation of nociceptor causes the release of various neurotransmitters, leading to the activation of specialised neurons located in the posterior horns of the spinal cord. The secondary axons arising from the dorsal horn travel through the opposite spinothalamic tract, which terminate in the thalamus that projects to the postcentral gyrus which is responsible for localisation of pain. Although the thalamus is responsible for the perception of pain, the cerebral cortex is essential for its discriminative and meaningful interpretation and for its emotional components. The other intermingled fibres, which form an ascending multisynaptic pathway, terminate in the thalamus and from there project to the frontal and limbic systems, and the hypothalamus. This system is concerned with the emotional component of pain.

Clinically the sensation of pain has several components including the emotional and psychic reaction. PH 1.19

Analgesics are the drugs which relieve pain without causing the loss of consciousness.

Classification of Analgesics

I. **Opioid analgesics:**
   The opioids are further subclassified as follows:

a. **Agonists** such as morphine and compounds which resemble it in most of their actions, such as derivatives of morphine; codeine and its derivatives; synthetic compounds such as pethidine, methadone, propoxyphene, levorphanol and tramadol.
b. **Partial agonists,** e.g. buprenorphine and meptazinol. They have partial agonist action only on the mu receptors (see section, Synthetic morphine substitutes).
c. **Mixed agonist–antagonists** which act as agonists at one type of opioid receptors and as competitive antagonists at another type of receptors, e.g. nalbuphine, pentazocine and butorphanol. Patients who have received repeated doses of a morphine-like drug to the point of physical dependence may experience an opioid withdrawal reaction when given a mixed agonist–antagonist.

II. **Nonopioid analgesics** do not interact with opioid receptors and relieve pain without CNS depression, e.g. NSAID (Chapter 11).

OPIOID ANALGESICS

The word **opiate** refers to the products obtained from the opium poppy. The term **opioid** (opiate-like) is used to denote all naturally occurring (endogenous and exogenous) semisynthetic and synthetic drugs which have an analgesic action, such as relief from pain and depression of the CNS, both reversed by naloxone. These drugs were formerly called 'narcotic' analgesics because some of them (such as morphine) induce sleep. The term 'narcotic' is no longer applied to opioids but is restricted in the legal sense to drugs capable of producing dependence.

Endogenous opioid peptides: Peptides with strong opiate-like analgesic and mu receptor binding activity are present in the CNS and other tissues. They act as

a. Endogenous analgesics
b. Neurotransmitters
c. Behaviour modulators

They are as follows:

- **Beta-endorphin,** a potent analgesic, is derived in the pituitary from a larger, parent molecule, proopiomelanocortin (POMC). It predominantly binds to mu receptors and acts as a pain modulator in the CNS.
- **Enkephalins,** derived from pro-enkephalin, are more widespread; they are found in the pituitary, brain, GI tract, spinal cord, pancreas and adrenal medulla. They predominantly bind to the delta receptors.
- **Dynorphins** A and B, derivatives of pro-dynorphin, have been found to be widely distributed in the CNS. They predominantly bind to k receptors.
- **Nociceptin/orphanin** FQ is a peptide with behavioural and pain-modulating effects that are complex. It is also implicated in learning, cough reflex and Parkinson disease.
- **Endomorphins 1 and 2,** tetrapeptides with high, selective affinity for mu receptors.

Endorphins, enkephalins and endomorphins are released during stressful conditions such as pain or in anticipation of pain and serve as **natural pain modulators.**

Milk and milk products contain opioid peptides such as **beta-casomorphins,** which are released from casein in the intestine during the digestion of milk and may modulate GI function.

OPIUM ALKALOIDS

Opium is the milky exudate obtained by incising the unripe seed capsule of the poppy plant *Papaver somniferum*. The poppy seeds, however, are devoid of pharmacological activity and are in fact used in food preparations. On drying, the exudate forms a gummy, brownish mass. The pharmacologically active alkaloids of opium (Table 10.1) are divided chemically into **phenanthrene group** and **benzylisoquinoline group** (Fig 10.1)

The benzylisoquinoline alkaloids are devoid of analgesic activity but act as smooth muscle relaxants. They are described later.

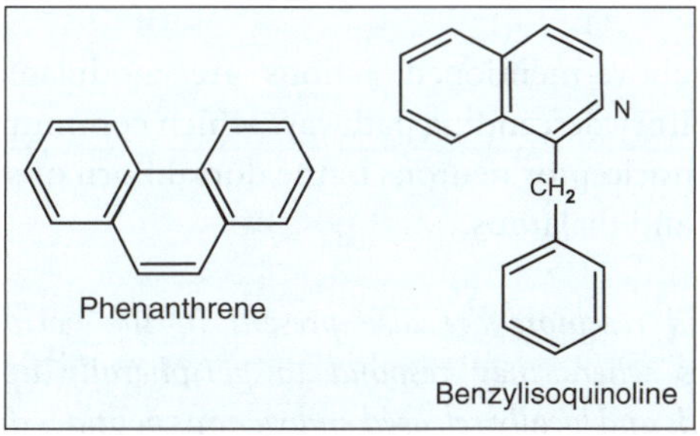

FIG. 10.1 Phenanthrene and Benzylisoquinoline

Table 10.1 Opium Alkaloids

	Name	Percentage
Phenanthrene series	Morphine	9.0–14.0
	Codeine	0.5–2.0
	Thebaine	0.2–1.0
Benzyl iso-quinoline series	Papaverine	0.8–1.0
	Noscapine	3.0–10.0
	Narcine	0.2–0.4

Mechanism of action of opioids: The opioid drugs produce their effects by **binding to opioid receptors** (Table 10.2) which are widely distributed in the CNS and other tissues. In the CNS, they are localised to

a. The periaqueductal grey matter of the brainstem, and the thalamus.
b. The area postrema which has the chemoreceptor trigger zone (CTZ) and the solitary nuclei which receive visceral sensory fibres from the vagus and glossopharyngeal nerves.
c. The amygdala which may be responsible for the influences of the opioids on the emotional reactions.
d. The spinal cord substantia gelatinosa, the first site in the CNS which integrates the sensory information.

Opioid receptors are a part of family of G-protein-coupled receptors. They have been classified into **mu** (mu_1, mu_2), **delta** ($delta_1$, $delta_2$), **kappa** (k_1, k_2, k_3) and **nociceptin** (orphanin) types. When activated, they

a. Open K^+ channels to inhibit postsynaptic neurons.
b. Close Ca^{++} channels on the presynaptic neurons to inhibit the release of the neurotransmitters from nociceptive nerve terminals. These actions reduce neuronal excitability.

The above-mentioned actions are modulated by inhibitory descending pathways which communicate with nociceptor neurons in the dorsal horn of spinal cord and thalamus.

Opioid receptors are also present in the peripheral nerves where they respond to peripherally applied opioids and locally released endogenous peptides during inflammation.

Table 10.2 Pharmacological Effects Associated with Opioid Receptor Types

Receptors	Effects
MOR (mu)	Supraspinal/spinal analgesia, euphoria, respiratory depression, sedation, miosis, decreased GI motility, smooth muscle spasm, physical dependence, release of prolactin and growth hormone, nausea and vomiting, feeding
KOR (kappa)	Supraspinal/spinal analgesia, sedation, miosis and decreased GI motility (of lesser degree), less physical dependence, dysphoria, psychotomimetic effects, diuresis, feeding
DOR (delta)	Supraspinal/spinal analgesia, less respiratory depression, decreased GI motility, release of growth hormone, feeding
NOR	Drug reward and reinforcement, stress responsiveness, learning and memory

MOR, mu opiod receptor; KOR, kappa opiod receptor; DOR, delta opiod receptor; NOR, nociceptin opiod receptor

The pharmacological effects associated with these receptor subtypes and selectivity of the various opioid drugs for these receptors are summarised in Tables 10.2 and 10.3.

The vast majority of opioid drugs used as analgesics are agonists at mu receptors. Similarly, the opioid antagonists, naloxone and naltrexone, show a high selectivity for mu receptors. Drugs with mixed agonist–antagonist properties bind to more than one receptor class at the usual clinical doses.

MORPHINE is the most important alkaloid of opium and is used as sulphate or hydrochloride; both salts are soluble in water.

Pharmacological actions: Morphine acts predominantly on **mu receptors** situated both in the CNS and other tissues such as the GI tract. The exact mechanism of pain relief is not known. However, opioids and endogenous opioid-like peptides decrease the release of glutamate from nociceptive nerve terminals, and also of acetylcholine, NA, 5-HT and substance P.

Table 10.3 Selectivity of Common Opioid Analgesic Drugs for Different Receptors

Compound	Receptor Type	
	MOR	KOR
Pure agonists		
Morphine	+++	+
Methadone	+++	0
Codeine	+	+
Partial agonists		
Buprenorphine[a]	(+++)	?
Agonist/antagonists		
Butorphanol	(++)/−	+++
Pentazocine	(+)/−	++
Nalbuphine	−	++

Notes: +, agonist; (+), partial agonist; –, antagonist; 0, no action. MOR, mu opioid receptors; KOR, kappa opioid receptors.
[a]Antagonist of mu receptors in high doses.

Central nervous system:

- **Analgesia:** Morphine, by acting on mu_1 receptors, produces relief of pain in a dose that usually does not cause motor incoordination. Other modalities such as touch, vibration and hearing are not obtunded.

  In subanaesthetic doses, morphine and its analogues have little effect on pinprick sensation and the withdrawal reflex, although pain arising from the tissues is well suppressed. **In moderate doses,** it is effective in relieving continuous, dull pain. **Larger doses** relieve sharp intermittent pain caused by trauma and by visceral pathology. *Morphine, pethidine, methadone and the other agonists do not have a ceiling dose as far as their analgesic effect is concerned*; the dose can be increased to a level just short of causing toxicity (as in the treatment of terminal cancer).

  Morphine raises the pain threshold, reducing the perception of pain, and also causes the feeling of well-being.
- **Euphoria, sedation and hypnosis:** Morphine produces a sense of emotional well-being termed 'euphoria' (mu_1 receptors). Euphoria eliminates the normal fear, panic, withdrawal and flight response to pain and aids the analgesic action of morphine. *The ability to produce euphoria even in the absence of pain makes morphine one of the worst drugs of abuse.* Rarely, it may produce a sense of anxiety or fear termed dysphoria, particularly in pain-free individuals.

  Sedation induced by morphine is characterised by drowsiness, difficulty in concentration and mental apathy. Thoughts may lack a logical sequence, and imagination becomes extravagant, producing vivid and colourful daydreams. Larger doses induce sleep. The normal NREM and REM cycle is disrupted.
- **Respiratory depression:** Morphine **in therapeutic doses** depresses all phases of respiratory activity. It acts (a) by direct depressant action on the respiratory centre (mu_2 receptors) and (b) by reducing its sensitivity to increased plasma CO_2 concentration.

  Retention of CO_2 brought about by initial respiratory depression by morphine increases the rate and depth of respiration to the predrug value. At a later stage, the hypoxic drive tends to maintain the minute volume despite diminished sensitivity of the respiratory centre to accumulated CO_2. The respiratory rate and minute volume, therefore, are not adequate monitors of respiratory depression caused by morphine. Bronchoconstriction as a result of histamine released by morphine enhances respiratory difficulties.

  With toxic doses, breathing is entirely maintained by the 'hypoxic drive' mediated through the carotid and the aortic body chemoreceptors, and this may result in *Cheyne–Stokes respiration.* Inhalation of pure oxygen at this stage abolishes the hypoxic drive and produces apnoea. *Hence, in such cases controlled, assisted ventilation and moderate concentrations of oxygen are indicated.*

  Chronic administration may cause tolerance to respiratory depressant effect.
- **Cough suppression:** Morphine depresses the cough reflex as a result of direct depression of the cough centre.
- **Pupillary constriction:** Morphine produces characteristic pin-point pupils. The miosis is due to an action on the Edinger–Westphal nucleus of the oculomotor nerve.

- **Nausea and emesis:** Morphine produces vomiting by the stimulation of the CTZ in the area postrema of the medulla. Morphine-induced vomiting is abolished by nalorphine and by prochlorperazine (5−10 mg 4−8 hourly), metoclopramide (10 mg 4−8 hourly) and haloperidol (1−2 mg daily) but not by antihistaminics.
  In large doses, it depresses the vomiting centre. *Thus, in cases of morphine poisoning, vomiting is absent and emetics are ineffective.*
- **Vagus stimulation:** Morphine stimulates the medullary vagal nucleus and may cause bradycardia.
- **Spinal cord excitation:** Morphine increases the reflex excitability of the spinal cord. This action is, however, usually masked by the depression of the higher centres in the CNS. Therapeutic doses of morphine may produce a significant increase in the CSF pressure.
- **Miscellaneous:** Morphine in large doses lowers the body temperature by the central action.
  Morphine depresses the respiratory and cough centres and stimulates the vagal and oculomotor centres and the CTZ.

Gastrointestinal tract: Morphine induces:

a. spasm of the smooth muscle of the gut, the ileocolic and the anal sphincters, and reduces the propulsive peristaltic movements (mu$_2$ receptors). There is a reduction in the secretion of saliva, gastric acid and the intestinal secretions. Desiccation of the faeces, abolition of the peristaltic movements, spasm of the sphincters, particularly the anal sphincter, and inattention to normal sensory stimuli from a loaded rectum as a result of the psychological effect of morphine all lead to constipation. *Atropine partially antagonises the spasmogenic action of morphine on the colon.* Patients on long-term use of morphine should receive a high-fibre diet and a laxative such as senna regularly. Lubiprostone (Chapter 39) may also be helpful.
b. Morphine increases the intrabiliary pressure by producing a spasm of the sphincter of Oddi. Hence, although it may relieve the biliary colic because of its analgesic action, the underlying disease is exacerbated. Atropine partially antagonises this action.

In mice, morphine produces a severe spasm of the anal sphincter resulting in erection of the tail. This test, termed **Straub's test**, was formerly employed to detect morphine in biological fluids.

Other smooth muscles: Morphine produces:

- *An increase in the tone of the ureters and the detrusor muscle of the bladder.* The vesical sphincter is contracted. These effects are augmented by inattention to stimuli arising from the bladder and may cause urinary retention.
- *An increase in the tone of the bronchi and the bronchioles.*

Except in large doses, it has no significant effect on the normal human uterus at full term.

Cardiovascular system: Therapeutic doses of morphine have negligible effect on the myocardium, the BP or the heart rate. Morphine produces dilatation of the peripheral blood vessels, particularly the cutaneous blood vessels. This may reduce the preload on the heart (see under Therapeutic uses). Large doses may produce hypotension.

Neuroendocrine system: Morphine inhibits the release of GnRH and CRH from the hypothalamus. It thus decreases the plasma concentration of FSH, LH and ACTH. The plasma prolactin increases.

Morphine produces a release of ADH with a resultant decrease in the urinary output. Administration of morphine reduces the efficacy of diuretics in patients with CHF.

Immune system: Opioids suppress the various immune functions and increase the susceptibility to infection in experimental animals, both by a direct action and an indirect action mediated by the CNS.

Absorption, fate and excretion: Given orally, morphine is adequately absorbed. It is extensively metabolised during first pass through the liver; hence its oral bioavailability is about 20%−40%. Sustained-release preparations have a longer duration of action. The drug can also be given rectally. Given subcutaneously, it produces analgesic effect within 15–20 min with the peak effect at 60–90 min; it persists for 3–5 h. Morphine, given intravenously, produces an immediate effect.

Morphine circulates in the plasma partly protein-bound and partly in the free form. It enters the brain rapidly. It crosses the placental barrier readily and is also secreted in milk. It is metabolised by the liver and the kidney. Morphine is conjugated with glucuronic acid to form both active and inactive products; *morphine-6-glucuronide, the active metabolite, is more potent than morphine*. In adults, the plasma t½ of morphine is about 2−3 h, whereas that of the glucuronide is longer.

Approximately 90% of the administered dose is eliminated in urine within 24 h, mainly in conjugated form. Biliary excretion of this form accounts for approximately 7% to 10% of the dose.

Preparations and dosage:

i. Morphine tablets (10, 20, 30 and 50 mg).
ii. Modified release tablets (5, 10, 15, 30, 60, 100 and 200 mg), modified release capsules (30, 60, 90, 120, 150 and 200 mg) and modified release granules (20, 30, 60, 100 and 200 mg) of morphine for prolonged action.
iii. Morphine solution (2−20 mg/mL) for oral use. Dose in adults is 10−30 mg. Larger doses (up to 200 mg) are needed in patients with terminal cancer. Orally, it is only about one-sixth as effective as parenteral administration.
iv. Morphine hydrochloride or sulphate injection 10, 15, 20 and 30 mg/mL. Dose: 10−20 mg SC or IM; 2.5−5 mg IV over 5 min. It has also been used by a continuous, low dose, IV infusion (10 mg is infused over the first 1 h and 10 mg over the next 4 h) and by epidural and intrathecal administration.
v. Suppository (10, 15 and 30 mg) of morphine sulphate. Dose is 15-30 mg 4 hourly.

Adverse reactions:

- **Intolerance:** These reactions include allergic skin rashes, pruritus and contact dermatitis. It is a histamine liberator. Anaphylactoid reaction with fall in BP has been reported after morphine injection.
- **CNS and respiratory depression:** It causes nausea, vomiting, dysphoria, mental clouding, vertigo, headache, fatigue and paraesthesia. Morphine may occasionally produce tremors and delirium. Respiratory depression occurs even in small doses (see Pharmacological actions).
  All opioids decrease respiratory drive and can cause apnoea in opioid naive patients, especially those with COPD, cor pulmonale and preexisting respiratory depression/poor respiratory reserve.
- **Constipation** following morphine may be dangerous in old people as it may precipitate intestinal obstruction. It may also cause abdominal distension and an increased biliary pressure.
- **Hypotension:** Morphine occasionally produces hypotension as a result of peripheral vasodilatation, more so in patients with a reduced blood volume.
- **Urinary retention:** Morphine may cause urinary retention postoperatively and in old people with prostatic hyperplasia. *Patients taking anticholinergic drugs are more prone to develop urinary retention.*
- **On the fetus:** Morphine administered to the mother during labour can depress fetal respiration. This asphyxia can be reversed by naloxone 10 mcg/kg given intravenously, intramuscularly or subcutaneously.
- **Tolerance:** Repeated administration of morphine at short intervals results in the loss of its effectiveness (tolerance). With an intermittent use, however, tolerance to analgesic and sedative effects does not develop. Tolerance also develops to the respiratory depressant, emetic, hypotensive and euphoriant effects of morphine as well as to urinary retention, *but the pupils and the GIT do not share this tolerance*. A morphine addict has thus characteristically pinpoint pupils and is habitually constipated.
  Tolerance to morphine is attributed primarily to the ability of the cells of the central nervous system to withstand large doses of the drug.
  Persons tolerant to morphine exhibit cross-tolerance to other opioid analgesics and even to compounds such as barbiturates and alcohol. Tolerance does not develop to antagonistic actions of pure or mixed agonist−antagonist. PH 1.22
- **Drug dependence:** This is a major drawback of morphine. Opium has been in use as a drug of abuse for several centuries and has precipitated wars. Dependence on morphine and morphine-like drugs results mainly from their euphoriant effects. In addition, these drugs produce a variety of sensations such as a 'turning in the stomach', a

feeling of warmth in the epigastrium and other parts of the body due to flushing; and sensations in the lower abdomen described by addicts as akin to sexual orgasm, and known as 'kick' or 'thrill'.

Morphine addicts are usually malnourished and debilitated. Even though they do not suffer from motor incoordination and are capable of performing complex motor and intellectual tasks, their productivity and utility to the society usually suffer. As the drug is commonly self-injected, the incidence of injection abscesses, tetanus, AIDS and serum hepatitis is high among the addicts.

Manifestations of **opioid withdrawal syndrome** are summarised in Table 10.4.

In order to prevent morphine dependence, morphine should not be prescribed readily for chronic pain except in cases of terminal cancer pain. Such patients rarely develop psychological dependence on morphine.

To decrease the misuse of opioids, opioid abuse deterrent formulations have been developed. (See under 'Opioid abuse deterrent formulations').

Table 10.4 Manifestations of Opiate Withdrawal

Abstinence Period	Manifestations
6–12 h	Intense craving for the drug, lethargy and weakness
12 h	Yawning, lacrimation, perspiration, rhinorrhoea, tremors and anorexia
48 h	Peak of the withdrawal syndrome; fever, rise in BP, increase in heart rate, dilatation of the previously constricted pupils and intestinal cramps
7–10 days	Symptoms clear up but the patient may complain of restlessness, insomnia, weakness and back and leg pains for several weeks

PH 1.23

Treatment of morphine dependence: In principle, it is similar to that of alcohol or barbiturate dependence. The results, however, are unsatisfactory because of the severity of withdrawal syndrome and the high relapse rate. Its gradual withdrawal with the substitution of another opioid analgesic to decrease the severity of withdrawal syndrome is usually advocated.

Buprenorphine (5-15 mg OD), a mixed agonist-antagonist, either alone or in combination with naloxone remains the drug of choice. Its efficacy is comparable to methadone but is much safer.

Methadone, which has longer t½ than morphine is an another alternative. Once the patient is stabilised on methadone, its dose is gradually reduced by 10%–20% daily and the drug can be completely stopped from 6th to 10th day. Though it reduces craving, its overdose has effects similar to morphine and can be life threatening.

Another alternative can be opioid antagonist like **naltrexone**, but it diminishes only euphoria and not the craving.

Acute opiate withdrawal symptoms and signs can be controlled to a certain extent by drugs such as **clonidine** and **propranolol** which counter the noradrenergic overactivity.

FM 10.1, IM 21.2

Acute morphine poisoning: Acute morphine poisoning may occur from clinical overdosage, accidental overingestion by an addict or from suicidal or homicidal intention. It is difficult to define the lethal dose of morphine. A dose of 60 mg is usually toxic, but rarely fatal, in a normal adult who is not in pain. Doses of 250 mg are usually fatal. Larger doses are generally required to produce toxicity in individuals with pain, whereas in addicts, the toxic as well as the fatal doses are much higher.

Morphine poisoning is characterised by respiratory depression, pinpoint pupils, cyanosis, reduced body temperature, decreased urinary output, hypotension, shock and coma. Convulsions may occur in infants. Death is usually due to respiratory depression, or shock and pulmonary oedema.

If a toxic dose of morphine has been ingested, even late gastric lavage is justified as the spasmogenic action of morphine frequently delays its absorption.

Naloxone and **nalorphine** are the specific morphine antagonists. They produce dramatic reversal of morphine-induced respiratory depression. Naloxone is usually preferred because of its specific antagonistic and negligible agonistic action (See section, Opioid antagonists). They should be administered with caution in treating acute morphine poisoning in addicts as they may produce a severe withdrawal syndrome. *The duration of action of opioid antagonists is shorter than that of opioids, and the patient has to be carefully monitored to prevent relapse into coma.*

Drug interactions: CNS depressants, phenothiazines, monoamine oxidase inhibitors and tricyclic antidepressants enhance the sedative effects of morphine and increase the respiratory depression. Use of opioids with serotonergic drugs can cause serotonin syndrome. Opioids can delay and decrease oral absorption of P2Y12 inhibitors and increase platelet activity.

Indications:

- **For relief of pain:** Morphine is one of the most potent analgesics, employed to alleviate severe pain in various conditions (Box 10.1). For relief of sudden excruciating pain, it is usually administered intravenously; prompt relief of pain minimises shock. *Morphine SC is not advocated in the presence of shock, as its absorption is hampered.* Repeated SC administration of it under these conditions may result in a sudden absorption of toxic quantities into the systemic circulation after the correction of hypotension.

  Parenteral morphine has been used to reduce postoperative pain; thoughtless use for this purpose should be avoided as it can produce respiratory depression, urinary retention and constipation; it reduces coughing and may mask the signs of recovery and of complications.

  Because opiate receptors are located within the spinal cord, **intrathecal and epidural morphine** produces long-lasting analgesia. Such analgesia is essentially segmental in distribution, the pain relief being remarkable and it is assumed to be selective without any interference with motor function or autonomic changes. However, respiratory depression, nausea, vomiting and pruritus may occur. Because of greater safety and ease of administration, most investigators prefer the epidural route to the intrathecal route. *Not all types of pain respond to opioids. For example, the deafferentation pain is relatively resistant (Chapter 11).*

Box 10.1 Analgesic uses of morphine

- Acute myocardial infarction
- Fractures of long bones
- Burns
- Cancer pain
- In palliative care e.g. terminal stage of malignancy
- Pulmonary embolism
- Acute pericarditis
- Renal and biliary colic (along with smooth muscle relaxant, atropine)
- Postoperative pain e.g. after thoracic and upper abdominal surgery

- **In acute left ventricular failure:** Morphine is valuable in the treatment of acute left ventricular failure and pulmonary oedema. It acts by reducing apprehension and the effort of breathing. Morphine-induced peripheral vasodilatation results in shunting of the blood from the pulmonary arteries to the dilated peripheral vasculature, and this in turn reduces preload. Thus, it reduces the cardiac work load, and relieves dyspnoea, provided oxygenation is maintained.
- **Sedation:** Morphine is a valuable sedative in the presence of severe pain.

  Although morphine was routinely for sedating patients with internal bleeding such as haematemesis, fentanyl or a sedative such as diazepam is safer for this purpose.
- **As a preanaesthetic medication:** See Chapter 7.

Precautions and contraindications with morphine therapy:

1. **Chronic obstructive pulmonary disease (COPD):** Morphine should be administered with caution to persons with diminished respiratory reserve, e.g. individuals with emphysema, kyphoscoliosis and COPD. Such patients are already on the verge

of hypoxia, which they avert by increasing their respiratory rate. Opioids decrease ciliary activity, depress cough reflex, cause bronchospasm and depress respiration, all of which can precipitate respiratory failure in such individuals. Deaths have been reported in patients with COPD following therapeutic doses of morphine.

2. **Myxoedema:** The lower BMR and reduced rate of metabolic disposal of drugs make such patients more sensitive to opioids and sedatives, and frank coma may be precipitated by even their conventional therapeutic doses. Patients with hypopituitarism and Addison disease are also more sensitive.
3. **Elderly and infants:** They are more prone to develop respiratory depression with morphine.
4. **Head injury:** Morphine should be avoided in such cases as it produces an increase in the CSF pressure, stimulates the spinal cord and produces respiratory depression, vomiting and miosis. Mental clouding and miosis may interfere with the diagnosis.
5. **Acute abdomen:** In this condition, morphine relieves pain symptomatically without modifying the underlying pathological process. It does not alter the physical signs such as abdominal rigidity. It may, therefore, facilitate clinical evaluation and permit diagnostic procedures. It may be helpful *provided the pain is not forgotten.* However, morphine-induced vomiting and its spasmogenic action on the GI and biliary tracts are its drawbacks.
6. **Shock:** Morphine IV may produce hypotension if administered during hypovolemic shock. Restoration of blood volume is more important in that condition.
7. **Severe impairment of liver and/or kidney function:** Cumulative toxicity can occur.
8. Use of morphine (or opioids) during pregnancy has been associated with still birth, IUGR and birth defects such as neural tube defects and congenital heart defects.

Other phenanthrene alkaloids of opium

CODEINE: Codeine, by itself, is:

a. A much less potent analgesic than morphine (weak agonist)
b. In therapeutic doses, it does not produce significant depression of respiration
c. It has a low dependence liability
d. It may produce excitement and convulsions in toxic doses

It enhances the analgesic effect of aspirin and is often combined with it. Unlike morphine, it is much better absorbed when given orally, with the bioavailability of about 50%. About 10% codeine is converted to morphine in the liver by CYP2D6, and which is responsible for its analgesic property. For drug interactions with inducers and inhibitors of CYP2D6, see Chapter 3. Extensive metabolisers are more susceptible to its toxicity. It is often used as an antitussive. Its main disadvantage is constipation. Codeine phosphate is available for oral and IM use.

Indications:

- **As an analgesic,** 30−60 mg t.i.d.
- **As an antitussive,** for suppression of dry cough (Chapter 26)
- **As an antidiarrhoeal agent** (Chapter 39)

Contraindication:

Codeine is contraindicated in all children <12 years and those <18 years who have undergone tonsillectomy or adenoidectomy. It should be avoided in children (12-18 years) having serious respiratory problems and breast feeding mothers.

Hydrocodone and **oxycodone** are other opioids used orally for treating cancer pain and also as antitussives. **Hydromorphone**, the active metabolite of hydrocodone is also available. Bioavailability of oxycodone is better than that of morphine. Both hydrocodone and oxycodone can be combined with paracetamol or ibuprofen for a synergistic effect. However, they are misused as a drug of abuse.

TRAMADOL: This synthetic codeine derivative is a weak agonist of the central mu receptors and also exerts a part of its analgesic action by inhibiting NA and 5-HT uptake. It is rapidly absorbed and is metabolised in the liver by CYP2D6 to an active compound with analgesic action. Its t½ is 6 h, and 30% is excreted unchanged in urine. It is as effective as pethidine in mild to moderate pain and causes less respiratory depression and constipation. It has a low addiction potential. It can be used in labour pains.

The drug causes dizziness, sedation and nausea, and rarely seizures. It can cause psychological and physical dependence. It should not be used concurrently with agents that enhance monamine activity or lower the seizure threshold, e.g. MAO inhibitors, TCA and SSRI. Its contraindications are same as codeine. The dose is 25–100 mg/day.

Tapentadol: This structural analogue of tramadol has similar mechanism of action and ADR profile as tramadol.

Benzylisoquinoline Alkaloids of Opium

PAPAVERINE: Papaverine is devoid of opioid and analgesic activities. It is a smooth muscle relaxant and causes vasodilation. Intracavernosal injection of papaverine causes penile erection and was used for the symptomatic treatment of erectile dysfunction (Chapter 67).

NOSCAPINE: This alkaloid has a significant antitussive action in therapeutic doses, without disadvantages of morphine. It is a potent releaser of histamine, and large doses can cause bronchospasm and hypotension. For its therapeutic use, see Chapter 26.

SEMISYNTHETIC DERIVATIVES OF NATURAL OPIUM ALKALOIDS

Codeine derivatives are mainly antitussive (see section, Other phenanthrene dervatives of opium). Only the derivatives of morphine are described as follows:

HEROIN (diacetylmorphine): It is a more potent analgesic than morphine, produces greater euphoria and consequently has a higher dependence liability. It is now rarely employed therapeutically because of this drawback but is extensively used (as *brown sugar*) as a drug of abuse.

Hydromorphone, oxymorphone and **methyldihydromorphinone** are effective analgesics with 4–5 h of duration of action. Their toxicity is similar to that of morphine.

Sustained-released hydromorphone is administered once daily for treating cancer pain.

Oliceridine is the first novel 'G protein-biased' mu receptor agonist. It is developed to have better analgesic effect with reduced risk of respiratory depression. Analgesic effects of opioids are mediated predominantly via G-protein signaling, whereas adverse effects are mediated by the β-arrestin pathway. Oliceridine activates G-protein signaling preferentially over β-arrestin. Though it is reported to possess favourable benefit-risk profile (less respiratory depression and vomiting) than conventional IV opioids for management of acute pain, more evidence is needed.

SYNTHETIC MORPHINE SUBSTITUTES

These are as follows:

1. **Pethidine and its congeners**
2. **Methadone and its congeners**
3. **Morphinan compounds and congeners,** e.g. levorphanol and butorphanol
4. **Benzomorphan derivatives,** e.g. pentazocine
5. **Miscellaneous:** Nalbuphine and buprenorphine

PETHIDINE (meperidine): As the pharmacological actions of this synthetic opioid (Fig 10.2) closely resemble those of morphine, only the salient differences between these two compounds are pointed out. Thus:

- On a weight basis, it is about one-tenth as potent as morphine as an analgesic when given intravenously, but it has a rapid onset and shorter duration of action ($t_{1/2}$ 4 h).
- In equianalgesic doses, pethidine produces as much sedation, euphoria and respiratory depression as morphine. However, unlike morphine, it reduces the tidal volume without significantly affecting the respiratory rate. Therefore, respiratory depression may be missed if respiratory rate alone is watched.

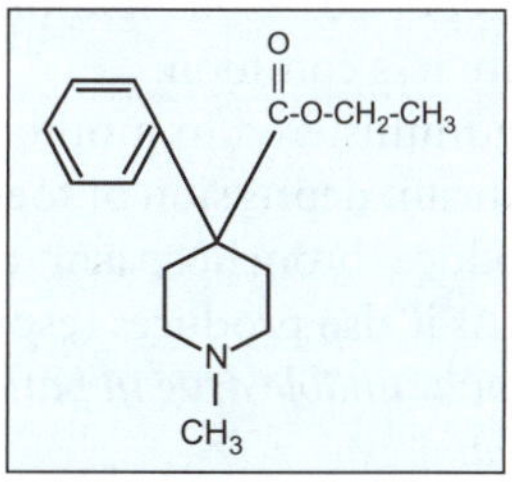

FIG. 10.2 Pethidine.

- The incidence of nausea and vomiting is higher than with morphine.
- Pethidine exerts an autimuscarinic effect. Compared to morphine, it is less spasmogenic and causes less constipation. It may, however, raise intrabiliary pressure by producing spasm of the sphincter of Oddi.
- Pethidine is devoid of antitussive activity.
- It may produce hypotension and syncope due to peripheral vasodilatation. Unlike morphine, however, IV pethidine may produce tachycardia and dryness of the mouth due to its vagolytic effect.

Absorption, fate and excretion: Oral bioavailability of pethidine is about 50%; the analgesic effect appears within 10–15 min. On parenteral administration, the action lasts for 2–4 h as compared to 3–5 h with parenteral morphine. It crosses the placental barrier and is also secreted in milk. It is highly irritant to tissues and can cause muscular fibrosis. It is mainly metabolised by the liver; *the metabolite norpethidine possesses a significant excitatory action on the CNS*. Only a small portion of pethidine is excreted unchanged in the urine. Its urinary excretion is enhanced when the urine is acidic.

Preparations and dosage

i. Pethidine hydrochloride tab, 50 mg. Dose: 50–150 mg 4 h.
ii. Pethidine hydrochloride injection 10 mg/ml or 50 mg/mL. Dose: IM/SC 25 to 100 mg IV 25 to 50 mg to be repeated, if necessary, after 4 h.

Adverse reactions

- The adverse effects, apart from local irritation on parenteral administration, include sweating, euphoria, dizziness, dry mouth, vomiting, dysphoria, visual disturbances, weakness and palpitation. Anaphylactoid shock following pethidine has been reported. Constipation and urinary retention are less common.
- Pethidine administered to mothers at term produces significant depression of foetal respiration.
- It can produce bronchospasm and drying of secretions. As it also produces respiratory depression, *it is not a suitable drug in patients with bronchial asthma.*
- Pethidine overdose causes respiratory depression and coma, or convulsions. Naloxone can antagonise the respiratory depression and coma but fails to modify the convulsant action of pethidine which probably is due to norpethidine. Acute pethidine poisoning should be treated on similar lines as acute morphine poisoning.
- **Tolerance and dependence:** Tolerance to analgesic and emetic effects develops on prolonged administration. The pethidine addict often shows dilated pupils, tremors, mental confusion, twitchings and occasionally convulsions.

Dependence on pethidine is fairly common. The **withdrawal syndrome** usually develops within 3 h after the last dose, reaches a peak by 8 to 12 h and declines by 4 to 5 days. There is little nausea, vomiting or diarrhoea, but the patient may show more excitement than during morphine withdrawal. The treatment is similar to that of morphine addiction. Methadone is employed initially as a substitute. One milligram of methadone can substitute for 20 mg of pethidine.

Drug interactions: Phenytoin increases the biodegradation of pethidine. Cimetidine (but not ranitidine) reduces the clearance of pethidine (but not morphine). Thus, morphine is a safer drug than pethidine to use in patients who are on cimetidine. Its administration to patients receiving imipramine or an MAOI may result in confusion, cerebral excitement and collapse.

Contraindications to the use of pethidine are similar to those for morphine.

Indications:

- **Analgesia:** It is particularly useful when a *short duration of action* is required, as in gastroscopy, cystoscopy or ascending pyelography. It serves as a morphine substitute for the relief of acute visceral pain, as short term remedy (24-48 hrs) e.g. in myocardial infarction, particularly the one that is associated with bradycardia, and in burns. The precautions to be observed with morphine for the treatment of shock also apply to pethidine.
- **Preanaesthetic medication:** Chapter 7.
- **Epidural and intrathecal analgesia** (see Chapter 7).

PETHIDINE CONGENERS:

FENTANYL (See Chapter7)

It is the most widely used agent. Its pharmacological profile is similar to morphine but it offers the following advantages:

- **It is 80 to 100 times more potent than morphine** and therefore microdoses are needed to produce analgesia and sedation
- It permits **lower anaesthetic drug concentrations with haemodynamic stability**
- **Reflex effects to pain are abolished**
- It exhibits **synergism when combined with BZD, to be used for minor procedures in poor risk patients for anaesthesia**
- It has less emetic activity and rarely causes clinically significant histamine release
- Given intramuscularly or intravenously (2–20 mcg/kg), it rapidly produces profound analgesia lasting for about 30-60 min.

Preparations and dosages

i. Fentanyl Citrate Inj. 50mcg/mL for IV or IM injection. Dose to be individualized.
ii. Fentanyl transdermal patches: The patches are designed to deliver approximately 12, 25, 50, 75, and 100 mcg/h fentanyl to the systemic circulation, which represent about 0.3, 0.6, 1.2, 1.8, and 2.4 mg / day respectively for a period 72 hours.
iii. Fentanyl citrate sublingual tablet: 100, 200,300, 400, 600, 800 mcg.
iv. Fentanyl citrate: available as lozenges (lollipop; 200, 400, 600, 800 1200, 1600 mcg/ lozenge), buccal tablet (100, 200, 400, 600, 800 mcg) and soluble film (200, 400, 600, 800, 1200 mcg)for transmucosal absorption.
v. Fentanyl citrate nasal spray: 50,100,200 mcg in single-dose container.

Indications:

- **Acute severe visceral pain:** An IV loading dose 1 to 2 mcg/kg, followed by maintenance dose of 0.35 to 0.5 mcg/kg every 0.5 to 1 hour intermittently is sufficient to control the pain.
- **Intraoperative analgesia:** It serves as an adjunct to general / regional Anaesthesia in the dose of 50 to 100 mcg slow IV when additional analgesia is required.
- **Postoperative analgesia:** In the recovery room, fentanyl may be administered intramuscularly for the control of pain, tachypnea and emergence delirium.
- **Cancer pain:** Fentanyl transdermal patches are used to control persistent, moderate to severe chronic pain in opioid-tolerant patients when continuous analgesia is needed.
- **Anaesthesia:** In combination with droperidol it is used as an anaesthetic agent (Chapter 7).
- **Preanaesthetic medication:** See Chapter 7.

The **fentanyl** congeners **alfentanil**, **sufentanil** and **remifentanilare** used mainly as anaesthetic adjuncts (Chapter 7). Remifentanil has a rapid onset of action and is metabolised rapidly by esterases in the plasma and muscles. As a result, its duration of action is extremely short with less respiratory depression

Alphaprodine has a shorter duration of action (1/2 to 2 h) on SC administration and causes emesis less frequently than other opioid analgesics.

Diphenoxylate and its metabolite **difenoxin** are used in the treatment of diarrhoea. In therapeutic doses, they do not produce morphine-like subjective effects, but large doses cause typical opioid symptoms.

Loperamide, a piperidine derivative, is used for its **selective GI mu receptor antidiarrhoeal effect** (Chapter 39). It is also used for neuropathic pain. Loperamide 5% ointment is used to relieve pain in diabetic neuropathy.

METHADONE: Methadone has analgesic potency almost equivalent to that of morphine.

Pharmacological actions: These are more or less similar to those of morphine but have a longer duration of action. A single therapeutic dose, however, exerts much less hypnotic activity than an equianalgesic dose of morphine. The drug depresses respiration to the same degree as morphine and has a marked antitussive effect. The actions of the drug on the GIT and the cardiovascular system are similar to those of morphine.

In addition, methadone inhibits the reuptake of noradrenaline and 5-HT; further, it also blocks the action of NMDA receptors, the known **modulators of neuropathic pain.**

Absorption, fate and excretion: Unlike morphine, methadone has the bioavailability of about 80%. The analgesic effect occurs within 10 to 15 min following parenteral, and 20–30 min after oral medication. It is highly bound to plasma proteins and also to the tissue proteins, including those in the brain. Plasma t½ of a single oral dose is 15 h, which increases up to 24−36 h following repeated administration. It crosses the placental barrier.

Methadone is slowly metabolised in the liver, which may explain its longer duration of action. Less than 10% of the drug is excreted unchanged by the kidneys.

Preparations and dosage:

i. Methadone hydrochloride, 5 mg tablets. Dose: 5–10 mg.
ii. Methadone hydrochloride, oral solution 1, 10 and 20 mg/mL. Dose: 10-30 mg daily and increased in doses of 5-10 mg until no signs of withdrawal. Usual dose is 60-120 mg daily.
iii. Methadone hydrochloride injection, 5, 10, 25 and 50 mg/mL. Dose 5 to 10 mg by IM/SC injection.

Adverse reactions: They are similar to those of morphine. Its repeated administration can result in cumulative toxicity. Methadone shares the respiratory depressant action of morphine. It causes dose-dependent lengthening of the QTc interval, which may precipitate cardiac arrhythmia. Acute methadone intoxication responds to naloxone.

Tolerance and the withdrawal syndrome develop more slowly and are less intense. The symptoms, however, persist much longer, approximately 10–15 days. Codeine is often used as a substitute during the treatment of methadone addiction.

Indications: It is used for the management of chronic pain. It can be used:

- In the **treatment of opioid abstinence syndrome** because it reduces the severity of withdrawal symptoms. Its longer duration of action, analgesic potency and lack of marked hypnosis make it a useful choice.
- As a substitute for morphine and pethidine for the **relief of severe visceral pain.**

METHADONE CONGENERS: These are levomethadyl acetate and propoxyphene.

Levomethadyl acetate exhibits a slow onset and prolonged duration of action, contributed partly by its active metabolite. A single dose every 72 h is used in the long-term management of heroin addicts to prevent protracted withdrawal syndrome.

d-Propoxyphene has been claimed to produce less depression of respiration, and fewer GI side effects. As an analgesic, it is only 1/25th to 1/50th as potent as morphine and is half as potent as codeine. The drug has little advantage over codeine.

MORPHINAN COMPOUNDS: The compound, **levorphanol,** is a more potent analgesic than morphine, is better absorbed orally and produces less constipation. It can cause drug dependence. It is administered orally or intramuscularly/subcutaneously in the dose of 2–3 mg.

BUTORPHANOL, a morphinan congener, is a **mixed agonist−antagonist.** It is a competitive antagonist at mu and exerts an agonistic action on kappa receptors. Its agonist activity (on a weight basis) is 4–7 times that of morphine and it is 20 times as potent as pentazocine. It is administered intramuscularly or intravenously in the dose of 2 mg, as well as intranasally.

PENTAZOCINE: This benzomorphan derivative is a mixed agonist−antagonist. It has a **potent analgesic (agonist)** action at the kappa receptors in the spinal cord and a **weak opioid antagonist activity** at the mu receptors. Compared to morphine

- It is half as effective as an analgesic and has a shorter duration of action
- It does not cause euphoria
- It has lower dependence liability
- Constipation is uncommon
- It causes less respiratory depression
- It raises the systemic and pulmonary arterial BP

with the resulting increase in the cardiac load; *hence it is not recommended in MI*

Absorption, fate and excretion: Pentazocine is given oral, rectal, SC, IM and IV routes. Although it is well absorbed orally, only 20% is bioavailable due to first pass metabolism. It is extensively metabolised by the liver and is excreted as glucuronide. *Smokers metabolise 40% more pentazocine than nonsmokers.*

Preparations and dosage:

It is available as 25 mg tablets and as 30 mg (lactate) per mL injection. The oral dose is 25–100 mg every 3–4 h. The parenteral dose (SC, IM and IV) is 30–60 mg every 3–4 h, as necessary.

Adverse reactions: These include the follows:

- **CNS:** Sedation, sweating, dizziness and nausea
- **Psychomimetic reactions,** hallucinations and unpleasant dreams. This is an important limitation to its use
- **Precipitation of acute withdrawal syndrome** in a morphine addict because of its antagonist action at mu receptor
- **Tolerance and physical dependence** have been reported, although the incidence is low

Nalorphine is valueless as an antidote to pentazocine but naloxone is useful.

Indications:

- **Visceral pain:** Pentazocine is used to control acute moderate to severe visceral pain in the dose of 30 mg every 3 to 4 hours. Maximum dose: 360 mg/day.
- **Labour pain** as 30 mg IM once a dayor 20 mg IV every 2 to 3 hours as needed (maximum dose: 60 mg)
- **Intraoperative analgesia:** It is used in a dose of 30 mg IM/IV/SC every 3 to 4 hours (maximum: 360 mg/day)

NALBUPHINE: This synthetic compound is chemically related to oxymorphone and the opioid antagonist naloxone. Like pentazocine, it is a **mixed agonist–antagonist** (kappa agonist and mu antagonist). As an agonist, it is 3–4 times more potent, while its antagonistic property is about 10 times more than that of pentazocine. The adverse effects are similar to those of pentazocine.

MEPTAZINOL: This partial agonist opioid is given orally or by injection. It is 1/10th as potent as morphine as an analgesic and has a shorter duration of action. It does not cause euphoria, and its respiratory depression is lesser than morphine.

BUPRENORPHINE: Buprenorphine, a highly lipophilic semisynthetic derivative of thebaine, has mainly **partial mu agonist properties. It is a weak antagonist at the kappa receptors.**

Pharmacological actions: As an analgesic, it is:

- More potent than morphine on a weight basis and has a longer duration of action (6 h)
- It causes less respiratory depression
- It has similar cardiovascular actions as morphine and can be used in MI
- It has a much less abuse potential than morphine

Naloxone does not precipitate acute withdrawal syndrome.

When it is given following the induction of anaesthesia with nitrous oxide and fentanyl, it reverses the anaesthetic and respiratory depressant effects of fentanyl but prolongs the analgesia.

Absorption, fate and excretion: It is inactive orally because of the first pass effect and hence given sublingually, intramuscularly or intravenously. The drug is highly protein bound and is excreted largely unchanged in the faeces.

Adverse reactions: It can cause respiratory depression similar to morphine at equianalgesic doses. *However, unlike morphine, the action is not readily reversed by naloxone.* Doxapram, a respiratory stimulant, may be useful. Other adverse effects are drowsiness, nausea, vomiting, constipation, miosis, headache bradycardia and hypotension. It prolongs QT interval, if used in high doses.

Preparations and dosage:

Buprenorphine is available as tablets 0.2 mg, as injections 0.3 mg/mL and as transdermal patches. The dose is 0.2–0.4 mg sublingually every 8 h and 0.3–0.6 mg IM or slow IV every 6–8 h. Transdermal patches of buprenorphine though effective in reducing chronic back pain, are not useful for severe cancer pain because the maximum content in patch is less (20 mcg/hr).

The other available formulations are oral transmucosal formulations (with or without naloxone), subdermal implants and once a month injection.

> *All partial agonists and mixed agonist/antagonists have a ceiling on their analgesic effect roughly equivalent to that of moderate doses of morphine.*

Indications:

- **As an analgesic:** It is given in a dose of 0.3 mg IM or IV every 6 h. for mild-moderate pain
- **Treatment of opioid dependence:** It is used alone or in combination with naloxone
- **To antagonize respiratory depression produced by anaesthetic doses of fentanyl:** The advantage is pain relief is not completely reversed

Pregnancy and opioids: Use of opioids by pregnant women affects the fetus causing birth defects, growth retardation, stillbirths and preterm births. Opioid withdrawal in these women also can cause spontaneous abortions and preterm labour. Hence such pregnant women who are physically dependent on opioids should receive maintenance therapy with buprenorphine or methadone.

Opioids excreted in milk can cause neonatal toxicity and deaths especially in breast fed infants.

Buprenorphine, hydrocodone, pethidine, methadone, oxycodone and tramadol are metabolised by CYP3A4. Concurrent use of drugs that induce/inhibit CYP3A4 can increase or decrease serum concentration of these drugs leading to respiratory depression or decreased analgesic effects respectively.

NONANALGESIC USES OF OPIOIDS

- **Antidiarrhoeal:** Diphenoxylate and loperamide (Chapter 39)
- **Central cough suppressant:** Codeine dextromethorphan (Chapter 26)
- **Emetic:** Apomorphine (Chapter 39)
- **Acute left ventricular failure:** Morphine (Chapter 31)

OPIOID ANTAGONISTS PH 1.19

Drugs that antagonise the effects of morphine and other opioid analgesics act mainly as competitive antagonists. Some of them also exert other actions not related to morphine receptors.

Classification:

i. **Pure antagonists** such as naloxone and naltrexone
ii. **Partial agonists of nalorphine type,** e.g. nalorphine, levallorphan and cyclazocine
iii. **Partial agonists of the morphine type,** e.g. propiram and profadol

Pure opioid antagonists, by themselves, produce few effects unless an opioid agonist has been administered previously. However, when endogenous opioids are activated as in shock or stress, an opioid antagonist does produce visible effects.

Partial agonists produce similar agonistic actions as morphine, which are antagonised by nalorphine or naloxone. However, they precipitate withdrawal symptoms in subjects maintained on very potent agonists such as morphine and heroin.

NALOXONE: This drug, N-allyl analogue of oxymorphone (Fig. 10.3), is a pure antagonist. It selectively antagonises the respiratory depressant action of morphine and other opioids. By itself, it is not a respiratory depressant, analgesic or euphoriant. It is not effective orally because of its first pass metabolism in the liver. One milligram of naloxone given intravenously completely blocks the effects of 25 mg of heroin. Its duration of action is 3–4 h. It is almost completely metabolised in the liver.

Preparations and dosage:

It is available in 1 mL vials containing 0.02, 0.4 mg/ml or 1 mg/mL and is the antagonist of choice in the treatment of opioid poisoning. It is administered

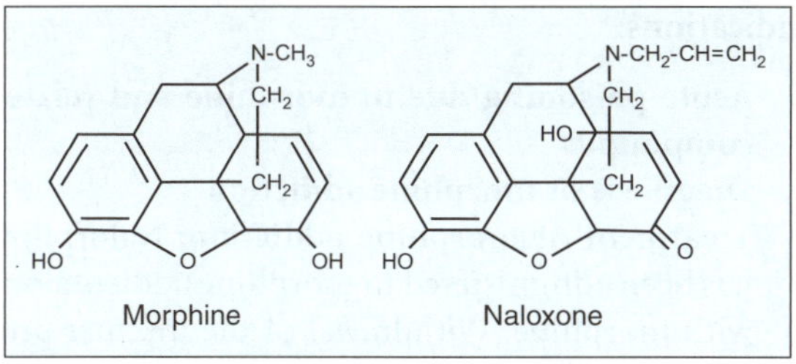

FIG. 10.3 Morphine and Naloxone.

as an IV bolus in the dose of 0.8–2.0 mg every 2–3 min to a total maximum dose of 10 mg. It can be administered intramuscularly or subcutaneously. It is also available as nasal spray as 4 and 8 mg / spray.

The IV dose in children is 10 mcg/kg (bolus); if there is no response, inject a 100 mcg/kg (bolus). Alternatively, it can be given in a dose of 0.4-0.8 mg i.m or s.c, repeated as necessary.

Adverse reactions: Hypersensitivity reaction may occur. The others are related to withdrawal syndrome precipitation in opioid-dependent patients and include nausea, vomiting, sweating, tachycardia, hypertension, tremulousness and pain. Acute pulmonary oedema has been reported in patients with heart failure. It lowers the seizure threshold in patients with seizure disorder. In neonates, shrill cry or failure to take feed may be observed.

Indications: Apart from its use in morphine poisoning, it is also used to reverse the residual respiratory depressant effects of an opioid analgesic at the end of an operative procedure. Low doses of naloxone are used to treat ADR associated with epidural opioids.

Endogenous opioid peptides, released by stress, may be responsible for hypotension observed in shock. Naloxone IV has been reported to correct the hypotension in septicaemic shock, although the effect is short lived.

NALTREXONE: This is an orally administered, *long-acting (24 h), pure opioid antagonist*. Its t½ is 3 h, whereas its active metabolite, 6-naltrexone, has t½ of 13 h. Naloxone, on other hand, is short acting and is ineffective orally. Naltrexone is well tolerated and has no euphoric effect, does not cause physical dependence and consistently blocks the effects of heroin and other addictive opiates for up to 4 days.

Naltrexone is available as 50 mg scored tablets. For treating heroin addiction, small doses (25 mg/day) are used initially, followed by 50 mg/day. For better compliance, the total weekly dose (350 mg) may be given on three days of the week (e.g. 100 mg on Monday and Wednesday, and 150 mg on Friday). Since naltrexone blocks the euphoric action of opioid agonists, it is given to former addicts to prevent re-addiction. For its use in alcoholism, see Chapter 6. A combination of naltrexone and bupropion is used in the treatment of obesity (Chapter 38).

Naltrexone in a much smaller dose (nearly in one-tenth of the dose used in addiction) is being used (not yet approved) in patients with multiple sclerosis and other degenerative diseases. It is claimed to arrest their progression.

Adverse reactions: The drug can cause GI disturbances, nervousness, sleeping difficulty and muscular pain. Rarely, thrombocytopenia and liver function abnormalities may occur.

Methylnaltrexone bromide is a peripherally acting mu receptor antagonist. In a dose of 8–12 mg SC *it is used to treat opioid-induced constipation in patients receiving palliative care*, when laxative therapy fails to produce adequate response.

The other two peripherally acting mu receptor antagonists include **naloxegol** and **naldemedine**.

Nalmefene is a pure mu receptor antagonist, more potent than naltrexone.

Samidorphan is an analogue of naltrexone. It is a mu receptor antagonist with partial agonistic action at kappa and delta receptors. It is used in combination with olanzapine in the treatment of schizophrenia to reduce weight gain due to the former.

NALORPHINE (N-allyl normorphine): Nalorphine is a semisynthetic congener of morphine. It can be used in the treatment of acute morphine poisoning.

By itself, it acts as a **partial agonist** and produces analgesia and respiratory depression. When administered after morphine, it acts as **competitive antagonist,** reversing the effects of morphine (Fig. 10.4).

Pharmacological actions:

Nalorphine shares many pharmacological actions of morphine such as analgesic, spasmogenic antitussive effect, miosis, respiratory depression. However, it does not cause drug dependence.

- **Administered after morphine,** nalorphine promptly abolishes the effects produced by morphine. Nalorphine is also a potent antagonist of codeine, heroin and synthetic morphine substitutes. *However, it is much less effective against pethidine.*
- **Administered to a morphine addict**, nalorphine precipitates the typical morphine withdrawal syndrome within 3–15 min. In normal individuals, nalorphine produces miosis, but, in an addict, it either dilates the pupils or fails to produce any demonstrable effect.

Nalorphine precipitates withdrawal syndrome in patients addicted to heroin and methadone.

Absorption, fate and excretion: Given orally, it is absorbed poorly, but more rapidly than morphine on SC administration. The drug is metabolised in the liver by conjugation.

Preparations and dosage: Nalorphine injection 10 mg/mL, administered by SC, IM or IV routes in the dose of 5–10 mg. The dose may be repeated to a total of 40 mg.

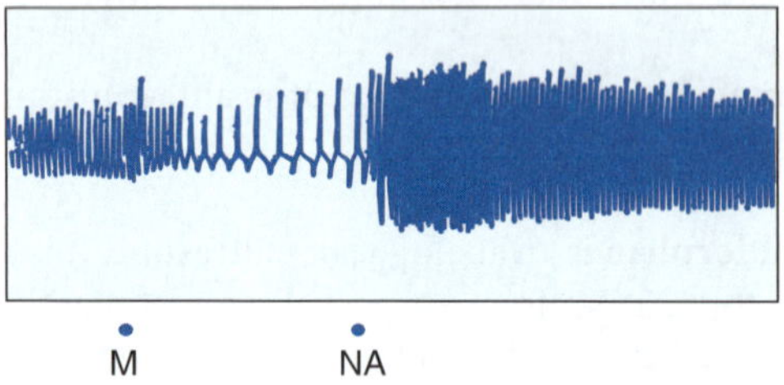

FIG. 10.4 Effect of nalorphine (NA) on morphine (M) induced respiratory depression in an anaesthetised cat.

Indications:

- **Acute poisoning due to morphine and related compounds**
- **Diagnosis of morphine addiction**
- **Treatment of morphine addiction:** Nalorphine has been administered to morphine addicts along with morphine. Withdrawal of the mixture produces a milder withdrawal syndrome than that observed after withdrawal of morphine alone.

Levallorphan: This opioid antagonist is similar to, but more potent than, nalorphine.

ALVIMOPAN: This drug, a **selective opioid-mu receptor antagonist,** is given orally. It is not much absorbed and blocks the GI effects of opioids by binding to GI opioid-mu receptors, without blocking the central analgesic action of opioids. It accelerates the return of GI motility and reduces the risk of paralytic ileus. It has been used for treating postoperative ileus after bowel resection. It is given 30 min to 5 h before surgery and continued for 7 days. The drug is not likely to be useful unless started before, paralytic ileus develops. It also helps to achieve early recovery of opioid-induced bowel dysfunction. It is usually well tolerated.

Opioid abuse deterrent formulations: These are developed because opioid formulations carry the risk of misuse by opioid addicts. They render the intentional non-therapeutic use more difficult or less awarding in addicts. For example, the extended release tablets of oxycodone and hydrocodone when dissolved in water form viscous gel and hence are difficult to inject and misused by addicts.

Similarly, formulations containing opioid agonist with antagonist are also developed e.g. extended release morphine capsule contains a sequestered core of naltrexone. If the capsule is taken orally then morphine is gradually released while naltrexone core passes through the GIT without getting absorbed. However, if the contents of the capsule are crushed or dissolved naltrexone gets released, and blocks euphoric effects of morphine.

ANALGESICS

Opioid analgesics

Agonists

- Morphine
- Codeine
- **Synthetic:**
- Pethidine
- Methadone
- Propoxyphene
- Llevorphanol
- Tramadol

Partial agonists

- Buprenorphine
- Meptazinol

Mixed agonist-antagonists

- Nalbuphine
- Pentazocine
- Butorphanol

Nonopioid analgesics

- NSAID

OPIOID ANTAGONISTS

Pure antagonists

- Naloxone
- Naltrexone
- Nalmefene

Partial agonists of nalorphine type

- Nalorphine
- Levallorphan
- Cyclazocine

Partial agonists of the morphine type

- Propiram
- Profadol

CHAPTER 11

Analgesic–Antipyretics and Nonsteroidal Anti-Inflammatory Drugs (NSAIDs)

Learning Objectives

This chapter will enable the reader:

1. To be aware of mechanisms for temperature regulation and inflammation.
2. To state properties of nonopioid analgesics as a group.
3. To classify NSAIDs giving examples of drugs.
4. To explain mechanism of action of NSAIDs that is responsible for their analgesic, antipyretic and anti-inflammatory effects as well as for their ADR.
5. To compare various NSAIDs with respect to their pharmacological effects, ADR and indications.
6. To outline management of paracetamol poisoning.
7. To compare and contrast selective COX-2 inhibitors with nonselective COX-inhibitors.
8. To discuss therapy for symptomatic relief of (a) acute pain, (b) chronic dull aching pain, (c) pain due to inflammatory condition, (d) cancer pain and (e) chronic neuropathic pain emphasising on principles of management and choice of drugs with basis for their selection.
9. To explain the role of topical analgesics and their combinations in pain management.
10. To describe toxic renal effects of NSAIDs and state precautions to be taken to minimise them.

KEY TERMS

fever and heat illness, p. 167
inflammation, p. 167
NSAIDs, classification, p. 167
cyclooxygenase (COX), p. 168
NSAIDs and renal damage, p. 170
salicylates, actions, p. 171
COX-2 inhibitors, p. 179
pain, pharmacotherapy, p. 181
adjuvant analgesics, p. 184
cancer pain, p. 184
deafferentation pain, therapy, p. 185
patient controlled analgesia, p. 185

Nonopioid analgesics are the most extensively used drugs in therapeutics as they are easily available as over-the-counter (OTC) products and are often self-administered. In contrast to the opioid analgesics, these analgesics as a group:

- *Relieve pain without interacting with opioid receptors.*
- *Reduce elevated body temperature (antipyretic effect).*
- *Possess anti-inflammatory property* and are known as *nonsteroidal anti-inflammatory drugs* (NSAIDs).
- *Have antiplatelet activity* to varying degrees.
- *Do not cause sedation and sleep.*
- *Are nonaddicting.*

In the last chapter, pain pathophysiology has been outlined. The temperature regulation and inflammatory responses are described below.

Temperature regulation: The hypothalamus controls the body temperature by two mechanisms: (i) cutaneous vasodilatation and (ii) increase in sweat gland activity through sympathetic cholinergic fibres. Normally, 60% of the body heat loss occurs by radiation, 20% by evaporation of water and the rest by convection and conduction.

Although the **body surface temperature** is ordinarily measured in clinical practice, the **body core temperature** is physiologically important. The rectal temperature (which reflects core temperature closely) is about 0.6°C (10°F) higher than oral temperature and about 1.4°C (2.5°F) higher than axillary temperature. The generally accepted normal limits of rectal temperature in adults are 36.1°C–37.8°C (97°F–100°F). The body temperature is higher in infants.

The commonest manifestation of increase in the core temperature is 'fever'. It can cause mental changes and an individual with high fever is often confused and delirious. The working of many tissue enzymes is adversely affected and **hyperpyrexia** (core temperature >41°C or >106°F) may result in death.

Fever is brought about by raising the hypothalamic set point from normothermic to febrile state. It involves a decrease in the heat loss by peripheral vasoconstriction and increase in the heat production by inducing shivering. Fever is usually caused by exogenous or endogenous pyrogens. **Exogenous pyrogens** are products from microbes or their toxins (endotoxins), which are lipopolysaccharides. Endotoxins are highly pyrogenic and act directly on vascular endothelial cells in the hypothalamus.

Several bacteria, fungi and viruses induce the synthesis of IL-1, IL-6, TNF-α and IFN-α from the inflammatory cells (Chapter 25). These are **endogenous pyrogens** (pyrogenic cytokines). They enter the circulation and act on the endothelial receptors of hypothalamic vessels to cause fever.

Pyrogens induce the synthesis of prostaglandin (PG) PGE_2. **Elevation of brain PGE_2 is the key event in raising the hypothalamic set point.** Peripheral actions of PGE_2 are responsible for myalgia and arthralgia, which usually accompany the fever.

Fever can also be caused in the absence of microbial infections, e.g. trauma, tissue necrosis, allergy, which can induce the production of **IL-1, IL-6** and **TNF-α.** Blocking the activity of cytokine reduces inflammation and fever.

In practice, as with pain, relief from fever with drugs adds to the comfort of the patient. However, fever (as caused by infections, inflammatory disorders, malignancies, tissue infarction and trauma) must be distinguished from **heat illnesses/hyperthermia** (due to malignant hyperthermia, heat stroke, atropine overdose and the use of street drugs). *Heat illness is due to failure of the thermoregulatory mechanisms; the body temperature rises to 106°F or higher and does not respond to the antipyretic drugs. Heat illness can be fatal and needs urgent lowering of the body temperature with external cooling including bath with cool water and use of fans.* On the other hand, in fever, the core temperature rarely exceeds 41°C (106°F), and the drugs described in this chapter are effective in lowering the body temperature.

Antipyretics include paracetamol and NSAIDs (See below).

Inflammation: It is a complex process which acts as a body defence against invading foreign agents. It helps to protect, repair and remodel tissues and involves innate immune components with multiple effectors such as leucocytes, mast cells, macrophages and locally produced cytokines. It comprises

(a) **systemic response** (involving nervous and hormonal adjustments and proliferation of the lymphoreticular system) and
(b) **local response** (pain, redness, warmth and swelling). These inflammatory responses are usually beneficial but often they cause functional impairment requiring drug therapy to prevent/suppress tissue damage and chronicity.

The important aspects of inflammation that can be readily measured are as follows:

1. Erythema (local vasodilatation)
2. Oedema (increased capillary permeability)
3. Increase in local temperature (secondary to increased blood supply)
4. Pain (local irritation secondary to inflammatory mediators and exudate)

Classification of NSAIDs PH 1.16

I. **Nonselective cyclooxygenase (COX) inhibitors:**
- **Salicylates and their congeners**
- **Pyrazolone derivatives**, e.g. phenylbutazone and oxyphenbutazone
- **Indoles and related drugs**: Indomethacin, sulindac
- **Heterocyclic arylacetic acid derivatives**: Diclofenac, tolmetin, ketorolac
- **Propionic acid derivatives:** Ibuprofen, fenoprofen, naproxen, ketoprofen and pirprofen
- **Fenamates**, e.g. flufenamic acid and mefenamic acid
- **Oxicams**, e.g. piroxicam

Box 11.1 General Properties of NSAIDs

- They are weakly acidic compounds with ionisation constants ranging from 3.0 to 5.0.
- They have varying degrees of lipid solubility and are absorbed almost completely orally.
- They are highly albumin bound and have small volumes of distribution.
- They are metabolised by the liver.

II. **Preferential COX-2 inhibitors:** Nimesulide, nabumetone, etodolac, meloxicam

III. **Selective COX-2 inhibitor:** Celecoxib

General properties of NSAIDs are given in Box 11.1.

Mechanism of action: Though these drugs have different chemical structures, they produce qualitatively similar analgesic, antipyretic and anti-inflammatory effects. During inflammation, pain or fever, arachidonic acid (AA) is liberated from phospholipid fraction of the cell membrane by phospholipase A_2. AA is then converted by COX-1 and -2 to PGs (Fig.11.1). The steps are as follows:

1. Oxidation of AA to the endoperoxide PGG_2
2. Its subsequent reduction to the hydroxy-endoperoxide PGH_2
3. Transformation of PGH_2 into the **primary prostanoids** PGE_2, PGF_2, PGD_2, PGI_2 and TXA_2 (Chapter 25).

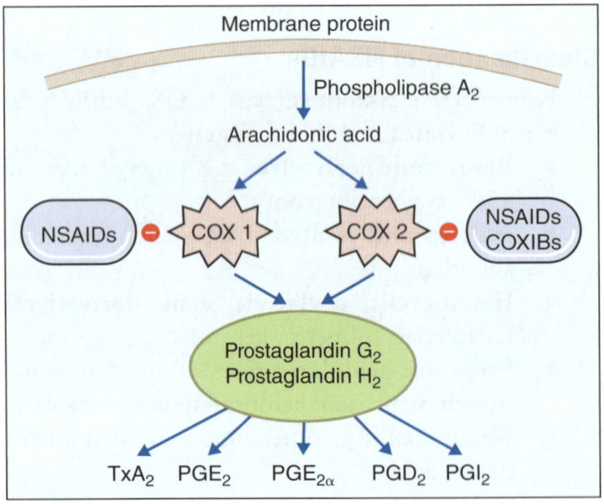

FIG. 11.1 **Mechanism of action of NSAIDs.**

PGs sensitise blood vessels to the effects of other inflammatory mediators that increase permeability. PGs particularly PGE_2 and PGI_2 produce hyperalgesia associated with inflammation and sensitise the chemical receptors of the afferent pain endings to other mediators such as bradykinin and histamine. Further, release of PGs in the CNS may lower the threshold of the central pain circuits.

COX-1 and COX-2, both, use the same endogenous substrate AA and form the same products by the same catalytic mechanism. Their major difference lies in the pathophysiological functions:

- **COX-1 activity is constitutively present in nearly all cell types at a constant level and is involved in tissue homeostasis**, whereas
- **COX-2 activity is normally absent from cells (except those of kidneys and brain) but is inducible** by bacterial liposaccharides, IL-1 and TNF-α in activated leucocytes and other inflammatory cells.

Thus, COX-1 is physiological while COX-2 is usually (but not always) pathological.

Aspirin and aspirin like NSAIDs mainly act by inhibiting COX-1 and 2 and block the synthesis of PGs. (Fig. 11.1). Inhibition of PG synthesis is the main mechanism of analgesic, anti-inflammatory and antipyretic action of NSAIDs.

In addition to its conversion to PGs via the COX pathway, AA is also converted via lipooxygenase pathway to leukotrienes (Chapter 25). Most NSAIDs do not inhibit the production of leukotrienes; in fact, by blocking the synthesis of PGs, they may make more AA available for synthesis of leukotrienes. This might explain the symptoms of bronchospasm in some subjects following the ingestion of aspirin and other NSAIDs.

Although inhibition of PG biosynthesis can explain many effects of NSAIDs, **other mechanisms may** also play an important role. Thus, indomethacin inhibits phosphodiesterase and increases the intracellular concentration of cAMP. Cyclic AMP has been shown to stabilise membranes, including lysosomal membranes in polymorphs. This prevents the release of enzymes important in the inflammatory response.

Further, some anti-inflammatory drugs also inhibit the activation of T-lymphocytes which, are abundant in the inflamed tissues and release proinflammatory cytokines (Chapter 25). Aspirin causes both PG synthesis inhibition and inhibition of T-lymphocyte activation.

Diclofenac and indomethacin also inhibit the lipo-oxygenase pathway, thus decreasing the production of leukotrienes by the leucocytes and the synovial cells.

NSAIDs may also unmask T cell suppressing activity, thereby suppressing the production of rheumatoid factors.

Pharmacological actions of NSAIDs:

Analgesic effects: Unlike the opioid analgesics,

- NSAIDs produce relief of pain without hypnosis or impairment of mental activity.
- Their analgesic action is mainly peripheral and only partly central.
- They do not affect the emotional reaction to pain.

Therapeutically it may be rational to combine aspirin with opioid analgesic like codeine for a synergistic analgesic effect. They are effective as analgesics only in pathological states where PGs are synthesized locally. Thus they are mainly useful for relieving (1) dull aching, throbbing pain of low intensity arising from integumental structures such as muscles and joints; (2) dysmenorrhoea; and (3) toothache. They are not very effective in sharp 'stabbing' pain caused by direct stimulation of sensory nerves (neuropathic pain of neuralgias and diabetic neuropathy). *They are not also useful in visceral pain.*

Antipyretic action: NSAIDs act centrally and reset thermostatic mechanism to the normal level and thereby reduce the temperature; they do not lower the body temperature in a normal individual.

NSAIDs act by inhibiting brain PG synthesis and release. They do not reduce heat production but increase dissipation of heat mainly by producing cutaneous vasodilatation. Accompanying sweating assists the reduction of body temperature. They, however, do not affect the pathological process responsible for fever.

Anti-inflammatory effects:

NSAIDs reduce the 'inflammatory component' of these diseases by:

- *Inhibiting PG synthesis in the peripheral tissues.*
- *Reducing the capillary permeability*, thereby minimising the exudation of fluid and development of inflammatory oedema.
- *Inhibition of neutrophil aggregation and activation.*

During inflammation, neutrophils release proteases, leukotrienes and cytokines (Chapter 25) and injure the tissues. Prostaglandins present in the inflammatory exudate are potent vasodilators and can cause oedema, erythema and pain. NSAIDs by inhibiting the synthesis of PG, prevent sensitisation of the pain receptors to mediators of pain and inflammation such as histamine, 5-HT and bradykinin.

The acidic mucopolysaccharides such as hyaluronic acid, chondroitin and mucoitin sulphuric acid constitute the ground substances of the extracellular matrix. NSAIDs inhibit the mucopolysaccharide biosynthesis and may, thereby, reduce oedema and tissue swelling.

Adverse reactions to NSAIDs:

All NSAIDs can precipitate asthma like symptoms and anaphylactoid reactions in aspirin sensitive patients.

Gastrointestinal effects: The commonest ADR of all NSAIDs (including parenteral formulations) are dyspepsia, nausea, vomiting, heartburn, ulceration and bleeding. The mucosal damage occurs in stomach (gastropathy) as well as in small intestine (enteropathy). NSAID induced enteropathy is mostly subclinical or may cause vague symptoms. PPI which block the gastric acid secretion prevent the gastropathy but are not useful in enteropathy. There is no drug that can prevent NSAID induced enteropathy. High doses and prolonged use of NSAIDs, presence of peptic ulcer disease, concomitant use of systemic corticosteroids, excessive alcohol intake, and advanced age increase the risk of GI effects.

Cardiovascular effects: NSAID users may show some rise in BP and/or heart failure due to retention of sodium and water. Hence NSAIDs can decrease the effectiveness of antihypertensive drugs such as diuretics, beta blockers, ACE inhibitors.

Bleeding: All NSAIDs except COX-2 inhibitors can interfere with platelet function and cause bleeding, especially in those with preexisting platelet defects or thrombocytopenia or those taking anticoagulants concurrently.

Renal effects: The relation between analgesic use and renal damage has been confirmed. Phenacetin was the first drug proven to cause 'analgesic nephropathy'. But, *all NSAIDs (including selective COX 2 inhibitors) can cause acute or chronic renal damage following repeated use*, sometimes as short as two weeks.

Drugs with a long half-life (e.g. naproxen, diclofenac and piroxicam) are more likely to cause renal damage than those with shorter half-life (e.g. ibuprofen).

Clinically, the **renal injury** can present itself in several forms:

- Acute renal failure
- Mild asymptomatic renal impairment
- Chronic renal impairment
- Hypertension
- Serious hyperkalaemia

The first three are due to NSAID- induced inhibition of intrarenal PG synthesis. Locally produced PGE_2 acts as intrarenal vasodilator to counteract the vasoconstricting effect of angiotensin II and noradrenaline (as in shock); PGE_2 also influences the tubular transport of ions and water. Inhibition of synthesis of PGs within the kidney has several adverse effects:

1. The protective intrarenal vasodilator effect of PGE_2 is lost.
2. Renal blood flow and GFR are reduced (in preexisting renal impairment).
3. The natriuretic effect of PGE_2 on the renal medulla is lost with consequent sodium retention. *This may precipitate oedema and CHF.*

Hyperkalaemia is due to diminished aldosterone synthesis secondary to inhibition of renin synthesis by NSAIDs (hyporeninimic hypoaldosteroism). Hyperkalaemia is likely to particularly occur in patients with diabetes mellitus (DM), renal disease and in those on potassium sparing diuretics.

Apart from nephropathy, NSAIDs can cause allergic and type of interstitial nephritis and urate nephropathy.

Renal toxic effects are often overlooked because their onset is insidious and the patients may forget to inform the doctor that they are taking an NSAID. The risk of renal damage due to NSAIDs is increased by the concurrent presence of: old age; hypertension; congestive heart failure; cirrhosis of liver; diabetic nephropathy; gout; renal or renovascular disease and salt/volume depletion (e.g. with diuretics). Studies indicate that **aspirin, in less than full anti-inflammatory doses, is perhaps safer** as its chronic use is less associated with analgesic nephropathy.

Remember that all NSAIDs can cause renal toxicity in the elderly. The possibility of chronic ingestion of analgesics, especially OTC preparations, should always be borne in mind when dealing with unexplained albuminuria/ chronic renal damage.

Effects in pregnancy and neonates: Taken at term, NSAIDs by inhibiting PG synthesis in the uterus may delay the onset of labour and cause greater blood loss at delivery. The administration of aspirin or indomethacin at term has been reported to cause premature closure of the ductus arteriosus with resultant serious pulmonary hypertension in the newborn. Not only at term, even during pregnancy NSAIDs can cause fetal renal dysfunction that could lead to oligohydramnios and neonatal renal impairment. Hence repeated use of NSAIDs in pregnant women should be avoided.

Indications:

- **As analgesic–antipyretic:** NSAIDs are beneficial in a variety of conditions such as arthralgias, myalgias, neuralgias, toothache, headache, backache and dysmenorrhoea.
  They are also very useful as antipyretics in the symptomatic treatment of fever.
- **As anti-inflammatory:** NSAIDs are used locally and orally to treat inflammatory conditions such as arthritis and fibromyositis; they

diminish but do not arrest the inflammatory response.

- **Miscellaneous:**
  a. PGs have been implicated in the maintenance of patency of ductus arteriosus. Indomethacin has been used for the closure of persistent patent ductus in neonates.
  b. Bartter syndrome: This rare condition associated with hypokalaemia and increased plasma renin and aldosterone levels can be treated with aspirin successfully.
  c. Prophylactic doses of aspirin (600–900 mg), indomethacin or ibuprofen have been shown to prevent symptoms of food intolerance inpatients who showed acute GI symptoms after eating specific foodstuffs; it may exert the beneficial effect in radiation induced and other diarrhoeas. These symptoms are probably mediated through PG release.
  d. NSAIDs have been used locally in the treatment of ocular inflammation (see later).
  e. PGD_2 release from the mast cells in the tissues causes vasodilatation and hypotension in patients with mastocytosis. Addition of an NSAID to antihistaminic for the treatment of this condition gives better results.
  f. For prolongation of gestation, see Chapter 42.
  g. For aspirin as antiplatelet drug, see later.

There is an inverse correlation between the chronic use of aspirin/NSAIDs and colorectal cancer. This is probably due to inhibition of COX-2, which is upregulated in this condition.

SALICYLATES

PH 1.16

Salicylates are esters of salicylic acid, e.g. methyl salicylate and sodium salicylate; or alternatively, also occur as salicylate esters of organic acids such as acetyl salicylic acid (**aspirin**), the most commonly used salicylate (Fig. 11.2). Aspirin was synthesised by Felix Hoffman in 1897 and is still being used in therapeutics after more than a 100 years!

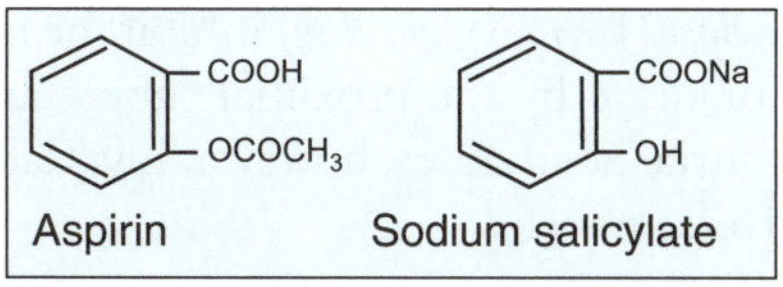

FIG. 11.2 Chemical structures of Aspirin and sodium salicylate.

Pharmacological actions:

Local actions: Salicylic acid and methyl salicylate are irritants; salicylic acid also has keratolytic, antiseptic and fungistatic actions (Chapters 60 and 69). The salts of salicylic acid do not irritate the intact skin but when ingested, may release free salicylic acid in the stomach causing local irritation.

Central nervous system:

- **Analgesia:** Aspirin inhibits the biosynthesis of PGs by **irreversible acetylation** and inactivation of COX in contrast to other NSAIDs which cause its **reversible** inhibition.

In smaller doses (325-650 mg 4-6 hourly), salicylates exert mainly analgesic action. With larger doses (1–4 G/day), they exert anti-inflammatory activity as well and relieve vascular congestion and oedema. Toxic doses (> 4G/day) produce stimulation of the CNS followed by depression (see later).

- **Antipyretic action:** As described under section Pharmacological actions of NSAIDs.
- **Respiratory stimulation:** Salicylates stimulate respiration in a dose dependent manner as a result of direct and indirect actions.

A plasma level of 35 mg% of salicylates is usually associated with hyperventilation and severe dyspnoea occurs when the level approaches 50 mg%.

Acid–base disturbances and hypokalaemia: The mild respiratory alkalosis produced by therapeutic doses of salicylates is countered by excretion of alkaline urine containing bicarbonate along with Na^+ and K^+. This is the stage of *compensated respiratory alkalosis.*

Hypokalaemia as a result of urinary loss of potassium is accompanied by water loss, through lungs due to hyperventilation, through skin via augmented sweating and through urine as a result of alkalosis. This may lead to dehydration and hypernatraemia.

With acute toxic doses of salicylates, hypokalaemia is aggravated, the respiratory centre is depressed and metabolic acidosis develops (see later).

Gastrointestinal system: Depending on the dose, salicylates may produce

- **Dyspepsia, nausea and vomiting** as a result of gastric irritation
- **Gastrointestinal erosions and bleeding**, leading to haematemesis or melena

The acid pH of the stomach favours the existence of salicylate in nonionised form. The nonionised form is, however, relatively water insoluble; hence, it tends to adhere to the gastric mucosa thereby producing irritation. Further, local absorption into the mucous cell causes inhibition of local COX-1 leading to decreased PGE_2 and PGI_2 synthesis, thus, causing a loss of the protective effect of PGE on the stomach. Salicylates also reduce the gastric motility and prolong the gastric emptying time. These effects increase the period of contact of salicylate with the gastric mucosa.

Alkalies induce ionisation of salicylates and thereby reduce their gastric absorption and local irritant effect. As the ionised salicylate is more water soluble, it leaves the stomach more quickly. Thus, to avoid gastric irritation, salicylates are administered:

i. *With plenty of water, after food.*
ii. *With milk.*
iii. *As soluble or buffered aspirin.*
iv. *With an alkali such as sodium bicarbonate.*
v. *With misoprostol, a PGE_1 analogue* (Chapter 41).

Hepatic effects: Salicylates have *choleretic action* but reduce the total concentration of cholates. *Large doses, particularly in children, can cause hepatic damage and even necrosis.*

Anti-inflammatory and antirheumatic effect: Salicylates suppress the clinical signs and improve the clinical picture in acute rheumatic fever and rheumatoid arthritis.

Aspirin by inhibiting the synthesis of PG, prevents sensitisation of the pain receptors to mediators of pain and inflammation such as histamine, 5-HT and bradykinin.

Immune system: Salicylates suppress a variety of antigen–antibody reactions *in vivo* including serum sickness in man. However, such effects occur at high dose; and their contribution to the antirheumatic activity is not clear.

Antiplatelet activity: Aspirin inhibits platelet aggregation. *It is unique in that it irreversibly inhibits COX by acetylation.* Platelets play an important role in thrombus formation. **Aspirin, by inhibiting COX suppresses the synthesis of thromboxane A_2 (TXA_2) in the platelets**. Platelets, being non-nucleated are unable to regenerate the enzyme, which explains the prolonged action of aspirin. *Thus, daily doses of 75–150 mg almost completely suppress the synthesis of TXA_2 for 7–10 days (Chapter 33)*. Other NSAIDs inhibit the enzyme reversibly so that the platelet function is restored when the drug is eliminated.

Salicylates reduce the leucocytosis and lower the high ESR observed in acute rheumatic fever. The latter effect is due to a reduction in the plasma fibrinogen content.

Cardiovascular system: Therapeutic doses of aspirin do not produce any deleterious effects on the CVS.

Renal effects: Salicylates in therapeutic doses do not modify renal functions significantly in normal individuals. *They can, however, affect renal function in compromised kidneys by inhibiting COX-1.*

Urate present in the glomerular filtrate is reabsorbed by the proximal tubules of the kidney and the main excretion of urate in urine occurs due to its secretion by the distal tubule. Aspirin exerts *biphasic* action on the excretion of urate.

- *Aspirin, in small doses* (*1–2 g per day*), interferes with urate secretion by the distal tubule, thereby elevating the plasma urate level, and block the action of other uricosuric drugs such as probenecid.
- *Large doses* (*over 5 g per day*) inhibit the reabsorption of urate by the proximal tubule and cause uricosuria. Such doses, however, invariably result in adverse effects.

Endocrine effects: Salicylates interfere with the binding of thyroid hormones to their binding proteins, especially thyroxine binding albumin. This comes in the way of interpretation of serum thyroxine and tri-iodothyronine values.

Metabolic effects: Salicylates uncouple oxidative phosphorylation (Chapter 62). The energy derived from oxidation is converted into heat. Toxic doses of salicylates may, thus, lead to hyperpyrexia, increased protein catabolism, aminoaciduria and a negative nitrogen balance.

In certain diabetic individuals, salicylates may reduce the blood sugar level and glycosuria, probably due to an enhanced peripheral utilisation of glucose and inhibition of neoglucogenesis. However, large doses cause hyperglycaemia and glycosuria in normal individuals.

Salicylates reduce lipogenesis and at the same time inhibit adrenaline induced lipolysis in the fat cells. Toxic doses lead to formation of ketone bodies.

Absorption, fate and excretion: Both salicylic acid and methyl salicylate are absorbed from intact skin, especially when applied in alcohol, petrolatum, lard or lanolin base and systemic poisoning in children has been reported following such local applications. Salicylates are absorbed from the stomach and largely from the upper small intestine. Factors such as particle size, pH of the GI tract, solubility of the salicylate preparation and presence of food in the stomach modify the absorption.

After absorption, approximately 80% of the salicylate (but only 50% of aspirin) is bound to plasma albumin. It is rapidly distributed to achieve significant concentration in various body fluids and organs and smaller amounts in the brain.

Aspirin, even though absorbed as such, is subject to rapid metabolism (50%–60%) to salicylate by deacetylation during first pass and is further hydrolysed in the blood and tissues to salicylic acid (t½ of 15 min).

Like phenytoin, aspirin exhibits dose dependent pharmacokinetics:

- **At lower dose levels** (300–600 mg individual doses), the plasma level increases in proportion to the dose ***(first-order kinetics)***.
- **At higher dose levels** (1–2 g individual doses), the increase in the plasma level is disproportionate and severe toxicity can occur ***(zero-order kinetics)***.

Salicylates are mainly excreted in urine in the form of conjugates with glycine and glucuronic acid.

An alkaline urine, by ionising the salicylate to a water soluble and indiffusible form, prevents salicylate back-diffusion in the distal tubule and enhances its excretion. Its excretion *is reduced* by probenecid, oliguria and kidney failure and is *augmented* by diuresis and alkaline pH.

Adverse reactions:

Allergic or pseudoallergic reactions: These include skin rashes, urticaria, pruritus, bronchospasm angioneuroticoedema, anaphylaxis-like shock or thrombocytopenic purpura. Angioedema and anaphylactoid reaction respond to adrenaline.

Salicylic acid and its derivatives are ingredients of a large number of substances including fruits like apples, grapes, oranges, peaches and plums, soaps containing oil of wintergreen, perfumes, beverages (especially birch beer), tooth pastes, gum and lozenges. *Individuals with idiosyncrasy to salicylates should also be warned against taking proprietary drug mixtures, which often contain salicylates.*

Gastrointestinal tract: In subjects taking 3–4 g of aspirin daily, the blood loss may be about 3–6 mL per day. Occasionally, aspirin can cause haematemesis. **Prolonged therapy even with low dose aspirin can also lead to anaemia**. The incidence of major GI bleeding due to aspirin is estimated at 15 per 100,000 chronic aspirin users per year. The bleeding is due to (a) local mucosal action; (b) inhibition of platelets; and (c) hypoprothrombinaemia.

Haemopoietic system: Salicylates but not the newer NSAIDs, **in large doses**, reduce the plasma prothrombin level by interfering with action of vitamin K in the liver. Salicylate-induced hypoprothrombinaemia can be reversed by administration of vitamin K. *Salicylates exert a synergistic effect with the coumarin anticoagulants, and hence, these drugs should be avoided in patients receiving oral anticoagulants.*

Kidneys: See section, Adverse reactions to NSAIDs, renal effects.

Reye syndrome: This serious and often fatal complication occurs a few days after a viral infection, especially influenza, in children below the age 12 years. There occurs anicteric liver dysfunction due to hepatic mitochondrial injury and a consequent metabolic encephalopathy. There is epidemiological evidence to associate administration of aspirin during the initial viral infection and the subsequent occurrence of this serious disease. *Aspirin should, therefore, be avoided in infants and in children <12 years, unless specifically indicated, e.g. for juvenile rheumatoid arthritis.*

Pregnancy and neonates: Salicylates readily cross the placental barrier and may prove toxic to the newborn. The toxic manifestations in newborn include hyperpnoea and haemorrhages. Hypoglycaemia after prolonged salicylate therapy has also been reported in infants. However, low dose aspirin is probably safe.

Salicylism: High doses of salicylates may produce a condition of mild salicylate intoxication termed **salicylism**. The syndrome usually develops when the plasma salicylate level exceeds 25 mg% and is characterised by headache, dizziness, vertigo, tinnitus, difficulty in hearing and dimness of vision; drowsiness, lethargy and mental confusion, nausea, vomiting and diarrhoea may also occur. These symptoms may be associated with tachypnoea and respiratory alkalosis. It is reversible on cessation of therapy. FM 9.1, FM 10.1

Acute salicylate intoxication: Acute salicylate intoxication may be due to overzealous therapy in infants or following an accidental ingestion. A serum salicylate level of 50 mg% indicates mild toxicity; levels above 75 mg% are potentially fatal. The characteristic features of acute intoxication are acid–base and electrolyte disturbances, hyperglycaemia, dehydration, hyperpyrexia, GI irritation and occasional haemorrhages. The stimulation of CNS causes restlessness, vertigo, tremor, apprehension, hallucinations and convulsions.

With toxic doses, the respiratory centre is depressed resulting in CO_2 accumulation and true metabolic acidosis.

Box 11.2 Principles of Management of Salicylate Poisoning FM 10.1

- Hospitalisation
- Activated charcoal 50 g orally
- Correct hyperthermia, dehydration (5% dextrose), hypokalaemia, acid–base disturbances, ketosis
- Increase elimination by alkalinisation, peritoneal dialysis or haemoperfusion
- Vitamin K, blood transfusion
- Exchange transfusion in very small children

Box 11.2 gives the principles of management of salicylate poisoning. Correction of acidosis and urinary alkalinisation should be carried out cautiously using normal saline containing 2% dextrose and 2% sodium bicarbonate, at the rate of 2 L/h, with frequent determination of blood pH and plasma bicarbonate, to prevent metabolic alkalosis.

Sedatives like barbiturates are dangerous when the patients show excitement with salicylate intoxication. These agents, by producing respiratory depression, may aggravate metabolic acidosis and precipitate coma.

Preparations and dosage:

i. Acetylsalicylic acid (Aspirin 75 and 300 mg tablets; also available as dispersible tablet and gastro-resistant formulations; suppository 150 and 300 mg). Dose: 0.3–0.6 g 4–6 hourly (maximum 4 g/day) orally or rectally in a dose of 0.45–0.9 every 4 hourly, for relief of integumental pain.
ii. Soluble aspirin tablet contains aspirin (300 mg), citric acid (30 mg) with calcium carbonate (100 mg) and saccharin sodium (3 mg). When mixed with water, citric acid reacts with calcium carbonate to form calcium citrate solution and this dissolves aspirin forming calcium acetyl salicylate.
iii. Buffered aspirin tablets contain aspirin and an antacid like magnesium hydroxide, aluminium hydroxide or aluminium glycinate.
iv. Methyl salicylate (oil of Wintergreen): liniment 25% v/v in peanut oil and, methyl salicylate ointment 50% in white bees wax and hydrous wool fat.

v. Salicylic acid: ointment contains 2%–6% salicylic acid w/w. Whitfield ointment contains 6% benzoic acid and 3% salicylic acid.

Indications:

- **Local application:** Salicylic acid is used for its keratolytic, fungistatic and mild antiseptic activity (Chapter 69). Methyl salicylate is used as a counter irritant. For local use of 5-aminosalicylic acid in the treatment of inflammatory bowel disease, see Chapter 43.
- **As analgesic–antipyretic:** For analgesia, combination of aspirin with an opioid analgesic like codeine is synergistic. In single doses of 300–1200 mg, aspirin shows graded responses. *Doses higher than 1200 mg, however, simply increase the risk of toxicity and should be avoided.*
  Aspirin is valuable in primary dysmenorrhoea. Treatment is started on the first day of the menstrual period and is continued for 2–3 days.
- **Acute rheumatic fever:** This autoimmune inflammatory condition is a delayed sequela of Group A Streptococcal (GAS) infection. It manifests as fever and affects multiple organs and tissues like heart, joints, subcutaneous tissue and CNS. The pharmacotherapy of rheumatic fever is discussed in Chapter 44 (Box 44.3). Therapy for fever and inflammation is given below.
  Aspirin in a dose of 4–8 g daily given at intervals (as 1 g dose) produces a dramatic relief of pain and inflammation of the involved joints within 24–48 hours. The fever is reduced, the pulse rate slows down and further joint involvement is prevented. *It, however, cannot prevent or reverse the cardiac complications, chorea, subcutaneous nodules or encephalopathy and fail to shorten the duration of the disease.*
  For children, the recommended daily dose is 120 mg per kg of body weight per day (with a maximum of 8 g) given in 4–6 divided doses. A plasma salicylate level of 25–40 mg% usually achieves adequate control. Full doses are continued for at least 2 weeks after disappearance of symptoms and signs of inflammation, and then gradually reduced over a period of 7–10 days. Sudden discontinuation may produce a relapse. Naproxen can also be administered in the dose of 10–20 mg/kg/day.
  Glucocorticoids (prednisolone 1–2 mg/kg/day) are useful in cases not responding to salicylates and appear to be more effective in the severely ill patients with high fever, rheumatic pericarditis and concomitant congestive cardiac failure or cardiac arrhythmias. The incidence of relapse after stoppage of corticosteroid therapy is relatively high. Some authorities recommend combined aspirin and glucocorticoid therapy.
  Concurrent penicillin therapy is recommended for eradication of streptococcal infection. See Chapter 44.
- **Rheumatic diseases:** In SLE, aspirin may ameliorate arthritis and serositis, but the vasculitic component caused by immune complex deposition is not affected. For use of aspirin in RA, see Chapter 75.
- **As antiplatelet agent:** Aspirin is used to prevent platelet aggregation. It blocks COX activity, inhibiting the platelets for 8–10 days after a single dose of 75–100 mg (Chapter 33).

Diflunisal and salsalate are nonacetylated salicylates which have analgesic and anti-inflammatory properties with weak antipyretic and antiplatelet activity. These drugs are only rarely associated with GI bleeding, are well tolerated by asthmatic patients and have longer duration of action than aspirin.

PYRAZOLONE DERIVATIVES

These are as follows:

- *Phenylbutazone* and *oxyphenbutazone*
- Other drugs like *metamizole sodium* or *dipyrone*

PHENYLBUTAZONE: It is a potent anti-inflammatory drug. Its anti-inflammatory activity exceeds that of salicylates. However, the drug is poorly tolerated by patients and causes various GI, hepatic, renal and fatal haematologic adverse effects. It gives rise to various drug interactions. Hence it is now obsolete.

OXYPHENBUTAZONE: This metabolic degradation product of phenylbutazone, is claimed to cause less gastric irritation than phenylbutazone. It shares all the toxic effects of phenylbutazone. It is sometimes used in the symptomatic treatment of ankylosing spondylitis.

Metamizole/Dipyrone: This potent analgesic and antipyretic injectable NSAIDs can cause fatal agranulocytosis and hence is banned.

INDOLES AND RELATED DRUGS

INDOMETHACIN: This indole acetic acid derivative (Fig. 11.3) is a potent analgesic, antipyretic and anti-inflammatory agent.

Pharmacological actions: In patients with RA with swollen joints, it brings about a quick relief of pain and reduction in the joint swellings. However, it is not superior to aspirin.

Absorption, fate and excretion: Given orally, it is absorbed rapidly and almost completely, with a peak plasma concentration within 1–2 h. It is mainly metabolised by the liver and is rapidly eliminated by the kidneys as glucuronide. Nearly 50%–90% of a single dose is excreted in urine within 24 h. Its action is more prolonged than is suggested by its t½ (2 h).

Adverse reactions: The reported incidence of ADR has ranged from 15% to 20%, even with low doses. Headache is most common, followed by giddiness, mental confusion, blurring of vision, depression and psychotic disturbances. *Such neuropsychiatric adverse reactions are more frequent with indomethacin than with other NSAIDs.*

Less common adverse effects are nausea, vomiting, dyspepsia, diarrhoea, skin rashes and rarely blood dyscrasias. Peptic ulceration associated with bleeding and liver damage have been reported. It may cause sodium retention, oedema and nephrotoxicity.

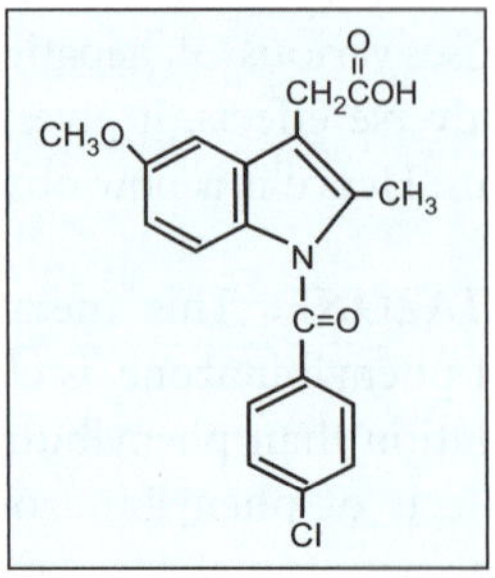

FIG. 11.3 Indomethacin.

Preparations and dosage: Indomethacin available as 25, 50 mg capsules and as 75 mg modified release capsules. Total daily dose recommended is 50–200 mg in divided doses, after food. Indomethacin can be given rectally in a dose of 100 mg as suppository twice daily if required.

Indications: It may be used in the treatment of acute gouty attacks and in ankylosing spondylitis *for short-term therapy. It should be avoided in treatment of mild and moderate pain.*

SULINDAC is a fluorinated derivative of indomethacin. It is a prodrug and has a longer duration of action. Its active metabolite is claimed to be much less nephrotoxic. It is given orally in the dose of 100–200 mg twice a day.

HETEROCYCLIC ARYLACETIC ACID DERIVATIVES

DICLOFENAC: This drug (Fig. 11.4) probably has substantially greater activity than indomethacin, naproxen and other NSAIDs because of its higher COX-2 inhibiting property. Fifty per cent of the sodium salt is metabolised during the first pass through the liver. It is extensively bound to plasma proteins, with a t½ of 1–2 h. It accumulates in the synovial fluid, which probably is responsible for its longer duration of action in arthritis. Its relative selectivity for COX-2 also explains the increased cardiovascular risk associated with this drug.

Adverse reactions: The incidence of ADR is high, about 20%. They are similar to indomethacin. GI symptoms including bleeding and elevation of liver enzymes can occur. Hence, liver enzymes should be evaluated in the first few weeks of long-term therapy. Other adverse effects include CNS effects, fluid retention, and cardiac toxicity. The drug may cause severe

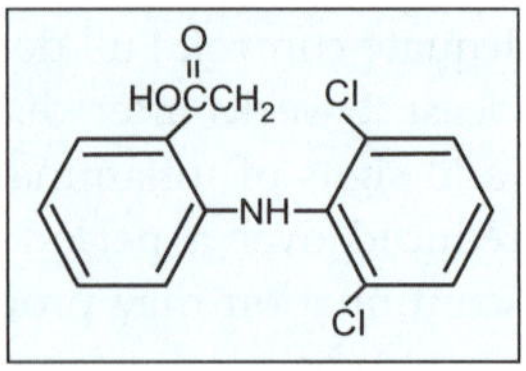

FIG. 11.4 Diclofenac.

oliguria due to marked reduction in renal blood flow and GFR and cause renal damage. *Its use should be avoided in children, pregnant women and nursing mothers, and in patients with suspected renal disease, such as diabetic nephropathy and in cardiac damage. Its long-term use should be avoided.*

Both topical application and systemic administration may cause hypersensitivity reactions.

Diclofenac is commonly used in veterinary practice and has been found to be highly toxic to vultures which consume caracass of animals previously treated with diclofenac.

Indications:

- **As an anti-inflammatory agent** in rheumatoid arthritis, severe osteoarthritis and in ankylosing spondylitis. **It is not the drug of choice.** Its dose is 75–100 mg orally, daily, in 2–3 divided doses after food and 75 mg by deep IM injection once or twice a day.
- **As eye drops 0.1% for the inhibition of intraoperative miosis** (but it does not possess intrinsic mydriatic activity) and to prevent postoperative inflammation in cataract surgery.
- **For postoperative analgesia**, the drug is used rectally as suppositories in the dose of 75–100 mg per day in divided doses.
- **As gel or ointment locally for joint pain and muscle pain.**

Studies confirm that dipyrone is a major cause of agranulocytosis and that phenylbutazone, indomethacin and diclofenac can cause aplastic anaemia. They may be used only when other NSAIDs are ineffective and that too for a short term.

KETOROLAC: Ketorolac IM 20–30 mg (single dose), is a moderately effective analgesic in patients with moderate to severe postoperative pain. Ketorolac IM/IV has been reported to be as effective as, and have fewer side effects than, morphine in surgical and chronic cancer pain. It has a longer duration of action (t½ of 5 h). IV ketorolac is frequently used in the emergency department to reduce opioid use. Parenteral administration can cause as much gastric mucosal injury as oral administration. The initial dose of 20–30 mg IM may be followed by 10–15 mg by the same route 6–8 hourly, to a maximum of 80–120 mg daily, for 2 days; IV doses are similar to IM doses. *The use of ketorolac is limited to 5 days because of a high risk of adverse effects, particularly GI toxicity.* **Ketorolac promethamine** is available as nasal spray.

Tolmetin: This drug, a pyrrole acetic acid derivative, has a t½ of 1–2 h. It resembles ibuprofen in its actions and its toxicity. It is, however, less potent than indomethacin.

PROPIONIC ACID DERIVATIVES

These compounds like **ibuprofen, naproxen** (Fig. 11.5), **fenoprofen, flurbiprofen** and **ketoprofen** have potent analgesic–antipyretic and anti-inflammatory properties similar to aspirin but are *better tolerated orally*. The incidence of adverse reactions is lower than that after high doses of aspirin, indomethacin and diclofenac.

Ketoprofen inhibits both COX and lipooxygenase, whereas flurbiprofen also inhibits TNFα and nitric oxide synthesis.

They are highly bound to plasma albumin (92%–99%) and, like aspirin, can displace drugs such as hydantoins, sulphonylureas and warfarin. They, however, differ in their pharmacokinetics and hence, in their duration of action.

Adverse reactions: They may cause GI disturbances such as epigastric pain, nausea, sensation of fullness in the stomach and heartburn. Occult blood loss is less common. Less frequently, they may cause CNS symptoms such as headache, dizziness, blurred vision and tinnitus. In a few cases, fluid retention

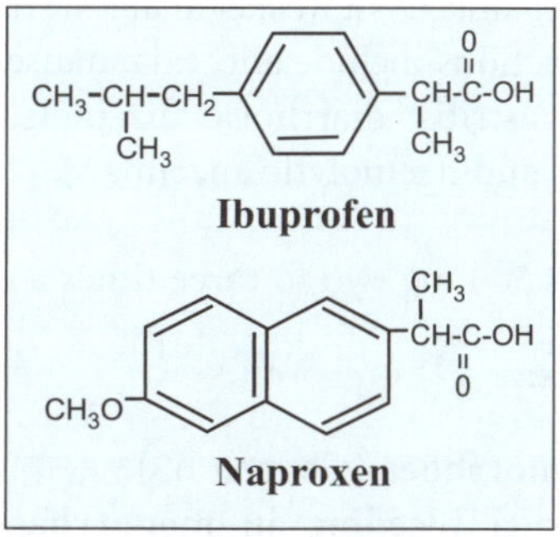

FIG. 11.5 Chemical structures of Ibuprofen and Naproxen.

and oedema of the feet may occur. Risk of cardiotoxicity is far less than diclofenac. Rarely, they cause hepatitis, impairment of renal function and thrombocytopenia. Risk of cardiotoxicity is lesser than diclofenac.

Any patient who is intolerant to aspirin may also suffer a severe reaction following administration of propionic acid derivatives.

Indications: They are used as substitutes for aspirin particularly in patients with RA, osteoarthritis and ankylosing spondylitis. *In general, ibuprofen is the better tolerated drug among the propionic acid derivatives, is cost effective and is a good substitute for aspirin, indomethacin and diclofenac as an anti-inflammatory agent.* Flurbiprofen is also available as eye drops for eye inflammation.

The use of ibuprofen simultaneously with aspirin reduces the anti-inflammatory effect of the latter. Further, ibuprofen, indomethacin, naproxen interfere with the antiplatelet action and hence reduce the cardioprotective effect of low dose aspirin. In patients who are taking antiplatelet doses of aspirin, sulindac and celecoxib may be preferred as anti-inflammatory drugs.

FENAMATES

These agents have a fenamic acid core structure and include mefenamic acid, tolfenamic acid, meclofenamic acid, and flufenamic acid. They have shown no clear advantages over other NSAIDs.

MEFENAMIC ACID: This is useful in chronic and dull aching pains. It is a weaker analgesic than aspirin. Adverse reactions include anorexia, nausea, abdominal pain, gastritis, diarrhoea, dizziness, headache, skin rashes and haemolytic anaemia.

The dose is 500 mg two to three times a day.

Indications:

- **Dysmenorrhoea** (Chapter 65)
- **Menstrual bleeding in menorrhagic women** may diminish by up to 50% with the use of PG inhibitors such as ibuprofen and mefenamic acid when used during menses.

Flufenamic acid has similar properties.

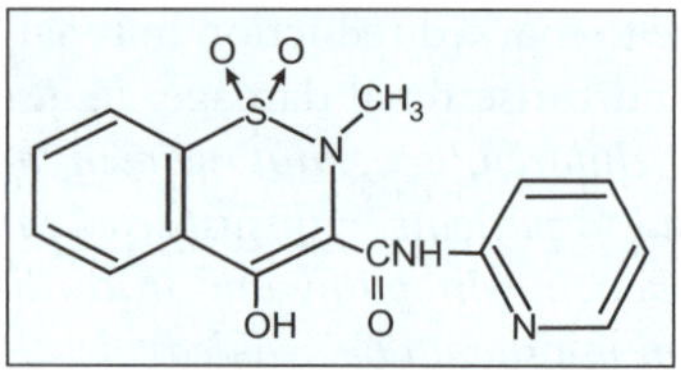

FIG. 11.6 Piroxicam.

OXICAMS

PIROXICAM: This NSAID is structurally different from other agents (Fig. 11.6).

Given orally, it is well-absorbed and has a *long half-life* (38–45 h). It is therefore administered once a day. Doses between 10 and 20 mg produce analgesic–antipyretic effect, whereas larger doses (20–40 mg) are needed for the anti-inflammatory effect. It commonly causes GI upset, peptic ulceration and CNS disturbances. It is used to treat RA, ankylosing spondylitis, osteoarthritis and acute gout. It has no special advantage except a longer duration of action.

Tenoxicam, meloxicam and **lornoxicam** are the other oxicams.

The NSAIDs commonly used as anti-inflammatory agents are listed in Table 11.1.

Table 11.1 Anti-Inflammatory Doses of Non-selective NSAIDs PH 1.16

Name	Available As	Dose/Frequency
Ibuprofen	200, 400 mg tab	400–600 mg t.i.d.
Fenoprofen	300 mg tablets	300–600 mg t.i.d.
Ketoprofen	50 mg capsules	50 mg t.i.d.
Naproxen	250 mg tablets	250–500 mg b.i.d.
Flurbiprofen	100 mg tablets	100–150 mg b.i.d.
Diclofenac	50 mg tablets	50 mg b.i.d.
Indomethacin	25 mg capsules	25–50 mg t.i.d.
Sulindac	100 mg tablets	200 mg b.i.d.
Etodolac	200 mg tablets	200–400 mg t.i.d
Piroxicam	10, 20 mg capsules	10–20 mg o.d.

PREFERENTIAL AND SELECTIVE COX-2 INHIBITORS

Drugs belonging to this group selectively block COX-2 activity more than COX-1 activity, thus interfering less with the protective action of COX-1 in the stomach (stomach-friendly), blood vessels and kidneys. The group includes **nimesulide, meloxicam, nabumetone** and **celecoxib** (Table 11.2).

Celecoxib is a highly selective COX-2 inhibitor. Other highly selective COX-2 inhibitors include **etoricoxib, parecoxib, lumiracoxib.**

Given orally, their absorption is complete. They are as effective as the nonselective analgesic–anti-inflammatory NSAIDs in the treatment of osteoarthritis and rheumatoid arthritis. Their major advantage is that they cause fewer gastric ulcers ('stomach-friendly') and do not inhibit platelet aggregation. Celecoxib is a CYP2D6 inhibitor and can increase serum concentrations of CYP2D6 substrates.

Adverse reactions: The most common adverse reactions are nausea, vomiting, dyspepsia, abdominal pain, diarrhoea, skin reactions and the renal adverse effects such as decrease in renal blood flow, oedema and dose-related worsening of hypertension. *Nimesulide has been reported to cause nephrotoxicity and hepatotoxicity. The drug was not licensed for use in some developed countries, and it has been banned/withdrawn from others (e.g. paediatric formulation in India). The use of nimesulide should be avoided in old persons.*

Studies in animals suggest that inhibiting COX-2 may interfere with wound (ulcer) healing, bone remodelling, ovulation and prenatal renal development. Their use is not recommended in children and women of child bearing age, and during lactation, as they are excreted in breast milk. Celecoxib is contraindicated in patients allergic to sulphonamides.

Table 11.2 Preferential and Selective COX-2 Inhibitors PH 1.16

Drug	Dose (mg)	Frequency
Nabumetone	500	b.i.d.
Nimesulide	100	t.i.d.
Meloxicam	7.5–15	o.d.
Celecoxib	100	o.d. or b.i.d.

Theoretically, selective inhibition of endothelial COX-2 would decrease the synthesis of PGI_2, which is a vasodilator and inhibitor of platelet aggregation; the continual production of COX-1, however, would produce TXA_2.This may increase the risk of thrombosis (**prothrombotic effect**).

It is now established that selective COX-2 inhibitors, rofecoxib and valdecoxib although **stomach-friendly**, *confer dose-related increased risk of heart attack and stroke.* Hence, they have been withdrawn by the manufacturers. *Currently, all the selective COX-2 inhibitors are under suspicion regarding their cardiovascular toxicity. They have been described as drugs with 'marginal efficacy, heightened risk and excessive cost as compared with traditional NSAIDs'. Among nonselective NSAIDs, the risk of prothrombotic effect appears to be highest with diclofenac and lowest with naproxen.*

Curcumin: It is an active constituent of Indian spice, turmeric roots (*Curcuma longa*), which is advocated by Ayurveda to treat inflammation. Curcumin has been demonstrated to possess antioxidant and anti-inflammatory activities. It probably acts inhibiting inflammatory cytokines. However, it has low solubility and poor bioavailability. It is not an analgesic.

ANALGESIC-ANTIPYRETIC DRUGS

Some drugs, which are non-opioids are devoid of anti-inflammatory activity but they exhibit analgesic and antipyretic properties. They are not NSAIDs and may or may not act through PG inhibition.

PARA-AMINOPHENOL DERIVATIVES

The commonly used drug is paracetamol (Fig. 11.7).

PARACETAMOL (Acetaminophen): This compound exerts analgesic and antipyretic effects like salicylates. It has weak activity on COX in the

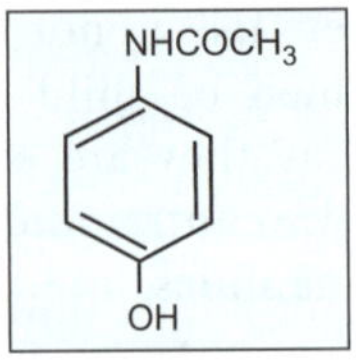

FIG. 11.7 **Paracetamol.**

inflamed peripheral tissues, which have high concentration of peroxides; however, it equals the blocking effect of aspirin on this enzyme in the brain. Therefore, *paracetamol is a potent antipyretic and is equianalgesic with aspirin in therapeutic doses but devoid of significant anti-inflammatory effect.* Compared to salicylates, *it does not produce GI irritation, acid–base imbalance nor does it affect platelet activity.*

Absorption, fate and excretion: It is rapidly absorbed orally and peak plasma levels are reached within ½ to 1 h. It is metabolised in the liver by CYP2E1 and excreted in urine, conjugated with glucuronic and sulphuric acids. The ability of infant liver for glucuronidation of paracetamol is poor, and this may enhance its toxicity.

Adverse reactions: At the recommended therapeutic doses (500–1000 mg given 6 hourly; maximum 3 g/day) in healthy subjects, paracetamol is generally well tolerated and causes minimal adverse effects.

FM 10.1, PE 14.4

- **Hepatic and renal toxicity:** Large doses (>6 g) of paracetamol as in acute poisoning produce extensive hepatocellular damage and renal tubular necrosis and death.
  The liver and renal toxicity is due to the metabolite ***N*-acetyl-*P*-benzoquinoneimiene** which is normally turned harmless by conjugation with glutathione. Depletion of hepatic and renal glutathione potentiates its toxicity whereas treatment with sulphhydryl compounds such as cysteamine, l-methionine and ***N*-acetyl cysteine** (NAC) is beneficial. In acute poisoning, NAC is administered by infusion initially, in the dose of 150 mg/kg in 15 min, and then 50–100 mg/kg slowly to total maximum of 300 mg/kg in 20 h. It can be combined with methionine. NAC has also been used orally. Prior liver damage as in chronic alcoholics and concurrent use of isoniazid increases the liability to hepatotoxicity.
- Paracetamol may cause skin reactions, fever, neutropenia, thrombocytopenia and nephropathy.
- It may produce anaemia as a result of haemolysis in individuals with G6PD deficiency.

Drug interactions: Concomitant use of drugs that induce CYP2E1, such as carbamazepine, phenobarbital, isoniazid, can increase concentrations of the hepatotoxic metabolite of paracetamol. Similarly administration of paracetamol with drugs that compete for glucuronidation, such as zidovudine, can increase the risk of hepatotoxicity.

Preparations and dosage:

i. Paracetamol 500 mg/650 mg tablets. In addition, it is available in various dosage forms such as effervescent tablet; soluble tablet; dispersible tablet; capsule; oral suspension; suppository and powder in varying doses. It is given in a dose of 0.5-1 gm every 4-6 hours via oral or rectal route. The total daily dose should not exceed 3 g in adults.
ii. Injection paracetamol (available as 10 mg/ml) to be given intramuscularly and intravenously. IV infusion dose (wt < 50 kg) is 15 mg/kg 4–6 hourly upto a maximum of 3 g daily. For patients with weight > 50 kg, the dose is 1 g 4–6 hourly; to a maximum of 4 g daily.

Indications: It is preferred to aspirin for mild pain, for fever in children and for treating osteoarthritic pain in the elderly.

BENZOXAZOCAINE DERIVATIVES

Nefopam: It is a nonopioid *centrally acting* analgesic drug. Its mechanism of action is not known but blockade of voltage gated sodium channel and inhibition of serotonin, dopamine and NA reuptake may contribute to its effects. At high doses, it causes sweating, dizziness and nausea. It is used as an alternative to or an adjunct with opioid analgesics.

Table 11.3 summarises the effects of commonly used analgesic–antipyretic agents.

Table 11.3 Effects of Commonly Used Analgesic–Antipyretic Agents

	Aspirin					
	Low Dose	Intermediate Dose	High Dose	Sodium Salicylate	Other NSAIDs[a]	Paracetamol
Antipyretic	0	+	+	+	+	+
Analgesic	0	+	+	+	+	+
Anti-inflammatory	0	0	+	+	+	Minimal
Inhibition of platelet PG synthesis	+	+	+	0	+	0
Inhibition of PG synthesis systemically	0	+	+	±	+	0

Low dose, 75–300 mg/day; intermediate dose, 500 mg–3 g/day; high dose, more than 3 g/day.
[a]Other NSAIDs are indomethacin, ibuprofen, naproxen, diclofenac, piroxicam.

PH 1.1, AS 8.3

PHARMACOTHERAPY OF PAIN

Pain is not simply a perception. It is a complex phenomenon , and the boundaries between normal discomfort and pathologic pain are often obscure.

It has two components one of which is the sensation described by the subject as pain. The other component, the emotional and psychological one, contributes considerably to the 'suffering', an affective reaction. *The intensity of pain suffered differs enormously with the personality, intelligence and culture of the individual.* Tribal people often display a stoic disregard for pain. As a generalisation, pain is complained of more vehemently by people belonging to the more affluent and elite sections of the society.

Emotional stress and anxiety adversely affect the pain response, while other factors which enhance its severity are debility and fatigue. Pain often becomes worse during the night when the distractions of daytime are absent and the patient has time to ruminate his ailment. Protracted severe pain can become so dominant a factor in a patient's life that it can eventually lead to both physical and psychological exhaustion. *The management of pain is always multidisciplinary, multimodal and involves pharmacotherapy, physiotherapy and cognitive behavioural therapy.* The choice of therapy depends upon the following:

- **The type of pain, its severity and underlying cause**
- **The mechanism of the pain**
- **Associated conditions**
- **Physical and psychological condition of the patient**
- **The risk of toxicity**

An attempt should always be made to find out the probable cause, and if possible, treat it. Thus, pain due to an abscess can be relieved by appropriate chemotherapy and surgery or that of duodenal ulcer by antacids and antisecretary drugs.

Patients in whom, the cause cannot be immediately treated, relief of pain can be obtained by *modifying the mechanism by which pain is produced*, e.g. use of nitrates in angina pectoris, miotics in glaucoma and muscle relaxants in certain musculoskeletal disorders. Mechanism of production of abdominal pain is often obscure and a demonstrable cause is absent. Individuals with 'functional dyspepsia', are known to be benefited by 'carminatives' which have been used for ages. It is a common experience that a few seeds of cardamom, fennel or a little ginger can make the stomach comfortable after a sumptuous meal! These agents form the traditional ingredients of many stomach ache powders and 'gripe waters'sold in the market. Ureteric, intestinal or biliary colic, however, needs administration of an antimuscarinic drug like atropine or its substitutes. Some drugs are relatively specific in that they act in a specific, inflammatory, painful condition, i.e. colchicine in acute gout (Chapter 73).

For the symptomatic relief of acute pain, opioid and nonopioid analgesics (NSAIDs) are the most commonly employed agents. It is important to administer

Table 11.4 Equianalgesic Doses of Opioids

Drug	Dose (mg) IM	Oral Dose (mg)
Morphine	10	60
Pethidine	75	300
Methadone	10	60
Codeine	–	120
Pentazocine	60	180
Buprenorphine	0.4	0.8*

*Sublingual, not oral.

analgesics at the very onset of pain. If the pain remains untreated, the analgesics become less effective, e.g. in migraine(Chapter 24).

The World Health Organisation issued the step wise selection of analgesics (Fig 11.8) for cancer pain in 1986, but this approach has been validated to be used for acute and chronic pain conditions. The selection of the initial analgesic drug is based on *pain severity scores (on rest and on movement). The severity of pain is measured on a visual analogue scale (VAS), where in 0 is no pain score and 10 is excruciating pain. The patient is asked to mark on this scale to get the score. The VAS score up to 4 indicates mild pain, 4.1 to 7 is moderate pain and above 7 indicates severe pain.*

For mild pain non-opioids such as paracetamol or NSAID are preferred. In moderate pain, weak opioids like tramadol and for severe pain, strong opioids like morphine or fentanyl are indicated. Modified adaptation of this WHO ladder includes the fourth step as neurosurgical procedures such as nerve blocks, epidural analgesia, spinal stimulators etc. for pain management

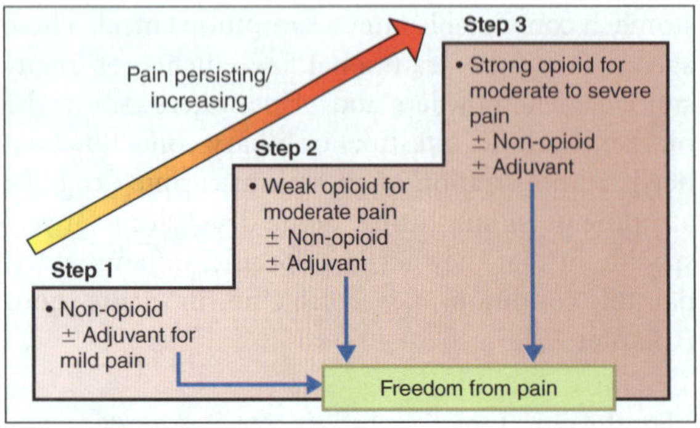

FIG. 11.8 **Step-wise selection of analgesics (WHO analgesic ladder)**

Mild acute pain like headache due to common cold, influenza or other fevers respond to paracetamol or NSAIDs. Single full doses of drug like ibuprofen are more effective than aspirin or paracetamol in such cases. Caffeine in the dose of 50–200 mg may enhance the analgesic effect of aspirin, paracetamol and ibuprofen.

For moderate pain, NSAIDs (e.g. naproxen) are more effective than paracetamol and may be as effective as oral opioids combined with paracetamol or even injected opioids.

In the treatment of **severe pain**, **morphine** is more **efficacious** than aspirin. Starting equianalgesic doses of opioids are given in Table 11.4; the optimum dose for each patient is determined by titration.

Severe pain of sudden onset, particularly the visceral pain (e.g. MI), can produce shock. In such cases, opioids are indispensable and should be administered immediately, e.g. in acute MI, fractures and pneumothorax. The opioids also induce a state of tranquillity, thus creating an indifference towards residual discomfort. When used with skill and discrimination, the adverse effects are not very bothersome.

Opioids should be administered in full doses, if necessary intravenously as patients with severe pain are remarkably tolerant of full therapeutic doses of morphine. When morphine is to be administered intravenously, it is injected slowly, the dose being 2.5–5 mg over 5 min. Pethidine or pentazocine have a shorter duration of action than morphine; this can lead to unsuspected under treatment. Conditions in which morphine or pethidine is recommended and the frequency of doses suggested make the possibility of drug addiction very remote. However, patients with acute pain treated with opioids for more than 5–7 days are likely to develop tolerance to the analgesic effects.

As the onset of pain relief by *NSAIDs* is much slower than that by the opioids, the latter may be combined with NSAIDs with synergistic effect. Fixed dose combinations of opioids and NSAIDs are also available e.g. tramadol with celecoxib.

The affective reaction to pain is also of overriding importance. In such cases, analgesics alone may not be adequate and adjuvant drugs as well as nondrug therapy may be more important. *The concurrent use of a phenothiazine, an anxiolytic or an antidepressant (Chapters 13 and 14) helps to relieve the pain by modifying the affective component of the pain.* Used in combination with analgesics, these drugs reduce the doses of the latter as well as relieve the suffering and improve the quality of life in chronic pain.

For the symptomatic relief of dull aching, chronic pain, nonopioid, nonaddicting analgesics like paracetamol and NSAIDs are preferred. Usually in mild to moderate cases paracetamol is the initial choice of drug. In *single smaller doses*, NSAIDs have analgesic activity comparable to that of paracetamol. They may, therefore, be used on demand to treat mild or intermittent pain or to supplement regular treatment.

In regular *full doses*, NSAIDs also have an anti-inflammatory effect and are effective in treating continuous or regular pain associated with inflammatory arthritis such as RA and ankylosing spondylitis. NSAIDs are also useful in the pain of advanced osteoarthritis when paracetamol fails to work; even in such cases much smaller doses of a mild drug such as ibuprofen are needed to control pain than those required in RA.

Clinical studies show no substantial difference in the therapeutic benefits of various NSAIDs, although the tolerability and individual preference may vary. Further, the duration of action (e.g. for relief of early morning stiffness of arthritis) and the availability in injectable form may determine the choice of an NSAID. Table 11.5 gives the plasma half-lives of NSAIDs. In most instances, the selection of an NSAID is dictated by response of an individual patient. Generally naproxen and Ibuprofen are commonly employed NSAIDs are also useful in *pain associated with injury to soft tissues*, e.g. sprains and postoperative pain.

Indomethacin, diclofenac and related compounds are potent NSAIDs but are more likely to cause GI bleeding, increase CVS risk and damage kidneys. *Routine use of these drugs in any dosage in treatment of mild to moderate pain is unjustified.* Most of the NSAIDs including diclofenac, flurbiprofen, ibuprofen, indomethacin, meloxicam, naproxen, piroxicam and celecoxib,are CYP2C9 substrates; dosage reductions may be required in CYP2C9 poor metabolizers and patients taking a CYP2C9 inhibitor.

Sustained release (SR), NSAID formulations are used especially in chronic pain to decrease tablet burden but are not 'superior' to individual active agents. Their only advantage is that they have longer duration of action. In fact, often individual agent is superior to 'slow releasing'one for prompt relief of pain. Such formulations are always expensive. Moreover, the drug remains in the body for longer time. The patients may 'self-administer'such formulations repeatedly for chronic pain. This is dangerous, as *NSAIDs can cause 'silent and irreparable' kidney damage, more so in elderly and in those with DM.*

In chronic pain, the abnormal activity of the pain-mediating afferent system may continue irrespective of the original cause, and blocking of the neural pathways may not be helpful. *This is because chronic pain is caused by several mediators* (e.g. cytokines, bradykinin, substance P, etc.).

Table 11.5 Plasma Half-lives of NSAIDs

<5 h	Aspirin, diclofenac, ketoprofen, flurbiprofen, indomethacin, tolmetin, flufenamic acid
10–30 h	Diflunisal, fenoprofen, naproxen, sulindac, nabumetone
>50 h	Phenylbutazone, piroxicam, tenoxicam

Countering their effects is useful. In some of these patients use of TCA like amitriptyline in small doses (5–10 mg/day) is often useful.

The cause of **chronic headache** is often obscure in practice and needs detailed investigations. Many headaches are, however, caused by anxiety, tension, fatigue or depression, and use of proper psychotherapeutic drugs like benzodiazepines or antidepressants can give dramatic results. Realisation of this psychic aspect of pain will prevent other unnecessary therapy. In such cases some minor adjustments in patient's life can be more therapeutic than even drugs. Headaches due to chronic sinusitis and eyestrain need specific treatment.

Backache presents similar diagnostic problems as headache. It can be due to many causes. *The commonest causes are faulty posture and lack of exercise.* Mental depression and nervous tension can often produce backache. Non pharmacological therapy (posture correction, physiotherapy) is recommended as a first line option for low back pain. Mild backache of vertebral osteoporosis may be relieved by oral calcium, vitamin D, bisphosphonates and physiotherapy, while unremitting pain may respond to calcitonin (Chapter 68).However, severe pain of ankylosing spondylitis needs treatment with NSAIDs, whereas acute vertebral fracture in osteoporosis needs a short period of bed rest followed by physiotherapy, in addition to an NSAID. **In inflammatory conditions such** as RA and gout, the NSAIDs relieve pain without affecting the basic disorder (Chapter 73).

PH 1.1, AS 8.4, AS 8.5

Cancer pain: Pain is a major problem in cancer patients and 70% of patients with advanced cancer have it. It can be caused by the cancer itself or by other associated conditions such as osteoarthritis, bedsores or surgery. It may be related to bones, nerve compression, metastases in soft tissues; further, psychological reactions to the illness including depression and a sense of helplessness (distress) may worsen the pain. Unremitting pain itself can cause secondary symptoms such as anorexia, disturbed sleep, irritability and impaired concentration. *It is, therefore, necessary to assess the causes of pain, as well as its effects, at the very outset in a patient with cancer; further, periodic reassessment of both is necessary so as to offer the patient appropriate treatment, to make life comfortable.*

The therapy consists of drug treatment and other methods like local radiation to a painful bony metastasis. Irradiation of the metastases by beta rays from injected ^{89}SrCl alleviates the bone pain.

Classification of drugs used in the treatment of cancer pain

I **Analgesics:**
   a. **Nonopioids** (paracetamol and NSAIDs)
   b. **Weak opioids** (codeine and dextropropoxyphene)
   c. **Strong opioids** (morphine, buprenorphine, pethidine and methadone)

II **Adjuvant analgesics:** These are the drugs used primarily for indications other than pain. They have analgesic properties in some painful conditions such as cancer or nonmalignant chronic pain. Hence they are used as 'add-on'drugs and serve as 'opioid-sparing'drugs. Sometimes, they are used as 'first-line'therapy, e.g. carbamazepine in trigeminal neuralgia. They are described elsewhere.
   a. **Antidepressants**
   b. **Antiepileptics** (carbamazepine and gabapentin)
   c. **α_2 Agonists** (clonidine, tizanidine)
   d. **Glucocorticoids**
   e. **Local anaesthetics** (transdermal lignocaine, mexiletine)
   f. **Topical agents** (capsaicin)
   g. **NMDA antagonists** (dextromethorphan, methadone, amantadine, ketamine)
   h. **Cannabinoid-Δ-9-THC**
   i. **Bisphosphonates** and **calcitonin**
   j. **GABA agonists** (baclofen)
   k. **Neuroimmunomodulatory agents** (thalidomide and its newer analogues).

They are described elsewhere.

In chronic cancer pain analgesics are used in a step ladder fashion, commencing with NSAIDs, and changing to weak and finally strong opioids as the drugs from the earlier used group cease to be effective. Ibuprofen or other NSAIDs may be useful in relieving pain of bony metastases and that due to mechanical compression of tissues other than nerves. The opioids are added sequentially when the need arises.

Glucocorticoids are very often prescribed in the palliative treatment of cancer pain. They have anti-inflammatory action, reduce oedema around damaged nerves, reduce nausea and improve appetite and the quality of life in general. Dexamethasone may be used 1–2 mg b.i.d.

In severe cancer pain especially in terminally ill patients, morphine is used by the clock, and one does not wait till the pain returns and the patient demands relief. The oral route is to be preferred; a commonly used dose is 5–30 mg every 4 h; but much larger doses may be needed. It has no ceiling dose but dosage may be limited by ADR. Nausea may be common at the beginning of treatment with morphine and is treated with a drug such as prochlorpromazine (5–10 mg 4–8 hourly), metoclopramide (10 mg 4–8 hourly) or haloperidol (1–2 mg daily). Constipation may be troublesome. Physical dependence and tolerance may develop during treatment with morphine; but psychological dependence rarely, occurs in cancer patients receiving opioids. Metastases in the liver are not a contraindication to opioids; but care should be exercised in patients with concomitant hepatic dysfunction. *In cancer patients, the use of potent analgesics is dictated by the intensity of pain and not by the brevity of prognosis.* The starting doses of other strong opioids are: buprenorphine (0.2–0.4 mg sublingually); methadone (5–10 mg orally) and pethidine (50–100 mg orally), on a 4-hourly basis. *Being a mixed agonist-antagonist, buprenorphine can reverse the analgesia caused by other strong opioids and, therefore, should not be combined with drugs such as morphine.* **Extended release oral preparations of hydromorphone** are available for treating severe cancer pain. Its effect lasts for 24 h. *The tablet must not be crushed or chewed but swallowed.* A self- adhesive skin patch which releases the opioid **fentanyl transdermally** can also be used. Its effects last for 72 h.

Patient-controlled analgesia: This is an approach where the patient himself injects small programmed dose of morphine, fentanyl or hydromorphone through an intrathecal or epidural catheter to produce analgesia without sensory loss. This has been shown to deliver better pain control. The effect lasts for 12–15 h. Careful monitoring is however needed. Low doses of local anaesthetic agents (bupivacaine or ropivacaine) are also given in combination with opioid analgesics (Chapter 16).

Chronic neuropathic (deafferentation) pain occurs in diabetic neuropathy as well as following herpes zoster. It is due to altered neuronal excitability resulting in abnormal spontaneous discharge. The drug used in the initial treatment of this shooting or stabbing pain occurring in these conditions can be a tricyclic antidepressant (TCA), a serotonin and norepinephrine reuptake inhibitor (SNRI), or an antiseizure drug.

Tricyclic **antidepressants** like amitriptyline (25–100 mg /day), nortriptyline (75–100 mg / day), and imipramine(50–100 mg /day) have been shown to relieve many types of neuropathic pain, including diabetic neuropathy, postherpetic neuralgia, polyneuropathy, and nerve injury or infiltration with cancer. The analgesic effects of these drugs is probably due to their inhibition of norepinephrine and serotonin reuptake. **Duloxetine** (60 mg /day), a SNRI (Chapter 14) has been used in the treatment of diabetic peripheral neuropathy pain, fibromyalgia, and chronic musculoskeletal pain.

Milnacipran (100 mg /day), is moderately effective in decreasing pain and improving function in fibromyalgia.

Antiseizure drugs (chapter 9) such as **gabapentin** (600-1200 mg bid) and **pregabalin** (75–300 mg bid) are approved for treating postherpetic neuralgia and diabetic neuropathy. Both these drugs can cause fatal respiratory depression especially in elderly patients with respiratory risk factors (e.g. presence of COPD, concurrent use of opioids or other CNS depressants). Routine use of gabapentin and pregabalin can lead to physical dependence.

Carbamazepine (100-600 mg bid) is approved for treatment of pain associated with trigeminal neuralgia.

Pain resistant to amitriptyline may respond to **capsaicin** derived from chillies (hot peppers). Capsaicin is applied to the concerned skin area as a 0.025%–0.075%cream. It is believed to act by interfering with pain transmission in the peripheral neurons by depleting and inhibiting the reuptake of substance P. It may cause local burning sensation. **Transdermal patches** of 8% capsaicin and 5% lignocaine are available for post- herpetic neuralgia. Application of the patch for one hour for postherpetic neuralgia or for 30 minutes for peripheral neuropathy has been modestly effective in reducing pain for up to 3 months. **Lignocaine** ointment 5%, can also be applied locally.

Ziconotide, a synthetic neuronal N-type calcium channel blocker, is administered intrathecally via a programmable microinfusion device for treatment of severe refractory chronic pain including neuropathic pain. It has been effective, both as monotherapy and as an add-on to standard therapy. Unlike opioids, ziconotide does not cause tolerance, dependence, or respiratory depression

Miscellaneous pains: *Obstetric analgesia* is achieved by the use of nitrous oxide (Chapter 7) or pethidine (Chapter 10). Analgesics are often used prior to surgery (pre-emptive analgesia) as they are known to reduce postoperative pain. Relief of *postoperative pain* not only increases the patient's comfort but can also remove an impediment to adequate ventilation in major upper abdominal surgery. If an NSAID such as paracetamol, ketorolac or diclofenac does not give adequate relief, buprenorphine (0.2–0.4 mg sublingually every 6–8 h) may be used.

The use of phenazopyridine to relieve *lower urinary tract pain* is discussed in Chapter 50.

Local treatment of pain: Topical NSAIDs should be considered before oral NSAIDs for treatment of localized pain (e.g., sprains, knee or hand osteoarthritis). Counterirritants such as turpentine or methyl salicylate, applied as a liniment, relieve dull-aching, localised musculoskeletal pain. They do not mask the underlying internal disease.

Several NSAIDs (such as methyl salicylate, diclofenac) in the form of gels/creams/ointments **get absorbed** after topical application and are available as OTC products for treatment of sprains, arthritis and post-extraction dental pain. *They can induce photosensitivity reaction and should not be applied to broken or inflamed skin.*

Eye drops containing diclofenac 0.1%, flurbiprofen 0.03%, suprofen 1% and nepafenac 0.1% are useful in patients undergoing cataract surgery. When started before surgery, they act synergistically with local mydriatics to prevent miosis (Chapter 70).

Nonpharmacological therapy: Such therapies as cognitive behavioural therapy, structural education and exercise programme, massage, acupuncture, Yoga, meditation have all produce beneficial effects in the treatment of chronic pain. Further, such treatments are unlikely to cause harm and in fact, will help to improve the quality of life.

NSAIDs

Nonselective cyclooxygenase (COX) inhibitors

Salicylates and their congeners

- Aspirin
- Methylsalicylate
- Salicylic acid

Pyrazolone derivatives

- Phenylbutazone
- Oxyphenbutazone

Indoles and related drugs

- Indomethacin
- sulindac

Heterocyclic arylacetic acid derivatives

- Diclofenac
- Tolmetin
- Ketorolac

Propionic acid derivatives

- Ibuprofen
- Fenoprofen
- Naproxen
- Ketoprofen
- Pirprofen

Fenamates

- Flufenamic acid
- Mefenamic acid

Oxicams

- Piroxicam

Preferential COX-2 inhibitors

- Nimesulide
- Nabumetone
- Etodolac
- Meloxicam

Selective COX-2 inhibitors

- Celecoxib
- Etoricoxib
- Parecoxib
- Lumiracoxib

DRUGS USED IN THE TREATMENT OF CANCER PAIN

Analgesics

Nonopioids
- Paracetamol
- NSAIDs

Weak opioids
- Codeine
- Dextropropoxyphene

Strong opioids
- Morphine
- Buprenorphine
- Pethidine
- Methadone

Adjuvant analgesics

Antidepressants

Antiepileptics
- Carbamazepine
- Gabapentin

α_2 Agonists
- Clonidine
- Tizanidine

Glucocorticoids

Local anaesthetics
- Lignocaine
- Mexiletine

Topical agents
- Capsaicin

NMDA antagonists
- Dextromethorphan
- Methadone
- Amantadine
- Ketamine

Cannabinoids
- Δ-9-THC

Bisphosphonates and calcitonin

GABA agonists
- Baclofen

Neuroimmunomodulatory agents
- Thalidomide
- Lenalidomide
- Pomalidomide

CHAPTER 12

Central Nervous System Stimulants

Learning Objectives

This chapter will enable the reader:

1. To classify central nervous system stimulants with examples.
2. To describe mechanism of action, pharmacological effects, ADR and indications for clinically relevant xanthine alkaloids.
3. To state uses of doxapram.
4. To state the drugs to be used for (a) narcolepsy and (b) attention-deficit hyperactivity disorder (ADHD).
5. To describe pharmacotherapy of strychnine poisoning.

KEY TERMS

Unlike central nervous system (CNS) depressants, CNS stimulants in general, lack selectivity of action. Hence they have fewer therapeutic applications. Further, excessive stimulation of CNS is followed by its depression. Some of the CNS stimulants are mainly used as **analeptics**. Analepsis is a Greek word which can be loosely translated as 'picking up those who have been cast down'. *Analeptics stimulate the CNS particularly the respiratory centre and, in large doses, they cause generalised convulsions.*

Classification of CNS Stimulants

I. **Those acting directly on the CNS**
   - **Predominantly cortical stimulants** like xanthine alkaloids, amphetamine, methyl amphetamine, methylphenidate and pipradrol
   - **Predominantly medullary stimulants**, e.g. picrotoxin, pentylenetetrazol, camphor and carbon dioxide
   - **Predominantly spinal stimulants**, e.g. strychnine

II. **Those which stimulate the CNS reflexly,** e.g. lobeline, ammonia and nicotine

The above classification is arbitrary and a CNS stimulant can stimulate the entire CNS. Only few of these agents have therapeutic utility in clinical practice (discussed below).

STIMULANTS OF THE CEREBRAL CORTEX

METHYLXANTHINE ALKALOIDS: **Caffeine, theophylline** and **theobromine are** three naturally occurring alkaloids (Fig. 12.1) present in several plants. These alkaloids leave behind a yellow residue when heated with nitric acid and hence the term xanthine, derived from the Greek word 'xanthos' meaning yellow. Coffee prepared by grinding the seeds of *Coffea arabica* contains caffeine; tea from leaves of *Thea sinensis* contains caffeine and small amounts of theobromine and theophylline; while cocoa obtained by grinding seeds of *Theobroma cacao* contains caffeine and theobromine. The cola-flavoured soft drinks also contain caffeine.

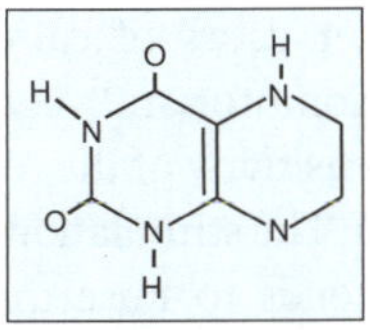

FIG. 12.1 **Xanthine.**

Mechanism of action: Methylxanthines act by:

- **Inhibiting phosphodiesterase** (PDE), thus preventing the conversion of cAMP to inactive 5′ AMP and thereby increasing tissue concentration of cAMP. This is its main action. The catecholamines, which also increase the concentration of cAMP by a different mechanism, act synergistically with methylxanthines.
- **Changing the distribution of calcium at the intracellular sites**
- **Blocking adenosine receptors which modulate adenylyl cyclase activity**

Pharmacological actions:

Central nervous system: Of the three xanthine alkaloids, caffeine possesses the most significant action on CNS, followed by theophylline and theobromine. Caffeine mainly acts on the cerebral cortex; larger amounts stimulate the medullary centres and toxic doses may cause convulsions.

- **Cerebral cortex:**
  a. Caffeine is a recreational drink. In small doses it facilitates clarity of thoughts, increases mental alertness and delays fatigue and drowsiness. *It stimulates mental activity when it is below normal* following fatigue or boredom; *it does not raise it above normal.*
  b. It also reduces reaction time, improves motor activity and augments conditioned responses. Thus, *it improves physical performance.* The cortical effects may be produced by ingestion of one or two cups of coffee, one cup containing 100–150 mg of caffeine.
  c. Larger doses of caffeine (exceeding 300 mg) produce irritability, nervousness, confusion, insomnia, headache and tremors. Recently acquired motor skills that require precise muscle coordination and accurate timing may be affected adversely as a result of nervousness and tremors. Toxic doses cause focal and generalised convulsions in animals.
- **Medulla:** Larger doses of caffeine stimulate the respiratory, vasomotor and vagal centres. Caffeine increases the sensitivity of the respiratory centre to carbon dioxide. The stimulation of vasomotor and vagal centres tends to raise the BP and induces bradycardia, respectively.
- **Spinal cord:** Very large doses of caffeine increase the reflex excitability of the spinal cord and may produce clonic convulsions and death in animals. In man, no fatalities after caffeine administration have been reported.

Cardiovascular system: Theophylline has the most prominent action on the CVS.

- **Heart:** Theophylline directly stimulates the myocardium and increases the heart rate, the force of contraction (**ionotropic effect**) and the myocardial oxygen consumption. *Large doses of theophylline as well as caffeine, can cause palpitation, tachycardia and rarely cardiac arrhythmias.* The increased force of contraction by theophylline assures a better emptying of the heart and reduces the central venous pressure. In individuals with congestive heart failure, the lowered venous pressure produces an increase in the cardiac output.
- **Blood vessels:** Theophylline produces peripheral vasodilatation by a direct action on vascular smooth muscle and *cause a decrease in cardiac preload.*
  Coronaries: are dilated and the coronary blood flow is increased.
  Cerebral blood vessels: Caffeine produces **a marked increase in the cerebral vascular resistance and reduces the cerebral blood flow** and the CSF pressure. This constriction may be responsible for the relief of migraine headache.
  Pulmonary blood vessels: Theophylline reduces the pulmonary artery pressure by relaxing the pulmonary arteries.
  Blood pressure: The direct cardiac stimulant action of xanthines tend to raise the BP. This action is aided by the stimulant action on the vasomotor centre and is antagonised by the central vagal stimulation and vasodilation. Changes in BP are, therefore, unpredictable. The combination of vasodilatation and increased cardiac output, however, raises the pulse pressure and the velocity of blood flow and helps to improve circulation. Aminophylline IV may produce a fall in BP.

Kidneys: Theophylline reduces tubular reabsorption of sodium and causes moderate diuresis (Chapter 37).

Smooth muscle: Xanthines are smooth muscle relaxant, particularly for the bronchial smooth muscle.

Theophylline abolishes bronchospasm produced by histamine, pilocarpine and anaphylactic shock.

Skeletal muscles: Xanthines, particularly caffeine, strengthen the contraction, increase the metabolism and postpone fatigue of skeletal muscles by both central and peripheral actions. Improved contractility of the diaphragm may contribute to the efficacy of aminophylline in asthma.

Miscellaneous actions: The xanthines increase the gastric acid secretion. Decaffeinated coffee also has similar effect.

Absorption, fate and excretion: The xanthines are readily absorbed on oral, rectal or parenteral administration.. They are metabolised in the liver, mainly by demethylation and oxidation by mixed function oxidases and xanthine oxidase. *Caffeine metabolism varies widely among individuals; its t½varies from 2 to 12 h. Beverages containing xanthines are not contraindicated in gout.*

Adverse reactions: In the usual doses, caffeine does not cause serious toxicity.

- **CNS:** Excessive, prolonged use of the methylxanthines may produce confusion, tremors, insomnia and excitement. The individual may complain of ringing in the ears, headache and may develop tachypnoea, tachycardia, emesis, fever and occasionally extrasystoles. *Hence, a patient with recurrent headache, should be asked about excessive tea or coffee drinking.* The symptoms are reversible and can be treated with sedatives.
- **Gastrointestinal (GI) tract:** The xanthine alkaloids and beverages should be administered with caution in patients with peptic ulcer. Theophylline, may produce hyperacidity, nausea, vomiting and epigastric pain even when it is given parenterally. GI irritation can be reduced by its administration with food.
- **Cardiovascular system:** Aminophylline, on parenteral administration, may produce dizziness, hypotension, severe precordial pain and even ventricular fibrillation. Fatalities have been reported following rapid IV use. In children, aminophylline intoxication is characterised by vomiting, severe thirst, dehydration, delirium, convulsions and shock.
- **Tolerance:** Tolerance develops after prolonged use of xanthines, mainly to their cortical stimulant, diuretic and peripheral vasodilator effects. It is usually abolished after abstinence from xanthine beverages.
- **Habituation:** Habituation to xanthine beverages such as tea, coffee and cola is extremely common. However, it does not seem to be harmful.

Though there is a wide interindividual variation in benefits and risks associated with different doses of caffeine, for healthy adults, daily consumption of caffeine up to 400 mg (~5.5 mg/kg for a 75 kg individual or 4-5 average cups of brewed coffee) does not pose a health risk. *Tea, coffee and cola drinks are better avoided in small children as they are thought to be less tolerant of the stimulant effects of caffeine.*

Preparations and dosage:

i. Caffeine citrate dose: 50-100 mg in divided doses; Maximum dose: 400 mg/day
ii. Aminophylline: (Chapter 27)
iii. Deriphylline (Chapter 27)

Indications:

- **As a CNS stimulant:** Caffeine in the form of coffee or tea is often employed for relief from fatigue. Theophylline and caffeine are used to treat neonatal apnoea.
- **Migraine:** Because of its constrictive action on the cerebral blood vessels, caffeine is used along with ergotamine tartrate for relief of migraine (Chapter 24).
- **Acute left ventricular failure (LVF):** *Aminophylline* is an adjuvant in the treatment of paroxysmal nocturnal dyspnoea due to LVF. Aminophylline increases the cardiac output, reduces the pulmonary artery pressure and the cardiac preload, induces bronchodilatation, stimulates the respiratory centre and causes diuresis. When the distinction between dyspnoea due to acute LVF (cardiac asthma) and bronchial asthma is not clear, it is safer to administer IV aminophylline rather than adrenaline (which is dangerous in the former condition) or morphine (which is dangerous in the latter condition). It is administered *slowly* intravenously in the dose of 500 mg along with other treatment such as morphine and oxygen. Its use has now declined because of the availability of more specific preload reducing drugs (Chapter 31).

- **In bronchial asthma** (Chapter 27).
- **As a diuretic** (Chapter 37).
- **Strong coffee is used in orthostatic hypotension of autonomic failure** (Chapter 30). PH 1.22

AMPHETAMINE: It is a sympathomimetic amine (See Fig. 18.6). Amphetamine is available in racemic and dextro forms. The d-isomer is approximately 3–4 times as potent as the levo form in its central effects.

Mechanism of action: Amphetamine exerts its effects indirectly by releasing NA and DA from their storage sites in the central and peripheral neurons and also blocks their reuptake (Chapter 17).

Pharmacological actions: Its central actions are similar to xanthines but peripherally it produces adrenaline-like actions (Chapter 18).

CNS: It is a potent CNS stimulant and can act as a 'psychic energizer'; it is not a true antidepressant. It neither corrects the depressive state nor prevents suicidal tendencies.

In therapeutic doses (10–30 mg orally), amphetamine produces euphoria, wakefulness and insomnia. It also decreases fatigue, and improves the physical performance, alertness and confidence. The psychic effects of amphetamine are determined by the personality of the individual and the dose. Larger doses cause tremors, restlessness, confusion, agitation and headache. Repeated and excessive stimulation by amphetamine is followed by fatigue and depression.

CVS: It increases the systolic and diastolic BP but does not elevate the cardiac output significantly. Repeated administration leads to tachyphylaxis to the hypertensive effect.

Smooth muscles: It contracts the sphincter of the bladder and relaxes the bronchial smooth muscle.

Appetite suppression: It is an anorexiant (Chapter 38).

Absorption, fate and excretion: Amphetamine is well absorbed on oral and parenteral administration and readily enters CNS. It is relatively resistant to inactivation by MAO and has t½ of 10 h. Approximately, 40% of the dose is excreted unchanged in urine.

Adverse reactions:

- Excessive sympathetic stimulation generally causes palpitation, restlessness, headache, tremors and agitation. CNS stimulation causes marked anxiety, confusion, erratic behaviour, paranoid psychosis and visual hallucinations.
- **Acute intoxication** causes
  a. *CNS effects* such as restlessness, dizziness, tremors, hyperactive reflexes, irritability and insomnia, followed by fatigue and depression.
  b. *Behavioural symptoms* such as delirium, confusion, acute neurotic or psychotic episodes, and suicidal/homicidal tendencies.
  c. *ANS instability* resulting in angina pectoris, cardiac arrhythmias, headache, chills, flushing, pallor, hypertension, excessive sweating and circulatory collapse. *Individuals on therapy with MAOI may develop an alarming rise in BP with therapeutic doses of amphetamine-like drugs.*
  d. *GI symptoms* including anorexia, nausea, vomiting, abdominal cramps and diarrhoea.
  e. *Hyperpyrexia* due to increased peripheral oxygen consumption. FM 10.1
- **Treatment of acute poisoning** is symptomatic. Sedation with diazepam is indicated to control the central stimulation. α-Adrenergic receptor blocking agents such as phentolamine are employed to control hypertension. Sodium nitroprusside can also be used. The urine should be acidified with ammonium chloride to promote its excretion. Peritoneal dialysis may prove useful.
- **Long-term consumption** results in irritability, aggressive and stereotyped behaviour, and paranoid psychosis. Marked weight loss is observed. PH 1.22
- **Dependence and withdrawal symptoms:** Amphetamine is a drug of abuse. It is misused by the students during examination period. It causes habituation, tolerance and psychic dependence. Withdrawal symptoms are listed in Box 12.1.

The focus of amphetamine deaddiction program is on gradual withdrawal of amphetamine, treatment of withdrawal symptoms, abstinence promotion and

Box 12.1 Amphetamine Withdrawal Symptoms

- Chronic fatigue, mental depression, asthenia, tremors.
- Gastrointestinal disturbances.
- Drowsiness, prolonged sleep or lethargy.
- Intense craving.

prevention of relapse. Psychosis may respond to antipsychotics or craving may be less with topiramate, buprenorphine or methadone but consistent effects cannot be guaranteed. There is no drug approved to treat amphetamine addiction. Counselling and psychotherapy (cognitive-behavioural therapy) play a crucial role.

Preparations and dosage: Dextroamphetamine sulphate as 5 mg tablets.

Indications: It is no more used for its peripheral effects; but its use is restricted to:

- **Attention Deficit Hyperactivity Disorder (ADHD):** Dextroamphetamine has been used in children with ADHD. The diagnosis of ADHD must be established properly as many other conditions in children which superficially resemble ADHD. Linear growth may be hampered during long-term treatment, probably because of its anorectic action.
- **Narcolepsy:** Amphetamine prevents attacks of sleep.

Methamphetamine, a congener of amphetamine, has more central than peripheral actions. It is less expensive and therefore is a **major drug of abuse**.

PIPRADROL and **METHYLPHENIDATE**, are piperidyl derivatives which are mild psychomotor stimulants. These drugs act by inhibiting reuptake of central NA and DA. Their actions are similar to those of amphetamine. Thus, they reduce fatigue and produce a feeling of well-being and alertness. The ADRs include headache, decreased appetite, weight loss, insomnia, tachycardia, abdominal pain, rarely priapism and peripheral vasculopathy. In large doses, they cause restlessness, tremors, palpitation, ataxia and even convulsions. Possibility of drug dependence is a drawback. The effects of methylphenidate last for 5 h; hence, several long-acting analogues of methylphenidate are also available now. In addition, fixed dose combinations containing immediate-release (**dexmethylphenidate**) and delayed- or extended-release components (prodrug **serdexmethylphenidate**) are also available . Their effects generally begin within 20-60 minutes after administration and persist for 8-16 hours. Methyphenidate is used in treatment of narcolepsy and ADHD. Pipradrol has *no place in the treatment of depression and is considered as a drug of abuse.*

MODAFINIL is a nonamphetamine drug used in the treatment of narcolepsy as it reduces Daytime Excessive Sleepiness (DES) and improves daytime performance. It promotes wakefulness in normal people and may help to work for longer time. Its mechanism of action is not known. Its main side effects are headache, nervousness, dizziness and insomnia. It is a reinforcing drug but with low abuse potential. It should not be used in persons with severe hepatic impairment. The dose is 200 mg (single dose) in the morning. Its R-enantiomer **armodafinil** is also available.

PHARMACOTHERAPY OF NARCOLEPSY

Narcolepsy is a heritable neurologic disorder with varied manifestations which begin to appear in late teens to 20s. The manifestations are as follows:

a. DES and poor or disturbed sleep at night.
b. Sudden sleep attacks during any day time activity.
c. Cataplexy: sudden onset of flaccid paralysis precipitated by anticipation, anger or surprise.
d. Hypnagogic hallucinations: frightening hallucinations at the onset of sleep.
e. Sleep paralysis: Muscle paralysis on awakening.

Type 1 narcolepsy is caused by selective and extensive damage of orexin (Chapter 8) producing neurons. This leads to reduced excitation of neurons that produce wakefulness-promoting neurotransmitters such as histamine. The cause for Type 2 narcolepsy is unknown and it does not have cataplexy.

The treatment of narcolepsy is symptomatic; the drug of choice is **modafinil** given as single daily dose. **Methylphenidate** or **dextroamphetamine** is used as an alternative to modafinil. They are more potent but also more toxic. Cataplexy, hypnagogic hallucinations and sleep paralysis are related to REM sleep and are treated with REM suppressing **antidepressants such as TCA**(protriptyline) or **SSRI**(fluoxetine).

DES, sleep attacks and cataplexy also may respond to **sodium oxybate**, a sodium salt of α-hydroxybutyrate. It is taken at bedtime and again during the night. The drug causes headache, nausea, dizziness, confusion, sleep walking , respiratory depression and coma. Its abuse has been associated with 'date rape'. In addition mixed-salt oxybate oral solutions are also available now to reduce the sodium content of the salt.

Recently **solriamfetol**, a dopamine and norepinephrine reuptake inhibitor and **pitolisant**, a H_3 receptor antagonist are approved for narcolepsy. Pitolisant binds selectively to H_3 receptors and acts as an antagonist/inverse agonist to increase histamine levels.

PHARMACOTHERAPY OF ATTENTION-DEFICIT HYPERACTIVITY DISORDER

This paediatric condition is characterised by inattentiveness and impulsiveness with or without hyperactivity, impaired learning and emotional liability. These children are easily distracted and accident prone.

One has to be sure of the diagnosis of ADHD. Assessment of the child's behaviour is dependent on social and psychological trends. There are no well defined standards for normal or desired behaviour. *Training the parents in behaviour management with behavioural classroom interventions are recommended as first line therapy to preschool age children and used as adjunct to medication in school age children and adolescents. Family counselling and psychotherapy are more effective than drug therapy in many cases.*

Drug therapy consists of stimulants which are preferred over nonstimulants as they are less effective. Nonstimulants are used to treat hyperactivity but less effective for inattention. Nonstimulants can be used in combination with stimulants or when stimulants are contraindicated, ineffective or not tolerated.

Psychomotor stimulants like, **methylphenidate, its analogue dexmethylphenidate, d-amphetamine and its prodrug lisdexamfetamine** cause beneficial effects when given for 1–3 months. Long acting methylphenidate formulations administered once a day are preferred. A short acting formulation is added to improve symptom control early in the morning or prolong duration and smooth withdrawal in late afternoon.

Stimulants are contraindicated in CV disorders, hypertension, hyperthyroidism, psychosis, mania and glaucoma.

Nonstimulant drugs include antihypertensive drugs such as **clonidine** and **guanfacine**(Chapter 30) and a NA reuptake inhibitor, **atomoxetine**, which probably acts by increasing NA and DA in frontal cortex. Atomoxetine is less effective than methylphenidate. The adverse effects include somnolence, nausea, vomiting, delayed growth, hypertension and suicidal tendencies. **Viloxazine**, another selective NA reuptake inhibitor is also approved for treatment of ADHD. It is a strong CYP1A2 inhibitor.

TCA, especially desipramine and nortriptyline, are sometimes used as alternative drugs. They may improve the core symptoms of ADHD in 2–6 weeks, but their effect on CVS and tolerance on long-term therapy are the important clinical concerns. **Fluoxetine**(Chapter 14) may also be used as an alternative for refractory ADHD.

STIMULANTS OF THE BRAIN STEM AND MEDULLARY CENTRES

DOXAPRAM: This is a nonspecific analeptic used mainly as a respiratory stimulant in the postanaesthetic period and in patients with hypoventilation. It is also used in patients of COPD with hypercapneic respiratory failure and in whom mechanical ventilatory support is contraindicated. Doxapram given as IV infusion or slow IV injection in these patients may tide over the crisis. It has a reasonable margin of safety. It is administered by IV drip in the total dose of 0.5–1.5 mg/kg at the rate of 5 mg/min. It may be repeated after 1 h. A single IV injection (0.7 mg/kg) produces peak action in 1 min lasting for 5–10 min. Adverse reactions include vomiting, hypertension, tachycardia, arrhythmias, muscle twitchings, tremors and convulsions.

MEDROXYPROGESTERONE ACETATE: Like progesterone, this drug has respiratory stimulant action. It is effective orally. It has been used with some success in patients with chronic ventilatory failure due to pathological obesity (**Pickwickian syndrome**).

CARBON DIOXIDE: Chapter 75.

STIMULANTS OF THE SPINAL CORD

STRYCHNINE: Strychnine is an alkaloid obtained from the button-shaped seeds of the plant *Strychnos nux vomica*. Strychnine acts mainly on the spinal cord but it stimulates the entire neuraxis in large doses. It acts as a competitive antagonist of the inhibitory NT glycine at the postsynaptic inhibitory sites and produces seizures leading to asphyxia and death. It has no therapeutic value.

REFLEX STIMULANTS OF THE CENTRAL NERVOUS SYSTEM

Lobeline: Lobeline, an alkaloid from the leaves of *Lobelia inflata*, stimulates the CNS through the chemoreceptors of the carotid sinus. It is now rarely used.

Other reflex stimulants of the CNS such as nicotine (Chapter 21), and apomorphine (Chapter 15) are discussed elsewhere. **Liquor ammonia**, camphor and **smelling salts** (ammonium carbonate) inhalation in syncope is a common household procedure which stimulates the respiratory and vasomotor centres reflexly.

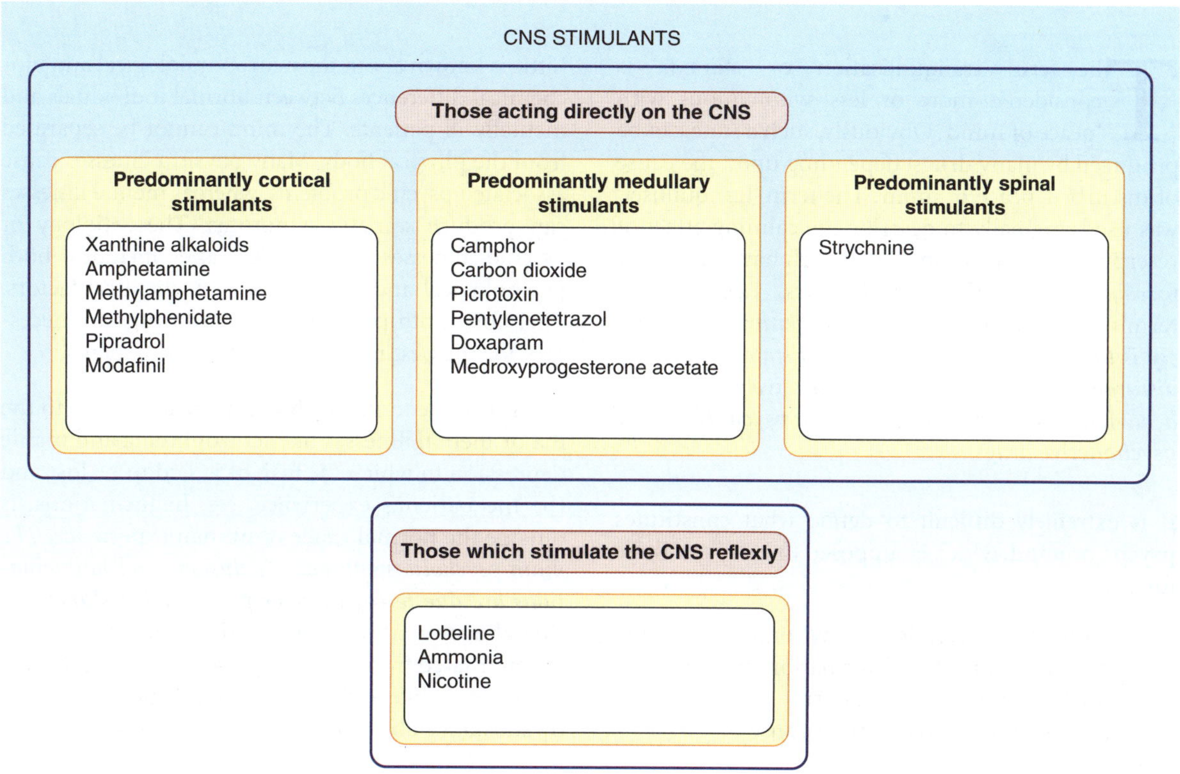

CHAPTER 13

Psychopharmacology – 1: Introduction, Antipsychotic Drugs, Pharmacotherapy of Psychosis and Psychotogenic Drugs

Learning Objectives

This chapter will enable the reader:

1. To be aware of the types of psychiatric disorders and methods used to evaluate psychotropic drugs.
2. To classify antipsychotic drugs giving examples.
3. To explain mechanism of action of typical antipsychotics and based on it describe their pharmacological effects, ADR and indications.
4. To compare and contrast typical and atypical antipsychotics.
5. To discuss principles of management of schizophrenia giving examples of drugs used.
6. To enlist psychotogenic drugs and describe their mechanism of action, pharmacological effects, and adverse reaction profile.
7. To enlist drug-induced psychiatric syndromes giving examples of drugs causing them.

KEY TERMS

psychotic disorders, p. 196
neurotic disorders, p. 197
antipsychotics, conventional and atypical, p. 197
chlorpromazine, p. 198
extrapyramidal reactions, p. 200
clozapine and other atypical antipsychotics, p. 202
schizophrenia, treatment, p. 205
psychotogenic drugs, p. 207
lysergic acid diethylamide, p. 207
cannabis, p. 208
drug-induced psychiatric syndromes, p. 210

The term 'tranquillisation' or 'ataraxia' is considered more or less synonymous with 'peace of mind'. Obviously, such a state can be produced by many drugs, depending upon the cause of disturbed 'peace of mind'. The term 'tranquilliser' was used originally to describe the calming effect of reserpine and chlorpromazine which have the ability to *calm without affecting wakefulness.* Regardless of terminology, *the objective of drug therapy in psychiatry is to induce an improved mental state in mentally disturbed patients. Drugs which selectively modify the behavioural pattern are known as* ***psychotropic*** *or* ***psychoactive*** *drugs.*

It is extremely difficult to define what constitutes **psyche** or **mind**, which is supposed to carry out three functions:

- **Cognition**, the reception of environmental stimuli
- **Affect**, analysing the information received and formation of a reaction pattern
- **Conation**, the behavioural response

Little is known about the neurophysiological and biochemical differences between normal individuals and mentally ill patients. The mind cannot be separated from the physical body. Many physical illnesses cause associated psychic problems, whereas mental illnesses can produce somatic symptoms. The aetiology of psychic illnesses is complex and includes both psychological and physiological/biochemical factors. Therefore, both psychotherapy and drugs are necessary for the best results in most of the patients.

Clinically, the term **psychotic disorders** refers to the major mental illnesses like schizophrenia and manic depression in which (a) insight is said to be lost and (b) the patient's experience, e.g. hallucinations, is outside the normal range of human experience. *The main psychotic symptoms, "delusions and hallucinations are due to cognitive or perceptual dysfunction".* The above-mentioned psychotic disorders must be differentiated from psychosis due to neurodegenerative diseases like Alzheimer's disease and that caused by substance abuse and prescribed medications.

In contrast, the term **neurotic disorders** implies the rest of recognised psychiatric conditions in which insight is preserved and the patient's experience, although unpleasant and extreme, is within the range of normal human experience. A major **affective disorder of mind** is the syndrome of mental depression.

For the evaluation of psychotropic drugs in man, a large number of rating scales have been designed to obtain an overall assessment of the mental state and to quantify the drug-induced modification of parameters such as anxiety, depression and the adverse effects. Rating scales can be used to assess both objective and subjective features of the condition. PS 18.1

Classification of Psychoactive Drugs

I. **Antipsychotic drugs (APD),** used mainly in major psychoses like schizophrenia and MDP. These drugs are also called **neuroleptics** because they reduce the agitation and disturbed behaviour often associated with delusions and hallucinations in schizophrenia.

II. **Antianxiety drugs (anxiolytics),** mainly useful in anxiety states and neurosis, e.g. benzodiazepines and buspirone. See Chapter 14
They have a calming effect in anxiety states associated with neurotic personality, situational crisis or physical disease.

III. **Antidepressants** also called *mood elevators or psychic energisers*. For detailed classification, e.g. Tricyclic antidepressants, Selective serotonin reuptake inhibitors etc. See Chapter 14.

IV. **Mood stabilisers,** mainly useful in manic depressive psychosis. e.g. lithium carbonate. See Chapter 14

V. **Psychomotor stimulants:** See Chapter 12.

VI. **Psychotogenic drugs,** which induce behavioural abnormalities resembling psychosis. See later

PH 1.19, PS 5.5

ANTIPSYCHOTIC DRUGS

Introduction of APD revolutionised the treatment of schizophrenia, the most common of the serious mental illnesses.

Classification

I. **Conventional/typical antipsychotics (1st generation)**
- **Phenothiazines**, e.g. chlorpromazine, trifluoperazine, fluphenazine
- **Butyrophenones**, e.g. haloperidol, trifluperidol
- **Diphenylbutylpiperidines**, e.g. pimozide, penfluridol and fluspirilene
- **Thioxanthenes**, e.g. chlorprothixene, flupentixol and zuclopenthixol
- **Indolic derivatives**, e.g. molindone, oxypertine

II. **Atypical antipsychotics (2nd generation)**
- **Di-Benzodiazepine,** e.g. Clozapine
- **Thieno-Benzodiazepine,** e.g. Olanzapine
- **Di-Benzothiazipine,** e.g. Quetiapine
- **Benzixazole,** e.g. Risperidone, paliperidone
- **Benzisothiazoles,** e.g. Ziprasidone, lurasidone
- **Quinolones,** e.g. Aripiprazole, brexipiprazole
- **Benzamide,** e.g. Amisulpride
- **Miscellaneous,** e.g. Zotepine, asenapine, brexiprazole, cariprazine, iloperidone, pimavanserin

PH 1.19

Mechanism of action of APD: They produce beneficial effects probably by affecting three of the major integrating systems in the brain, i.e.

1. Mesolimbic system
2. Mesocortical system
3. The hypothalamus

The conventional APDs:

- Block mainly postsynaptic dopaminergic D_2 receptors (D_2 -antagonists) and to some extent 5-HT receptors.
- Modify the function of the mesolimbic system.
- Reduce the incoming sensory stimuli by acting on the brainstem reticular formation.

Their therapeutic efficacy is mostly related to their ability to bind and to block the dopaminergic (D_2) receptors in the mesolimbic system. Dopamine receptor subtypes (D_1-D_5) are distributed in the limbic region, the frontal cortex, the basal ganglia, the midbrain and the medulla. Although several of these subtypes need to be blocked simultaneously for the maximum benefit, **the predominant action appears to be at the D_2.** Blockade of dopamine action in the corpus striatum is responsible for the extrapyramidal reactions (EPR) often associated with these drugs.

Atypical APDs have affinities for other receptors which are comparable or even higher than those to D2 receptors. They:

- Cause D_2 **receptor blockade** but also dissociate rapidly from D_2 binding, which explains the low risk for EPR with these drugs. Amisulpiride is D_2 and D_3 antagonist and can cause higher extrapyramidal reactions and hyperprolactinaemia (Table 13.4).
- Have **potent 5-HT$_{2A}$ antagonist** action. Some atypical antipsychotics block 5-HT$_{1A}$ (e.g. aripiprazole) and 5-HT$_{1C}$ (e.g. clozapine, olanzapine, risperidone) receptors. This alters relationship between dopamine and serotonin. 5-HT$_{2A}$ antagonism increases dopaminergic neurotransmission in the nigrostriatal pathway, reducing the risk of EPR.
- Serve as **5-HT$_{1A}$ agonists**, which results in increased dopamine release in the prefrontal cortex and also reduction of glutamate release. This may be responsible for improvement in negative and cognitive symptoms of schizophrenia. 5HT$_{1A}$ agonism is exhibited by ziprasidone, quetiapine and clozapine.
- Block **alpha-2 adrenoreceptors** e.g. by risperidone, clozapine, olanzapine, paliperidone, quetiapine. This may explain their usefulness in improving negative symptoms.
- Cause **blockade of NMDA receptors**.

The action profile of conventional and atypical APDs and their adverse reactions can be explained to some extent on the basis of their affinity to multiple receptors. For example, drugs like chlorpromazine and clozapine **block muscarinic receptors** and cause less EPR. **Blocking H_1 receptors** produces sedation or sleep.

PHENOTHIAZINE COMPOUNDS

Phenothiazines have a three-ring structure, in which two benzene rings are linked by sulphur and nitrogen atoms (Fig. 13.1). According to the chemical structure, phenothiazines could be predominantly antipsychotic, anticholinergic or antihistaminic (Table 13.1).

CHLORPROMAZINE: Introduction of chlorpromazine into psychiatric practice by Delay and Deniker in 1952 marked the beginning of modern psychopharmacology. Since chlorpromazine is the most extensively studied antipsychotic phenothiazine, pharmacological actions of the group are discussed taking chlorpromazine as a prototype. Other antipsychotic phenothiazine drugs differ from chlorpromazine mainly in potency and to a certain extent in their profile of actions (Table 13.1).

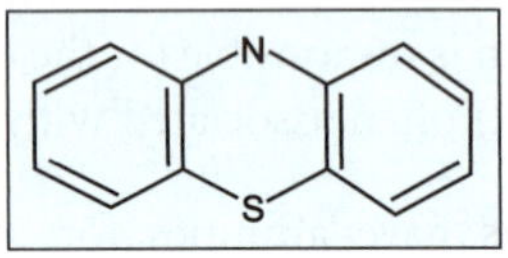

FIG. 13.1 Phenothiazine nucleus.

Pharmacological actions: It acts on multiple receptors, the predominant action being D_2 receptor blockade. It has multiple effects.

Central nervous system (CNS) actions:

Behavioural effects:

In patients with major psychosis with agitation, chlorpromazine produces psychomotor slowing, emotional quietening, **diminution of hallucinations delusions, initiative and anxiety, without affecting wakefulness** (**neurolepsis**). The patient sits in silence and shows indifference to the events around him, responding minimally to external stimuli. Although tolerance develops rapidly to its sedative action, the antipsychotic effect continues.

Other CNS effects: It causes the following:

- **Diminution of spontaneous motor activity.** It produces a state of catalepsy where the body and limbs are moulded into various postures and remain immobile for prolonged periods. **Catalepsy** resembles but is not the same as **catatonia** seen in some schizophrenics; the latter is relieved by phenothiazines.
- **Induction of sleep** with characteristic slow wave pattern on the EEG and normalisation of sleep in schizophrenics.
- **Improvement of cognitive and intellectual functions** but impairment of vigilance and motor response required in a variety of tests.
- **Antiemetic action:** Chlorpromazine depresses the chemoreceptor trigger zone (CTZ) and thus acts as a potent antiemetic. It counters the effects of apomorphine (a dopamine agonist) on the CTZ in the medulla. It, however, is not effective in vomiting due to vestibular stimulation or that caused by local GI irritation.
- **Potentiation of the action of opioid analgesic drugs.**

Table 13.1 Some Commonly Used Phenothiazine Derivatives PH 1.19

Compound and Side Chain	Pharmacological Properties	Daily Dose (mg[a])
Group I (propyldimethylamino)		
Chlorpromazine	Marked sedative and autonomic effects	100–1000
Promazine	Marked autonomic, moderate EPR and antiemetic effects	100–800
Triflupromazine	Marked EPR, high-antiemetic and low-autonomic effects	5–50
Group II (piperidine)		
Thioridazine	Moderate sedative and autonomic, less EPR but more cardiotoxic	50–300
Group III (piperazine)		
Fluphenazine	Moderate sedative, marked EPR and less autonomic effects	2.5–10
Trifluoperazine	Same as Above	5–10
Perphenazine	Less sedative, less autonomic and marked EPR effects	12–24
Prochlorperazine	Moderate sedative, marked EPR and less autonomic effects	10–30
Thiethylperazine maleate	Antiemetic	10–30
Group IV (ethyldiethylamino)		
Diethazine, ethopropazine (Profenamine)	Antiparkinsonian agents	
Promethazine	Antihistaminic (see Chapter 23)	Chapter 23

Notes: Gp I, II and III are used as APD and sometimes as antiemetics. EPR, extrapyramidal reactions.
Less potent APD such as chlorpromazine tend to cause sedation and ANS adverse effects but have a lower propensity to cause EPR whereas potent APD such as haloperidol, fluphenazine and trifluoperazine are more selective in binding to the D_2 receptors. Hence, they cause EPR more often but less sedation.
[a]In divided dose

- Phenothiazines with an aliphatic side chain (Group I, Table 13.1) **can precipitate seizures in epileptic patients.**

Autonomic nervous system: It acts as an **autonomic suppressant**. Because of its alpha adrenergic blocking action, it blocks certain actions of adrenaline and noradrenaline (NA). It also has moderate antimuscarinic and anti-5HT actions. It has a central depressant action on the hypothalamic centre controlling sympathetic activity.

Cardiovascular system: Chlorpromazine may produce orthostatic hypotension due to inhibition of centrally mediated pressor reflexes along with peripheral adrenergic blocking action. It also dilates the blood vessels directly.

It is a myocardial depressant and may cause defects in intraventricular conduction, prolongation of QT interval and blunting of T waves in the ECG.

Hypothalamic pituitary–gonadal axis: Dopamine receptor blockade in the hypothalamus and the pituitary causes

a. an **increase in serum prolactin levels**, leading to galactorrhoea,
b. inhibition of ovulation and amenorrhoea,
c. diminution of libido in men and
d. blockade of the release of growth hormone.

Miscellaneous effects: It has a potent local anaesthetic action. It prevents the shivering response to cold and thus favours the development of hypothermia.

Tolerance: In practice, patients develop tolerance to the sedative effect of phenothiazines. However, tolerance to the antipsychotic effect has not been observed.

After sudden cessation of treatment with phenothiazines, withdrawal nausea and vomiting may develop in as many as 30% of patients. Muscular discomfort, exacerbation of the psychotic state and insomnia may also occur. Although some degree of dependence on phenothiazines has thus been accepted, real drug dependence has not been demonstrated. The characteristic craving is absent and the withdrawal symptoms are essentially mild.

Absorption, fate and excretion: Phenothiazines are well absorbed orally and parenterally. After absorption, they are distributed in all the body tissues. Brain concentrations are much higher than the plasma concentrations. *An active enterohepatic circulation prolongs the biological half-life of chlorpromazine and its duration of action.* Thus, chlorpromazine or its metabolites can be detected in urine even 6–12 months after discontinuation of therapy.

Phenothiazines are metabolised in the liver by hydroxylation and subsequent glucuronide conjugation, sulphoxidation and demethylation.

Adverse reactions: The phenothiazines are divided into three major groups (Table 13.1) based on their adverse effects (Table 13.2).

Apart from **common effects** such as nasal stuffiness, dryness of mouth and palpitation, the adverse reactions include the following:

- **Intolerance:** Skin eruptions of various types, photosensitivity and contact dermatitis are common. Rarely, yellowish brown or purple discoloration of the exposed skin may develop on prolonged therapy. The colour is due to melanin or a melanin-like substance formed by the phototoxic action of sunlight acting on the phenothiazines deposited in the skin. Visual impairment due to pigmentary retinopathy is known. FM 10.1
- **Extrapyramidal reactions (EPR):** Many patients receiving phenothiazines show EP symptoms of parkinsonism, e.g. tremor, muscular rigidity, excessive salivation and akinesia. These are due to blocking of dopamine receptors in the basal ganglia *and can be countered by anticholinergic drugs such as benzhexol but not by levodopa or amantidine* (Chapter 15). Motor restlessness, akathisia (inability to sit still), acute dystonic reactions, perioral tremors (rabbit syndrome) and dyskinesias can also occur. **Tardive dyskinesia** is a late-appearing neurological syndrome in patients on long-term therapy. It is characterised by repetitive involuntary movements of lips and tongue with/without choreoathetosis (Chapter 15).
- **Behavioural reactions:** These include drowsiness, impaired psychomotor function, restlessness, excitement, psychotic reactions and toxic confused states. However, such reactions are rarely serious. *Endogenous depression may develop after the patient has been on therapy for many weeks, and the patient may commit suicide. Such depression should be watched for and should be treated.*
- **CNS:** The phenothiazines and other neuroleptics *in large doses* may occasionally produce epileptic seizures (particularly in individuals with history of seizures).
- **Autonomic nervous system:** The phenothiazines, by virtue of their:
  1. *Antimuscarinic activity* may produce dryness of mouth blurring of vision, tachycardia, constipation, difficulty in micturition and sometimes inhibition of ejaculation.
  2. *Adrenergic system blockade* can cause postural hypotension and prolongation of QT_c interval. *Chlorpromazine should not be given intravenously, as fatalities due to a sudden fall in BP have been reported.*
- **Haemopoietic system and the liver:** These drugs may rarely produce agranulocytosis, thrombocytopenia and aplastic anaemia.
  Reversible intrahepatic obstructive (cholestatic) jaundice occurs in about 0.5%–2% of the patients receiving chlorpromazine. It is probably allergic in origin.

Table 13.2 Phenothiazines Grouped According to Adverse Effects

Sedation	Antimuscarinic	Extrapyramidal
Group I[a]	+++	++
Group II[a]	++	+++
Group III[a]	+	+

[a]Refer Table 13.1.

Administration of phenothiazines during pregnancy has been associated with increased incidence of neonatal jaundice.

- **Endocrine and metabolic disturbances:** Long-term therapy may occasionally produce gynaecomastia and impotence, galactorrhea and menstrual irregularities. Aggravation of diabetes mellitus and weight gain as a result of increased food intake has been reported with most classical APD. FM 10.1
- **Neuroleptic malignant syndrome:** This is a rare but potentially fatal reaction to the neuroleptic drugs. The manifestations include hyperthermia, fluctuating level of consciousness, muscular rigidity and autonomic dysfunction with tachycardia, sweating, urinary incontinence and labile BP. The offending drug should be discontinued immediately as there is no proven effective treatment.

Preparations and dosage (Table 13.1):

i. Chlorpromazine hydrochloride tablets 10, 25, 50, 100 and 200 mg; syrup 20 or 25 mg/(for adults) and 5 mg/mL (paediatric) and suppositories. Dose 25–100 mg 3 times a day; maximum dose 1g when administered orally while the rectal dose is 100 mg every 6–8 hours.
ii. Chlorpromazine injection 25 mg/mL. It is usually administered intramuscularly in the dose of 25–50 mg. The patient should be confined to bed for 30 min following IM injection in order to avoid postural hypotension.
iii. **Depot phenothiazines:** Esters (such as decanoate, enanthate and palmitate) of fluphenazine, perphenazine, flupentixol and oxyprothepine, given intramuscularly or subcutaneously, release the active drug slowly. Satisfactory therapeutic response in schizophrenia can be obtained by injecting **fluphenazine decanoate** (available as 25 and 100 mg/ml) in the dose of 12.5–100 mg every 2–4 weeks.

Drug interactions: See Box 13.1.

APD from other chemical groups tend to resemble Group III phenothiazines. They include the butyrophenones (droperidol, haloperidol and trifluperidol); diphenylbutylpiperidines (fluspirilene and pimozide); thioxanthenes (flupentixol), oxypertine; and loxapine.

Box 13.1 Interactions of Phenothiazines with Other Drugs

- Prolongation and intensification of the CNS depressant effect of barbiturates, morphine, pethidine and alcohol
- Precipitation of bizarre and dangerous reactions if used simultaneously with MAO inhibitors
- Precipitation of serious hypotension if used together with such drugs as reserpine, methyldopa and phentolamine
- Neutralisation of the hypotensive action of guanethidine and clonidine

HALOPERIDOL: This butyrophenone is a very potent APD. It is more effective in highly agitated or manic patients and has less prominent sedative and autonomic effects.

It is given orally in the dose of 1.5–7.5 mg b.i.d. It can also be given intramuscularly in the dose of 2–10 mg, repeated every hour up to a total of 30 mg, in highly agitated and violent patients. Depot injectable preparations of haloperidol are also available.

Its ADR are similar to chlorpromazine. However, the incidence of EPR with haloperidol is high. Apart from use in psychosis, it is a preferred drug for Huntington disease. The other drugs of this series are **trifluperidol** (Triperidol) and **droperidol** which are used in combination with fentanyl for neuroleptanalgesia (Chapter 7).

DIPHENYL BUTYL PIPERIDINES: Pimozide 2–10 mg once daily may have the advantage in that the prescribed dosage can be administered under supervision. **Penfluridol,** structurally related to haloperidol, has a long duration of action. It is given orally in the dose of 20–100 mg once a week. Such oral preparations are useful in practice to ensure patient compliance.

Other APD such as chlorprothixene, clopenthixol, centbutandol, molindone and prothipendyl mainly differ from the phenothiazines in their pharmacokinetic properties and in their sedative, autonomic and extrapyramidal effects.

Table 13.3 Actions of Typical and Atypical Antipsychotic Drugs on Various Receptors

Drug	Receptors Blocked				
	D_2	5-HT_{2A}	α_1	H_1	M_1
Chlorpromazine	+++	+	+++	++	++
Haloperidol	+++	+	0	+	0
Clozapine	+	++	+++	+++	+++
Olanzapine	+	+++	+	+++	+++
Quetiapine	++	+	++	+++	++
Risperidone	+++	+++	+++	++	+
Ziprasidone	++	+++	++	+	+
Sertindole	++	+++	+++	+	+
Aripiprazole	partial agonist	+++	+	0/+	+
Asenapine	++	+++	+++	++	–
Brexpiprazole[a]	Partial agonist	+++	+	+	–
Cariprazine	Partial agonist	+++	+	+	–
Iloperidone	++	++	+	–	–
Lurasidone	++	++	[illegible]	[illegible]	[illegible]
Paliperidone	+++	+++	++	+	–
Lumateperone	++	+++	++	–	–
Amisulpride	++	–	–	–	–
Pimavanserin	–	Inverse agonist	–	–	–

a, also blocks α_2 receptors. 0, absent; 0/-, minimal; number of + indicate degree of blockade
Note: D, dopamine; 5-HT, 5-hydroxytryptamine; H, histamine; M, muscarinic

ATYPICAL ANTIPSYCHOTICS (SECOND GENERATION)

The classical APD described above can cause EPR even in therapeutic doses. Further, they are less effective against negative symptoms. 'Atypical' APD in general:

- **Have greater affinity for other neuroreceptors** such as 5-HT_2, α adrenergic, histaminergic and muscarinic, than the classical APD (Table 13.3)
- **Help to improve negative symptoms**
- **Have lower propensity to cause EPR and tardive dyskinesia** than phenothiazines and haloperidol; however, all of them can cause akathasia
- **Are less likely (except risperidone) to cause hyperprolactinemia**
- **Cause dose-dependent ADR** which include sedation (more with clozapine, olanzapine), anticholinergic effects and postural hypotension
- **Cause metabolic syndrome** *including weight gain, hyperglycemia and hyperlipidemia*
- *Have been found useful* **as an adjunctive in the treatment of major depressive disorders** *(MDD)*

CLOZAPINE: This APD was found to cause agranulocytosis and hence its use was abandoned. It has now staged a comeback for a specific indication, i.e. in the treatment of schizophrenia resistant to classical APD. It has selective effects in the limbic, dopaminergic systems wherein it blocks dopamine receptors. However, it has more potent action in blocking the $5HT_2$ receptors than D_2 receptors. Its other actions include antiadrenergic and anticholinergic actions. *It differs from phenothiazines in that it causes fewer EPRs and does not cause hyperprolactinemia.*

Given orally, it produces antipsychotic effects similar to those of haloperidol. Its major advantage is that the drug improves not only the positive symptoms but also the negative symptoms such as emotional withdrawal, blunted affect, retardation and social withdrawal. It is started in the dose of 12.5 mg once daily and gradually increased to 200–450 mg/day in divided doses.

Adverse reactions: These include nausea, vomiting, sedation, postural hypotension, marked tachycardia, paralytic ileus, sialorrhoea, confusion and delirium. It may cause hypomotility of GIT resulting in toxic megacolon. Therefore, prophylactic laxatives are advocated with clozapine. Its main drawback is the relatively high incidence of grand mal seizures, myocarditis and agranulocytosis. *Because of its toxicity, the drug should be used only in patients resistant to standard therapy (see above) and that too under supervision* with regular monitoring of blood counts.

OLANZAPINE: This drug causes less EPR and cardiovascular toxicity. Orally, it is absorbed well but about 40% is metabolised during first pass through the intestinal wall. In dose of 5–25 mg, once daily, the drug is as effective as haloperidol in reducing psychotic symptoms and also acts against negative symptoms. The incidence of hyperprolactinemia and sexual dysfunction is also lower than with risperidone. The drug may also be useful in children with developmental CNS disorders and in patients with Tourette syndrome.

Adverse reactions: These include dry mouth, sedation, nausea, postural hypotension and constipation. Among atypical APD, olanzapine has the highest propensity to cause metabolic syndrome. Hence recently a fixed dose combination of olanzapine and **samidorphan**, a new opioid antagonist, has been approved as samidorphan is intended to mitigate the weight gain that occurs with olanzapine.

It should be avoided in elderly patients, especially hypertensives, because of increased risk of cerebrovascular accidents.

QUETIAPINE: It has effects similar to those of olanzapine; but it is less likely to cause weight gain. It has a short t½ and is administered b.i.d.

RISPERIDONE: This atypical APD though less effective has a profile similar to that of clozapine in respect of negative symptoms. It has action on D_2, 5-HT, alpha adrenergic and histaminergic receptors. It is as effective as haloperidol. However, it causes dyskinesias such as akathisia and hyperprolactinemia. Other adverse reactions include postural hypotension, dizziness, insomnia and constipation. It does not cause blood dyscrasias. The starting dose is 2 mg/day in divided doses increased gradually to 4–6 mg/day. A depot preparation is also available.

The drug also appears to be effective and well tolerated for the treatment of tantrums, aggression and self-injurious behaviour of children with autistic disorders.

Paliperidone is the primary active metabolite of risperidone.

LUMATEPERONE: This recently approved atypical antipsychotic has a unique receptor binding profile. It modulates all the 3 NTs *viz.* serotonin, dopamine and glutamate. It is a:

- Potent 5-HT_{2A} receptor antagonist and also a serotonin reuptake inhibitor (SERT inhibitor).
- Partial agonist at presynaptic D_2 and antagonist at postsynaptic D_2 receptors. It reduces dopamine signalling.
- Agonist at D_1 receptors, which modulates NMDA mediated glutamate signalling.

It shows a moderate binding affinity for dopamine D_4, and α_{1A} and α_{1B} adrenergic receptors but has low affinity for muscarinic and histaminergic receptors.

It can alleviate both positive and negative symptoms of schizophrenia and is claimed to have better tolerability. ADR are mild and include headache, somnolence, dizziness, sedation, fatigue, and constipation. It carries a low risk of EPR and cardiometabolic side effects. No prolactin increase is observed during short-term treatment.

Lumateperone on oral administration gets absorbed from small intestine, has wide distribution throughout the body, undergoes liver metabolism by CYP family and conjugated metabolites are excreted in urine. Some amount is excreted in feces. Its t½ is 13–18 hours.

It can be used for patients with treatment-resistant schizophrenia and for patients with schizophrenia who are vulnerable to developing metabolic dysfunction

Table 13.4 Relative Efficacy and Toxicity of Second Generation Antipsychotics PH 1.19

Drug	Efficacy	Postural Hypotension	EPR	Hyperpro-lactinaemia	QTc prolong-ation	Blood glucose increase	Weight gain
Clozapine[a]	++++	+++	+/–	+/–	+	++++	++++
Olanzapine	+++	+	+	+	+	++++	++++
Quetiapine	++	+++	+/–	+/–	+	++	+++
Risperidone	+++	+++	+++	+++	+	++	+++
Sertindole	+++	+++	++	+	+++	+	++
Ziprasidone	++	+	+/–	+	++	+/–	+/–
Aripiprazole	++	+	++	–	+/–	+/–	+
Amisulpride	+	+	+++	+++	+	++	++
Zotepine	++	+	+	+	++	++	++
Asenapine	+++	++	++	++	+/–	+	++
Brexpiprazole	+++	++	+	+/–	–	+	++
Cariprazine	++	+	+++	–	–	+/–	+
Iloperidone	++	++	+/–	+/–	++	++	++
Lurasidone	++	–	++	+/–	+/–	+/–	+/–
Paliperidone	++	+++	+++	+++	+	++	+++
Lumateperone	++	+	+/–	–	–	+/–	+/–

[a]Can cause agranulocytosis, myonecrosis.
–, absent; +/–, minimal; +, mild; 2+, moderate; 3+, moderately severe; 4+, severe.

and movement disorders. The dose is 42mg once a day administered orally with food. However it is expensive and needs further evaluation.

Pimavanserin is a potent $5HT_{2A}$ inverse agonist but shows no binding to D_2 receptors. It is indicated for psychosis associated with Parkinson's disease (Chapter 15) and is used as a single daily dose. The effects are seen after 2–6 weeks of therapy.

For other second-generation APD, see Table 13.4.

Carbamazepine, an antiepileptic, is useful as an adjunct in the treatment of schizophrenic patients with aggressive or violent behaviour or agitation, who show resistance to the usual APD (Chapter 9).

RESERPINE: It is obtained from the plant *Rauwolfia serpentina* (Benth), so called because of the resemblance of its root to a snake.

Mechanism of actions: It depletes endogenous catecholamines and 5-HT from the brain and peripheral sites by interfering with amine storage. Such depletion can last for days or weeks. The depletion of cerebral monoamines is responsible for its calming effects.

Reserpine has antipsychotic action resembling that of chlorpromazine; however, it has no antihistaminic, anticholinergic or direct antiadrenergic action. It is less effective than chlorpromazine in the treatment of schizophrenia. It can also cause mental depression precipitating suicidal tendencies; hence, it is not used as an APD. Reserpine lowers BP and was in use as an antihypertensive drug (Chapter 30).

Indications for antipsychotics:

- **Schizophrenia:** This is discussed in the section on management of schizophrenia.
- **Manic depressive psychosis (MDP): Chlorpromazine** and **haloperidol** are both effective in the treatment of mania (see section, manic depressive psychosis-management).
- **Other psychotic disorders:** Apart from classical schizophrenia, APD are also used to treat other psychotic disorders characterized by delusions, hallucinations, disorganised thinking and abnor-

mal psychomotor behaviour e.g. schizoaffective disorders, senile psychosis, postpartum psychosis and for psychotic symptoms associated with neurodegenerative disorders.

- **Drug dependence:** They are used in the management of psychosis associated with chronic alcoholism but may not be always effective. They are *contraindicated* in acute withdrawal syndromes (alcohol, opiates and other sedatives) for fear of precipitating seizures.
- **Behavioural disorders in children:** Phenothiazines are sometimes used to control the excessively aggressive and destructive behaviour in children and exert a quietening effect. *In such cases, other causes of aggressiveness such as temporal lobe epilepsy, schizophrenia, hypoglycaemia and drug (amphetamine) abuse should be ruled out.*
- **Antiemetic and antihiccup: Chlorpromazine** in small, nonsedating doses, is useful to control vomiting due to uraemia, radiation sickness and certain drugs. It can also be employed to treat nausea and vomiting of pregnancy; but the **other phenothiazines (e.g. prochlorperazine)** are preferred. *It is not effective in motion sickness.* Chlorpromazine is sometimes effective in the treatment of intractable hiccups.
- **Miscellaneous:** Some phenothiazines are used as preanaesthetic medication (Chapter 7). PS 5.3

MANAGEMENT OF SCHIZOPHRENIA

Schizophrenia (idiopathic psychosis) is a serious mental disorder characterised by persistent disturbance in the perception and evaluation of reality, leading to characteristic changes in the perception, thinking, affective responses and behaviour **(cognitive abilities)**.

The disease is mainly genetic but can be sporadic. It is dominated by one set of ideas or a complex to the exclusion of others. Thus, the harmonious working of the mind is split. The schizophrenic patient, therefore, lives in his own world, dissociated from reality (**psychosis**). He is a victim of **illusions** (perception falsified, e.g. mistaking a rope for a snake), **hallucinations** (perception without a stimulus or false perceptions, e.g. hearing God talking) and **delusions** (false beliefs, not based on cultural mores, that cannot be corrected by logic and reasoning) and believes that only his behaviour and actions are rational, without realising that he is ill (**lack of insight**). The motor behaviour and speech are disorganised and the patient has **flattened affect** (restricted range ofemotions). The mental functioning is sufficiently impaired (**cognitive deficits**) to interfere grossly with his capacity to meet the ordinary demands of life. It may exist in several varieties, and the paranoid form (delusional disorder), in which the individual becomes suspicious of and belligerent towards the entire society, is perhaps the most dangerous. *The disease is neither preventable nor curable and has a high recurrence rate.* The aetiology of schizophrenia is complex and still unknown. It is believed to be due to disturbances in hippocampus, midbrain, corticostriatal-thalamic-prefrontal circuit. Many studies indicate that excess synaptic levels of dopamine and glutamate cause increased postsynaptic stimulation, responsible for psychotic symptoms. Other brain neurotransmitters such as 5HT, ACh, and GABA are likely to be involved in its pathogenesis.

The symptoms of schizophrenia can be both positive and negative. The **positive symptoms** include hallucinations, delusions, agitation, repetitive behaviour and thought disorder. The **negative symptoms** include psychomotor slowing, marked social withdrawal, anhedonia (inability to experience pleasure), paucity of speech, apathy, as well as lack of energy and motivation.

PH 1.1

Several randomised controlled studies have reported no significant differences in overall effects between typical and atypical APD. All APD are effective in controlling the core symptoms of schizophrenia and schizophrenia like illness. The possible advantage of an atypical APD is that they may cause fewer EPR and may show more activity against negative symptoms. However, they may cause:

a. weight gain, hyperglycaemia, hyper-prolactinaemia and disturbed lipid metabolism.
b. Some of them are associated with increased cardiovascular risk (prolongation of QTc).
c. As a group atypical APD are not more efficacious, have no clearly different ADR profile as compared to typical APD and
d. are much more expensive.

Box 13.2 Factors Determining Selection of APD

- Symptom profile of the patient
- Past responses to treatment if any
- ADR profile of APD
- Concomitant diseases
- Potential drug-drug interactions
- Patient preferences
- Treatment compliance

Their use should be reserved for some selected patients.

Thus an evidence-based algorithmic approach to antipsychotic selection is not possible and several factors play a role in the initial selection of the APD (Box 13.2). potential drug.

Selected APD is started in the **smallest possible dose and increased gradually as needed.** Full remission requires 6-8 weeks.

Risperidone, haloperidol, trifluoperazine (high potency) or **chlorpromazine** (medium potency) may be preferred. Risperidone is started at the dose of 2 mg /day then gradually increased at weekly intervals to a maximum of 8 mg/day based on patient symptom profile and tolerability. **Haloperidol** is administered orally in the dose of 2.5–7.5 mg/day and increased gradually up to 20 mg/day whereas trifluoperazine is started with 5 mg tablet b.i.d with gradual increase to 50 mg/day. The oral dose of chlorpromazine varies widely from 100 to 1000 mg per day. The initial dose usually is 25 mg three times a day in adults, increased gradually to 300 mg a day. In these doses more than 80% D_2 receptors are blocked and no additional benefits are achieved with higher doses. If patient presents with negative symptoms or cognitive impairment, risperidone or other atypical APD is the initial APD.

Clozapine is considered the most effective atypical APD but because of its toxicity it is reserved for refractory disease and patients at increased risk for suicide attempts or suicide remains substantial despite other treatments. Prior to initiating clozapine treatment a baseline CBC is warranted and CBC should be repeated even during the treatment. The treatment is initiated with 12.5 mg o.d/b.i.d, increase in 25-50 mg/day increments for 2 weeks, then further increments not exceeding 100 mg up to twice weekly. The typical daily dose of clozapine is 300-450 mg to a maximum of 900 mg /day.

In elderly care should be taken to use small doses as they can cause postural hypotension and falls. In addition, an increased risk of stroke and transient ischaemic attacks has been reported in elderly patients with dementia receiving atypical APD for the treatment of behavioural disorders.

Schizophrenia is a relapsing disease; hence, after the therapeutic response is obtained, the drug should be continued in smaller maintenance doses for a long time (sometimes lifelong) even after the first episode of illness. **Although relapse rates may be lower in patients maintained on what are regarded as standard doses, those maintained on lower doses may have the advantage of improved social and vocational functioning.** Chlorpromazine may cause more drowsiness and depression. Daytime drowsiness may interfere with the patient's ability to work, but this could be reduced if he takes most of his daily dose at night. Haloperidol may cause more EPR. Some authorities routinely combine phenothiazines with benzhexol for preventing EPR. However, combinations of antipsychotic drugs do not increase the efficacy.

A longer maintenance period is recommended, particularly in patients with a history of relapse. The withdrawal should be slow (6–12 months) as reappearance of symptoms following withdrawal is not uncommon. Patients having a history of relapse or a frequent hospitalizations due to poor adherence to oral maintenance therapy can be treated with either weekly, biweekly, monthly or yearly injectable extended release formulations of atypical antipsychotics (depot antipsychotics). e.g. risperidone IM once in 2 weeks or SC once a month, aripiprazole / olanzapine IM once in a month, paliperidone IM once every month/ once in 3 months/ once in 6 months.

Table 13.5 Equipotent Oral Doses of Classical and Atypical Antipsychotics PH 1.19

Drug	Oral Dose (mg)
Classical APD	
Chlorpromazine	100
Chlorproxithene	100
Trifluoperazine	2-5
Haloperidol	2
Fluphenazine	5-10 mg weekly dose
Atypical APD	
Sertindole	16
Clozapine	50-100
Olanzapine	4-5
Risperidone	1-2
Quetiapine	75-100
Ziprasidone	40-60
Aripiprazole	6-8
Amisulpride	100
Asenapine	4-5
Iloperidone	3-6
Lurasidone	16-20
Paliperidone	1.5-2
Zotepine	60

Table 13.5 gives the equipotent oral doses of various classical and atypical APD.

Highly agitated, rowdy and violent patients need larger doses of APD, sometimes given parenterally. Short-acting parenteral APD are used intramuscularly for acute treatment of agitation associated with schizophrenia and bipolar mania. *High doses of APD offer little advantage over smaller doses, at least in the majority of acute psychotic episodes.* **Acute schizophrenic reaction** needs initiation of treatment with Haloperidol 2-5 mg IM every 4 to 8 h, or olanzapine in the dose of 2.5-10 mg IM, with maximum dose of 30 mg/day; or ziprasidone 20 mg IM. These doses are equivalent of 400 mg of chlorpromazine per day given in four divided doses. On subsequent days, the daily dose is increased by the equivalent of 200 mg of chlorpromazine till the acute reaction is controlled. The maintenance dose for preventing recurrence in chronic cases is the equivalent of 50–200 mg of chlorpromazine per day.

Box 13.3 Causes of Nonresponse to Neuroleptic Therapy

- Inadequate doses
- Poor patient compliance
- Pharmacokinetic factors
- Persistent and severe psychosocial stress
- Poor family support
- Substance abuse

Causes of nonresponse to treatment: They are listed in Box 13.3. Irrespective of the drug used, many chronic schizophrenics discontinue the medication probably because of lack of efficacy, adverse reactions or lack of supervision; and hence, cooperation of patient's relatives is vital.

The APD that stimulate the secretion of prolactin are better avoided in patients with established breast cancer. Both typical and atypical APD may provoke seizures in susceptible subjects, e.g. epileptic patients. *Most APD, if consumed in very high doses, do not cause life-threatening coma, and the lethal dose is very high.* D_2 receptor antagonists are not consistently useful for psychotic symptoms caused by other medical conditions or drug abuse/toxicity.

PSYCHOTOGENIC DRUGS

These drugs, when consumed, produce psychosis – 'a state characterised by maladaptive behaviour in which an individual reacts inappropriately to his environment'. They produce depersonalisation, changes in mood and a variety of effects on memory and learned behaviour. As some of these effects resemble those observed in psychosis such as schizophrenia, these drugs are also called **psychotomimetic**, and because of their ability to produce hallucinations, they are sometimes designated as **hallucinogens/psychodysleptics.** PH 1.22

Classification of Psychotogenic Drugs

- **Indolic** such as lysergic acid diethylamide (LSD) and psilocybine
- **Nonindolic** such as mescaline, phencyclidine, tenamphetamine and cannabis

LYSERGIC ACID DIETHYLAMIDE: LSD is an amine alkaloid, synthesised from ergot by Stoll and

Hoffmann in 1938. It has some resemblance to ergometrine and possesses oxytocic action.

Mechanism of action: The exact mechanism of the central action is not known. But, **LSD is a potent agonist at central DA receptors, central presynaptic 5-HT$_{1A}$ autoreceptors and 5-HT$_{2C}$ receptors;** its hallucinogenic action is probably related to its 5-HT$_2$ receptor action. The drug also blocks peripheral 5-HT$_2$ receptors.

Pharmacological actions: The drug is rapidly absorbed on oral administration and produces its actions in doses as low as 20–25 mcg.

(a) Behavioural actions: Generally, LSD has a disintegrating effect on both inborn and learned behaviour patterns. Individuals under LSD effect exhibit marked changes in mood with emotional outbursts; they may laugh or cry on slightest provocation. Motivation is impaired. The person experiences visual hallucinations, accompanied by a kaleidoscopic-like play of colours. There is a cognitive distortion of time and space. If the dose is not large, the consciousness and memory are retained. Many subjects experience a fear of disintegration of the self. The syndrome clears up after about 12 h.

(b) Sympathomimetic actions: These include such as dilatation of pupil, tachycardia, tremor, piloerection and hyperglycemia. It may cause nausea and frequency of micturition.

Tachyphylaxis to behavioural effects of LSD is known, and a cross-tolerance exists between LSD, mescaline and psilocybine. The drug causes psychic but not physical dependence.

Adverse reactions: The margin of safety between effective dose and lethal dose appears to be wide. Sometimes, it produces suicidal tendencies. Although the psychotic changes are generally reversible, the drug can cause permanent psychosis and personality changes. LSD may produce 'flashback' reactions in which events associated with drug use are suddenly thrust into consciousness in the non-drugged state and can occur many months after the last use.

Phenothiazines such as chlorpromazine, a D$_2$ blocker, can antagonise many acute effects of LSD.

Other agents chemically related to LSD such as **psilocybine, 5-hydroxy-dimethyl tryptamine** (bufotenine) and **harmine** produce similar psychotogenic actions.

MESCALINE: The cactus *Lophophora williamsii* was used to produce ecstatic states by the Red Indian tribes in Mexico and in North America on special religious occasions. This cactus contains an alkaloid mescaline. Effects of mescaline are similar to LSD. The effects of a single dose persist for about 12 h.

Uses: Both LSD and mescaline have been employed as an experimental tool to produce a model of psychosis.

Tenamphetamine: It is related to mescaline and amphetamine. It acts as central and peripheral adrenoreceptor stimulant. *It is often misused as 'dance' drug at rave parties.*

CANNABIS (MARIJUANA): Cannabis is one of the oldest herbal remedies, known since 4000 BC for its therapeutic and recreational properties. It is obtained from the hemp plants, *Cannabis sativa* and *Cannabis indica.* The active ingredients are present in the resinous exudate of the tops of the female plant. The resin is known as *Hashish* or *Charas. Bhang* is prepared from the dried leaves and the flowering shoots, while *ganja* is the resinous mass obtained from the small leaves and brackets of inflorescence. The term *Marijuana* is used to describe any plant part or extract containing the active principle.

The psychoactive principle of Cannabis is known as **Δ-9-tetrahydrocannabinol (THC)**. Its synthetic analogous are also available. Cannabidiol (CBD) and cannabidivarin are the two other cannabinoids. Unlike THC, they do not cause intoxication or euphoria.

Mechanism of action: Two cannabinoid G- protein coupled receptors, CB$_1$ and CB$_2$, have been identified. CB$_1$ receptors are widely distributed, with the highest concentration found in the brain neurons, particularly in hypothalamus, the limbic system, cerebellum and the basal ganglia.They are also located in the GI tract and adipocytes. CB_1 receptors present on the on excitatory glutamatergic and inhibitory γ-aminobutyric acid (GABA)-ergic interneurons and glial cells inhibit the release of both NTs and are responsible for euphoria. CB_2 receptors are present in the cells of the immune system.

CB_1 and CB_2 receptors are effectors of the endogenous system *viz.* endocannabinoid system, which has two physiological ligands, 2-arachidonoylglycerol (2-AG) and anandamide. THC is a partial agonist at both the receptors.

Pharmacological actions:

Acute effects: When smoked, THC is rapidly absorbed and effects appear within minutes and last for about 2–3 h. Taken orally, the onset of action is delayed up to 30 min–2 h. The pulse rate increases, conjunctiva becomes red and BP may fall slightly; at higher doses, orthostatic hypotension occurs. Muscle strength is decreased; appetite may increase, leading to increase in food intake.

CNS and behavioural effects vary according to the dose, the route of administration and the individual personality. There is initial euphoria or 'high', which is followed by drowsiness. It produces a dreamy state, feeling of well-being, excitement and joyousness. An individual under its influence may become garrulous and hilarious, exhibiting uncontrollable laughter even with minimal stimuli. Violent or aggressive behaviour, however, is rare. Time sense is altered and hearing becomes less discriminating. Vision becomes apparently sharper with many visual distortions. The drug causes difficulty in concentrating and thinking. Motor coordination, memory and judgement may be impaired. It often causes nausea, vomiting, increased urinary frequency and dryness of mouth.

Chronic effects: The effects of chronic use are less certain. These are more marked in adolescents. Some degree of **tolerance** is known to develop rapidly and **psychic dependence** can occur in daily users. *The withdrawal syndrome includes dysphoria, irritability, insomnia and anxiety. However, physical dependence is rare.*

Heavy chronic cannabis users can develop an *amotivated syndrome*, with apathy and loss of academic performance in students. Such an effect is expected since cannabis is concentrated in the limbic system, the motivational centre of the brain, and also interferes with memory, cognition and psychomotor performance.

Those who smoke regularly in adolescence may have impaired neuronal connectivity in hippocampus and prefrontal region (regions important for learning and memory).

Even social doses can impair car driving ability because of distortions of time and space estimations, reduced vigilance and coordination. Effects persist for many hours because the drug is eliminated slowly.

Absorption, fate and excretion: The crude oily resinous extracts contain many ingredients, the THC being most active. Its content in various preparations varies widely depending upon the source. It is well absorbed following inhalation or ingestion. Cannabinoids are extensively metabolised to various active metabolites. They are highly lipid soluble and are stored in body fat. Their slow release prolongs their action. Acute administration of THC inhibits hepatic metabolising enzymes and chronic intake may induce them.

Adverse reactions: Large doses of cannabis may cause an acute panic reaction, a toxic delirium, an acute paranoid state or acute mania. Cannabis can unmask latent psychiatric disorders and can aggravate schizophrenia.

Unlike LSD, the flashback reaction is mild with cannabis.

Chronic cannabis users may have decreased sperm production. Women may have anovulatory menstrual cycles associated with decreased LH. The drug may cause aggravation of diabetes mellitus. 'T'cell function may be inhibited.

Chronic cannabis smokers, like tobacco smokers, often develop significant airway obstruction, bronchitis, cough and precancerous mucosal changes. Cross-tolerance with alcohol is known.

Cannabinoids might increase the incidence of low birth weight, preterm birth, and stillbirth but teratogenic effects are not conclusively reported. However, it is better to avoid cannabis use in pregnancy. There are reports of impaired neurocognitive development of the fetus if exposed to it *in utero*. This may result in attention deficits, increased hyperactivity and impulsivity as well as increased incidence of tremors, exaggerated startles and diminished crying in the neonates.

Indications: Although cannabis possesses antiemetic, mild analgesic, muscle relaxant, anticonvulsant and sedative-hypnotic actions, it cannot be recommended for these purposes because of its adverse effects. The uses are:

- **Small doses** of oral THC can stimulate appetite without causing serious psychotropic effects and have been used to treat chronic wasting in AIDS.
- Synthetic cannabinoids, **nabilone** and **dronabinol** are useful as **antiemetics** in patients receiving cancer chemotherapy (Chapter 39). They have been used to relieve pain.
- **Nabiximol,** an oromucosal spray, has shown some beneficial effects in the treatment of neuropathic pain and against spasticity of multiple sclerosis.
- **Cannabidiol** oral solution has been approved as an antiepileptic drug to treat seizures associated with Lennox-Gastaut syndrome or Dravet syndrome.

DRUG-INDUCED PSYCHIATRIC SYNDROMES

Psychiatric disturbances are often attributed to concomitantly administered drugs; yet, it is generally difficult to establish the causal relationship between the two. Such a drug-induced reaction should, however, be suspected whenever an unexpected psychiatric disturbance arises suddenly in a person of good previous personality, after a new drug has been consumed. The psychiatric reactions to drugs can be broadly categorised into the following:

1. **Delirium** (acute brain syndrome, toxic confusional state): This is characterised by a fluctuating clouding of consciousness, restlessness, emotional changes usually fear and perplexity and, in severe cases, paranoid delusions or visual hallucinations. The elderly are particularly susceptible. They may follow overdose or drug withdrawal, or may be due to intolerance to a normal therapeutic dose. Although many drugs can cause such states, CNS depressants, anticholinergics and cimetidine are the ones implicated most frequently.
2. **Psychotic states:** Hallucinogens such as LSD can induce a psychotic state with clear consciousness, paranoid delusions and visual hallucinations. States closely resembling schizophrenia with auditory hallucinations, thought disorder, aggressive behaviour and occasionally violence and suicide are seen with the CNS stimulants (cocaine and amphetamine), sympathomimetic nasal sprays, anorexiants and beta adrenergic agonists. Other drugs which can cause psychotic states are beta-adrenergic blockers, anticholinergics, opioids, dopamine agonists, glucocorticoids and rarely NSAID.
3. **Manic states** are sometimes observed with antidepressants, anticholinergics, high doses of corticosteroids, isoniazid, levodopa, dexamphetamine and clonidine.
4. **Depression** can occur with antihypertensive drugs (reserpine, methyldopa, clonidine and propranolol), levodopa, chloroquine, anticonvulsants and OC pills.
5. **Behavioural disorders** reported are withdrawal syndrome after cessation of BZD and akathisia during treatment with APD. **Pathological gambling and other compulsive behaviours** such as compulsive eating and drinking have been reported in patients on nonergoline dopamine agonists, particularly **pramipexole** (Chapter 15).

PSYCHOACTIVE DRUGS

Antipsychotic drugs (APD)
- Conventional antipsychotics (Neuroleptics)
- Atypical antipsychotics

Antianxiety drugs (anxiolytics)
- Benzodiazepines
- Buspirone

Antidepressants
- TCA
- SSRI
- Newer antidepressants

Mood stabilisers
- Lithium carbonate

Psychomotor stimulants
- Methylphenidate
- Dextroamphetamine
- Pemoline

Psychotogenic drugs
- LSD
- Cannabis
- Hallucinogens

ANTIPSYCHOTIC DRUGS

Conventional / typical antipsychotics (1st generation)

Phenothiazines
- Chlorpromazine
- Trifluoperazine
- Fluphenazine

Butyrophenones
- Haloperidol
- Trifluperidol

Diphenylbutylpiperidines
- Pimozide
- Penfluridol
- Fluspirilene

Thioxanthenes
- Chlorprothixene
- Flupentixol
- Zuclopenthixol

Indolic derivatives
- Molindone
- Oxypertine

Atypical antipsychotics (2nd generation)

Di-Benzodiazepine
- Clozapine

Thieno-Benzodiazepine
- Olanzapine

Di-Benzothiazipine
- Quetiapine

Benzixazole
- Risperidone
- Paliperidone

Benzisothiazoles
- Ziprasidone
- Lurasidone

Quinolones
- Aripiprazole
- Brexipiprazole

Benzamide
- Amisulpride

Miscellaneous
- Zotepine
- Asenapine
- Brexiprazole
- Cariprazine
- Iloperidone
- Pimavanserin

PSYCHOTOGENIC DRUGS

Indolic

- Lysergic acid diethylamide (LSD)
- Psilocybine

Nonindolic

- Mescaline
- Phencyclidine
- Tenamphetamine
- Cannabis

CHAPTER 14

Psychopharmacology – 2: Anxiolytics, Antidepressants and Pharmacotherapy of Depression and Manic-Depressive Psychosis

Learning Objectives

This chapter will enable the reader:

1. To classify antianxiety drugs.
2. To compare mechanism of action, adverse effects, drug interactions, advantages of various antianxiety drugs.
3. To describe nonpharmacological and pharmacological modalities for (a) panic disorders, (b) phobic anxiety and (c) general anxiety disorder giving rationale for use of selected drugs.
4. To be aware of neurochemical changes in depression.
5. To classify antidepressants giving examples of drugs.
6. To describe mechanism of action, pharmacological effects, ADR, drug interactions and indications of MAO inhibitors, tricyclic antidepressants and selective serotonin reuptake inhibitors.
7. To compare and contrast atypical antidepressants with above-mentioned antidepressants.
8. To outline management of depression emphasising pharmacotherapeutic principles.
9. To describe mechanism of action, pharmacological effects, ADR, drug interactions and indications for lithium.
10. To state the drug(s) of choice and alternatives to be used in various phases of MDP, i.e. acute mania, depressive phase, depression with psychosis and long-term prophylaxis giving rationale for their selection.
11. To recognise advantages and problems associated with psychotropic drug combinations.

KEY TERMS

anxiolytics, p. 213
benzodiazepines, p. 213
selective serotonin reuptake inhibitors, p. 214
monoamine oxidase inhibitors, p. 218
hypertensive crisis, p. 219
Serotonin syndrome, p. 223
lithium carbonate, p. 231
manic depressive psychosis, treatment, p. 231
psychotropic drug combinations, p. 232

Anxiety disorders are perhaps the most common psychiatric illness encountered in general practice. **Anxiolytics** are the drugs used for the treatment of anxiety disorders. Their central nervous system (CNS) depressant effect is dose dependent: PH 1.19, PS 8.6, PS 18.1

1. **In smaller doses,** they relieve anxiety.
2. **In larger single doses,** they induce sleep and can, therefore, be grouped together with sedative hypnotics.
3. Because of their depressant effect on the motor cortex, many of them also act as **muscle relaxants** and anticonvulsants (Chapter 9).

Classification of Antianxiety drugs

I. **Benzodiazepines** (BZD)
II. **Azapirones** e.g. Buspirone
III. **Selective serotonin reuptake inhibitors** (SSRI)
IV. **Adjuvants:** Sympatholytics, e.g. beta-blockers sedative antihistaminics, sedative tricyclic antidepressants

BENZODIAZEPINES (BZD): They are the most commonly prescribed antianxiety agents and provide immediate relief of symptoms. All anxiolytic BZD have similar properties; however, they differ in their pharmacokinetic profiles (Chapter 8).

Mechanism of action: The exact mechanism of antianxiety action is not known though they act at many levels of the neuraxis. Experimentally, they have been shown to act on the limbic system, the hypothalamus and the brain stem reticular system. They bind to BZD binding sites on GABA receptors and facilitate the action of GABA (Chapter 8). BZD also reduce the turnover of brain 5-HT and NA (for details, see Chapter 8).

Pharmacological actions: BZD produce sedation, reduce aggressiveness and thus have a calming (taming) effect. Clinically, they produce beneficial effects in anxious, neurotic patients. Such benefits are, however, difficult to assess.

BZD can cause memory impairment (anterograde amnesia) and other cognitive impairment; this is their major drawback (see Chapter 8).

SELECTIVE SEROTONIN REUPTAKE INHIBITORS (SSRI): These are recommended in the treatment of anxiety but improvement in symptoms may occur over a period of 4 to 6 weeks. Even serotonin norepinephrine reuptake inhibitor (SNRI) e,g. duloxetine and venlafaxine are used as antianxiety agents. For detailed pharmacology see under the section, Antidepressant drugs.

BUSPIRONE: This azaspiro decanedione (azapirone) is an anxiolytic not related to BZD and lacks the sedative-hypnotic, muscle relaxant and anticonvulsant properties of BZD.

It acts as a partial agonist of inhibitory, presynaptic autoreceptors, 5-HT_{1A} receptors and reduces the release of 5-HT which probably explains its anxiolytic action. It also has a weak D_2 receptor antagonistic action. The drug does not potentiate the CNS depressant effect of the commonly used depressant medications and, therefore, may be particularly useful in anxious, elderly patients. It causes less cognitive and psychomotor impairment than diazepam.

It has a short t½ (2–5 h), and is prescribed in the dose of 30 mg/day in divided doses. *It does not cause tolerance/dependence nor interacts with alcohol. It has a wide margin of safety. Its major drawback is that its onset of action is slow, requires thrice a day dosing and may take as much as two weeks for its anxiolytic effect. This effect is weaker than that of BZD. Furthermore, it is not useful in severe anxiety with panic disorder and in alcohol withdrawal syndrome. It is mainly used as an adjunctive therapy.*

Adverse reactions include GI disturbances, nervousness, dizziness, confusion and tachycardia. Patients on monoamine oxidase inhibitors (MAOI) can develop hypertension when given buspirone. Co-administration of buspirone and SSRI or SNRI is common but the risk of serotonin syndrome increases.

Gepirone, ipsapirone and **trospirone** are the analogues of buspirone.

Sedative-antihistaminics (hydroxyzine hydrochloride, diphenhydramine and buclizine; Chapter 23) are promoted as OTC drugs for treating insomnia due to anxiety. They do not cause muscle relaxation and can cause dryness of mouth, palpitation, daytime sedation and confusion.

Pregabalin, has been used as an anxiolytic and is claimed to be as effective as SSRI. Its antianxiety effect is due to inhibition of release of glutamate from PQ type voltage gated calcium channels. Gabapentin also has antianxiety effects. Both the drugs cause respiratory depression and bear abuse potential.

Sedative tricyclic antidepressants *such as amitriptyline and doxepin in low doses (5–10 mg) are also promoted for the treatment of anxiety. However, none of them is superior to BZD, either as anxiolytic or hypnotic. TCA have been used to treat anxiety that has not responded to SSRI or SNRI. Similarly, quetiapine, an antipsychotic drug has been used as a second or third line drug in the treatment for anxiety.*

Beta blockers have been used to prevent performance anxiety. A single dose of propranolol taken one hour before a performance is effective in reducing anxiety symptoms without affecting the quality of the performance.

PH 1.1, PS 8.4

TREATMENT OF ANXIETY DISORDERS

Some amount of anxiety (fear of the known or unknown) is a normal physiological response that assists the individual in solving various problems in life. Amygdala modulates fear and anxiety. *Pathological anxiety is that which has no apparent external cause and exhibits heightened amygdala responses, resulting in high intensity of symptoms which persist over time and lead to the development of harmful behavioural strategies (avoidance, compulsions, etc.) that impair function.* Anxiety may be secondary to stressful situations, bodily disease or the use or withdrawal of drugs/substances of abuse. It is a cardinal symptom of many psychiatric disorders.

Primary anxiety disorders are those in which no cause is discernible. Depending on the manifestations, these disorders are given such names as: **stress-related adjustment disorders, phobias, panic disorders, and generalised anxiety disorder (GAD).**

Anxiety-associated disorder is a common condition in which anxiety is the most prominent symptom. The patient is generally aware of his/her symptoms and the probable cause. These reactions have been considered as the maladaptive results of conflict between unfulfilled desires and repressive tendencies.

SSRI do not cause sedation, but they have a slow onset of action and can delay orgasm. Once started, these drugs must not be stopped suddenabruptlyly, but withdrawnand should be tapered slowly over 4–8 weeks., if needed. These drugs are preferred forin patients who also also have depression associated with anxiety.

Anxiety has two components: (1) **a psychological component** (dread, unpleasant anticipation or a feeling of impending doom) and (2) **a physical component** (autonomic arousal).

The reactions and emotions of a patient suffering from anxiety disorder are usually an exaggeration of those experienced by normal persons in day to day life. Subjects generally complain of headache, tension, feeling of a tight band round the head, palpitation, tremulousness, dryness of mouth, hyperhidrosis, coldness of extremities, spasm of back muscle giving rise to vague bodyache and insomnia. They may also suffer from bowel disturbances and phobias such as fear of dying, insanity and heart disease. *The appetite and libido, however, are less affected, and thoughts of committing suicide are absent unless there is underlying severe depression or major psychosis.*

In practice, many patients complain of 'mental tension' with vague symptoms without any obvious signs of illness. These are due to minor maladjustments in day-to-day life and **do not really need drug therapy**. However, in the highly technical age that we live in, one always seeks a technical solution to every problem. Unfortunately, such ideas are encouraged by drug firms and further enhanced by media by publishing confusing reports. *Drugs can temporarily modify the patient's emotional response to environmental factors. They are not expected to influence the environment or socioeconomic situations.* Hence in today's world, one should learn to cope actively and constantly to ever changing outer environment. One must also remember that emotions are expressions of mind and can be wide and variable, indicating its normal functioning. **Anxiolytics should not be used to modify such normal cyclic behavioural changes without assessing the disability produced.**

Principles of Pharmacotherapy

- **Antianxiety drugs** can reduce the somatic and autonomic disturbances, abolishing physical malaise, bodyache and anxiety. None of them, however, produces permanent benefit which can come only from realisation by the patient of the nature of his problems and his adjustment to them. *Counselling and psychotherapy are more effective.* Effective treatment of anxiety needs patient co-operation. **The majority can be helped more by an empathetic approach of the doctor and relatives than by drugs.**
- Drugs should be used only for a short term to lessen the patient's distress. Antianxiety agents are particularly useful in treating acute stress reactions.
- Since insomnia is a common complaint of these patients and as most antianxiety drugs (not buspirone) induce sleep, the dose should be given at bedtime.
- Since anxiety is often episodic and varying in intensity, drugs should be used to treat each episode and not be given continuously for prolonged periods. It must be emphasised that in anxious patients, placebo responses are frequent.
- *Indiscriminate use of antianxiety agents for pro-*

longed periods may kill all the initiative in the individual and may cause drug dependence.

- Effective treatment of anxiety needs patient co-operation. The majority can be helped more by an empathetic approach of the doctor and relatives than by drugs.

BZD are usually preferred drugs to initiate treatment of anxiety disorders due to their rapid effects. There is little difference among the various BZD as anti-anxiety agents. They can be safely administered in patients with suicidal tendencies.

However, they can cause dependence and interaction with alcohol. Hence, they are not recommended for chronic disorders.

SSRI do not cause sedation, but they have slow onset of action and can delay orgasm. Once started, these drugs must not be stopped abruptly, but should be tapered slowly over 4–8 weeks, if needed. These drugs are preferred for patients who also also have depression associated with anxiety.

Severe anxiety can be extremely disabling and associated with marked autonomic overactivity. *Often it may be the presenting symptom of a more serious psychiatric disorder such as schizophrenia or depression. In such cases appropriate treatment of the underlying disorder is important, and a short course of fast-acting, high-potency BZD such as* **alprazolam, clonazepam** or **lorazepam** is preferred along with antidepressants or APD. Oxazepam in small, divided doses may be preferred in the elderly and in those with hepatic dysfunction, because of its short t½.

In some patients with severe anxiety, somatic symptoms such as palpitation, trembling and giddiness dominate the clinical picture. In such cases, the **beta-adrenergic blocking agent**, like **propranolol** may be useful.

Phobic anxiety is observed in specific situation. Its intensity increases as the person approaches the feared situation such as air or ship travel, public speaking, interviews, etc. and it remains as long as the exposure to that situation lasts. The person will try to avoid the situation if possible. Patients with phobic anxiety may suffer from **panic attacks** when suddenly or overwhelmingly exposed to the feared situation.

The term **panic disorder** is used to describe a condition in which *panic attacks appear to occur spontaneously and repeatedly.* Because of marked somatic symptoms, its diagnosis is likely to be missed. Panic disorder has distinct symptoms. The patient abruptly develops a feeling of intense fear, impending disaster or death accompanied by various physical symptoms such as palpitation, sweating, trembling, feeling of choking, abdominal distress, chills or hot flushes, etc. **Panic attacks are many times associated with agoraphobia, a morbid fear, and avoidance of being alone or being in a public place, resulting in a marked restriction on travel.** Medical conditions that are commonly noted in subjects with panic attacks include episodic high blood pressure, acute dyspepsia, cardiac arrhythmias and mitral valve prolapse. *Unfortunately such patients often receive treatment for the secondary disorder and not the primary anxiety state.*

Not all panic attacks constitute panic disorder. Often, a similar picture may be observed in *specific phobias*, e.g. at heights or on seeing a snake; or in *social phobias* such as facing a stranger or appearing for an examination (where a person is likely to be scrutinised). However, patients with panic disorder may not be aware of the source of their fearfulness. *Furthermore, the panic disorder is often associated with underlying major depression.*

The drugs used in panic disorder are as follows:

i. Antidepressants: The treatment should be started with these drugs given in lower doses than that required for the treatment of depression.
   - **Selective serotonin reuptake inhibitors (SSRI)** such as fluoxetine (5–10 mg/day), paroxetine (10 mg/day) or sertraline (25-50 mg/day) are effective in inducing response and remission. Though considered as first line therapy, they take 2-6 weeks to act (see section, Selective serotonin reuptake inhibitors). They help to control the comorbid depression. Fluoxetine appears to be the most efficacious but sertraline is better tolerated.
   - **Selective serotonin-norepinephrine reuptake inhibitor** (**SNRI**) e.g. venlaflaxine (37.5 mg/day) is an alternative.

- **Tricyclic antidepressants (TCA)** such as imipramine or amitriptyline are also as effective as the SSRI and are less expensive. They also have a sedative action which is helpful. However, TCA with prominent anticholinergic effects such as amitriptyline are less tolerated by the elderly.
- **Monoamine oxidase inhibitors (MAOIs):** They are useful if the patient has comorbid features of atypical depression (hypersomnia and weight gain).

ii. **High potency BZD, such as alprazolam**, in the starting dose of 0.25 mg 2–4 times a day orally, works faster (in days, unlike antidepressants which take weeks) to relieve anxiety and panic symptoms. It is therefore used early in the course of treatment and if required, sporadically later on. It causes sedation. Other BZD are equally effective, and the long acting ones such as clonazepam (t½ = 18–50 h) are easier to withdraw and hence preferred.

BZD given alone are not useful in depression, phobic or obsessional states and chronic psychosis. However, they may be used initially, concurrently with SSRI/TCA for a speedier response. They are tapered over 4–12 weeks while SSRI is continued. In children, anxiolytics should only be used to relieve acute anxiety caused by fear, e.g. before surgery.

iii. The **β-adrenergic blocker**, propranolol, isused as an adjunct for controlling tachycardia, palpitation and tremors during social phobia. By itself, it does not counter the basic anxiety.

Drug therapy should be maintained for 1-2 years and combined with **cognitive-behavioural therapy** (CBT). CBT alone may not be as helpful; but it enhances the long-term well-being of the patient. For resistant panic attacks, short course with aripiprazole, divalproex sodium (sodium valproate and valproic acid in a 1:1 ratio) is useful.

Generalised anxiety disorder (GAD): This term is used when excessive anxiety (tension) and persistent worry *are present on most the days in a week for at least six months.* The symptoms are restlessness, difficulty in concentrating, easy fatiguability, irritability, muscle tension and disturbed sleep, along with symptoms such as palpitation, dry mouth and sweating. Such symptoms are gradual in onset and do not create life-threatening fear but relapses are common. *Major depression is the most commonly coexisting psychiatric disorder in patients with GAD,* occurring in almost 60% of the patients. The treatment of GAD is very difficult. The current therapy includes a combination of BZD, SSRI/TCA and CBT. The initial therapy should be with a combination of BZD and SSRI; the dose of BZD is tapered after 2–3 weeks when SSRI become effective. Severe, intractable GAD may need MAO inhibitors. Atypical antipsychotics such as quetiapine are also used in some patients. Some patients will need maintenance drug therapy almost lifelong.

Emphasis should be on counselling, exercise, mental relaxation/meditation and behavioural therapy. Excessive intake of stimulants in any form should be avoided, and diseases such as thyrotoxicosis should be excluded.

Drugs should be used only if symptoms interfere with normal social functioning. Even in these, many patients are likely to respond to the minimum therapy, and one should not rush into treatment approaches that involve long-term risk and expense. PH 1.19, PS 6.6

ANTIDEPRESSANT DRUGS

The syndrome of depression is a major affective disorder, and though common is often underdiagnosed. Its causes are complex and its pathophysiology is not well understood. It is associated with depletion of brain monoamines, 5-HT and NA.

Despite the availability of several antidepressants (**psychoanaleptics/mood elevators**) the treatment of major depression, in general, is far from satisfactory. The drugs take long time to act. They act mainly by increasing the intrasynaptic availability of the monoamines (NA, 5-HT and to some extent DA) in the brain. This is achieved by:

1. Inhibition of the neuronal reuptake of such amines
2. Receptor blockade
3. Inhibition of amine metabolism by enzyme inhibitors such as MAOI

Classification of Antidepressants PS 18.1

I. **Monoamine oxidase inhibitors (MAOI)**
- **Irreversible:**
  i. **Hydrazine MAOI**, e.g. isocarboxazid, iproniazid and phenelzine
  ii. **Nonhydrazine MAOI**, e.g. tranylcypromine
- **Reversible:** e.g. moclobemide

II. **Tricyclic antidepressants (TCA)** *mainly act by inhibiting reuptake of both, NA and 5HT. They can be*:
  i. *Predominantly NA-reuptake inhibitors*, e.g. desimipramine, amitriptyline, protriptyline, etc.
  ii. *Predominantly 5-HT-reuptake inhibitors*, e.g. clomipramine

These agents are termed '**nonselective**' as they also interact with H_1, α_1 and muscarinic receptors to a variable extent.

III. **Selective serotonin (5-HT) reuptake inhibitors (SSRI):** Fluoxetine, paroxetine, fluvoxamine, sertraline, citalopram, escitalopram

IV. **Newer antidepressants:** These include:
- **Selective 5HT-NA reuptake inhibitors (SNRI):** Venlafaxine, duloxetine, milnacipran desvenlaflaxine, levomilnacipran
- **Selective NA reuptake inhibitor (NARI):** Reboxetine
- **5-HT$_2$ receptor antagonists:** Trazodone, nefazodone, mirtazapine, mianserin, vortioxetine
- **Miscellaneous:**
  i. **Unicyclic:** Bupropion
  ii. **Tetracyclic:** Amoxapine, maprotiline
  iii. **Atypical antipsychotics:** Quetiapine, olanzapine, aripiprazole, brexpiprazole
  iv. **Others:** Tianeptine, esketamine, brexanolone

MONOAMINE OXIDASE INHIBITORS (MAOI)

This heterogeneous group of drugs acts by inhibiting the oxidative deamination of naturally occurring amines such as NA, 5-HT and DA.

Mechanism of action: Relatively large amounts of 5-HT and NA are present in the hypothalamus and in other subcortical regions of the brain. These amines are stored in granules in the neurons and are released following neuronal stimuli. The active amines thus liberated act on the postsynaptic receptors but do not accumulate as they are rapidly metabolised by the MAO. It is present intracellularly in most of the tissues, particularly the CNS, gut and liver. The two types, MAO-A and MAO-B, differentially affect the metabolism of neurotransmitters.

- **Inhibition of the MAO-A** *decreases the deamination of NA and 5-HT. This causes increase in local NA and 5-HT which is associated with both antidepressant action* and hypertensive interactions with foods containing tyramine and with sympathomimetic drugs.
- **Selective inhibition of MAO-B**, which preferentially decreases the deamination of dopamine, *is not associated with antidepressant action* or hypertensive interactions, but is useful in treating parkinsonism (Chapter 15).

Given orally, these drugs exert a considerable effect on liver MAO enzymes because of their high concentration in portal circulation.

Pharmacological actions:

Behavioural effects: These drugs produce antidepressant effect similar to TCA though the mechanism of action is different. MAOI are potent REM sleep inhibitors.

Cardiovascular effects: There is no specific action on heart or the coronary flow. Some MAOI may, however, cause hypotension.

Potentiation of action of sympathomimetic amines: MAOI potentiate the sympathomimetic actions of other amines which are metabolised by MAO, e.g. amphetamine and ephedrine.

In animals pretreated with MAOI, administration of reserpine produces agitation and excitement due to accumulation of amines. This is known as 'reserpine reversal'.

Miscellaneous: As these drugs also inhibit MAO and other enzymes present in the liver, they prevent the metabolism of many drugs and prolong their actions. This may precipitate toxicity.

Box 14.1 Some Drugs Whose Action is Potentiated by MAOI

- Alcohol
- Sympathomimetics: Amphetamine, ephedrine
- Anaesthetics
- Anticholinergics
- Antihistaminics
- Narcotics: Morphine, pethidine, barbiturates
- Antidepressants: TCA, SSRI

Absorption, fate and excretion: They are well absorbed orally. The effect of MAOI continues for 10–14 days after the drug is withdrawn. This is due to their irreversible action on the MAO, which may take over 2 weeks to normalize.

Adverse reactions:

- **Behavioural effects:** These include headache, excitement, agitation, hallucinations and disturbed sleep. These drugs **may activate latent psychosis**; hence, their use alone in cases of schizophrenia is contraindicated.
- **CNS effects:** They may cause insomnia and CNS stimulation as observed by tremors, twitching, ataxia, hyper-reflexia, hyperthermia and even convulsions.

  Iproniazid and isocarboxazid sometimes cause peripheral neuritis which responds to pyridoxine.
- **Hypertensive crisis:** This can be precipitated by concurrent administration of *sympathomimetic pressor amines* like amphetamine and ephedrine. Sudden rise in BP may cause subarachnoid haemorrhage. Hypertensive crisis can also occur in patients taking MAOI, if they consume *cheese* or *red wine* which contain tyramine. Normally, tyramine is metabolised in the liver by MAO enzymes. MAOI, by inhibiting its metabolism, lead to tyramine accumulation which releases NA from binding sites causing a marked rise in BP. Eating of *broad beans* which contains DOPA, can also produce a similar complication. *Yeast extract* contains both tyramine and histamine. Some other foodstuffs which are incompatible with MAOI include *yoghurt, buttermilk, meat extracts, soyabeans, chocolates, ripe bananas and figs.*

  A hypertensive crisis arising due to this food-drug interaction should be treated with IV phentolamine 5 mg slowly or sodium nitroprusside infusion. (Chapter 30)
- **Autonomic effects:** Hydrazine compounds can cause antimuscarinic effects such as constipation, dry mouth, blurring of vision, impotence, difficulty in micturition and orthostatic hypotension.
- **Miscellaneous effects:** They induce weight gain. Hydrazine compounds, particularly iproniazid, may cause hepatocellular jaundice.
- **Acute toxic effects** following overdosage include agitation, hallucinations, hyperpyrexia and convulsions. BP may be low or high. The treatment is mainly symptomatic. Vasopressor agents should be administered cautiously.

Drug interactions: By blocking drug degradation, *MAOI* potentiate the action of several drugs (Box 14.1). Thus, the normal dose of pethidine in a patient receiving *MAOI* can cause shock, collapse, respiratory. depression and death. *The effects of adrenaline, noradrenaline and isoprenaline, however, are not enhanced as they are inactivated by catechol-o-methyl transferase, another enzyme present in the liver and blood.*

Preparations and dosages:

i. Isocarboxazid 10 mg tablet, usual daily dose 10–30 mg increased up to 60 mg
ii. Phenelzine sulphate 15 mg tablet. Usual daily dose 45–60 mg. Maximum daily dose recommended is 90 mg
iii. Tranylcypromine 10 mg tablet, 10–20 mg daily increased up to 30 mg

With all these drugs, smaller doses should be used for maintenance therapy and in the elderly.

MOCLOBEMIDE: This drug acts by selective, reversible inhibition of MAO-A enzyme and, hence, is termed as reversible inhibitor of MAO (**RIMA**). It causes less potentiation of pressor amines and lower incidence of drug interactions than irreversible MAOI.

TRICYCLIC ANTIDEPRESSANTS (TCA)

Structurally, TCA differ from phenothiazines in that the sulphur is replaced by an ethylene linkage

(Fig. 14.1). **Imipramine**, a dibenzazepine derivative, is a well-studied TCA.

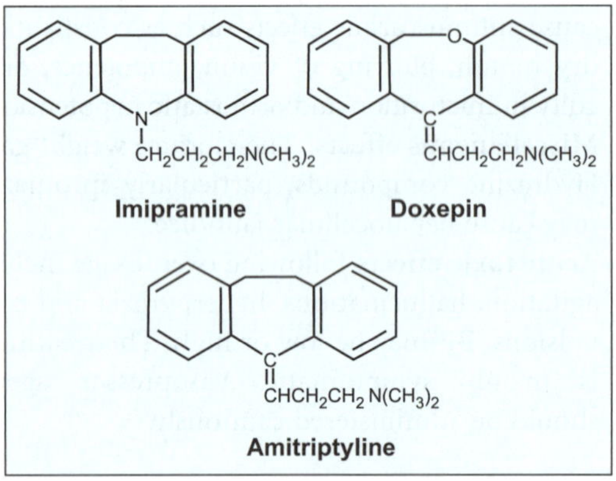

FIG. 14.1 Chemical structures of commonly used TCA

Mechanism of action: Normally, a large proportion of 5-HT/NA liberated at the nerve endings is inactivated by reabsorption into its storage sites (Fig. 17.4 and Fig. 24.3) TCA:

- *Inhibit neuronal NA and to a variable extent, 5-HT reuptake in the brain* by binding to their transporters (SERT and NET). This causes a localised increase in NA/5-HT in the synaptic gap. Uptake blockade occurs quickly but antidepressant action occurs after weeks. In the initial period, presynaptic α_2 and 5-HT_1 auto receptors get activated by increased amount of NA and 5HT in the synaptic cleft resulting in decreased secretion of NT. But over a period, autoreceptors get desensitized and down regulated and amine turnover is increased with enhanced NA and 5HT neurotransmission.
- *Cause variable blockade of α_1* and to a lesser extent, presynaptic α_2 adrenoreceptors.
- *Possess central antimuscarinic properties.*

Table 14.1 Half-lives of Antidepressants and their Metabolites

Drug	Drug t½ (h)	Metabolite, t½ (h)
Tricyclics		
Imipramine	12	14–62
Amitriptyline	31	20–92
Doxepin	16	30
Protriptyline	80	–
Clomipramine	32	54–77
SSRI		
Fluoxetine	50	180
Paroxetine	20	–
Fluvoxamine	15	14–16
Sertraline	22	62–104
Citalopram	32	–

In addition, the different TCA also block other receptors such as H_1, 5HT_2 and DA to differing degrees. This may explain the differences in their action profiles.

Pharmacological actions:

Behavioural effects: These drugs elevate the mood of depressed individuals. Patients feel more energetic, less sleepy and more fresh. Tendency for suicidal rumination diminishes. In some patients there may be agitation, talkativeness and restlessness. *Their are observed after a latent period of a few days to 3–4 weeks.* TCA can reverse the depressant action of reserpine without restoring brain monoamines. They also have some anxiolytic action.

Central nervous system: TCA produce some degree of sedation, enhance sleep and disrupt obsessive rumination. They suppress REM sleep but increases stage 4 sleep. Repeated use may produce difficulty in concentration and thinking. They have no euphoriant effect, no abuse potential and drug dependence is rare.

They lower the seizure threshold in animals and, hence, should be prescribed with caution in patients with history of seizures.

Autonomic nervous system: They exert antimuscarinic effects (see below).

Cardiovascular system: See section on Adverse reactions.

Absorption, fate and excretion: Given orally, TCA are well absorbed. They are highly lipophilic, widely distributed and get strongly bound to proteins in the various tissues. Antidepressants in general are metabolised by hepatic CYP3A4 and CYP2D6, and some of them are converted to an active metabolite having longer duration of action (Table 14.1).

Table 14.2 Antidepressant Drugs PH 1.19

Drugs	Adverse Reactions due to Blockade of Receptors: H_1 Sedative Activity	M Antimuscarinic Activity	α_1 Orthostatic Hypotension	Total Daily Dose: Out Patients	Hospital Patients
I. Tricyclic antidepressants					
Imipramine	+ +	+ +	+ +	50–200	75–300
Trimipramine	+ + +	+ + +	+ +	50–100	75–300
Desipramine	0/+	+	+	100–120	
Amitriptyline[a]	+ + +	+ + +	+ + +	50–100	75–200
Nortriptyline	+	+	+	25–50	50–100
Doxepin	+ + +	+ +	+ +	50–100	75–300
Dothiepin	++	+		50–100	100–200
II. Selective serotonin (5-HT) reuptake inhibitors (SSRI):					
Fluoxetine	0/+	0	0	20	20–60
Fluvoxamine	0/+	0	0	50–100	100–300
Paroxetine	0/+	0/+	0	20–40	20–50
Sertraline	0/+	0	0	100–150	100–200
Citalopram	0/+	0	0	10–40	20–40
III. Selective serotonin-NA reuptake inhibitors (SNRI)					
Venlafaxine	0	0	0	75–150	75–375
Duloxetine	0/+	0	0/+	60–120	
IV. Selective NA reuptake inhibitor (NARI):					
Reboxetine	0/+	+	0	8–12	8–12
IV. $5\text{-}HT_2$ receptor antagonist:					
Trazodone	+ + +	0	0	150–300	150–600
Nefazodone	+ + +	0	0	200–400	
Mirtazapine	++++	–	0/+	15	15–45
VI. Miscellaneous:					
(a) Unicyclic compound					
Bupropion	0	0	0	200–300	200–450
(b) Tetracyclic compounds					
Amoxapine	+	+	++	50–200	100–600
Maprotiline	++	+	+	75–150	100–225

Note: 0, negligible; +, minimal; ++, moderate; +++, marked. H_1, histaminic; M, muscarinic; α_1, alpha$_1$ adrenergic.
[a]Injections 100 mg/10 mL for IM use.

Imipramine is converted in the liver to its active metabolite desmethylimipramine. Some patients are poor metabolisers of TCA and may not tolerate standard doses.

It is important to note that there is a marked variation in steady state plasma levels between individuals following similar doses. Furthermore, Asian-Americans and African-Americans are known to require much lower doses than Caucasian Americans. This may be true for Indians.

Most tricyclics are completely eliminated within 7–10 days.

Adverse reactions: Some of these can be explained on the basis of *blocking of various neurotransmitter receptors* in the brain (Table 14.2). Blocking of D_2 receptor

Box 14.2 Drug Interactions of Imipramine

- MAOI: Severe reactions like atropine poisoning (hyperpyrexia, convulsions and coma)
- Orthostatic hypotension with antihypertensives
- CYP3A4 inducers and inhibitors can change serum levels
- CYP2D6 inhibitors like fluoxetine increase serum levels of TCA
- Potentiation of action of phenylephrine, adrenaline and NA with potentially fatal accidents
- Phenothiazines and thyroid preparations enhance its effects
- Anticholinergics and antihistaminics potentiate ADRs

is responsible for the endocrine adverse effects, e.g. galactorrhoea following clomipramine, amoxapine, trimipramine, etc. Usually, TCA are well tolerated.

- **Allergic reactions** like urticaria, skin rashes, pruritus and photosensitivity.
- **Antimuscarinic effects:** These are relatively common and include dryness of mouth, difficulty in accommodation, tachycardia, constipation, difficulty in micturition, impotence, and delayed ejaculation. TCA should be used cautiously in patients with glaucoma or enlarged prostate. Rarely, they can cause paralytic ileus. Central antimuscarinic action may cause confusion, disorientation or psychosis.
- **Central nervous system:** Feeling of tiredness, lethargy, headache and weight gain may be observed. Because of their strong affinity for H1 receptors, amitriptyline, trimipramine, doxepin, trazodone and mirtazepine are potent sedatives and can cause sleep. This may be beneficial. Like MAOI, these drugs can cause tremors, muscle jerking, ataxia and hyper-reflexia. They are best avoided in epileptics.
- **Cardiovascular system:** Both imipramine and amitriptyline may rarely cause inverted or flattened T wave, prolongation of QT interval and depressed ST segment in the ECG. Postural hypotension, cardiomyopathy and heart failure have been reported following long-term therapy. With overdosage, they can precipitate cardiac arrhythmias.
- **Miscellaneous:** Like chlorpromazine, imipramine can cause cholestatic jaundice, agranulocytosis and oedema.

  TCA cross the placental barrier and can cause jitteriness, suckling problem, hyperexcitability and rarely cardiac arrhythmias in the neonate.

  Sudden discontinuation of TCA may rarely lead to cholinergic crisis and a flu-like syndrome. FM 10.1
- **Acute poisoning** with TCA produces hyperpyrexia, hypertension or hypotension, convulsions and coma. Cardiac arrhythmias may be present. It may also cause metabolic acidosis. The treatment is symptomatic. Sodium bicarbonate IV is preferred for TCA-induced cardiotoxicity and BZD for seizure suppression.

Drug interactions: See Box 14.2.

Preparations and dosage: See Table 14.2.

Indications:

- **Major depression**, discussed in the section Treatment of major depression.
- **Acute panic attacks, anxiety disorders, social phobias** (see section, Treatment of anxiety disorders).
- **Obsessive compulsive neurosis:** This disorder is characterised by obsessional pattern of thinking and ritualistic compulsive behaviour as a defence against anxiety. If such thoughts or action is prevented or interrupted, the patient becomes anxious. The treatment is either with a TCA or with a SSRI.
- **Nocturnal enuresis:** Enuresis is defined as bedwetting that occurs after the age at which bladder control should have been achieved, usually between the ages 2–3 years. The disorder exists in two forms: (a) primary (persistent) and (b) secondary (acquired or regressional). Primary enuresis is more common. The main treatment consists of bladder training and correction of psychopathologic factors. Imipramine, in a single bedtime dose of 10–75 mg, has been used with variable success. The exact mechanism of action is not known. The other drugs used are amitriptyline and desmopressin (Chapter 37).
- **Bulimia nervosa:** This is a behavioural disorder characterised by episodes of overeating, usually followed by self-induced vomiting, cathartic or diuretic abuse or fasting to undo the threat of weight gain. Antidepressants such as imipramine and SSRI are the favoured drugs treatment for this condition.
- **Migraine**, see Chapter 24.
- **Deafferentation pain**, see Chapter 11.

- **Attention-deficit hyperactivity disorder** *(ADHD)* (Chapter 12).
- **Nonspecific fibromyalgias.**
- **Pruritus:** Topical doxepin is used because of its antihistaminic effects.
- **Insomnia:** Small doses of doxepin are used (Chapter 8).

Imipramine and amitriptyline are still the most cost-effective TCA for general use.

SELECTIVE SEROTONIN REUPTAKE INHIBITORS (SSRI)

Drugs belonging to this group are listed in Tables 14.2 and 14.3.

Mechanism of action: As the name suggests, the selective serotonin reuptake inhibitors (SSRI) act mainly by inhibiting the reuptake of serotonin by the tryptaminergic neurons. They bind to the serotonin transporter (SERT) at a site other than the binding site of 5-HT and inhibit the transporter.

This causes stimulation of 5HT autoreceptors (1A, 1D and 5HT7), which initially reduces net synthesis and release of 5HT. But later on with continued treatment, downregulation and desensitization of autoreceptors occurs resulting in enhanced 5HT neurotransmission. Downregulation of postsynaptic $5HT_{2A}$ receptors or heteroreceptors on NA neurons and may also contribute to their antidepressant effects. Post-receptor cellular effects are responsible for long-lasting antidepressant effects. SERT expression reduces with prolonged treatment resulting in decreased clearance and increased 5 HT neurotransmission.

Pharmacological action: Because of their selective receptor action, **they cause less:**

- *Antimuscarinic effects.*
- *Antihistaminic effects, including sedation.*
- *Cardiovascular effects* (bradycardia, hypotension, conduction disturbances)

They *are generally safer than the TCA in the elderly.*

Absorption, fate and excretion: SSRI are well absorbed orally and have long t½, which permits their once-a-day administration. In general, like TCA, many of these are metabolised in the liver. Some of the metabolites are also active, with t½ longer than those of the parent drugs (Table 14.1). All SSRI except citalopram and escitalopram inhibit one or more CYP450 and may cause increased toxicity of TCA, tramadol, methadone, type 1C antiarrhythmics, alcohol and theophylline; sertraline inhibits CYP3A4 and alters blood levels of digoxin. On the other hand, antiepileptics, e.g. carbamazepine which induces CYP 450 can cause decreased efficacy of SSRI.

Adverse reactions: These include the following:

- **Gastrointestinal:** Anorexia, nausea, abdominal pain and diarrhoea.
- **CNS:** Anxiety, agitation, akathisia, headache, transient insomnia, vivid dreams and weight gain.
- **Anorgasmia:** They decrease sexual thoughts and desire, decrease libido and may delay orgasm in both sexes (anorgasmia). This side effect, however, makes them useful in the therapy of paraphilias and sexual obsession associated with increased suicidal tendencies. Derangement in sexual function can be treated by reducing the dose, giving weekend drug holidays.
- **Increased risk of bleeding** may be observed as SSRI inhibit serotonin uptake by platelets.
- **Hyponatremia**, particularly in elderly patients.
- **QT interval prolongation** has been reported with all SSRI; the risk appears to be greatest with citalopram and escitalopram.
- **Serotonin syndrome:** This may be due to hyperstimulation of $5\text{-}HT_{1A}$ receptors in brain stem. It is necessary to monitor patients closely if taking serotonergic drugs in combination. It comprises the following:
  a. ***Cognitive-behavioural symptoms***: mainly agitation, insomnia, anxiety hypomania and seizures. Some of them may increase the risk of suicide in children and adolescents.
  b. ***Autonomic symptoms***: nausea, salivation, diaphoresis, diarrhoea, abdominal cramps, flushed skin, hypertension and hyperthermia

c. *Neuromuscular symptoms*: hyper-reflexia, shivering, twitching, rigidity. The reaction may be rarely fatal. The treatment is symptomatic.

The administration of an MAOI concurrently with or immediately prior to one of these drugs can cause serotonin syndrome. Other drugs which cause this syndrome are listed in Box 14.3.

Like other antidepressants, the SSRI may cause mania when used in patients with undiagnosed bipolar depression.

Sudden stoppage of any of the SSRIs can produce variety of **withdrawal symptoms** such as a flu-like reaction, anxiety, depressed or irritable mood, agitation, confusion, insomnia, sweating, tremor, dizziness, strange sensations of vision and touch, electric shock like sensations and vomiting. The incidence is generally greater with potent, short-acting SSRI-like paroxetine than fluoxetine which has a longer t½.

Preparations and dosage: See Table 14.2.

Fluoxetine is used initially in the dose of 20 mg once a day, in the morning, increased by 20 mg once in several weeks, to a maximum of 80 mg daily (less in the elderly). *Doses higher than 20 mg should be given in two divided doses in the morning and at noon.* **Fluvoxamine** and **sertraline** are used initially in the dose of 50 mg once a day, increased by 50 mg once a week, to a maximum of 200 mg daily (less in the elderly).

Box 14.3 Some Drugs which May Induce Serotonin Syndrome

- MAOI
- Pethidine
- Dextromethorphan
- Clomipramine
- Amphetamine
- Lithium
- Levodopa
- Buspirone
- Bromocriptine
- Two or more SSRI (especially fluoxetine)

Indications: They should be given in the morning hours as they can disturb sleep. They are preferred in patients who have:

- **Major depression disorder** and especially those who:
  a. **Have a high risk of suicide.**
  b. **Are accident prone,** as the older antidepressants have sedative and autonomic adverse effects.
  c. **Cannot tolerate the TCA.**
  d. **Are elderly:** as TCA can cause dizziness, postural hypotension, constipation and difficulty in micturition in these patients.
- **Obsessive compulsive disorder (OCD):** A major role for serotonin system in mediation of OCD has been suggested, which explains clinical effectiveness of SSRI and also their better safety and tolerability profile than tricyclics.
- **Bipolar depression:** In moderate-severe bipolar depression SSRI are used in combination with mood stabilisers (see under the section Pharmacotherapy of Bipolar Depression)
- **Panic disorders, Social Phobia:** see under the section Panic disorder
- **Bulimia nervosa:** See under the section Indications for TCA

If used concurrently, they may increase the TCA, lithium and carbamazepine plasma levels.

SSRI should not be used:

- In the manic phase of bipolar depression.
- Together with MAOI.
- Concurrently with ECT.

Choice of SSRI: All SSRIs are almost equally effective as antidepressants. Patients who do not respond to one drug may respond to another. Because of the differences in their hepatic metabolism, they differ in their potential for drug interactions. **Fluoxetine, sertraline** and **escitalopram** are currently considered the drugs of choice for routine use. Fluoxetine can also be used to treat depression in children and adolescents. **Paroxetine** exerts more antimuscarinic effects, may cause more weight gain as well as pose a high risk of mood changes and withdrawal syndrome. **Sertraline** has relatively lower risk of drug interaction than the former drugs. However, all the

Table 14.3 Newer Antidepressants

Group Name (t½)	Mechanism of Action	Metabolism	Important ADR	Drug Interactions
		SNRI		
Venlafaxine (8–11 h)	Potent 5-HT and less potent NA inhibitor	Hepatic CYP2D6 Active metabolite (desvenlafaxine); Lowest protein binding	Serotonergic: hypertension, tachycardia, insomnia; Intense withdrawal syndrome; constipation, urinary retention	Few
Duloxetine (12–15 h)	As above	Hepatic CYP2D6 and CYP1A2; High protein binding	Nausea, somnolence, constipation, hepatic damage	With CYP2D6 inhibitors and itself elevates TCA and other substrate levels
		NA reuptake inhibitors (NARIs)		
Reboxetine (13h)	Selective inhibitor of NA reuptake	Hepatic	Tachycardia, dry mouth, constipation, sexual dysfunction	Few
		5-HT_2 receptor antagonists		
Trazodone (2–6 h)	Blocks post synaptic 5-HT_{2A} and presynaptic α_2	Hepatic CYP3A4 Active metabolite; High protein binding	Nausea, orthostatic hypotension, priapism	Few
Nefazadone (2–6 h)	As above	Hepatic CYP3A4; High protein binding	Nausea, dose dependent antimuscarinic effects, orthostatic hypotension, sedation, hepatotoxic	Many with CYP3A4 inhibitors
Mirtazapine (20–40 h)	As trazodone. Also high affinity for H_1 receptors	Hepatic; High protein binding	Marked sedation, increased appetite, weight gain	Few. With CNS depressants
		Miscellaneous		
Bupropion (11–14 h)	Inhibits NA and to a lesser extent DA reuptake. Weak antidepressant	Hepatic, Active metabolite; High protein binding	Insomnia, anorexia, agitation, lowers seizure threshold	With CYP2D6 inhibitors

Note: For tetracyclic compounds amoxapine and maprotiline, see Table 14.2.

three drugs prolong QTc interval, the risk is highest with citalopram and escitalopram.

SSRI with additional 5-HT_{1A} receptor agonist activity have been developed for the treatment of major depressive disorder. These include **vilazodone**, which inhibits reuptake of serotonin and acts as a 5-HT_{1A} receptor partial agonist and **vortioxetine** which is 5-HT_{1A} receptor agonist activity and 5-HT_3 receptor antagonist.

Newer Antidepressants

These drugs (Table 14.3) have diverse structures, mechanisms of action and ADR profile but they have efficacy similar to SSRI. Because of their selective profile, they may be useful in matching individual patient's needs in terms of efficacy and tolerability. For example, sexual dysfunction is less common with mirtazapine while weight gain is not a problem with venlafaxine and reboxitine. *They should not be used with MAO inhibitors. Because of suspected effect on mood fluctuations and possible suicidal thoughts, paroxetine, mirtazapine, venlafaxine and nefazodone should be avoided in children.* Drugs like trazodone, nefazodone, venlafaxine and bupropion require frequent dosing. All are expensive.

Tianeptine is an atypical TCA, which was earlier thought to increase 5-HT uptake . However, now it is known that it modulates glutamatergic neurotransmission, which is responsible for its antidepressant effects. It is however is a mu-opioid receptor agonist. This action results in dopamine release, causing euphoria and a risk of overdose. It has a potential for abuse and dependence when ingested at high doses. It is claimed to be effective in anxiodepressive state.

Esketamine is the S-enantiomer of ketamine (Chapter 7). It also modulates the glutamatergic transmission by inhibiting the NMDA receptor on GABA interneuron. This reduces the GABA release and therefore frees the glutamatergic neuron from GABA inhibition. Released glutamine acts on the postsynaptic AMPA receptors and bring about cellular responses that restore disturbed glutamatergic neurotransmission to produce antidepressant effects. Esketamine produces rapid and long lasting effects. It is used as nasal spray along with oral antidepressants in patients with resistant depression. However, it is administered under the direct supervision and the patient is monitored for at least 2 hours after administration. ADR include sedation, increase in BP for prolonged time, impairment of memory and concentration and dissociation symptoms that cause anxiety and confusion. These risks and the abuse potential makes it a drug of restricted access as ketamine.

Brexanolone is structurally identical to allopregnanolone, the endogenous neurosteroid. It is a modulator of the $GABA_A$ receptor and enhances ligand gated Cl- current to mediate inhibitory neurotransmission. The restoration of dysregulated neural activity is responsible for antidepressant effects. It is used only for postpartum depression. It is administered by continuous IV infusion over 60 hours under constant pulse oximetry monitoring to detect hypoxia. It can cause sedation and dizziness. It is very expensive.

Studies indicate that **atypical antipsychotics** which are $5HT_2$ receptor antagonists are useful as an *adjunct therapy in major depressive disorders even without psychotic features especially in treatment resistant patients.* They are given along with fluoxetine or SSRI or SNRI. A fixed-dose combination of olanzapine and fluoxetine is available for treatment-resistant depression. atypical antipsychotics are also used in bipolar depression or major depression with psychotic feature. Their main disadvantage is metabolic syndrome and weight gain (Chapter 13)

St. John's Wort: This herbal product is derived from the plant *Hypericum perforatum.* Many phytoconstituents probably contribute to its action. Given orally, it has variable beneficial effects in mild to moderate depression. The ADR include GI disturbances, dry mouth, dizziness, sedation and confusion. It is an inducer of hepatic CYP450.

Patients with reduced folate levels may less likely to respond to antidepressant treatment and more likely to experience relapses. Folate is necessary for endogenous synthesis of 5-HT, NA, and DA, and increased levels of these NT have been associated with an improved response to the antidepressant treatment. Hence L-methylfolate, is used in the treatment of depression as a medical food. PH 1.1, PS 6.4

TREATMENT OF MAJOR DEPRESSION

Depression is a major disorder of mood (affect) prevalent in a significant percentage of the population and has a strong familial predisposition. It is a serious condition as it can disrupt the normal social life and may drive the individual to commit suicide. Hence, it is essential that it is diagnosed early as antidepressant drugs can alleviate the majority of depressive illnesses.

Although there is no unanimity about the clinical classification of depression, it can be broadly divided into **two main groups**:

- **Unipolar depressive disorders** which include major depressive disorder (MDD). Depression is considered as MDD, when a person has 'depressed mood on a daily basis for a minimum duration of two weeks.
- **Bipolar disorder or Manic depressive psychosis (MDP):** Patients with MDP have different pathologies.

Unipolar depression can be thought of as of two types.

1. *Reactive, neurotic or psychological* depression, is an exaggerated reaction to adversity, manifested as gloom, unhappiness and tearfulness. It is precipitated by such factors as sudden monetary loss, failure in examinations or an accident. *The individual blames the situation rather than himself.* It is usually associated with marked anxiety. It responds favourably to moral, spiritual and social support from friends and relatives, who can share the problems and discuss the possibilities of solution. In such **situational crises**, *anxiolytics like BZD help to tide over the crisis. The patient improves with the change of situation.*
   Death of a close person normally results in a **grief reaction**, which resolves in course of time. Short-term use of anxiolytics can be helpful immediately after such loss; but their prolonged use may actually hinder its resolution. If severe, the grief reaction may be complicated by depression, physical ill health and even suicide. The use of antidepressants in such a situation helps the depressive symptoms.
2. *Melancholic, earlier known as endogenous, depression* produces a varied picture. The dictionary meaning of melancholia is 'a mental state characterised by dejection and misery'. It usually occurs in the middle or later years of life.

The symptoms may vary markedly and are probably related to relative deficiency of NA, DA and/or 5HT (see below). In its classical form, an individual shows retardation of thoughts, movement and speech; he remains withdrawn from the usual activities. It is associated with early-morning waking, occasional nightmares, anxiety, feeling of guilt and unworthiness. *There is a tendency for self-blaming.* The patient generally complains of various aches and pains, tiredness, loss of appetite, loss of libido, lack of concentration and loss of weight. **There is a greater tendency to commit suicide.**

Pathophysiology of major depression is complex and not well understood. It may have a biochemical basis which is related to decreased synthesis and turnover of brain 5-HT, NA and DA as well as an increased accumulation of ACh. Reserpine, which depletes brain catecholamines and 5HT, causes depression.

Studies in depressed persons indicate decreased metabolic activity in the caudate nuclei and frontal lobes and altered NA activity in various parts of the brain. Patients who have attempted suicide have significantly lower CSF levels of the 5-HT metabolite, 5-hydroxyindolacetic acid (HIAA) than those who have not. *However, there appears to be no definite biological markers/test for depression.* Other systems such as HPA axis may also be involved in its genesis. *Clinically, majority of depressive disorders are multifocal, and disturbances in brain chemicals/neurotransmitters are only the part of the mechanism.* Hence, treatment is guided mainly by patient's history and symptom profile.

The **aims of therapy** are to:

1. Reduce the symptoms and prevent suicidal tendency.
2. Prevent relapse/recurrence of symptoms.
3. Improve cognitive and functional state.
4. Help in rehabilitation.

For the successful treatment of depression, the **doctor-patient relationship** is important. The doctor must try to boost confidence of such patients. The relatives should be counselled not to increase the patients' guilt feeling. It is worth searching for possible external factors contributing to the depressive illness and trying to reduce their impact by modifying the environment or by psychotherapy and exercise. *Cognitive behavioural and interpersonal therapies and exercises are effective in mild depression. Counselling or patient education alone may be sufficient.*

Drug therapy: Pharmacotherapy is useful for moderate to severe episodes of depression. Therapeutic response to antidepressants is variable and delayed. There is no way to decide who will respond better to which drug – TCA or SSRI. Since both, catecholamine and 5HT deficiency, appear to be involved in its pathogenesis, it is perhaps prudent to start with a drug which modulates both these central amines. In this respect, none of the newer antidepressants appears to be consistently therapeutically superior except in a few selected subgroups of patients. The choice among antidepressants is made based on the age, other medications, comorbidity, previous treatment response and side effects, cost, safety in overdose and availability.

Many current treatment guidelines recommend SSRI because of their acceptable ADR profile as compared to TCA. However, they all can cause GI disturbances, sleep impairment, sexual dysfunction, anxiety and rarely serotonin syndrome. They should be avoided in children. Commonly used drugs are fluoxetine, sertraline and escitalopram. **Fluoxetine, paroxetine** and **sertraline** have been reported to cause drug dependence. SSRIs may not be effective for treatment of depression in patients with chronic nonpsychiatric disorders such as heart failure or chronic kidney disease.

The advantages of SSRI are:

a. They are given in a single daily dose.
b. They cause less sedation and have no antimuscarinic or cardiovascular effects; hence, compliance is better.

The choice of TCA is determined by the adverse effects it produces e.g. sedation, orthostatic hypotension and antimuscarinic effects. They are relatively cheap and cost-effective. *They are contraindicated in patients with serious cardiovascular risk factors.* They are relatively cheap and cost-effective.

Patients with agitation or anxiety are best treated with a TCA having sedative effects. Amitriptyline, doxepin and dothiepin are more sedative than imipramine. Nortriptyline and desipramine have negligible sedating action. Treatment with amitriptyline is often associated with substantial weight gain.

The elderly metabolise TCA more slowly and may achieve therapeutic plasma concentrations with doses as low as 25–50 mg daily. Because of pharmacokinetic considerations, the entire daily dose of imipramine or amitriptyline may be given at bedtime; their sedative effect may eliminate the need for an additional hypnotic. Wide variations are known to occur in the serum concentration in different people on the same dose. *Asians generally require lower doses than Caucasians.*

Although the list of ADR following TCA is formidable, in the doses recommended their incidence is not high and they usually occur during the first few days of treatment. Tolerance may develop to the sedative and autonomic effects (but not to its antidepressant effects). TCA are well tolerated and have dose related ADR.

An antidepressant should be started in a low dose, which is gradually increased depending on the response. Improvement is usually observed after 3-4 weeks (therapeutic lag). In majority of the cases, remission occurs within 8-12 weeks. *A trial for this period should be given before the prescribed antidepressant is judged ineffective;* in that case, a drug from a different class is prescribed either alone or in combination with the first agent. Some patients may respond to SNRI like extended release venlafaxine. Maintenance treatment is needed for 6–12 months to prevent relapse. *Some cases with high risk of relapse (having depression for more than 2 years) may need lifelong maintenance treatment.* Attempts are made to achieve lower doses for maintenance by trial and error.

Bupropion is an alternative to an SSRI or SNRI for treatment of major depressive disorder when anxiety is not a prominent symptom. It is not sedating and has not been associated with weight gain, sexual dysfunction, or an increased risk of bleeding. It may be helpful in patients with impaired concentration, hypoactive sexual desire disorder, or antidepressant-induced sexual dysfunction.

Similarly mirtazapine may be particularly useful in patients with insomnia or marked weight loss. Mirtazapine may also be helpful in patients who experience significant nausea with SSRIs, SNRIs,or bupropion.

Combining two antidepressants (but not two serotonergic drugs) from different classes, such as bupropion and an SSRI, or adding another drug

Box 14.4 Important Points to Remember about Depression and Its Therapy

- Depression is quite common in practice and affects daily functioning and well-being.
- It recurs in 25%–30% of cases in 1 year.
- Up to 25% of the patients develop chronic depression needing long-term therapy.
- Many depressed patients either remain undiagnosed or receive inadequate therapy.
- Treatment is initiated after assessing symptoms and functioning. Rule out any another cause responsible for the symptoms of a patient, such as a medical condition, a side effect from a medication, or related to the use of illicit substances. Imminent risk of suicide should also be assessed.
- There may be co-existing medical and psychiatric comorbidities, which are associated with poor prognosis and increased chances of recurrence.
- In 60–70% of patients, symptoms ameliorate after 6–8 weeks of drug therapy given at a therapeutic dose.
- Once remission is achieved, antidepressants should be continued for 6–9 months. Early dose reduction leads to a higher risk of relapse.
- Gradual tapering of drug should be done to terminate the therapy. Patients must be monitored carefully after that since relapse is common.
- In patients with two or more episodes of depression it should be considered for indefinite period, even lifelong.
- Meta-analysis has revealed little evidence that any particular antidepressant or class of antidepressants is more efficacious than others, and choice of drug/s is guided by their profiles of other actions.
- Most of the antidepressants increase the risk of suicidal tendencies and behaviour in children, adolescents and adults. They can also induce mania, most often in patients with undiagnosed bipolar disorders.

for augmentation are additional alternatives to manage resistant depression.

A less common ADR of all antidepressants is *hyponatremia*. It should be suspected in patients who develop drowsiness, confusion or convulsions while on antidepressants. Subjects with erectile dysfunction may benefit from trazodone or citalopram.

Withdrawal of TCA and SSRI should be gradual as sudden stoppage can cause withdrawal symptoms (see earlier).

In pregnant ladies with depression, nonpharmacologic treatment must be considered as first line treatment for mild depression, but untreated depression may be more harmful to the fetus than pharmacotherapy. Discontinuation of antidepressants during pregnancy may increase the risk of relapse.In general, **TCA appear to be safe during pregnancy.** They are, however, secreted in the breast milk. **SSRI** are the most frequently prescribed drugs during pregnancy as it has been demonstrated that the risk of congenital malformations after taking an SSRI during pregnancy appears to be very low with no increase in perinatal mortality.

SSRI are also used to treat postpartum depression. They are, however, secreted in the breast milk. Brexanolone has been approved for treatment of postpartum depression.

MAOI, though faster acting and highly effective in atypical depression, are potentially more hazardous. Although it is claimed that younger patients do better with MAOI, these compounds cannot be recommended as drugs of choice. *Combination of TCA or SSRI with MAOI should not be used concurrently or within 2 weeks of each other as it is hazardous and can cause agitation, convulsions, coma and death* (**serotonin syndrome**).

Similarly other concomitant drugs with MAOI activity e.g. linezolid, triptans, opioids (dextromethorphan, tramadol and methadone) and St. John's Wort can cause serotonin syndrome when taken concurrently with an SSRI or SNRI and their concomitant use must be avoided.

Antianxiety agents like BZD (e.g. alprazolam) may be combined to lessen anxiety in early stages. A sedative like diazepam and flurazepam may be given at bedtime to those who complain of early awakening. *Phenothiazines can be combined with TCA in bipolar depression with agitation or psychotic symptoms.*

For depression resistant to drug and psychotherapy, neurostimulation in form of ECT is used.

In severe cases with delusions, suicidal ruminations, marked retardation or severe agitation, ECT is preferred to drug therapy, as the beneficial results can be obtained more quickly. Repetitive transcranial magnetic stimulation (rTMS) and vagus nerve stimulation are also used for treatment-resistant depression. Unlike ECT, rTMS does not require anesthesia and does not appear to have cognitive adverse effects. However, efficacy of ECT is better than rTMS.

A history of suicidal attempt or strong suicidal thoughts points to the need for immediate hospitalisation. Finally, safety of self-administration of large doses with suicidal intention must be a major determinant in the choice of an antidepressant in such patients.

As mentioned earlier **atypical APD** (risperidone, olanzapine, aripiprazole) can be used in patients with MDD who do not respond adequately to monotherapy even after 6–8 weeks. However, atypical APD may cause unwanted effects such as weight gain, akathesia, hyperglycemia and hyperprolactinaemia. Other adjunctive drugs used are thyroxine and triiodothyronine.

The relationship between depression and anxiety is complex. Depression can be precipitated as a reaction to severe anxiety. Both can coexist in a patient with neurotic illness, schizophrenia or an organic syndrome.

Finally, it is important to remember that depression often coexists with chronic illnesses, such as cancer and worsens the quality of life. It is often missed and needs to be diagnosed to treat.

In addition to drugs, psychotherapy, particularly cognitive-behavioral therapy and interpersonal therapy, are effective for treatment of moderate to severe, non-psychotic depression and can achieve remarkable therapeutic results. *The kindness from relatives and friends is of immense benefit, and the patient should be made to feel that s/he is useful to the family and community and not an unwanted, useless burden.*

It must be realised that mild anxiety/depression is a normal manifestation of cyclic variations in mood. It is usually transient and self-limiting. In such patients euphoriants should not be prescribed as they are potentially toxic. The important points to remember about depression are listed in Box 14.4.

PH 1.19, PS 7.6

MOOD STABILISERS

LITHIUM CARBONATE: The use of lithium carbonate in mental illness was described by Cade in 1949.

Lithium is useful as a mood stabiliser in manic depressive psychosis (MDP). As compared to chlorpromazine, lithium causes less drowsiness while controlling the marked psychomotor overactivity in about 75% of the patients.

Mechanism of action: Its exact mechanism of action is not known. It causes:

1. Inhibition of phospholipase C synthesis with resultant decrease in brain inositol triphosphate and diacylglycerol concentration; this reduces the sensitivity of some neurons to the action of various neurotransmitters.
2. Modification of GABA concentration in the brain and modulation of synaptic glutarnate availability.
3. Decrease in the synthesis of DA and NA in the brain and facilitation of their neuronal reuptake.
4. Decrease in the function of brain protein kinases, leading to alterations in the release of neurotransmitters and hormones.

Absorption, fate and excretion: It is well absorbed on oral administration and gets distributed throughout the total body water. Being a metallic ion, it is not metabolised nor gets protein-bound, but is mostly excreted in the urine. *Lithium decreases the sodium reabsorption by the renal tubules* leading to sodium loss. *Patients on lithium treatment, therefore, should maintain adequate salt and water intake.*

FM 10.1

Adverse reactions: Lithium toxicity is closely related to its serum level and the therapeutic window is narrow. Hence, *the drug must be administered, with facilities for estimating serum lithium levels.* Blood levels exceeding 2.0 mEq/L are associated with dangerous toxic effects. *Salt depletion from any cause, including a diuretic, increases its renal tubular reabsorption and plasma level, thus precipitating toxicity.*

1. **Mild toxicity** includes GI disturbances, drowsiness, muscular weakness and alopecia. It can also cause allergic reactions, blurred vision, glycosuria and polyuria.
2. **Large doses** (level >1.5 mmol/L) cause **sodium depletion**, cerebellar ataxia, tremors, cardiac arrythmias seizures, hypotension and coma.
3. **Chronic administration** may give rise to goitre formation, hypothyroidism (rare) and ECG changes.
4. **Embryotoxicity:** Lithium is embryotoxic.
   Because of toxicity and narrow therapeutic window, lithium should be prescribed only by a specialist who will also be responsible for monitoring it.

Indications: The uses are as follows:

- **To prevent the recurrence of mania and of depressive episodes in bipolar disorder.** Lithium salts are the first choice for long-term prevention of MDP.
- **To treat acute episodes of mania** it is **combined with an APD** like haloperidol.
- **To treat alcohol dependence** (Chapter 6).

MANIC DEPRESSIVE PSYCHOSIS (MDP) – MANAGEMENT

MDP, a bipolar disorder, is a highly recurrent and heterogeneous illness. It has a strong genetic propensity. The central features of MDP consist of unpredictable swings in mood as **mania** followed by **depressive episodes**, with near normal behaviour in between.

Mania is characterised by elevation of mood and overactivity. A manic patient is energetic, cheerful and optimistic. Sleep is reduced; speech is often rapid and copious. Appetite and sexual desire may increase. The patient believes that his ideas are brilliant and that his work is of outstanding quality. This may be accompanied by grandiose delusions and occasionally hallucinations. It may also be presented as **hypomania**, which is less dramatic but with similar features. Subject may be over talkative and mildly reckless. This is followed by a brief episode of **depression**, characterised by low mood, poor appetite and insomnia. Many patients, however, can control their symptoms, for a short period, and often remain undiagnosed.

Pharmacotherapy of Bipolar Depression (Table 14.4): PH 1.1, PS 7.4

The main objectives of treatment are

- immediate control of acute mania or depression and
- long-term prevention of recurrences.

If patients presents with severe agitated state (psychotic) the therapy is initiated with haloperidol as it controls hyperactivity and psychotic features of mania. **Lorazepam**(1–2 mg every 4 hourly) is used in severe cases to control overactivity. Once the patient is able to cooperate, kidney and thyroid function should be tested and **lithium** or other antimanic drugs can be started. Adjuvant therapy with other BZD helps to calm the patients and induce sleep.

For moderately severe euphoric patients, the immediate **treatment** of acute mania includes either **lithium, sodium valproate** or **carbamazepine.** However, all the three drugs have delayed onset of effects.

SODIUM VALPROATE: This antiepilectic drug (Chapter 9) acts faster and produces beneficial effects in 3–5 days. It is preferred as first choice drug. It is as effective as lithium during early weeks and is often effective in patients not responding to lithium. Its mechanism of action in psychosis is not known. It can be combined with lithium and is much less toxic.

PS 7.6

Lithium salts also remain the treatment of choice in acute manic state and are effective as monotherapy in mild to moderate mania. They should be used only in patients with normal sodium intake. Lithium carbonate is usually given initially in the loading dose of 600 mg followed by 300 mg b.i.d. or t.i.d. The dose is increased by 300 mg every 2–3 days till plasma levels are 1–1.5 mEq/L. It takes 2–3 weeks for full therapeutic effect. TDM is mandatory. In patients resistant to lithium, sodium valproate or atypical APD may be added.

CARBAMAZEPINE: Response rate to carbamazepine is lower than that seen with lithium or sodium valproate but it can be used as an alternative to lithium (Chapter 9).

Lamotrigine though may be useful (Table 14.4) it takes longer time for titrating the effective dose.

In severe and refractory bipolar depression, lithium or sodium valproate is combined with either conventional / atypical APD. *However, in such cases, ECT is preferred because of its proven, rapid antidepressant effect.*

For patients in depressive state or those having severe depression with psychosis, refer Table 14.4 for choice of drug therapy.

For long-term prophylaxis of MDP, lithium or carbamazepine are the preferred agents. **Sodium valproate or lamotrigine** are also used for maintenance.

Psychotropic drug combinations: It is rational to combine various psychotropic drugs when psychiatric illnesses are associated with a comorbid condition which needs to be treated. Thus, schizophrenia is often associated with depression which needs combined therapy with an APD and antidepressant. Combinations are also needed in the treatment of MDP and BZD are often combined with antidepressants in patients with associated insomnia. However, such combinations must be chosen with specific goals in mind. The dangers of combinations are:

- *The opposing effects may attenuate the desired therapeutic effect.*
- *The summation of the anticholinergic effects of phenothiazines, the tricyclics and antiparkinsonian agents may produce bladder or bowel paralysis, precipitate an attack of acute glaucoma or cause mental symptoms.*
- *There exists a possibility of increased potential drug interactions.*

Several psychotropic drugs and other drugs are substrates for CYP2D6, e.g.: citalopram, desipramine, chlorpromazine, risperidone, etc. or to CYP3A4, e.g. alprazolam, diazepam, carbamazepine, etc. or to both, e.g. fluoxetine, sertraline, amitriptyline, imipramine, haloperidol, etc. Moreover, drugs like fluoxetine inhibits CYP3A4 or CYP2D6. When these drugs are co -administered, they may compete for the same

Table 14.4 Pharmacotherapy of Bipolar Depression (MDP)

	Preferred Drugs	If No Response
I Acute mania		
Moderate, euphoric	Sodium valproate/carbamazepine/lithium/ atypical APD; if agitation/insomnia: add lorazepam/clonazepam	Two drug combination: (a) lithium+ sodium valproate/atypical APD and (b) sodium valproate + atypical APD
Severe, psychotic	Lithium/sodium valproate + APD-either conventional or atypical	Lithium + haloperidol; lorazepam + lamotrigine. If refractory, add clozapine; ECT
II Depressive state		
Moderate	Lithium/quetiapine[a] ± SSRI	Lamotrigine (+bupropion if needed)
Severe	Lithium/quetiapine+ SSRI/bupropion/ venlafaxine	*Levothyroxine in supraphysiological doses*
III Severe depression with psychosis	Lithium + APD + SSRI/bupropion/ venlafaxine; *levothyroxine in supraphysiological doses*	ECT
IV Long-term prophylaxis	Lithium or carbamazepine as monotherapy; lamotrigine for depressive symptoms	Valproic acid + olanzapine; *levothyroxine in small doses*

Notes: Levothyroxine is used *only* as an adjunctive drug along with other definitive drugs.
APD, antipsychotic drug; ECT, electroconvulsive therapy; SSRI, selective serotonin reuptake inhibitors; fluoxetine/sertaline/paroxetine may be preferred.
[a]Other second-generation APD like olanzapine and lurasidone can be used.

enzyme and if one of them is an inducer or inhibitor of the enzyme then it may enhance or inhibit the metabolism of others leading to either its therapeutic failure or toxicity.

ANTIANXIETY DRUGS

Benzodiazepines

- Diazepam
- Lorazepam
- Clonazepam
- Alprazolam
- Oxazepam

Azapirones

- Buspirone
- Gepirone
- Ipsapirone
- Trospirone

Selective serotonin reuptake inhibitors

- Fluoxetine
- Paroxetine
- Sertraline

Adjuvants

- Beta blockers (Propranolol)
- sedative antihistaminics (Hydroxyzine, Diphenhydramine, Buclizine)
- Sedative tricyclic antidepressants (Amitriptyline, Doxepin)

ANTIDEPRESSANTS

Monoamine oxidase inhibitors (MAOI)

Irreversible

Hydrazine MAOI
- Isocarboxazid
- Iproniazid
- Phenelzine

Nonhydrazine MAOI
- Tranylcypromine

Reversible (RIMA)

- Moclobemide

Tricyclic antidepressants

NA+ 5HT reuptake inhibitors
- Imipramine
- Doxepine

Predominantly NA reuptake inhibitors
- Desimipramine
- Amitriptyline
- Protriptyline

Predominantly 5HT reuptake inhibitor
- Clomipramine

Selective serotonin (5-HT) reuptake inhibitors (SSRI)

- Fluoxetine
- Paroxetine
- Fluvoxamine
- Sertraline
- Citalopram
- Escitalopram

Newer antidepressants

Selective 5-HT-NA reuptake inhibitors (SNRI)

- Venlafaxine
- Duloxetine
- Milnacipran
- Desvenlaflaxine
- Levomilnacipran

Selective NA reuptake inhibitor (NARI)

- Reboxetine

5-HT_2 receptor antagonists

- Trazodone
- Nefazodone
- Mirtazapine
- Mianserin
- Vortioxetine

Miscellaneous

Unicyclic

- Bupropion

Tetracyclic

- Amoxapine
- Maprotiline

Atypical antipsychotics

- Quetiapine
- Olanzapine
- Aripiprazole
- Brexpiprazole

Others

- Tianeptine
- Esketamine
- Brexanolone

CHAPTER 15

Drug Therapy of Parkinsonism and Other Neurodegenerative Disorders

Learning Objectives

This chapter will enable the reader:

1. To be aware of pathophysiology of parkinsonism and neurotransmitters involved.
2. To enumerate drugs inducing parkinsonism, giving rationale for its manifestation.
3. To state the therapeutic goals.
4. To classify anti-parkinsonian drugs based on their mechanism of action giving examples of drugs.
5. To describe mechanism of action, pharmacological effects, salient pharmacokinetic features, ADR and drug interactions of levodopa, MAO-B inhibitors, COMT inhibitors, dopamine releaser, D_2 agonist and anticholinergics.
6. To explain pharmacological basis for use of combination of carbidopa and levodopa, highlighting the advantages and limitations of such use.
7. To justify treatment strategies for parkinsonism.
8. To state various extrapyramidal reactions and treatment for the same.
9. To mention the drugs used in the treatment of following diseases giving rationale for their use: (a) motor neuron disease, (b) Alzheimer's disease and (c) multiple sclerosis.
10. To enumerate drugs used to treat (a) tremors, (b) chorea, (c) dystonia and (d) myoclonus.

KEY TERMS

Parkinsonism as a clinical entity was first described by James Parkinson in 1817 (Parkinson disease; PD; paralysis agitans). *It is a syndrome of varied aetiology and its important features are bradykinesia, muscular rigidity, postural instability, loss of associated movements and tremor.* Excessive salivation, seborrhoea, depression and liver damage may occur.

Besides the idiopathic PD, arteriosclerotic and post-encephalitic forms, the syndrome is seen in hepatolenticular degeneration of Wilson disease and can be induced by drugs like haloperidol, triperidol, chlorpromazine, other halogenated phenothiazines and reserpine.

Pathophysiology: The basal ganglia consist of the corpus striatum (the caudate nucleus and the putamen), globus pallidus and substantia nigra. They modulate **the extrapyramidal (EP) control of motor activity.** The substantia nigra pars compacta (SNpc, which is rich in dopaminergic neuronal cell bodies), projects to the corpus striatum where dopamine is released. Corpus striatum, in turn, projects back via the globus pallidus and substantia nigra pars reticulata (SNpr) to the thalamus and finally to the cerebral motor cortex, and regulates their involvement in voluntary movement (Fig. 15.1). The nigro-striatal neurons make efferent connections with the striatum where they make contact with two types of striatal neurons bearing: (a) **excitatory D_1 receptors** and (b) **inhibitory D_2 receptors.**

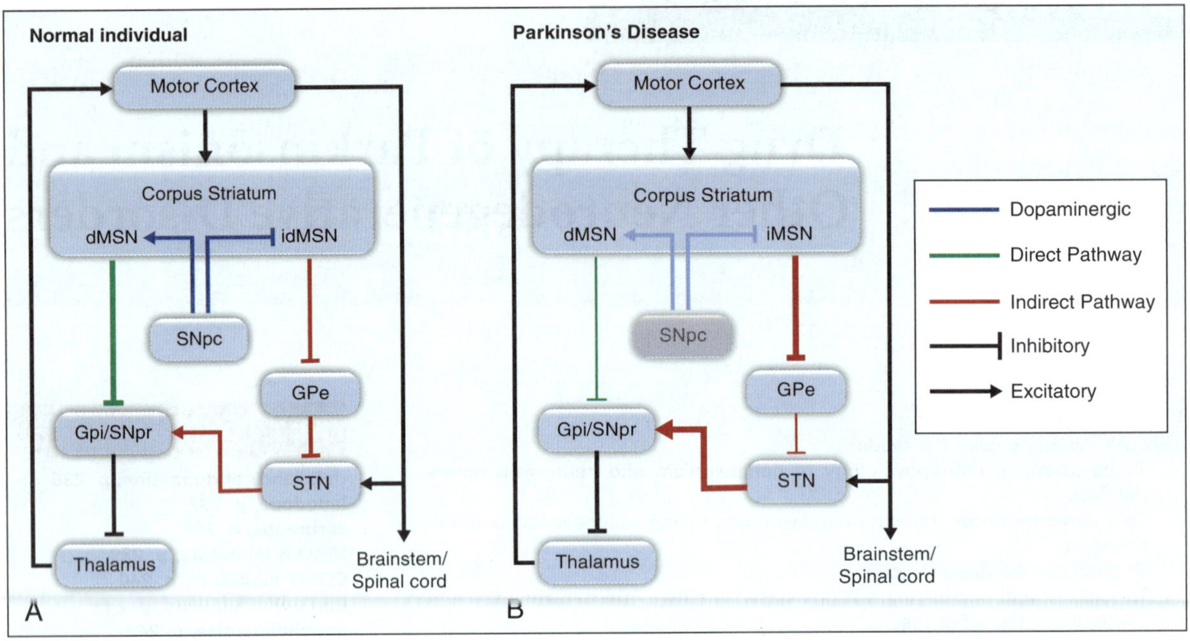

FIG. 15.1 Dopaminergic pathway in basal ganglia in a normal individual and in a patient with Parkinson's disease SNc = Dopaminergic neurons of pars compacta; MSN= Medium Spiny neurons having GABAergic Inhibitory Cells; GPi = Globus pallidus pars interna; Gpe= Globus pallidus pars externa; SNr =Substantia nigra pars reticulata; STN = Subthalamic nucleus

The neurons which possess D_1 receptors relay impulses via a **direct excitatory pathway**; on the other hand the neurons which bear D_2 receptors relay impulses via an **indirect inhibitory pathway** to the same cerebral motor cortical neurons.

As shown in Fig 15.1A, in **normal individuals,** dopamine (DA) from the dopaminergic neurons of SNpc activates direct (excitatory) pathway and inhibits indirect (inhibitory) pathway in the straitum. This effect decreases globus pallidus par interna (GPi) output, releasing inhibition on the thalamus and cortex and promoting movement. Degenerative changes in the dopaminergic neurons of SNpc in PD causes deficiency of DA. This results in hypoactivity of the direct pathway and hyperactivity of the indirect pathway, which leads to excessive GPi output (Fig 15.1B). The resulting over-inhibition of the thalamus and cortex suppresses movements. This accounts for the major symptoms and signs of PD. Other defects may account for the unrelieved symptoms and signs, e.g. degeneration of the noradrenergic locus coeruleus may contribute to autonomic symptoms and depression; and degeneration of the cholinergic nucleus basalis may account for the dementia. Thus, the clinical features of PD can be explained by a combination of:

- Predominantly dopamine deficiency
- Relative cholinergic preponderance
- Increased activity of GABAergic neurons in basal ganglia
- NA deficiency

As no drug can halt the progressive loss of the nigrostriatal neurons, the disease is progressive and incurable. PH 1.19

Classification of Antiparkinsonian Drugs:

I. **Those that increase the dopaminergic (DA) activity:**
   - **Precursors of DA,** e.g. Levodopa
   - **Drugs that inhibit DA metabolism**
     i. MAO-B inhibitors, e.g. Selegiline
     ii. COMT inhibitors, e.g. Tolcapone, entacapone
   - **Drugs that release DA,** e.g. Amantadine
   - **DA receptor agonists**

i. Ergot derived: Bromocriptine
ii. Nonergot: Pramipexole, ropinirole

II. **Those that suppress the cholinergic activity:** Atropine, Benztropine, benzhexol, procyclidine and antihistaminics with anticholinergic properties.

LEVODOPA: Levodopa, 3–4, dihydroxyphenylalanine (Fig. 15.2), is a 'universal anti-Parkinsonian drug'.

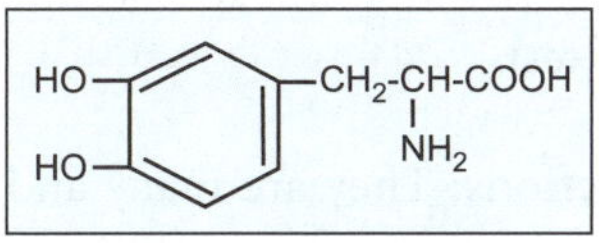

FIG. 15.2 **Levodopa.**

Mechanism of action: Levodopa, a prodrug, is a metabolic precursor of DA (Chapter 18). It crosses the BBB by an active process and is taken up by the dopaminergic neurons and is decarboxylated to DA. Levodopa can, thus, be looked upon as a 'replacement therapy'. *Dopamine itself does not cross the BBB and hence is ineffective.*

In advanced PD, as there are few dopaminergic neurons remaining, levodopa becomes less and less effective. In the peripheral tissues, such as the liver and the kidneys, it is converted to DA which accounts for its peripheral effects.

Pharmacological actions:

CNS actions: Levodopa improves all the major manifestations of PD. Bradykinesia responds first, followed by rigidity and tremor. Other manifestations such as seborrhoea, sialorrhoea and aphonia may also improve. The drug improves mood, memory and makes the patients more alert and interested in themselves and in their surroundings. About 30% of the patients show 'impressive' improvement, whereas another 30% show 'worthwhile' improvement. In general, younger patients with milder symptoms derive greater benefit than elderly, debilitated patients.

Levodopa has also been found to ameliorate idiopathic dystonia in children and adolescents.

Cardiovascular actions: It produces its cardiovascular effects by being converted peripherally to DA which,

- *Acts on specific dopaminergic receptors to cause renal and mesenteric vasodilatation* which causes fall in BP following small doses.
- *Stimulates beta-adrenergic receptors in the heart (positive inotropic action).* This effect can be blocked by beta blockers
- *Stimulates alpha-adrenergic receptors in blood vessels* to produce vasoconstriction. Thus, *large doses* of levodopa may cause rise in BP which can be countered by alpha-adrenergic blocking agents such as prazosin.

These effects can be prevented following prior administration of a decarboxylase (DC) inhibitor such as carbidopa, which does not cross the BBB.

Endocrine actions: Levodopa inhibits prolactin secretion and suppresses lactation by acting on the D_2 receptors on the pituitary lactotropes.

Absorption, fate and excretion: The drug is rapidly absorbed from the small intestine by active transport with peak plasma levels at ½–2 h, and its plasma t½ is 1–3 h. As more than 95% of orally taken levodopa is rapidly decarboxylated to DA in the lumen of the GI tract, liver (first pass effect) and other tissues, less than 1% is left to enter the CNS. Hence, large doses of levodopa are needed to raise brain DA level. Pyridoxine accelerates its peripheral decarboxylation as the DC is pyridoxine dependent.

The blood levels of levodopa can be increased by inhibiting the DC by using **DC inhibitors** (see section on Dopa decarboxylase inhibitors). Since the DC inhibitors do not penetrate the BBB, conversion of levodopa to DA in the brain is not affected.

As high protein content of a meal interferes with the absorption of l-DOPA, the drug is taken 1 h before or 1 h after a meal. Only in patients difficult to control, who need frequent doses and who have a fluctuating motor response, protein intake should be restricted.

It is metabolised by both MAO and COMT. The drug is excreted in the urine partly unchanged and partly as DA and mainly as its metabolite, homovanillic acid. Some of the drug is also converted to NA. The dose of l-DOPA generally needs no adjustment in patients with renal or hepatic disease.

Adverse reactions: Almost every patient may show some adverse effect. Behavioural and CNS effects occur during prolonged treatment, and as tolerance does not develop to these symptoms, they prove dose-limiting.

1. **Early ADR:**
   - **GI:** Nausea, vomiting and anorexia are common. Due to its action on CTZ and are minimised by taking levodopa with food, by increasing the dose slowly and by domperidone 10 mg t.i.d. *Carbidopa, in addition to that present in the levodopa–carbidopa combination, in the dose of 25 mg three times a day may help in resistant cases.*
   - **Cardiovascular:** It causes:
   a. Postural hypotension, generally asymptomatic, by its central action; *this is not prevented by DC inhibitors;* instead it can be helped by fludrocortisone.
   b. Peripherally, DA causes palpitation, sinus tachycardia, increased A-V conduction and ventricular arrhythmias; these can be countered by a DC inhibitor and by adrenergic beta blocker such as atenolol. Tolerance develops over weeks to postural hypotension as well as to the cardiac effects.
2. **Late ADR:**
   - **Behavioural:** This includes agitation, confusion, restlessness, hypomania, hallucinations, delusions and depression with attempted suicide. The drug exacerbates latent or active psychotic states, making it necessary to abandon treatment. *The use of conventional antipsychotics may worsen PD. Patients with history of psychiatric disturbances should not be treated with levodopa.*
   - **CNS:** On prolonged therapy, abnormal movements (dyskinesia, e.g. **choreoathetosis**) involving head, neck and sometimes even the extremities may occur. They can be quite disturbing and even incapacitating. *They are not prevented by a DC inhibitor(see section management of PD).*

     Parkinsonian patients suffer from insomnia but do not complain of it because their daytime symptoms are more disabling. An improvement in their daytime symptoms can make them more aware of their insomnia.

     A syndrome similar to the **neuroleptic malignant syndrome** (Chapter 13) can occur rarely after rapid reduction in dosage or abrupt discontinuation of levodopa.
3. **Miscellaneous:** Blood urea nitrogen and serum SGOT may show a transient rise. Rise in plasma cholesterol levels and a decrease in carbohydrate tolerance can occur.

   The urine is red coloured when passed and becomes dark on exposure to air or alkali. It gives a false positive test for ketone bodies with the dip-stick test.

Drug interactions: They are many and are listed in Box 15.1.

Anticholinergics, benzodiazepines, tricylic antidepressants, diuretics, oral hypoglycemic agents, antibiotics, glyceryl trinitrate, digoxin, propranolol and antiarrhythmic agents may, however, be safely used along with levodopa.

Preparations and dosage: Levodopa tablets as 100, 200, 250 and 500 mg. The initial dose is 50 mg t.i.d. in combination with carbidopa increased progressively (see section, Management of parkinsonism).

As the drug has a short plasma t½, frequent dosage is necessary to maintain asteady therapeutic effect and to minimise ADR. *Concurrent administration of a DC*

Box 15.1 Drug Interactions of Levodopa

- MAOI may precipitate severe hypertension. They should be stopped two weeks before starting levodopa therapy
- Pyridoxine accelerates the peripheral decarboxylation of levodopa
- Reserpine and phenothiazines antagonise the effects of levodopa
- Methyldopa intensifies the adverse effects of levodopa
- Anticholinergics increase the stay of levodopa in the stomach and increase its degradation. They should be taken, if needed, 2 h before levodopa
- Sympathomimetics such as adrenaline and isoprenaline should be avoided in patients on levodopa
- Coadministration of an antihypertensive drugs could increase the risk of orthostatic hypotension.
- Levodopa increases the cardiac toxicity of halothane anaesthesia

inhibitor permits a 75% reduction in the daily dose of levodopa. Hence, combination is always preferred.

In patients with advanced PD, gastric emptying may be delayed and unpredictable, which can affect the rate and extent of levodopa/carbidopa absorption and its efficacy. Hence formulations have been developed to overcome this difficulty, e.g. levodopa/carbidopa enteral suspension/ intestinal gel formulation, which is administered as a continuous 16-hour infusion via a percutaneous endoscopic gastrostomy with jejunal tube connected to a portable infusion pump. The infusion rate and total dose administered can be customized to control symptoms and minimize dyskinesia, and patients can self-administer extra doses to manage acute off symptoms.

Only Levodopa dry powder inhaler is another such formulation for intermittent treatment of off episodes in patients with PD.

DECARBOXYLASE INHIBITORS (DCI): By themselves, these drugs are inactive. *They do not enter the brain. Their concurrent administration decreases the peripheral decarboxylation of levodopa to DA, thus increasing l-DOPA plasma level. This endows certain advantages* (Box 15.2).

Postural hypotension, abnormal involuntary movements and psychiatric disturbances, all of which are central in origin, are not prevented or eliminated by use of DC inhibitors.

Carbidopa (methyl DOPA hydrazine) and **benserazide** hydrochloride are the two DC inhibitors available in combination with levodopa. They are available as:

1. **Carbidopa and levodopa in the ratio of 1:10.** Approximately 75–100 mg of carbidopa is needed to totally block the effect of DOPA-DC. Sustained release preparations and disintegrating tablets are also available.
2. **Benserazide and levodopa in the ratio of 1:4.** The dose, expressed as levodopa, is initially 50–125 mg 3–4 times a day; the maintenance dose is 0.75–1.0 g per day.

Box 15.2 Advantages of Adding DCI to Levodopa

- The dose of levodopa can be reduced by as much as 75%
- Nausea, vomiting and cardiac effects are largely prevented
- This permits more rapid increase in the dose of levodopa to optimum level
- Pyridoxine does not antagonise the effects of levodopa and can be given concurrently
- The control of symptoms is smoother and wide diurnal fluctuations are avoided
- The number of daily doses can be reduced without loss of control

MAO-B INHIBITORS

SELEGILINE: *It is a relatively selective, irreversible inhibitor of MAO-B.* It prevents DA from degradation and thus increases the concentration and storage of DA within the striatum. Hence, it prolongs the duration of improvement brought about by levodopa. Further, it diminishes the diurnal fluctuations in physical strength and reduces the end-of-dose 'wearing-off' effects. It has no antidepressant action.

Adverse reactions: They are due to an increase in the incidence of central dopaminergic effects, e.g. dyskinesia, nausea and hallucinations. As selegiline is a MAO inhibitor, the drug should be discontinued for some time before starting an antidepressant.

Selegiline is generally well tolerated in mild PD. However, in advanced disease, it may accentuate the adverse motor and cognitive effects of levodopa. Metabolites of selegiline include amphetamine and methamphetamine, which may cause anxiety and insomnia. Its use with pethidine or an SSRI can precipitate serotonergic reaction.

The daily dose is 10 mg, administered as 5 mg at breakfast and at lunch. Administration later in the day can cause insomnia. Higher doses can cause inhibition of MAO-A as well and should be avoided.

Rasagiline is another MAO-B inhibitor, claimed to be more potent and selective. The dose is 0.5-1 mg every morning.

Clinical studies have indicated that the mortality due to hypertensive crises may be higher in patients treated with levodopa–carbidopa–selegiline combination than in those with levodopa–carbidopa combination. *Hence, newly diagnosed patients should not be treated with such triple drug regimens.*

Both rasagiline and selegiline can be used as monotherapy in early disease and can delay initiation of levodopa/carbidopa treatment. Added to levodopa in advanced disease, it can permit use of lower doses of levodopa. Recently, reversible MAO-B inhibitor **safinamide** is approved for use in a dose of 100 mg every morning as an adjunct to carbidopa/ levodopa in patients with PD.

COMT INHIBITORS

TOLCAPONE: When levodopa is administered with DCI, it gets metabolised mainly by COMT. The resultant metabolite 3, O methyldopa competes with levodopa for a carrier required for its transport across GI mucosa and BBB and decreases its bioavailability. This affects therapeutic response to levodopa. Tolcapone inhibits COMT and reduces the central and peripheral, metabolic degradation of levodopa, which prolongs its plasma t½. *Given alone, it is not useful.* Adverse effects reported are nausea, orthostatic hypotension, dyskinesia, diarrhoea, urine discoloration, induction of hallucinations due to increase in the serum level of levodopa and serious hepatotoxicity. It is used as an adjunct to l-DOPA in a dose of 100-200 mg tid.

Entacapone, an analogue, is claimed to be less hepatotoxic than tolcapone. *Its action is primarily peripheral and is of shorter duration as compared to tolcapone.* It has been effective in decreasing daily off time by about 1 hour, improving motor scores, and reducing levodopa requirements in patients with motor fluctuations. It is available both alone to be given as 200 mg with each levodopa dose and in a fixed dose combination with carbidopa and levodopa **Opicapone** acts peripherally and appears to be similar in efficacy to entacapone; it offers the advantage of once-daily administration in a dose of 50 mg (at night).

Coadministration of a COMT inhibitor and a nonselective MAOI can result in decreased metabolism of catecholamines and toxicity. Additive CNS depressant effects could occur if COMT inhibitors are used concurrently with any drug that causes CNS depression or sedation.

Concomitant use of methylphenidate, amphetamines, and an MAO-B inhibitor can result in severe hypertension.

DOPAMINE RELEASERS

AMANTADINE: This drug, developed originally as an antiviral agent, has been found to ameliorate bradykinesia, rigidity and tremor in parkinsonism. **It acts by liberating DA from the residual intact nerve terminals.** It also inhibits the activity of NMDA receptors and has some antimuscarinic action. Its therapeutic efficacy is 15%–20% that of levodopa. However, it produces a more rapid response (2–5 days) than levodopa and is less toxic. The drug is well absorbed orally and is excreted unchanged in urine (Chapter 57).

Adverse reactions: In general, the drug is well tolerated. The ADR are similar to those of anticholinergic drugs whose adverse effects it potentiates. Nausea, dizziness, myoclonus, insomnia, confusion, hallucinations, peripheral edema, and livedo reticularis (net-like reddish-blue skin discoloration) can occur. QT-interval prolongation and torsades de pointes have been associated with amantadine overdose. In toxic doses, it causes convulsions and mania. Sudden withdrawal of amantadine may cause severe exacerbation of parkinsonian symptoms, confusion, neuroleptic malignant syndrome, and acute delirium. Patients taking amantadine should be advised not to consume alcohol. Elimination of amantadine is enhanced in acidic urine, hence drugs that alkalinize the urine, such as carbonic anhydrase inhibitors, can increase amantadine concentrations and the risk of adverse effects.

The dose is 100 mg per day, increased to 100 mg twice a day after 7–10 days. As restlessness is one of its major adverse effects, the second dose should not be taken late in the day. Extended release formulations are also available to permit single dosing.

Addition of amantadine in patients receiving near maximum benefit from levodopa causes little further improvement. It is used as an adjunct to l-DOPA; tolerance to it develops quickly. It is also used as antidyskinesia agent in patients with advanced disease.

DOPAMINE (D_2) AGONISTS

In general, the dopamine agonists used in the treatment of PD (Table 15.1):

1. Do not require functional nigrostriatal neuron.
2. Do not need conversion to active metabolite.
3. Have substantially longer duration of action than levodopa.
4. Are better tolerated.
5. Are administered in higher doses in parkinsonism than in hyperprolactinemia.

Dopamine agonists are less effective than levodopa/carbidopa treating the motor symptoms of PD, and the possibility of motor fluctuations and dyskinesia is less. They are effective as monotherapy in early, mild disease, but as disease advances, most patients require addition of levodopa/carbidopa. In advanced disease, dopamine agonists can be used as an adjuncts to reduce motor fluctuations. This allows the use of lower doses of levodopa.

BROMOCRIPTINE: This synthetic ergoline acts as a specific dopamine D_2 receptor agonist (Chapter 65). It crosses the BBB. It is slower acting than levodopa. It causes nausea by its dopaminergic action on the medullary CTZ. This can be treated by domperidone (Chapter 39). Bromocriptine causes serious long term adverse effects like pleural as well as retroperitoneal fibrosis and digital spasms It is no longer recommended for the treatment of PD.

Table 15.1 Dopamine Agonists Used in Parkinsonism

Drug	Dose
Ergot derived (ergolines)	
Bromocriptine	20–30 mg/day
Nonergot derived	
Ropinirole	Up to 24 mg/day
Pramipexole	Up to 4.5 mg/day
Rotigotine	4–6 mg/day, transdermal patch
Apomorphine	Parenteral dose as needed (2-8 mg), after priming with an antiemetic such as domperidone

Note: All drugs except rotigotine and apomorphine are given orally.

ROPINIROLE: This synthetic nonergoline, a selective D_2 agonist, is well absorbed and its actions are similar to those of bromocriptine. However, it is effective within a week or less. The adverse reactions include nausea (40%), edema, somnolence, vomiting, dizziness and fatigue. It may cause sudden sleep attacks, postural hypotension, confusion and psychosis. Pathological gambling and other compulsive behaviours have been reported. The drug causes embryonic loss in animals.

Pramipexole has properties similar to those of ropinirole. It particularly induces impulse control disorders including pathologic gambling, hypersexuality, uncontrollable spending, and excessive computer use. When such symptoms are detected, dopamine agonists should be tapered and stopped, and treatment with levodopa, which is less likely to cause these adverse effects, should be initiated.

Rotigotine, a nonergot DA agonist, is available as transdermal patch. Application-site reactions and nail dyschromia have occurred with this patch.

All the dopamine agonists in large doses can cause severe neuropsychiatric adverse effects. Withdrawal of dopamine agonists should be done gradually because it can lead to development of physical and psychological symptoms in some patients, particularly those with impulse control disorders; these include anxiety, dysphoria, irritability, fatigue, suicidal ideation, generalized pain, and drug cravings.

For pharmacological effects of **apomorphine**, see Chapter 10. Subcutaneous injection of apomorphine, a dopamine agonist, is effective for intermittent acute treatment of off episodes in PD patients with motor fluctuations. Apomorphine sublingual film is also effective in relieving off episodes, but chances of discontinuation of therapy are higher because of oropharyngeal adverse effects. Serotonin receptor antagonists such as ondansetron are contraindicated for use with apomorphine because the combination can cause severe hypotension with loss of consciousness.

ISTRADEFYLLINE: This is a selective adenosine A_{2A} receptor antagonist, approved for use as an adjunct to levodopa/carbidopa in patients with PD who experience off episodes. The exact mechanism of action of the drug in PD is unknown. Adenosine A_{2A} receptors are located on neurons in the striatum that form the indirect output pathway from the striatum to the globus pallidus. Hence, adjunctive treatment with istradefylline decreases off time and increases on time without troublesome dyskinesia. Istradefylline is administered orally in a dose of 20-40 mg per day and metabolized primarily by CYP1A1 and 3A4.

Adverse effects include dyskinesia, nausea, constipation, dizziness, hallucinations, and insomnia. It may increase the risk of impulse control disorders. It is an expensive drug.

ANTICHOLINERGICS

By their antimuscarinic action, these drugs diminish the cholinergic preponderance and can relieve, to some extent, rigidity, tremor, hyperhidrosis, seborrhoea and sialorrhoea. Further some atropine substitutes (e.g. benztropine) inhibit active DA reuptake in the striatum and increase the local DA concentration. In general, anticholinergics are less effective but safer than levodopa. They are in use since many years in the treatment of Parkinsonism; they are often the only drugs patients can afford for prolonged periods. **Benzhexol** is discussed below in detail as a prototype.

BENZHEXOL HYDROCHLORIDE (Trihexyphenidyl): Benzhexol is the most commonly used atropine substitute for parkinsonism. It has weaker peripheral anticholinergic actions and is well tolerated.

Pharmacological actions: The drug is useful in controlling muscular rigidity, tremor, sialorrhoea and seborrhoea. It improves the mood. It does not improve bradykinesia and loss of postural reflexes significantly. Like atropine, larger doses cause cerebral stimulation.

Absorption, fate and excretion: Benzhexol is well absorbed orally. It rapidly disappears from the tissues but its fate is unknown.

Adverse reactions: It is free from serious adverse reactions; however, atropine-like side effects may develop even in therapeutic doses in 10%–20% of patients. These include xerostomia, blurred vision, nausea, dizziness, restlessness and urinary retention in the presence of prostatic enlargement. Overdosage causes confusion, hallucinations and delirium.

Preparations and dosage: It is available as 2 and 5 mg tablets and 5 mg sustained release capsules. Oral solution as 1 mg/ml is also available. The initial dose is 1–2 mg, increased gradually up to 10–15 mg per day. A single dose of the sustained release capsule maintains the effect for 15 h and may be employed after initial stabilisation. The central stimulation produced by the drug can be countered by combining it with diphenhydramine.

Indications: It is generally used in combination with l-DOPA. It can be used even in the presence of hypertension and cardiac disease. *It is effective in drug-induced parkinsonism and is helpful in postencephalitic parkinsonism.*

It is also useful in certain forms of dystonias. The other drugs used are listed in Table 15.2.

Table 15.2 Drugs with Atropine-Like Action Used in Parkinsonism

Drug	Dosage (mg/day)
Synthetic atropine substitutes:	
Benzhexol	2–10
Cycrimine HCl	5–20
Procyclidine HCl	7.5–30
Biperiden HCl	2–10
Benztropine mesylate[a]	1.5–4
Antihistaminics	
Diphenhydramine HCl	50–100
Promethazine HCl[b]	25
Orphenadrine HCl	150–250

[a]A potent blocker of reuptake of dopamine; has a prolonged action and a sedative effect.

[b]Useful intravenously, in rapidly controlling drug-induced acute dystonic reactions. Other doses are oral.

MISCELLANEOUS

Certain **phenothiazines/antihistaminics** (Table 15.2) used to treat parkinsonism also have anticholinergic action. **Diphenhydramine** (50–100 mg/day) is well tolerated. It relieves rigidity but not tremor or sialorrhoea. It can cause drowsiness and giddiness. **Promethazine** (25 mg intravenously) is useful in rapidly controlling acute drug induced dystonic reactions (Chapter 23).

MANAGEMENT OF PARKINSONISM

The aims of therapy in PD are outlined in Box 15.3 and include:

- **Relief of rigidity, tremors and bradykinesia:** Most of the drugs reduce rigidity more than tremor and bradykinesia. Tremor, in fact, may be aggravated after reduction in rigidity. Levodopa ameliorates all the three. Tremor is best relieved by anticholinergic drugs. Physiotherapy acts as a valuable adjunct in such cases.
- **Correction of mood changes:** Most parkinsonian patients have a mild intellectual disability as a result of frontal lobe dysfunction. **Depression** is often a marked feature of arteriosclerotic parkinsonism. If the primary drug employed fails to correct it, a SSRI may be helpful.
- **Treatment of other symptoms** such as excessive salivation, seborrhoea and of complications like oculogyric or sweating crisis.
- **Treatment of the cause, if possible:** Parkinsonism following drugs is completely reversible after stopping the drugs. Reduction in high tissue copper levels associated with Wilson disease also results in some relief.

Successful management of parkinsonism depends on a multidisciplinary approach, and demands compassionate care of the patient. The various forms of treatment available are (i) drug therapy; (ii) nonpharmacologic therapy comprising education, support, physiotherapy, nutrition; and (iii) surgery. PH 1.19, IM 19.8

Box 15.3 Aims of Therapy of Parkinsonism

- Relief of rigidity, tremor and bradykinesia
- Correction of mood changes and control of psychotic symptoms
- Treatment of other symptoms
- Treatment of cause, when possible

DRUG THERAPY

Levodopa still remains the most effective drug in the treatment of Parkinson disease. However, its adverse effects make continued close supervision mandatory. In general, l-DOPA should be started as soon as the patient's symptoms interfere with the quality of life. Many patients derive substantial benefit from l-DOPA over the entire course of their illness. Levodopa increases life expectancy in patients with PD, and survival is significantly reduced if the administration is delayed until greater disability develops. Hence, some authorities advocate early treatment with l-DOPA or dopamine agonist such as ropinirole to provide improved quality of life. However, dopamine agonists are expensive.

Levodopa is commonly used in combination with a DC inhibitor, carbidopa. **This combination promotes active life, and should be prescribed for patients who are incapacitated due to severe disease.** It is preferred in elderly patients (older than 70 years) who tolerate anticholinergics poorly.

Usual starting dose is 50 mg of l-DOPA with 12.5 mg of carbidopa given 8 hourly. Dose is then gradually increased till maximum benefit is achieved without serious toxicity; this may be 500–1000 mg daily in 3–4 divided doses. If no benefit is observed even with a dose of 1000 mg, the clinical diagnosis of PD should be reviewed. Its withdrawal, if necessary, must be gradual as sudden withdrawal may precipitate symptoms resembling neuroleptic malignant syndrome. Levodopa can be combined with amantadine, dopaminergic agonists or COMT inhibitors.

Some experts recommend MAO-B inhibitor for patients with mild symptoms considering its good safety profile. It is also advocated to start therapy with multiple drugs (levodopa, dopamine agonist, COMT Inhibitor, MAO-B Inhibitor) used at lower doses. This may avoid ADR associated with high doses of any single agent.

Drawbacks of long term levodopa treatment are as follows:

- **Dyskinesias** involving involuntary choreoform movements, and rapid fluctuations in motor strength (dystonia).
- **Motor symptoms** that include:

a. ***Predictable 'off' periods of immobility*** or greater severity of Parkinsonian signs, when the medication effect 'wears off'. This has a relation to the timing of the anti-Parkinsonian medication and can be helped by a COMT inhibitor (entacapone).

b. ***Unpredictable 'on–off' fluctuations*** which are of sudden occurrence (lasting for seconds) of shifts between on and off periods that are apparently not related to the timing of medication. With the passage of time, 60% of initial responders start experiencing 'end-of-dose' wearing effect (advanced disease).

They are managed by combination therapy and if refractory, treatment options like surgery, DBS or infusion devices for continuous dopaminergic drug delivery are opted for.

- **Psychiatric complications** are due to the stimulant action of levodopa on dopamine receptors in the mesolimbic and mesocortical dopamine systems. An atypical antipsychotic such as clozapine may be helpful. **Pimavanserin** (Chapter 13), a 5-HT_{2A} inverse agonist and antagonist, has been approved for treatment of hallucinations and delusions associated with PD psychosis. It does not block dopaminergic, muscarinic, adrenergic and histaminergic receptors and therefore is devoid of the undesirable effects associated with antipsychotics. It appears to be effective for the short term for treatment of psychotic symptoms without exacerbating motor symptoms.

Dopamine agonists especially the nonergot derivatives are better tolerated and less toxic, but, have limited efficacy. In addition, with prolonged use, their effect diminishes.

Synthetic atropine substitutes are still important in the treatment of parkinsonism, **benzhexol** being the most effective. They, in combination with physiotherapy, may be sufficient and cost effective in the relatively inactive patients with minimal disease and no functional impairment. They are particularly well tolerated by and hence preferred in the 'younger' patients (younger than 50 years), in whom cognitive impairment is rare. However, early levodopa/carbidopa therapy is indicated even in these younger patients. Treatment with benzhexol should be started with a small dose and increased gradually. *As maximally tolerated doses do not give much more benefit than slightly smaller and better tolerated doses, no attempt should be made to push the dose to the limit of tolerance.* Anticholinergics can be combined with either amantadine or levodopa. *However, it is better to avoid such combination if there is history of psychosis or dementia.*

Diphenhydramine, an **antihistaminic** is particularly useful in elderly patients with mild disease, who cannot tolerate the anticholinergic drugs. Further, they help to counter the insomnia in patients on levodopa or anticholinergics.

Amantadine is a useful alternative to anticholinergic drugs in patients with mild PD. It can also be used as an adjunct in patients who are unable to tolerate levodopa. It may help in dyskinesias.

Disease-slowing benefit observed following selegiline given initially is now thought to be due to the amelioration of symptoms. *The initial effect following selegiline was not sustained and the drug did not delay the development of dyskinesias.*

The drug therapy in PD are outlined in Box 15.4.

Acute infections and surgery tend to cause rapid deterioration in the patient's health. Hence, surgery should be avoided unless it is absolutely necessary. Further, levodopa should be continued postoperatively and during an infectious illness.

Other symptomatic treatment: Treatment with

Box 15.4 Pharmacotherapy in PD PH 1.1

- Therapy is initiated only when the manifestations of the disease begin to interfere with daily life
- Selegiline with or without an anticholinergic may be used in mild cases
- In patients *under* 70 years, with intact cognitive function, dopamine agonists are used. Anticholinergics can be used as an alternative
- In younger patients with severe disease, add levodopa with or without amantadine
- In patients over 70 years, start treatment with levodopa or a nonergot dopamine agonist
- In patients over 70 years and in those with dementia, avoid anticholinergics

central anticholinergics/antihistaminics (trihexyphenidyl and orphenadrine) can prevent oculogyric crises. They are also effective in preventing and treating the rarer sweating crises.

Depression is common in PD and can occur especially in patients on levodopa. It can be treated with an **SSRI antidepressant**.

Sialorrhoea is usually controlled by atropine substitutes. If dryness of the mouth is bothersome, it can be relieved by the use of hard candy.

Limitations of drug therapy:

- *Drugs do not cure the disease nor retard its progression.* All that can be expected is 20%–70% symptomatic improvement in 60%–80% of the patients. Tremor is not relieved by most drugs except l-DOPA.
- *Tolerance develops to most of the drugs.*
- *Drugs with prominent anticholinergic actions must be used cautiously* in patients with glaucoma and prostatic enlargement.
- *Levodopa is not recommended during pregnancy, lactation or in children below 18 years.*
- *Levodopa therapy is expensive, has many adverse effects* and needs regular monitoring.

TREATMENT OPTIONS FOR ADVANCED PD OR MOTOR COMPLICATIONS

Deep brain stimulation (DBS), ablative or lesioning procedures (pallidotomy, thalamotomy, subthalamotomy), and dopaminergic medication infusion devices are the treatment options for patients with advanced PD and those having motor complications (refractory tremor/intolerable dyskinesia/motor fluctuations) with levodopa. These therapies reduce levodopa dosage requirements, which may be maintained for several years and improve dyskinesias, off-medication motor function, medication -refractory tremors and quality of life. DBS i.e. high-frequency electrical stimulation of the subthalamic nucleus or globus pallidus is used in some patients with early motor complications. Generally it is preferable to surgery because it can be performed bilaterally and stimulation effects are adjustable and reversible. Magnetic resonance-guided focused ultrasound subthalamotomy (MRgFUS) which permits the ablation of deep brain structures without the need for craniotomy is an another treatment option. For patients with poor cognitive functions, unstable psychiatric symptoms or significant comorbidities levodopa/carbidopa enteral suspension/ intestinal gel formulation or continuous subcutaneous apomorphine infusion should be preferable rather than DBS or surgery.

Education of the patient and his family is important to ensure **compliance** and **emotional** and **social support** to the patient. **Exercise**, especially stretching and strengthening exercises, can prevent or alleviate secondary orthopaedic effects of rigidity and flexed posture and may improve function.

Nutrition: High fibre diet and adequate hydration can prevent constipation. Large, high fat meals which slow gastric emptying and interfere with drug absorption should be avoided.

Coenzyme Q10 has been shown to produce some beneficial effects in Parkinsonian symptoms (Chapter 77).

DRUG THERAPY OF OTHER EXTRAPYRAMIDAL SYNDROMES

Tremor: Mild cases need no treatment. Propranolol in the total daily dose of 30–120 mg is helpful in alleviating essential tremor. Primidone may be combined with propranolol in resistant cases.

Chorea: Haloperidol may be used. However, it may increase rigidity. In severe cases, sodium valproate and carbamazepine are preferred over haloperidol. Treatment should be continued for 1–2 weeks till symptoms subside.

Dystonias: Drug therapy (e.g. carbamazepine, diazepam, baclofen) has variable results. For the use of botulinum toxin type A, in muscle spasticity see Chapter 22.

Myoclonus: Valproic acid and clonazepam can alleviate myoclonus.

DRUG-INDUCED EXTRAPYRAMIDAL REACTIONS (EPR)

Certain drugs used in therapeutics (phenothiazines, butyrophenones, thioxanthenes, metoclopramide, reserpine, methyldopa and levodopa) cause a variety of EPR. These reactions can be broadly grouped into four syndromes:

1. **Parkinsonism:** It is almost indistinguishable from idiopathic parkinsonism but tremor is an infrequent feature. It has been reported with all drugs mentioned above except levodopa. In drug induced parkinsonism, the DA receptors in the striatum are blocked; there is no deficiency of DA. *Hence it is reversible following withdrawal of the offending agent or is treated by adding a synthetic atropine substitute.* Anticholinergics, however, impair cognitive function and have peripheral antimuscarinic effects. They also exacerbate tardive dyskinesia. Alternatively, amantadine is recommended as treatment. It reduces parkinsonian symptoms without increasing psychotic symptoms.
2. **Akathisia** (Inability to sit still at one place): In this syndrome, the patient exhibits a compulsive motor restlessness, is constantly on the move and is apprehensive. It needs to be distinguished from psychotic agitation which it resembles, because unlike the latter it is aggravated by an increase in the dose of the antipsychotic drugs.
   It has been reported with the antipsychotic drugs including atypical antipsychotics and with metoclopramide. The anticholinergic benztropine and small doses of propranolol or clonazepam may be helpful.
3. **Acute dystonic reactions:** These are characterised by painless, spasmodic contraction of one or more muscle groups resulting in trismus, torticollis, opisthotonus or oculogyric crisis. **They are seen mainly with phenothiazines, haloperidol, metoclopramide and prochlorperazine.** Acute dystonic reactions respond well to an IV injection of an antihistaminic such as diphenhydramine 10 mg or promethazine 25 mg, followed by 25 mg of the same drug orally.
4. **Tardive dyskinesia:** This syndrome, reported to occur late during typical antipsychotic drug therapy, develops gradually and consists of involuntary movements such as repetitive sucking, smacking of lips, grimacing and movements of the tongue and extremities. It may persist indefinitely even after stopping the drug and is presumed to be related to DA receptor supersensitivity.

There is no satisfactory treatment. Atypical antipsychotics may be used as replacement, especially **risperidone** or **olanzapine**. It has been reported that **clonazepam** improve TDS and should be used. Amantadine with APD as short term therapy is also used. Tetrabenazine, a vesicular monoamine transporter Type 2 (VMAT-2) inhibitor, has been used "off label" but plasma fluctuations, frequent dosing, and adverse effects limit its use. Recently two VMAT-2 inhibitors, **valbenazine** and **deutetrabenazine** have been approved for tardive dyskinesia. Further evaluation is needed for their long term benefits and safety.

Episodes of EPR can be prevented by:

1. Prescribing the antipsychotic drugs in the minimal, effective doses.
2. Concurrent administration of low doses of benzhexol with antipsychotic drugs.
3. Using less toxic drugs such as benzodiazepines for sedation or cyclizine for vomiting. Anticholinergics, however, fail to prevent the development of tardive dyskinesia.
   Keeping a watch for the ADR during therapy is mandatory. At the first sign of EPR, the dose of the offending drug should be reduced or if possible, replaced by a less toxic drug. PH 1.19

MOTOR NEURON DISEASE (MND) DRUG THERAPY

Amyotrophic lateral sclerosis or motor neuron disease (MND) is one of the most severe degenerative neurological disorders. The aetiology of the disease is unknown. The currently favoured hypothesis centres around glutamate.

Glutamate is the principal excitatory amino acid (EAA) neurotransmitter in the brain and the spinal cord. Excessive stimulation of glutamate receptors (excitotoxicity) may cause neuronal injury or death in various neuropathological conditions. Experimentally, selective inhibition of glutamate in the culture medium results in slowing of degeneration of motor neurons. It is suggested, therefore, that a drug that reduces the effect of glutamate may help in MND.

RILUZOLE: This 2-amino-6 trifluoro-methoxy benzothiazole, given orally, is rapidly absorbed and crosses the BBB. It is largely metabolised in the liver. It blocks the release of glutamate from the neuronal cells as well as blocks the postsynaptic NMDA receptors and thus may protect against the excitotoxicity. The adverse effects include nausea, diarrhoea and elevation of liver enzymes.

> Riluzole retards the progression of MND and increases the duration of survival by a few months.
>
> **Baclofen, tizanidine** and **dantrolene** (Chapter 22) have been tried for symptomatic treatment of spasticity in MND. In general, treatment of MND is unsatisfactory.

DRUGS AND MEMORY

In recent years, attempts have been made to develop drugs for improving memory in disorders of cognitive deterioration such as Alzheimer's disease and other dementias. PH 1.19

Alzheimer's disease is a chronic, progressive, degenerative, nonpsychiatric disorder of the brain. There is damage to cortical and subcortical areas of the brain, resulting into disturbances of multiple higher functions such as thinking, memory, judgment and orientation. It is characterised by cognitive deficit and debility but consciousness is not affected. Its aetiology is not known.

Cholinergic system is essential for normal behaviour and cognition. The disease is associated with degeneration of cholinergic neurons in the basal ganglia, frontal cortex and hippocampus, resulting in a significant loss of choline acetyl transferase, the enzyme responsible for formation of ACh. This results in decreased central cholinergic transmission. There is a genetic predisposition. Treatment with currently available drugs is unsatisfactory, unreliable and disappointing; there is no cure.

Alzheimer's disease must be differentiated from other types of dementia such as due to depression, vitamin deficiency and hypothyroidism, DM, etc., which are treatable. Before starting treatment, other causes of cognitive impairment such as intracranial lesions and cardiovascular disease have to be ruled out.

Classification of drugs used in Alzheimer's disease

1. **Cholinesterase inhibitors,** e.g. donepezil, rivastigmine, galantamine
2. **NMDA receptor antagonist:** Memantine
3. **Antipsychotics and antidepressants:** for treatment of neuropsychiatric symptoms

Selective cholinesterase inhibitors are now used and include

1. **Rivastigmine** (noncompetitive inhibitor; t½ 1.5 h; duration of action 8 h)
2. **Donepezil** (noncompetitive inhibitor; t½ 70 h; duration of action 24 h)
3. **Galantamine** (competitive inhibitor; t½ 8 h; duration of action 8 h)

They may produce moderate improvement in cognition and mood. *However they do not have a sustained effect on disease progression or an improvement in the quality of life.* They are also used to treat vascular dementia and mild cognitive impairment. Donepezil and rivastigmine have been found to be effective in dementia due to PD.

These drugs are generally well tolerated and less hepatotoxic than tacrine (the first ChE inhibitor which has been discontinued because of hepatotoxicity), but can give rise to GI adverse reactions, muscle cramps and abnormal dreams infrequently. GI related ADR appear to be lesser with transdermal formulations of rivastigmine and donepezil.

NMDA Receptor Antagonist

Memantine is a weak noncompetitive, NMDA receptor antagonist. *It selectively inhibits excessive, pathological NMDA receptor activation and reduces glutamate-induced excitotoxicity.* It has a t½ of 40–60 h. ADR includes headache, drowsiness, dizziness, constipation, shortness of breath and hypertension. It is recommended for moderate to severe Alzheimer's disease.

Anticholinesterases can be combined with memantine. The decline in cognitive function has been found to be lesser with the combination than with individual agents.

Table 15.3 depicts the doses of the drugs used in Alzheimer's disease. *None of these drugs stop neurodegeneration and their clinical utility is limited.*

Low dose second generation antipsychotics are commonly used to treat agitation, aggression and psychosis in patients with dementia. However somnolence, gait changes and extrapyramidal effects can occur. The latter are more severe if the patient is taking an anticholinesterase inhibitor. **Pimavanserin**, a second generation antipsychotic is devoid of these effects. It may prolong QT interval.

There is an increased risk of mortality among elderly patients with dementia taking second generation antipsychotic drugs.

Agitation but not other behavioural symptoms can be improved by antidepressants such as sertraline and citalopram.

Drug therapy is combined with nonpharmacological treatment such as social interaction and person-centred care training, which are more important than the drugs. PH 1.19

Table 15.3 Drugs Used to Treat Alzheimer's disease

Drug	Dose
Rivastigmine	1.5 mg bid; to be increased after 2 weeks by 1.5 mg bid to maximum of 6 mg bid
Donepezil	5 mg once a day; to be increased after 4-6 weeks to 10 mg and if required after 3 months to 23 mg/day
Galantamine	4 mg bid; to be increased after 4 weeks to 8 mg bid and if required after another 4 weeks to 12 mg bid
Memantine	5 mg once a day; to be increased gradually by 5 mg/week to 10 mg bid

Rivastigmine and donepezil are available as transdermal patch.

MULTIPLE SCLEROSIS (MS)

Multiple sclerosis (MS) is a complex inflammatory disease of the brain and spinal cord, characterised by focal lymphocytic infiltration, leading *to damage of the oligodendrocytes (which synthesise myelin) and axons.* Initially the inflammation is reversible and remyelination can occur but later episodes cause permanent damage. Inflammation is driven by IL-17 secreting T-lymphocytic-subtype. This allows the T-helper 17 (Th-17) cells to cross the BBB and enter the brain, where they attack the neurons.

The therapy includes:

1. **Rest, physiotherapy,** family/social support
2. **Symptomatic treatment**, e.g. carbamazepine and gabapentin to treat paroxysmal symptoms
3. **Treatment with disease-modifying drugs:**
   - **Acute attacks: Methylprednisolone** in pulse doses is useful (Chapter 64).
   - **Relapsing form:** Immuno-modulators such as *interferon beta* (Chapter 57) and **glatiramer acetate** (Chapter 72) are considered as first-line drugs to reduce the frequency of relapses. Their usefulness for delaying or preventing long-term disability is, however, unpredictable.

Second-line drugs are usually reserved for severe disease. They are as follows:

1. **Natalizumab**, a humanised anti α-4, β-1 integrin antibody acting against the α-4, β-1 integrin on the surface of lymphocytes.
2. **Alemtuzumab**, a humanised monoclonal antibody which targets CD52 on the surface of T cell population, B cells and monocytes.
3. **Ocrelizumab and ofatumumab** are humanized anti-CD20 antibodies, approved for the treatment of adults with relapsing forms of MS. Ocrelizumab is given by IV infusion every 6 months and ofatumumab is injected SC once monthly.
4. **Fingolimod**, an oral sphingosin 1-phosphate receptor modulator, interferes with T cell migration, and thus helps to sequester circulating T lymphocytes to lymph nodes. Other oral sphingosin 1-phosphate receptor modulators include **ozanimod**, **siponimod** and **ponesimod**.
5. **Mitoxantrone**, an anticancer drug with immunomodulatory properties, it slows the progression of MS. But it is cardiotoxic.
6. **Teriflunomide**, an active metabolite of leflunomide (Chapter 73), inhibits mitochondrial enzyme dihydroorotate dehydrogenase and blocks pyrimidine synthesis, which results in reduction in T and B cell activation. It is orally active and indicated in relapsing MS.
7. **Dimethyl fumarate**, an antioxidant induces expression of antiinflammatory proteins and reduces relapse rate.
8. **Cladribine**, a purine antimetabolite selectively depletes B lymphocytes, particularly memory B cells which are implicated to play a role in MS. The drug is administered orally in patients of relapsing –remitting MS. ADR include serious infections, lymphopenia and increased risk of malignancy.

All these drugs provide varied benefits; however, they are toxic and expensive. There is no cure.

ANTIPARKINSONIAN DRUGS

- **Those that increase the dopaminergic (DA) activity**
  - **Precursors of DA**
    - Levodopa
    - *Peripheral dopa decarboxylase inhibitors* (administered with Levodopa)
      - Carbidopa
      - Benserazide
  - **Drugs that inhibit DA metabolism**
    - *MAO-B inhibitors*
      - Selegiline
      - Rasagiline
    - *COMT inhibitors*
      - Tolcapone
      - Entacapone
  - **Drugs that release DA**
    - Amantadine
  - **DA receptor agonists**
    - *Ergot derivatives*
      - Bromocriptine
    - *Non ergot derivatives*
      - Pramipexole
      - Ropinirole
- **Those that suppress the cholinergic activity**
  - Benztropine
  - Benzhexol
  - Procyclidine
  - *Antihistaminics*
    - Diphenhydramine
    - Promethazine
    - Orphenadrine

Drugs effective in extrapyramidal disorders

- **Parkinsonism**
  - Antiparkinsonian drugs
- **Tremors**
  - Propranolol
  - Primidone
- **Chorea**
  - Haloperidol
  - Sodium valproate
  - Carbamazepine
- **Dystonia**
  - Carbamazepine
  - Diazepam
  - Baclofen
  - Botulinumtoxin type A
- **Myoclonus**
  - Sodium valproate
  - Clonazepam

Drug induced EPR

- *Parkinsonism, akathasia, acute dystonia*
  - Anticholinergics
  - Antihistaminics with anticholinergic effects
- *Tardive dyskinesia*
  - Diazepam
  - Amantadine
  - Valbenazine
  - Deutetrabenazine

Drugs used in Alzheimer's disease

- **Cholinesterase inhibitors**
  - Donepezil
  - Rivastigmine
  - Galantamine
- **NMDA receptor antagonist**
  - Memantine
- **Antipsychotics and antidepressants**
  - *For treatment of neuropsychiatric symptoms*
    - Atypical antipsychotics
    - SSRI

3
SECTION

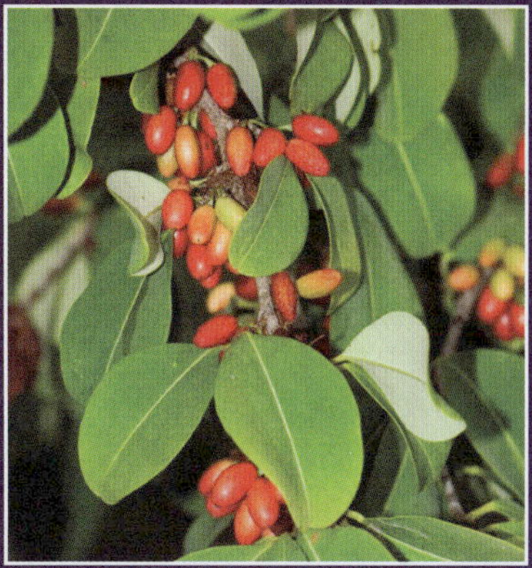

Erythroxylon coca

Local Anaesthetics

Section Outline

This section consists of the following chapter:

CHAPTER 16

Local Anaesthetics

Learning Objectives

This chapter will enable the reader:

1. To classify local anaesthetic drugs with examples.
2. To explain their mechanism of action illustrating various pharmacological effects and ADR.
3. To enumerate precautions to be taken for prevention of local anaesthetic-induced toxicity.
4. To discuss different techniques used for local anaesthesia with respect to their advantages and limitations and choice of agents used.
5. To explain the pharmacological basis for combining lignocaine with (a) adrenaline and (b) prilocaine and state uses of such combinations.
6. To state the adverse effects of spinal anesthesia and their management.

KEY TERMS

sodium channel block, p. 254
membrane stabilising effect, p. 254
lignocaine, p. 257
infiltration anaesthesia, p. 258
surface anaesthesia, p. 258
nerve block, p. 258
spinal anaesthesia, p. 258
lignocaine/prilocaine, eutectic mixture, p. 259
epidural anaesthesia, p. 259
local anaesthetic combinations, p. 259
patient- controlled analgesia, p. 259

Local anaesthetics are drugs which, when applied directly to peripheral nerves, block nerve conduction and abolish all sensations in the part supplied by the nerve. They are applied to somatic nerves and act on axons, cell body, dendrites and synapses. PH 1.17

Miscellaneous drugs with local anaesthetic action are discussed elsewhere. Local anaesthesia can also be produced by physical methods such as refrigeration which is achieved through application of ice or ethyl chloride spray.

Classification of Local Anaesthetics

I. **Natural:** Cocaine

II. **Synthetic nitrogenous compounds:**
- **Derivatives of para-aminobenzoic acid**
  - i. Freely soluble: Procaine and amethocaine
  - ii. Poorly soluble: Benzocaine and orthocaine
- **Derivatives of acetanilide**, e.g. lignocaine (lidocaine)
- **Quinoline derivatives**, e.g. cinchocaine (nupercaine)
- **Acridine derivatives**, e.g. bucricaine

III. **Synthetic non-nitrogenous compounds:** Benzyl alcohol and propanediol.

IV. **Miscellaneous drugs with local action,** e.g. clove oil, phenol, chlorpromazine, antihistaminics like diphenhydramine. Miscellaneous drugs with local anaesthetic action are discussed elsewhere.Local anaesthesia can also be produced by physical methods such as refrigeration which is achieved through application of ice or ethyl chloride spray.

General Properties of Local Anaesthetics

Synthetic local anaesthetic drugs have many properties in common. They possess varying degrees of water and lipid solubility; as the nervous tissue is rich in lipid, lipophilicity of the drug helps to move it into the neuronal fibre, whereas water solubility helps to get the drug to the site of action from the site of injection or application. Thus, the local anaesthetic with high lipid

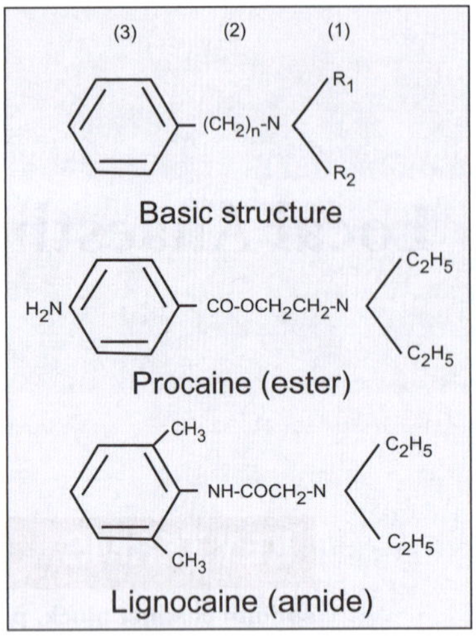

FIG. 16.1 **Structure of local anaesthetics.**

but low water solubility will not be much useful because of difficulty in transportation through the aqueous phase surrounding the neuronal fibre. Chemically, the local anaesthetics consist of three parts (Fig. 16.1):

1. **Hydrophilic amino group**
2. **Intermediate chain**
3. **Lipophilic aromatic group**

Due to presence of amino nitrogen, these drugs are bases and form water soluble salt with acids (pH 4.6) and are generally dispensed as hydrochlorides. In the tissues where the pH is alkaline (pH 7.4), the free base is liberated and produces its pharmacological action.

Majority of the clinically useful local anaesthetics are nitrogenous compounds:

1. **Esters,** e.g. procaine, tetracaine, benzocaine
2. **Amides,** e.g. lignocaine, prilocaine, bupivacaine, ropivacaine

Mechanism of Action

Local anaesthetics block both the generation and the conduction of the nerve impulse. They bind to receptors near the intracellular end of the voltage gated sodium channels. *This prevents the increase in permeability of the cell membrane to Na^+ion*, the first event in depolarisation (**sodium channel block**). Thus, an action potential is not generated. This action affecting the process of depolarisation, leading to failure of impulse propagation without affecting the resting potential, is known as **membrane stabilising effect**. Increased extracellular calcium antagonises the action of local anaesthetics on nerves and muscles, whereas potassium facilitates the same (Fig. 16.2). The local anesthetics have affinity for open channels than inactivated ones while resting are not affected.

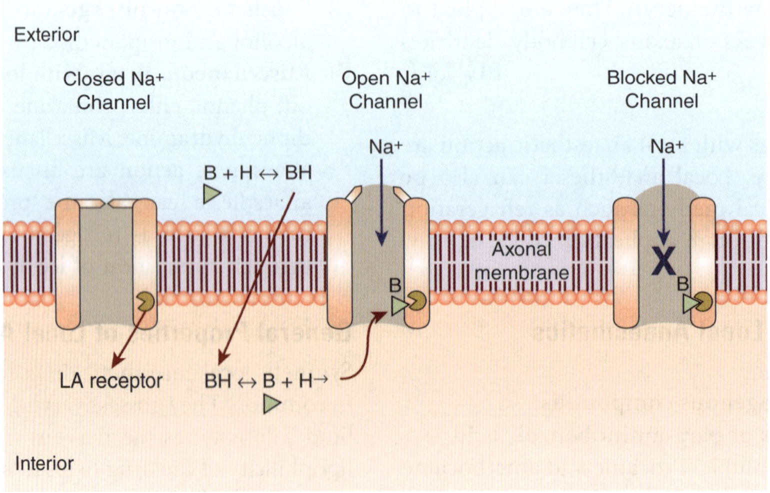

FIG. 16.2 **Mechanism of action of local anaesthetics.**

A smaller nerve fibre presents a greater surface area per unit volume for the action of an anaesthetic drug rather than a larger fibre. Smaller fibres are, therefore, blocked first. Thus, the various fibres are blocked in the following order:

- Autonomic fibres
- Sensory fibres conducting temperature and pain
- Sensory fibres carrying touch, pressure and vibration sensations
- Motor fibres

Recovery of function occurs in the reverse order.

Local anaesthetics are less effective when injected into an inflamed area. The exact cause for this phenomenon is not known.

Pharmacological Actions

Besides the local anaesthetic properties, cocaine and the other nitrogenous synthetic substitutes have important actions on other systems.

Central nervous system: They **stimulate the CNS** and cause restlessness, tremors and in toxic doses, convulsions. Central stimulation is followed by depression; death is usually due to respiratory depression.

Cocaine in smaller doses acts more prominently on the higher centres causing euphoria, mental alertness and hallucinations. It is a drug of abuse.

Cardiovascular system: These drugs are **myocardiac depressants**. They decrease heart rate and the amplitude of contraction; increase the excitability threshold and the refractory period while slowing down conduction (**membrane stabilising effect**). Higher concentrations may lead to cardiac arrhythmias and cardiac arrest. Procainamide (related to procaine) and lignocaine are used therapeutically for their cardiac depressant properties (see Chapter 28).

Except cocaine, which is not used therapeutically, all the other drugs produce **hypotension**, by a direct action on the vessel wall. Cocaine is a vasoconstrictor.

Other actions: Synthetic nitrogenous local anaesthetics have a direct **spasmolytic action** on smooth muscle and in large doses, they can produce neuromuscular blockade.

Absorption, Fate and Excretion

Local anaesthetics are not absorbed from unbroken skin. Applied to the mucous membrane, the absorption varies with the mucous surface. Thus, absorption is more rapid from the trachea than from the pharynx, whereas it is poor through the urinary bladder. A large amount of drug can be absorbed from a raw granulating surface and can precipitate toxicity.

When used by infiltration, the absorption can be retarded by combining it with a vasoconstrictor agent like adrenaline. It must be emphasised that a latent period of several minutes elapses between drug application and therapeutic effect. Failure to allow sufficient time for establishment of block may convey the erroneous impression that the dose employed is inadequate; this may lead to use of unnecessarily large toxic doses.

Local anaesthetics, which are esters are metabolised by hydrolysis in both the liver and plasma. The amide-like local anaesthetics such as lignocaine are dealkylated. Cocaine is excreted unchanged in human urine.

Anticholinesterases increase the duration of action of procaine by inhibiting its degradation by plasma pseudocholinesterase.

Adverse Reactions

- **Allergic reaction:** This may manifest as a mild allergic dermatitis, a typical asthmatic attack or a severe fatal anaphylactoid reaction. It is generally seen with the local anaesthetics of the ester type and may show cross sensitivity with chemically related compounds. *Intradermal sensitivity test is recommended before using these drugs.* A negative response, however, does not rule out drug sensitivity.
- **CVS:** Fall of BP and cardiac arrest can sometimes occur. Hypotension should be treated with vasoconstrictor drugs such as noradrenaline and phenylephrine. If the heart stops, external cardiac massage is indicated. (see Chapter 18).
- **CNS:** This toxicity can be countered to a certain extent by preanaesthetic administration with diazepam. If convulsions occur, IV diazepam is used. Oxygen is given to prevent hypoxia.

Box 16.1 Prevention of Toxicity of Local Anaesthetics

- Enquire about the history of allergy
- Drugs should be given cautiously in the presence of liver and myocardial damage
- Avoid food at least 4 h prior to nerve block / spinal anaesthesia to prevent vomiting.
- Preanaesthetic medication, diazepam may be given.
- Select the proper site; correct knowledge of the nerve course is needed before attempting a nerve block
- Use minimal effective dose, well diluted, preferably with the vasoconstrictor drug, adrenaline. Avoid intravenous injection
- Wait after injection; remember the latent period
- Observe the face for any twitching, excitement, and pulse for tachycardia
- Observe postoperatively for allergic reactions; warn the patient against using the drug again, if allergy is observed

Prevention of toxicity: See Box 16.1.

In case of systemic toxicity of local anaesthetics, attention should be given to airway management, treatment of hypotension, arrhythmias and seizures. IV infusion of 20% lipid emulsion can reverse cardiac and neurologic effects of local anaesthetics by extracting lipid soluble local anaesthetic agents in it.

The salient pharmacological features of individual local anaesthetics are described below:

COCAINE is an alkaloid from the leaves of the coca tree (*Erythroxylon coca*) and other species. It is the methylbenzoyl ester of ecgonine which is chemically closely related to atropine. *Cocaine is not used as a local anaesthetic*, but it is an important drug of abuse for its psychotropic effects.

Pharmacological actions:

Local anaesthetic action: At concentrations used to produce local anaesthesia it is poisonous to many cells.

Central nervous system: It is a **central stimulant**. It blocks the reuptake of DA in mesolimbic and mesocortical pathways leading to euphoria. Its euphoric effect following smoking lasts for 20 min whereas that following intranasal administration may last for 1–1½h. Later, depletion of DA from the nerve endings gives rise to dysphoria so characteristic of cocaine withdrawal.

It also blocks the uptake of tryptophan and 5-HT. This accounts for the striking alteration of the sleep-wake cycle and may enhance the central excitatory effect of dopamine.

Cardiovascular system: It impairs the reuptake of adrenaline and NA by presynaptic nerve endings and thus **activates the adrenergic system leading to hypertension and tachycardia.**

Adverse reactions: These are as follows:

- **Acute**
  a. Allergic reactions.
  b. Activation of adrenergic nervous system produces vasoconstriction, an acute rise in BP, tachycardia and a predisposition to acute myocardial infarction, ventricular arrhythmias and convulsions. It may also result in mydriasis, hyperglycaemia and hyperthermia.
  c. Sudden death after administration by any route. As it is metabolised by plasma and liver cholinesterases, people with deficiency of these enzymes (liver disease), infants, pregnant women and old persons are at greater risk of cocaine toxicity.
- **Chronic**
  a. Although at low dose levels cocaine delays ejaculation and orgasm and causes heightened sensory awareness, its chronic use can cause sexual dysfunction and sexual disinterest. *It is not a true aphrodisiac.*
  b. Anorexia, emaciation, tremors, disturbances of sensation and emotion, hallucinations and insanity are observed in cocaine addicts.
  c. Cocaine when used by pregnant women may cause prematurity, intrauterine growth retardation and microcephaly. **It has teratogenic effects on brain development**. It can cause neurological symptoms including sudden death in the newborn.
- **Drug dependence:** Persons dependent on cocaine show paranoid and suicidal tendencies. *Cocaine is one of the major drugs of abuse* and its withdrawal can cause severe CNS depression.

PROCAINE: This diethyl aminoethyl ester of para-aminobenzoic acid is non-irritant and as effective as cocaine, but is much less toxic. It is a vasodilator. However it is poorly absorbed from the mucous membranes and, therefore, has no topical use. Procaine is rapidly hydrolysed by esterases in the plasma and liver and is partly excreted in the urine, conjugated with glucuronic acid and glycine.

AS 5.4, PM 3.5

LIGNOCAINE (Lidocaine): This is the most commonly employed local anaesthetic.

- It is stable, can be stored for a long time at room temperature and can be autoclaved.
- It has a quick onset of action and a high degree of penetration.
- It is also an excellent surface anaesthetic.
- Its toxicity is similar to that of other local anaesthetics in equipotent doses.

Lignocaine may cause drowsiness but has no vasoconstricting action. Topical formulations should not be applied on the wounds or denuded skin as it can undergo absorption and produce adverse cardiac or neurological effects.

Preparations and dosage:

i. . Lignocaine injection as 5 mg/mL (0.5%), 10 mg/mL (1%), 15 mg/mL (1.5%), 20 mg/mL (2%), 40 mg/mL (4%), 100 mg/mL (10%), 200 mg/mL (20%). Dose: 4.4 mg/kg (not more than 300 mg total). Maximum recommended dose in paracervical block is 200 mg and for IV regional anaesthesia is 4 mg/kg.
ii. Lignocaine 0.5%, 1%, 1.5%, 2%, 4%with adrenaline. Dose: 7 mg/kg (not more than 500 mg total). Doses are reduced for children, elderly, debilitated patients, and patients with cardiac or liver disease. *Formulations containing preservatives should not be used for spinal, epidural, or caudal block or IV injection.*
iii. Lignocaine topical formulations: Spray: 0.5%, 10%; solution: 2%, 4%; cream: 0.5%; gel: 0.5%, 2.5%; jelly: 2%; ointment: 2.5%, 5%.
iv. Lignocaine transdermal patch: 5%.

Following infiltration of 0.25%–0.5%solution, the duration of action varies between 30 and 60 min. Addition of adrenaline (1 in 200,000) prolongs the action for about 2 h. Analgesia is complete within a few minutes and recovery occurs quickly, within 2–3 h after spinal anaesthesia.

Indications:

Lignocaine is recommended for topical use, nerve blocks, infiltration and epidural injection and for dental analgesia. Analgesic effect of lidocaine used in patient-controlled analgesia varies with type of pain. Nociceptive pain requires higher doses than neuropathic pain. It can be used in patients allergic to procaine and other ester-type local anaesthetics. Its use in cardiac arrhythmias is discussed in Chapter 28.

Prilocaine has similar actions as lignocaine. It does not require adrenaline. CNS toxicity is less and is used for IV regional blocks. It is used in dentistry.

BUPIVACAINE: This local anaesthetic is about four times as potent as lignocaine and has more prolonged action (up to 8 h). Its toxicity is similar to that of lignocaine but it is more cardiotoxic. It is used for spinal anaesthesia and epidural analgesia.

Mepivacaine has *N*-methyl substituent in the place of the butyl group of bupivacaine. **Ropivacaine** is less potent than bupivacaine and is also claimed to be less cardiotoxic. It is used for epidural and regional anaesthesia and is more motor sparing. Duration of action is 2–4 h.

Both bupivacaine and ropivacaine are effective analgesics for **labour pain** and are given either as continuous low-dose infusion via epidural route or with fentanyl as combined spinal–epidural route (patient-controlled analgesia, see below).

AMETHOCAINE (Tetracaine) is a potent long acting local anaesthetic, used topically; its absorption from the vascular mucous membranes is very rapid and deaths have occurred following its use in urethra and respiratory tract. *It should never be used on inflamed, injured or vascular surfaces.*

Cinchocaine (dibucaine and nupercaine) is a potent but toxic local anaesthetic. It can be used locally (1%ointment) for anorectal conditions.

Benzocaine is poorly water soluble and is used topically as ointment, gel or liquid spray.

Articaine is an amide type of local anaesthetic agent. It has a short duration of action and is of intermediate potency. It is widely used for dental anaesthesia.

BUCRICAINE: This acridine derivative, and is used locally in ophthalmic, dental and general surgical procedures in much the same way as lignocaine. Bucricaine has a longer duration of action than lignocaine. Further, the drug has some inherent vasopressor activity and, therefore, does not require the addition of a vasopressor for infiltration anaesthesia. Its CNS and cardiac toxicity appears to be less than that of lignocaine, and it **can be used in patients allergic to lignocaine**.

Types of local anaesthesia with their indications

The choice of the local anaesthetic for a particular type of local anaesthesia depends upon its desired duration of action. Procaine is short acting, lignocaine and mepivacaine are intermediate, whereas tetracaine and bupivacaine are long acting.

- **Surface anaesthesia**: In this type, local anaesthetic is applied directly to the skin or mucous membrane. For example, amethocaine is used as a surface anaesthetic for the eye (e.g. adjuvant in cataract surgery, eyelid surgical minor procedures), throat (e.g. pharyngitis,endoscopy) urethra (e.g. cathterisation), rectum (e.g. proctoscopy)and skin (e.g. venipuncture, intra-arterial catheterization). Similarly, benzocaine and lignocaine hydrochloride are used as all-purpose surface anaesthetics except for the eye. Dibucaine is used for the ear, rectum and skin. **Proparacaine** and **tetracaine** are used exclusively for the eye as eye drops to anaesthetize the ocular surface prior to eye examination e.g. application tonometry to measure intraocular pressure/ minor procedures.
- **Infiltration anaesthesia:** In this procedure, the nerve endings are anaesthetised by their direct exposure to the drug, infiltrated subcutaneously (e.g prior to suturing a lacerated wound). **Procaine 2% and lignocaine 2%** are most commonly used. They are mixed with adrenaline (1:200,000) to prolong the action. Lignocaine acts longer than procaine. Adrenaline should be avoided when local anaesthetics are used to produce ring block to anaesthetise the digits or penis, in order to avoid local ischaemia and in patients with known myocardial disease.

AS 5.4

- **Nerve block or conduction block** where the drug is injected very close to the nerve, e.g. brachial plexus block administered as adjuvant to general anaesthesia for surgery on upper extremity. Choice of the anaesthetic is determined by the duration of anaesthesia needed.
- **Spinal anaesthesia:** In this procedure the local anaesthetic without adjuvants is injected into the subarachnoid space. Its level in the space is adjusted by using solutions with higher (hyperbaric) or lower (hypobaric) specific gravity than that of CSF, as vehicles. Usually, the injection is made 'heavy' by adding dextrose or 'light' (approximately isotonic) by adding saline. **The position of the patient is important in limiting the block to the desired level.**

  Lignocaine and **bupivacaine** are the most commonly used drugs for spinal anaesthesia needed for surgery involving lower abdomen e.g. hernia, hydrocele. They give good muscle relaxation and allow the use of cautery and electrical appliances during surgery. These drugs, however, are not suitable for surgery above the diaphragm and in apprehensive and mentally disturbed patients.

Complications of spinal anaesthesia:

1. Due to sympathetic blockade these drugs produce arteriolar dilatation, decreased venous tone and diminished venous return to the heart. The cardiac output and the BP are reduced. Thus, *hypotension is one of the most important complications of spinal anaesthesia.* It is treated by:
   i. *Elevation of the legs or wrapping the legs* in elastic bandages to increase venous return.
   ii. *Rapid intravenous infusion of fluids* for filling the dilated vascular bed.
   iii. *Use of vasopressor drugs*, e.g. methoxamine to restore arteriolar and venous tone.

   Failure to block the vagus may precipitate hypotension and hiccough due to reflex stimulation during abdominal surgery.

Table 16.1 Some Injectable Local Anaesthetics

Drug	Infiltration (%)	Nerve Block (%)	Spinal (%)	Epidural (%)
Procaine	0.25–0.5	1.0–2.0	10.0	–
Amethocaine	–	–	1.0	–
Lignocaine	0.5	0.5–2.0	1.5–5.0	1.0–2.0
Bupivacaine	0.25	0.25–0.5	0.5–0.75	0.25–0.75
Prilocaine	0.5	1–2	–	–

2. Postoperative urinary retention and intestinal atony. Treatment of these is discussed in Chapter 19.
3. Headache, which is commonly observed following spinal anaesthesia, is probably due to leakage of CSF from site of puncture; it responds to analgesic drugs.

- **Epidural anaesthesia:** The local anaesthetic is injected outside the dura. Hence, its spread is restricted to a specific region thereby, causing fewer complications.

Combined spinal–epidural analgesia is induced by injecting local anaesthetic intrathecally with additional doses given by epidural route. The former provides rapid analgesia without any significant motor block of the lower extremities. An epidural route ensures further maintenance of analgesia. Spinal, epidural and their combination are termed as **neuraxial analgesia**.

*Thus **local anaesthesia** includes surface and infiltration anesthesia while **regional anaesthesia** includes peripheral nerve blocks and neuraxial anesthesia i.e. spinal and epidural anaesthesia.*

The concentrations in which various local anaesthetics are used are given in Table 16.1.

Non-anaesthetic indications of local anaesthetics:

- **Lignocaine in the treatment of cardiac arrhythmias** (see Chapter 28).
- **As IV analgesics** in the treatment of severe pruritus and pain due to malignancy.

Local anaesthetic combinations: Prilocaine (3%) in combination with felypressin (0.03 IU/mL; AVP analogue) is preferred to lignocaine + adrenaline combination in patients with past history of vasospasm, hypertension and heart failure. **Felypressin** produces vasoconstriction by acting on V1 receptors. In the concentrations used, it acts on veins and exerts no effect on arteries or heart. Its vasoconstricting effect is lesser than adrenaline but it has no arrhythmogenic potential.

Lignocaine and prilocaine are solid bases but the combination of equal quantities (by weight) of the two agents results in a **eutectic mixture of local anaesthetics (EMLA)**. This means that the mixture has lower melting point than of either solid ingredient alone. The **lignocaine/prilocaine mixture** (either 2% or 7% of each) exists as oil with the melting point as 180°C. It can be emulsified with water to form a cream that can penetrate intact skin. This also allows higher concentrations of anaesthetic agent in the cream. Applied topically under occlusive dressing 30–60 min prior to any procedure, it serves as an alternative to infiltration anaesthesia for procedures such as venipuncture, cannulation, skin graft harvesting or minor dermatological procedures. The common ADR include mild skin blanching and erythema. However, application to abraded skin and mucous membranes results in rapid absorption with systemic toxicity.

Patient-controlled analgesia (PCA): PCA pumps have been developed, which allow the patient to self-administer drug for pain control as per the need in post-operative period, for cancer pain (Chapter 11) or in labour pain. Low doses of a local anaesthetic (lignocaine, bupivacaine or ropivacaine) without epinephrine are used with either fentanyl, morphine, or hydromorphone (Chapter 10). Adverse effects of PCA include sensory and motor deficits, low blood pressure and urinary retention.

LOCAL ANAESTHETICS

- **Natural**
  - Cocaine
- **Synthetic nitrogenous compounds**
  - **Derivatives of para-aminobenzoic acid**
    - Freely soluble
      - Procaine
      - Amethocaine
    - Poorly soluble
      - Benzocaine
      - Orthocaine
  - **Derivatives of acetanilide**
    - Lignocaine (Lidocaine)
  - **Quinoline derivatives**
    - Cinchocaine (Nupercaine)
  - **Acridine derivatives**
    - Bucricaine
- **Synthetic non-nitrogenous compounds**
  - Benzyl alcohol
  - Propanediol
- **Miscellaneous drugs with local action**
  - Clove oil
  - Phenol
  - Chlorpromazine
  - Antihistaminics (e.g. Diphenhydramine)

4
SECTION

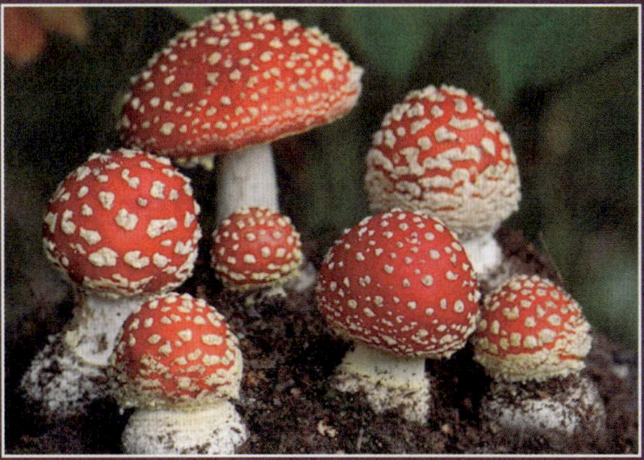

Amanita muscaria

Autonomic Nervous System

Section Outline

This section consists of the following chapters:

SECTION 4

Autonomic Nervous System

CHAPTER 17

General Considerations

Learning Objectives

This chapter will enable the reader:

1. To be aware of functions, distribution and neurotransmission involved in sympathetic and parasympathetic nervous system.
2. To enumerate sites of action of ACh and noradrenaline.
3. To describe the synthesis, storage, release and fate of ACh and noradrenaline.
4. To explain how drugs can modulate adrenergic and cholinergic neurotransmission giving suitable examples.

KEY TERMS

Autonomic nervous system (ANS) was so named by Langley (1898), because of the fact that unlike the somatic nervous system of the skeletal muscles, it is independent of volitional control and, thus, enjoys some degree of autonomy.

The ANS comprises the **parasympathetic** (**cholinergic**), the **sympathetic** (**adrenergic**) and the **enteric nervous system (ENS)**. The parasympathetic system mainly participates in tissue building reactions, whereas the sympathetic system enables the individual to respond to stress and prepares the body for 'flight or fight'. An animal can survive complete elimination of sympathetic but not of parasympathetic nervous system. Usually, these systems are in a state of dynamic equilibrium.

The autonomic functions are regulated through the reticular formation and its constituents, along with the cranial nerve nuclei. In the **hypothalamus,** the posterior and the lateral nuclei modulate sympathetic activity, whereas the midline nuclei modulate parasympathetic function. The thalamus, the relay station for sensory perception, can modify the autonomic activity. The limbic system co-ordinates the autonomic reactions with emotions, but the ultimate synchronisation of the somatic and vegetative functions is achieved in the cortex.

The autonomic innervation consists of a myelinated **preganglionic fibre** which forms a synapse with the cell body of a nonmyelinated, second neuron, termed the **postganglionic neuron**. The postganglionic fibre in turn terminates in a synapse with the receptors of the organ supplied by it. The **synapse** may thus be defined conceptually as a structure that is formed by the close apposition of a neuron either with another neuron or with effector cell. The synapse merely transmits impulses from one neuron to another; the effect (excitation or inhibition) on the second neuron depends upon the type of neurotransmitter (NT) released and the types of receptor on which it acts. The synapse between the preganglionic and postganglionic fibres is termed as a **ganglion,** whereas that between the postganglionic fibre and the receptors is termed the **neuroeffector junction**. It must be emphasised that the synapse is a physiological and not an anatomical entity.

DISTRIBUTION OF PARASYMPATHETIC NERVOUS SYSTEM

The parasympathetic nervous system serves two important functions:

- It carries from the viscera the afferent impulses (**visceral afferents**) which reflexly modify the autonomic functions.
- It supplies **motor fibres** to smooth muscle, glands, heart and viscera through its **craniosacral outflow** (Fig. 17.1).

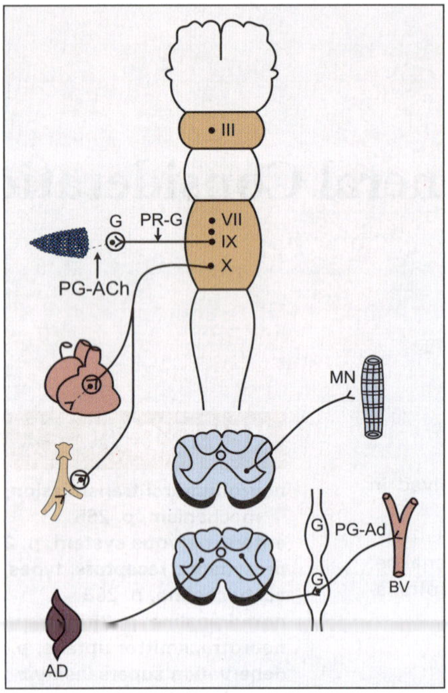

FIG. 17.1 **Schematic representation of the sites of release of neurohumoral transmitters acetylcholine (ACh) and noradrenaline (NA). ACh is released at all the ganglia (G), postganglionic cholinergic nerve endings (PG-ACh), myoneural junctions (MN) and the adrenal medulla (AD). Noradrenaline is released at postganglionic adrenergic nerve endings (PG-Ad). Adrenaline is released from the adrenal medulla. PR-G, preganglionic.**

The **important afferents** are as follows:

- **Afferents from the carotid sinus and carotid body carried through the glossopharyngeal nerves:** Stimulation of these afferent fibres occurs as a result of local elevation of BP or decrease in blood pH respectively; this results in a fall in BP and bradycardia (**carotid sinus reflex**) and stimulation of respiration (**carotid body reflex**) respectively.
- **Afferents from the aortic arch, carried through the vagus nerve:** Their stimulation also produces hypotension.
- **Afferent fibres from the lungs, heart and the GI tract carried through the vagus:** These afferents mediate visceral sensations. The reflex responses vary from hypotension (**Bezold Jarisch reflex**) to vomiting (afferents from stomach).

Craniosacral outflow: The craniosacral outflow, mainly *efferent in nature*, consists of

- **Midbrain or tectal outflow** through the Edinger Westphal nucleus of the oculomotor (III) nerve. The postganglionic fibres supply the ciliary muscle and the circular fibres of sphincter pupillae (Fig. 17.1).
- **Medullary outflow** comprising parasympathetic components of the facial (VII), glossopharyngeal (IX) and vagus (X) nerves.
  a. The facial nerve supplies secretomotor and vasodilator fibres to the submandibular and sublingual salivary glands and probably also to the lacrimal glands.
  b. The glossopharyngeal nerve carries the parasympathetic supply of the parotid glands via the otic ganglia.
  c. The vagus provides secretomotor and vasodilator fibres for the thoracic and the abdominal viscera with the exception of the lower third of the GI tract.
- **Sacral outflow** consists of axons arising from the second, third and fourth sacral segments of the spinal cord and forms the pelvic nerves (*nervi erigentis*) which synapse near or within the bladder, the lower third of the GI tract including the rectum, and the sexual organs, and supplies secretomotor and vasodilator fibres.

The distribution of the parasympathetic system is much more limited than that of the sympathetic system. Usually, a single preganglionic parasympathetic fibre synapses with a single postganglionic cell body of the same system. An exception to this rule is the vagus nerve

DISTRIBUTION OF SYMPATHETIC NERVOUS SYSTEM

The sympathetic division consists of the **thoracolumbar outflow**. The cells of the preganglionic sympathetic fibres are situated in the intermediolateral column of the spinal cord and extend from the 8th cervical to the 2nd or 3rd lumbar segments.

The sympathetic ganglia are of five types.

1. **Paravertebral ganglia** consist of 22 pairs of ganglia that form a lateral chain on either side of the vertebral column.
2. The **prevertebral ganglia** lie in the abdomen and the pelvis. They are the coeliac, superior and inferior mesentric and aorticorenal ganglia. The postganglionic fibres from these supply the abdominal viscera, the urinary bladder and the external genitalia.
3. The **terminal ganglia** are few and are distributed in close proximity to the viscera such as urinary bladder and the rectum.
4. The **intermediate ganglia** are closely associated with the anterior spinal roots and lie outside the paravertebral ganglia.

   A **preganglionic adrenergic** fibre may end in any of these ganglia. Thus, many preganglionic fibres arising from the

5th to the 12th thoracic segment form the splanchnic nerves which synapse into the coeliac ganglion.

The **postganglionic** adrenergic fibres from the upper thoracic ganglia (1st to 4th) form cardiac, oesophageal and pulmonary plexuses and end as arborisations in these organs.

5. The **adrenal medulla** is anatomically, embryologically and functionally a sympathetic ganglion. However, it does not have a postganglionic continuation and serves a secretory function. *It secretes mainly adrenaline and small amounts of noradrenaline (NA).*

ENTERIC NERVOUS SYSTEM (ENS)

The ENS, the third division of the ANS, consists of collections of highly organised neurons situated in the wall of the GI tract. It includes the myenteric plexus (**Auerbach plexus**) and the submucosal plexus (**Meissner plexus**). This network receives preganglionic fibres from the parasympathetic system and from the postganglionic sympathetic neurons (Fig. 17.2). Auerbach plexus is principally responsible for the peristaltic movement of the bowels. The Meissner's plexus is an inner plexus that innervates cells in the epithelial layer and the smooth muscle of the muscularis mucosa and is involved in controlling the GIT secretions and local blood flow. ENS controls GI motility, secretions and the mucosal blood flow. Stimulation of the ENS causes release of other putative transmitters, leading to relaxation or stimulation of smooth muscles. Some of the neurons have been identified as containing peptides (**vasoactive intestinal peptide [VIP]), nucleotides (ATP) and nitric oxide** (**NO**), which cause inhibition. On the other hand, noncholinergic, excitatory transmitters such as **substance P**, released locally, have also been identified in the enteric plexus. They play a modulatory role in controlling ENS functions. *Some enteric neurons acts as mechanoreceptors or chemoreceptors providing local reflex pathways that can control the secretory and motor GI function without external inputs.*

Although the adrenergic and cholinergic systems are traditionally believed to act antagonistically, their actions on specific tissues may be either discrete and independent or integrated and interdependent. Thus, they act as complementary in an integrated fashion on the male sexual organs to promote sexual function.

NEUROHUMORAL TRANSMISSION

Transmission of an impulse across the synapse occurs mainly as a result of release of a neurohumoral transmitter into the synaptic cleft. Electrical

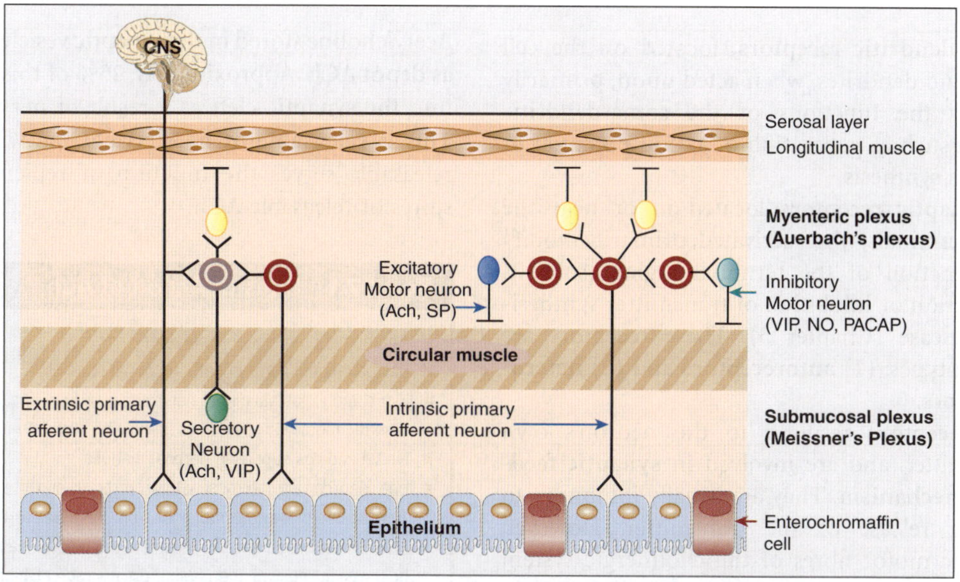

FIG. 17.2 Enteric nervous system. ACh, acetylcholine; VIP, vasoactive intestinal peptide; NO, nitric oxide; SP, substance P; PACAP, pituitary adenylatecyclase activating polypeptide. Diagram modified from: Tally NJ. *Serotoninergic neuroenteric modulators.* The Lancet, 2001; 358:2061–8.

transmission of impulses has, however, been demonstrated in lower organisms like crayfish and annelids.

The work of Dale, Gaddum, Feldberg and others led to the extension of the chemical transmitter hypothesis to the autonomic ganglia and myoneural junctions where ACh was identified as the transmitter.

Barger and Dale (1910), while describing the pharmacological actions of adrenaline and related substances, employed the term **sympathomimetic** as these actions resembled those seen following sympathetic stimulation; similarly, the actions of pilocarpine, muscarine and related substances were described by them as **parasympathomimetic**. Dale in his later work (1914) used the term **Nicotinic action** to describe the ganglionic and neuromuscular actions of ACh and **Muscarinic action** to describe the actions at the postganglionic parasympathetic nerve endings, because of their resemblance to those observed following the alkaloids, nicotine and muscarine, respectively. Since the terms sympathetic and parasympathetic do not give any idea about the chemical transmitter at the nerve endings, Dale classified autonomic nerves as (a) **adrenergic,** which release NA and (b) **cholinergic,** which release ACh, as transmitters.

A neuron can receive chemical messages at various active sites called **receptors** (Chapter 5), three groups of which are considered important:

- **Soma-dendritic receptors,** located on the cell body and dendrites, when acted upon, primarily modify the functions of the soma-dendritic region such as generation of action potential or protein synthesis.
- **Presynaptic receptors** located in or near the axon terminals, when activated, primarily modify the function of the terminal region, such as facilitation or inhibition of transmitter synthesis and release (Chapter 5). These receptors are of two types: (1) **autoreceptors** and (2) **heteroreceptors**.
  Autoreceptors respond to the neuron's own transmitter, and are involved in **synaptic feedback mechanism**. They are usually inhibitory to further release of the transmitter. However, somatic motor fibres of the cholinergic system have excitatory presynaptic receptors.
  The nerve terminals also have regulatory receptors that are activated by blood-borne agents or NTs from the neighbouring cells. They are termed **heteroreceptors**, e.g. angiotensin II type 2 (AT_2) receptors on adrenergic cells.
- **Postsynaptic receptors** are associated with the target organs/tissues (Fig. 17.1).

NEUROHUMORAL TRANSMITTERS

ACh, NA, dopamine (DA), gamma-aminobutyric acid (GABA) and 5-hydroxytryptamine (5-HT) are considered as the classical NTs.

Steps involved in the synthesis and the storage of the **neurohumour,** its metabolism and its interaction with the receptors are potential points where a drug can act. The latter can thus mimic or antagonise the action of the corresponding neurohumor.

Acetylcholine: an ester of choline, acts as the neurohumoral transmitter at sites shown in Box 17.1.

ACh is synthesised inside the nerve fibre by combination of choline taken up from the ECF with an acetyl group. The acetyl group is obtained from acetylcoenzyme A, a product of the intermediary metabolism. The axon terminals contain a large number of mitochondria where acetylcoenzyme-A is synthesised.

Acetylcholine stored in the synaptic vesicles is termed as **depot ACh**. Approximately, 25% of this is released into the synaptic cleft as a result of nerve impulse. This is **releasable ACh**. Acetylcholine which is not releasable serves the function of replenishing the stores of releasable ACh.

Box 17.1 Sites of Action of ACh

- Autonomic preganglionic nerve endings
- Postganglionic parasympathetic nerve endings
- Sympathetic postganglionic nerve endings, supplying sweat glands
- Somatic motor nerve endings, supplying skeletal muscles
- Nerve endings supplying adrenal medulla
- Between certain neurons within the brain and the spinal cord. Transmission from the motor neuron collateral to the Renshaw cells is cholinergic and the receptors are predominantly nicotinic. In contrast, most of the cholinergic neurons at higher levels of the CNS have muscarinic receptors
- Noninnervated receptors on vascular endothelium

ACh released as a result of nerve impulse produces a change in permeability of the effector cell, leading to its depolarisation by ionic fluxes. Thus, with inward flux of sodium and outward flux of potassium, the negativity of the intra-axonal voltage diminishes, and this produces a **nerve action potential (NAP)**. The NAP leads to either conduction of the nerve impulse along the axon or activation of the effector organ resulting in a secretory or a motor response.

Acetylcholine released into the synaptic cleft is rapidly degraded by the true cholinesterase into choline and acetic acid. This reverses the ionic changes and enables the postsynaptic membrane or the receptor site to get repolarised.

Two main types of cholinesterase have been identified:

- **Acetylcholinesterase (AChE) or true cholinesterase,** present in neurons, ganglia and at myoneural junctions, which rapidly hydrolyses ACh and another choline ester, methacholine but not benzoylcholine.
- **Butyrocholinesterase (BuChE) or pseudocholinesterase,** present mainly in the plasma, RBCs, liver, ganglia and other organs, which hydrolyses ACh slowly, but not methacholine.

Noradrenaline and **dopamine:** NA and DA are monoamines and act as neurohumoral transmitters at the postganglionic sympathetic nerve endings and certain regions within the brain. These amines are present in the highest concentration in the terminal axonal processes of specific neurons, where they are synthesised and stored in the vesicles within the terminals.

The enzymes participating in the formation of NA are synthesised in the cell bodies of the adrenergic neurons and are transported to the axon terminals. These enzymes are not completely specific as they also play a part in the synthesis of 5-HT.

The three **NTs**, i.e. **DA**, **NA** and **adrenaline**, are sequentially synthesised from the amino acid phenylalanine (Fig. 17.3).

The hydroxylation of tyrosine by tyrosine hydroxylase to dihydroxyphenylalanine (DOPA) and decarboxylation of DOPA to DA occurs in the cytoplasm. About 50% of DA is then actively transported into the vesicles containing DA-beta-hydroxylase enzyme, where it is converted to NA, which is stored as granules.

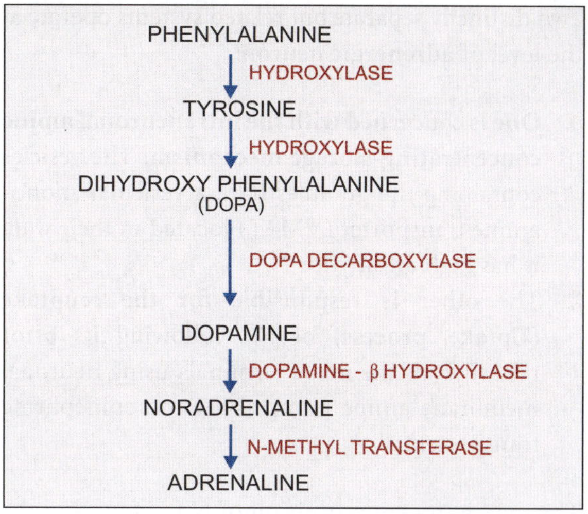

FIG. 17.3 Biosynthesis of catecholamines.

Catecholamine content of adrenal medulla normally is 85% adrenaline and 15% NA. DA serves as a precursor of NA and also acts as a neurohumoral transmitter. **Adrenaline** is formed in the **adrenal medulla** by methylation of NA and is stored in the chromaffin granules. The adrenaline and NA forming cells in the adrenal medulla are two distinct cell types. Because of their unique blood supply, the adrenal chromaffin cells are exposed to high concentrations of cortisol in the venous drainage from the adrenal cortex. Glucocorticoids cause induction of the enzyme noradrenaline-N methyl-transferase and thus control the rate of synthesis of adrenaline. It is released into the blood stream on stimulation of the adrenal medulla.

The hypothalamus plays an important role in the regulation of catecholamine secretion by adrenal medulla. Stress stimulates the release of cortisol from the adrenal cortex (via ACTH) and of adrenaline from the adrenal medulla (via neuronal impulses). In addition, adrenaline secretion increases in response to various circulating substances such as glucagon, histamine, angiotensin II and bradykinin.

Two distinctly separate but related systems operate at the level of **adrenergic neuron**:

1. **One is concerned with the intraneuronal amine concentrating-storage mechanism.** The vesicles containing the granules have a vesicular monoamine transporter (VMAT) located in their wall; it has high affinity for NA.
2. The **other is responsible for the reuptake** (**Uptake$_1$ process**) of NA following its prior release from the nerve terminals using neuronal membrane amine pump (NET; norepinephrine transporter).

The maximum concentration of NA is found in the adrenergic nerve terminals in the brain as well as the peripheral adrenergic neurons. NA in the adrenergic nerve terminals exists in several pools, the major portion, over 60%, being present in protein bound form as granules. In the granules, it exists with calcium and ATP. An influx of Ca^{++} into the axonal terminals results in fusion of the vesicles with the plasma membrane and exocytosis of NA. Its movement from the extracellular space back to the cytoplasm, however, involves active transport mechanisms (**Uptake$_1$** in Fig. 17.4).

Presynaptic NA release is regulated through a negative feedback mechanism mediated by **adrenergic presynaptic α_2 receptors** (Fig. 17.4) and a positive feedback mechanism mediated by **presynaptic β-receptors**. According to this hypothesis, beta-receptors are more sensitive to agonists so that during the initiation of release, low concentrations of NA in the synaptic cleft accelerate the release process. *When the concentration of NA reaches high levels, the presynaptic α_2 receptors are stimulated, and the secretion is terminated by a negative feedback mechanism*. The combined effects of the positive and negative feedback mechanism may thus control the 'need-oriented' release of the transmitter. It appears that a presynaptic regulating mechanism similar to that described in the periphery operates in the CNS as well. Drugs could produce actions by altering the release of these NTs centrally or peripherally, by modifying the presynaptic regulatory mechanisms (Chapter 5).

A part of released NA is metabolised outside the cell by the enzyme **COMT** but a large part (75%–80%) is taken back into the cell by an active process and restored mostly in mobile pool. Only a small portion is metabolised intracellularly by **MAO.** *Rebinding of NA with the granules represents a way by which it is immobilised but can be used again. In fact, unlike Ach,*

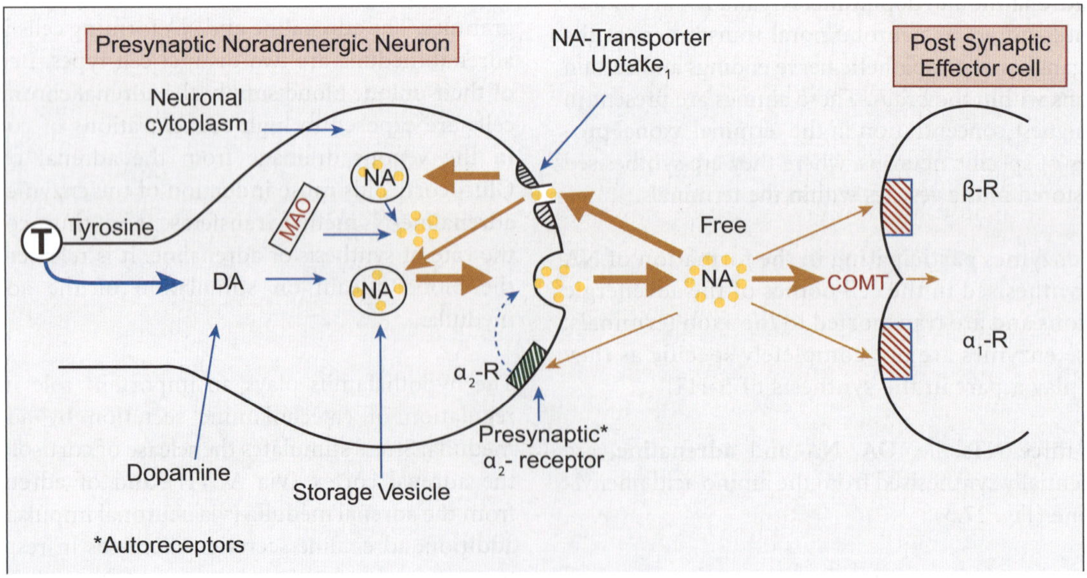

FIG. 17.4 Synthesis and metabolism of NA at adrenergic neuronal endings. Dotted line indicates the inhibition of release of transmitter

uptake and restorage are the major routes of NA inactivation and enzymatic destruction plays only a minor role (Fig. 17.4).

The enzymes MAO and COMT are widely distributed throughout the body including the brain, with the highest concentrations in the liver and the kidneys. It is also present in the intestinal mucosa. There are two types of MAO:

1. '**MAO-A**', which oxidises mainly NA and 5-HT, can be selectively inhibited by very low concentration of inhibitors, clorgyline and moclobemide.
2. '**MAO-B**', which oxidises DA in the brain, can be selectively inhibited by selegiline (Chapter 15).

The liver contains both forms in equal amounts, whereas the brain MAO is predominantly type B.

The mechanism of NA metabolism is discussed in Chapter 18. The end-products of NA and adrenaline metabolism are excreted in urine in a free form and as conjugates of glucuronic and sulphuric acids.DA is degraded predominantly by monoamine oxidase-B (MAO-B) in the brain and by MAO-A outside the CNS, and partly by catechol-O-methyl-transferase (COMT).

For details about adrenergic, DA and cholinergic receptors, see Chapters 18 and 19.

NEUROTRANSMISSION MECHANISMS AND DRUGS PH 1.13

A) Drugs acting on cholinergic system

In **cholinergic neurons**, the transport mechanism is for transmitter precursor choline rather than for ACh. Various agents which act on the **cholinergic system** (Fig. 17.5) produce their effects by:

- **Blocking synthesis of ACh**, e.g. hemicholinium which blocks the uptake of precursor, choline
- **Blocking the uptake of ACh into synaptic vesicles**, e.g. vesamicol
- **Inhibiting the release of ACh**, e.g. botulinum toxin
- **Increasing the release of ACh**, e.g. black widow spider toxin
- **Preventing the destruction of ACh by cholinesterase**, e.g. anticholinesterases
- **Interacting with postsynaptic receptors**
  a. ***Muscarinic receptors:*** e.g. muscarine (as an agonist) and atropine (as an antagonist)
  b. ***Nicotinic receptors on ganglia*** **(N_n):** e.g. DMPP (as an agonist) and hexamethonium (as an antagonist)
  c. ***Nicotinic receptors on N–M junction*** **(N_m):** e.g. nicotine (as agonist) and *d*-tubocurarine (as an antagonist)

B) Drugs acting on the adrenergic systems

Many studies have defined the properties of the catecholamine 'uptake' mechanisms involved and their modification by drugs.

1. **Uptake$_1$** *is the taking up of catecholamines from the synaptic cleft into the adrenergic neurons and in other extraneuronal cells.* This process demonstrates a greater affinity for NA than for adrenaline. Catecholamines taken up by 'Uptake$_1$' are then transferred to the storage vesicles in the adrenergic neurons by a separate process; both these processes are carrier-mediated transport system.
2. **Uptake$_2$** *is the taking up of catecholamines* by an organic cation transporter (OCT_3) located on *the effector cells in the peripheral tissues* such as the vascular smooth muscle, the heart and the exocrine glands. Such uptake is followed by rapid degradation of the catecholamines. In contrast to 'Uptake$_1$', 'Uptake$_2$' demonstrates a higher affinity for adrenaline and isoprenaline than for NA.

'Uptake$_1$' may be looked upon as 'uptake with retention'; by contrast, 'Uptake$_2$' is an 'uptake followed by metabolism'. Noradrenergic Uptake$_1$ and Uptake$_2$ transport systems can be blocked selectively by a number of drugs (Box 17.2).

Box 17.2 Inhibitors of NA Inhibitors of NA Uptake$_1$ and Uptake$_2$

Inhibitors of Uptake$_1$: Cocaine, tricyclic antidepressants, phenoxybenzamine, amphetamine, MAO inhibitors and chlorpromazine
Inhibitors of Uptake$_2$: Normetanephrine, glucocorticoids, phenoxybenzamine

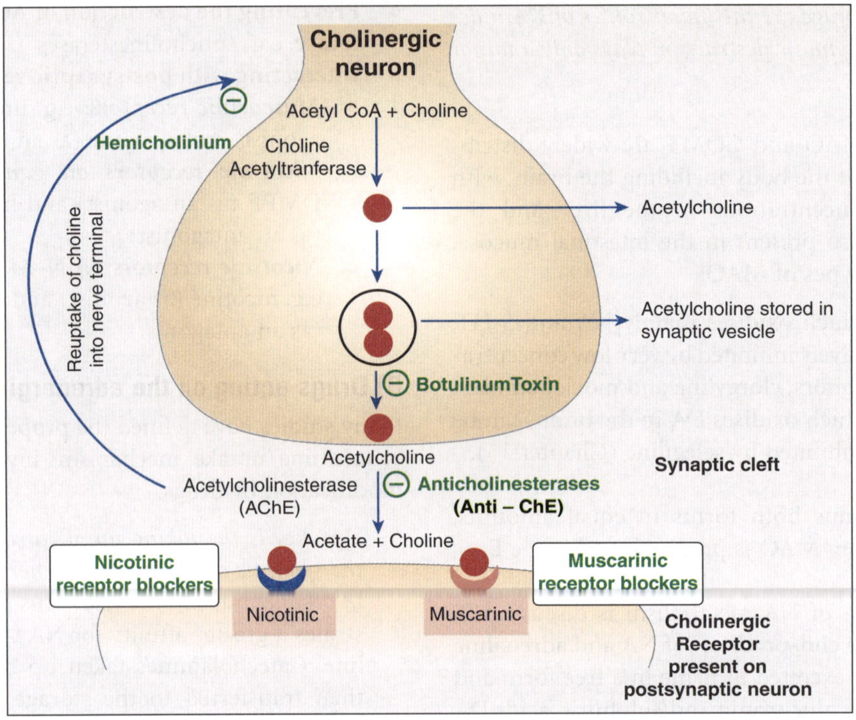

FIG. 17.5 Target sites for drug action on cholinergic system. ⊖ denotes inhibition

Many sympathomimetic amines are also taken up by 'Uptake$_1$' process and, hence, can act as competitive substrates, thus inhibiting the NA uptake. Other important drugs which are known to inhibit the 'Uptake$_1$' mechanism are listed in Box 17.2. *Drugs that inhibit 'Uptake$_1$'* potentiate and prolong the responses of sympathetically innervated organs to nerve stimulation. The drug 6-hydroxydopamine accumulates selectively through 'Uptake$_1$' process and produces selective destruction of adrenergic neurones (*chemical sympathectomy*) in both peripheral and central nervous system.

Various drugs which act on the **adrenergic neuron** produce their effects by modifying the synthesis, storage, 'Uptake$_1$' mechanism and blocking receptors as well as (Fig. 17.6) by:

- **Supplying an amine precursor**, e.g. levodopa used in Parkinson disease is a precursor of DA
- **Blocking the Uptake$_1$ of NA by inhibiting NET**, e.g. TCA like imipramine used in the treatment of mental depression; cocaine
- **Interfering with the synthesis of NA**, e.g. α-methyltyrosine
- **Inhibiting the transport into the vesicles, thus interfere with the storage of NA, leading to its depletion from the sites**, e.g. antihypertensive reserpine
- **Blocking the release of NA from the binding stores in the terminals**, e.g. guanethidine, a drug used in the treatment of hypertension
- **Promoting a synthesis of a false transmitter** which displaces NA, e.g. alpha methyldopa
- **Promoting the release of NA from the storage sites**, e.g. tyramine
- **Inhibiting the intraneuronal degradation of NA**, e.g. MAO inhibitors used as antidepressants
- **Blocking postsynaptic receptors**, e.g. adrenergic receptor blocking drugs

The above mechanisms are discussed elsewhere.

Specialised uptake mechanisms, similar to that described for NA neurons, are also known to exist in DA and 5-HT neurons in CNS and in cholinergic neurons in the periphery and CNS. PH 1.14

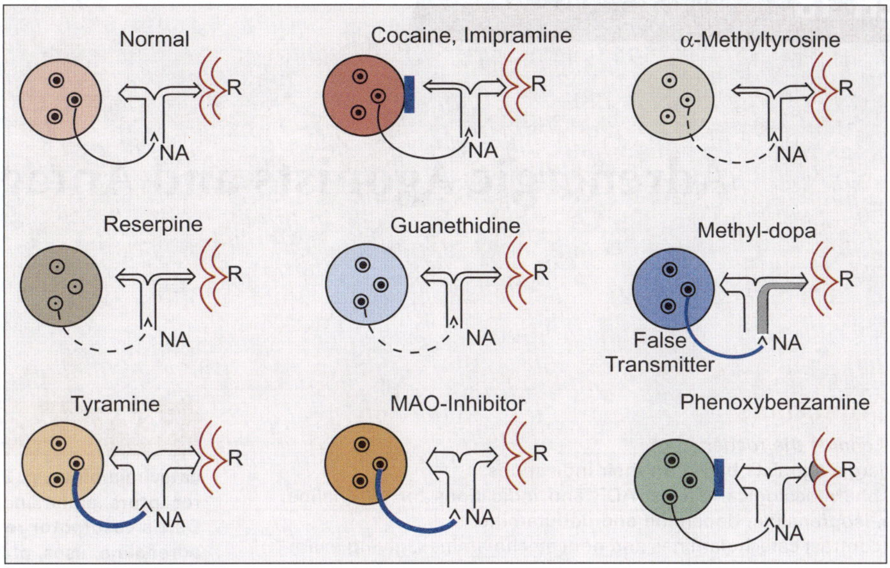

FIG. 17.6 Schematic diagram showing the effect of some drugs on noradrenaline (NA) uptake and release mechanisms. Drugs may act by inhibiting its Uptake$_1$ process (imipramine, cocaine), by interfering with the synthesis of transmitter (methyltyrosine), by depletion of NA from storage site (reserpine), by blocking the release from the storage site (guanethidine), by producing a false transmitter (methyl-DOPA), by promoting the NA release (tyramine), by inhibiting the destruction of NA by MAO (MAO-inhibitor) and by blocking both alpha Uptake$_1$ and Uptake$_2$ mechanisms (phenoxybenzamine).

Both ACh and NA are also termed as **local hormones** because they act at the site of their synthesis. Although ACh and NA are the main classical NTs at the autonomic nerve endings, the neurons may also possess other chemical messengers such as VIP, neuropeptide Y, etc., which function as primary NTs, co-transmitters or neuromodulators. Thus, autonomic transmission may, therefore, be mediated by the release of multiple neurochemicals.

Supersensitivity: Interruption of the nerve supply of an effector organ (denervation) makes it more sensitive to the neurohumor of the system supplying it. Thus, a skeletal muscle, after sectioning the motor nerve, becomes highly sensitive to ACh and the nictitating membrane becomes highly sensitive to NA after sectioning its postganglionic sympathetic supply. This phenomenon is termed **denervation supersensitivity**. Its mechanism is not known. It may be related to the elimination of the neuronal uptake mechanism. It could also partly be due to degeneration of the nerve terminals after sectioning, leading to disappearance of associated enzymes that normally inactivate the transmitter. It may also be due to an increase in receptor number (**upregulation**) induced by the fall in the catecholamine concentration within the synaptic cleft (also Chapter 2). Supersensitivity to transmitter substances has also been observed after prolonged administration of blocking agents.

CHAPTER 18

Adrenergic Agonists and Antagonists

Learning Objectives

This chapter will enable the reader:

1. Classify adrenergic agonists based on their indications.
2. Compare the pharmacological effects, ADR and indications for adrenaline, noradrenaline, isoprenaline, dopamine and dobutamine.
3. Compare and contrast catecholamines and noncatecholamines, giving examples of the latter.
4. State indications and ADR of noncatecholamines.
5. Classify the sympathetic blocking drugs with examples.
6. Discuss pharmacological effects, ADR and indications for α adrenergic blockers.
7. Enumerate various classes of β adrenergic receptor antagonists with examples.
8. Describe the pharmacological effects, salient pharmacokinetic features, ADR and contraindications of β adrenergic receptor blockers.
9. State various cardiovascular and noncardiovascular uses of β blockers giving the pharmacological basis for their use.

KEY TERMS

catecholamines, p. 273
receptors, alpha and beta, p. 273
Dale's vasomotor reversal, p. 276
adrenaline, uses, p. 279
noncatecholamines, p. 283
α receptor agonists, p. 284
nasal decongestants, p. 284
β_2 receptor stimulants, p. 285
α receptor blockers, p. 286
β adrenergic blockers, p. 288
labetolol, p. 291

The sympathomimetic or adrenergic drugs mimic the responses obtained after stimulation of the sympathetic or adrenergic nerves. Majority of these substances contain an intact or a partially substituted amino (–NH_2) group and, hence, are also called sympathomimetic amines. PH 1.13

Classification of Adrenergic Drugs based on their Therapeutic Use

I. **Adrenergic drugs used for raising blood pressure,** e.g. noradrenaline (NA), metaraminol and phenylephrine
II. **Those used for their inotropic actions on the heart,** e.g. dopamine (DA), dobutamine and isoprenaline
III. **Those used as central stimulants,** e.g. amphetamine, dextroamphetamine and methylphenidate
IV. **Those used as smooth muscle relaxants,** e.g. (a) *nonselective* β *stimulants* such as adrenaline, isoprenaline and (b) *selective* β_2 *stimulants*, e.g. isoxsuprine, salbutamol and terbutaline
V. **Those used in allergic reactions,** e.g. adrenaline and ephedrine
VI. **Those used for local vasoconstrictor effect,** e.g. adrenaline
VII. **Those used for nasal decongestion,** e.g. naphazoline, phenylephrine and xylometazoline
VIII. **Those used for suppressing the appetite (anorectic),** e.g. fenfluramine and phenteramine

These drugs can also be structurally classified as follows:

- **Catecholamines**, which are compounds containing a catechol nucleus (i.e. a benzene ring with two adjacent OH groups) and an amine-containing side-chain (Fig. 18.1)
- **Noncatecholamines** which lack the hydroxyl groups, e.g. amphetamine, ephedrine

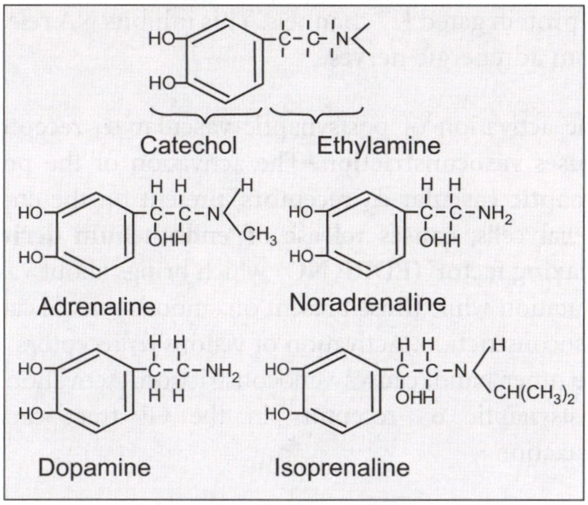

FIG. 18.1 **Catecholamines.**

CATECHOLAMINES

The catecholamines include the *neurohumoral transmitters* (a) **noradrenaline (NA)** and **dopamine (DA)***;* (b) *the main hormone of the adrenal medulla* **adrenaline;** *and* (c) *the synthetic compound* **isoprenaline** *(isoproterenol, isopropylarterenol)*.

The word 'nor' in NA was originally coined to indicate nitrogen (N) without (O – Ohne) a radical (R), in this case a methyl (CH_3) group.

Mechanism of action of catecholamines: The catecholamines produce their action by direct interaction with receptors located on the cell membrane. This drug–receptor combination leads to either an increase (*excitation*) or a decrease (*inhibition*) in the tissue activity. In order to explain these differences in responses by different tissues, the concept of two different receptors, **alpha** and **beta**, was proposed by Ahlquist (1948). Thus, (a) the α receptor stimulation is mainly responsible for the **excitatory effects**, whereas (b) the β receptor stimulation usually produces **inhibitory effects.** A given tissue may contain either α or β, or both types of receptors. Of the catecholamines:

1. **NA specifically acts on the α and β_1 receptors**
2. **Adrenaline acts nonspecifically on both α and β receptors**
3. **Isoprenaline acts only on β receptors**

Even though α receptors are generally excitatory and β receptors inhibitory in character, there are certain exceptions. Thus, β receptors, predominantly present in the heart, are excitatory in character; their stimulation increases the rate and force of cardiac contraction. Similarly, both the α and β receptors of the GI tract are inhibitory and their stimulation produces smooth muscle relaxation.

Adrenergic receptors are further subclassified according to their selective sensitivity to agonists and antagonists. At the molecular level, the adrenergic receptor–effector mechanism involves three interacting proteins: (i) Receptor(ii) G-protein (iii) Effector enzyme-ion channel.

Three distinct **β receptor subtypes** are as follows:

- **β_1 receptors** responsible for myocardial stimulation and renin release.
- **β_2 receptors** responsible for bronchial muscle relaxation, skeletal muscle vasodilation and uterine relaxation.
- **β_3 receptors** expressed primarily in brown and white adipose tissue. They regulate NA-induced changes in energy metabolism and thermogenesis. β_3 agonists stimulate metabolic rate and induce weight loss without reducing food intake in animals. It is relatively resistant to blockade by β antagonists.

Generally, β adrenergic responses appear to result from binding of the catecholamine to β receptors (β_1 and β_2) which via the mediation of a stimulatory G-protein (G_S) **stimulate a plasma membrane enzyme, adenylyl cyclase**. This results in a rise of the intracellular cyclic AMP (see Fig. 2.2 in Chapter 2). The cyclic AMP alters the cellular function by stimulation of a protein kinase, which causes phosphorylation of certain enzyme proteins, resulting in activation of some and inactivation of others. This may explain the stimulatory and inhibitory actions of drugs acting on the β receptors.

Phosphodiesterase, another enzyme, promotes the breakdown of cyclic AMP. Drugs like caffeine, theophylline and other methyl xanthines inhibit this enzyme and potentiate the β receptor stimulant action of adrenaline.

Presynaptic β receptors facilitate the release of NA at the adrenergic nerve terminals. (Chapter 17).

α Adrenergic receptors are of two types: α_1 and α_2, with *three subtypes* each (α_{1A}, α_{1B}, α_{1D}, and α_{2A}, α_{2B}, α_{2C}).

- **α_1 Adrenergic receptors** (**postsynaptic**) are predominantly in the vascular smooth muscles and are excitatory in nature:
  a. Their activation increases the intracellular concentration of calcium by activation of phospholipase C in the cell membrane via stimulatory G-protein (G_S).
  b. The phospholipase C then hydrolyses membrane bound phosphoinositides with the generation of two second messengers, diacylglycerol and inositol triphosphate.
  c. This results in an increase in the intracellular Ca^{++} which accounts for the vasoconstrictor effect.
- **α_2 Adrenergic receptors** are found both in effector tissues (**postsynaptic**) and on the neuronal endings (**presynaptic**) where they act as **autoreceptors.**

Activation of the **presynaptic α_2 receptors** by agents acting through the **inhibitory G protein** (**Gi**) inhibits adenylyl cyclase and **reduces the intracellular concentration of cyclic AMP.** These receptors activate G-protein gated K^+ channels. This inhibits NA release from adrenergic nerves.

The activation of postsynaptic **vascular α_1 receptors causes vasoconstriction.** The activation of the **postsynaptic vascular α_2 receptors**, present on the endothelial cells, **causes release of 'endothelium derived relaxing factor'** (**EDRF, NO**) which brings about vasodilatation while those present on smooth muscle cause vasoconstriction. Activation of venous α_2 receptors, on the other hand, causes venoconstriction. Activation of postsynaptic α_2 receptors in the GI tract causes relaxation.

α_2 Adrenergic receptors are also present at the postjunctional or nonjunctional sites in several tissues such as the brain. Activation of postjunctional α_2 receptors in the brain by clonidine causes the antihypertensive effect (Chapter 30).

The presence of α receptors has been also demonstrated on human leukocytes and platelets.

The predominant receptors in various organs and the usual responses to their activation are given in Table 18.1; however, such responses in isolated tissue

Table 18.1 Distribution and Responses of Adrenergic Receptors

Tissue	Response
Predominantly α receptors	
a. Medulla oblongata (α_2)	Reduction of BP and heart rate
b. Blood vessels: (α_1)	
Skin and mucosa	Constriction
Cerebral	Constriction (slight)
c. Skin:	
Pilomotor muscle (α_1)	Contraction
Apocrine sweat glands	Secretion increases
d. Radial muscle of iris (α_1)	Contraction (mydriasis)
e. Salivary glands, except parotids	Thick, viscous secretion
f. Sex organ, male (α)	Emission
Predominantly β receptors	
a. Heart: (β_1, α_1)	
S-A node – β_1	Increased heart rate (positive chronotropic action)
Atria – β_1	Increased contraction (positive inotropic action)
A-V node – β_1	Faster conduction
Ventricles – β_1	Increased contractility and conductivity, increased automaticity (positive dromotropic action)
b. Bronchial muscle – β_2	Relaxation
c. Skeletal muscle changes – β_2	Changes in contractility

Table 18.1 Distribution and Responses of Adrenergic Receptors—cont'd

Tissue	Response
d. Skeletal muscle blood vessels – β_2	Dilatation
e. Kidney: JG apparatus – β_1	Renin secretion
Both α and β receptors	
a. GI tract:	
Motility and tone (α_2 β_2)	Decreased
Sphincters (α_1)	Contraction
Pancreas:	
α_2	Inhibiting insulin release
β_2	Stimulation of insulin release
b. Urinary bladder:	
Trigone – α_{1A}	Contraction
Detrusor – β_2	Relaxation
c. Blood vessels:	
Coronary – α, β_2	Constriction; dilatation
Pulmonary – α, β_2	Constriction; dilatation
Abdominal viscera – α, β_2	Constriction (mainly); dilatation
Renal – α, β_2	Constriction; dilatation
Skeletal muscle – α, β_2	Constriction; dilatation
d. Adipocyte:	
α_2	Inhibit lipolysis
β_3	Lipolysis
Liver – α_1, β_2	Glycogenolysis, neoglucogenesis, inhibition of glycogen synthetase
e. Leukocyte (human) – β_2	Inhibits chemotaxis and lysosomal enzyme release
Platelet (human) – α_2	Platelet aggregation
f. Uterus:	
α_1	Contraction
β_2	Relaxation

Table 18.2 Drugs Acting on Adrenergic Receptor Subtypes

	α_1	α_2	β_1	β_2
Agonists	Phenylephrine Methoxamine Metaraminol Mephentermine	Clonidine Apraclonidine Methyldopa Guanfacine	Dobutamine Isoprenaline	Orciprenaline Salbutamol Terbutaline Isoetharine
Antagonists	Prazosin Indoramin	Yohimbine	Propranolol Pindolol Atenolol Metoprolol	Propranolol Pindolol
Location of receptors	Postsynaptic (vessels, glands and smooth muscles)	Presynaptic Postsynaptic (vessels and brain tissue) Nonsynaptic (platelets, leucocytes and lipocytes)	Postsynaptic (heart, brain and JG cells and lipocytes Presynaptic adrenergic and cholinergic nerve terminals)	Presynaptic Postsynaptic (heart and smooth muscles) Nonsynaptic (lymphocytes and polymorphonuclear cells)
Mechanism of action	Alteration of cellular calcium-ion fluxes	Inhibition of adenylyl cyclase	Stimulation of adenylyl cyclase	Stimulation of adenylyl cyclase

preparations may differ from those in the intact animal owing to the presence of compensatory reflex activity in the latter. Table 18.2 lists the **agonists** and **antagonists** of the adrenergic receptor subtypes.

Adrenaline and Noradrenaline

Pharmacological actions: Adrenaline is a nonselective α and β receptor agonist, whereas NA acts more selectively as α and β_1 agonist.

Cardiovascular system:

- **Heart: Adrenaline stimulates the β_1 receptors** in the heart and increases the:
  a. Rate
  b. Force of contraction
  c. Conduction velocity

This is associated with increased metabolism of the myocardium and increased oxygen consumption. It also increases cardiac output by stimulating venoconstriction, thus increasing the venous return, and increasing the force of atrial contraction which augments the ventricular diastolic volume. Very high cardiac rate, however, prevents proper diastolic filling and may produce fall in the cardiac output. *Enhanced conduction across the A-V node may cause ventricular arrhythmias.*

NA, though β_1 stimulant does not usually increase the heart rate but tends to produce bradycardia due to compensatory vascular reflex activity. It should be noted, however, that NA is the physiological transmitter in the heart and its capacity to stimulate cardiac β_1 receptors is of vital importance.

The myocardial effects of adrenaline and NA can be blocked by the β receptor blockers.

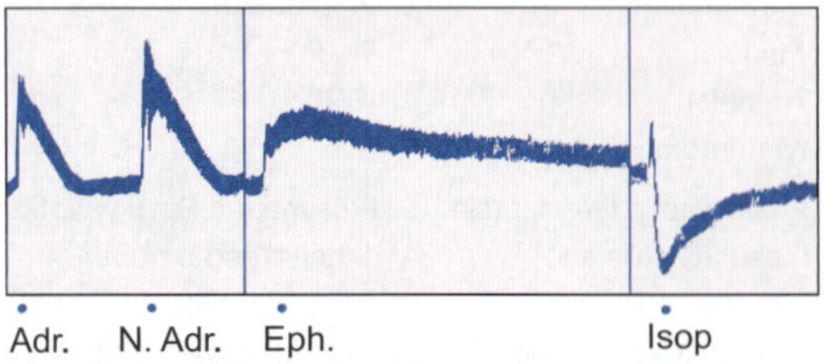

FIG. 18.2 Effect of adrenaline (Adr), noradrenaline (N.Adr), ephedrine (Eph) and isoprenaline (Isop) on blood pressure in anaesthetised dog.

- **Blood vessels and blood pressure** (Fig. 18.2): Adrenaline and NA constrict the blood vessels of the skin and mucous membranes.

PH 4.2

Adrenaline *dilates the blood vessels of the skeletal muscles* on account of the preponderance of β_2 receptors; and decreases the total peripheral resistance. Hence, although *adrenaline raises the systolic BP mainly by its cardiac actions, it lowers the diastolic pressure by its peripheral actions*; and therefore, **it is not suitable for routine use in hypovolemic shock**.

As the rise in systolic BP with adrenaline is only of moderate magnitude, compensatory reflexes do not antagonise its cardiac actions and the rise in systolic BP is accompanied by tachycardia, increased cardiac output and increased stroke volume.

The rise in systolic BP produced by moderate doses of adrenaline is often followed by a fall. This is because stimulation of α receptors produces a rise in BP. However, its action on β receptors is more persistent and hence, when the action on α receptors wears off, the action on β receptors gets unmasked producing a fall in BP. **This response to moderate doses of adrenaline is termed as biphasic response.** Sir Henry Dale noted that this **biphasic response** was converted to a depressor response by prior administration of ergot extract which blocks the α receptor, leading to stimulation of peripheral β_2 receptors by adrenaline, resulting in a fall in BP. This phenomenon is termed as **Dale's vasomotor reversal** (Fig. 18.3). Such reversal is not seen with NA.

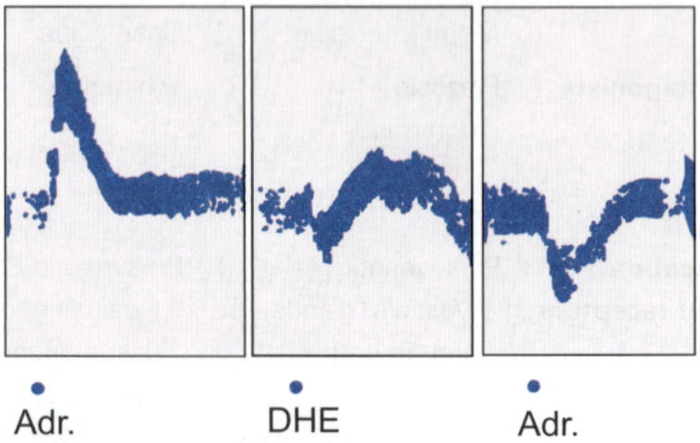

FIG. 18.3 Dale's vasomotor reversal. Note the fall in BP with adrenaline after injection of dihydroergotamine (DHE).

NA produces a rise in both systolic and diastolic BP, which is associated with reflex bradycardia. The pulse pressure increases. Its β_2 receptor actions are very feeble. PH 4.2

Renal blood flow is reduced by both, adrenaline and NA, even in doses that have no significant effect on BP. The urine output and urinary excretion of sodium, potassium and chloride decreases. Renin secretion is increased by direct β_1 receptor effect, independent of renal vascular changes, whereas α_2 receptors are responsible for inhibition of renin release from the kidney.

Both adrenaline and NA constrict the hepatic and mesenteric blood vessels and raise the portal venous pressure. The pulmonary arterial and venous pressures are raised by both. Constriction of the musculature of the great systemic veins tends to push the blood from the periphery into the pulmonary circulation and this may occasionally cause pulmonary oedema.

Adrenaline in moderate doses increases the coronary and cerebral blood flow and oxygen consumption.

Smooth muscle: Table 18.1.

- **Bronchi:** Adrenaline by its **β_2 receptor agonist action causes relaxation of the bronchial smooth muscle** and act as a bronchodilator. It antagonises the bronchospasm produced by vagal stimulation, choline esters, histamine or an antigen–antibody reaction, bradykinin, leukotrienes or prostaglandin $F_2\alpha$.
- **Gastrointestinal tract:** Adrenaline and NA relax the smooth muscle of the gut and reduce its motility; the sphincters are constricted.
- **Uterus:** The response of the uterus to the catecholamines varies according to species, the phase of oestrous cycle, presence or absence of gestation, period of gestation and the dose administered. The rat uterus is relaxed irrespective of all these factors. The human nonpregnant uterine strip is stimulated to contract by adrenaline. *In the last month of pregnancy adrenaline inhibits uterine contraction and causes relaxation.*
- **Other smooth muscles:** Adrenaline contracts the pilomotor muscle of the hair follicle, vesical sphincter and the trigone (α receptor), however, it relaxes the detrusor muscle (β receptor). Adrenaline and NA produce contraction of the splenic capsule producing a release of erythrocytes into the circulation. This probably serves as a protective mechanism during stress such as hypoxia and haemorrhage.

Eye: Sympathetic stimulation causes **mydriasis** due to contraction of the radial muscle fibres of the iris, and exophthalmos due to contraction of the orbital muscles. Adrenaline and NA, on topical application, do not readily penetrate the eyeball.

Respiration: Adrenaline is a weak stimulant of respiration. Given intravenously, both adrenaline and NA may induce apnoea partly by stimulating the baroreceptors and mainly by a direct central action. Adrenaline, particularly in aerosol form, constricts the pulmonary vessels and relieves bronchial congestion.

Metabolic effects: Adrenaline **increases**:

- **Blood sugar level** by enhancing hepatic glycogenolysis (β_2 effect) and by decreasing peripheral glucose uptake.
- **Blood lactate** by enhancing the breakdown of glycogen to lactate in the skeletal muscles.
- **Plasma-free fatty acid concentration** by increasing lipolysis in adipose tissue.
- Serum K^+ level transiently, followed by a more sustained **hypokalaemia.** Both adrenaline and NA promote cellular uptake of K^+.

Activation of pancreatic α_2 adrenergic receptors by adrenaline and by severe stress (via activation of adrenergic nervous system) inhibits insulin release; β_2 adrenergic receptor agonists and vagal nerve stimulation enhance it.

Central nervous system: The catecholamines do not cross the BBB satisfactorily and hence, their central actions are limited. Adrenaline may produce excitement, tremor stupor, vomiting and restlessness.

NA and DA are important neurotransmitters in the CNS (Chapter 5).

Skeletal muscle: The **α effect** on the motor nerve endings increases the amount of ACh released and is probably the main factor in the improvement of neuromuscular transmission by adrenaline. **The β action** on the muscle fibre itself probably contributes to the improvement of muscle contractions and tremor, sometimes observed following these drugs.

Antiallergic action: Adrenaline and related compounds prevent the release of mediators of allergy such as histamine from the tissue mast cells (Chapter 27).

Miscellaneous: Adrenaline produces thick viscid secretion from salivary glands, leucocytosis and eosinopenia and accelerates blood coagulation. It also stimulates platelet aggregation through α_2 receptors.

The important pharmacological actions are summarised in Table 18.3.

Absorption, fate and excretion: Catecholamines are not effective orally because they are rapidly inactivated by monoamine oxidase (MAO) in the gut and the liver. On inhalation as aerosol, small quantities may be absorbed into circulation.

Adrenaline and NA are rapidly metabolised by:

- **Catechol-O-methyl transferase** (COMT) located extracellularly
- **Monoamine oxidase** (MAO), located inside the mitochondria of the adrenergic neurons

These enzymes are also present in the liver and kidney. They act sequentially as shown in Fig. 18.4 and convert them into the final urinary excretory products: VMA, metanephrine (metadrenaline) and normetanephrine (normetadrenaline). A small quantity of catecholamines is excreted unchanged.

Table 18.3 Comparison of the Pharmacological Actions of Catecholamines

Effector Organ	Adrenaline	Noradrenaline	Isoprenaline
Heart			
Rate	+ +	–	+ +
Stroke volume	+ + +	+ +	+ + +
Cardiac output	+ + +	0, –	+ + +
Arrhythmias	+ + +	+ +	+ + +
Coronary blood flow	+ +	+	+ +
Blood pressure			
Systolic	+ + +	+ + +	+, 0, –
Diastolic	+, 0, –	+ +	+, 0, –
Pulse	+, 0	+ +	0, +
Mean	+, 0	+ +	0
Peripheral blood flow			
Muscle	+ +	+, 0	+ +
Skin and mucous membrane	–	+, 0, –	+
Renal	–	–	?
Splanchnic	+ +	0, +	+ +
Cerebral	+	0, –	+
Total peripheral resistance	–	+ + +	–
Smooth muscles			
Bronchi	+ + +	+, 0	+ + +
Metabolism			
Oxygen consumption	+ +	0, +	0
Blood sugar	+ + +	0, +	0
Eosinopenic response	+	0	0

Note: +, increase; 0, no change; –, decrease.

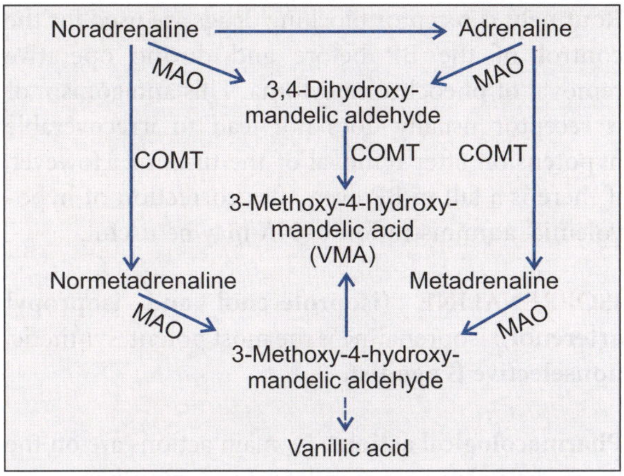

FIG. 18.4 **Metabolism of adrenaline and noradrenaline.**

The normal 24-h urinary excretion of VMA and free catecholamines is 4–8 mg and 50–100 mcg, respectively. A significant increase in these values is considered diagnostic of pheochromocytoma, an adrenal medullary tumour, producing excessive catecholamines.

Adverse reactions: These are **mostly cardiovascular** and are due to extension of the pharmacological actions. Adrenaline, given subcutaneously, may produce palpitation, throbbing headache and tremors. NA, employed in the form of IV drip, may cause anxiety, pallor and headache.

- Both adrenaline and NA, injected rapidly, intravenously, may cause a sudden, marked increase in BP, precipitating subarachnoid haemorrhage and occasionally a stroke.
- They can cause ventricular arrhythmias including fatal ventricular fibrillation. In individuals with cardiac decompensation, adrenaline may precipitate acute pulmonary oedema.
  NA infusion has to be carefully titrated, and BP has to be checked at least every 15 min to prevent the above mentioned complications. *The infusion must never be left unattended.* NA infusion, if stopped suddenly, may result in alarming hypotension.
- NA infusion, if extravasated, produces local vasospasm and sloughing.
- Adrenaline and NA (particularly the former) may precipitate anginal pain in persons with ischemic heart disease. Thyrotoxic or hypertensive individuals are more sensitive to the pressor effects of these agents.

Preparations and dosage:

i. Adrenaline injection: 0.5 or 1 mL ampoules containing 1:1000 adrenaline (1 mg/mL) in water. Dose: 0.2–0.5 mL subcutaneously or intramuscularly. Rarely, the drug is administered intravenously, in the dose of 0.25 mg, further diluted with saline and given slowly, under monitoring and supervision for cardiac arrest. Adrenaline 1mg/10ml (1 in 10,000) dilute solution is available.
   Similarly adrenaline as 0.5 mg/ml and 0.15mg/0.3ml (1 in 2,000) is also available as autoinjectors for immediate treatment of anaphylactic shock.
ii. Adrenaline inhalation; is a nonsterile, 1:100, aqueous solution of adrenaline tartrate.
iii. NA injection; 0.2% solution of NA bitartrate in 2-mL ampoules. It is administered as an i.v. infusion. For this purpose, 2 mL of NA bitartrate (equivalent to 4 mg of the salt and 2 mg of the base) is added to 500 mL of 5% *dextrose solution (which is generally acidic)* resulting in a concentration of 4 mcg of the base per mL. After judging the cardiovascular response with a test dose of 2–3 mL, the drug is administered at the rate of 0.5–1 mL/min. The dose is controlled according to the blood pressure response. NA *is unstable at the neutral pH of normal saline and vitamin C (500–1000 mg) should be added to the infusion*, if NA needs to be infused in normal saline.

Indications for adrenaline:

- **Anaphylaxis and angioneurotic oedema:** Adrenaline is the **drug of choice** in the treatment of anaphylactic shock. (Chapter 23). It is life-saving in angioneurotic oedema of the larynx.
- **Cardiopulmonary resuscitation (CPR):** Cardiac arrest is an emergency and 70% cardiac arrest occur at home or on the road. Measures to resuscitate the victim should be started within 3 minutes by anyone nearby, diagnosed if the patient collapses suddenly and becomes unconscious, is not breathing, and the carotid pulse absent. Box 18.1 summarises the general guidelines for CPR, which comprises **attention to: C (circulation), A (airway) and B (breathing)** . Indian Society of Anaesthesiologists (ISA) have developed guidelines for resuscitation by layperson – the compression-only life support (COLS).

Box 18.1 Steps of Cardiopulmonary Resuscitation

- Tap on the shoulder and confirm unconsciousness (no verbal response or by purposeful movement), absent carotid pulse and apnoea
- Shout for help or call on pan- India emergency contact number-108
- Initiate CPR sequentially as Compressions (C), Airway (A), Breathing (B) in that order (CAB approach).
- Apply external cardiac massage (C) i.e. initiate precordial chest wall compressions (chest wall must depress by at least 5 cm) at the rate of at least 120/min.
- Tilt the victim's head by the forehead back and lifting the chin to open the airway. Clear the oropharynx. Pinch shut the victim's nose using the forefinger and thumb
- Give mouth to mouth breathing; deliver breaths over 1 second while looking for the victim's chest to rise.
- The cycle of 30 compressions and 2 breaths should be continued until there is a sign of return of spontaneous circulation (movement of any part of the body, coughing or vocalizing), the rescuer is physically unable to do so or professional rescuers arrive (i.e.compression: breath ratio as 30:2).
- As soon as an automatic external defrillator becomes available it should be turned on and its instructions should be followed to connect it to the patient.
- Hospitalise

It involves chest compression for 5 consecutive cycles (30 compressions in each) without any mouth to mouth breathing.

The therapy of cardiac arrest comprises (1) **basic life support**, to be administered at the site of the occurrence and (2) **advanced life support**, to be provided in the intensive care facility of a hospital.

- **Control of haemorrhage:** Adrenaline in the concentration of 1:1000 to 1:20,000 is sometimes used *topically* for controlling bleeding, e.g. epistaxis and bleeding after tooth extraction.
- **Other local uses:** Adrenaline, because of its vasoconstrictor effect, is infiltrated in the concentration of 1:50,000 to 1:100,000 along with local anaesthetics. It reduces the systemic absorption of the local anaesthetic, thus prolonging its action and minimising its toxicity.

Indications for NA:
NA is mainly used to combat refractory hypotension following **shock** (Chapter 32), or spinal anaesthesia (Chapter 16).

Routinely, α receptor blocking drugs are used for the control of the BP before and during operative removal of pheochromocytoma. This antagonism of α receptor usually does not lead to irrecoverable hypotension after removal of the tumour. However, if there is a fall in BP even after correction of hypovolemia, administration of NA may be useful.

ISOPRENALINE (isoproterenol and isopropyl arterenol): Isoprenaline is the most potent, synthetic, **nonselective β agonist.**

Pharmacological actions: Its main actions are on the heart, skeletal muscle vasculature and smooth muscles. It:

a. **Stimulates the heart** to increase myocardial contractility and causes tachycardia.
b. **Lowers the peripheral vascular resistance** in skeletal, renal and mesenteric vascular beds and produces a fall mainly in the diastolic pressure.
c. **Relaxes the smooth muscles** particularly those of bronchi and GI tract.
d. Has **calorigenic and FFA releasing actions** are similar to those of adrenaline.

Absorption, fate and excretion: Isoprenaline is inconsistently absorbed sublingually and orally. Absorption is quicker after IM injection and by inhalation. It is rapidly inactivated by uptake into tissue and metabolised by COMT.

Adverse reactions: are mainly cardiac, e.g., palpitation, tachycardia, arrhythmias, anginal pain, headache and flushing.

Preparation and dosage:

i. Isoprenaline injection, 2 mg/mL to be diluted for IV infusion.

Indications:

- **Stokes–Adams syndrome:** Isoprenaline, because of its lesser liability to produce cardiac arrhythmias, is preferred to adrenaline in this condition. It may be administered either intravenously or orally in the dose 30–120 mg 6–8 hourly.
- **To counter cardiotoxicity due to β blocker overuse.**

Table 18.4 Pharmacological Effects of Dopamine

Dose (by Infusion mcg/kg/min)	Effects
2–5 (Dopaminergic range)	Renal, mesenteric and cerebral *vasodilation by action on dopamine (D_1)* receptors
5–10 (Dopaminergic + β_1 range)	Same as above. Plus increase in myocardial contractility with increase in heart rate and cardiac output, by action on dopamine (D2) and β_1 receptors. This is of advantage in the treatment of shock. The peripheral resistance is lowered or unchanged.
11–20 (β_1 range)	*Predominantly cardiac action*
More than 20 (α_1 range)	*Vasoconstriction*, Decrease in renal blood flow and urine output, and sometimes aggravation of heart failure, by action on α_1 adrenergic receptors

Precautions and contraindications for catecholamines: Catecholamines should be administered cautiously in the presence of hypertension, hyperthyroidism, angina pectoris (ischaemic heart disease; IHD), acute left ventricular failure and hypotension during halothane anaesthesia.

DOPAMINE (DA): This naturally occurring precursor of NA acts on dopaminergic and other adrenergic receptors.

Postsynaptic DA receptors are of two types: **D_1-like** (D_1 and D_5) and **D_2-like** (D_2, D_3, D_4). Refer Table 5.3. **Presynaptic receptors** or **autoreceptors for DA are present in the brain**. DA is also a weak α and β adrenergic receptor agonist.

It is metabolised by MAO and COMT. It has extremely short half-life. Its effects can be blocked, by the use of α blocker phentolamine. DA does not cross the BBB.

Table 18.4 and Fig. 18.5 summarise the pharmacological effects of DA, at different doses.

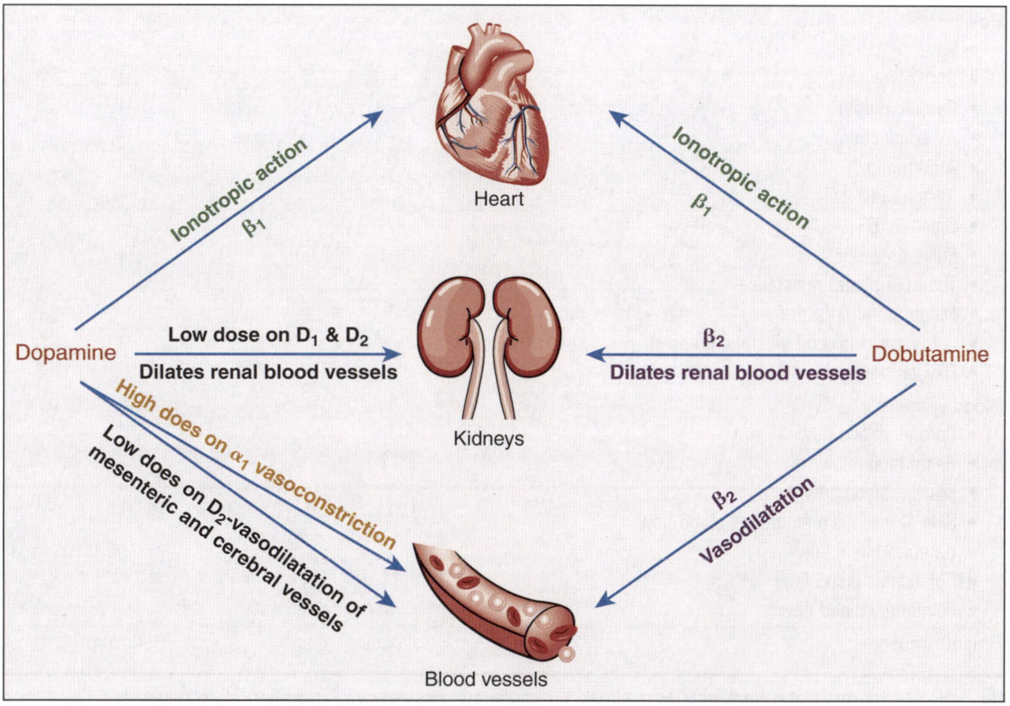

FIG. 18.5 Actions of dopamine and dobutamine.

Adverse reactions: These include nausea, vomiting, palpitation, ectopic beats and anginal pain. A sudden rise in BP may occur. Small doses occasionally precipitate a fall in BP. Infusion of large doses for long time may cause ischemia and gangrene of limbs.

> *Reduction in urine output, tachycardia and development of arrhythmias indicate toxicity.*

Indications:

- **Shock:** Chapter 32.
- **Severe CHF in patients with oliguria:** Chapter 31.
- **Threatened acute renal failure:** In low dose (less than 5 mcg/kg/min), it preferentially dilates the renal vessels and may produce diuresis. If the patient does not respond in 10–12 h, the drug should be discontinued.

FENOLDOPAM: This **D_1 receptor agonist** acts as a peripheral vasodilator and is used in hypertensive crises (Chapter 30).

D_2 receptor agonists (e.g. bromcriptine) are described in Chapter 65.

DOBUTAMINE, though structurally related to DA, has a **selective β_1 receptor agonist action with predominant effect on cardiac contractility.** DA receptors are not involved in its action. It has negligible chronotropic and peripheral vascular actions. Unlike DA, it does not cause renal vasodilatation. In patients with low-output cardiac failure, it increases the cardiac output without increasing the heart rate. The comparison of pharmacological effects of dopamine and dobutamine is presented in Fig 18.5 and Table 18.5.

It has a short duration of action and is given by slow IV infusion in 5% dextrose, at the rate of 2.5–15 mcg/kg/min. Its ADR is similar to that of DA. *Like other catecholamines, dobutamine loses its effect in an alkaline medium.*

It is particularly useful as an ionotropic agent in refractory, chronic, congestive heart failure,

Table 18.5 Comparison of Pharmacological Effects of Dopamine and Dobutamine

Effector Site	Dopamine	Dobutamine
Heart		
• Rate	++	+
• Stroke volume	+	+
• Cardiac output	++	+
• AV conduction	+	+
• Arrhythmia	+	+
• Systolic BP	++	+
• Diastolic BP	−/+	−
• Pulse pressure	++	+
• Total peripheral resistance	−	−
• Mean aortic pressure	↑	−
• Left ventricular end diastolic pressure	++	+
• Oxygen demand		
Blood vessels		
• Coronaryblood flow	↑	↑
• Renal blood flow	↑↑	−
• Muscle blood flow	↑	↑
• Skin & mucous membranes blood flow	↑	↑
• Cerebral blood flow	↑	−/↑
• Splanchnic blood flow	↑↑	−
• Pulmonary blood flow	↓	−
Smooth muscle	Relaxation	Relaxation

Note: −/+, May or may not have effect; +, minimal; ++ moderate; No change; ↑ increase; ↑, decrease unresponsive to digoxin. It may also have beneficial hemodynamic effects in patients with bacteremic shock.

Dopexamine is another inotropic agent used in heart failure associated with cardiac surgery.

NONCATECHOLAMINES

The sympathomimetic amines devoid of the catechol nucleus comprise compounds like **ephedrine, amphetamine** and other **vasopressors** as well as **smooth muscle relaxing compounds.**

Both, ephedrine and amphetamine, have limited use in clinical practice.

Mechanism of action: These drugs:

- **Release NA and/or DA from the sympathetic neurons**. Noncatecholamines are taken up in the neuron by norepinephrine transporter (NET) and are concentrated in the vesicles by vesicular monoamine transporter (VMAT). They displace NA, which is subsequently released into the synaptic cleft. This *indirect action* produces mainly α adrenergic effects resembling those of NA.
- **Inhibit the reuptake of neurotransmitters** *DA, NA and 5-HT by membrane transporters, e.g. amphetamine and ephedrine.*
- **As partial agonists of NA,** they *directly* stimulate the adrenergic α and/or β receptors. This explains the relaxation of the bronchial smooth muscle by ephedrine, uterine smooth muscle by isoxsuprine and vascular smooth muscle by nylidrin and stimulation of the myocardium by mephenteramine.

Compared to catecholamines, they:

1. Are effective orally.
2. Cross the BBB and therefore have significant CNS effects.
3. Are relatively resistant to the action of MAO; and hence
4. Have longer duration of action.

EPHEDRINE is an alkaloid (Fig 18.6) obtained from plants of the genus *ephedra*. Although used as an indigenous medicine in India and China for over 5000 years, it has not been studied extensively in humans.

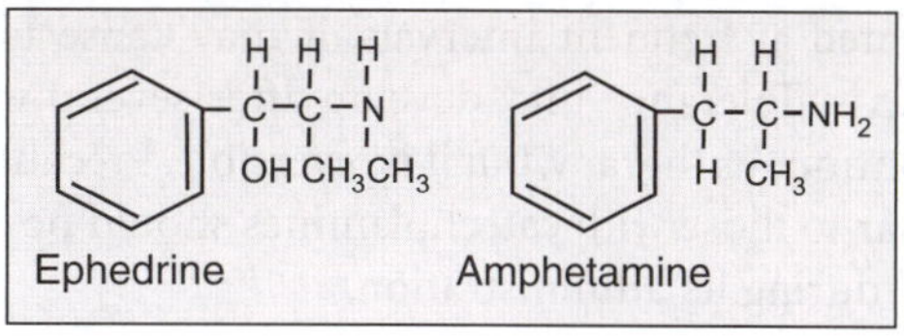

FIG. 18.6 **Chemical structure of noncatecholamines.**

Pharmacological actions: As stated above, ephedrine acts indirectly as well as directly.

CVS: Effects of ephedrine are similar to those of adrenaline but it is a less potent agent. Repeated administration at short intervals decreases the pressor response, (**tachyphylaxis**).

Smooth muscles: The bronchial relaxation is less prompt than with adrenaline but persists for a longer time.

CNS: Ephedrine stimulates the CNS probably by acting on the reticular activating system. Therapeutic doses, often cause increases in mental activity, restlessness, insomnia, anxiety and tremors. It enhances the monosynaptic and polysynaptic reflexes of the spinal cord and increases the depth and rate of respiration.

Eye: It produces mydriasis.

Metabolic effects: Like adrenaline, it increases the metabolic rate and oxygen consumption but is less effective in raising the blood sugar level.

Absorption, fate and excretion: Ephedrine is well absorbed orally. As it is relatively resistant to MAO, it has a longer duration of action than adrenaline. It is deaminated to some extent in the liver, but largely (60%–75%) is eliminated unchanged in urine.

Adverse reactions: The adverse reactions are similar to those encountered with catecholamines. However, in therapeutic doses ephedrine is usually well tolerated. Being a nonselective sympathomimetic, it may cause CNS stimulation, insomnia, tremors, palpitation, rise in BP and difficulty in passing urine, particularly in the elderly and rarely psychotic symptoms.

Repeated at frequent intervals, it may cause tachyphylaxis. Tolerance may develop after several weeks of continuous therapy, but it is reversible. Precautions similar to those with catecholamines should be exercised during its administration.

Indications: Ephedrine is now replaced by other drugs. It is misused by bodybuilders, weight lifters and athletes for weight loss and performance enhancement. It appears to play role in exercise addiction and eating disorders. Hence it is considered as a drug of abuse and is banned.

Pseudoephedrine hydrochloride, a stereoisomer of ephedrine (30 and 60 mg tablets, and syrup 30 mg in 5 mL) is used as a nasal decongestant. It is less liable to produce tachycardia, increase in BP and CNS stimulation. PH 1.22

AMPHETAMINE, which is structurally related to ephedrine (Fig. 18.6), For details see Chapter 12.

OTHER NONCATECHOLAMINES

1. Vasopressor Agents

The vasopressor agents increase the BP either by increasing the peripheral resistance or by increasing cardiac output or by a combination of both. They can be classified as:

1. **Nonselective**, acting on both, α and cardiac β receptors, e.g. NA (discussed earlier)
2. **Selective**, acting only on α_1 adrenergic receptors, e.g. **mephentermine, metaraminol, phenylephrine** and **methoxamine**

These agents are used parenterally:

- **To correct hypotension due to cardiogenic shock and to prevent and treat hypotension due to neurogenic shock**, e.g. during or after spinal anaesthesia.
- **To correct cardiac arrhythmias** associated with hypotension.

METARAMINOL: Metaraminol, α receptor agonist, is less potent than NA. It has a gradual onset and longer duration of action. A part of its effect is mediated indirectly through release of NA.

Rise in BP is usually accompanied by reflex bradycardia. It increases the coronary blood flow, probably as a result of increased BP, but reduces the cerebral, splanchnic, renal and limb blood flow.

It is used to treat hypotension in the dose of 2–10 mg intramuscularly. The IV dose is 0.5–10 mg. It can also be given as a slow infusion. It is also used as a nasal decongestant.

MEPHENTERMINE acts directly, as well as indirectly by releasing NA. Its actions resemble those of ephedrine. It causes CNS stimulation.

PHENYLEPHRINE: This vasopressor agent has a potent selective α_1 receptor stimulant action. The pressor response is accompanied by reflex bradycardia. It has minimal action on the CNS. It is used as a **nasal decongestant** (0.25%–0.5%) and as a mydriatic (1%–2%).

METHOXAMINE: This α-adrenergic agonist, raises BP purely by peripheral vasoconstriction accompanied by reflex bradycardia. Its haemodynamic actions are similar to those of phenylephrine. A 0.25% solution is used as a **nasal decongestant**.

MIDODRINE: This prodrug acts through its active metabolite, **desglymidodrine**, on α_1 receptors. It is used to treat postural hypotension resulting from impaired autonomic function (Chapter 30). As it causes supine hypertension, it is administered to a patient in upright position.

When using vasopressor agents, the BP should be raised only moderately above the critical level (100/70 mm Hg) necessary for adequate tissue perfusion. Excessive vasoconstriction jeopardises tissue perfusion and defeats the very purpose of vasopressor therapy.

2. Nasal Decongestants

In addition to the vasopressor agents mentioned above, other sympathomimetic amines are available for use topically as nasal decongestants. Also, see Chapter 27.

Nasal vasculature tone is influenced by the sympathetic nervous system. Alpha-adrenoceptor sympathomimetic drugs act on postjunctional alpha-adrenergic receptors found on precapillary and postcapillary blood vessels of the nasal mucosa. Due to their vasoconstrictor action, they oppose vasodilation, causing decongestion. This reduces nasal airway resistance and thus facilitates nasal breathing.

An ideal nasal decongestant should:

a. produce a prompt, prolonged and reliable effect
b. be free from tachyphylaxis, local irritation and damaging effect on nasal cilia
c. not produce after-congestion and systemic adverse effects

Only a *few drugs in very dilute solution are safe*; majority of them can produce temporary or even permanent damage to ciliated respiratory epithelium after repeated use, with the possibility of atrophic changes. *It is important to remember that they may blunt effects of antihypertensive drugs.*

For nasal decongestion, often simple decongestants like **Xylometazoline hydrochloride** 0.1%, and oxymetazoline 0.05% are used. Their effect lasts for 8-10 hrs. **Ephedrine hydrochloride** 0.5% in normal saline also produces symptomatic relief for several hours.

Pseudoephedrine and phenylephrine are common constituents of various **oral preparations** promoted for the relief of nasal congestion.

3. Selective α_2 Receptor Stimulants

Clonidine and **methyldopa**, α_2 adrenergic receptor agonists, are used for the treatment of hypertension; they act by stimulating central α_2 adrenergic receptors (Chapter 30).

Apraclonidine and **brimonidine** are used to decrease IOP in glaucoma (Chapter 70). **Tizanidine** is used as central muscle relaxant (Chapter 22).

4. Selective β_2 Receptor Stimulants

Nonselective βreceptor stimulants like isoprenaline stimulate both β_1 and β_2 receptors and, therefore, when used as bronchodilator or tocolytic cause adverse cardiac effects. Hence drugs with predominant action on β_2 receptors were developed. Selective bronchodilators are either short acting, e.g. **salbutamol (albuterol), fenoterol, terbutaline,** or long acting e.g. **salmeterol**. Given by inhalation, they act as promptly as isoprenaline but have a longer duration of action (2–12 h) with less stimulant action on the heart. These drugs are used in the treatment of bronchial asthma (Chapter 27).

Tocolytics (Uterine relaxants) are **isoxsuprine** and **ritodrine**.

ISOXSUPRINE: This has β_2 receptor actions as well as direct action on vascular and uterine smooth muscle. It is used in the treatment of threatened abortion and premature labour (Chapter 42). It is also used in the treatment of peripheral vascular disease. It is available as 10 mg tablets and as IM/IV injection.

5. Anorexiants

The use of these agents in the treatment of obesity is discussed in Chapter 38.

SYMPATHETIC BLOCKING DRUGS PH 1.13

The actions produced by stimulation of the sympathetic nervous system can be blocked by peripherally acting drugs:

1. **Drugs that induce depletion of catecholamines from the various body tissues**, e.g. reserpine and tetrabenazine (Chapter 30).
2. **Drugs that interfere with synthesis of the adrenergic transmitter** either in the adrenergic neuron or in the adrenal medulla, e.g. alpha methyl paratyrosine (Chapter 30).
3. **Drugs that interfere with transmission of impulses across the postganglionic adrenergic neurons**, e.g. adrenergic neuron blockers like guanethidine (Chapter 30).
4. **Drugs which block the adrenergic receptors**, e.g. α and β adrenergic receptor blocking agents. They are described below.

ADRENERGIC RECEPTOR BLOCKERS

Adrenergic receptor blocking agents prevent the response of effector organs to endogenous as well as exogenous adrenaline, NA and other sympathomimetics. These drugs block either or receptors, or both.

Alpha receptor blockers

These drugs are more effective in antagonising the α receptor effects of exogenously administered adrenaline and NA than direct adrenergic stimulation. They are classified as follows:

I. **Nonselective α adrenergic blockers:**
   a. **β Haloalkylamines**, e.g. dibenamine and phenoxybenzamine
   b. **Natural and hydrogenated Ergot alkaloids**
   c. **Imidazoline derivatives**, e.g. tolazoline and phentolamine

II. **Selective α_1 adrenergic blockers:** Quinazolines, e.g. prazosin, terazosin, doxazosin and indoramin

III. **Selective α_2 adrenergic blockers,** e.g. yohimbine

PHENOXYBENZAMINE: It binds to α receptors and causes prolonged and stable nonequilibrium (noncompetitive) type of blockade, termed as irreversible blockade. It also blocks both, the $Uptake_1$ and $Uptake_2$ mechanisms.

Pharmacological actions: Phenoxybenzamine is a prodrug with an active metabolite. It nonselectively **blocks both postsynaptic α_1 and presynaptic α_2 receptors**. The blocking effect is established only after 1–2 h, even on IV administration and persists for 3–4 days. The usual doses cause slight lowering of diastolic BP in normal individuals but significant lowering of BP in patients with pheochromocytoma (Fig. 18.7). It can prevent cardiac arrhythmias induced by sympathomimetic amines like adrenaline.

In clinically effective doses, phenoxybenzamine causes orthostatic hypotension due to α_1 blockade in the blood vessels. Accumulated NA at the adrenergic neuronal endings would normally be reduced by action of presynaptic α_2 receptors (autoreceptors); but as they too are blocked, the released NA stimulates cardiac β receptors, **causing tachycardia** (Fig. 18.7). It also antagonises the actions of ACh, 5-HT and histamine. Slow IV infusion often produces sedation and drowsiness, probably by its antihistaminic activity.

Absorption, fate and excretion: Phenoxybenzamine is given orally or by IV infusion .Its oral absorption

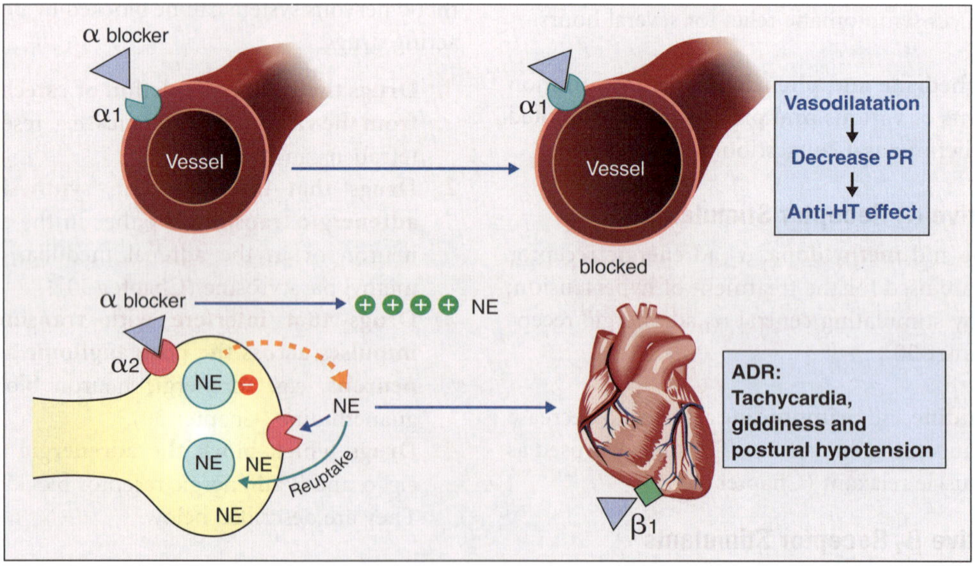

FIG. 18.7 Effect and ADR of nonselective alpha blockers. Note that these drugs (e.g. phenoxybenzamine) act on post-synaptic α1 receptors of the vessel causing vasodilatation, which is responsible for its therapeutic effect. They also block pre-synaptic α2 receptors, leading to increased release of NA. The released NA cannot act on post-synaptic α1 receptors which are already blocked. However, it acts on the cardiac β1 receptors causing adverse reaction.

is irregular. It is highly lipid soluble. Approximately 50% of the IV dose is excreted within 12 h and 80% within 24 h.

Adverse reactions: Phenoxybenzamine may cause palpitation, giddiness and postural hypotension. Other ADR include miosis, dryness of mouth, nasal stuffiness and inhibition of ejaculation. Large doses produce nausea, vomiting, increased excitability and even convulsions. It can cause cumulative toxicity as it accumulates in the body fat.

Preparations and dosage: Phenoxybenzamine 10 mg capsules. The usual daily maintenance dose is 20–60 mg. It is also available as 50 mg/ml solution for injection.

Indications: It is used orally to prepare a patient suffering from pheochromocytoma for surgery and in its long-term treatment. (Chapter 30).

NATURAL AND DIHYDROGENATED ERGOT ALKALOIDS: The detailed pharmacology of the ergot alkaloids is discussed in Chapter 42. However, their α adrenergic receptor blocking activity is of no therapeutic value.

TOLAZOLINE and **PHENTOLAMINE:** They cause competitive nonselective α adrenergic blockade. They also increase the force of myocardial contraction and cause tachycardia. They dilate the peripheral blood vessels, particularly the arterioles and capillaries of the skin, and increase the gut motility and the gastric secretion.

Tolazoline is a partial α_1 agonist and because of its predominant cardiac effect, often evokes a mild rise in BP, whereas **phentolamine** usually produces a moderate fall due to peripheral vasodilatation.

Absorption, fate and excretion: Tolazoline is well absorbed on oral and parenteral administration and eliminated mainly unchanged in urine. Phentolamine is poorly absorbed on oral administration; approximately one-tenth of its total parenteral dose is eliminated in urine, whereas the rest is probably metabolised.

Adverse reactions: These include palpitation, flushing and apprehension. Other ADR are nasal congestion, postural hypotension, piloerection, nausea, vomiting, epigastric distress and diarrhoea.

Preparations and dosage: Phentolamine mesylate injection 5 mg/mL. Dose: 1–10 mg intravenously, repeated if necessary.

PRAZOSIN: It (Fig. 18.8) acts selectively by blocking postsynaptic α_1 receptors.

Thus, it:

- **Dilates the arteries** (lowering blood pressure) *and* **the veins** (reducing the venous return and cardiac output)
- **Reduces the tone of the internal sphincter of the bladder** thus decreasing the resistance to urinary outflow in patients with benign prostatic hyperplasia (BPH; Chapter 67)
- It **does not cause tachycardia** as it does not block presynaptic α_2 receptors. For details, see Chapter 30.

TERAZOSIN: This selective α_1 adrenergic blocker is used in the treatment of BPH. The drug is longer acting than prazosin and is used once a day in the dose of 1 mg (at bed time), increased at weekly intervals to 2–10 mg (administered as a single dose per day).

Doxazosin, alfuzosin, bunazosin and **tamsulosin** are the other α_1 adrenergic blockers. Tamsulosin acts more selectively on the prostatic α_{1A} and α_{1D} adrenergic receptors and hence is used in benign hypertrophy of prostate (Chapter 67).

INDORAMIN: This selective α_1 blocker can be used to treat BPH. For its use in hypertension, see Chapter 30.

URAPIDIL, an α_1 antagonist, has weak α_2 agonist

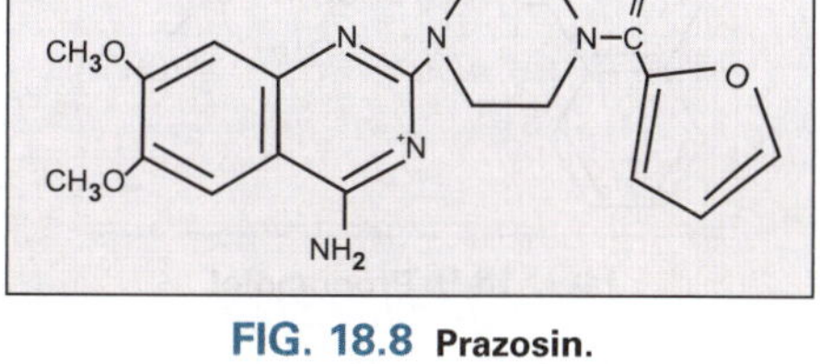

FIG. 18.8 Prazosin.

and 5-HT_{1A} agonist actions. It is also a weak β_1 antagonist. It is used as an antihypertensive and for BPH.

YOHIMBINE, an alkaloid from the West African tree *Pausinystalia chimbe*, is a competitive **α_2 receptor antagonist** with short duration of action. Stimulation of the presynaptic α_2 receptors inhibits the release of NA from the peripheral adrenergic nerve endings. Their blockade by yohimbine increases the sympathetic outflow and potentiates the release of NA. The drug once promoted for erectile dysfunction (aphrodisiac), is no more used.

Indications for α adrenergic blockers: These drugs have limited therapeutic applications, mainly owing to their adverse effects like tachycardia and postural hypotension. The important uses are:

- **Hypertension and pheochromocytoma:** See Chapter 30
- **Peripheral vascular disease:** See Chapter 28
- **Benign prostatic hyperplasia:** See Chapter 67
- **Scorpion sting:** See Chapter 71
- **Prevention of cutaneous necrosis due to extravasation of NA:** Phentolamine is infiltrated in the dose of 2.5–5 mg

Ketanserin, a 5-HT receptor antagonist, also blocks α_1 adrenergic receptors (Chapter 24).

α Adrenergic blocking action of chlorpromazine and haloperidol is discussed in Chapter 13.

Beta receptor blockers

The first β blocker was discovered by James Black (Nobel Prize, 1988). These drugs selectively and competitively block the actions of catecholamines on the β receptors. They inhibit the activity of the cell membrane enzyme adenylyl cyclase and decrease the production of cyclic AMP.

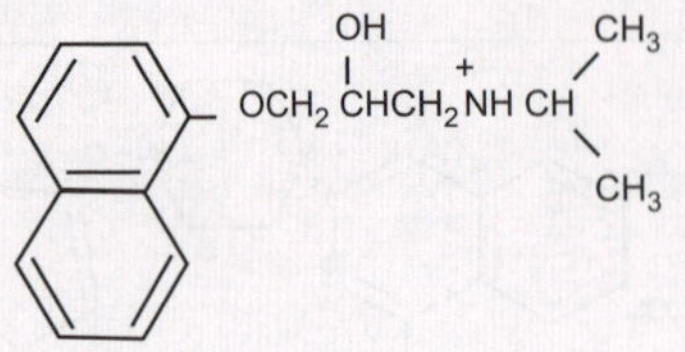

FIG. 18.9 **Propranolol.**

Classification of β blockers

I. Nonselective β_1 and β_2 blockers:
  a. **With membrane stabilising activity,** e.g. propranolol (Fig 18.9)
  b. **With intrinsic sympathomimetic activity,** e.g. carteolol
  c. **With membrane stabilising activity and intrinsic sympathomimetic activity,** e.g. oxprenolol, pindolol
  d. **Without membrane stabilising activity,** e.g. timolol, nadolol and sotalol

II. Cardioselective β_1 blockers, e.g. acebutolol, atenolol, metoprolol, bisoprolol, and esmolol. Acebutolol has intrinsic sympathomimetic activity

III. β Blockers with additional properties
  a. **Nonselective with α blocker activity:** Labetalol, bucindolol, carvedilol
  b. **Cardioselective:** Betaxolol, nebivolol, celiprolol

Pharmacological actions (Table 18.6):

Cardiovascular system:

- **Heart:** These drugs do not produce any marked effect on the normal heart in the individual at rest. In the presence of increased sympathetic tone, the cardiac β receptor blockade:

1. Reduces the automaticity and prevents the rise in heart rate
2. Reduces the myocardial contractility, cardiac output and stroke work
3. Slows A-V conduction
4. Reduces myocardial oxygen requirement and improves exercise tolerance

The cardiac response to exercise and to other situations in which sympathetic tone is increased, is attenuated.

- **Blood pressure:** They reduce BP probably by their action on the heart and reduction in cardiac output. They reduce renin release and lower the plasma renin activity (PRA), but cause an increase in natriuretic peptide secretion (Chapter 30). They also reduce central sympathetic outflow and have a central hypotensive action. *They do not cause postural or exercise induced hypotension as the α_1 adrenergic receptors are not blocked.*

Table 18.6 Properties of Some β Adrenergic Blockers

Drugs	Relative Lipid Solubility	β_2 Agonist Activity	Protein Binding (%)	Liver Metabolism	Kidney Excretion	Plasma Half-life (h)
I. Nonselective:						
Propranolol[c]	+ + +	0	90	+ + +	<5	3–6
Oxprenolol	+ +	+ +	–	+ + +	5	1–2
Pindolol[c]	++	+ + +	40	+ +	30–40	3–4
Nadolol	+	0	30	+	76	20–24
Timolol	+ +	0	<10	+ + +	10	4–6
Labetolol[a]	++	+	50	+ + +	<5	3–4
Carteolol[c]	+	+ +	25–30	0	80	6
Carvedilol[a]	+ + +	0	98	+ + +	<5	7–10
II. Cardioselective:						
Atenolol	0	0	6–16	+	85	6–8
Metoprolol[c]	+ +	0	12	+ +	10	3–6
Bisoprolol	+	0	30	+ +	50	9–12
Acebutolol[c]	+	+	26	+	30–40	3–4
Esmolol[b]	+	0	55	+ + +	2	0.15
Celiprolol	+	+	4–5	0	12–8	5–6
Nebivolol	+ +	0	98	+ + +	40	11–30

Note: +, present; 0, absent. [a]αReceptor blocking also. [b]IV infusion only, in emergency management of unstable angina, threatened infarct, cardiac arrhythmias and thyrotoxic crisis. [c]Local anaesthetic action.

Bronchial effects: The blockade of β_2 receptor sites in bronchi and bronchioles causes increase in airway resistance which could be harmful in patients with asthma. Celiprolol may be preferred in them as it is a weak bronchodilator due to its partial B_2 agonist and weak smooth muscle relaxant properties.

Membrane-stabilising action: Propranolol and some other β blockers (celiprolol) have a variable direct myocardial depressant effect on the heart similar to that of lignocaine. *It occurs only with high doses, which are not used therapeutically.*

Intrinsic sympathomimetic action: Some of the β blockers possess β receptor stimulating activity (**partial agonist property**). It has been *suggested but not proved*, that β blockers with additional intrinsic sympathomimetic activity may cause less cardiac depression and are thus less likely to precipitate congestive heart failure in the presence of damaged heart.

It should be noted that the pharmacological actions of β receptor antagonism are always present at lower concentrations of the drug than either membrane stabilising or paradoxical agonist effect. *The primary β blocking action of all these drugs is in fact mostly responsible for their beneficial as well as adverse effects.*

Effects on the CNS: Lipid soluble propranolol, metoprolol and labetalol readily cross the BBB. Propranolol alters mood and has been used in anxiety states. Atenolol, with the lowest lipid solubility, has fewer central side effects.

Metabolic effects: β Blockers are capable of modifying carbohydrate and lipid metabolism. **Nonselective Beta Blockers**, prevent catecholamine-induced glycogenolysis and mobilisation of glucose during hypoglycaemia, and delay recovery. Further, they decrease the release of free fatty acids (FFA) from the adipose tissue. Long-term use increases LDL cholesterol and triglycerides, and decreases HDL cholesterol. However, selective β_1 blockers such as celiprolol, carvedilol and carteolol may improve the lipid profile.

Ocular effects: β Blockers, used topically or orally,

cause a reduction in IOP due to a reduction in the secretion of aqueous humour (Chapter 70).

Some β blockers have additional actions, e.g. through NO production (celiprolol, carteolol), calcium channel blocking (carvedilol), and potassium channel opening (tilisolol). Their contribution to the therapeutic effects, however, is not clear.

Absorption, fate and excretion: The effective oral dose ranges of the β-blocking drugs are wide. Plasma concentrations vary markedly between individuals receiving the same dose. This is because although most of these compounds are completely and rapidly absorbed, some of them like propranolol and metoprolol are rapidly metabolised by the liver (*first pass metabolism* (Table 18.6). Thus, for propranolol, the relative oral bioavailability is low and variations in plasma levels are marked (almost up to 20-fold). Those which are largely excreted by the kidney, i.e. atenolol, nadolol tend to accumulate in the presence of kidney damage. Pindolol, acebutolol, atenolol and timolol are eliminated to variable extents by both routes.

The plasma half-life of the β blockers that are mostly metabolised by the liver is short (2–3 h), whereas that of drugs excreted unchanged is longer (8–12 h). Duration of effect is modified by liver and kidney diseases (Table 18.6) and by the active metabolite(s), e.g. the active metabolite of propranolol, 4-hydroxypropranolol, makes twice a day administration of propranolol possible. *The plasma t½, however, does not correlate well with the duration of their therapeutic effects.* This is because the plasma level declines exponentially, as it follows first order kinetics, whereas the effect decreases linearly, outlasting the plasma levels. Hence, *most agents can be given orally at much longer intervals than is suggested by their plasma half-lives.*

Adverse reactions: In general, they are well tolerated and are reasonably safe.

- **Cardiovascular effects:** These are mostly due to the *extended cardiac actions.* Thus, *propranolol may cause hypotension and pronounced bradycardia.* The ventricular function depends on increased contractility due to sympathetic activity, and β blockade prevents this homeostatic response leading to clinical heart failure in patients with cardiac damage.

Some of these drugs *can aggravate A-V conduction defects.* However, prolonged AV conduction may be beneficial in patients with atrial fibrillation. Excessive bradycardia due to overdose can be countered by IV atropine 0.6–2.4 mg in divided doses (Chapter 32).

If β blocker therapy is to be discontinued in angina, the dosage should be reduced gradually, as myocardial infarction may be precipitated following its abrupt withdrawal.

Cold extremities and absent pulses may sometimes be observed after β blockade. Raynaud phenomenon may occasionally be troublesome and intermittent claudication may be aggravated.

- **Metabolic effects:** Nonselective β blockers mask the symptoms indicative of hypoglycaemia such as palpitation and tremor and prevent its recognition by the patient (**hypoglycaemia unawareness**) and as mentioned earlier they may delay recovery from hypoglycemia. *In clinical practice cardioselective β blockers may be used safely* in most patients with T2DM (Chapter 63).
- **Bronchospasm:** This may occur particularly in patients with bronchial asthma. Cardioselective β blockers in low doses may be preferred but none is absolutely safe.
- **CNS effects:** Prolonged use of beta blockers that cross BBB (e.g. propranolol) can cause fatigue, sleep disturbances (insomnia and nightmares), muscle cramps, lethargy and rarely mental depression.
- **Miscellaneous:** These include allergic reactions, thrombocytopenia and sexual dysfunction. In patients with severe renal failure, their dose needs to be adjusted. β Blockers can be used during pregnancy. However, they can cross placental barrier and may cause hypoglycaemia and bradycardia in neonates. Drugs such as NSAIDs that cause sodium retention attenuate the antihypertensive effect of β blockers. A combination of β blockers with verapamil and amiodarone may be dangerous as the combination aggravates bradycardia and depression of AV conduction.

β Blockers may increase the severity and possibly the frequency of anaphylactic reactions to drugs, biologicals, insect stings and foods, and the reaction may prove resistant to treatment with adrenaline.

Table 18.7 depicts the dosage schedules of the commonly used β blockers.

Indications: Clinically, in terms of β-blocking activity, no drug is superior to others. The choice is guided by safety, pharmacological properties, ease of administration and cost. *For routine use, a cardioselective β blocker such as atenolol may be preferred*, keeping in mind that cardioselectivity is not absolute.

1. **Cardiovascular uses:**
   - **Angina pectoris:** β Blockers are the mainstay of the chronic, prophylactic treatment of patients with angina of effort (Chapter 29)
   - **Myocardial infarction:** Chapter 29
   - **Cardiac arrhythmias:** β Blockers can be used to treat tachyarrhythmias precipitated by sympathetic overactivity as during exercise, emotion and anaesthesia. (Chapter 28)
   - **Hypertension:** Chapter 30
   - **Heart failure with reduced ejection fraction (HFrEF):** Chapter 31
   - **Hypertrophic obstructive cardiomyopathy** is characterised by a marked hypertrophy of the ventricular musculature, commonly of the left ventricle, leading to palpitation, angina, dyspnoea or syncope. Propranolol causes symptomatic improvement.
   - **Pheochromocytoma:** α Adrenergic blocking agents are routinely used prior to surgery in patients with pheochromocytoma. In some patients, however, α blockade leads to a severe tachycardia. Propranolol, in the dose of 1–5 mg intravenously, prevents this complicatio.

2. **Noncardiovascular uses:**
   - **Chronic open-angle glaucoma:** Timolol maleate 0.25%–0.5% is used as eye-drops in lowering IOP (Chapter 70).
   - **Thyrotoxicosis:** β Blockers are valuable adjuncts to antithyroid drugs in the treatment of thyrotoxicosis, where they produce rapid symptomatic relief (Chapter 62).
   - **Portal hypertension:** Propranolol and nadolol used orally prevent variceal bleeding by lowering the pressure in the portal circulation (Chapter 33).
   - **To control the withdrawal symptoms in alcohol addicts.** (Chapter 6).
   - **Miscellaneous:** Increased adrenergic activity is prominent in anxiety states and propranolol can reduce the associated symptoms such as palpitation, tachycardia and sweating β blockers may be used to decrease cardiac symptoms prior to important meetings and public speaking engagements in susceptible individuals. Propranolol is also useful in the prevention of migraine and treatment of essential tremor.

Contraindications to β blockers: are listed in Box 18.2.

α and β receptor blockers

LABETALOL: Labetolol is a nonselective β blocker. It exhibits different relative affinity for the receptors accounting for the complex drug effects:

Table 18.7 Dosage Range of Some β Adrenergic Blocking Drugs

Drug	Total Daily Dose (mg)	Schedule
Propranolol	80–240	6–12 hourly
Metoprolol	100–200	12 hourly/single
Atenolol	25–100	Daily
Timolol	10–60	12 hourly
Pindolol	10–45	6 hourly
Labetalol	200–600	12 hourly
Carvedilol	20–50	12 hourly

Box 18.2 Contraindications to β Blockers

Absolute:
- Severe bradycardia
- Pre-existing high grade heart block
- Overt left ventricular failure (untreated)
- Cardiogenic shock
- Severe bronchospasm
- Severe depression
- Raynaud phenomenon (active disease)

Relative: Prinzmetal angina; concomitant use of verapamil, diltiazem or digoxin; mild asthma; diabetic patients on insulin

1. Blockade of the β_1 and β_2 receptors
2. Partial agonistic activity at β_2 receptors
3. Selective blockade of α_1 receptors
4. Inhibition of neuronal uptake of NA

These actions prevent the vasoconstriction observed following nonselective β blocker. Given orally, it is less effective than atenolol.

The drug undergoes extensive first pass metabolism with t½ of 4 h. It is given b.i.d.

Adverse reactions: Labetalol may cause GI disturbances, dryness of mouth and fluid retention. Cardiac effects are similar to those of other β blockers. Postural hypotension may occur. Other reactions include nervousness, sexual dysfunction, muscle cramps and depression. The drug accumulates in tissues with high melanin content such as the choroid, and periodic eye examination is recommended.

Indications: It is mainly used by infusion (1 mg/min titrated at ½ hourly interval) to treat hypertensive emergencies, as the effect is rapid due to concurrent α_1 blockade (Chapter 30).

CARVEDILOL: Like labetalol, this drug is a non-selective β blocker with selective α_1 blocking action. It also has other additional properties such as antioxidant activity, anti-inflammatory activity, membrane stabilizing effect and calcium entry blockade action.

Absorption, fate and excretion: Carvedilol is rapidly absorbed on oral administration with peak plasma concentrations occurring in 1–2 hours and highly plasma protein bound (95 %). It is metabolized by CYP2D6, CYP2C9 with an elimination half life of 7–10 hours.

Adverse reactions: Orthostatic hypotension and dizziness due to α_1 blockade and like other β blockers, initial exacerbation of heart failure, renal failure may occur.

Indications:

- **Hypertension:** See Chapter 30.
- **Heart failure:** It decreases lipid peroxidation and vascular wall thickening, effects that are beneficial in heart failure. It also helps to reduce the workload on the heart by blocking sympathetic stimulation.
- **Ischaemic heart disease:** See Chapter 29.

Bisoprolol and **Nebivolol** are cardioselective β blockers (Table 18.6) with NO-mediated vasodilator properties. They are effective in hypertension as well as CHF and improve left ventricular function (Chapter 31). They have t½ of 10–11 h. They are more expensive.

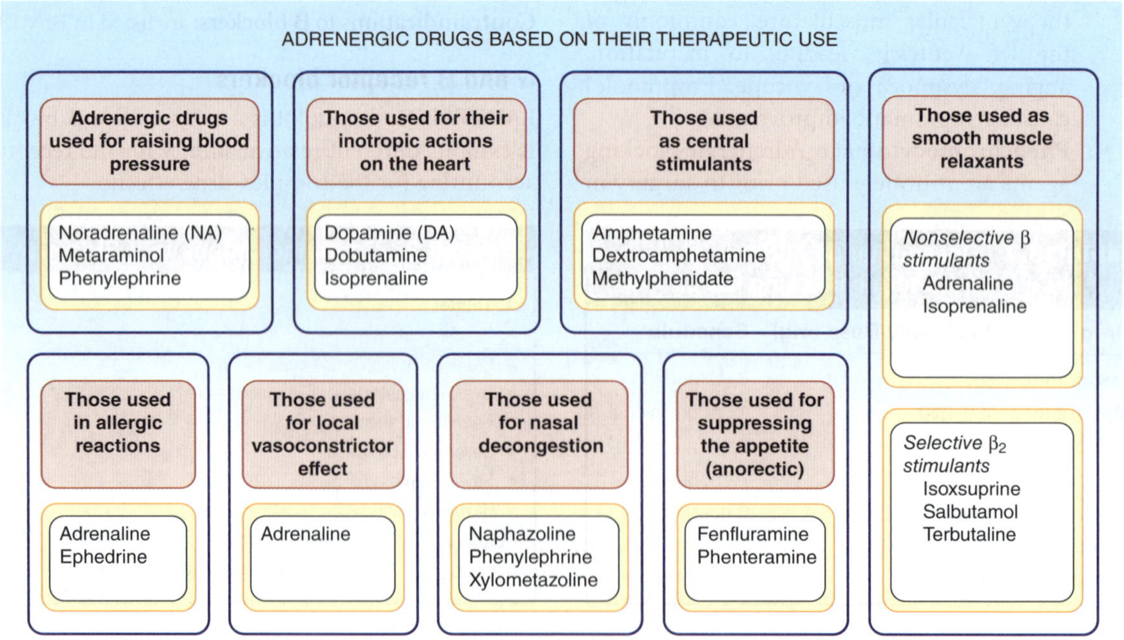

ALPHA ADRENERGIC RECEPTOR BLOCKERS

Nonselective α adrenergic blockers

β Haloalkylamines
- Dibenamine
- Phenoxybenzamine

Natural and hydrogenated Ergot alkaloids

Imidazoline derivatives
- Tolazoline
- Phentolamine

Selective α_1 adrenergic blockers

- Quinazolines
  - Prazosin
  - Terazosin
  - Doxazosin
  - Indoramin

Selective α_2 adrenergic blockers

- Yohimbine

BETA ADRENERGIC RECEPTOR BLOCKERS

Nonselective β_1 and β_2 blockers

With membrane stabilising activity
- Propranolol

With intrinsic sympathomimetic activity
- Carteolol

With membrane stabilising activity and intrinsic sympathomimetic activity
- Oxprenolol
- Pindolol

Without membrane stabilising activity
- Timolol
- Nadolol
- Sotalol

Cardioselective β_1 blockers

- Acebutolol
- Atenolol
- Metoprolol
- Bisoprolol
- Esmolol

β Blockers with additional properties

Nonselective with α blocker activity
- Labetalol
- Bucindolol
- Carvedilol

Cardioselective
- Betoxolol
- Nebivolol
- Celiprolol

CHAPTER 19

Cholinergic Drugs

Learning Objectives

This chapter will enable the reader:

1. To classify cholinergic drugs, giving examples.
2. To describe the pharmacological effects of acetylcholine and explain why it is not used in therapeutics.
3. To compare and contrast acetylcholine and other cholinomimetic alkaloids used in clinical practice.
4. To classify cholinesterase inhibitors explaining the basis for the classification.
5. To describe pharmacological effects, salient pharmacokinetic features, ADR and indications for reversible anticholinesterases.
6. To outline the management of myasthenia gravis.
7. To discuss the principles and treatment of acute organophosphorous poisoning.

KEY TERMS

choline esters, p. 294
receptors, muscarinic and nicotinic, p. 294
pilocarpine, p. 297
anticholinesterases, reversible and irreversible, p. 298
neostigmine, p. 299
myasthenia gravis, p. 301
organophosphorus compound poisoning, p. 303
pralidoxime, p. 305

Cholinergic or parasympathomimetic drugs stimulate the effector cells innervated by postganglionic parasympathetic cholinergic nerves. In general, their actions are similar to those seen following the stimulation of the parasympathetic nervous system. PH 1.14

Classification of Cholinergic Drugs

I. **Esters of choline,** e.g. acetylcholine, carbachol and bethanechol
II. **Cholinomimetic alkaloids,** e.g. pilocarpine, muscarine and arecoline
III. **Cholinesterase inhibitors (anticholinesterases),** e.g. physostigmine, neostigmine and organophosphorus compounds

ESTERS OF CHOLINE

Acetylcholine (ACh) is an ester of choline with acetic acid, whereas **carbachol** and **bethanechol** are esters of choline and betamethylcholine respectively with carbamic acid. The base choline also possesses properties similar to ACh. Its esterification augments the cholinergic activity.

Chemically, ACh and related substances are quaternary ammonium compounds and their unique specific action is attributed to the trimethylammonium [R-N^+ $(CH_3)_3$] groupings.

ACETYLCHOLINE (Fig. 19.1). Although it is not useful in therapeutics it is important to know its actions for understanding the actions of other cholinergic drugs. *There is no circulating ACh in the blood.*

Mechanism of action: ACh acts on two subtypes of cholinergic receptors:

1. **Muscarinic (M),** located *on tissues supplied by postganglionic parasympathetic nerves, CNS and noninnervated receptor on vascular endothelium*

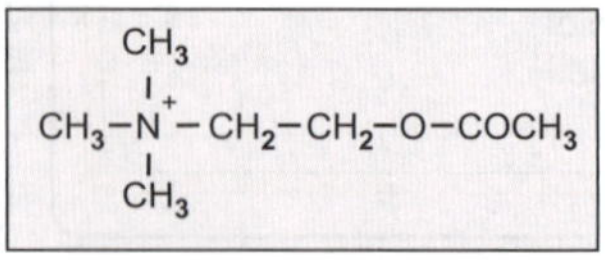

FIG. 19.1 Acetylcholine.

2. **Nicotinic (N),** situated in *all sympathetic ganglia, adrenals, CNS (Nn) and skeletal neuromuscular junction (Nm)*

Muscarinic actions: The actions produced as a result of ACh released from the postganglionic parasympathetic nerve endings in various tissues are termed as *muscarinic actions, e.g. secretory glands, smooth muscles and the heart.* They are blocked by atropine. The designation muscarinic action comes from the fact that these actions are similar to those produced by the poisonous mushroom alkaloid muscarine.

Currently, five subtypes of the muscarinic receptors M_1, M_2, M_3, M_4 and M_5 have been identified (Table 19.1).

M_1, M_3 and M_5 receptors act through Gq protein, which **stimulates** phospholipase C. This leads to the hydrolysis of phosphatidylinositol polyphosphate (PIP) to form inositol 1-4-5 triphosphate and diacylglycerol. The former causes release of intracellular calcium from endoplasmic reticulum, whereas the latter activates protein kinase C.

The M_2 and M_4 receptors interact with Gi proteins with resultant **inhibition** of adenylyl cyclase and activation of K^+ channels, particularly in the heart, and modulation of the activity of calcium channels in certain cell types. These effects account for both the negative chronotropic and the inotropic effects of ACh.

Nicotinic actions: The actions of ACh at the nicotinic receptors (Table 19.1) are termed nicotinic actions, as they resemble those produced by the alkaloid nicotine present in tobacco. Receptor activation causes a rapid increase in cell permeability to Na_+ and K_+ ions that results in depolarization.

These actions, on blood pressure and splenic volume are depicted in Fig 19.2.

Pharmacological actions: Given orally, ACh is rapidly destroyed in the GI tract and hence, it has to be administered by IV infusion to elicit its actions. *Even large IV bolus doses of ACh have no appreciable action in man because it is rapidly metabolised by the plasma pseudocholinesterase, and at the site of action by the specific true cholinesterase.* The only important actions seen after IV injection of ACh are flushing and transient fall in BP due to vasodilatation.

Cardiovascular system:

- **Heart:** The effect of ACh on the heart is similar to that obtained by stimulation of the vagus which is a cholinergic nerve. Thus, it
  a. Depresses the SA node, causes bradycardia (**negative chronotropic action**) and may cause cardiac arrest.
  b. Decreases the contractility (**negative inotropic action**).
  c. May cause A-V block.
  d. Increases the conduction velocity in the atria.
  These changes are transient and can be blocked by atropine.
  ACh reduces the cardiac rate. However, in the presence of atropine, a large dose of ACh due

Table 19.1 Cholinergic receptors - subtypes and location

Cholinergic Receptor	Location	Type of receptors
M_1	CNS and ganglia	Gq protein coupled receptor
M_2	Heart, presynaptic CNS neurons, autonomic nerve terminals	• Gi protein coupled receptor • Presynaptic receptors: autoreceptors
M_3	CNS, GI smooth muscle, detrusor muscles of bladder	Gq protein coupled receptor
M_4	CNS	Gi protein coupled receptor
M_5	Substantia nigra, Ventral tegmentum area	Gq protein coupled receptor
Nn	CNS neurons	Ligand gated ion channels
Nm	Neuromuscular junction	Ligand gated ion channels

PH 4.2

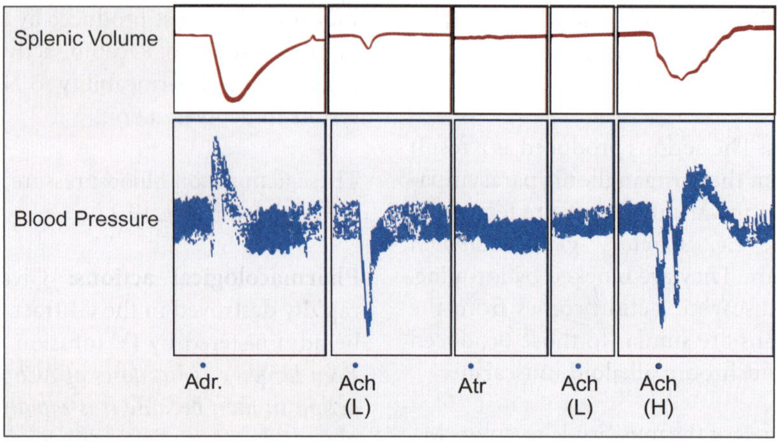

FIG. 19.2 Blood pressure and spleen volume (upper tracing) in anaesthetised dog. Note the fall of B.P. following a low dose (L) of acetylcholine (ACh) which is blocked by atropine (muscarinic action). High dose (H) of ACh in this atropinised animal produced rise in B.P. and contraction of the spleen (nicotinic action), resembling the action of adrenaline (Adr).

to its nicotinic action, stimulates the heart, causing ventricular arrhythmias.

- **Blood vessels:** ACh **dilates the blood vessels** mainly of the skin and the mucous membranes by acting on the M_3 receptors located on the endothelial cells of the vessel wall. Their stimulation causes release of nitric oxide (NO) which results in vascular relaxation. If the endothelium is damaged, ACh causes vasoconstriction. It also dilates the coronary arteries ACh given intravenously results in transient flushing, a sense of warmth in the skin and throbbing headache.

Smooth muscles: ACh:

- Increases (stimulates) the tone and the rhythmic activity of the smooth muscle of the GI tract and enhances peristalsis. The sphincters are, however, relaxed resulting in a rapid forward propulsion of the intestinal contents.
- Contracts the smooth muscle of the gall bladder.
- Contracts the detrusor muscle of the urinary bladder, whereas the smooth muscle of the trigonal sphincter is relaxed.
- Constricts the bronchial smooth muscle and causes bronchospasm.
- Usually contracts the smooth muscle of the ureter whereas that of the uterus shows inconsistent response.

Secretions: Cholinergic **stimulation increases** the gastric, intestinal; pancreatic, bronchial, salivary, lacrimal and nasopharyngeal **secretions.** The increased bronchial secretions, accompanied by bronchospasm, may result in cough and dyspnoea. The salivary secretion is profuse and watery. *As the postganglionic sympathetic fibres supplying the sweat glands are cholinergic, ACh enhances sweating.*

Eye: Instillation of ACh in the eye is without any effect as it is not absorbed. However, intra-carotid injection after sectioning of the postganglionic fibres from superior cervical ganglion (removal of sympathetic tone) produces:

- **Constriction of the pupil** (miosis) by contracting the circular fibres of sphincter pupillae, resulting in **reduction in intraocular tension** by increasing the drainage of ocular fluid through the canal of Schlemm.
- **Contraction of the ciliary muscle** which results in relaxation of the suspensory ligament (zonule) of the lens. This reduces the tension on the lens and allows the lens to bulge into the anterior chamber thereby increasing its thickness and reducing the focal length. Vision is, therefore, fixed for a short distance. This is termed **spasm of accommodation.**

Autonomic ganglia: ACh -induced ganglionic stimulation results in an increased output of ACh and NA from the postganglionic parasympathetic and sympathetic nerve endings respectively. The released NA causes rise in the BP. In addition, large doses of ACh also stimulate the adrenal medulla and increase the secretion of adrenaline (Adr) which further augments and sustains the rise in blood pressure (Fig. 19.2).

Myoneural junction: Ach released as a result of **stimulation of the somatic nerves** induces contraction of the skeletal muscle. However, a very high concentration of ACh at the myoneural junction can produce paralysis of the skeletal muscles by keeping the muscle in a persistently depolarised state in which it is refractory to further stimuli.

The action of ACh on the autonomic ganglia is blocked by ganglion blocking agents like hexamethonium whereas the action on the myoneural junction is antagonised by tubocurarine (Chapter 22).

Miscellaneous actions: ACh is a neurohumoral transmitter in the CNS. *Most of the cholinergic neurons at the cortical and subcortical levels of the CNS have predominant muscarinic receptors. However, being a quaternary ammonium compound, ACh does not cross the BBB and hence, IV ACh exerts no significant central actions.*

Indications: Owing to its extremely transient action, ACh cannot be used systemically in clinical practice. However, it is sometimes used as 1% solution for direct irrigation of anterior chamber during ophthalmic surgeriesto induce rapid miosis.

Hence, its substitutes have been synthesised which are:

- Effective orally.
- More selective in their actions.
- Act directly as ACh receptor agonists.

CARBACHOL: Carbachol is resistant to both true and pseudocholinesterase. It has a more sustained miotic effect on topical application and is used 0.01-3 % solution in ophthalmic surgeries. *The muscarinic effects of carbachol are not adequately antagonised by atropine.*

BETHANECHOL: Like carbachol, this choline ester is resistant to hydrolysis by both true and pseudocholinesterase. It is given orally and is better absorbed. It has predominantly muscarinic actions. Its cardiovascular effects are negligible. The muscarinic effects are well antagonised by atropine. *Bethanechol should never be administered intravenously.*

Preparations and dosage: Bethanechol 25 mg tablets. Available outside India as 5, 10, 25 and 50 mg. Dose: 10–50 mg 3–4 times daily. It is also available as SC injection administered in a dose of 5 mg and repeated after 30 minutes if necessary.

Adverse reactions:

These are mostly an extension of the pharmacological actions.

- **Minor effects:** Flushing, salivation, sweating and bradycardia
- **GI** and **urinary tracts:** Increased activity may produce a desire for defaecation and micturition, abdominal cramps, diarrhoea
- **Eye:** Difficulty in visual accommodation
- **Serious reactions:** Hypotension, syncope, bronchospasm, and occasionally cardiac arrhythmias

Indications

- **Gastrointestinal and urinary tracts: Bethanechol** has been employed for the treatment of postoperative paralytic ileus and abdominal distension and for urinary retention. In chronic urinary retention 10 mg of the drug may be given 3–4 times a day till voluntary or automatic voiding is established.

Contraindications

- Asthma, COPD
- Gastritis, peptic ulcer
- GI or urinary obstruction
- Bradycardia, hypotension
- Hyperthyroidism

CHOLINOMIMETIC ALKALOIDS

PILOCARPINE: Pilocarpine, an alkaloid obtained from the South American shrubs *Pilocarpus microphyllus* and *Pilocarpus jaborandi*, **directly stimulates cholinergic receptors** (agonist) and produces both muscarinic and nicotinic actions of ACh. Applied topically to the eye, it produces miosis, followed by a sustained fall in intraocular pressure (IOP) and a spasm of accommodation.

Adverse reactions: It has all the adverse effects of choline esters. *The drug is too toxic for systemic use.*

Indications: Pilocarpine alone (0.5%–4% aqueous solution) or in combination with 1% physostigmine is used to reduce intraocular tension in acute congestive glaucoma. (Chapter 70).

MUSCARINE and **ARECOLINE:** Muscarine is an alkaloid from the poisonous mushroom *Amanita muscaria*. Acute mushroom poisoning is characterised by diarrhoea, dyspnoea, abdominal pain, lacrimation, salivation, weakness, confusion, convulsions and coma. These muscarinic effects can be antagonised by large doses of atropine. *Delayed poisoning* which develops within 6–15 h after ingestion of another mushroom *Amanita phalloides is characterised by nausea, vomiting, diarrhoea, jaundice and vasomotor collapse; this is attributed to other toxins and does not respond specifically to atropine.* Muscarine has no therapeutic application.

Arecoline, the alkaloid of betel nut *Areca catechu*, has cholinergic actions. It has no therapeutic application in humans. Betel nut is commonly used by chewing and may have mild euphoriant effect.

Cevimeline, a quinuclidine derivative, is an **M_3 receptor agonist** which increases salivary and lacrimal secretions on oral administration. It is long acting and is claimed to be less toxic than pilocarpine. It can be used in the treatment of xerostomia (dry mouth).

CHOLINESTERASE INHIBITORS

Anticholinesterase (anti-ChE) **drugs inhibit the enzymes, true and pseudocholinesterase** and thus **prevent inactivation of ACh**. Their pharmacological effects resemble those of stimulation of cholinergic nervous system. In addition, some anti-ChE have independent pharmacological actions.

Classification of Cholinesterase Inhibitors

I. **Reversible:** These produce reversible inhibition of cholinesterase
   - **Naturally occurring**, e.g. physostigmine
   - **Synthetic:** Neostigmine, pyridostigmine, ambenonium, demecarium, edrophonium, tacrine and rivastigmine

II. **Irreversible:** These induce almost irreversible inhibition of cholinesterase, e.g. di-isopropylflurophosphate (DFP), octa methyl pyrophosphotetramide (OMPA) and other organophosphorus compounds and carbamates.

Mechanism of action: ACh is inactivated by combination with two sites on the enzyme cholinesterase: *an anionic site* bearing a negative charge which attracts the quaternary nitrogen atom (N^+) of ACh; and an *esteratic site* which attracts the carboxylic acid group (COOH) of the ACh molecule (Fig. 19.3). As a result of the union of ACh with cholinesterase, the esteratic site of the enzyme is acetylated, and this results in splitting off of choline. The acetyl group combined with the esteratic site is, however, immediately removed as a result of hydrolysis, forming acetic acid. This sets the esteratic site of the enzyme free for inactivation of another molecule of ACh.

The **reversible anticholinesterases** bear a structural resemblance to ACh and combine with the anionic and esteratic sites of cholinesterase as well as with ACh receptor. However, the complex which they form with the esteratic site of cholinesterase is much less readily hydrolysed than the acetyl-esteratic site complex formed with ACh. This produces a temporary inhibition of the enzyme. In contrast to other reversible anticholinesterases, edrophonium forms reversible complex only with the anionic site and hence, has a shorter duration of action.

The irreversible anticholinesterases, *organophosphorus compounds, combine only with esteratic site of cholinesterase and consequently the esteratic site is phosphorylated*. The hydrolysis of the phosphorylated site, however, is slow and in certain cases does not occur at all. This produces an almost irreversible inhibition of cholinesterase. In contrast to other organophosphorus compounds, echothiophate forms complexes with both anionic and esteratic sites and hence, is much more potent than other compounds.

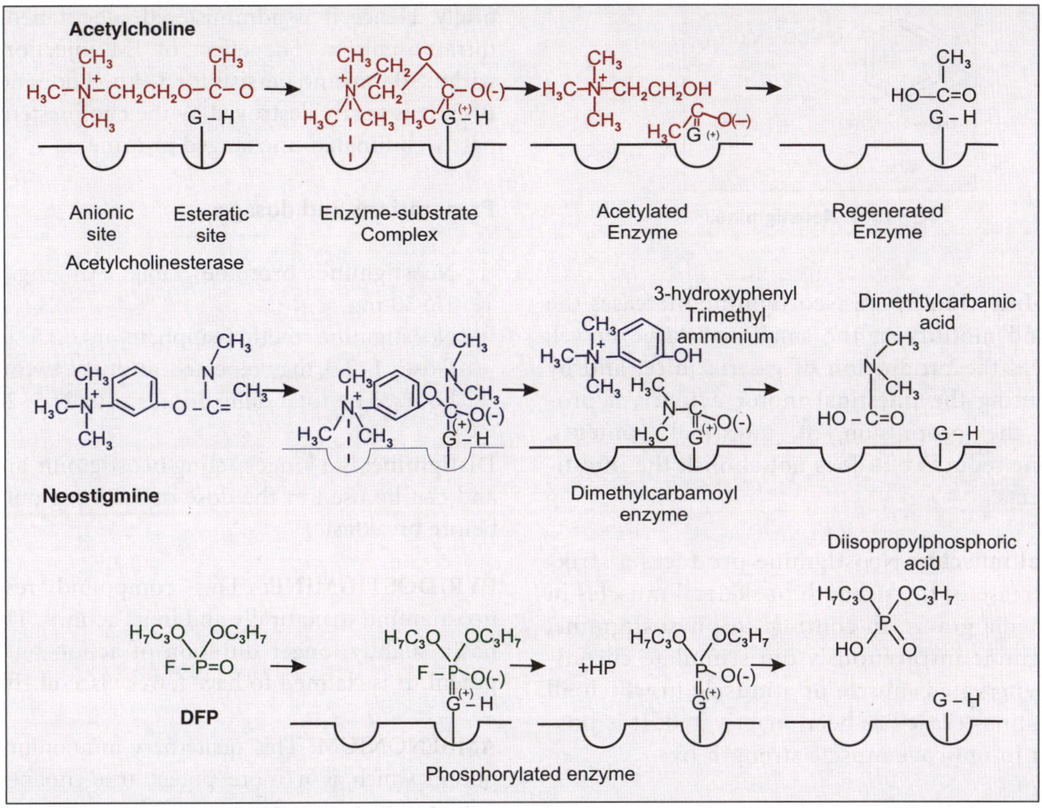

FIG. 19.3 The inactivation of acetylcholine by cholinesterase and the mechanism of action of reversible anticholinesterase drug, Neostigmine, and irreversible anticholinesterase drug, DFP. G-H: a protonated acidic group of the esteratic site.

I. Reversible Anticholinesterases

PHYSOSTIGMINE: This is an alkaloid obtained from the calabar bean, the dried ripe seed of an African woody climber *Physostigma venenosum.*

Pharmacological actions: The pharmacological effects of physostigmine are similar to those of other cholinergic agents.

Topical instillation into the eye produces miosis, spasm of accommodation and a fall in intraocular tension.

It is rapidly absorbed on oral or parenteral administration and has a short duration of action. It crosses the BBB and exerts central cholinergic actions.

Preparations and dosage: Physostigmine salicylate is used in eye as 0.25%–0.50% aqueous solution or as an ointment. On storing, the solution becomes pink owing to decomposition. Physostigmine salicylate inj. 2 mg/2 mL.

Indications:

1. As miotic
2. In the treatment of anticholinergic drug (atropine) intoxication
3. In poisoning with phenothiazines and tricyclic antidepressants

NEOSTIGMINE: This synthetic, quaternary ammonium compound (Fig. 19.4) that inhibits both true and pseudocholinesterases.

Pharmacological actions: In addition to its anticholinesterase activity, **neostigmine also directly stimulates certain organs having cholinergic receptors.** Its actions are:

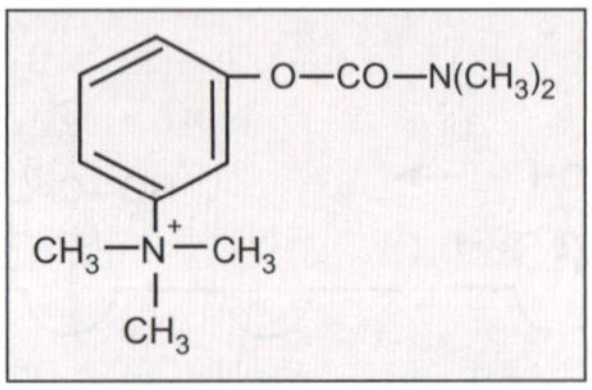

FIG. 19.4 **Neostigmine.**

Gastrointestinal tract: Neostigmine increases the tone and motility of the small and large bowel, enhances the production of gastric juice; and by augmenting the intestinal motor activity, it promotes the propulsion of intestinal contents. Atropine reduces but does not abolish the intestinal effects.

Skeletal muscles: Neostigmine produces a striking increase in the strength of skeletal muscles in myasthenia gravis. In contrast to physostigmine, neostigmine intravenously can stimulate chronically denervated muscle or a muscle in which all the cholinesterase has been inactivated. It is postulated to improve muscle strength by:

- *Its anti-ChE activity* causing greater accumulation of ACh at the motor end plates
- *Increasing the amount of ACh released* during each nerve impulse
- *Directly stimulating the nicotinic receptors sites on the motor end plate* by virtue of its structural similarity to ACh. It thus acts *as a partial agonist.* Administration of neostigmine to normal individuals may cause twitchings and fasciculations of skeletal muscles but these are not encountered in myasthenic patients. It reverses the neuromuscular blockade produced by d-tubocurarine, but it actually enhances the paralysis of skeletal muscles caused by persistent depolarisers like succinylcholine (Chapter 22).

Cardiovascular system: The drug causes bradycardia and fall in BP by peripheral vasodilatation.

Secretions: It increases bronchial secretions and causes bronchospasm.

Absorption, fate and excretion: Being a quaternary ammonium compound, it is absorbed incompletely orally. Hence it is administered subcutaneously or intramuscularly. The effect of IM injection starts within 10 min and persists for 3–4 h. It does not cross BBB. It is partly destroyed by the cholinesterase and partly eliminated unchanged in urine.

Preparations and dosage:

i. Neostigmine bromide tablet 15 mg. Dose: 15–30 mg.
ii. Neostigmine methyl-sulphate inj. 2.5 mg/mL. Dose: 1–2.5 mg, repeated at every two to four hours. The total daily dose is usually 5–20 mg.

Distigmine: is a longer acting neostigmine analogue and can be used in the dose of 5–20 mg once daily before breakfast.

PYRIDOSTIGMINE: This compound resembles neostigmine structurally and in its actions. The drug has a slightly longer duration of action but is less potent. It is claimed to have fewer visceral effects.

AMBENONIUM: This quaternary ammonium compound which is a more potent true-cholinesterase-inhibitor than neostigmine and has a more marked direct stimulant effect on the skeletal muscle. The action is more sustained with a lower incidence of GI side effects. It is available as 10 mg tablets. Dose: 5–20 mg 3–4 times a day as required.

DEMECARIUM: Structurally, demecarium is made up of two neostigmine molecules joined through 10 methoxy groups. It is a potent miotic. This effect may last for 3–10 days. It is accompanied by a spasm of accommodation. *It is used as 0.125%–0.25% eye drops once or twice weekly for treating glaucoma when shorter acting miotics provide inadequate control.*

EDROPHONIUM: It is structurally related to neostigmine. It has a weak anticholinesterase activity as compared to neostigmine. But it enhances neuromuscular transmission with a dose that is too low to affect the smooth muscles, the myocardium and the glands. *It has a quicker onset of action than neostigmine, and the effects of a single IV dose persists only for 10 min*. The muscarinic side effects are mild.

Preparations and dosage: Edrophonium chloride 10 mL vials containing 10 mg/mL.

Rivastigmine: See Chapter 15.

Adverse reactions:
The reversible anticholinesterases produce effects attributable mainly to their muscarinic actions.

These are:

- **Gastrointestinal**: Epigastric distress, nausea, abdominal cramps and diarrhoea
- **Secretions**: Increased salivation, sweating and lacrimation
- **Neurological**: Paraesthesia, tremors, fasciculations particularly around the mouth and superior extremities, tremors
- **Miscellaneous**: Hypotension
  Demecarium and physostigmine eyedrops, may pass into the nose through the nasolacrimal duct and produce muscarinic side effects.
  When used in the treatment of myasthenia gravis, an overdose of these compounds may produce skeletal muscle paralysis by persistent depolarisation. This phenomenon, termed **cholinergic crisis,** has to be differentiated from the sudden exacerbation of muscular weakness in myasthenia often associated with severe upper respiratory infection, termed **myasthenic crisis**. *In myasthenic crisis, the requirement of the anti-ChE agent is increased* and occasionally the patient becomes resistant to anticholinesterase medication. **Edrophonium** 2 mg intravenously (ameliorative test) is used to differentiate between these two crises. It brings about a prompt improvement of muscle strength in myasthenic crisis, whereas it exacerbates muscle weakness in cholinergic crisis. Edrophonium is preferred because of its extremely short duration of action. This ensures immediate reversal in case of cholinergic crisis of edrophonium. FM 9.5

The cholinergic crisis is treated by administration of large doses of atropine, oximes and artificial respiration.

Indications:

- **Myasthenia gravis:** See under Myasthenia Gravis—Pharmacotherapy
- **Glaucoma:** Chapter 70 AS 4.1
- **For decurarisation** following the use of neuromuscular blockers like d-tubocurarine in anaesthetic procedures.
- **Paralytic ileus and urinary retention:** Neostigmine can be employed parenterally to treat postoperative paralytic ileus and urinary retention. It is now rarely used for this purpose.
  Benzpyrinium is also employed for similar purpose. FM 10.1
- **Curare poisoning:** Edrophonium is preferred to neostigmine to antagonise curare induced skeletal muscle paralysis because of its short latent period of action.
- **Alzheimer's disease** (see Chapter 15).
- **Snake venom poisoning:** An anti-ChE may be beneficial in the management of neurotoxicity of Asian-cobra-venom. For this purpose, atropine sulphate (0.6 mg) is given intravenously, slowly, for blocking muscarinic action, and is followed immediately by edrophonium 10 mg/neostigmine 1.5 mg intravenously over 2 min. Edrophonium/neostigmine reverses oculomotor and glosso-pharyngeal paralysis as well as respiratory paralysis as the pathophysiological nature of paralysis after cobra bite is very similar to that of myasthenia gravis. The improvement can be maintained by neostigmine 0.5 mg with atropine every 30 minutes for 5 doses. Neostigmine and glycopyrolate as a fixed dose combination can also be used. usually positive response to "AN" trial occurs in 1 hour as 50% or more recovery of the ptosis. If there is no response after 3 injections then this trial is stopped. AN trial should not delay antivenom treatment or endotracheal intubation. *However,* anti-AchE are not useful against *Krait beta-bungarotoxin, which causes presynaptic blockage* (Chapter 71).

Myasthenia Gravis—Pharmacotherapy

Myasthenia gravis is a disease characterised by easy fatiguability and progressive weakness of striated muscles and with intermittent periods of exacerbation. Pregnancy usually leads to an improvement or even temporary remission of this condition.

Myasthenia gravis is an autoimmune disease caused by a deficiency of the postsynaptic neuromuscular ACh receptor complex. Circulating immunoglobulin G (IgG) antibodies to post-synaptic ACh receptors or other components of NM junction have been demonstrated in 70%–90% of patients with myasthenia gravis. This results in impairment of ACh dependent signal transmission at NM junction and causes internalization and degradation of Ach receptors. Many patients with this disorder have thymic hyperplasia or a thymoma.

Another myasthenic syndrome (**Lambert–Eaton syndrome**) of autoimmune nature occurs in association with small cell carcinoma of the lung. *The defect is presynaptic and does not respond to anticholiesterases.*

Treatment: **Neostigmine** was formerly used in the treatment of myasthenia. However, because of its relatively short duration of action (<4 h), development of tolerance and waxing and waning of muscle strength, drugs with longer duration of action and fewer side effects, e.g. **pyridostigmine** (4–6 h) and **ambenonium** (4–8 h) are now preferred. These drugs may, however, be combined with neostigmine as the onset of action of neostigmine is quicker. The therapy is initiated with neostigmine 7.5–15 mg or pyridostigmine 30–60 mg or ambenonium 2.5–5 mg orally, at a time, and the dose is gradually increased until the maximal benefit is obtained.

The **reversible anti-ChE** are usually administered 3–4 h, orally or parenterally to ensure a smooth and sustained effect. Parenteral medication is indicated before meals so as to enable the patient to swallow his food. Approximately, 80%–90% recovery occurs in 25% individuals. Further increase in dosage precipitates toxic actions without appreciable increase in clinical improvement. *It is, therefore, wiser to accept minor disability rather than overdose the patient. Infection increases the requirements of anticholinesterases.*

Because of the autoimmune basis of myasthenia, **prednisolone**, a glucocorticoid has been used in the dose of 25–100 mg once a day. Dose should be regulated slowly. *Alternate day regimen is preferred. It causes remission or improvement in 80% of cases.* Such therapy may, however, cause exacerbation of weakness in the early stages.

Immunosuppresants such as azathioprine, cyclosporine as well as plasmapheresis have been used as adjunctive therapy in resistant cases. **Eculizumab** is also used intravenously for severe, generalised anti -ACh receptor antibody positive myasthenia gravis. It is a complement inhibitor. Recently for such patients, intravenous **efgartigimaod**, a human IgG1 antibody fragment which binds to Fc receptor has been approved. The neonatal Fc receptors prolong the life-span of IgG by preventing its lysosomal degradation. Efgartigimaod blocks Fc receptors and causes IgG catabolism thus reducing circulating ACh receptor antibodies. This first-in-class neonatal Fc receptor antagonist is also undergoing testing against variety of other autoimmune diseases. However, its long term efficacy and safety is not known.

Thymectomy can help patients with thymoma.

Box 19.1 Drugs which Aggravate Myasthenic Symptoms

- ***Antibiotics:*** Aminoglycosides, polymyxins, norfloxacin, ciprofloxacin, erythromycin, tetracyclines
- ***Antiarrhythmics:*** Procainamide, quinidine, lignocaine, propranolol
- ***CNS depressants*** may depress respiration
- ***Miscellaneous:*** Chlorpromazine, lithium, thyroid hormones, phenytoin, methoxyflurane, d-tubocurarine and penicillamine

Box 19.1 lists the drugs which aggravate the symptoms in myasthenic patients.

II Irreversible Anticholinesterases: PH 1.14

ORGANOPHOSPHORUS COMPOUNDS (OPC), the organic esters of phosphoric acid, are **potent irreversible inhibitors of cholinesterase**. Unlike the quaternary ammonium anti-ChE, most of these compounds have high lipid solubility, and hence:

- *Are absorbed by practically all the routes* including the GI tract, the intact unbroken skin, mucous membranes and lungs
- *Cross the BBB and affect the functions of the CNS*

Box 19.2 lists the important organophosphorus compounds.

Box 19.2 Important Organophosphorus Compounds

- ***Therapeutically useful:*** Diisopropyl flurophosphate (DFP), metrifonate, echothiophate
- ***Insecticides:*** Fenthion (Dalf), malathion (diazone), octamethylpyrophosphphotetramide (OMPA), sumithion (Tik-20), monocrotophos (Nuvaeron)
- ***Highly toxic nerve gases:*** Tabun, sarin, soman synthesised for chemical warfare

The **pharmacological actions** of these compounds are those of ACh which accumulates in the tissues due to prolonged inhibition of the true and pseudocholinesterases.

The OPC compounds are inactivated in the body almost entirely by oxidation and hydrolysis, and the end products are eliminated in urine.

Indications: The OPC have limited therapeutic uses owing to high toxicity. They are used **mainly as insecticides** and are of toxicological importance.

- **Glaucoma:** Echothiophate 0.06% reduces the intra-ocular tension; the action persists for 1–3 weeks. The drug, however, produces a marked ciliary spasm, browache, headache and blurring. See Chapter 70.
- **Worm infestation:** Metrifonate, a prodrug owes its effect to its metabolite, dichlorovas, an OPC, which is effective against *S. hematobium* (Chapter 58).

PH 1.51, PE 14.3 and FM 9.5

ORGANOPHOSPHORUS COMPOUND POISONING

Poisoning with organophosphorus compounds may be:

- *Occupational* as in persons engaged in spraying insecticides
- *Accidental*, e.g. by consumption of the agricultural products sprayed with these insecticides
- *Suicidal* due to intentional ingestion of any of these compounds

Acute organophosphorus pesticide poisoning is an important cause of morbidity and mortality all over the world. Of these, 99% of the fatal poisonings occur in the developing countries, mostly among agricultural workers.

Symptomatology: The effects of acute intoxication are:

- **Muscarinic effects:**
  a. Localised exposure of the eyes produces miosis, spasm of accommodation, headache and conjunctival hyperaemia.
  b. Inhalation results in bronchospasm, cough and augmented bronchiolar secretions and a sense of 'tightness in the chest'.
  c. On ingestion, the GI symptoms are the earliest to appear and consist of anorexia, nausea, vomiting, abdominal cramps, tenesmus and diarrhoea. The other muscarinic effects are severe bronchospasm and pulmonary oedema.
- **Nicotinic effects:** These are characterised by fasciculations, twitching, generalised weakness and a depolarisation type of paralysis. There may be either tachycardia or bradycardia.
- **Central effects:** These include giddiness, anxiety, confusion, ataxia, hypotension, respiratory depression, convulsions and coma. Death is usually due to paralysis of respiratory muscles and respiratory failure.
  The duration of effect is longest with DFP, and shorter with echothiophate and tetraethyl pyrophosphate (TEPP). It appears that even single episodes of clinically significant organophosphorus intoxication are associated with *persistent decline in neuropsychological function.*
- **Neurotoxic effects:** In addition to the acute toxic manifestations, DFP and mipafox may produce *delayed symptoms due to demyelination of the nerve tracts in the central and peripheral nervous systems* such as the spinocerebellar tract, pyramidal tract and the sciatic nerve, producing permanent functional derangements. *This is not related to ChE inhibition.* It produces weakness, fatiguability, twitching and loss of tendon reflexes, leading to paralysis. Adulteration of edible olive oil with lubricating oil containing triorthocresyl phosphate (TOCP) caused thousands of deaths in a tragedy that occurred in North Africa. No treatment is available. PH 1.1, PH 1.52

Treatment of acute poisoning: Box 19.3 summarises the **principles of treatment** of acute OPC poisoning.

As recommended by the WHO, 'The treatment must be instituted rapidly in order to prevent a fatal outcome. In intoxication by mouth, rapid gastric lavage is imperative. For removal of secretions and maintenance of a patent airway, place the patient in a prone position with head down and to one side, the mandible elevated and the tongue pulled forward. Clear the mouth and pharynx with finger or suction. Use an oropharyngeal or nasopharyngeal airway or endotracheal intubation if airway obstruction persists. If the body is soiled with the insecticides or if vomiting

Box 19.3 Principles of Treatment of Acute Organophosphorus Poisoning PH 1.1

- Remove soiled clothes
- Wash soiled skin, eyes
- Nurse in prone position
- Clear mouth and throat
- Insert an airway/intubate
- Gastric lavage
- Atropine in sufficient quantities
- Cholinesterase activator such as pralidoxime
- Supportive measures such as oxygen, treatment of shock, prophylactic antibiotics
- Treatment of convulsions (diazepam)
- Continued vigilance as delayed toxicity may occur as late as 2–4 weeks after apparent recovery

Mechanism of action – oximes.

or hypersalivation has occurred, clothes must be removed and the skin washed with soap and water for at least 10 min. Contamination of the eyes is treated by washing of the conjunctiva'.

Mouth to mouth respiration is to be avoided when it is suspected that the patient has been intoxicated by mouth since vomited material may contain toxic amounts of substances.

Drug Therapy: On signs of systemic absorption, both **atropine** and **reactivators of cholinesterase** (see below) must be given parenterally. Persons without signs of respiratory insufficiency who manifest peripheral symptoms should be treated with 2–4 mg of atropine sulphate and 1–2 g of a soluble salt of **pralidoxime** (P-2-AM) or 250 mg of **obidoxime chloride** (See under Oximes) by slow IV injection. More atropine (with or without the reactivator) may be given depending upon the severity of the intoxication and the response to the first dose. After the administration of oximes, less atropine may be required. **Reactivators of cholinesterase should not be used before atropine administration, as given alone they may increase muscle weakness.**

Atropine *is effective in antagonising the central and peripheral muscarinic effects but does not modify the ganglionic action and the neuromuscular paralysis. It should not be given to a cyanosed patient until the cyanosis has been overcome, since it may cause ventricular fibrillation.* Convulsions are treated with diazepam.

In severe intoxication, 4–6 mg of atropine sulphate should be given initially, followed by repeated doses of 2 mg or as much as required to maintain full atropinisation at 5-10 minutes interval. The patient's condition, including respiration, convulsions, blood pressure, pulse, and salivation should be monitored as a guide to further administration of atropine. *Usually however, it is not necessary to exceed 50 mg.* **Tachycardia may occur and watch must be kept on salivary secretion in order to prevent over-atropinisation.** *The pulse rate should not be allowed to exceed 120/min.*

Because most intoxications occur after exposure of the skin or after ingestion, *any deterioration in the patient's condition due to delayed absorption must be carefully watched for. Reactivators are excreted fairly rapidly if kidney function is normal (in the case of pralidoxime 80% in 2–3 h) and repeated doses of 1 g may be needed.*

Pralidoxime (chloride or methanesulphonate) should be started within two hours of ingestion of the poison. Studies from India have shown that in 'moderately severe' poisoning, a loading dose of 2 g (base) of pralidoxime by IV infusion over 30 min, followed by 1 g/h by **continuous IV infusion** for 48 h, is highly effective. This is followed by pralidoxime (base) 1 g IV infusion every 4 h till the patient is weaned from the ventilator. This regimen appears to be well tolerated and mortality is low. However, extent of therapeutic usefulness of oximes, in general, is not yet well defined.

After the resolution of the initial symptoms, some patients may develop the **'intermediate syndrome'**. It is characterised by flaccid, proximal paralysis. Later, after a gap of 2–4 weeks, a **'delayed polyneuropathy'** with sensory and motor, impairment, usually of the lower limbs, may manifest. Unfortunately, there is no specific treatment.

OXIMES (Cholinesterase reactivators): The irreversible inhibition of cholinesterase produced by the OPC is due

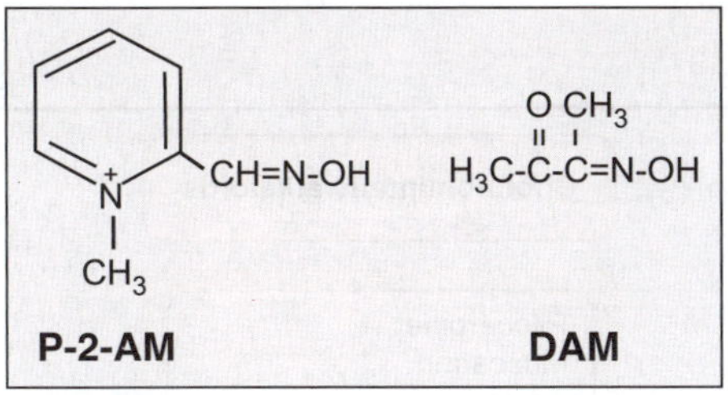

FIG. 19.5 Chemical structure of oximes

to phosphorylation of the esteratic site of the enzyme (Fig. 19.3). Oximes are nucleophilic (Fig. 19.5). They orient themselves in close proximity to phosphorus at the esteratic site and form a soluble phosphoryloxime complex . This results in setting free the esteratic site and reactivation of the enzyme.

The oximes are particularly effective in reversing the neuromuscular paralysis where atropine is ineffective. Their effects on the autonomic ganglia and the CNS are not significant, except probably in the case of DAM which crosses the blood brain barrier. *As mentioned earlier, these compounds are effective only when administered within a short time after poisoning.* Late administration fails to produce the expected results because of aging of enzyme. In this case, the phosphorylated enzyme undergoes a chemical change, in which one of the alkyl (alkoxy) group of the bound OPC is lost. This strengthens the stability of the phosphorylated enzyme. OPC with secondary (DFP) and tertiary (Soman) alkoxy groups are more prone to lose their alkoxy group. Oximes are mainly metabolised in the liver.

Preparations and dosage:

i. Pyridine-2 aldoxime chloride (P-2-AM, pralidoxime) by IV infusion. Dose: 1–2 g; can be repeated, as needed. It can also be given intramuscularly. It is also available for oral use.
ii. Diacetylmonoxime (DAM) administered by IV infusion. It crosses the BBB.
iii. Obidoxime chloride is more potent than pralidoxime. It is given intravenously in a dose of 250 mg as a bolus, followed by continuous infusion of 750 mg/24 h.

Adverse reactions: The oximes are not free from toxicity. They may produce local irritation, drowsiness, giddiness, blurred vision, diplopia, tachycardia and hypotension. *Pralidoxime has weak anti-ChE activity and hence is contraindicated in the treatment of overdosage with neostigmine or physostigmine. It also does not antagonise the effects of carbamate type (Baygon/Carbaryl) of anticholinesterases (Chapter 60).* High doses of oximes can themselves cause neuromuscular blockade.

CHOLINERGIC DRUGS

Esters of choline

- Acetylcholine
- Carbachol
- Bethanechol

Cholinomimetic alkaloids

- Pilocarpine
- Muscarine
- Arecoline

Cholinesterase inhibitors (Anticholinesterases)

Reversible

Naturally occurring

- Physostigmine

Synthetic

- Neostigmine
- Pyridostigmine
- Ambenonium
- Edrophonium
- Tacrine
- Rivastigmine

Irreversible

Therapeutically useful

- Di-isopropylflurophosphate (DFP)
- Metrifonate
- Echothiophate

Insecticides

- Octa methyl pyrophosphotetramide (OMPA)
- Fenthion
- Malathion
- Sumithion
- Monocrotophos

Highly toxic nerve gases

- Tabun
- Sarin
- Soman

CHAPTER 20

Muscarinic Receptor Blocking Drugs; Pharmacotherapy of Bladder Dysfunction

Learning Objectives

This chapter will enable the reader:

1. To describe pharmacological effects, ADR, contraindications and indications for belladonna alkaloids.
2. To compare and contrast atropine and scopolamine.
3. To classify atropine substitutes based on their indications, giving examples of drugs
4. To justify drug/s of choice for various functional abnormalities of micturition

KEY TERMS

belladonna alkaloids, p. 307
muscarinic blockade, p. 307
pre-anaesthetic medication, p. 311
atropine substitutes, p. 311
dicyclomine, p. 312
flavoxate, p. 312
bladder dysfunction, treatment, p. 313

Cholinergic–muscarinic receptor blocking drugs include **atropine and related alkaloids** obtained from the plants *Atropa belladonna* (the deadly nightshade), *Atropa acuminata, Hyoscyamus niger* (henbane), *Scopola carniolica* and *Datura stramonium* (Datura) and **synthetic or semisynthetic atropine substitutes.** They block the muscarinic actions of ACh; the ganglionic and skeletal neuromuscular actions of ACh are not affected. PH 1.14

Atropine is more effective in blocking the effects of externally administered ACh than that of cholinergic nerve stimulation. The dose of the drug required to produce muscarinic blockade varies from organ to organ. Thus, salivary and bronchial secretions are extremely sensitive to atropine blockade, whereas the heart, the smooth muscle of the GI tract, gastric acid secretion and the eye are less affected even after relatively large doses. *In the CNS, cholinergic transmission*

BELLADONNA ALKALOIDS

The two important belladonna alkaloids are: **atropine** (dl-hyoscyamine) and **scopolamine** (hyoscine). Atropine is an ester of an aromatic organic acid 'tropic acid' with a complex organic base 'tropine', whereas hyoscine is an ester of tropic acid with another base 'scopine' (Fig. 20.1).

Mechanism of action: The belladonna alkaloids block both the peripheral and central muscarinic effects of ACh. The antagonism between ACh and atropine is of *competitive* type which can be reversed by an increase in the concentration of ACh at the muscarinic neuroeffector site.

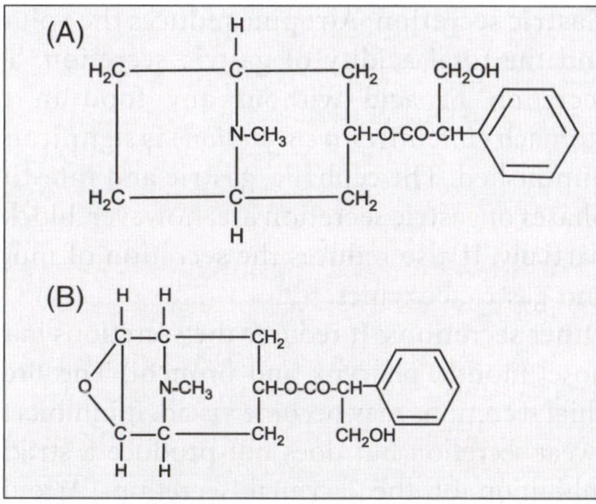

FIG. 20.1 **(A) Atropine and (B) Scopolamine.**

at subcortical and cortical levels is predominantly muscarinic (M_1) and can be blocked by atropine.

Although atropine can completely abolish the effects of choline esters on the GI tract, it does not completely abolish the effects of vagal stimulation. This is so because it neither blocks noncholinergic, neurohumoral transmitters nor responses to GI peptide hormones.

In large doses, atropine blocks the nicotinic action of ACh at the autonomic ganglia; it is more marked following atropine substitutes containing the quaternary ammonium ($-NH_4$) ion.

Pharmacological actions: The pharmacological actions of **atropine** and **scopolamine** are qualitatively similar except that:

a. *Atropine is a central nervous system stimulant, whereas scopolamine is a central depressant* and can act as a sedative
b. Atropine is more active on the heart, the gut and the bronchial smooth muscle
c. Scopolamine has more prominent effects on the iris, the ciliary body and the salivary, bronchial and sweat secretions
d. Atropine has a longer duration of action than scopolamine

Secretions: The secretions of the exocrine glands except the production of milk are reduced.

- **Salivary secretion**: Atropine blocks the watery salivary secretion giving rise to dryness of mouth and difficulty in swallowing.
- **Gastric secretion**: Atropine reduces the volume and the total acidity of gastric secretion. The secretion of acid without any food in the stomach (*interdigestive secretion*) is significantly diminished. The cephalic, gastric and intestinal phases of gastric secretion are, however, blocked partially. It also reduces the secretion of mucin and gastric enzymes.
- **Other secretions:** It reduces the secretions in the nose, mouth, pharynx and bronchi. The bronchial secretions may become viscid. It inhibits the sweat secretion but does not produce a striking inhibition of the lacrimal secretion. Atropine has little effect on the pancreatic and intestinal secretions.

Smooth muscle:

- **Gastrointestinal tract:** Atropine reduces both the tone and the motility of the gut, and acts as an **antispasmodic**. It antagonises the spasmogenic action of morphine on intestine and can also completely abolish the excessive motility induced by the cholinergic agents. It is, however, only partially effective in blocking the effects of vagus nerve stimulation, and *it does not interfere significantly with normal peristalsis.*
- **Biliary tract:** Atropine exerts a weak antispasmodic (relaxant) action on the biliary tract and the gallbladder.
- **Urinary tract:** Atropine produces reduction in normal as well as in drug induced ureteral peristalsis. Therapeutic doses reduce the tone of the fundus of the bladder and enhance the tone of the trigonal sphincter and hence can cause urinary retention.
- **Bronchi:** Atropine relaxes the smooth muscles of the bronchi and bronchioles. It is particularly effective in relieving bronchoconstriction produced by cholinergic agents but is much less potent than adrenaline in relieving histamine induced bronchoconstriction. Since it dries up the secretions, it is not recommended in the treatment of bronchial asthma.
- **Uterus:** Atropine and scopolamine have no significant effect on the uterine muscle.
- **Eye:** On local instillation, atropine produces:

a. **Mydriasis** by blocking the cholinergic nerves supplying the smooth muscle of the sphincter of the iris. Photophobia is manifested in response to bright light because of the sphincter paralysis.
b. **Cycloplegia** as the ciliary smooth muscle is paralysed by atropine. This produces a tightening of the suspensory ligament resulting in flattening of the lens with a consequent increase in its focal length. The individual, therefore, is able to see things clearly only at a distance owing to fixing of lens for far vision. This *paralysis of accommodation is termed as **cycloplegia**.*
Local instillation of 1% atropine drops produces maximum mydriatic response within 30–40 min and recovery occurs within 7–10 days. Maximum cycloplegia with atropine is seen within 1–3 days; it persists for 7–11 days.
Atropine does not alter the intraocular tension in

the normal eye but in individuals with *shallow anterior chamber and in those with narrow angle glaucoma,* a precipitous increase in intraocular tension may occur. It is due to relaxation of the ciliary muscle and crowding of the iris in the angle of the anterior chamber interfering with the drainage of aqueous humour.

- **Cardiovascular system:** Atropine, in therapeutic doses, may initially decrease the heart rate owing to stimulation of the medullary vagal nuclei, followed by tachycardia, particularly in young individuals who have a high vagal tone and in whom the heart rate may increase by 30–40 beats per minute. Tachycardia is due to blocking of M_2 receptors in the SA nodal pacemaker. This action is sometimes not observed in old people and in infants probably because of the lower vagal tone. Atropine abolishes the effects of cholinergic agents on the heart rate and also the bradycardia induced by manoeuvres like carotid massage and pressure on an eyeball.

In **therapeutic doses,** atropine completely counters the vasodilatation and hypotension produced by cholinergic agents. However, by itself, it has insignificant effect on the vasculature and does not modify the BP. **Toxic doses** cause dilatation of the cutaneous blood vessels resulting in 'atropine flush' and hypotension.

- **Central nervous system:** Atropine causes a **mild stimulation of the medullary vagal nuclei and higher cerebral centres.** This occasionally produces bradycardia and an increase in the rate and depth of respiration. Respiratory depression produced by toxic doses of anticholinesterases can be antagonised appreciably by atropine. In **moderate doses**, it controls the tremors and rigidity in Parkinsonism. **In toxic doses,** it produces marked excitation.

In contrast to atropine, therapeutic doses of scopolamine depress the reticular activating system and usually produce euphoria, drowsiness, amnesia and dreamless sleep which last for 1–2 h.

Scopolamine owes its antimotion sickness effects to its direct action on the vestibular function (Chapter 41).

Absorption, fate and excretion: The belladonna alkaloids are satisfactorily absorbed from the GI tract, from parenteral sites and from mucous membranes. The absorption from the eye and intact skin, however, is not significant. Atropine is partly detoxified in liver and partly excreted unchanged by kidneys. It has plasma t½ of 4 h. Approximately, 50% of the parenterally administered drug appears in the urine in free form within 24 h, whereas 33% is excreted as metabolites. Scopolamine is mostly metabolised.

Atropine crosses the placental barrier and is secreted in milk and saliva.

Adverse reactions: Majority of these are due to extension of its pharmacological actions. Infants, young children and elderly are particularly susceptible to atropine toxicity and may show adverse effects at therapeutic doses.

Mild reactions include dryness of mouth (xerostomia), flushing and constipation. Atropine can precipitate glaucoma and urinary retention, especially in the elderly. Locally, atropine can give rise to allergic reactions such as dermatitis, conjunctivitis and swelling of eyelids. IM 21.2

- **Acute atropine poisoning:** Atropine has a wide margin of safety. The lethal dose of atropine is not known but is believed to be 10–20 mg in children and 80–130 mg in adults, although survival after doses over 200 mg in adults has been reported. Scopolamine is claimed to be more toxic than atropine. Poisoning may also occur following ingestion of leaves or seeds of *Datura* species or berries of solanaceous plants.

  The **symptoms** and **signs** are due to:

  a. ***Peripheral muscarinic blockade.*** Dryness of mouth, difficulty in swallowing, intense thirst, tachycardia, palpitation, flushing, hyperpyrexia due to inhibition of sweating, dilatation of pupils, blurred vision and photophobia are the cardinal manifestations. Difficulty in micturition and urinary retention may occur due to spasm of the trigone. A rash may appear over the face, neck and upper part of the trunk, leading to desquamation of the skin.

b. ***Central effects*** which are attributed to initial stimulation and subsequent depression of the CNS. The patient shows excitement, restlessness, motor incoordination, slurring of speech, disturbance of memory, confusion, hallucinations, and occasionally mania and delirium. Nausea and vomiting are infrequent. Severe poisoning depresses the vasomotor centre, leading to vasomotor collapse.

The cardinal features of atropine poisoning can be remembered with the mnemonic *"Red as a beet, dry as a bone, hot as hare, blind as a bat, mad as a hatter, full as a flask"* referring to flushing, dry skin and mucous membrane, fever, mydriasis with loss of accommodation, CNS excitement and urinary retention.

These symptoms may sometimes be mistaken for an exanthematous fever.

The other drugs which cause a syndrome like acute atropine intoxication include drugs possessing muscarinic blocking action such as: tricyclic antidepressants, phenothiazine antipsychotics and the antihistaminics like promethazine and diphenhydramine.

FM 10.1

Treatment: If the poison has been ingested, prompt attempts to remove it by gastric lavage should be made. Alkaloidal inactivators like universal antidote should be administered before and after gastric lavage.

The **muscarinic effects can be countered** by administration of slow IV physostigmine 1–4 mg (0.5–1 mg in children) or neostigmine 2–5 mg subcutaneously. The drugs may be repeated at intervals of 1–2 h till satisfactory control over muscarinic blockade is established. *Physostigmine is preferred in patients with CNS symptoms as it crosses the BBB. Restlessness and delirium may be treated with diazepam, but this drug may augment the respiratory depression seen in later stages of atropine intoxication.*

A dark room to alleviate photophobia, catheterisation for urinary retention, tepid sponging for pyrexia, good nursing care, oxygen and artificial ventilation, when necessary, constitute the supportive treatment.

- **Chronic use of belladonna** is manifested by dryness of mouth, skin eruptions, tremors and speech disturbances.

Preparations and dosage:

i. Atropine sulphate 0.6 mg tablets. Dose: 0.3–2.4 mg.
ii. Atropine sulphate injection 0.2, 0.3, 0.4, 0.5, 0.6 in 1 mL. Dose: 0.25–2 mg subcutaneously or intramuscularly.
iii. Atropine eye ointment 1%.
iv. Scopolamine hydrobromide tablets 0.3–0.6 mg. Dose 1–2 tablets 4 times daily. It is also available as injection: 400 mcg/ml, 600 mcg/ml
v. Scopolamine-*N*-butylbromide: Tablets 10 mg; injection 20 mg/mL. Dose: 10–20 mg 3–4 times a day orally; 20 mg intramuscularly.
vi. Scopolamine hydrobromide skin patch 1 mg (TTS) releases the drug over 72 h. It is to be applied behind the ear 5–6 h before journey and repeated after 72 h, if required.

Indications for atropine:

For many of the below-mentioned conditions, atropine derivatives and substitutes, which are more selective, are now preferred. **Atropine has retained its therapeutic place only in organophosphorus compound poisoning and treatment of A-V block.**

- **Organophosphorus poisoning:** See Chapter 19. Atropine is also useful in certain mushroom poisoning. These mushrooms contain muscarine and cause muscarinic effects on ingestion. Atropine 1-2 mg intramuscularly or intravenously blocks these effects.
- **Cardiovascular conditions:** Atropine may be useful in abolishing A-V block due to excessive vagal activity. It is also occasionally useful in countering the syncope and bradycardia due to hypersensitive carotid sinus.
- **Gastrointestinal colic:** Atropine is used as **intestinal antispasmodic** to control colicky pain. Constipation due to spastic state of the bowel may be relieved after atropine. It also controls spasticity induced by lead and morphine.
  Relaxation of smooth muscles by atropine

facilitates procedures like GI endoscopy and GI radiology. Its antispasmodic action is useful in **IBS and colonic diverticular disease.**

- **Other colics:** Atropine is usually administered along with morphine in the treatment of **biliary colic.** Morphine tends to increase the intrabiliary pressure, and this effect is countered by concomitant atropine administration. Atropine–morphine combination is also used for relief of **renal colic.**
  Atropine and its substitutes are often used to allay the frequency and **urgency of micturition** accompanying cystitis. They act probably by increasing the capacity of the bladder as a result of its relaxant effect on the bladder wall. Frequency of micturition associated with paraplegia is also controlled with atropine.
- **Ocular conditions:** Atropine is used to produce mydriasis and cycloplegia. Mydriasis is necessary for a fundoscopic examination and in the treatment of acute iritis, iridocyclitis and keratitis. Atropine reduces pain in these conditions by relaxing the inflamed musculature of iris and the ciliary body. It also reduces the chances of adhesion formation.
- **As preanaesthetic medication:** See Chapter 7. It is administered at least 30 min before general anaesthesia. Atropine:
  a. Prevents the development of laryngospasm by reducing the respiratory secretions and does not directly abolish the laryngospasm during anaesthesia
  b. Blocks vagal reflexes induced by surgical manipulation of viscera. It also inhibits oculocardiac reflex associated with ophthalmic surgery.
  c. Counters the cholinergic effects of neostigmine used for decurarization after surgery.
  However, reduction in the bronchial secretion can lead to inspissation of the residual secretions and formation of thick bronchial plugs.

Indications for scopolamine

- **Motion sickness: Scopolamine hydrobromide** in the dose of 0.5–1 mg by mouth is used in the treatment of motion sickness. Dryness of mouth signifies the onset of effect and the protection conferred lasts for 4–6 h. Larger doses may produce excessive sedation. Atropine is much less effective than scopolamine. Scopolamine can also be given by transdermal route (Chapter 39).

Relative contraindications to atropine therapy: Atropine should be administered with caution in:

1. Patients older than 40 years, as it may precipitate an attack of acute congestive glaucoma
2. Individuals with enlarged prostate, as retention of urine may develop
3. Chronic lung conditions as it may reduce the secretions and produce drying
4. Congestive heart failure with tachycardia

SYNTHETIC AND SEMISYNTHETIC ATROPINE SUBSTITUTES

PH 1.11

The need for atropine substitutes arises mainly because of the lack of its selectivity in action. Thus, the dose of atropine required to produce the therapeutic effects on GI tract invariably produces many adverse effects. Drugs have been synthesised, therefore, to produce more therapeutic selectivity. Chemically, atropine substitutes are as follows:

1. **The quaternary ammonium compounds**, which are not satisfactorily absorbed orally, **do not cross the BBB and generally exhibit a greater degree of nicotinic (ganglionic) blocking action.**
2. **The tertiary amine drugs,** which are better absorbed orally, cross the BBB and act more selectively at the muscarinic receptors.

Atropine substitutes are employed mainly for their predominant actions:

- As **mydriatics** and **cycloplegics** e.g., Cyclopentolate, tropicamide. See Chapter 70.
- As **antispasmodics** (particularly for GI and urinary bladder muscles). See below.
- In **Parkinsonism** e.g, Benzhexol, benztropine, biperiden See Chapter 15.
- As **bronchodilators** in chronic bronchitis, chronic obstructive pulmonary disorder (COPD) and bronchial asthma e.g., Ipratropium bromide and tiotropium (Chapter 27).
- As **preanaesthetic medication: Glycopyrrolate,**

a quaternary ammonium compound, is structurally unrelated to atropine but reduces GI tone and motility. Given intravenously, it decreases salivary secretion. Tachycardia is lesser than atropine. It is also used to abate cholinergic effects of neostigmine, when the latter is given post-operatively to reverse effects of skeletal muscle relaxant.

- In **peptic ulcer** e.g., pirenzepine, but it is now rarely used. See Chapter 41.

Atropine Substitutes Mainly Used as Spasmolytics

(a) Mainly for GI tract

These atropine substitutes are commonly used in the treatment of colics. Some of them are quaternary ammonium atropine substitutes which do not cross the blood brain barrier and are relatively free from the central effects. They are more liable to produce ganglionic blockade, resulting in impotence, postural hypotension and urinary retention. They may also block neuromuscular transmission by a curarimimetic action.

ATROPINE METHONITRATE: Besides its ophthalmic use, it is administered orally in the dose of 0.2–0.4 mg 4–6 times a day to treat congenital hypertrophic pyloric stenosis.

METHSCOPOLAMINE BROMIDE: This quaternary ammonium compound is devoid of the central effects of scopolamine and is used in the treatment of renal colic and frequency of micturition associated with cystitis. Dose: 2–5 mg orally, three times a day, or parenterally in the dose of 0.25–1 mg. **Hyoscine-N-butyl bromide** has potent smooth muscle relaxant action and similar use.

METHANTHELINE: It is a synthetic quaternary ammonium compound with a high ratio of ganglion blocking to muscarinic blocking activity. The GI effects and the duration of action of this drug are greater than those of atropine. The drug may produce impotence, postural hypotension, urinary retention and neuromuscular blockade. Rarely, it can cause restlessness and acute psychosis.

PROPANTHELINE: It is related to methantheline and possess more potent ganglionic and muscarinic blocking actions than methantheline. It has been used as a muscle relaxant in irritable bowel syndrome and for relieving pain of diverticulitis. It is administered orally in the dose of 15 mg t.i.d.

OXYPHENONIUM: This quaternary ammonium compound has a higher ratio of ganglion blocking to antimuscarinic activity than majority of other synthetic atropine substitutes. It is a potent antispasmodic. The usual dose is 10 mg orally.

DICYCLOMINE: This tertiary amine has relatively weak antimuscarinic effect but, it is a **direct relaxant for GI smooth muscles.** It is better tolerated and is safe. Dicyclomine hydrochloride is available as 10 mg tablets and as a syrup containing 10 mg per 5 mL. Dose: 10–20 mg t.i.d. Smaller doses are used in children. *It is commonly used to treat dysmenorrhoea, colic and diarrhoea especially in irritable bowel syndrome (IBS).*

(b) For urinary bladder

FLAVOXATE: This tertiary amine has a direct relaxant action on smooth muscles especially of urinary tract. It also possesses weak anticholinergic, local anaesthetic, antihistaminic and analgesic properties. It is used to treat dysuria, nocturia, suprapubic pain, and urinary urgency and frequency associated with cystitis, prostatitis and urethritis. The dose is 100–200 mg 3–4 times a day.

OXYBUTYNIN: This compound has antimuscarinic (selective M_3), direct antispasmodic and some local anaesthetic effects on the urinary bladder. It has been used in the treatment of urinary urgency, urge incontinence and urinary frequency except that following transurethral surgical procedures. The oral dose in adults in 5 mg t.i.d. However, incidence of ADR is more. Hence topical gel formulations and transdermal system have been developed.

TROSPIUM is a nonselective antimuscarinic with efficacy similar to those of oxybutynin.

TOLTERODINE: This tertiary amine acts as a selective M_3 receptor antagonist and is used to treat bladder detrusor instability in the treatment of urinary incontinence. It is metabolised in the liver to active metabolites with actions similar to the parent compound. Dose: 2 mg b.i.d. **Fesoterodine** is a prodrug of tolterodine.

Box 20.1 lists some drugs which may cause antimuscarinic side effects when used in therapy.

Anti-Parkinsonian drugs are themselves antimuscarinic, whereas others exert antimuscarinic effects in addition to their primary pharmacological effects.

Box 20.1 Some Drugs with Antimuscarinic Side Effects

- **Anti-Parkinsonian drugs,** e.g. benzhexol
- **Antipsychotics,** e.g. chlorpromazine
- **Antidepressants,** e.g. TCA
- **Antihistaminics,** e.g. diphenhydramine

BLADDER DYSFUNCTION – PHARMACOLOGY

Normal urinary bladder function and the act of urination (micturition) are well coordinated, involving several neurotransmitters and neuromodulators. Normal urination involves higher centres (pons), spinal cord and peripheral autonomic, somatic and afferent sensory innervation of the lower urinary tract. Disorders of any of these can contribute to the symptoms of bladder dysfunction.

Acetylcholine, by acting on the M_3 receptors, causes detrusor muscle contraction, whereas adrenergic activation causes its relaxation through the **stimulation of β_3 adrenergic receptors.** Stimulation of **dopamine D_1 receptors** suppresses bladder activity, whereas D_2 stimulation facilitates voiding. Other neurotransmitters such as GABA, encephalin, glutamate and 5-HT are also involved in the regulation of bladder function.

The internal sphincter at the bladder neck is rich in α_1 adrenoreceptors; their activation causes sphincter contraction; their inhibition by α_1 antagonists is helpful in benign prostate hyperplasia (BPH) (Chapter 67). PM 7.6

The **common functional abnormalities of micturition** that call for treatment are as follows:

1. **Overactive bladder**
2. **Hypotonic bladder**
3. **Nocturia/nocturnal enuresis**

Drugs used in disturbances of bladder function are summarised in Table 20.1.

1. **Overactive bladder,** a symptom complex, includes urinary urgency with or without urge incontinence, urinary frequency and nocturia (awakening more than once at night to void urine). It is observed in the elderly with prevalence rate of 30%–40% in subjects over 75 years of age. There is no identifiable cause nor any local abnormality.

   Among the types of chronic urinary incontinence, **urge incontinence** is the most common. It is characterised by sudden urgency with leakage of urine, and may be **associated with increased frequency and nocturia.**

   Stress incontinence, the next common type, is more common in the older females. It is associated with weakened pelvic floor muscles and consequent increased mobility of the bladder outlet and urethra. Leakage of urine occurs with increased abdominal pressure as during coughing, sneezing and laughing.

   The **nonpharmacological treatment** of these conditions includes education about bladder function in cognitively intact, motivated patients, pelvic floor exercises and bladder training. The latter involves teaching of urge suppression and regular, scheduled voiding. This is more important than drugs and is considered as first line therapy. Some patients can be helped by biofeedback-assisted training. An extended-release anticholinergic drug or a β-$_3$ agonist can be tried in patients who do not respond to nonpharmacologic therapy.

   Functional urinary frequency, urgency and incontinence are treated with **antimuscarinic drugs** such as **oxybutynin, flavoxate, tolterodine** and **trospium.** They act by inhibiting the involuntary detrusor contractions and thus increasing the bladder capacity. They can be used for both neurogenic and non-neurogenic overactive bladder. These drugs are also useful in detrusor muscle spasm associated with cystitis due to bladder infection. However, they can cause anticholinergic side effects. Extended release

Table 20.1 Drugs Used in Bladder Dysfunction

Drugs	Mechanism of Action	Use	Dose (mg)
Antimuscarinics			
Oxybutynin	Decreases bladder contraction	Overactive bladder	2.5–5.0 t.i.d.
Tolterodine	Do	Do	2 b.i.d.
Trospium	Do	Do	20 b.i.d.
Flavoxate	Do	Do	100–200 t.i.d.
Darifenacin	Do	Do	7.5–15 o.d.
Fesoterodine	Do	Do	4–8 o.d.
β_3 adrenergic agonist			
Mirabegron	Relaxes detrusor smooth muscle	Do	25–50 o.d.
Vibegron	Relaxes detrusor smooth muscle	Do	50–75 o.d.
Alpha$_1$ adrenergic antagonists			
Terazosin	Relaxes urethra and prostate capsule smooth muscle	Urge incontinence asso. with BPH	1–10/d
Doxazosin	Do	Do	1–8/d
Tamsulosin	Do	Do	0.4 o.d., HS
Cholinergic agonist			
Bethanechol	Stimulates bladder contraction	Hypotonic/atonic bladder	10–30 t.i.d.
Estrogen[a]			
Cream (vaginal)	Strengthens periurethral tissue	Urge/stress incontinence associated with vaginal atrophy	0.5–1.0 g/day for first 2 weeks; then twice weekly for 4 weeks.
Tablets (vaginal)	Do	Do	25 mcg/day as above
Antidepressants			
Imipramine	Anticholinergic ? Central action	Nocturnal eneuresis	Chapter 14

[a]Long acting and transdermal estrogen preparations are available.

formulations cause less dryness of mouth and are preferred.

Solifenacin and **darifenacin** are the new drugs, claimed to be relatively 'bladder specific' in their antimuscarinic action (M_3 antagonist) for use in overactive bladder. However, there is no convincing evidence of their superiority over the older drugs.

Long-term use of anticholinergic drugs has been associated with a dose related increase in the risk of dementia hence should be used cautiously in elderly patients with demetia. Trospium or darifenacin have less risk of producing dementia as they have less CNS penetration. Further, obstruction due to enlarged prostate, carcinoma of the prostate and bladder stone must be ruled out.

Anticholinergic drugs should be avoided in patients with narrow-angle glaucoma or gastric retention.

All bladder active anticholinergics are CYP3A4 substrates and are hence prone to cause drug interactions with CYP3A4 inducers and inhibitors. Darifenacin is a CYP2D6 inhibitor and can increase serum concentrations of tamsulosin, which is metabolised by CYP2D6. Concurrent use of solifenacin or tolterodine with a drugs that prolongs the QT interval can increase the risk of QT prolongation.

Mirabegron, a β_3 adrenergic agonist is used for overactive bladder. It causes relaxation of detrusor smooth muscle and increases bladder capacity.

It may cause GI symptoms, headache, dizziness and nasopharyngitis. Mirabegron can increase blood pressure; it should not be used in patients with severe uncontrolled hypertension. Tachycardia, urinary retention and rarely, leukocytoclastic vasculitis have also been reported.. It is moderate inhibitor of CYP2D6.

Vibegron is another β_3 adrenergic agonist which does not inhibit any of the CYP enzymes and hence less likely to cause drug interactions. It does not penetrate BBB and can be given to elderly with cognitive dysfunction.

β_3 agonists are better tolerated than anticholinergic drugs. In case of non responders to monotherapy, antimuscarinic drugs can be combined with β_3 adrenergic agonists. Concurrent use of an anticholinergic drug and a β_3 agonist ((use as beta symbol and 3 subscript) can increase the risk of urinary retention.

Onabotulinum toxin A (Botox) is another drug used as single intradetrusor injection, to treat severe refractory overactive bladder (Chapter 22) or if any of the above drugs cannot be used.

Tibial nerve stimulation and sacral neuromodulation are options for some patients with refractory symptoms not responding to drug therapy.

Postsynaptic α_1 adrenergic blockers such as **terazosin** and **tamsulosin** are **used to treat urinary frequency due to BPH** (Chapter 67).

2. **Bladder hypotonicity** sometimes causes urinary retention. It may be treated by cholinergic drugs such as **bethanechol**, neostigmine or distigmine (Chapter 19). *Urinary retention due to BPH, however, will be worsened by these drugs.*

3. **Nocturia,** a symptom of overactive bladder, can be due to detrusor overactivity, nocturnal polyuria or a primary sleep disorder-nocturnal eneuresis. Antidepressant **imipramine** has anticholinergic action, and possible central effect on voiding reflexes. It is useful in some patients with stress-urge incontinence and nocturnal eneuresis (Chapter 14).

*Finally, it should be remembered that the distal part of the female urethral epithelium possesses estrogen receptors. Their degeneration after menopause can cause urinary incontinence. Such patients may be helped by **topical (vaginal) or oral estrogen** therapy.*

CHAPTER 21

Ganglion Stimulating and Blocking Drugs; Treatment of Tobacco Dependence

Learning Objectives

This chapter will enable the reader:

1. To describe the pharmacological effects of nicotine.
2. To outline the management of acute and chronic nicotine poisoning.
3. To discuss the pharmacotherapy of tobacco dependence.
4. To enlist pharmacological effects of ganglion blocking agents.

KEY TERMS

nicotinic receptors, p. 316
nicotine, p. 316
varenicline, p. 320
ganglion blocking agents, p. 320

The ganglion stimulating agents have hardly any place in therapeutics. The important agents belonging to this group are the alkaloids nicotine and lobeline. Although nicotine has no therapeutic utility, it is the important constituent of tobacco. Lobeline is described in Chapter 12. In addition, synthetic compounds like tetramethylammonium (TMA) and dimethylphenylpiperazinium (DMPP) are mainly used as experimental tools. PH 1.22

NICOTINE: Nicotine was isolated from leaves of the tobacco plant, *Nicotiana tabacum* in 1828. It is a tertiary amine consisting of a pyridine ring and a pyrolidine ring.

Mechanism of action: Nicotine acts as an **agonist at cholinergic receptors present in the brain, autonomic ganglia and neuromuscular junctions,** which explains its multiple effects. Nicotinic receptors are of two types:

1. N_n in the CNS and the autonomic ganglia
2. N_m in the skeletal neuromuscular junction

Activation of nicotinic receptors facilitates the release of ACh, NA, DA, 5-HT and beta-endorphin in the CNS. It also causes release of GH, prolactin and ACTH.

Pharmacological actions: The amount of nicotine absorbed during smoking is sufficient to produce measurable pharmacological and psychopharmacological effects.

Behavioural effects: These vary according to the dosage used and are probably linked to DA release. High density of nicotinic–ACh receptors is present in the mesolimbic system, the reward centre of the brain. Their stimulation by **small doses** of nicotine improves attention, learning, reaction time and problem solving. Smokers often report pleasure and relaxation and reduction in anger, tension, depression and stress. However, large doses cause mental depression. It is a drug with addition potential.

Central nervous system: Nicotine stimulates the CNS and produces tremor, whereas large doses may produce convulsions. Small doses reflexly stimulate respiration through aortic and carotid body chemoreceptors. Large doses directly stimulate the medullary respiratory centre, followed by its depression.

Stimulation of the chemoreceptor trigger zone (CTZ) causes vomiting. It stimulates the supraoptic nuclei of the hypothalamus and induces the release of AVP and exerts an **antidiuretic effect.** In sensitive individuals, this effect may become apparent after smoking two or three cigarettes.

Autonomic ganglia: Like ACh, nicotine initially stimulates the autonomic ganglia leading to stimulation of postganglionic nerves.

However, in large doses, it produces persistent depolarisation of the ganglionic cell bodies resulting in ganglionic blockade.

Adrenal medulla: Initially nicotine stimulates adrenal medulla, leading to discharge of adrenaline into the blood. Larger doses block the secretory response to splanchnic nerve stimulation.

Cardiovascular system: The most consistent effects of smoking are an increase in the heart rate and peripheral vasoconstriction. Carotid chemoreceptors are very sensitive to low levels of nicotine. Blood pressure may rise and skeletal muscle and coronary blood flow may increase. Cardiac work and O_2 consumption are increased. *These effects are due to increased release of catecholamines following stimulation of the sympathetic ganglia and adrenal medulla.* Tolerance to increase in the heart rate develops fairly rapidly. It increases the platelet adhesiveness.

GI tract and secretions: Nicotine increases the motility, tone and secretion of the GI tract and may cause colonic evacuation due to stimulation of the parasympathetic ganglia. Stimulation is usually followed by decrease in motility and tone, leading to constipation. Nicotine initially increases the salivary and bronchial secretions, followed by their inhibition. Salivation accompanying smoking, however, is due to irritant nature of the smoke rather than its nicotine content.

Myoneural junction: Nicotine produces a transient depolarisation of the motor end plate, resulting in a stimulation of skeletal muscles and twitchings. In large doses, this stimulant effect is followed by blockade of myoneural transmission. It is usually the cause of death in nicotine poisoning. Its actions on the autonomic ganglia are more prominent than on the myoneural junction.

Liver enzymes: Nicotine **itself does not induce or inhibit hepatic microsomal enzymes significantly**. Inhalation of cigarette smoke (not nicotine) induces CYP1A2, CYP2E1 and glucuronosyl transferases, hence the metabolism of several drugs including nicotine is enhanced.

Metabolic effects: Nicotine increases the metabolic rate slightly at rest but almost doubles it during light exercise. The increase in BMR, along with appetite suppression, leads to weight loss. Nicotine, via catecholamine release, causes lipolysis and release of free fatty acids (FFA) into the circulation. Excessive release of cortisol following nicotine could affect mood and may contribute to osteoporosis.

Miscellaneous: Intradermal injection or local application of nicotine produces local sweating and vasoconstriction. This effect is attributed to cutaneous axon reflexes mediated by sympathetic nerves and serves as a basis for testing the integrity of the postganglionic sympathetic fibres. It is blocked by local anaesthetics, atropine and ganglionic blocking agents.

Tolerance and dependence (addiction): One-third to one-half of occasional smokers develop physical dependence. Most tobacco-dependent persons never achieve lasting abstinence and one half of all smokers die prematurely of tobacco-related diseases. A regular smoker is able to withstand large amounts of nicotine in contrast to a nonsmoker. **The addictive effects of tobacco smoking are largely due to nicotine.**

Withdrawal syndrome manifests as craving, depression, nervousness, restlessness, irritability, anxiety, impaired concentration, increased appetite and weight gain.

Absorption, fate and excretion: Nicotine is well absorbed from all mucous membranes and even from intact, unbroken skin. It undergoes extensive first pass metabolism when administered orally. It is concentrated in the liver, lungs and the brain. A major portion is metabolised mainly in liver by CYP2D6 to inert cotinine which is then glucuronidated and excreted by the kidney. Its t½ is 2 h. An acidic urine enhances the excretion of ionised nicotine. Nicotine may be secreted in the milk.

Adverse reactions:

- **Acute nicotine poisoning** occurs in workers engaged in spraying nicotine as an insecticide and in children from accidental ingestion of cigarettes. It is, however, one of the most toxic agents and can produce death with the rapidity of cyanide.

Acute nicotine poisoning is characterised by nausea, salivation, vomiting, abdominal pain and diarrhoea. Dizziness, headache, confusion and marked weakness develop. The pupils initially constrict but dilate subsequently. The initial rise in BP is followed by a fall and initial bradycardia is followed by tachycardia. Cold sweat is a prominent feature. Respiration, after brief stimulation, becomes irregular. Convulsions may appear and death occurs from respiratory paralysis.

The **treatment** consists of gastric lavage with 1:10,000 solution of potassium permanganate. As nicotine is rapidly metabolised in the body, attempts should be made to tide over the crisis by symptomatic therapy. Paralysis of respiration should be treated by artificial ventilation with oxygen. *The use of analeptics for respiratory paralysis is dangerous.*

- **Chronic nicotine toxicity and tobacco smoking:** Tobacco, the dried leaf of *Nicotiana tabacum*, is used in various forms as snuff, as plug for chewing and for smoking. The nicotine content of tobacco varies from 0.5% to 8%. Large quantities of nicotine are absorbed from the inhaled smoke and a person who 'drags' on his cigar or cigarette absorbs larger quantities. A cigarette contains 6–11 mg of nicotine, of which, the smoker typically absorbs 1–3 mg irrespective of the nicotine yield rating provided by the tobacco companies. *The other ingredients of tobacco smoke include tar, pyridine, volatile acids, furfural, carbon monoxide and carcinogens.* They too contribute to the adverse effects of tobacco smoking.

Cigarette smoking is associated with increase in morbidity and a shortening of life expectancy. It is higher in older than in younger persons, is seen especially in those who start smoking early in life and in those who inhale the smoke deeply. *Most of the increase in mortality is from cancer of various organs, chronic bronchitis, emphysema and ischaemic heart disease.*

- **Carcinoma of the lung:** The risk of carcinoma of the lung is 15–20 times higher in cigarette smokers than in nonsmokers. Tobacco smoke contains several cancer initiators (carcinogens) and cancer promoters (co-carcinogens); all have not been identified, but the best known is **benzapyrene**.
- **Chronic bronchitis and emphysema:** The incidence of chronic bronchitis is higher in habitual smokers than in nonsmokers. **A smoker's respiratory syndrome** characterised by cough, dyspnoea, wheezing, pain in chest and frequent infection of the upper respiratory tract has been described.

  A number of irritants in tobacco smoke cause bronchoconstriction, damage to the ciliary epithelium and hypertrophy of the mucus glands. Prolonged, heavy smoking is the main cause of **chronic obstructive pulmonary disease (COPD)** which has two components, chronic bronchitis and emphysema. Emphysema is due to hyperinflation of the lungs coupled with destruction of the alveolar walls causing loss of elastic tissue. Lung function is reversible if young smokers give up smoking early. The benefit is less dramatic in older persons with established chronic bronchitis and emphysema.
- **Ischaemic heart disease:** Mortality from IHD and the frequency of angina pectoris are more in smokers than in nonsmokers. Further, atherosclerotic changes are more extensive in smokers than in nonsmokers. These effects are probably due to release of catecholamines from the adrenal medulla by nicotine. Catecholamines increase (a) platelet adhesiveness, (b) the concentration of blood lipids and (c) the tendency to hypertension and cardiac arrhythmias. Further, smoking increases the concentration of carboxyhaemoglobin in the blood. Thrombosis is an important mechanism of smoking-induced cardiac events.
- **Peripheral vascular disease:** Nicotine causes prolonged vasoconstriction in the hands and feet with intermittent claudication. Thromboangiitis obliterans (TAO) occurs far more frequently in smokers than in nonsmokers.
- **Tobacco amblyopia:** Tobacco amblyopia causes decrease in the visual acuity, particularly in the central field, is attributed to a spasm of the retinal blood vessels.
- **GI disturbances:** Nicotine causes excessive salivation, gastric acidity, aggravation of peptic ulcer

disease and constipation. Increased incidence of cancers of the mouth, larynx and oesophagus has been reported in association with smoking and tobacco chewing.

- **Miscellaneous:** Women who smoke heavily are at risk for a premature menopause. Those who smoke during pregnancy have a higher incidence of abortions and give birth to babies with low birth weights. *It is an important cause of impotence in men and infertility in women.*
  The polycyclic hydrocarbons present in the cigarette smoke accelerate the metabolism of many drugs by inducing hepatic microsomal enzymes (Chapter 3).

E-cigarettes: These are electronic nicotine delivery Systems (ENDS) commonly known as E-cigarettes. These battery operated devices look like traditional tobacco cigarettes, cigars, or pens or USB memory sticks. Majority of the e-cigarettes contain nicotine, which is inhaled as an aerosol. They may also contain flavoring agents such as diacetyl, a chemical linked to a serious lung disease; volatile organic compounds, cancer-causing chemicals and heavy metals such as nickel, tin, and lead. Other ENDS include e-sheesha and e-hookah, which like e-cigarettes, can pose risk to public health, mainly non-smokers.

ENDS are not safe for children, young adults, pregnant women, or adults who do not currently use tobacco products.

Prevention of tobacco use in any form is important. In this respect, education of children in the concept of positive health and in the harmful effect of smoking on health is of prime importance. This must be done as much by practice as by preaching since children tend to imitate the grown-ups around them and cannot be expected not to smoke as long as they see people, particularly family members, smoking or chewing tobacco all around them.

Doctors can help by inquiring about the smoking habits of all their patients, by educating them about its harmful effects, by strongly advising against smoking and by not smoking themselves!

Pharmacotherapy of Tobacco Dependence (Deaddiction Treatment): PH 1.23

Drugs are used to:

- **Reduce craving for nicotine** during abstinence period.
- **Inhibit reinforcing effects** of nicotine during smoking.

Tobacco produces both psychological and physical dependence. The dependence is likely to be mediated by mesolimbic $\alpha_4\beta_2$ sub units of N_n receptors which cause release of DA resulting in positive reinforcing effects of nicotine. Abrupt cessation of heavy smoking may cause irritability and drowsiness.

Box 21.1 lists the drugs used in treating tobacco dependence. Attention to any underlying psychological disturbances, thus may prove rewarding.

Nicotine substitution therapy for tobacco dependence increases the rate of success of quitting smoking. Reinforcing effect of smoking is maximum with inhalation, less with oral use and least with the slow-release, transdermal nicotine patch. Hence, the following preparations are used for **substitution therapy:**

i. Transdermally delivered nicotine (nicotine patches)
ii. Transmucosally delivered nicotine in form of gums and lozenges
iii. Inhaler and nasal spray

These preparations, in contrast to smoking, provide slower rise in, and lower and less variable plasma nicotine concentrations, thus helping the

Box 21.1 Drugs Used in Tobacco Dependence

I. **Nicotine receptor agonists**
   Nicotine transdermal patches
   Nicotine polacrylate gum/lozenges
   Nicotine nasal spray
   Nicotine oral inhaler
II. **Nicotine receptor partial agonist,** e.g. varenicline
III. **Dopamine/NA central reuptake inhibitor:** Bupropion (Chapter 14)
IV. **Miscellaneous:** Nortriptyline, clonidine, naltrexone

smoker to abstain from tobacco, resulting finally in cessation of smoking.

The possible mechanisms by which the smoker's cessation efforts are strengthened by this medication are as follows:

- **Nicotine substitution decreases withdrawal symptoms.**
- **It partially decreases the craving for cigarettes by sustaining tolerance**, in much the same way that methadone partially decreases the craving for morphine.
- **It may provide some euphoria.**

Transdermal patches may occasionally cause nightmares and insomnia.

All nicotine substitution therapies are equally effective; combining transdermal patch with rapid onset formulation (e.g. gum, lozenge, inhaler or nasal spray) is more effective then single agent alone. The optimal duration of treatment in most patients is at least 3 – 6 months.

E-cigarettes are not approved as substitution therapy. Long term benefits and safety of e-cigarettes, as substitute for regular cigarettes, is not known.

VARENICLINE is a partial agonist of $\alpha_4\beta_2$ sub units of cholinergic N_n receptors, which mediate dopamine release, decrease cravings and withdrawal symptoms during abstinence. Varenicline has greater affinity for $\alpha_4\beta_2$ receptors than nicotine, reducing the reward of smoking. Its t½ is 14–24 h. It should be started orally 7 days before the target quit date in low dose of 0.5 mg/day taken after meals with a full glass of water, and increased gradually over a week to 1 mg twice a day. It is continued for 12 weeks. It causes nausea, headache, abnormal dreams, sleep disturbances, constipation and weight loss. **Severe neuropsychiatric symptoms,** agitation, depressed moods and suicidal ideation have been reported. Cardiovascular risk is also suspected.

Varenicline is more effective than single nicotine substitution agent / bupropion and equieffective as combination nicotine substitution therapy. Recently nasal spray of varenicline is approved for treatment of dry eye disease.

CYTISINE: This alkaloid (also called baptitoxine and sophorine), obtained from leguminous family, is used mainly in Eastern Europe for several years to treat tobacco dependence. It acts as a **partial agonist at nicotinic receptors of ACh,** subtype $\alpha_4\beta_2$. It is well absorbed orally and has t½ of 4.8 h. It is used in the dose of 1.5–9 mg/day for 25 days. It is claimed to be as effective as varenicline. The ADR reported are nausea, vomiting and sleep disturbances. It is highly cost-effective and needs further evaluation.

BUPROPION, an antidepressant, helps some individuals to give up smoking. It is a selective blocker of NA and DA neuronal uptake and may help to reduce craving. It has additional nicotinic receptor blocking activity which may help in smoking cessation. Therapy with sustained release bupropion formulation is started 7 -14 days before the target quit date. The initial dose is 150 mg daily for 3 days, increasing to 150 mg twice a day for 8-12 weeks. It is as effective as single nicotine substitution agent. It can be used along with nicotine patches. It can cause dryness of mouth, insomnia, neuropsychiatric disorders and seizures (see Chapter 14). Bupropion and its active metabolite hydroxybupropion both inhibit CYP2D6 and can cause potential drug interactions. It has anorexigenic effects and is used in the treatment of obesity (Chapter 38).

Nortriptyline (TCA; 75–100 mg/day for 8–12 weeks) and **clonidine** (α_2 agonist; 0.15–0.75 mg/day) are considered as second-line options.

Some of the effects of nicotine perceived as positive effects such as performance enhancement, contribute to addiction and are opioid mediated. Hence **naltrexone**, an opioid antagonist, has also been used for smoking cessation.

GANGLION BLOCKING AGENTS

The ganglion blocking agents are drugs which selectively competitively block the transmission across the autonomic ganglia, both sympathetic and parasympathetic, by blocking the ACh receptors. They can cause adverse reactions due to:

1. **Parasympathetic blockade** (visual disturbances, dry mouth, urinary hesitancy, constipation and sexual impotence).
2. **Sympathetic blockade** (syncope from postural hypotension).

Once used to treat hypertension, these drugs are now obsolete (Chapter 30).

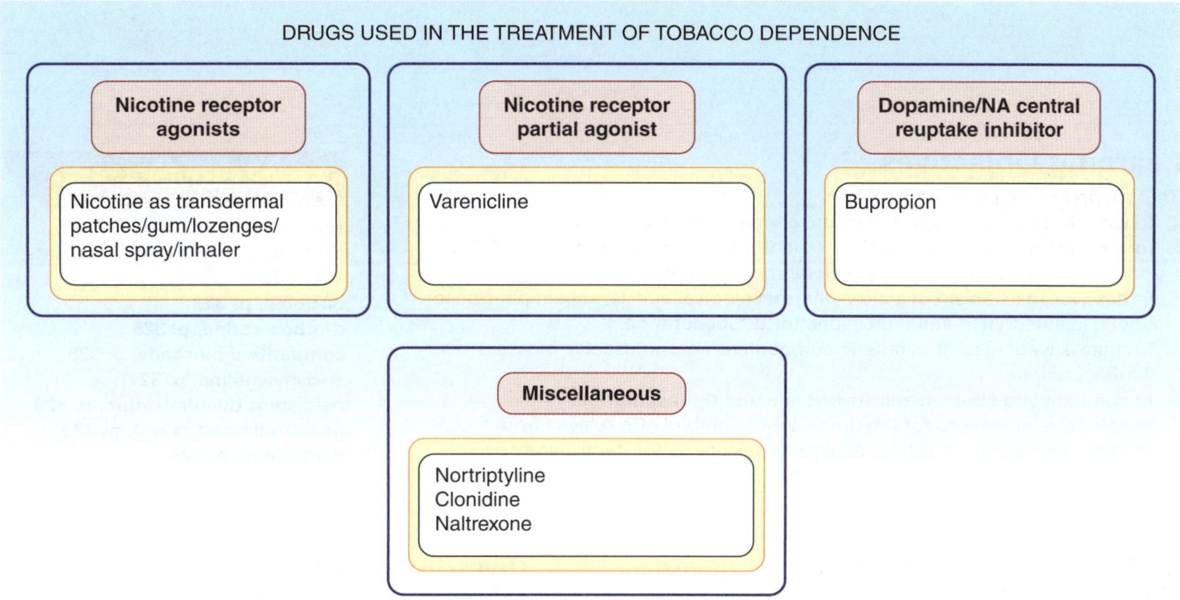

CHAPTER 22

Skeletal Muscle Relaxants

Learning Objectives

This chapter will enable the reader:

1. To classify skeletal muscle relaxants, giving examples of drugs.
2. To describe mechanism of action, salient pharmacological effects, ADR and indications for centrally acting skeletal muscle relaxants.
3. To describe mechanism of action, pharmacological effects, salient pharmacokinetic features, ADR and indications for d-tubocurarine.
4. To state advantages of synthetic competitive neuromuscular blockers over d-tubocurarine.
5. To compare and contrast succinylcholine and d-tubocurarine.
6. To enlist the indications for the drug/s which inhibits ACh release from motor.
7. To state mechanism of action, ADR and indications for dantrolene.

KEY TERMS

spasticity, p. 322
centrally acting muscle relaxants, p. 322
baclofen, p. 323
d-tubocurarine, p. 325
competitive blockade, p. 325
succinylcholine, p. 327
persistent depolarization, p. 328
onabotulinum toxin A, p. 329
dantrolene, p. 329

Skeletal muscle relaxants help to reduce unwanted spasm or spasticity without interfering with consciousness and normal voluntary movements; they are used in various neurological or painful musculoskeletal disorders and during surgery for achieving satisfactory muscle relaxation.

Spasticity is due **to increase in skeletal muscle tone** associated with decrease in muscle power due to damage to the corticomotoneuronic pathways as in cerebral palsy, multiple sclerosis, CNS injury or stroke. **Spasm**, on the other hand, is **an involuntary contraction of a muscle or group of muscles**, usually accompanied by pain and limited function.

Classification of Skeletal Muscle Relaxants PH 1.15

That do not cause loss of consciousness:

1. **Drugs acting centrally**, e.g. benzodiazepines (Chapter 8), baclofen and tizanidine
2. **Drugs acting peripherally at neuromuscular junction** e.g. d-tubocurarine, succinylcholine
3. **Drugs acting directly on muscle,** e.g. dantrolene
4. **Drugs effective in extrapyramidal disorders** such as Parkinsonism (Chapter 15)

CENTRALLY ACTING SKELETAL MUSCLE RELAXANTS

Centrally acting muscle relaxants (Table 22.1) cause muscular relaxation without loss of consciousness. They act on selective areas in the CNS like cortex, brain stem and spinal cord. The exact mechanism of action is not known. However, depression of polysynaptic spinal and supraspinal reflexes, especially of the reticular system, controlling the muscle tone appears to be responsible for their effects. They reduce the muscle tone without causing paralysis. Inhibition of pathways in ascending reticular formation, which are involved in maintenance of wakefulness, results in sedation, a common property of most of these drugs. Sedative anxiolytic agents like diazepam exhibit central muscle relaxant action.

Classification

1. **Antispastic agents:** Prescribed for conditions such as cerebral palsy and multiple sclerosis: diazepam, baclofen and dantrolene

Table 22.1 Centrally Acting Muscle Relaxants

Name	Preparation (Tab)	Total Daily Dose
Benzodiazepines	(e.g. see Diazepam. Chapter 8)	
Baclofen	5/10 mg	20 mg
Cyclobenzaprine	15/30 mg	15–30 mg
Tizanidine	2/4 mg	6–18 mg
Carisoprodol	0.35 g	0.7–1.4 g
Chlorzoxazone	0.25 g	0.5–1.5 g
Metaxalone	0.4 g	2.4–3.2 g
Methocarbamol[a]	0.75 g	4–8 g
Orphenadrine[a]	0.05 g	0.1–0.2 g

Note: Daily doses mentioned are usually given in divided doses.
[a]IM and IV preparations available.

2. **Antispasmodic agents:** Prescribed for musculoskeletal conditions: cyclobenzaprine, tizanidine, diazepam, metaxalone, methocarbamol, orphenadrine, carisoprodol and chlorzoxazone

DIAZEPAM: This BZD is useful alone, or in combination, for relieving spasticity especially in patients with lesions of the spinal cord, and occasionally in patients with cerebral palsy or multiple sclerosis. Painful spasms due to a spinal cord lesion are often reduced. It may be of benefit in the stiff-man syndrome, localised muscle spasms due to traumatic causes and for leg spasm that disturbs sleep. Oral dose is 2 mg twice daily, which is increased gradually to maximum of 5 mg 3–4 times daily. It has low muscle relaxant: sedation ratio, which limits the dose used for muscle relaxation. The drug has long t½ due to an active metabolite, and hence, it is better avoided in elderly patients and in patients with hepatic impairment. It is the drug of choice to control spasms in tetanus, where it can be given intramuscularly or intravenously. *Diazepam should not be mixed with other drugs for IV use* (see Chapter 8).

BACLOFEN: This compound, beta-4(chlorophenyl)-gamma aminobutyric acid, is structurally related to inhibitory neurotransmitter, GABA.

Mechanism of action: It is a **selective $GABA_B$ receptor agonist**, mainly acting, on presynaptic receptors in the spinal cord. It depresses the reflexes by reducing the calcium influx and thereby prevents release of excitatory neurotransmitters. It also appears to inhibit the release of substance P (neurokinin-1) in the spinal cord. It causes a dose-dependent 'antinociceptive' effect in the intact animal and may thus be useful in pain syndromes.

It is almost completely absorbed, and 80% is excreted unchanged in the urine within 72 h.

Clinically, it produces considerable relief of painful flexor (and sometimes extensor) spasms and of increased flexor tone in patients with spinal transection. It also reduces tonic flexor dystonias of the lower extremities in patients with spinal spasticity and may improve bladder and bowel control in patients with spinal lesions. It has no action on muscle power and it does not improve muscle function. *It is not useful in spasticity of cerebral origin.* It may be useful as a **'back up' drug** in the treatment of trigeminal neuralgia.

Adverse reactions: The drug is generally well tolerated. Adverse reactions include drowsiness, lassitude, hallucinations, depression, ataxia, blurred vision and GI disturbances. Baclofen should be tapered off slowly in epileptic patients as increased seizure activity has been reported on withdrawal.

CYCLOBENZAPRINE: This drug, structurally related to TCA, probably acts on descending 5-HT pathway to reduce tonic somatic motor activity. It has a long elimination t½. Adverse effects are dose-related and include sedation, dizziness and anticholinergic effects. It should be avoided in older patients and in patients with glaucoma. It is contraindicated in patients with arrhythmias, recent MI and CHF. It should be avoided in patients who are prone to seizures especially, those on tramadol.

TIZANIDINE: This drug, an **α_2 adrenergic agonist,** reduces muscle spasm by reinforcing both, the presynaptic and postsynaptic inhibition of the motor neurons. It serves as antispasmodic and antispastic agent and is used for the treatment of spasticity secondary to spinal cord injury and multiple sclerosis. It exhibits intrinsic analgesic activity. It is given in the dose of 2–8 mg t.i.d. but dose for optimal response varies markedly among patients. Its efficacy as skeletal muscle relaxant is comparable to diazepam, baclofen and dantrolene.

Adverse reactions: These include dizziness, drowsiness, asthenia, hypotension, dry mouth and hepatoxicity. Sudden stoppage of drug can result in rebound hypertension in patients on long-term therapy.

CARISOPRODOL: This drug has favourable muscle relaxant: sedation ratio. It is also weak analgesic, antipyretic and anticholinergic. It gets metabolised to meprobamate, which is a sedative-hypnotic with extensive abuse. Carisoprodol also exhibits addictive potential.

Adverse reactions: These include allergic reactions like rash, asthma and angioneurotic oedema. Rarely, idiosyncratic reactions (mental status changes and temporary loss of vision) may occur after first dose, which may need hospitalisation.

CHLORZOXAZONE: This synthetic benzoxazole is marketed as FDCs with NSAIDs. It inhibits degranulation of mast cells and cytokines from inflammatory cells. It is claimed to inhibit calcium and potassium influx, which causes neuronal inhibition. It causes dizziness, drowsiness, red- or orange-coloured urine, GI irritation and rarely GI bleeding and hepatic damage.

METAXALONE: This drug is moderately effective and produces less dizziness and drowsiness compared to other skeletal muscle relaxants. It should be used with caution in patients with liver failure.

METHOCARBAMOL: This is a carbamate of guaifenesin, but does not produce guaifenesin as a metabolite because the carbamate bond is stable. Its abuse potential is minimal. ADR include hypersensitivity reactions, discolouration of urine, nausea, anorexia, drowsiness, dizziness, restlesness, anxiety, confusion and convulsions. Parenteral administration may cause syncope, hypotension, bradycardia and anaphylaxis. It may exacerbate myasthenia gravis by inhibiting effects of pyridostigmine and should be used with caution with anticholinesterase agents. Fetal abnormalities have been reported. It is also marketed as FDC with NSAIDs like ibuprofen, paracetamol and diclofenac.

ORPHENADRINE: It is a **centrally acting anticholinergic agent** developed to treat EPR of antipsychotics. It is related to antihistaminic, diphenhydramine and also to the nonopioid analgesic, nefopam. It is used to treat pain of various aetiologies, from headaches to radiculopathy and also to relieve muscle spasm. It exerts several CNS and peripheral effects. It has long t½.

Adverse reactions: These include GI irritation, hypersensitivity reaction, anticholinergic effects like drowsiness, dry mouth, tachycardia, urinary retention, increased intraocular tension, and rarely aplastic anaemia.

The doses of centrally acting muscle relaxants are presented in Table 22.1. PM 3.5

Although various muscle relaxants mentioned above reduce the activity of polysynapic reflexes and resolve decerebrate rigidity in the spinal cat, these findings do not necessarily indicate their usefulness in cerebrate man. *Hence, though they are promoted for certain spastic neurological disorders, they are not useful. They may be of some use in cases with localised muscle spasm and are advocated as adjuvant analgesics (Chapter 11) in conditions such as fibrositis, myalgia, myositis and spasms associated with arthritis. The marginal beneficial effects observed with these agents are probably because of their central sedative and analgesic actions, and none of these compounds* **except diazepam and baclofen** *can be recommended as effective, reliable and specific muscle relaxants.*

The centrally acting skeletal muscle relaxants should be used with caution in pregnant women and in the presence of renal damage. They are contraindicated in myasthenia gravis.

PERIPHERALLY ACTING SKELETAL MUSCLE RELAXANTS

Physiology of Skeletal Muscle Contraction

The steps in neuromuscular transmission leading to skeletal muscle contraction consist of the following:

- Release of ACh in relatively *large amounts* from the synaptic vesicles of the motor nerve into the synaptic cleft as a result of a nerve impulse which is also called **nerve action potential** (NAP). Even in the absence of nerve impulse, *minute quantities* of ACh are released continually into the synaptic cleft.
- Acetylcholine thus released, binds to the nicotinic receptors (N_m) on the **motor end plate** (MEP), leading to the development of an end plate potential (EPP). Influx of sodium, into the MEP, causes depolarisation.
- When the EPP achieves sufficient magnitude, the surrounding area of the muscle fibre membrane is excited, resulting in the development of muscle action potential (MAP) which initiates contraction as a result of release of calcium into the sarcoplasm.
- Acetylcholine is rapidly hydrolysed by AChE enabling the repolarisation of the MEP and the muscle fibre membrane.

Calcium ions play a crucial role in excitation–contraction coupling in the skeletal muscle.

Skeletal muscle contraction can be blocked at several points as shown in Box 22.1.

In clinical practice, paralysis of skeletal muscles is usually induced by interfering with the function of MEP.

Box 22.1 Ways of Blocking Skeletal Muscle Contraction in Response to Nerve Impulse

- **Blocking the transmission of impulse across the motor nerve,** e.g. local anaesthetics
- **Inhibiting the synthesis of acetylcholine in the motor nerve,** e.g. hemicholinium
- **Inhibiting the release of acetylcholine,** e.g. botulinum toxin A and beta bungarotoxin
- **Modifying the MEP functional states** so that it does not respond to ACh, e.g. d-tubocurarine and succinylcholine
- **Interfering with sarcoplasmic reticulum function,** e.g. dantrolene

Classification of Peripherally Acting Skeletal Muscle Relaxants PH 1.15, AS 4.1

1. **Competitive blockers of ACh at the motor end plate**, e.g. d-tubocurarine, alcuronium, atracurium and vecuronium
2. **Persistent depolarizers of the motor end plate and the muscle fibre membrane**, e.g. succinylcholine
3. **Inhibitors of the release of ACh from the motor nerve terminals**, e.g. botulinum toxin Type A

1. Drugs Acting by Competitive Blockade

d-TUBOCURARINE: This is the dextrorotatory, quaternary ammonium alkaloid obtained from the plant *Chondrodendron tomentosum*, indigenous to the Amazon region, and plants of the Strychnos species. The prefix 'tubo' is derived from the fact that crude curare was transported by the South American Indians in bamboo tubes, who used it selectively as an arrow poison. Although the mechanism of this action was studied by Claude Bernard in 1856, the alkaloid was isolated by Harold King in 1935. PY 3.5

Mechanism of action: d-Tubocurarine selectively binds to the nicotinic receptors (N_m) on the MEP and thus blocks the action of ACh by **competitive blockade.** The muscle paralysed by d-tubocurarine still responds to direct electrical stimulation. If the concentration of ACh in the synaptic cleft is increased either by augmenting its release (stronger electrical stimulation of the motor nerve) or inhibiting its degradation (by an anti-ChE drug), d-tubocurarine blockade is reversed (Fig. 22.1).

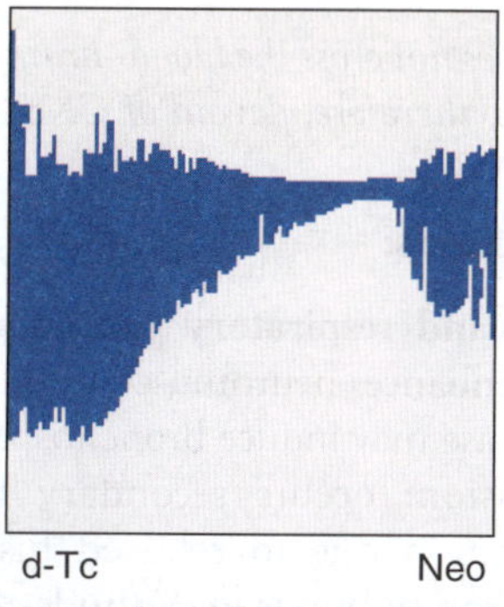

FIG. 22.1 Blocking effect of d-tubocurarine (dTc) on electrically stimulated rat phrenic nerve diaphragm preparation. Note the quick recovery following the addition of neostigmine (Neo).

Pharmacological actions:

Skeletal muscle: d-Tubocurarine, given parenterally, produces motor weakness initially, followed by flaccid paralysis. Small, rapidly moving muscles of the fingers, toes, ears and eyes are affected first, making it impossible to perform delicate motor tasks. The muscles of limbs, neck and trunk are affected later, followed by the intercostal muscles. Finally, the diaphragm is paralysed and death occurs from hypoxia. Consciousness and sensorium are unaffected. Recovery occurs in the reverse order, the diaphragm recovering first and the small muscles recovering last.

Autonomic ganglia: In the doses used it can produce partial blockade of both the autonomic ganglia and adrenal medulla resulting in fall of BP, after brief initial stimulation.

Histamine release: It produces histamine release from tissues by acting directly on mast cells. This may occasionally cause bronchospasm, increased salivary, tracheo-bronchial secretions and contributes to production of hypotension.

Absorption, fate and excretion: d-Tubocurarine, being a quaternary ammonium compound, is not significantly absorbed from the GI tract. The drug is well absorbed on IM administration and is widely distributed in tissues. The drug owes its brief duration of action to its rapid redistribution. About 33% of the dose is eliminated unchanged in urine within 24 h. Repeated administration can cause cumulative toxicity.

The drug does not cross the blood–brain or placental barrier. It is, therefore, devoid of CNS effects.

Adverse reactions: FM 10.1

- **Hypoxia and respiratory paralysis:** Respiratory acidosis enhances neuromuscular blockade. Histamine release may induce bronchospasm.
- **Hypotension:** occurs secondary to peripheral vasodilatation due to released histamine. This hypotension responds to IV fluids. Antihistaminics are also useful to counter bronchospasm and peripheral vasodilatation.
- **Miscellaneous:** There may be a regurgitation of gastric juice into the oesophagus and aspiration into the lungs due to paralysis of the oesophageal sphincter and the diaphragm.

Drugs which synergise with d-tubocurarine are general anaesthetics (ether, halothane, isoflurane and enflurane), aminoglycosides, trimethaphan, opioids, propranolol, glucocorticoids, digitalis, chloroquine, calcium channel blockers, quinidine, diuretics and catecholamines.

d-Tubocurarine has become obsolete in clinical practice and is described above as a prototype.

Synthetic competitive neuromuscular blockers: Currently, used drugs are classified in Table 22.2. Chemically, they are:

a. **Benzylisoquinolones**, e.g. atracurium, doxacurium and mivacurium
b. **Ammoniosteroids**, e.g. pancuronium, vecuronium and rocuronium
c. **Mixed**, e.g. gantacurium

They have similar properties but differ in their relative toxicities. Broadly, they differ from d-tubocurarine in that they:

- **Are more selective and do not block ganglionic transmission significantly.**
- **Have fewer cardiovascular adverse effects.**
- **Are less liable to release histamine.**

Table 22.3 summarises the properties of neuromuscular blocking agents.

Table 22.2 Competitive Neuromuscular Blocking Agents

Long acting (60–120 min)	Doxacurium, pancuronium, pipecuronium, vecuronium
Intermediate acting (20–50 min)	Atracurium, rocuronium
Short acting (10–20 min)	Mivacurium, rapacuronium
Ultra short acting (10 min)	Gantacurium

Table 22.3 Neuromuscular Blocking Agents

Drug	Onset	Duration (min)	Mode of Elimination	Other Actions	Require Reversal with Neostigmine
			Competitive		
d-Tubocurarine	4–6	80–120	Renal and hepatic clearance	Ganglionic blockade ++, vagal blockade ++, histamine release ++ (hypotension reflex tachycardia, cutaneous flushing and broncho-spasm)	Yes
Pancuronium	4–6	120–180	Renal	Ganglionic blockade +, vagal blockade ++, no histamine release (slight tachycardia and increase in BP)	Yes
Vecuronium	2–4	60–90	Hepatic (to active metabolites)	No ganglionic blockade, vagal blockade or histamine release (no tachycardia)	Yes
Rocuronium	1–2	30–40	Hepatic	Same as above	Yes
Doxacurium	4–6	90–120	Renal	No ganglionic or vagal blockade, histamine release + (transient hypotension)	Yes
Atracurium	2–4	30–40	Plasma ChE and Spontaneous degradation (Hoffman elimination)	Same as above. Preferred in renal/liver impairment	No
Mivacurium	2–4	12–18	Plasma ChE	Same as above	No
Rapacuronium	1–2	15–30	Hepatic	Bronchospasm; hence withdrawn	Yes
Gantacurium	1	5-10	Non-enzymatic ester hydrolysis	Histamine release ++	No
			Noncompetitive		
Succinylcholine	1–1.5	6–8	Plasma ChE	Ganglion stimulation, histamine release	No

The relaxant effect of synthetic muscle relaxants is reversed by neostigmine and edrophonium. However, they can cause hypotension and bradycardia, and hence concomitantly atropine or glycopyrrolate is administered.

2. Drugs Acting by Persistent Depolarisation

SUCCINYLCHOLINE: Succinylcholine is a quaternary ammonium compound with a structure resembling two molecules of ACh joined together. It has a short duration of action. PY 3.5

Mechanism of action: It is a **partial agonist of acetylcholine and produces skeletal muscle depolarisation, by acting on the membrane channel.** This can explain the fasciculations preceding skeletal muscle paralysis with this agent. However, in contrast to ACh, the drug is destroyed much more slowly, being susceptible only to plasma and liver pseudocholinesterase. This causes

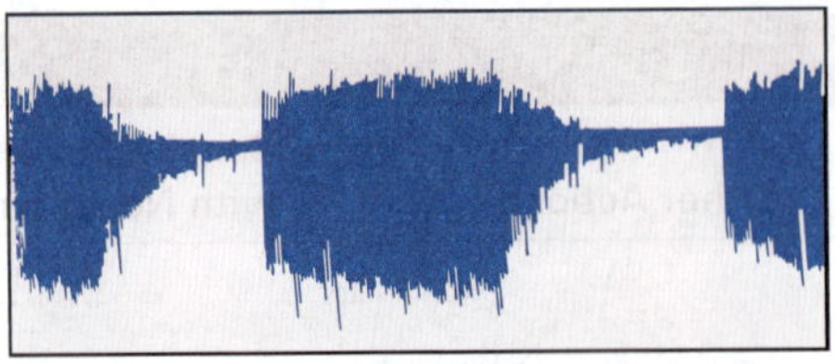

FIG. 22.2 **Blocking effect of succinylcholine (Sc) on electrically stimulated rat phrenic nerve diaphragm preparation. Note the worsening of the block following neostigmine (Neo) and recovery after wash (W).**

a **persistent depolarisation** during which the muscles remain insensitive to ACh released from nerve endings and remain paralysed (Fig. 22.2).

Pharmacological actions:

Skeletal muscle: Paralysis of skeletal muscle produced by succinylcholine is preceded by transient muscular fasciculations and twitching. Succinylcholine relaxes the limb and neck muscles in a dose that does not significantly affect respiratory muscles. Transient apnoea is, however, usually observed with the peak effect of succinylcholine. The skeletal muscle paralysis by succinylcholine is enhanced by anti-ChE neostigmine which increases the local concentration of ACh (Fig. 22.2).

Hyperkalaemia: Prolonged depolarisation may cause shift of intracellular potassium to the extracellular space. In patients with extensive soft tissue trauma or burns, as well as other condition which cause hyperkalaemia, this can be life-threatening.

Cardiovascular system: Repeated administration leads to stimulation of the vagal nuclei and sympathetic ganglia. The former produces bradycardia, cardiac arrhythmias, and hypotension. The latter causes persistent hypertension and tachycardia.

Miscellaneous: Large doses may cause hypotension as a result of muscarinic effect and to some extent by ganglionic blockade. *Because of its muscarinic action, atropine is generally given before its use.*

Absorption, fate and excretion: Succinylcholine IV produces fasciculations which last for 10–15 s. Peak effect develops within 1–2 min and muscle power recovers within 5 min. The drug is hydrolysed by plasma and liver pseudocholinesterase to succinic acid and choline. About 10% of the dose is excreted unchanged in the urine. It **can be used in obstetric cases.**

Adverse reactions: Apart from allergic reactions, the other adverse reactions are as follows:

- **Cardiac arrest and arrhythmias:** High incidence of cardiac arrhythmias with the use of succinylcholine–halothane combination has been reported. The drug may occasionally produce cardiovascular collapse. Changes in K^+ distribution may cause serious arrhythmias in patients on diuretics and digitalis. FM 10.1
- **Succinylcholine apnoea:** Apnoea needing respiratory support longer than 15 min is considered abnormal. It can be precipitated by metabolic acidosis. It is treated by artificial respiration and fresh frozen plasma transfusion. No antidote is available.
- **Malignant hyperthermia:** The drug can rarely trigger serious malignant hyperthermic crisis in patients receiving ether or halothane.
- **Miscellaneous:** Muscle soreness is a frequent complaint following succinylcholine.

Drug interactions: They are similar to those of d-tubocurarine. Anti-ChE drugs, however, act synergistically with depolarising blockers.

Preparations and dosage: Succinylcholine chloride 50 mg/mL. Dose: 1 mg/kg given slowly intravenously, followed by 0.3 mg/kg as needed.

Indications for peripheral skeletal muscle relaxants:

- **Adjuvant to anaesthesia:** The main use of skeletal muscle relaxants is to promote skeletal muscle relaxation during abdominal surgery, orthopaedic manipulations, and various brief procedures like laryngoscopy, bronchoscopy and oesophagoscopy. For the latter procedures **mivacurium** and **rocuronium** are preferred because of their rapid onset of action. Between the two, rocuronium has longer duration of action and is preferred for procedures that last for 30 min.
- **In electroconvulsive therapy:** Succinylcholine or

mivacurium is often administered along with diazepam to protect the patient from injury during electroconvulsive therapy.

PM 3.5

3. Drugs Which Inhibit ACh Release from Motor Nerve Terminals

BOTULINUM TOXIN TYPE A (Onabotulinum toxin A) is produced by *Clostridium botulinum.* **It binds irreversibly presynaptically, to its target site,** which is one of the proteins (SNAP-25) at the core SNARE complex. SNARE complex serves as a calcium sensor and is responsible for fusion of ACh containing vesicles and synaptic membrane, which precedes exocytosis. By binding to SNAP-25, **the toxin inhibits the release of ACh from the motor nerve terminals.** *Local injection* of the toxin weakens the overactive muscle and decreases the hypersecretion of glands innervated by cholinergic neurons. It has been used to treat:

IM 19.9

- Spastic conditions such as spasmodic torticolis, hemifacial spasm, strabismus, blepharospasm, dystonias, lower oesophageal spasm and painful anal fissure
- Wrinkles on the face and neck
- Palmar hyperhidrosis
- Overactive bladder (Chapter 20)

It appears to be safe and effective in these conditions. Its action lasts for 3–4 months.

Adverse reactions include ptosis, diplopia, reduced blinking leading to dry eyes, minor bruises and lid swelling; reversible muscle atrophy can occur after repeated administration.

BOTULINUM TOXIN TYPE B can be used in patients who have become resistant to Type A toxin.

Drugs Acting Directly on Skeletal Muscle

DANTROLENE: This phenytoin analogue relaxes the skeletal muscles by direct action.

Mechanism of action: It binds to the ryanodine receptors (RYR) on the sarcoplasmic reticulum, blocking their opening. This prevents the release of Ca^{++} from the sarcoplasmic stores. Thus, the muscle contraction is weakened without muscle paralysis. It does not alter the neuromuscular transmission. It has relatively little effect on cardiac and smooth muscle.

Given orally, it is incompletely (about one-third) absorbed and is largely metabolised in the liver. It can also be given intravenously.

Adverse reactions: These include generalised muscle weakness, dizziness, drowsiness, fatigue and diarrhoea. Rarely, it may cause serious hepatotoxicity.

Indications:

- **Spasticity:** The drug is particularly useful for the treatment of spasticity (especially cerebral spasticity) in patients in whom nursing care is made difficult by muscle spasm. Patients in whom spastic, dystonic stiffness is useful as a sort of protective endogenous crutch should not be treated with dantrolene.
- **Malignant hyperthermia:** Intravenous dantrolene (1 mg/kg, bolus, repeated if required to a maximum total dose of 100 mg) is life-saving in this rare, fatal and familial, genetic disorder of skeletal muscle. It causes muscle rigidity, hyperpyrexia (temperature > 42°C), hyperkalaemia, tachycardia and metabolic acidosis.

It must be noted that management of the patient with spasticity implies more than just treatment of the spasticity. For many patients the increased tone is not harmful and may even be helpful. Active measures to reduce spasticity are only justified where the reflex hyperexcitability interferes with function, making rehabilitation, physiotherapy and nursing care difficult.

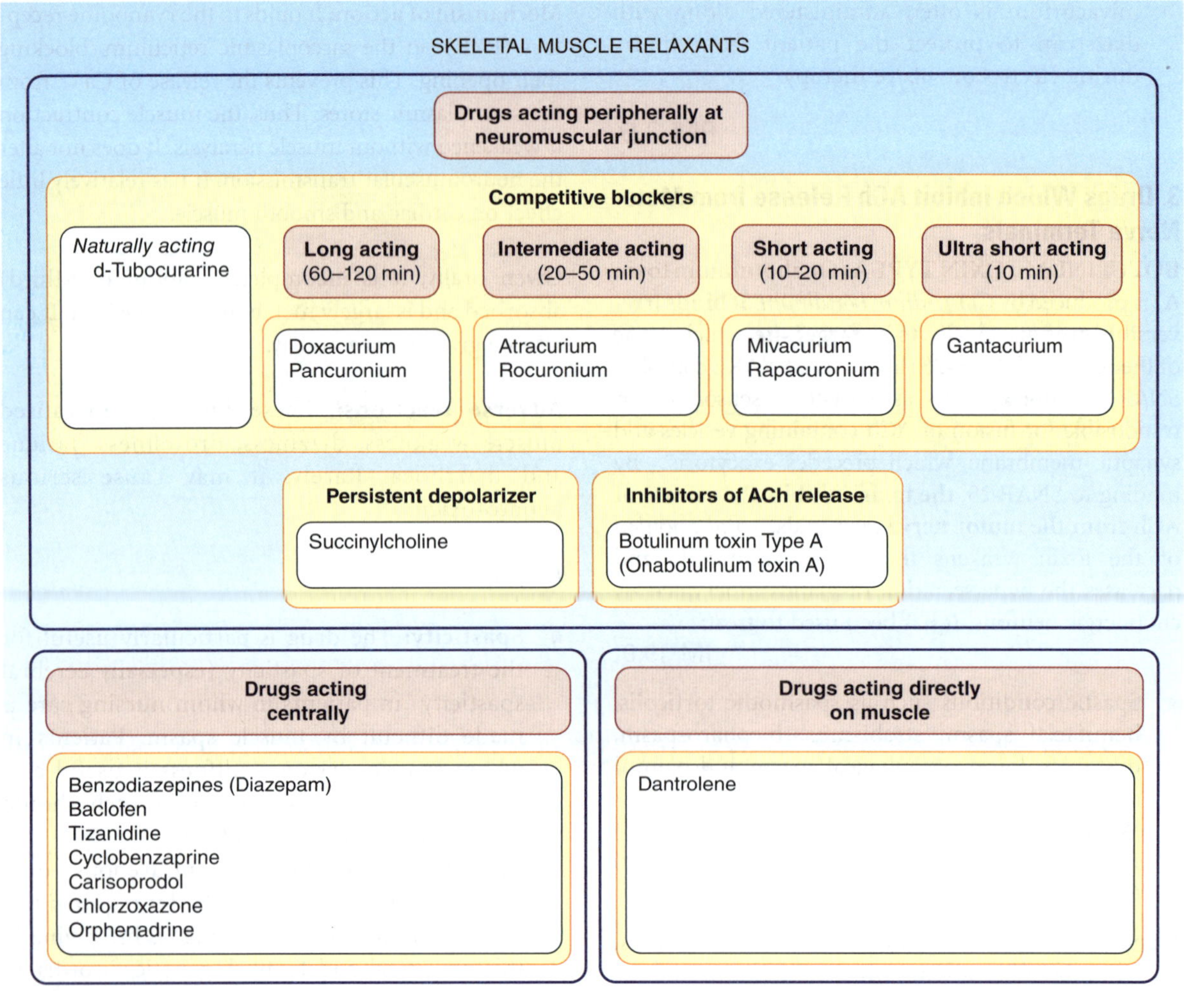
SKELETAL MUSCLE RELAXANTS
Drugs acting peripherally at neuromuscular junction
Competitive blockers
Naturally acting
d-Tubocurarine
Long acting (60–120 min)
Doxacurium
Pancuronium
Intermediate acting (20–50 min)
Atracurium
Rocuronium
Short acting (10–20 min)
Mivacurium
Rapacuronium
Ultra short acting (10 min)
Gantacurium
Persistent depolarizer
Succinylcholine
Inhibitors of ACh release
Botulinum toxin Type A (Onabotulinum toxin A)
Drugs acting centrally
Benzodiazepines (Diazepam)
Baclofen
Tizanidine
Cyclobenzaprine
Carisoprodol
Chlorzoxazone
Orphenadrine
Drugs acting directly on muscle
Dantrolene

CHEMICAL CLASSIFICATION OF NEUROMUSCULAR BLOCKERS

Benzylisoquinolones	Ammoniosteroids	Mixed
Atracurium Doxacurium Mivacurium	Pancuronium Vecuronium Rocuronium	Gantacurium

5

SECTION

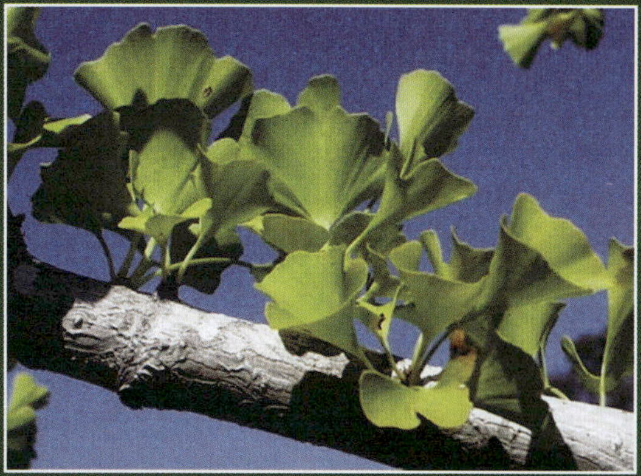

Ginkgo biloba

Other Biogenic Amines and Polypeptides

Section Outline

This section consists of the following chapters:

CHAPTER 23

Histamine and Antihistaminic Drugs

Learning Objectives

This chapter will enable the reader:

1. To describe distribution, synthesis, mechanism of action, pharmacological actions of histamine.
2. To outline the treatment of anaphylactic shock.
3. To classify H_1 receptor antagonists.
4. To describe pharmacological effects, salient pharmacokinetic features, ADR and indications for antihistaminics.
5. To compare and contrast first generation and second generation of antihistaminics.

KEY TERMS

histamine receptors, types, p. 335
triple response, p. 337
betahistine hydrochloride, p. 338
anaphylactic shock, treatment, p. 338
H_1 receptor antagonists, p. 340
allergic disorders, p. 342
ecallantide, p. 343
nonsedative H_1 antihistaminics, p. 344

HISTAMINE ('tissue amine'), a potent biogenic amine, was synthesised by Windaus and Vogt in 1907, even before its isolation from plants and animals. The role of this extremely potent natural substance in the genesis of allergic and anaphylactic manifestations was forecast by the brilliant work of Lewis.

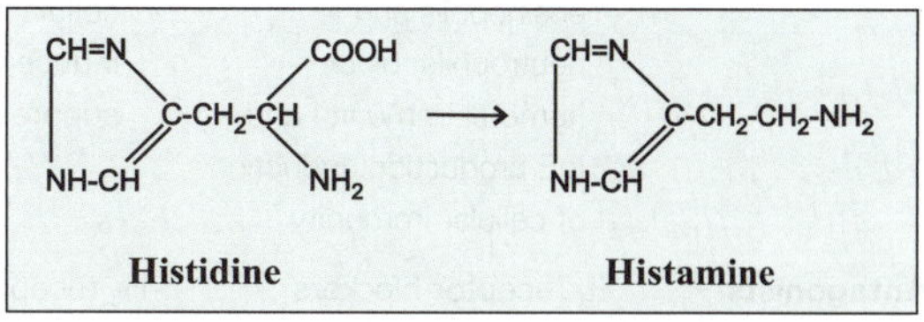

FIG. 23.1 **Biosynthesis of histamine.**

Distribution and synthesis: Histamine, an imidazole compound, is widely distributed in plant and animal tissues and is also present in the venom of bees and wasps. Almost all tissues in mammals synthesise histamine, from amino acid histidine by decarboxylation with the help of **histidine decarboxylase** (Fig. 23.1).

Histamine is present in various biological fluids, platelets, leucocytes, basophils and mast cells. A major portion of histamine is stored in mast cells and circulating basophils. These cells possess histidine decarboxylase and also contain specialised granules, wherein histamine is stored in an inactive form. Tissues devoid of mast cells, e.g. human epidermis, gastric mucosa, and CNS neurons also contain a significant concentration of histamine. Within the gut, the histamine concentration is highest in the stomach wall and gastric and intestinal glands. In the CNS, the area postrema, mast cells (histaminocytes) and histaminergic neurons of the pituitary stalk and the hypothalamus contain significant amounts of histamine.

Mechanism of action: Four types of receptors, H_1, H_2, H_3 and H_4, have been identified and cloned. All these receptors belong to the family of GPCR (G protein coupled receptors) (Table 23.1).

- **Activation of H_1 receptors** *causes pain, pruritus, bronchoconstriction, vasodilatation, increase in vascular permeability and in secretions.* In the tissues, histamine serves as a chemotactic agent for neutrophils and eosinophils. *H_1 receptor effects can be competitively blocked specifically by the conventional antihistaminics (H_1 receptor blockers).*
- **Activation of H_2 receptors** *increases the gastric acid secretion and myocardial contractility. These effects* are not blocked by the conventional

Table 23.1 Histamine Receptors and Their Functions

Receptor	H_1	H_2	H_3	H_4
Distribution	Widespread in the neuronal system, smooth muscles, endothelium and other cells	Widespread–gastric mucosa, smooth muscle, heart, brain and mast cells	Mainly in the histaminergic neurons of CNS and myenteric plexus	Mainly bone marrow and eosinophils, neutrophils and CD4 T cells
General role	On stimulation: itching, pain, vasodilatation, tachycardia, hypotension, increased permeability, bronchoconstriction, cough	Increased gastric acidity, vascular permeability (hypotension); chronotropic and inotropic actions on heart; increased airway mucus production	Prevent excessive bronchoconstriction; mediate pruritus	Differentiation of myeloblasts and promyelocytes
Role in CNS	Control: sleep–awake cycle, food intake, temperature regulation, emotional behaviour, memory and learning (feedback inhibitor)	Neuroendocrine regulation	Presynaptic auto-receptors; decrease histamine, NA, DA, 5-HT, ACh, GABA and glutamate release	Not known
Role in allergy and immune modulation	Increased release of histamine and other mediators; promote chemotaxis of eosinophils and neutrophils; block humoral immunity and IgE production. Induction of cellular immunity	Decrease neutrophil and eosinophil chemotaxis; induce humoral immunity; suppress cellular immunity; induce IL-10 and suppress IL-12	Control neurogenic inflammation; proinflammatory activity; decrease HCl secretion mediated by H_2 receptors	Increase eosinophil chemotaxis and IL-16 production
Antagonists (see text)	H_1 receptor blockers	H_2 receptor blockers	Under evaluation	Under evaluation

antihistaminics but *are specifically blocked by H_2 receptor antagonists* such as cimetidine.

Both H_1 and H_2 receptors appear to be involved in vascular dilatation, hypotension and oedema formation.

- **For H_3 and H_4 receptors**, see Table 23.1.

The exact physiological role of histamine in the body still remains unclear. However, its pharmacological actions are well known for several decades.

Pharmacological actions

Cardiovascular system:

- **Blood vessels: Histamine causes marked vasodilatation by:**

a. *Activation of H_1 receptors present on the endothelial cells which release of NO.* This vasodilatation is rapid and short-lived.

b. *Activation of H_2 receptors in the vascular smooth muscle leading to* slower but more prolonged vasodilatation.

c. *Direct relaxation of the smooth muscle of the arterioles and capillaries resulting* lfall in BP.

The pulmonary vessels are dilated by histamine, producing a fall in pulmonary artery pressure. It also dilates the cerebral blood vessels and produces throbbing headache, palpable temporal pulsations, and a transient increase in the CSF pressure. The headache is attributed to stretching of sensory nerve endings around the cranial arteries. Histamine causes marked flushing, a sense of warmth; and marked increase in capillary permeability after large doses, which causes oedema and reduction in plasma volume. Histamine constricts large veins.

- **Blood pressure:** Hypotension, induced by moderate doses of histamine, is transient. Large doses, however, produce prolonged hypotension. Histamine-induced hypotension can be prevented but only partially reversed by antihistaminic agents. However, it can be reversed by adrenaline (**physiological antagonism**).
- **Triple response:** When a pointed object is *drawn lightly* over the skin, the stroke line becomes blanched, i.e. white reaction, owing to contraction of the precapillary sphincters. It lasts for about 15 s. When histamine (20 mcg) is injected ID or the skin is stroked firmly with the pointed object, a triple response develops at the site. It comprises sequentially:
    a. **Flush** or red reaction which is a red line/spot developing within 10 s, owing to local dilatation of capillaries and venules.
    b. **Wheal** which is local swelling due to oedema, and mottled reddening around the injury, and lasts for about 1½ min; it is due to increased permeability of capillaries and post capillary venules, with consequent extravasation of fluid.
    c. **Flare** in which the redness with irregular margins spreads out from the injury.

  The triple response (Lewis response) is a part of the normal reaction to injury.
- **Heart:** Histamine increases the sinus rate (**positive chronotropic action**), increases the amplitude of ventricular contraction (**positive inotropic action**), decreases A-V conduction time and increases coronary blood flow. High concentrations induce ventricular fibrillation.

Smooth muscle: Histamine stimulates the smooth muscle of various tissues directly (H_1 action). *The bronchial and the uterine smooth muscle is highly sensitive to histamine.* Its action on the pregnant uterus is, however, not significant. Histamine-induced bronchospasm is antagonised by adrenaline, isoprenaline and aminophylline *but not by antihistaminics or atropine.*

The GI and the ureteral smooth muscles respond moderately to histamine. Histamine, through H_1 receptors, causes gall bladder contraction, whereas H_2 receptors mediate gall bladder relaxation.

Exocrine glands: Histamine is **an important physiological mediator of gastric acid secretion. It acts by activating H_2 receptors.** It is blocked by the specific H_2 receptor antagonists (Chapter 41).

Central nervous system: Histamine does not readily cross the BBB. The histamine receptors in the brain mediate the actions of locally synthesised, stored and released histamine. Histamine is thought to be **a waking amine** within the brain. It acts through H_1 receptors which release intracellular Ca^{++}, and H_2 receptors which release intracellular cyclic AMP. *Competitive blocking of H_1 receptors by the 'classical' antihistaminic drugs and of H_2 receptors by cimetidine causes drowsiness as an adverse effect.*

Histamine also modulates the release of neurotransmitters via presynaptic H_3 receptors located on histaminergic and non-histaminergic neurons in the central and peripheral nervous systems. **The evidence suggests a role of histamine as a neurotransmitter in the CNS.**

Immunomodulation: All the four histamine receptors are involved in immunomodulation (Table 23.1).

Miscellaneous actions: Histamine, on intraepidermal injection, evokes itching and pain.
Histamine has an effect on lymphocytes via H_2 receptors, and it also inhibits the secretory activity of the mast cells and the basophils by a negative feedback via H_3 receptors. It facilitates proinflammatory activity through H_4 receptors.

Absorption, fate and excretion: Histamine is a very stable compound and is absorbed from all sites. However, only a small quantity of oral histamine reaches the circulation because of its first pass metabolism. It is mainly converted into **N-methylhistamine** by an enzyme imidazole-*n*-methyltransferase and then further converted by MAO-B into N-methylimidazole acetic acid. It may be metabolised by oxidative deamination by the enzyme nonspecific diamine oxidase (histaminase) to imidazole acetic acid. The metabolites are eliminated in the urine. Estimation of urinary N-methylhistamine is a reliable indicator of histamine in circulation and therefore is used to diagnose mastocytosis.

Adverse reactions: These are due to its pharmacological actions and include hypotension, edema, flushing, angioedema, headache, visual disturbances, diarrhoea and dyspnoea due to bronchospasm. *Man and guinea pig are extremely sensitive to histamine, whereas rats and mice are highly resistant.* Large quantities of histamine may be formed by bacteria in the small intestine by acting on spoiled fish which may have high-histidine content. Ingestion of such fish may lead to severe nausea, griping, headache and sweating.

Uses: It was used to study gastric acid secretion. Now it is used as a control during skin sensitivity testing for various allergens.

BETAHISTINE HYDROCHLORIDE: is a histamine substitute, claimed to reduce the frequency of episodes of vertigo in some patients with Meniere syndrome. It is given in the dose of 8–16 mg t.i.d. The drug causes vasodilatation and improves blood flow to the labyrinth and brainstem. The improvement is short lived. The compound may aggravate peptic ulcer and bronchial asthma. It can cause drowsiness.

Histamine Liberators

Various agents can release tissue histamine and may thus cause histamine reactions. They are as follows:

I. **Those which release histamine mainly from the mast cells with minimal tissue damage:**
   - *Proteolytic enzymes* such as trypsin, certain venoms, food products, e.g. crabs, lobsters and fish
   - *Surface tension–reducing substances* e.g., bile salts, anionic and cationic surfactants
   - *Substances with high molecular weight* e.g., dextran and polyvinyl pyrrollidone
   - *Drugs***,** particularly organic bases such as quaternary ammonium compounds, e.g. d-Tubocurarine, morphine, pethidine, amphetamine, hydralazine, tolazoline, basic polypeptides (polymyxin B) and a few antihistaminic drugs
   - *The polybasic compound 48/40 and the compound 19/35 L*, the most potent histamine liberators, used in animal experiments

II. **Those which release histamine accompanied by substantial tissue damage:**
   - *Trauma* due to cold and chemical, thermal or radiant energy
   - *Antigen–antibody reactions* (Chapter 2)

HISTAMINE, ANAPHYLAXIS AND ALLERGY

The term **anaphylaxis** is used clinically to describe a severe, potentially life-threatening allergic reaction caused by a variety of agents such as drugs, foods, plants, chemicals, latex and insect/reptile bites. However, it can occur in some patients without any obvious triggering factor. It is mediated by IgE (Chapter 2), and histamine is the most important mediator involved in it. There is a sudden onset and rapid progression of clinical features (e.g. hoarse voice, wheeze, fatigue, low BP) due to **airway, breathing and cardiovascular (ABC) problems** that can be severe enough to manifest as laryngeal oedema (stridor), bronchospasm (cyanosis) and hypotension (**anaphylactic shock**). Skin and/or mucosal changes (e.g. urticaria, flushing, angioedema) may accompany. An anaphylactic reaction may progress either slowly or rapidly, the latter especially after parenteral drug administration. PH 1.7

The term **anaphylactoid** is used for a similar condition, commonly caused by vancomycin, quinolone antibiotics, opioids and iodine containing contrast dyes, but it *is not IgE induced*. However, it is safer to assume that all such reactions are immune mediated and avoid future exposure to the same agent. PH 1.27

Treatment of Anaphylactic Shock

Anaphylactic shock needs immediate treatment for laryngeal oedema, bronchospasm and hypotension:

- Withdraw the trigger, if recognized (e.g. stop the drug infusion)
- **Lay the patient flat and raise his legs** to maximize venous return. A change from supine to standing position can reduce venous return and myocardial perfusion. This may cause cardiovascular collapse and death.
- When possible, **apply a tourniquet** to obstruct

the draining blood flow from the site of deposition of the antigen or inciting medication

- **Administer adrenaline:** as soon as the features of anaphylaxis are developed. 0.5 ml (500 mcg) adrenaline (1 mg/mL), 1:1000 solution intramuscularly (on the anterolateral side of middle third of the thigh), produces a dramatic reversal of the hypotension, bronchospasm and laryngeal oedema and is life-saving. It may be repeated cautiously after 5 min, if necessary. Few patients may need second or even third dose of adrenaline. If the ABC problems are not resolved after 2 injections of adrenaline, it is considered as refractory anaphylaxis. It indicates continued release of inflammatory mediators, suboptimal adrenaline level or poor circulation. Critical care support is sought as early as possible and till that time IM adrenaline is injected every 5 min till the IV infusion is started by the specialist. When the patient is severely ill and there is doubt about the adequacy of circulation and absorption from the IM site, adrenaline (3-5 mL of **1:10,000; NEVER 1:1000; solution**) may be injected intravenously, slowly, in the dose of 500 mcg, at the rate of 100 mcg/min. However, this is to be given preferably by an experienced specialist (Box 23.1).

Rapid IV injection of adrenaline or IV injection of the 1:1000 solution can induce lethal cardiac arrhythmias like fibrillations.

In patients on a nonselective beta blocker, severe anaphylaxis may not respond to adrenaline and may need additional IV salbutamol.

- **Attend to the airway and use supportive measures:** These include oxygen and assisted ventilation. Monitor BP, ECG and pulse oximetry.

Box 23.1 Adrenaline 1:1000 solution (1mg/mL) intramuscularly

- ***Adults and children > 12 years:*** 0.5 mL (500 mcg)
- ***Children > 6-12 years:*** 0.3 mL (300 mcg)
- ***Children 6 months- 6 years:*** 0. 15 mL (150 mcg)
- ***Children < 6 months:*** 0.1-0.15 mL (100-150 mcg)

- **Intravenous fluids:** IV fluid (0.9% saline) administered as bolus is used as an adjunct if there is no response to adrenaline. Hypotension associated with anaphylactic shock should be corrected by immediate IV administration of 500-1000 ml of fluids (preferably colloids). If necessary, dopamine or norepinephrine can be infused intravenously. H_2 blocker has been used in refractory cases.
- **Antihistaminic drugs:** *These drugs have no role in the treatment of anaphylaxis as they do not adequately reverse the hypotension and bronchospasm or improve survival.* However, after administration of adrenaline, less sedating antihistaminic such as cetrizine may be given for symptomatic relief of skin features such as itching/urticaria.
  Injection of an H_2 receptor antagonist, e.g. ranitidine 50 mg, intravenously over 3–5 min may be helpful.
- **Glucocorticoids:** Glucocorticoids though routinely administered in the treatment of anaphylactic shock earlier, are no longer recommended. Their use is associated with increased morbidity. Steroids may be of benefit in anaphylaxis for patients with poorly controlled asthma (Chapter 27) and those with refractory anaphylaxis or ongoing shock. Hydrocortisone hemisuccinate 100 mg is given intravenously, followed by oral prednisolone. *They are not a substitute for adrenaline which is the drug of first choice.*
- **Refractory anaphylaxis:** is managed in the hospital setting by a specialist using a low dose intravenous fluid infusion of adrenaline along with fluid resuscitation. Nebulised and IV bronchodilators such as salbutamol may be required.

Anaphylaxis symptoms may recur after resolution of the earlier reaction, without any exposure to the same trigger. This is termed as biphasic reactions, which can be life-threatening. Hence based on the risk factors the period of observation after treatment of initial reaction varies. For example, the patients who respond to a single dose of adrenaline within 30 min and can be supervised at home need observation for 2 hr after complete

Box 23.2 Methods of Countering the Actions of Histamine

- **Preventing histamine release** from storage sites, e.g. cromolyn sodium, nedocromil
- **Using adrenaline** which has actions opposite to those of histamine and thus acts as a physiological antagonist
- **Hastening the destruction of histamine** by using histaminase, which is, however, clinically not effective
- **Blocking the actions of histamine on various receptors:** H_1 receptor antagonists and H_2 receptor antagonists

resolution of anaphylaxis. It is extended to 6 hr for those who needed 2 doses. Those having severe reaction or comorbidity like asthma, or continued exposure to allergen should be observed for at least 12 hr. The methods of countering the actions of histamine in the body are listed in Box 23.2.

PH 1.16

H_1 RECEPTOR ANTAGONISTS

Several *specific competitive H_1 receptor antagonists* with different chemical structures are now available. *The term antihistaminics, unless qualified, refers to these agents.* In addition to their antihistaminic activity, many of them also have CNS and ANS actions.

Clinical Classification

(Table 23.2):

I. **First Generation antihistaminics**
   - **Potent and sedative**
   - **Potent but less sedative**
   - **Less potent and less sedative**

II. **Second Generation (Nonsedative) antihistaminics:** They do not cross the BBB in significant amounts.

Most of the antihistaminic agents can be represented by the general structure (Fig. 23.2). Depending upon the configuration of X, the antihistaminic agents can be grouped into different chemical classes e.g. if X=O, then the class is ethanolamines, which includes antihistaminics like diphenhydramine and doxylamine. The chemical class, having X =nitrogen as a part of phenothiazine nucleus, includes promethazine, trimeprazine, which have potent antiemetic effect (See the flow chart at the end of the Chapter). The detailed chemical classification is presented in the 26th edition of the book.

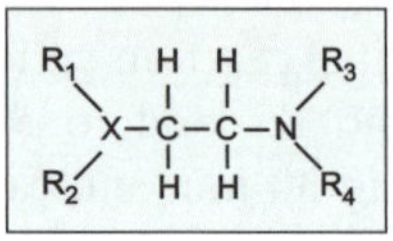

FIG. 23.2 **General structure of antihistaminics.**

Pharmacological actions:

Antihistaminic actions: These drugs competitively block histamine actions at many sites. Thus, they antagonise the stimulant action of histamine on the smooth muscle of the GI tract, the bronchi, the uterus and the blood vessels and inhibit histamine-augmented salivary secretion. They also reduce histamine-induced triple response and itching, but fail to produce resorption of the oedema fluid. Antihistaminics prevent the itching, oedema, urticaria and increased gastric motility and to a lesser extent, the hypotension produced by the histamine releasing drugs.

Antiallergic and anti-inflammatory actions involve (a) inhibition of the release of mediators from mast cells and basophils and (b) downregulation of H_1 receptors.

Pretreatment with an oral H_1 antihistamic reduces the early response to an allergen challenge in the conjunctiva, nose, lower airways and skin. However, *as described above, the bronchospasm and hypotension during anaphylaxis are not adequately reversed by them.* This is probably because of the other mediators released during the reaction. These agents do not antagonise the cardiovascular actions of histamine.

Other actions: These actions vary according to the drug used and are related to their blocking of muscarinic, 5-HT as well as α_1 adrenergic receptors. They are as follows:

Sedation and hypnosis: CNS depression is a common side effect with the **first-generation** antihistaminics. Blocking of central H_1 receptors induces sedation, drowsiness and sleep. Sedation is sometimes beneficial,

Table 23.2 H_1 Receptor Blocking (Antihistaminic) Agents PH 1.16

Drug	Adult Oral Dose (mg)	Remarks
	Potent and sedative[a]	
Diphenhydramine HCl[b]	25–50 (parenteral: 10)	Moderate antispasmodic, antimuscarinic
Dimenhydrinate[b]	25–100	Mainly used for motion sickness
Promethazine HCl[b]	12.5–25	Marked antimuscarinic action
Promethazine chlorotheophyllinate[c]	25–75	Marked antimuscarinic action; used mainly in motion sickness. Superiority over promethazine HCl is doubtful
Pheniramine maleate[c]	25–75	Antimuscarinic
Trimeprazine[c]	5–10	Mainly antipruritic
Doxylamine	25	Antiallergic. OTC sleep-aid
	Potent and less sedative[a]	
Chlorpheniramine maleate[b]	4–20 (parenteral: 5–20)	
Triprolidine[c]	2.5–5.0	
Cyclizine HCl[b]	50	Used in motion sickness
Meclizine HCl[c]	25–50	Mainly used for motion sickness
Buclizine	25–75	Antiemetic
	Less potent and less sedative[a]	
Mepyramine maleate[b]	50–100 (parenteral: 25–50)	
Antazoline HCl	50–100	Moderately active; antiarrhythmic
Cinnarizine[b]	25	Antivertigo; to treat EP reactions
Flunarizine	5–10	Antivertigo; to treat EP reactions
	Nonsedative (second generation)	
Loratadine[c]	10 (once daily)	Less antimuscarinic and relatively free from cardiac toxicity
Desloratadine	5 (once daily)	Less antimuscarinic and relatively free from cardiac toxicity
Fexofenadine[c]	120 (once daily)	Less antimuscarinic and relatively free from cardiac toxicity
Acrivastine[b]	8 (t.i.d.)	Less antimuscarinic and relatively free from cardiac toxicity
Cetirizine[c]	5–10 (once daily)	May cause some sedation
Mizolastine	10 (once daily)	Used in allergic rhinitis and chronic idiopathic urticaria
Ebastine	10-20 (once daily)	Active metabolite, carebastine Used in allergic rhinitis and chronic idiopathic urticaria
Rupatidine	10 mg (once daily)	Used in allergic rhinitis and chronic idiopathic urticaria
Azelastine	Eyedrops (0.05%) 1-2 drops twice daily. 140 mcg (into each nostril twice daily)	Used in the treatment of allergic conjunctivitis and rhinitis.

[a]First generation or classical.
[b]Short acting.
[c]Long acting.

particularly in the treatment of allergic reactions. *Drugs like promethazine and diphenhydramine are potent sedative-hypnotics*. Sedation is often accompanied by inability to concentrate, dizziness and disturbances of co-ordination, and thus may interfere with daily work.

Sedation is negligible with second-generation antihistaminics such as fexofenadine and desloratadine.

CNS stimulation: Conventional doses of a few drugs such as promethazine may occasionally produce paradoxical restlessness, tremors and insomnia. Stimulation is less commonly encountered than depression.

Antiemetic and antimotion sickness effects: *Motion sickness, attributed commonly to vestibular disturbances, is benefited to a considerable extent* by **dimenhydrinate, promethazine, cyclizine** and **meclizine**. They block the histaminergic signals from the vestibular nucleus to the vomiting centre. *Vomiting due to other labyrinthine disturbances, such as labyrinthitis and fenestration operation also responds to antihistaminics.* These agents, except the phenothiazine antihistaminics, however, are of limited value in treating emesis due to jaundice, radiation and alkylating agents (Chapter 39).

Anti-parkinsonian effect: Central antimuscarinic actions of some antihistaminics, such as **diphenhydramine** or **promethazine**, are useful in treating Parkinsonism (Chapter 15).

Autonomic nervous system: Majority of the **first-generation** antihistaminics exhibit **muscarinic blocking activity**. Dryness of mouth is common. Antihistaminics, such as antazoline and promethazine, exert an **alpha adrenergic blocking effect**. The **second-generation** antihistaminics usually do not have these actions.

Cardiovascular system: Although therapeutic doses of antihistaminics fail to affect the cardiovascular system, rapid IV administration of diphenhydramine, antazoline and tripelennamine may cause dose-related prolongation of QT interval due to their membrane stabilising action.

Local anaesthesia: Antihistaminics such as **promethazine** and **diphenhydramine** exhibit some local anaesthetic activity due to blockade of sodium channels.

Absorption, fate and excretion: They are absorbed well orally and parenterally; the antihistaminic effect starts within 15–30 min, peaks by 1 h and lasts for 3–6 h. *The actions of meclizine, however, persist for 12–24 h.* All first-generation compounds are mainly metabolised in the liver by CYP3A4, and the products are eliminated in urine. H_1 receptor antagonists can induce hepatic microsomal enzymes, facilitating their own metabolism.

Adverse reactions: They are as a rule mild and can be grouped as follows:

- **CNS:** *The first-generation antihistaminics commonly cause sedation, hypnosis and fatigue.* Individuals taking such antihistaminics should not drive vehicles because of drowsiness and impaired motor coordination. Extrapyramidal reactions (Table 23.2), excitement and delirium may occur rarely. In children less than 2 years, promethazine may cause fatal respiratory depression and must not be used.
- **Antimuscarinic effects:** The commonest effects are dry mouth, blurring of vision, bladder disturbances and rarely impotence, seen with *first-generation drugs.*
- **GIT:** Nausea, vomiting and epigastric distress may occur rarely.
- **Miscellaneous:** The antihistaminics, in spite of their antiallergic properties, may themselves produce allergic manifestations, especially after topical use.

Acute, first-generation antihistaminic poisoning is characterised by **marked central stimulation**. In children the clinical picture often resembles that of atropine intoxication, whereas in adults, fever and flushing are uncommon, and drowsiness often precedes the development of delirium and convulsion. Blood pressure and respiration are usually well maintained. Death is due to central depression leading to cardiorespiratory collapse and coma. *The treatment is symptomatic and supportive. Diazepam can control convulsions.*

Preparations and dosage: See Table 23.2. The number of antihistaminic drugs available in the market far exceeds their utility.

Indications:

- **Allergic disorders:** The antihistaminics are beneficial in the suppression of allergic manifestations like polinosis and urticaria. They are extremely effective in the treatment of seasonal hay fever, where they reduce the sneezing, rhinorrhoea and other manifestations associated with this condition. PH 1.52, IM 20.9

Antihistaminics effectively counter the pruritus and urticaria in atopic and contact dermatitis and that induced by various drugs, chemicals and plants (Chapter 69). They partially control the pruritus of eczema. Combination of a phenothiazine such as chlorpromazine with an antihistaminic may give better results in severe pruritus than the antihistaminic alone. Systemic administration also controls, to some extent, the pain and the itch due to bee or wasp stings. The antipruritic action of the antihistaminics is probably nonspecific. *Their topical use is not recommended owing to the risk of sensitisation and tendency to cause eczema.*

Antihistaminics, however, are ineffective in itching of clinically normal skin.

Antihistaminics are of some value in controlling mild blood transfusion reactions but not pyrexia or haemolysis (Chapter 32). Weak atropine like activity of the first generation antihistaminics may account for the beneficial effects of antihistaminic drugs on rhinorrhoea in a few cases of common cold (Chapter 27).

Urticaria and Angiodema. Urticaria may occur as acute episodes but is considered chronic when it lasts longer than six weeks. In some cases, an *allergen* (fish, seafood, nuts, eggs; food additives such as citric acid, preservatives and colouring agents like tartrazine; drugs such as aspirin and other NSAID; vegetable gums), an *offending physical agent* (mechanical trauma, cold, heat), insect bites and stings, or *underlying disease* (infection, connective tissue disorder) may be identified. However, no such factor is found in majority of cases. If a causative agent can be identified, it must be avoided if possible and treated if it is a systemic disease. But, a witch-hunt for a 'septic focus' is unrewarding.

The treatment of choice for severe acute urticaria (and acute angioedema) is SC injection of adrenaline (1:1000 aqueous solution) in the dose of 0.3 mL, repeated if necessary. If adrenaline is contraindicated, an antihistaminic (50 mg of diphenhydramine intramuscularly or intravenously) may be used.

Oral antihistaminics are the drugs of choice in **chronic urticaria**; they are more effective when given, prophylactically on a regular basis, than after urticarial lesions start; the nonsedative antihistaminics may be preferred. Alternatives to the antihistaminics are cyproheptadine, doxepin (an antidepressant with a potent antihistaminic action). In resistant cases, an H_2 blocker such as ranitidine may be added to the H_1 blocker. Very few patients need corticosteroids and then, they should be used for the shortest possible period.

Topical application of **calamine lotion** is useful for its cooling and soothing effects and can be used alone in mild cases.

Ecallantide, a selective and reversible Kallikrein inhibitor is approved for acute attacks of hereditary angioedema (Chapter 25).

Allergic conjunctivitis is a common condition and causes itching. Local treatment with H_1 receptor antagonists (**emedastine** 0.05%, **levocabastine** 0.05%), mast cell stabilisers (**cromolyn sodium** 4%, **nedocromil sodium** 2%; Chapter 27) and drugs having both actions (**ketotifen** 0.025%; Chapter 27) can give symptomatic relief. Their use is safe. The adverse reactions are mild and include ocular irritation, burning and stinging; headache may occur. *Routine long term use of local glucocorticoids (Chapter 64) is not justified for fear of causing raised intraocular pressure, and cataract.*

- **Mastocytosis:** This rare disease is characterised by an abnormal increase in mast cells in the body leading to an increase in the production of mast cell mediators mainly histamine. This gives rise to symptoms such as pruritus, diarrhoea and anaphylaxis. Partial symptomatic relief can be obtained by a combination of H_1 and H_2 receptor antagonists.
- **Other Indications:**
  a. **As hypnotics**, e.g. diphenhydramine and promethazine (Chapter 8)
  b. **As antiemetics**, e.g. dimenhydrinate and meclizine and doxylamine (Chapter 39)
  c. **In Parkinsonism**, e.g. diphenhydramine and promethazine (Chapter 15)
  d. **In motion sickness and vertigo** (Chapter 39)
  e. **As antitussives**, e.g. diphenhydramine
  f. **In drug-induced acute dystonias** diphenhydramine, promethazine (Chapter 15)

Drug interactions: Sedation is enhanced when the sedative antihistaminics are used concurrently with alcohol, barbiturates, benzodiazepines or tricyclic antidepressants. PH 1.16

Second generation (Nonsedative) H_1 antihistaminics are:

- *Highly specific H_1 receptor antagonists*
- *Nonsedating in therapeutic doses as they poorly cross the BBB*
- *Devoid of antimuscarinic, antiserotonergic and antibradykinin action*
- *Less prone to cause clinically relevant drug interactions*
- *More expensive*

Most of the second generation antihistaminics exert H_1 independent anti- inflammatory and anti-allergic actions mediated through mast cell stabilization, blockade of pro-inflammatory autocoids, antagonism of TNF- α etc. For example, cetirizine exerts anti-inflammatory action by reducing migration of neutrophils and eosinophils and by inhibiting release of LTB_4 and expression of VCAM-1.

Preparations and dosage: See Table 23.2.

Cetirizine is largely excreted as such in the urine; fexofenadine is primarily excreted in the faeces. **Fexofenadine** is an active metabolite of terfenadine, whereas cetirizine is an active metabolite of hydroxyzine. **Azalastine** and **mizolastine** are the newer antihistaminics which are used in allergic rhinitis.

Adverse reactions: Though claimed as nonsedative, sedation may occur in some individuals. Fexofenadine and desloratadine are relatively safer.

Indications:

- **Allergic disorders** (Chapter 27)
- **Urticaria**
- **Dermographia** PH 1.1

Choice of Antihistaminic: In practice, the choice of an antihistaminic drug depends upon efficacy, onset and duration of action, adverse effects and cost. These vary among different preparations, and among individuals. None of the preparations available is ideal for all conditions in all the patients.

Less sedating antihistamines are equally efficacious for allergic conditions and are preferred. Sedative-hypnotic property may be beneficial, particularly when sleep is disturbed. Sedative antihistaminics, because of their established safety, are used in pregnant women; the only exception is promethazine, which has shown adverse events in animal studies at very high doses.

H_2 RECEPTOR ANTAGONISTS

H_2 receptors (Table 23.1) are responsible for histamine induced gastric acid secretion and their antagonists are useful in the treatment of peptic ulcer (see Chapter 41). Experimentally, they block positive chronotropic action of histamine, counter the enhanced automaticity of atria and ventricles and prevent ventricular tachyarrhythmias induced by histamine.

H_3 AND H_4 RECEPTORS

H_3 receptors are thought to be presynaptic heteroreceptors that exert a tonic autoinhibitory control on histamine synthesis and release within the brain. Betahistine, a weak, partial agonist at H_1 and H_2 receptors, behaves as a weak H_3 receptor antagonist. For H_4 receptors, see Table 23.1.

H_1 RECEPTOR ANTAGONISTS (ANTIHISTAMINICS)

Clinical Classification

First generation

Potent and sedative
- Diphenhydramine HCl
- Dimenhydrinate
- Promethazine HCl
- Promethazine chlorotheophyllinate
- Pheniramine maleate
- Trimeprazine
- Doxylamine

Potent and less sedative
- Chlorpheniramine maleate
- Triprolidine
- Cyclizine HCl
- Meclizine HCl
- Buclizine

Less potent and less sedative
- Mepyramine maleate
- Antazoline HCl
- Cinnarizine
- Flunarizine

Second generation

Nonsedative
- Loratadine
- Desloratadine
- Fexofenadine
- Acrivastine
- Cetirizine
- Mizolastine
- Ebastine
- Rupatidine
- Azelastine

Chemical Classification

Ethanolamines
- Diphenhydramine
- Doxylamine

Ethylenediamines
- Tripelennamine
- Mepyramine
- Antazoline

Alkylamines
- Chlorpheniramine
- Triprolidine
- Acrivastine

Piperazines
- Hydroxyzine
- Buclizine
- Meclizine
- Cinnarizine
- Cetirizine

Phenothiazines
- Promethazine
- Trimeprazine

Piperidines
- Cyproheptadine
- Loratadine
- Fexofenadine
- Ketotifen

Dibenzoxepines
- Doxepin

HISTAMINE LIBERATORS

Those which release histamine mainly from the mast cells with minimal tissue damage

Biological substances

Trypsin
Certain venoms
Food products
- Crabs
- Lobsters
- Fish

Substances with high molecular weight

Dextran
Polyvinyl pyrrollidone

Surface tension–reducing substances

Bile salts
Anionic and cationic surfactants

Drugs

d-Tubocurarine
Morphine
Pethidine
Amphetamine
Hydralazine
Tolazoline
Basic polypeptides (polymyxin B)

The polybasic compound 48/40 and the compound 19/35 L

Those which release histamine accompanied by substantial tissue damage

Trauma due to cold and chemical, thermal or radiant energy

Antigen–antibody reactions

CHAPTER 24

5-Hydroxytryptamine (Serotonin), Its Agonists and Antagonists; and Treatment of Migraine

Learning Objectives

This chapter will enable the reader:

1. To describe distribution, synthesis, receptor types, physiological functions, role in pathological conditions and pharmacological actions of 5-hydroxytryptamine (5-HT).
2. To enlist clinically used 5-HT receptor agonists and antagonists along with conditions in which they are used.
3. To describe mechanism of action, pharmacological effects, ADR and indications for sumatriptan.
4. To discuss the management of acute attack of migraine highlighting target sites of various drugs used.
5. To state indications for preventive therapy of migraine enlisting the drugs used for prophylaxis.
6. To state the role of onabotulinumtoxin -A in the treatment of chronic migraine.
7. To list the monoclonal antibodies against CGRP or its receptors and their indications.

KEY TERMS

5-HT receptors, types and subtypes, p. 347
ondansetron, p. 353
migraine, treatment, p. 354
sumatriptan, p. 356
ergotamine, p. 358
migraine prevention, p. 358
menstrual migraine, p. 360

5-HYDROXYTRYPTAMINE (5-HT), also termed *serotonin* (Fig. 24.1), was isolated in 1948. It has a wide tissue distribution and a variety of pharmacological actions in CNS and peripheral tissues.

Distribution and synthesis: 5-HT is widely distributed in plants and in animal tissues, mast cells and platelets. In the mammalian tissues, the highest concentration is present in the pineal gland, where it serves as a precursor for the synthesis of the hormone melatonin. It is also present in the venoms of wasps, bees and scorpions. Fruits like pineapples, bananas, tomatoes, plums and various nuts contain considerable amounts of 5-HT. However, it largely undergoes metabolic degradation on entering the circulation.

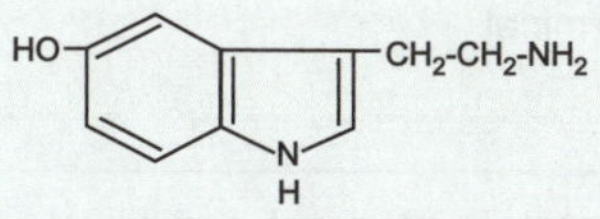

FIG. 24.1 **5-Hydroxytryptamine.**

The compound is synthesised from the essential amino acid tryptophan (Fig. 24.2). The enzyme L-aromatic amino acid decarboxylase also decarboxylates histidine to histamine and DOPA to dopamine. Within the CNS and the GI tract, 5-HT is stored in the chromaffin granules.

5-HT receptors: Seven 5-HT receptor groups have been identified; 5-HT_1, 5-HT_2, 5-HT_3, 5-HT_4, 5-HT_5,

L-Tryptophan
↓ **Tryptophan 5-hydroxylase**
1 -5-Hydroxytryptophan (5HTP)
↓ **l-Aromatic amino acid decarboxylase**
5-Hydroxytryptamine (Serotonin)

FIG. 24.2 **Synthesis of 5-hydroxytryptamine (5-HT).**

5-HT_6 and 5-HT_7. They are further subdivided into several subtypes. All the 5-HT receptors belong to G-protein-coupled receptor (GPCR) families, except 5-HT_3 which is a ligand-operated ion channel receptor.

The **5-HT_1 receptor** has six subtypes. Of these, 5-HT_{1A} is found in the raphe cell bodies and dendrites, and 5-$HT_{1B/1D}$ on the axon terminals (presynaptic). They function as **autoreceptors** and regulate 5-HT release. 5-HT_{1D} is also found in the substantia nigra and basal ganglia and they regulate release of DA.

The **5-HT_2 receptor** has three subtypes. Of these, 5-HT_{2A} receptors are found in the prefrontal, parietal and somatosensory cortex, GI tract and platelets. $5HT_{2B}$ are found in vascular smooth muscle and certain immune cells. 5-HT_{2C} receptors are present in CNS and regulate CSF production, feeding behaviour and mood.

The **5-HT_3 receptor** is a **monoamine neurotransmitter receptor**, located at the cholinergic terminals in the GI tract, nucleus solitarius and in the area postrema (CTZ). *Both the CNS and GI tract 5-HT_3 receptors participate in the process of vomiting.*

The **5-HT_4 receptor** is widely distributed throughout the body, including the CNS, smooth muscles, myenteric plexus and secretory cells. Their stimulation causes increased mucus secretion in the GI tract and facilitates the peristaltic process.

The **5-HT_{5A}** receptors are distributed widely in CNS and are responsible for circadian rhythm and cognition. The **5-HT_6** receptors are abundant in CNS especially cortex, limbic system and extrapyramidal system and regulate motor function and cognition. The **5-HT_7** receptors are also present in CNS and linked with depression.

The handling of 5-HT at the receptor level is similar to that of NA. Thus a large portion of 5-HT released from the neuronal endings is retaken up (Uptake 1) by a transporter, SERT and stored in the granules by the neurons (Fig. 24.3). It is metabolised by the enzyme MAO. The metabolite 5-Hydroxy-indole-acetic-acid (5-HIAA) is actively transported out of the brain by a process which can be blocked by probenecid.

Functions of first four 5-HT receptors are summarised in Table 24.1.

Significance of 5-HT: Generally 5-HT:

1. Acts as a central neurotransmitter
2. Plays a major role in the regulation of GI motility
3. Serves as an autocoid in the peripheral vascular system

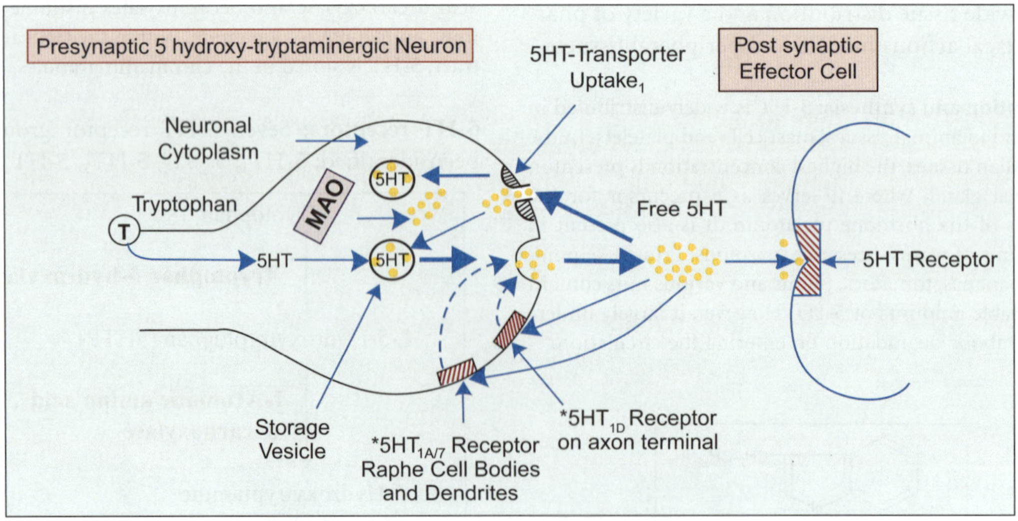

FIG. 24.3 Synthesis and metabolism of 5-HT at serotonergic neuronal endings. *Autoreceptors; Dotted line indicates inhibition of release of the transmitter.

Table 24.1 Important 5-HT Receptors and Their Functions

Receptor	Signal Transduction	Subtype	Location	Functions
5-HT$_1$	G-protein coupled. Inhibits AC	5-HT$_{1A}$	Raphe nuclei, cortex, hippocampus	Mood and behaviour: anxiety; sleep; feeding and thermo-regulation. Autoreceptor regulating 5-HT release
		5-HT$_{1B}$	Substantia nigra and basal ganglia; vascular smooth muscles	Autoreceptors (may be regulating dopamine release). Locomotor function; behaviour; pulmonary vasoconstriction
		5-HT$_{1D}$	Basal ganglia; cerebral vessels	Autoreceptors, cerebral vasoconstriction: migraine
5-HT$_2$	G-protein coupled. Activates PLC	5-HT$_{2A}$	Frontal cortex, platelets, smooth muscles, autonomic neurons	Neural excitation; behavioural effects (of LSD); platelet aggregation; smooth muscle contraction (GI tract, bronchi, bladder)
		5-HT$_{2B}$	Gastric fundus	Contraction
		5-HT$_{2C}$	Choroid plexus, basal ganglia	CSF secretion, neuronal excitation
5-HT$_3$	Ligand operated ion channels		Cholinergic terminals of GI tract; tractus solitarius; area postrema; hippocampus	Emesis Behaviour: anxiety, Neuronal excitation (autonomic, nociceptive neurons)
5-HT$_4$	G-protein coupled. Activates AC		Hippocampus; myenteric neurons; smooth muscles of esophagus, secretory cells	Neuronal excitation; contraction of muscle; stimulation of secretion

Note: AC, adenylyl cyclase; PLC, phospholipase C.

Pharmacological actions:

Central nervous system: 5-HT is considered as CNS neurotransmitter which is widely distributed in the brain. One of the important functions attributed to the tryptaminergic dorsal raphe neurons is dampening of over-reactiveness to various stimuli, and *5-HT is involved in some way in regulation of the state of consciousness.* Altered tryptaminergic function may be responsible for disturbances in sleep, appetite, mood, sexual behaviour, motor activity, perception and in development of migraine. These neurons are also involved in temperature regulation, endocrine control and extrapyramidal activity. 5-HT receptors have been identified in brain areas implicated in learning and memory. **Many centrally acting drugs are known to influence responses to 5-HT or alter its reuptake, synthesis and metabolism.** Prominent among these are antipsychotic drugs like chlorpromazine, reserpine, antidepressants, hallucinogens like lysergic acid diethylamide (LSD), mescaline and even analgesics like morphine.

- **Sleep**: 5-HT controls sleep–wakefulness cycle; depletion of 5-HT causes insomnia, which can be reversed by 5-hydroxytryptophan.
- **Behaviour**: Disturbances in the brain 5-HT metabolism are suspected as a cause of certain psychiatric disorders such as affective disorders. 5-HT$_2$ receptors present in brain in limbic and cortical areas are known to be involved in controlling mood, emotion, reward and memory. 5-HT$_2$ receptor antagonists reduce the increased psychomotor drive associated with a mesolimbic dopamine excess. Low CSF 5-HIAA is associated with

impulsive, violent and suicidal behaviour, and 5-HT reuptake inhibitors (SSRI) are used to treat mental depression (Chapter 14).

- **Emesis and migraine**: *Selective 5-HT$_3$ receptor antagonists can prevent emesis associated with anticancer drugs and radiotherapy.*

  5-HT metabolism is abnormal in patients with migraine and IV administration of 5-HT can alleviate migraine attacks. Sumatriptan, a 5-HT$_{1B/1D}$ agonist, is used to treat acute attacks of migraine (see section, Pharmacotherapy of migraine).

- **Gastrointestinal tract**: Enterochromaffin cells in the GI tract synthesise 5-HT which forms the major source of circulating 5-HT. A part of it is metabolised by the hepatic MAO during its first pass through the liver. 5-HT released by the neuronal endings acts locally to regulate the GI motility. **5-HT stimulates smooth muscles** (5-HT$_3$ receptors) and the most significant effect is seen on the small intestine. Both the tone and the motility are initially augmented followed by an inhibition of the spontaneous activity. *5-HT is believed to act as a local hormone for the initiation and sustenance of intestinal peristalsis.*

It reduces the volume, acidity, and pepsin content of the gastric juice and promotes the production of mucus.

Smooth muscle: 5-HT also evokes bronchoconstriction.

Cardiovascular system:

- **Blood vessels**: **5-HT constricts majority of blood vessels** including the renal, splanchnic, meningeal, cerebral and pulmonary arteries, **whereas it dilates the blood vessels of skeletal muscles**, the coronaries and the capillaries of the skin. It also constricts the veins and venules. Administration of 5-HT in humans results in cutaneous vasodilatation.
- **Heart**: Though 5-HT has weak direct positive inotropic and chronotropic effects on the myocardium; these, are not manifested because of reflex bradycardia.
- **Blood pressure**: A characteristic 'triphasic response' is observed in BP after IV injection of 5-HT. It consists of:
  a. ***Initial transient depression*** of BP due to increased vagal activity following stimulation of carotid chemoreceptors
  b. ***Rise in BP*** due to peripheral vasoconstriction
  c. ***Sustained hypotension*** which is due to dilatation of skeletal muscle blood vessels

Platelets: Platelets do not synthesise 5-HT but take it up from the circulation and store it. 5-HT release, following a vascular injury along with other mediators of injury, activates platelets, which then promote vascular occlusion and vasoconstriction.

Hormone secretion: Sex hormones may affect mood and the mental state by activating the central 5-HT receptors.

Unlike with histamine the human skin does not contain significant amounts of 5-HT and the 5-HT antagonists are not effective in controlling inflammation in human skin.

Absorption, fate and excretion: 5-HT is not significantly absorbed orally as it is degraded rapidly within the GI tract. Platelets have the capacity for its uptake and storage. 5-HT, administered exogenously, does not readily cross the BBB. It is mainly metabolised by the hepatic enzyme MAO and excreted as 5-HIAA in the urine(Fig. 24.4). The upper limit of normal urinary 5-HIAA in man is about 10 mg per day.

Uses: 5-HT is not used therapeutically. However, several drugs act by manipulating 5-HT at various

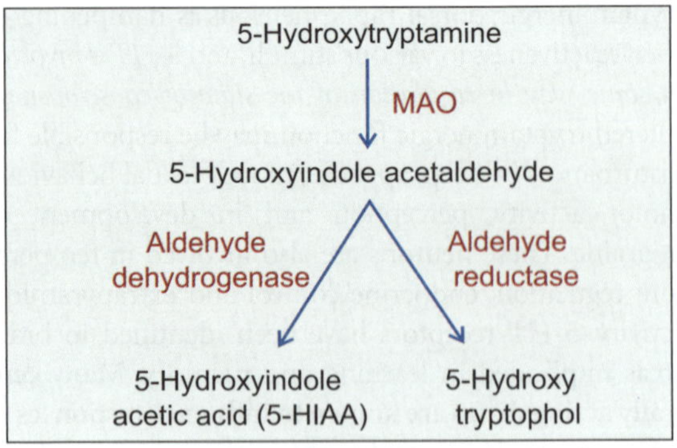

FIG. 24.4 **Metabolism of 5-HT.**

Table 24.2 5-Hydroxytryptamine and Drugs PH 1.16

Drug	5-HT Receptor Subtype	Other Receptors	Uses
Agonists			
Ergotamine	All 1, 2A, 2B	Dopamine; alpha-adrenergic agonist	Acute attack of migraine
LSD	2A, 2C, 1A	–	Hallucinogen
Triptans	1B,1D	–	Acute attack of migraine
Buspirone	1A (partial agonist)	–	Anxiety states
Cisapride	4	–	Gastroesophageal refux disease (GERD)
Metoclopramide	4	D_2 blocker	GERD, gastroparesis
Antagonists:			
Cyproheptadine	2A, 2C	H_1 blocker Antimuscarinic	Migraine prophylaxis; carcinoid syndrome; postgastrectomy dumping syndrome
Metoclopramide	3	D_2 blocker	Antiemetic
Methysergide	2A, 2C	–	Carcinoid syndrome; migraine prophylaxis
Ketanserin	2A, 2C	H_1 and α_1-adrenergic blocker	Migraine, hypertension
Mianserin	3, 2A, 2C	H_1 and α_2-adrenergic blocker	Antidepressant
Atypical antipsychotics:			
Clozapine	2A, 2C	D_2 antagonist	Schizophrenia
Risperidone	2A, 2C	D_2 antagonist	Schizophrenia
Others			
Alosetron	3	–	Irritable bowel syndrome
Ondansetron	3	–	Antiemetic
5-HT uptake inhibitors:			
a. Selective (SSRI) (Chapter 14)	–	H_1 blocker, antimuscarinic	Antidepressant; Obsessive compulsive disorder; Panic disorder
b. Nonselective (Chapter 14)	–	NA-reuptake inhibitor	Antidepressant; Obsessive compulsive disorder
5-HT depletors:			
Reserpine	Depletion of intraneuronal stores of 5-HT and NA	–	Antihypertensive; antipsychotic

Note: NA, noradrenaline; H, histamine; D, dopamine.

receptor sites, centrally as well as peripherally. Drugs can also act directly on 5-HT receptors as agonists or antagonists; because of multiple types of 5-HT receptors, their actions and therapeutic uses vary. Some drugs also act on histaminergic, dopaminergic and adrenergic receptors. Some of the drugs acting through 5-HT receptors are summarised in Table 24.2.

5-HT-Receptor Agonists PH 1.16

These compounds differ in their chemical structures and actions. The important agents are as follows:

1. **5-HT$_{1A}$ agonists**, e.g. buspirone used as an anti-anxiety agent (Chapter 14)
2. **5-HT$_{1B/1D}$ receptor agonists**, e.g. sumatriptan used in the treatment of migraine (see under the section Pharmacotherapy of migraine)
3. **5-HT$_4$ agonists**, e.g. Mosapride used in the

treatment of gastroesophageal reflux disease (Chapter 39)

4. **Nonselective 5-HT agonists**, e.g. ergotamine in migraine (see under the section Pharmacotherapy of migraine; (Chapter 42), LSD as a hallucinogen (Chapter 13)

5-HT Antagonists PH 1.16

Apart from PCPA, 5-HT synthesis can be inhibited by alpha methyldopa (Chapter 30), some halogenated tryptophans and phenylalanine.

A number of compounds antagonise the actions of 5-HT on the tissues. *Since there are multiple types of 5-HT receptors, a drug acting as an antagonist at one site may not act similarly at others.* **The 5-HT antagonists of therapeutic importance are:**

METHYSERGIDE: Methysergide, a congener of LSD, is a $5\text{-}HT_{2A}$ and $5\text{-}HT_{2C}$ antagonist. It was previously used as an effective prophylactic agent for patients with resistant migraine *but is of no value in treating an acute attack.* However because of its significant toxicity viz. peripheral arterial insufficiency, precipitation of angina, retroperitoneal fibrosis, pleuro-pulmonary fibrosis and cardiac valve damage it is now rarely used.

CYPROHEPTADINE: This compound (Fig. 24.5), with structural resemblance to phenothiazines, is a **potent antagonist** of **$5\text{-}HT_2$ receptors** and to a certain extent of histamine and acetylcholine. As a central depressant it exhibits anticonvulsant and antitremor activities. Cyproheptadine is satisfactorily absorbed from the GI tract. The metabolic fate of the compound is not known. PH 1.16

It stimulates appetite probably by acting directly on the hypothalamus. Weight is gained rapidly during the first few weeks of therapy and is lost when the drug is stopped. There is evidence that 5-HT is involved in the control of ACTH secretion, possibly by stimulating corticotropin releasing factor (CRF) secretion from the hypothalamus. Administration of cyproheptadine can **block the release of hydrocortisone** and has, in fact, been used in the treatment of ACTH dependent Cushing disease. It also **suppresses aldosterone production** in idiopathic aldosteronism.

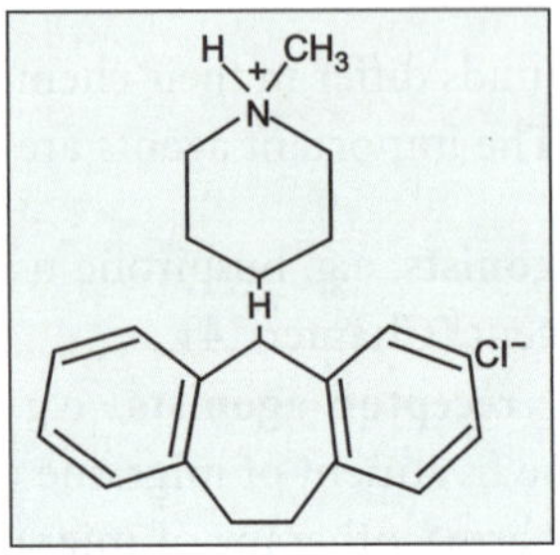

FIG. 24.5 Cyproheptadine.

The drug is available as 4 mg tablets. Dose: 4–20 mg/day in divided doses.

Adverse reactions: The common adverse effect is transient drowsiness which seldom necessitates withdrawal of the drug. Other adverse reactions include dryness of mouth, mental confusion, ataxia, dizziness, headache and visual hallucinations.

Indications:

- **Migraine prophylaxis:** See section, Pharmacotherapy of migraine
- **Treatment of postgastrectomy dumping syndrome and carcinoid syndrome;** its 5-HT antagonising action is probably useful.
- **Relief of pruritus** associated with allergic dermatitis, urticaria and neurodermatosis. This action is probably due to its antihistaminic effect.
- **Symptomatic relief in seasonal and perennial pollinosis**
- **Appetite stimulant** in certain conditions. *However, its promotion as a general appetite stimulant or tonic is not justifiable.*
- **Cushing disease:** Only in certain cases

PIZOTIFEN: This is an antihistaminic and 5-HT antagonist, structurally related to TCA. It is effective in the prophylaxis of migraine and other vascular headaches. It may cause drowsiness, weight gain and urinary retention due to antimuscarinic action.

KETANSERIN: Ketanserin blocks 5-HT receptors, mainly $5\text{-}HT_{2A}$ and thereby antagonises vasoconstriction, platelet aggregation and bronchoconstriction. It has affinity for adrenergic α_1 and H_1 receptors which it blocks. It can cause lowering of blood pressure. The drug is used to improve digital circulation in patients with vasospastic conditions such as Raynaud syndrome.

ONDANSETRON: This is a specific 5-HT_3 receptor antagonist and is particularly useful as an **antiemetic** in nausea and vomiting following cytotoxic drugs and radiotherapy. Its action is partly central and partly peripheral. **Granisetron, alosetron, palanosetron** and **tropisetron** have similar antiemetic properties as ondansetron but have longer t½. **Their antiemetic effects outlast their t½ permitting their once a day dosing.** (Table 24.3) **Dolasetron** is also available.

Table 24.3 Salient pharmacokinetics and doses of 5HT_3 antagonists

Drug name	Salient pharmacokinetics	Anti emetic dose and route
Ondansetron	• Complete and rapid absorption after oral administration • Bioavailability : 60% due to hepatic first-pass metabolism • Time to reach peak concentration: 0.5 – 2 hours after oral ingestion; the drug to be given at least 30 minutes before chemotherapy • Widely distributed • Plasma protein binding moderate: 70-76% • Elimination t1/2: 4 h • Hepatic metabolism: 95%	• *Oral route:* **Highly Emetogenic Cancer Chemotherapy:** 24 mg 30 minutes before the start of chemotherapy. **Moderately Emetogenic Cancer Chemotherapy:** 8 mg twice a day, with the first dose administered 30 minutes before the start of chemotherapy and the subsequent doses 8 hours later for 1–2 days after the completion of chemotherapy • *IV route:* 0.15 mg/kg (Max 16 mg /dose), with the first dose (infused over 15 minutes) 30 minutes before the start of emetogenic chemotherapy and subsequent doses given 4 and 8 hours after the first dose. **Postoperative Nausea/Vomiting:** • *Oral route:* 16 mg orally 1 hour before the induction of anesthesia • *IV route:* 4 mg (undiluted) immediately before induction of anesthesia or postoperatively within 2 hours after surgery **Radiation Induced Nausea/Vomiting** • 8 mg orally 3 times a day
Granisetron	• Rapid absorption • Bioavailability: 60% as a result of first-pass hepatic metabolism • Time to reach peak concentration: within 2 hours • Elimination t1/2: 6–10 h	*Oral route:* 1-2 mg 1 hr prior to start of chemotherapy, then 2 mg/day as a single or in 2 divided doses for up to 1 wk after chemotherapy. Max: 9 mg/day In case of radiotherapy induced nausea / vomiting, 2 mg once daily within 1 hr of irradiation. 1-3 mg 5 min prior to start of therapy; further doses may be given at least 10 min apart *Transdermal route*: Patch to be applied 24–48 h before chemotherapy; to remove at least 24 hr after the end of chemotherapy. May be worn for up to 7 days.
Alosetron	• Rapid absorption • Duration of action ~10 h • Elimination t1/2: 1.5 h • Hepatic metabolism	*Oral route:* 1 mg/d divided into two doses for the first 4 weeks and, if tolerated, advanced to a maximum of 1 mg twice daily if necessary.
Palonosetron	• Well absorbed and distributed • Hepatic metabolism • Elimination t1/2: 40 h	*Oral route:* 500 mcg 1 hr before therapy. *IV route:* 250 mcg over 30 sec approx 30 min before therapy

Adverse reactions: Ondansetron is well tolerated. Its ADR include headache, constipation, dizziness, allergic reaction and chest pain. Unlike phenothiazine, it causes neither sedation nor extrapyramidal reactions, this is an advantage.

The other $5\text{-}HT_3$ antagonists have similar safety profile. **As a group all can prolong QT interval.** They can precipitate serotonin syndrome in patients taking SSRI or SNRI.

Indications:
Nausea and vomiting due to:

1. **Cancer Chemotherapy:** They are mainly used for prevention of acute nausea and vomiting due to cancer therapy. But they are not very effective for delayed nausea and vomiting that occurs after 24 hours of chemotherapy. Hence they should be co-administered with dexamethasone or NK-1 antagonists.
2. **Radiation**
3. **Surgery**

CLOZAPINE: This atypical antipsychotic drug acts as $5\text{-}HT_{2A/2C}$ receptor antagonist and is used in the treatment of schizophrenia. Many other antipsychotic drugs have 5-HT antagonist action (Chapter 13).

Carcinoid syndrome: This clinical syndrome is associated with argentaffin cell tumours of the GI tract which secrete 5-HT. Carcinoid syndrome is characterised by intermittent attacks of flushing, hypotension, bronchospasm, colic and diarrhoea. Some of these manifestations are due to excessive production of 5-HT. The diagnosis is usually confirmed by demonstrating high plasma 5-HT and high urinary HIAA levels.

The drug, parachlorophenylalanine (PCPA) inhibits 5-HT synthesis by inhibiting tryptophan hydroxylase. Administration of PCPA results in almost complete inhibition of this enzyme leading to stoppage of diarrhoea, cramps and decreases in 5-HIAA excretion in urine. Some benefit may also be achieved by cyproheptadine and methysergide. However, treatment of choice is surgery.

PHARMACOTHERAPY OF MIGRAINE PH 1.1

Migraine is a common **neurovascular disorder** that presents with an episodic throbbing headache, unilateral or bilateral, and exacerbated by physical activity. It may be associated with GI, autonomic or behavioural disturbances. It is common in females and shows a strong hereditary tendency. Its onset is usually before 35 years of age and it remits with advancing age.

Attacks of headache may be triggered by factors like food (chocolate, nuts, cheese), visual stimuli, impending menstruation, stress, sleep disturbances, delay in eating despite feeling hungry and relaxation after emotional tension. However, the role of these triggers is limited.

Classically, the headache is unilateral, moderate-to-severe in pain intensity and may vary in duration from a few minutes to days. These attacks are often accompanied by nausea, vomiting, diarrhoea, prostration, photophobia, and phonophobia. In 10%–15% of cases, it is preceded by aura, which are visual and neurological phenomena such as scintillating scotomata and visual field defects. *Rarely, migrainous headaches are due to structural lesions in the CNS like an aneurysm or an angioma.*

Migraine is classified as follows:

- **Migraine with aura** (*classical migraine*)
- **Migraine without aura** (*common migraine*)

When migraine headaches occur for 14 days or less frequently in a month, then it is termed as **episodic migraine**. About 3% of patients with episodic migraine progress to chronic migraine each year. **Chronic migraine** is defined as ≥ 15 migraine days per month for 3 months with atleast 8 headache days showing the characteristics of migraine.

Pathophysiology: Migraine initiation depends on activation of first-order trigeminovascular neurons. Though, exact mechanism of activation is not known, migraine involves abnormal cortical activity. A self-propagating wave of depolarization across the cerebral cortex (cortical spreading depression) causes ionic gradient disruption and opens neuronal pannexin-1 channels which release inflammatory mediators (e.g., nitric oxide and prostanoids) which mediate their effects through cAMP–and cGMP – mediated pathways. Whichever is the pathway, they result in the opening of ATP-sensitive potassium (K_{ATP}) channels on the vascular smoothmuscle cells in the walls of the intracranial arteries. This causes hyperpolarisation and vasodilatation. Increase in extracellular potassium sensitizes and discharges the perivascular trigeminal primary afferents, generating nociceptive impulses, which are transmitted to cortical and subcortical brain regions through ascending trigeminal pain pathways, involving neurons in the brain stem and the thalamus.

During the pathogenesis of migraine and other vascular headaches calcitonin gene related peptide (CGRP), pituitary adenylate cyclase–activating polypeptide (PACAP-38) and nitric oxide are released. *They are potent vasodilators of the meningeal and cerebral blood vessels and are also capable of causing the release of proinflammatory cytokines from the meningeal mast cells. In addition, they are also involved in the genesis of pain.* The throbbing headache is mostly due to dilatation of pain-sensitive arteries. **Triptans, which block the release of CGRP rapidly relieve the headache.**

Chronic migraine is associated with many functional changes such as increased cortical hyperexcitability, central trigemino-thalamic sensitisation and dysfunction of descending pain modulatory activity. There is lowering of pain thresholds and atypical release of nociceptive molecules. All these events increase central sensitisation of trigeminal and thalamic neurons, with little recovery time in between causing continuous migraine attacks.

Cluster headaches share the same pathophysiological mechanisms as migraine but differ in signaling cascade. The attacks are of short duration (15–90 min), recur multiple times a day and there is pain-free interval between attacks. The trigger factors and response to triptans is similar.

The aims of treatment of migraine are to:

- *Produce quick symptomatic relief* by nonspecific analgesics.
- *Suppress the attack*, using a specific triptan.
- *Prevent further attacks* by behavioural or pharmacological therapy

Nonpharmacological therapy for prevention include:

1. Avoidance of precipitating factors such as loud noise, bright light, stress, certain foods and hypoglycaemia
2. The use of cognitive behaviour and relaxation therapy

The *behavioural approach* involves education of the patient about the precipitating causes of attacks and their avoidance; a regular lifestyle, regular meal hours, adequate but not excessive sleep, and minimising stress.

3. Noninvasive neuromodulatory devices have been introduced which help by either disrupting wave of cortical spreading depression by magnetic energy (Transcranial Magnetic Stimulation- TMS) or by modulating pain regulation centre in brainstem (Remote electrical Neuromodulation- REN) or by stimulating vagus nerve and thereby blocking pain signals. IM 17.11

Treatment of acute attacks: See Table 24.4. The target sites of drugs used in the treatment of acute attacks are depicted in Fig. 24.6.

A. NSAIDs

NSAIDs act by inhibiting PG synthesis, which prevents neurologically mediated inflammation in the trigemino-vascular system. **Aspirin** (600–900 mg) or **ibuprofen** (400–600 mg) are effective in relieving mild-moderate migraine pain in 2 hours. **Paracetamol (usually 1000 mg) is preferred for those who cannot tolerate aspirin or ibuprofen and is the drug of choice for pregnant woman having acute attack of migraine.** Many patients may not need additional medication, if NSAIDs are taken at the very onset of headache and repeated every 4 h till the headache subsides. Opioids such as codeine, tramadol, butorphanol etc. are considered unsuitable for routine use because of their dependence liability. If nausea is prominent, an antiemetic such as domperidone (10 mg orally or suppository) or metoclopramide (10 mg orally) may be added to the above medication. The NSAID may be used prophylactically.

If for 3 or more consecutive attacks, response to any one of the NSAIDs is absent or inadequate then triptan should be recommended.

PH 1.16

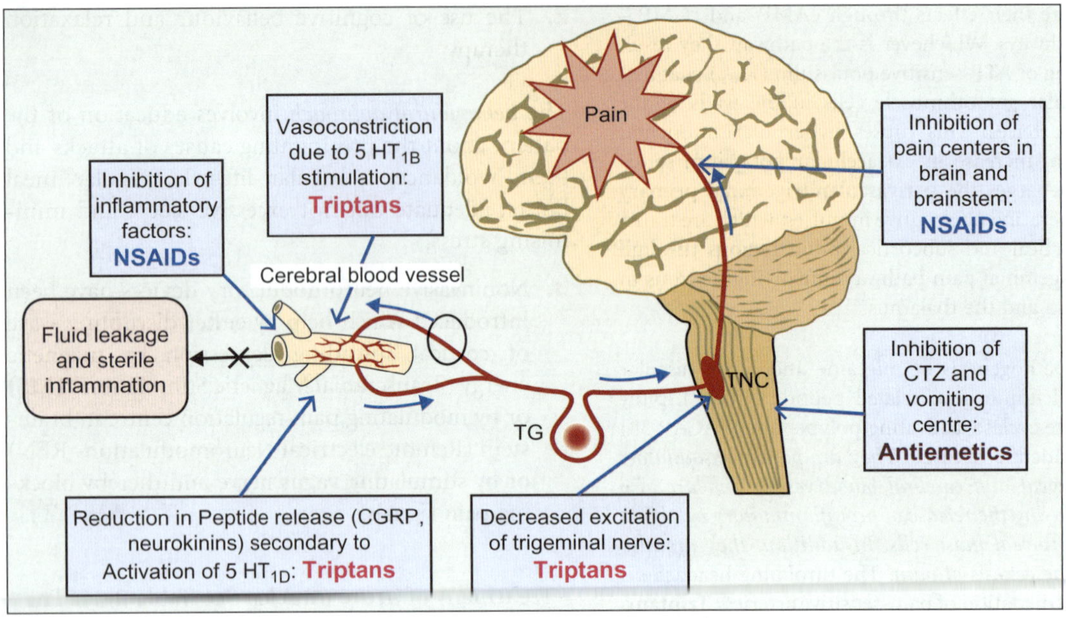

FIG. 24.6 Mechanism of action of anti-migraine drugs. CGRP, calcitonin gene related peptide; CTZ, chemoreceptor trigger zone; TG, trigeminal ganglion; TNC, trigeminal nucleus caudalis.

B. TRIPTANS ($5\text{-}HT_{1B/1D}$ receptor agonists) **The triptans, another group of antimigraine drugs, are highly effective in the specific treatment of an acute attack of migraine.** Sumatriptan, the prototype drug from this class is discussed below.

SUMATRIPTAN This drug, an indole derivative (Fig. 24.7), is a selective agonist of $5\text{-}HT_{1B/1D}$ receptors located in cranial blood vessels and nerve terminals (Fig. 24.6).

Mechanism of action:

Activation of $5\text{-}HT_1$ receptors by sumatriptan leads to:

1. Selective constriction of extracerebral and intracranial blood vessels. It also constricts other blood vessels such as the coronary arteries.
2. Inhibition of trigeminal neurons in the brain stem and upper spinal cord, which decreases pain transmission. Stimulation of $5\text{-}HT_{1B/1D}$ receptors is responsible for the same.
3. Inhibition of the release of several vasodilator neuropeptides through stimulation of presynaptic $5\text{-}HT_{1D}$ or $5\text{-}HT_{1F}$ receptors.
4. Reduction in the increased concentration of CGRP in migraine attacks (Fig. 24.8).

Given orally, sumatriptan is highly effective in treating acute attacks of migraine.

Absorption, fate, excretion: The oral bioavailability is only 14%. It can also be given by nasal spray and subcutaneously. The drug is metabolised in the liver by MAO-A enzyme to an inactive metabolite. Its t½ is about 2 h. It does not cross the BBB. Subcutaneous sumatriptan acts within 2 h.

Adverse reactions: These are usually mild to moderate in intensity. It may cause a sensation of flushing and heat at the injection site, neck pain, dizziness, asthenia and tingling in the hands. Occasionally, it may cause myocardial ischaemia due to coronary

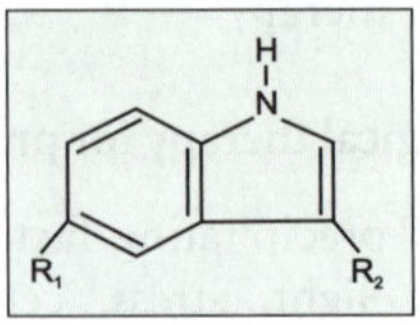

FIG. 24.7 Triptan nucleus.

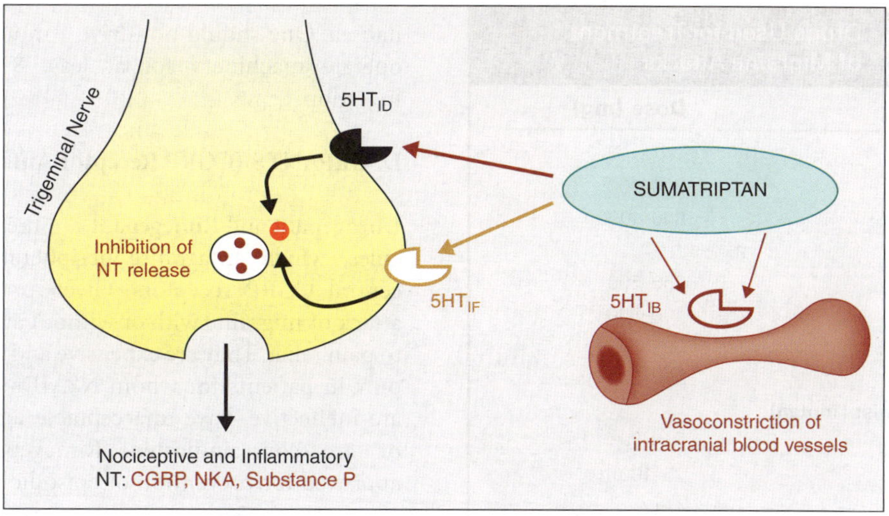

FIG. 24.8 Mechanism of action of sumatriptan. CGRP, calcitonin gene related peptide; NKA, neurokinin A; NT, neurotransmitter.

vasoconstriction. *It is, therefore,* **avoided** *in certain conditions (Box 24.1). It should not be combined with ergotamine and other vasoconstrictor drugs. A triptan should not be used until 24 h after the last dose of ergotamine.*

Preparations and Dosage: See Table 24.4

Although analogues of sumatriptan such as **Zolmitriptan, Rizatriptan, Almotriptan, Eletriptan, Frovatriptan** and **Naratriptan** have been introduced, their superiority over sumatriptan has not been established. They differ in their pharmacokinetic properties. Rizatriptan and zolmitriptan are available as mouth dissolving tablets.

Indication

1. **Acute attack of migraine: Sumatriptran** (25–50 mg) is the preferred triptan based on efficacy, safety profile and cost. It is given orally and may be repeated every 2 h, if necessary, to the maximum total dose of 300 mg within 24 h. It can also be given by nasal spray in the dose of 10–40 mg or subcutaneously. It is effective in 80% of patients within 2 h and the pain relief persists till 24 h.

Box 24.1 Avoid triptans in the presence of:

- Untreated arterial hypertension
- Coronary heart disease
- History of ischaemic stroke
- Basilar or hemiplegic migraine
- Raynaud's disease
- Severe liver or kidney failure
- Pregnancy, breastfeeding
- Age ≥ 65 years

If there is no effect after giving a triptan for 3 attacks, one should switch over to another triptan. One can also add naproxen.

Though triptans should be avoided in pregnancy, their use **during pregnancy is not associated with major teratogenic effects, low infant birth weight, or preterm delivery.** When indicated, sumatriptan is preferred.

In resistant acute attacks, combination therapy with Triptan and NSAID (preferably naproxen) may be tried. If all the triptans(+ naproxen) show no effect or insufficient effect for 3 or more consecutive migraine attacks, then either ditan or gepant should be advocated (See below).

PH 1.16

C. DITANS (5-HT$_{1F}$ receptor agonists)

Table 24.4 Drugs Used for Treatment of Migraine Attacks

Drug[a]	Dose (mg)
Analgesic	
Aspirin	600–900
Paracetamol	500–1000
NSAID	
Naproxen	250–500
Ibuprofen	400–800
Diclofenac (IM)	50
Ketorolac (IM)	30–120
$5\text{-}HT_{1B/1D}$ agonist (Triptan)	
Sumatriptan	
Oral	25–100
SC	4–12
Nasal spray	10–30
Nasal powder	22 mg (11 mg in each nostril)
$5\text{-}HT_{1F}$ agonist (Ditan)	
Lasmiditan	50–200
CGRP receptor antagonists (Gepants)	
Ubrogepant	50–100
Rimegepant	75
5-HT partial agonists/antagonists	
Ergotamine	
Oral	1–4
Sublingual	1–4
DHE (IV/IM / SC/Nasal spray)	1–2/1–3/2
Dopamine antagonists (oral/IV)	
Metoclopramide	10
Haloperidol	5–10
Prochlorperazine	25/10

[a]Oral, unless specified.

LASMIDITAN is a **selective serotonin 1F receptor agonist**. It lacks vasoconstrictor activity and hence preferable for those with relative contraindications to triptans due to cardiovascular risk factors. It is administered orally for acute attack in an initial dose of 50 or 100 mg. If no effect is seen, then there is no benefit of repeating same or higher dose. More than one dose should not be taken in 24 hours. In subsequent attacks, higher dose (100 or 200 mg) can be used.

Adverse reactions: It can cause dose dependent dizziness, paresthesia, somnolence, fatigue, and nausea. One should not drive a motor vehicle or operate machinery for at least 8 hours after ingestion.

D. GEPANTS (CGRP Receptor Antagonists)

Ubrogepant and **Rimegepant** are the small molecules, which antagonise peripheral as well as central CGRP receptors. Given orally in acute attack of migraine with or without aura, they lead to pain relief. They are expensive and are indicated only in patients for whom NSAIDs and triptans are ineffective, have unacceptable adverse effects or are contraindicated. Rimegepant is also approved for prevention of episodic migraine.

E. ERGOT PREPARATIONS

Ergotamine tartrate (1 mg) with or without caffeine (100 mg) is used in moderate- severe migraine. It is a **partial agonist of $5\text{-}HT_{1B/1D}$ receptors.** A tablet is chewed and swallowed early during an attack. Not more than four tablets should be taken in 24 h, nor more than 12 tablets per week. Ergotamine worsens the nausea of migraine; this may be pretreated with an antiemetic drug. It can cause leg cramps or tingling in the extremities.

Dihydroergotamine (DHE) 1 mg subcutaneously, with antiemetic pretreatment, is also effective. It is used to treat refractory migraine. **However it should be avoided for 24 hours after triptan.** *Persistent, chronic headache may be a symptom of overtreatment with ergot preparations.*

Ergot preparations are contraindicated in the presence of peripheral vascular disease or coronary artery disease (angina). They should be avoided in hypertension, during pregnancy, and in hepatic and renal disease. *Ergotamine should never be used in migraine prophylaxis.* IM 17.12

Migraine Prophylaxis: See Table 24.5. Preventive treatment is considered when attacks occur more than 2–3 times a month or are severe enough to limit normal activity; and when symptomatic therapy fails or causes serious ADR. It is also used for those having

Table 24.5 Drugs Used for Prevention of Migraine Attacks

Drug	Dose (mg)
Beta-adrenergic antagonists	
Metoprolol	450–100 mg oral twice daily or 200 mg modified-release oral once daily
Propranolol	40–240[a]
Atenolol	25–50 o.d.
Anticonvulsants	
Valproic acid	300–600[a]
Topiramate	25–100 b.i.d.
Antidepressants	
Amitriptyline	10–50 at night
Venlafaxine	37.5
Calcium channel blockers	
Verapamil	100–200[a]
Flunarizine	5–10 mg o.d.

[a]Daily divided.

prolonged, uncomfortable, or disabling aura. The objectives of preventive therapy are to:

- Reduce the frequency, duration, or severity of migraine attacks
- Prevent progression from episodic migraine to chronic migraine
- Improve the response to acute pain management
- Improve activities of daily living and quality of life

Medications containing vasodilators should be discontinued, if possible.

Drugs from different classes have shown ability to prevent migraine but the exact mechanism for their effect is not known.

The most commonly prescribed group is **beta blockers** (Chapter 18). They normalize the cortical evoked potentials and decrease the headache frequency by more than 50%. Most consistent effects are observed with **metoprolol** and **propranolol.** Propranolol is the drug of choice in patients with attacks related to stress. *Beta blockers with intrinsic sympathomimetic activity are not useful.*

Valproic acid and **topiramate** have been reported to be useful in some patients. Valproic acid prevents migraine possibly through GABAergic mechanisms whereas topiramate effects may be mediated through inhibition of neuronal voltage-dependent sodium channels. It may be enhancing the inhibitory activity of GABA and has weak carbonic anhydrase inhibitor activity.

Calcium channel blockers like **flunarizine** (non-selective CCB with antidopaminergic property) and **verapamil** probably prevent initiation and propagation of cortical spreading depression. They also inhibit serotonin release and neurovascular inflammation. They are more beneficial in patients with prolonged aura.

TCA, **amitriptyline** and SNRI, **venlafaxine** (Chapter 14) are also effective for migraine prophylaxis. Amitriptyline in the low dose of 5–10 mg at bedtime daily is especially useful in patients who have concomitant depression.

Lisinopril and **candesartan** have also shown to prevent migraine attacks but the evidence is low. The exact mechanism is unclear but they may be reducing renin/angiotensin mediated relay of pain in the brain.

Therapy is started with small doses with cheaper and easily accessible drug. The lowest effective maintenance dose should be used. The response should be assessed after 2–3 months. If the response is good, the medication may be tapered gradually after 9–12 months. If headaches recur, the treatment should be restarted. Propranolol, if used, should not be stopped abruptly.

ONABOTULINUM TOXIN- A (OBT-A)

This botulinum toxin- A (Chapter 22) is used in the treatment of chronic migraine. It acts on the on Soluble N-ethylmaleimide-sensitive fusion protein attachment protein receptor (SNARE) complexes (Chapter 19). Core SNARE complex has four

Table 24.6 Monoclonal Antibodies Targeting GCRP and its receptors

	Erenumab	Fremanezumab	Galcanezumab	Eptinezumab
Target	CGRP receptor	CGRP peptide	CGRP peptide	CGRP peptide
Type	Fully human murine	Humanised murine	Humanised murine	Humanised yeast
Dose and dosing	70-140 mg monthly SC	225 mg monthly SC or 675 mg12 weekly SC	240mg loading dose & then 120 mg monthly SC	100 -300 mg 12 weekly IV
Indications	EM, CM	EM, CM, eCH, cCH	EM, CM, eCH, cCH	EM, CM
Availability in India	Yes	Yes	Yes	Yes

EM, episodic migraine;CM, chronic migraine, eCH, episodic cluster headache; cCH, chronic cluster headache

α-helices, synaptobrevin, syntaxin and SNAP-25 and synaptotagmin. It serves as calcium sensor and mediates fusion of NT containing vesicles and synaptic membrane, resulting into exocytosis. OBT-A binds to C-terminus of SNAP-25 and cleaves it. Hence release of neuropeptides CGRP and substance P is prevented.

OBT-A IM injections (0.1 ml 5 units per site; total 155–195 units) across 30–39 sites on the head and neck are required. The procedure is repeated every 12 weeks. Response occurs after 9 months. The drug is extremely well tolerated provided aseptic precautions are taken to prevent infection.

MONOCLONAL ANTIBODIES TARGETING CGRP OR ITS RECEPTOR

Four monoclonal antibodies have been approved for migraine prophylaxis in adults. As against gepants, they have greater molecular weight and thus cannot cross BBB. Their action is thus restricted to peripheral CGRP and its receptors. Table 24.6 depicts their salient features. In general, they have rapid onset of action and long t½. But they are expensive and are to be used in episodic or chronic migraine who have been unsuccessfully treated with two or more preventive treatments and those who cannot use other preventive treatments because of comorbidities, side-effects, or poor compliance.

They are contraindicated in patients with a history of stroke, subarachnoid haemorrhage, coronary heart disease, inflammatory bowel disease, COPD, or impaired wound healing. Long term safety data is still awaited. They should not be used in pregnant or nursing women.

Menstrual migraine (attacks occurring during menses and are secondary to drop in estrogen levels) is generally refractory and may need prophylactic treatment with NSAID or triptans, which should be started from two days before expected date of menstruation and continued for five days after bleeding starts. Amitriptyline/beta blocker, plus NSAID/ergotamine at the onset of menses are other alternatives. Oral diuretics are sometimes helpful in such cases as they counter fluid retention.

Combined hormonal contraceptives are contraindicated in women with migraine with aura regardless of any association with their menstrual cycle, because their use is associated with increased risk of stroke.

DRUGS USED IN THE TREATMENT OF ACUTE ATTACKS OF MIGRAINE

Analgesic
- Paracetamol

NSAID
- Naproxen
- Ibuprofen

5-HT$_{1B/1D}$ agonist
- Sumatriptan
- Zolmitriptan
- Rizatriptan
- Almotriptan
- Eletriptan
- Frovatriptan
- Naratriptan

5-HT partial agonists/ antagonists
- Ergotamine
- DHE

Ditans (5-HT1F receptor agonists)
- Lasmiditan

Gepants (CGRP receptor antagonists)
- Ubrogepant
- Rimegepant

Dopamine antagonists (for vomiting)
- Metoclopramide
- Prochlorperazine

DRUGS USED IN THE TREATMENT OF PREVENTION OF MIGRAINE ATTACKS

5-HT antagonists
- Pizotifen

Beta-adrenergic antagonists
- Propranolol

Antidepressants
- Amitriptyline

Calcium channel blockers
- Verapamil
- Flunarizine

Anticonvulsants
- Valproic acid
- Topiramate

Monoclonal antibodies
- Erenumab
- Fremanezumab
- Galcanezumab
- Eptinezumab

ONABOTULINUM TOXIN-A (OBT-A)

CHAPTER 25

Angiotensin, Kinins, Leukotrienes, Prostaglandins and Cytokines

Learning Objectives

This chapter will enable the reader:

1. To state sites and steps involved in biosynthesis and describe physiological actions and pathological role of angiotensins, kinins, leukotrienes and prostaglandins.
2. To state uses of prostaglandin analogues giving examples of drugs.
3. To describe general properties of cytokines.
4. To classify cytokines according to their functions giving examples.
5. To discuss the role of IL-1, IL-2 and TNFα in defence mechanisms, inflammation and repair.

KEY TERMS

angiotensin II receptors, types, p. 362
ecallantide, p. 363
bradykinin, p. 364
leukotrienes, p. 364
5-lipooxygenase, p. 364
prostaglandins, p. 365
arachidonic acid, p. 366
interferons, p. 368
interleukins, p. 368
tumour necrosis factor, p. 368

ANGIOTENSINS are peptide hormones derived from a protein precursor angiotensinogen (a serum globulin, also called renin substrate) by the sequential actions of proteolyltic enzymes present in the circulation and several tissues. Angiotensinogen, synthesised by the liver, is converted by the circulating renin released from the kidney into **angiotensin I**, a decapeptide. It is converted by **angiotensin converting enzyme** (**ACE**) into the octapeptide **angiotensin II**, which is further converted to either angiotensin III or angiotensin IV. ACE is located in the plasma and the capillary endothelial cells, mainly in the lungs. It is also found in various tissues including the brain, kidney and the adrenals.

ACE is a nonspecific enzyme and it also inactivates other substrates such as bradykinin. **Angiotensin II** is **the most potent angiotensin.** It can also be synthesised by a pathway that does not require ACE. Both angiotensin II and III act through G protein coupled receptors, AT_1 and AT_2. .

Most of the classic actions of angiotensin are mediated by the AT_1 receptors. Thus:

- **AT_1 receptors:**
    a. Mediate the vasoconstrictor action.
    b. Stimulate aldosterone production.
    c. Promote cell growth and hypertrophy of the arterial and the ventricular wall muscle in the diseased and failing heart.
- **AT_2 receptors** ameliorate the adverse effects of AT_1 receptor activation by inhibiting cell growth and hypertrophy. AT_2 receptors are less abundant and are present in brain, adrenal medulla, vascular endothelium and reproductive tissues.

Actions of angiotensin II: It acts at several sites in the body (Table 25.1). It is a 40–50 times more potent vasoconstrictor than NA on molar basis:

- **It causes rapid regulation of arterial BP in response to an acute fall in BP,** by constricting the arterioles, and to a smaller extent, venules.
- *Long-term maintenance of BP (slow response) is mediated by regulation of Na^+* excretion by the kidney. **Angiotensin II directly promotes renal Na^+ reabsorption in the proximal tubules and also causes Na^+ retention through the release of aldosterone.**

Table 25.1 Actions of Angiotensin II via AT_1 Receptors

Tissue	Action(s)
• **Artery**	Contraction and growth
• **Heart**	Contraction and ventricular hypertrophy
• **Adrenal**	Stimulates aldosterone biosynthesis
• **Kidney**	Inhibits renin release; stimulates sodium reabsorption; stimulates vasoconstriction (efferent glomerular arterioles in low concentrations, and both afferent and efferent in higher concentrations); releases PGE
• **Sympathetic nervous system**	Increased release of NA and adrenaline from autonomic ganglia and adrenal medulla respectively. Facilitates peripheral transmission

- **It also causes hypertrophy of the heart and thickening of the blood vessels.** Angiotensin II contributes to the pathogenesis of hypertension, cardiac hypertrophy, heart failure and diabetic renal disease.
- **It stimulates vasopressin (AVP) and ACTH release. It increases the thirst.**

The ill effects of excess angiotensin II can be countered by drugs such as: PH 1.16

1. *Angiotensin converting enzyme inhibitors* (ACEI)
2. *AT_1 receptor blockers (ARBs)* (Chapter 30)

KININS

The kinins are vasoactive polypetides released from an α_2 globulin fraction of the plasma, termed as kininogens (Fig. 25.1), by the action of enzymes termed **kallikreins**. Kininogens are present in two forms:

- Low molecular weight kininogen (LMWK)
- High molecular weight kininogen (HMWK)

HMWK is limited to the blood stream, whereas LMWK can reach the tissues.

The kallikreins (*kallikreas*, the Greek name for pancreas) are highly specific proteases and exist in **two forms**:

- **plasma kallikreins**
- **tissue kallikreins.** Both normally exist in inactive forms called prekallikreins (PK).

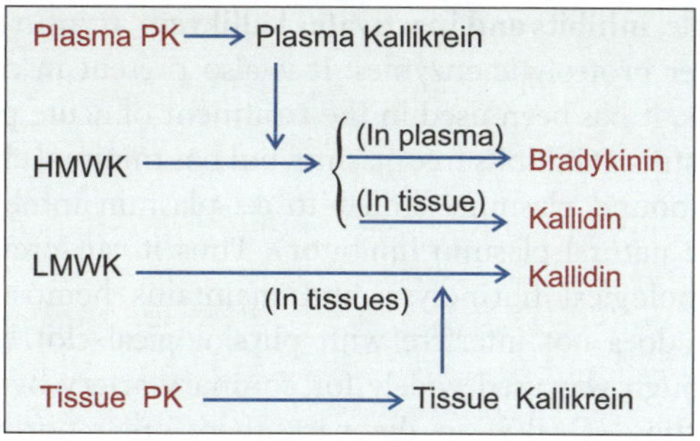

FIG. 25.1 Kinin generation.

Plasma prekallikrein is bound to its substrate HMWK. When this system binds to a receptor complex on the endothelial cell membrane, it gets activated to kallikrein. The generated kallikrein activates clotting factor XII and cleaves HMWK to a nonapeptide, **bradykinin**.

Tissue prekallikrein is present in epithelial or secretory cells of salivary glands, pancreas, prostate, distal nephron and human neutrophils. The active tissue kallikrein acts locally and converts HMWK and LMWK to a decapeptide, kallidin (lysyl bradykinin) (Fig. 25.1). PH 1.16

ECALLANTIDE: This recombinant human peptide is a *potent, selective and irreversible human plasma kallikrein inhibitor.* It is used for the treatment of hereditary angioedema, wherein there is an unregulated activity of kallikrein and excessive bradykinin production causing recurrent attacks.

Hereditary angioedema is a familial disorder due to a deficiency or malfunction of C1 esterase inhibitor and does not respond to usual treatment of angioedema (Chapter 23). It is manifested as painless, non-pitting and nonpruritic skin swelling.

Ecallantide dose is 30 mg SC as 3 separate injections or IV.

ADR include headache, nausea, fatigue and diarrhea. There can be a risk of potentially serious hypersensitivity reactions, including anaphylaxis.

For its use to prevent bleeding during cardiothoracic surgery, see Chapter 33.

APROTININ a high molecular weight polypeptide, extracted from the parotid glands and lymph nodes of cattle, **inhibits and inactivates kallikrein**, trypsin and other proteolytic enzymes. It is also present in mast cells. It has been used in the treatment of acute pancreatitis. It inhibits free plasmin but has minimal effect on bound plasmin, similar to α2-plasmin inhibitor (the natural plasmin inhibitor). Thus it can prevent pathological fibrinolysis and maintains hemostasis but does not interfere with physiological clot lysis. Though was used widely for coronary artery bypass grafting (CABG) in the past, there are reports of adverse cardiovascular, neurological and renal events associated with its use. Hence it was banned for few years but since 2011 it has been allowed to be used only in adult patients undergoing isolated CABG, who are at a high risk of major blood loss. It is also used to treat haemorrhage due to hyperplasminemia. Aprotinin-induced anaphylaxis is another major risk.

Both **kallidin** and **bradykinin** are referred to as **'plasma kinins'** and **have essentially identical pharmacological properties**. In addition to kallikreins, various other serine proteases like trypsin and certain snake venoms are capable of generating kinins. Preformed kinins exist in the venoms of wasps and hornets.

Physiological role: The kinins are:

- potent vasodilators
- the most potent activators of PG-release, including PGI_2 from vessels
- modulators of migration of leucocytes and tissue cells that take part in the inflammatory process

Bradykinin acts on two receptors. These are:

1. **B_1 receptors**,which are induced by inflammation and are absent in normal tissues.
2. **B_2 receptors**,which are constitutive and most of the actions of kinin are mediated through it.

Kinins have been incriminated in the processes of inflammatory and allergic reactions (asthma), shock, disseminated intravascular coagulation and inflammatory bowel disease.

Pharmacological actions:

Cardiovascular: The kinins have about 10 times the **vasodilator** activity as histamine. They produce mainly arteriolar dilatation in the skeletal muscle, heart, kidneys, intestines and liver, via the local release of nitric oxide and PGI_2. The kinins also have direct **positive chronotropic and inotropic actions** on the myocardium and in moderate doses, release adrenaline from the adrenal medulla. They increase vascular permeability and induce oedema.

Smooth muscle contraction: The kinins **stimulate** smooth muscles including those of the uterus, the bronchi and the GI tract. They promote epithelial ion transport and fluid secretion in the airways and GIT, leading to **cough/angioedema** in the former and diarrhoea in the latter.

Genesis of pain: The kinins evoke pain (algesia) and itching. NSAIDs can antagonise this pain.

Release of PGs and PAF: Kinins can cause the release of biologically active lipids such as platelet activating factor (PAF) and PGs from a variety of cells; some of the actions of kinins are indirect via the release of such mediators of inflammation.

The kinins are rapidly inactivated by the plasma and erythrocyte aminopeptidases and carboxypeptidases. They have *very short plasma t½ of 15 s. ACE converts angiotensin I to angiotensin II and also metabolises bradykinin.* The reaction is inhibited by ACEI.

ICATIBANT: It is a selective bradykinin- B2 receptor antagonist. It is used in the treatment of heredity angioedema in a dose of 30 mg SC on abdomen using a prefilled syringe. Maximum 3 injections can be given in 24-hours. Its ADR include injection site reaction, fever and dizziness.

LEUKOTRIENES (LTs)

Leukotrienes along with PGs, thromboxanes and lipoxins, are the major constituents of a group of eicosanoids. All the LTs are synthesised from arachidonic acid(cell wall constituent) by action of the enzyme 5-lipooxygenase (Fig. 25.2) which is present in neutrophils, eosinophils, monocytes, macrophages, mast cells, basophils and B-lymphocytes. LTs exert their biological actions through specific ligand–receptor interactions.They are produced locally and

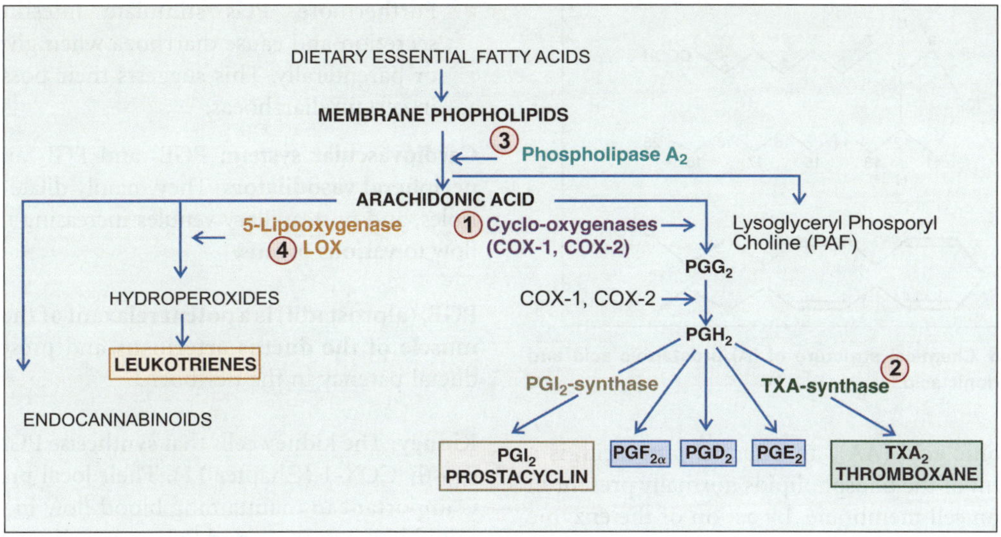

FIG. 25.2 Synthesis of leukotrienes and important mammalian prostaglandins. ① Aspirin and NSAID inhibit COX-1 and COX-2 ② Dazoxiben inhibits TXA synthase ③ Glucocorticoids inhibit generation of AA from cell membrane phospholipids by phospholipase A2 ④ Zileuton inhibits 5-lipooxygenase.

act as 'local hormones'. Their t½ is very short. Biologically active LTs are **LTB_4, LTC_4, LTD_4 and LTE_4;** the last three are also collectively known as **slow reacting substance of anaphylaxis** (SRS-A)/ **sulphidopeptides / cysteinyl LTs** .

Pharmacological/biological actions: LTs have several potent actions. Thus, **LTB_4:**

- Is the *most potent neutrophil chemotactic agent*
- plays an important *role in the induction of neutrophil–endothelial–cell adhesion*
- *Causes the release of substantial quantities of glucuronidase and lysozyme* from the neutrophils
- Stimulates myelopoiesis and proliferation of T lymphocytes
- Is an important *mediator of inflammatory pain*

Cysteinyl LTs (LTC_4, LTD_4 and LTE_4) **play an important role in the inflammatory process.** They cause:

- *Vigorous and sustained contraction of smooth muscle.* They are the most potent bronchoconstrictors.
- *Vasodilatation and modulation of vascular (venular endothelial) permeability, leading to the development of oedema.* They constrict the cutaneous and small coronary blood vessels.
- *Increased mucus secretion in the airways*
- *Immune modulation*

Clinical implications of cysteinyl LTs: Their release has been implicated in the pathogenesis of anaphylactic shock, asthma and various inflammatory diseases such as cystic fibrosis, glomerulonephritis, rheumatoid arthritis, psoriasis, inflammatory bowel disease and adult respiratory distress syndrome. Currently, LT synthesis inhibitors and antagonists are used in the treatment of asthma (Chapter 27).

PH 1.16

PROSTAGLANDINS (PGs)

PGs were originally identified in human semen and named as PG because of its probable origin from the prostate. The various PGs are closely related derivatives of the lipid soluble **prostanoic acid** (Fig. 25.3). PGs are also present in extracts of other tissues such as iris, lung, human menstrual fluid, brain, thymus, pancreas and kidneys.

Prostaglandin of the human semen is a mixture of six closely related substances belonging to the groups E, F, A and B. The other human tissues contain mostly groups E and F PGs, though PGD_2, PGG_2, PGH_2 and PGI_2 (prostacyclin) have also been described.

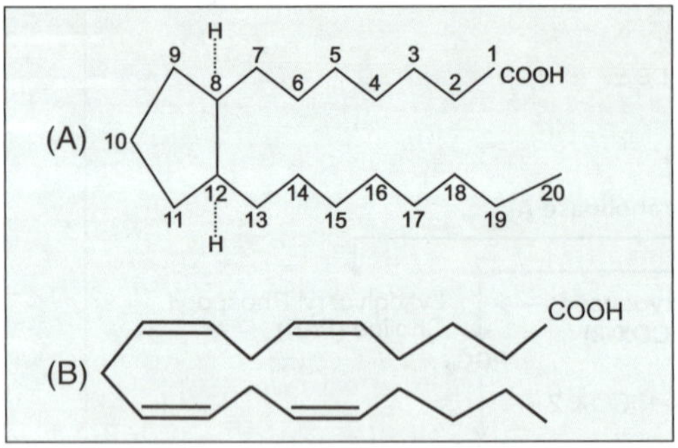

FIG. 25.3 Chemical structure of (A) prostanoic acid and (B) arachidonic acid.

Arachidonic acid (AA), an essential fatty acid, is a constituent of the phospholipids normally present in the human cell membrane. By action of the enzyme cyclo oxygenase (COX) on AA, PGs of PG-2 series (Fig 25.2), with marked proinflammatory activity are generated (Chapter 11). Under stimulation by mechanical, thermal, chemical and bacterial insults, PGs are released in large amounts locally to produce an inflammatory response. They have also been incriminated in the pathogenesis of chronic inflammatory disorders such as psoriasis and rheumatoid arthritis (RA).

Because of their instability, short duration of action and lack of tissue specificity, the natural PGs have limited clinical applications. Various synthetic derivatives available, however, overcome some of these limitations.

Pharmacological actions: PGs produce their effects by acting on PG receptors.

Smooth muscles: PGE_2, $PGF_{2\alpha}$ and TXA_2 stimulate the human myometrium and increase the intestinal motility. **PGE inhibits** the tone of tracheal and bronchial muscles and thus has a **bronchodilator action.**

Gastrointestinal system: PGs are distributed throughout the gut though their concentration varies in different parts.

- **PGE_2 and PGI_2** synthesised by COX-1 inhibit the gastric acid secretion, enhance the mucosal blood flow, and thus have a **cytoprotective effect** on gastric and duodenal mucosa.
- Both PGE and PGF cause contraction of the longitudinal muscle of the gut.
- Furthermore, PGs stimulate intestinal fluid secretion and cause diarrhoea when given orally or parenterally. This suggests their possible role in certain diarrhoeas.

Cardiovascular system: PGE_2 and PGI_2 are **potent peripheral vasodilators.** They mainly dilate the arterioles, and postcapillary venules increasing the blood flow to various organs.

PGE_1 (alprostadil) is a potent relaxant of the smooth muscle of the ductus arteriosus and preserves the ductal patency in the newborn.

Kidney: The kidney cells that synthesise PGs contain mostly COX-1 (Chapter 11). Their local production is important in maintaining blood flow in compromised kidneys. **PGE_2 and PGI_2 cause diuresis, natriuresis and kaliuresis by direct action on the renal tubules. PGE inhibits water reabsorption induced by ADH**; it also inhibits chloride reabsorption.

Reproductive system: Apart from their stimulant action on the uterine smooth muscle, PGs exert other actions on the reproductive system. COX-2 may play a role in the birth process and its excessive activity may be responsible for premature labour (Chapter 42). Functions of PGs present in the semen are not clear.

CNS: The role of PGs as neurotransmitters has been suggested. COX-1 is distributed in neurons throughout the brain, being most prevalent in the forebrain. COX-2 is also expressed constitutively in a few areas. PGs are probably involved in the central mechanisms that cause hyperalgesia. Furthermore, PGE_2 and $PGF_{2\alpha}$ are implicated in the pathogenesis of fever i.e. have pyrogenic activity (Chapter 11).

Platelet aggregation: In the platelets, the only isoform detectable is COX-1.

1. PG endoperoxide and **TXA_2**, cause *platelet aggregation and vasoconstriction.*
2. PGI_2 (**prostacyclin**) which is found in the vascular endothelium is a *potent inhibitor of platelet aggregation and causes vasodilatation.*

When the platelets are damaged they release PG endoperoxides which cause aggregation of platelets. However, the vascular endothelial PGI_2 has antiaggregatory effect. Damage to the endothelium reduces PGI_2 synthesis and increases the tendency to thrombosis because of the unopposed action of TXA_2. Aspirin blocks formation of both TXA_2 and PGI_2 but COX-1 in the vascular endothelial cells regenerates so that PGI_2 synthesis is re-established (Chapter 11). The TXA_2 synthesis, however, is irreversibly inhibited for the lifetime (8–10 days) of the platelets in circulation (Chapter 33).

Role in inflammation: Presence of PGE and kinins in the inflammatory exudates suggests their role in the genesis of inflammation. COX-2 is clearly associated with inflammation (Chapter 11).

Miscellaneous: PGE_1 and PGE_2 block the lipolytic effect of adrenaline, ACTH and glucagon. They also produce pain when applied to an exposed blister base.

Some PGs are potent bone resorbing agents which act by stimulating osteoclasts. Experimentally, bone destruction, induced by implanted metastasising tumours in rats and rabbits, can be reduced by PG inhibition by aspirin or indomethacin.

PGE_2 also stimulates the adrenal steroid production and insulin release.

Adverse reactions and **Indications:** These are presented in Table 25.2.

Endocannabinoids are the endogenous ligands for the cannabinoid receptors. They are derived from AA in the brain and mimic some of the pharmacological actions of Δ9-tetrahydro-cannabinol, dronabinol (Chapters 13 and 39).

CYTOKINES

Inflammation is an integral part of the body's defence mechanisms against foreign insults, and natural as well as acquired (specific) immunity play an important role in human defence. Several polypeptides act as mediators of the inflammatory process.

The effector phases of both natural and acquired immunity are in large part mediated by protein hormones called **cytokines**, which are released from a variety of cell types in response to a number of stimuli (**induced secretion**).

- In case **of natural immunity**, effector cytokines are mainly derived from the mononuclear phagocytes and the natural killer (NK) cells.
- Most cytokines in **acquired immunity** are released from activated T lymphocytes. T cells produce several cytokines that serve primarily to regulate the growth, differentiation and activation of various lymphocyte populations (**constitutive secretion**). They activate and regulate inflammatory cells such as monocytes, neutrophils and eosinophils.
- Both lymphocytes and mononuclear phagocytes also produce other cytokines such as colony stimulating factors (CSF) which stimulate the growth and differentiation of immature lymphocytes in the bone marrow.

Cytokines act by binding to specific receptors on the surface of target cells. Such target cells may be (1) the same cells that secrete the cytokine (**autocrine action**); (2) nearby cells (**paracrine action**); or (3) distant cells as in the case of classical hormones (**endocrine action**).

General Properties of Cytokines:

- **Cytokines are low molecular weight proteins** secreted mainly by white blood cells and other cells and are responsible for cell to cell communication. Many individual cytokines are produced by multiple types of cells.
- **They are produced during the effector phase of natural and acquired immunity** and play an important role in mediating and regulating the immune, inflammatory and erythropoietic responses, including the termination of the inflammatory response, angiogenesis, healing and repair.
- **They are not stored as preformed molecules.** Their constitutive secretion is brief and self-limited. Failure of termination of their induced secretion can lead to chronic inflammatory disorders.
- **A given cytokine has different biological effects on different cell types** *(pleotropism).*
- **Cytokines influence the synthesis of other cytokines**, which may affect the other cells in turn. Thus, even if small number of cells are involved in the beginning, this cascade induction leads to amplification of the biological effects and involves a larger cellular network.
- Two or more cytokines may interact with each other to **produce additive, synergistic or antagonistic effects**.

Table 25.2 Prostaglandin Analogues: Adverse Effects and Therapeutic Uses

PG Analogue	Pharmacological Name	Adverse Effects	Therapeutic Uses
PGE_1	Misoprostol (oral, intravaginal)	Diarrhea with or without abdominal pain and cramps	NSAID induced gastric ulcer (Chapter 41), Cervical ripening and induction of labour, and Therapeutic abortion (Chapter 42)
PGE_1	Alprostadil (IV, Intraurethral, Intracavernosal route)	Apnea in 10-12 %of neonates with congenital heart defects	Maintenance of patency of ductus arteriosus (Chapter 11), erectile dysfunction (Chapter 67)
PGE_1	Gemeprost (IV, Intraurethral, Intracavernosal route)	Vaginal bleeding, mild uterine pain, GI (nausea, vomiting, diarrhoea), CVS (flushing, shivering, headache, dizziness, hypotension), local tissue irritation and erythema following IV doses. Rarely, DIC	Therapeutic abortion (Chapter 42)
PGE_2	Sulprostone (IV)	Same as above	Therapeutic abortion (Chapter 42)
PGE_2	Dinoprostone (Intravaginal)	Uterine hyperstimulation, Rest same as above	Cervical ripening and induction of labour, Therapeutic abortion (second trimester), benign hydatidifom mole (Chapter 42)
$PGF_2\alpha$	Latanoprost, Travoprost, Tafluprost, Bimatoprost (eyedrops)	Growth of eyelashes, allergic conjunctival hyperemia, permanent brown pigmentation of iris, orbital fat atrophy, corneal epithelium irritation	Glaucoma (Chapter 70), Bimatoprost solution for eyelash hypotricosis
15 methyl $PGF_2\alpha$	Carboprost tromethamine(IM)	Nausea, vomiting, diarrhoea, fever, flushing, transient bronchoconstriction	Therapeutic abortion (second trimester), postpartum haemorrhage (Chapter 42)
PGI_2	Epoprostenol (IV infusion; t½ 3-5 min), Iloprost (IV, inhalation; t½ 30 min) Treprostinil (IV or SC infusion, oral; t½ 4h) Selexipag (Oral; prodrug)	Myalgias and pain in the extremities, jaw pain, headaches, nausea, abdominal discomfort, diarrhea, flushing, dizziness, and hypotension. Cough and insomnia with iloprost	Pulmonary artery hypertension (Chapter 30)

- For many target cells, **cytokines act as regulators of cell division** *(growth factors)*.

Classification of Cytokines

I. **Haematopoietin family,** e.g. GM-CSF, erythropoietin, IL-2, IL-4 (interleukin)

II. **Interferon family,** e.g. alpha, beta and gamma, IL-10

III. **Chemokine family,** e.g. IL-8, monocyte chemotactic protein, neutrophil activating protein, platelet factor 4

IV. **Tumour necrosis factor (TNF) family,** e.g. TNFα, TNFβ, TNFγ

Cytokines can also be **classified into four groups according to their functions** (Table 25.3).

Table 25.3 Cytokine Groups According to Functions

Group	Members	Major Sources
Mediators of natural immunity	Interferon α and β	Macrophages, fibroblasts
	TNF α	Macrophages
	IL-1	MNP, endothelial and epithelial cells
	IL-6	Macrophages, endothelial cells
	IL-8	Macrophages, epithelial cells
	IL-12	Macrophages, dendritic cells
Regulators of lymphocyte activation, growth and differentiation	IL-2	T cells
	IL-4	TH2 cells; mast cells
	IL-5	TH2 cells
	TGF β	T cells; macrophages; others
	Interferon γ	TH1 cells, NK cells
Regulators of immune-mediated inflammation and repair	Interferon γ	T cells; NK cells
	IL-5	TH2 cells
	IL-10, IL-17	T cells
	IL-12	Macrophages and dendritic cells
	IL-18	Macrophages
	Lymphotoxin	T cells
	MIF	T cells
Stimulators of immature leucocytes, growth and differentiation	IL-3, IL-9	T cells
	IL-7	Fibroblasts, bone marrow stromal cells
	GM CSF, M CSF, G CSF	MNP; endothelial cells; fibroblasts
Stimulation of erythropoiesis	Erythropoietin	Kidney
Stimulation of platelet production	Thrombopoietin, IL-11	Liver, bone marrow

Note: CSF, colony stimulating factor; G, granulocyte; GM, granulocyte macrophage; IL, interleukin; M, macrophage; MIF, migration inhibition factor; MNP, mononuclear phagocytes; TGF, transforming growth factor; TNF, tumour necrosis factor.

Functions of Cytokines

The target cell responses that require cytokines fall broadly into the:

1. *Defence role* of alerting the body to invasion and dealing with it.
2. *Repair role* of cleaning up the debris and replacing lost matrix and tissue.
3. *Controlling cellular proliferation and differentiation.* IL-1 also produces metabolic responses; thereby, the necessary energy resources and rebuilding materials are mobilised.
4. *Haematopoiesis.*

Role in body defence and regulation of inflammatory responses: *IL-1 and TNFα are mediators of biological responses to endotoxins and promote inflammation.* IL-1 causes erythema, oedema, chemoattraction, and adherence as well as migration of defence cells into the sites of inflammation. IL-1 is responsible for the immune component of inflammatory diseases. Both play an important role in killing the invading organisms using oxidative mechanisms. The cytokines activate the cells leading to release of hydrolytic enzymes and increase PG production. Inhibition and killing of stray tumour cells is yet another property of TNFα and to a lesser extent of IL-1. These cytokines inhibit the replication of certain RNA and DNA viruses and induce viral resistance in a variety of cell types. For pyrogenic cytokines, see Chapter 11.

TNFα and IL-2 are potent upregulators of several cell types including fibroblasts and T cells.

The cytokines secreted from subpopulation of helper T cells (TH1 and TH2) are important determinants of the immune response generated to eliminate the pathogens. TH1 cells secrete interferon gamma and

IgG which help in defence mechanisms against viral and intracellular pathogens. On the other hand, IL-4 and IL-5 secreted from TH2 cells induce production of IgE. IL-5 is also responsible for eosinophil differentiation and activation; these defence mechanisms help to tackle helminth infections.

Role in body repair: Both IL-1 and TNFα appear to have considerable **influence on the earlier repair events of debridement**, mitogenesis and differentiation. Release of enzymes including proteoglycanase, collagenase and gelatinase can be induced from fibroblasts, synoviocytes and chondrocytes by IL-1, and the same is true for TNFα. Enzyme release is accompanied by release of PGE_2, which may also contribute to the degradation process.

Biological actions of TNFα are concentration dependent.

- **At low concentrations:** TNFα acts as a paracrine and autocrine regulator of leucocytes and endothelial cells. These actions are useful in generating the inflammatory responses which help to counter the microbial infections. TNFα and IL-1 are endogenous pyrogens, and act on cells in the hypothalamus to produce fever.
- **Moderate amounts of TNFα**: enter the blood stream and may cause systemic effects, including an increase in the **acute phase proteins (APP);** further. TNFα may be the mediator of matrix destruction in RA.
- **High concentrations of TNFα**: on the other hand, cause depressed myocardial contractility, relaxation of vascular smooth muscle and intravascular thrombosis, leading to fall of BP, decreased tissue perfusion and metabolic acidosis; thus, **TNFα contributes in a major way to death in septic shock.** It also causes depletion of hepatic and muscle glycogen. TNFα and IL-1 both can induce bone resorption.

Metabolic role: It is likely that the body wasting (cachexia) seen with severe disease states is due to the catabolic properties of TNF.

PGE_2, like cytokines, causes a rise in APP by different mechanisms. The severity and outcome of connective tissue diseases such as RA, and number of ischemic heart events during atherosclerosis correlate with APP levels.

Other cytokines like IL-10 decrease cytokine and PGE_2 formation by monocytes. TGF beta, which also serves as immunosuppresant, reduces inflammation and increases extracellular matrix formation required for repair. This activity of TGF β is kept under control by interferon gamma which inhibits collagen production and also has myelosuppressive activity.

Although over 200 cytokines have been detected and shown to be involved in physiological functions, so far only a few have been shown to be clinically relevant. PH 1.16

HUMAN RECOMBINANT IL-2 (Aldesleukin): Though it is structurally different from native IL-2, it enhances lymphocyte proliferation, cytotoxic and killer cell activity and IFN gamma activity, all of which contribute to activation of cellular immunity. It is presently used in therapy of melanoma and metastatic renal cell carcinoma.

For uses of gamma interferon, see Chapter 57; of growth factors, GCSF and GM-CSF, Chapter 35; and of **TNFα antagonists**, Chapter 73.

Platelet-activating factor (PAF-acether): This ether-linked phospholipid is *released during mast cell degranulation* and is implicated in pathophysiological states including allergic inflammation, anaphylactic shock and bronchial asthma. It is also formed by eosinophils, macrophages, neutrophils, vascular endothelium and the renal medullary cells.

PAF is a potent vasodilator. It activates most inflammatory cells and is believed to be responsible for mobilisation of eosinophils, neutrophils and/or platelets in lungs after exposure to the allergen. Given by aerosol inhalation, it causes dose dependent bronchoconstriction and bronchial inflammation. Increased microvascular permeability causes oedema of the airways. Furthermore, it also induces nonspecific bronchial hyper-responsiveness in nonasthmatic subjects. It promotes platelet aggregation and release of TXA_2, acts as a chemotactic agent and is a gastric ulcerogen.

PH 1.16

A substance called **ginkgolide** isolated from the extract of the tree *Ginkgo biloba* has been used in China for the treatment of asthma and other disorders. It has been claimed to exert specific PAF receptor antagonistic activity. It causes inhibition of PAF induced platelet aggregation, of degranulation of isolated, human neutrophils, and of oxygen free radical production by the human neutrophils. Its possible use in the treatment of bronchial asthma and other allergic disorders is under investigation.

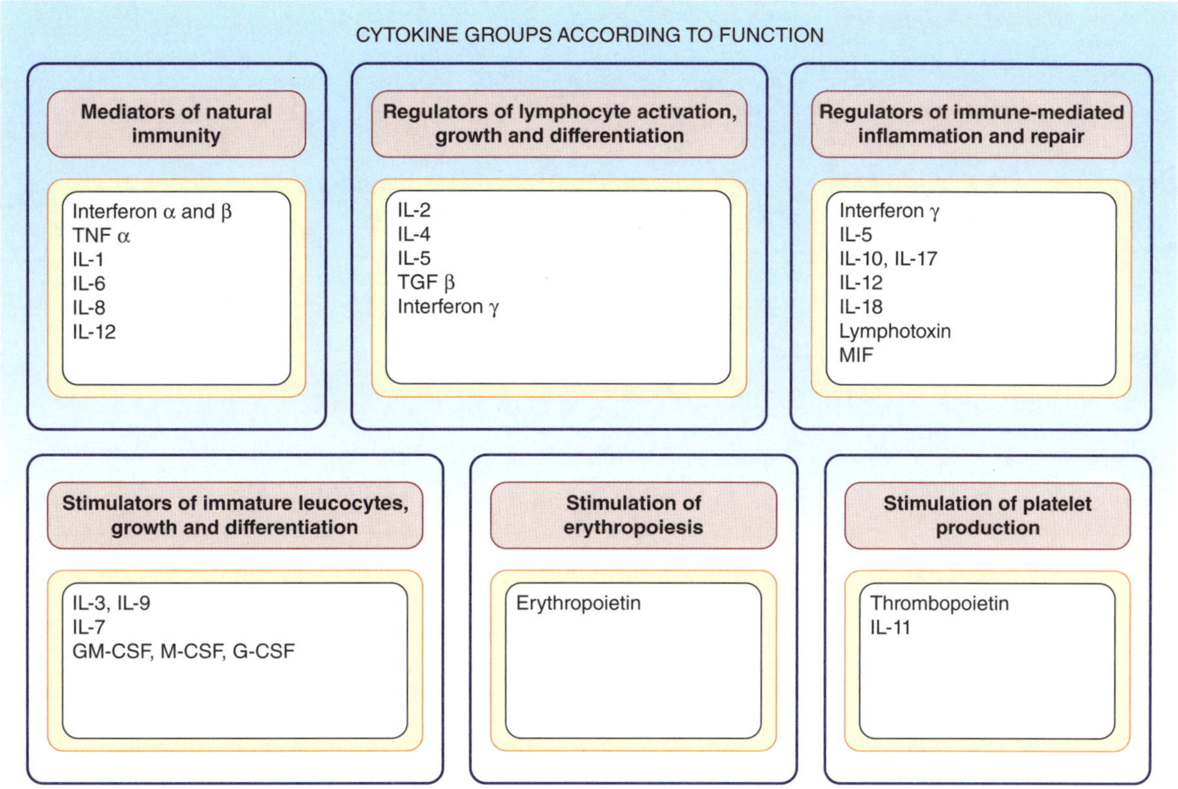

6 SECTION

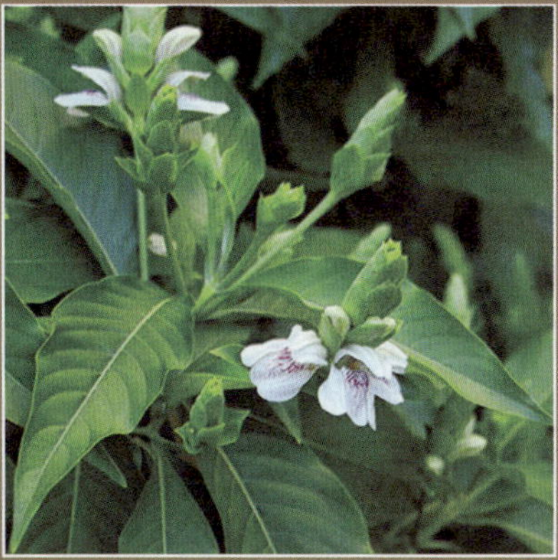

Athatoda vasaca

Drugs Used in Respiratory Disorders

Section Outline

CHAPTER 26

Pharmacotherapy of Cough

Learning Objectives

This chapter will enable the reader:

1. To discuss pathophysiology of cough.
2. To classify drugs used for symptomatic treatment of cough
3. To describe mechanism of action, clinical indication(s) and ADR of demulcents, expectorants, cough suppressants and mucolytics giving example of drug/s from each class.

KEY TERMS

cough centre, p. 375
pharyngeal demulcents, p. 376
antitussives, p. 376
expectorants, p. 377
mucolytics, p. 378
codeine, p. 379
dextromethorphan, p. 379

Cough acts as a protective reflex and helps to expel irritant matter from the respiratory tract. This is necessary for preventing any mechanical obstruction to breathing. Stimulation of the mucosal and C-fibre receptors in pharynx, larynx, trachea or bronchi generates tussal impulses. These are carried by afferent fibres in the vagus and sympathetic nerves to the brainstem nucleus solitarius, which is connected to the **medullary cough centre,** which initiates the act of coughing. C-fibre receptors are chemoreceptors, highly sensitive to medullary bradykinin, capsaicin and H^+ ions (pH).

The respiratory mucosa contains cells bearing cilia which transport the locally produced mucus towards the throat, from where it can be either coughed out or swallowed to keep the respiratory tract clean (*mucociliary clearance*). Defective mucociliary clearance leads to the retention of secretions in the respiratory tract and recurrent respiratory infections. In turn, respiratory infection impairs the mucociliary clearance further, with worsening of the infection. Chronic cough is an important symptom in such patients.

The act of coughing involves an initial deep inspiration followed by forced expiration against a temporarily closed glottis. Closure of the glottis causes an increase in intrathoracic pressure. When the glottis opens suddenly, the pulmonary air is forced through the trachea almost at the speed of sound, throwing out the respiratory tract secretions as expectoration. Most coughs are greatly in excess of that required to expel the particulate material. Furthermore, the strong expiration leads to a stronger succeeding inspiration and thus produces a vicious cycle in the form of a fit of coughing.

Cough may be

- **Productive,** associated with a large amount of sputum.
- **Nonproductive, dry and irritating.**

Environmental pollutants may cause cough by irritating the lungs, trachea or bronchi. Tobacco smoking is a well-known cause of chronic persistent cough. Cough due to the inhalation of allergens such as dust, chemicals and pollen is commonly observed in asthmatics.

Important causes of cough are:

- *Upper respiratory tract infections (URTI),* which may be self-limiting or persistent. The commonest cause of transient cough is viral URTI (common cold), and this leads to postnasal drip that stimulates receptors in the upper respiratory tract resulting in cough.

- *Allergic / obstructive diseases of respiratory tract:* allergic rhinitis, chronic sinusitis, and obstruction due to enlarged adenoids can cause cough. Enlarged, infected tonsils, an abnormally elongated uvula or nasal polyps can also cause chronic persistent cough.
- *Acute lung infections* and *pleural diseases* where therapy of the underlying cause will relieve cough.
- *Chronic pulmonary diseases* such as asthma, chronic bronchitis, bronchiectasis, tuberculosis and lung cancer.
- *Secondary to acute left ventricular failure (LVF),* which calls for immediate attention to the cardiac condition.
- *Gastroesophageal reflux disease* (GERD): See Chapter 41.
- *Drug-induced cough:* see Box 26.1.

Outside the respiratory tract, disorders of the external auditory canal and ear drum, pericardium and even of the stomach can give rise to chronic nonproductive cough. Thus, wax impacted in the ear, inflammation or eczema or even irritation of the drum by hair can cause dry cough. The entity called **'psychogenic cough'** induced voluntarily, is well known; it is nonproductive and is not present during sleep.

Cough can be:

- **Acute,** self-limiting (less than 3 weeks)
- **Subacute** (3–8 weeks)
- **Chronic** (more than 8 weeks)

Acute cough can occur in common cold, sudden exposure to allergens/ environmental pollutants/ occupational hazards. From the therapeutic point of view, chronic cough **with normal chest X-ray** can be either of the following:

Box 26.1 Some drugs which induce cough

- ACE inhibitors such as enalapril
- Beta blockers
- Inhaled corticosteroids and disodium chromoglycate
- Nebulised acetylcysteine
- Amiodarone
- Iodides
- Inhaled ether

1. **Glucocorticoid responsive,** due to eosinophilic disorders as in asthma, eosinophilic bronchitis and allergic rhinitis.
2. **Inhaled glucocorticoid resistant,** e.g. postnasal drip, GERD, postrespiratory infection and drug induced. PH 1.33

Classification of Drugs Used in the Symptomatic Treatment of Cough

I. **Pharyngeal demulcents and local sialogogues**, e.g. syrups and linctuses

II. **Mucoactive drugs** e.g. expectorants, mucolytics, mucokinetics and mucoregulators.

III. **Central cough suppressants**
   - **Opioids and related drugs**, e.g. codeine, dextromethorphan, pholcodeine, levopropoxyphene, noscapine
   - **Nonopioids**, e.g. caramiphene and pipezethate
   - **Antihistaminics**, e.g. diphenhydramine and chlorcyclizine

IV. **Peripheral cough suppressants**
   - **Local anaesthetics**, e.g. benzonatate, laevodropropizine and nebulised lignocaine

Fig. 26.1 illustrates the target sites and mechanism of action of above-mentioned drugs.

Antitussives (*tussis:* Latin for 'cough') or **cough suppressants** are used for immediate symptomatic relief of dry cough and are not substitutes for the specific therapy of the underlying cause. They act either centrally or peripherally.

PHARYNGEAL DEMULCENTS

Demulcents act by increasing the flow of saliva, the best natural demulcent which produces a protective and soothing effect. *They are useful in cough due to irritation of the pharyngeal mucosa above the larynx.* They are administered in the form of lozenges, troches, cough drops or linctuses. In practice, salivary secretion can be increased by such simple methods as using a few lemon drops, candy sugar, glycyrrhiza or drops of lemon juice in a thick syrupy base. Costly preparations like lozenges and troches, containing multiple ingredients such as menthol and antiseptics, are usually unnecessary and wasteful.

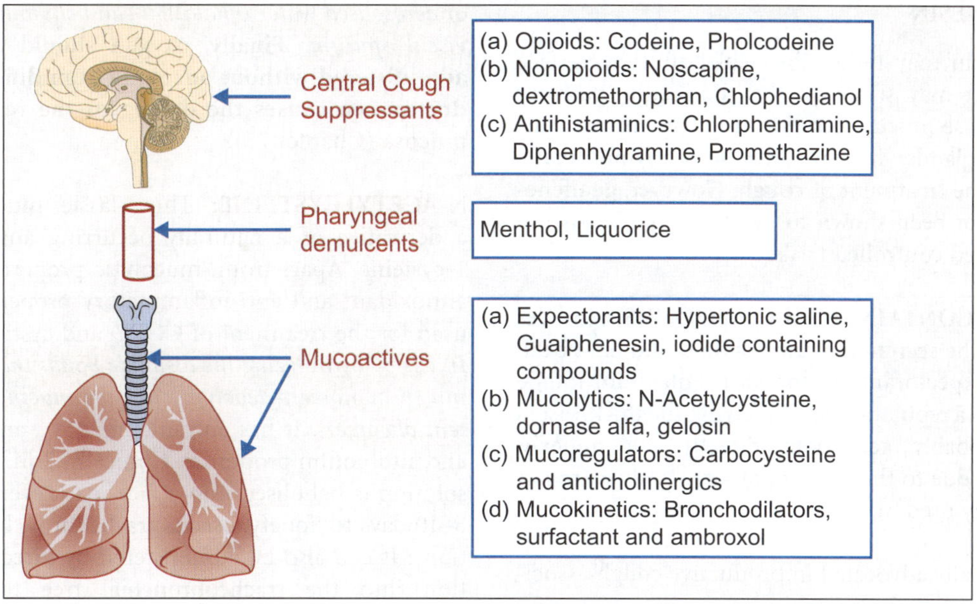

FIG. 26.1 **Target sites and mechanism of action of drugs used in treatment of cough.**

MUCOACTIVE DRUGS

These drugs are capable of modifying mucus production, its secretion, nature and composition, or its interactions with the mucociliary epithelium. *They alter the viscoelastic properties of mucus and also promote clearance of secretions.* Based on their mechanism of action, mucoactive drugs are classified as follows:

1. **Expectorants**, which increase the mucus secretion and cause its expulsion from the respiratory tract by inducing cough e.g. hypertonic saline, guaiphenesin and iodide containing compounds
2. **Mucolytics**, which reduce the viscosity of mucus, e.g., N-Acetylcysteine, dornase alfa, gelosin
3. **Mucokinetics**, which increase mucociliary clearance by acting on the cilia e.g., bronchodilators, surfactant and ambroxol
4. **Mucoregulators**, which regulate mucus secretion and suppress mechanism of hypersecretion or interfere with the DNA/F-actin network. e.g., carbocysteine and anticholinergics. PH 1.33

Expectorants

The Latin word 'expectorare' means 'to drive from the chest'. *Expectorants are the drugs which increase the production of the demulcent respiratory tract fluid that covers and protects the irritated mucosa.* They expel the mucus from the upper respiratory tract or lungs by a coughing or sneezing action. The exact mechanism of expectorants is unknown. They may act directly or indirectly as irritants to gastric vagal receptors to stimulate glandular exocytosis of a less viscous mucus (**reflex expectorants**). These drugs are useful in the treatment of cough due to neural irritation of the respiratory mucosa by the thick viscous mucus plugs below the larynx.

Volatile oils such as oil of eucalyptus, anise and lemon, administered orally or inhaled with steam, increase the respiratory secretions probably by a **direct action**. Alcohol and cedar wood oil (active ingredient terpene hydrochloride), added to steam inhalation, have a similar effect.

HYPERTONIC SALINE

Inhaled hyperosmolar saline is an inexpensive therapy that improves pulmonary function in patients with cystic fibrosis lung disease. However, hypertonic saline has an unpleasant taste and induces coughing, which may limit its acceptance and thus its efficacy as a long-term therapy.

GUAIFENESIN

Guaifenesin may reduce bronchial sputum surface tension. It may stimulate the cholinergic pathway and increase mucus secretion from the airway submucosal glands. It may offer some symptomatic relief in the treatment of cough. However, guaifenesin has not been shown to be clinically effective in randomised controlled trials.

IODIDE-CONTAINING COMPOUNDS: Iodides promote the secretion of airway fluid and have been used as expectorants in the past. Potassium iodide which has a reputation for liquefying the thick, viscid fluid probably acts both directly and reflexly. However, due to their potential toxicity they are not commonly used.

It is generally advocated in productive cough associated with chronic bronchitis, asthma and emphysema. It is administered orally in a dose of 300 mg thrice daily in mixture form. The mixture has a slightly bitter saline taste.

Potassium iodide can cause symptoms of iodism, characterised by nasal catarrh, conjunctival swelling, oedema of eyelids, lacrimation, oedema of the larynx, headache and various types of skin rashes. Chronic administration occasionally gives rise to goitre. It should be avoided in children and pregnant women.

VASICINE

The active alkaloid, **vasicine,** and its derivative **vasicinone,** from the leaves of *Adhatoda vasaca*, possess weak bronchodilator, expectorant and mucolytic properties. The **aqueous extract of leaves** of this plant has been used in India as an Ayurvedic medicine for the treatment of cough since ancient times. It appears to be safe and effective. PH 1.33

Mucolytics

These drugs make the sputum thin and less viscid, so that it can be easily expectorated. They are of two types – 'classic mucolytics' which depolymerise mucin glycoproteins and 'peptide mucolytics' that depolymerise DNA and F-actin polymer networks.

Many patients with chest disease become dehydrated, and adequate hydration along with steam inhalation or aerosolised water inhalation can help to liquefy the viscid sputum. **Finally, oxygen should never be administered without adequate humidification as dry oxygen causes the drying of the respiratory mucosa** (Chapter 75).

N-ACETYLCYSTEINE: This classic mucolytic is a derivative of a naturally occurring amino acid, 1-cysteine. Apart from, mucolytic properties it has antioxidant and anti-inflammatory properties. It is used for the treatment of COPD and cystic fibrosis. *It acts by hydrolyzing the disulfide bonds that link the mucin monomers depolymerizes the mucin glycoprotein oligomers.* It has antiinflammatory, antioxidant and antibiofilm properties. Clinically, 2mL of a 10% solution is nebulised into a face mask every 8 h for 5–10 days to liquefy viscous tracheobronchial secretions. It can also be administered by direct instillation into the tracheobronchial tree through a tracheostomy.

Adverse reactions include bronchospasm, fever, nausea, vomiting, stomatitis, rhinorrhoea and haemoptysis.

Carbocysteine and **methylcysteine** have similar properties as acetylcysteine. They can be given orally or by inhalation.

Dornase alpha: This phosphorylated, glycosylated, recombinant, human deoxyribonuclease (proteolytic enzyme) is a peptide mucolytic. It acts by breaking down the highly polymerised DNA released by degenerating neutrophils in purulent sputum. When administered by nebulization it decreases the viscosity and adhesiveness of infected sputum and modestly improves lung function in patients with cystic fibrosis. However, its cost and lack of evidence for benefit in the patients without cystic fibrosis, limits its use.

Mucokinetics

BROMHEXINE: This is a synthetic benzylamine derivative of alkaloid vasicine obtained from the plant *Adhatoda vasaca*. The mechanism of action of bromhexine is incompletely explored. *It reduces the viscosity of sputum by dissolving mucopolysaccharide fibres. It improves the mucociliary clearance and reduce cough.* It is given orally, parenterally and by inhalation. It is usually administered in doses of 8–16 mg thrice daily. Adverse reactions are mild and infrequent and include GI side effects and headache. It can be combined with bronchodilators.

AMBROXOL: This active metabolite of bromhexine is used orally (15 mg t.i.d.) as an alternative to bromhexine.

Bronchodilators: See Chapter 27

Surfactants: See Chapter 27 PH 1.33

CENTRAL COUGH SUPPRESSANTS

These drugs inhibit the cough reflex by *directly suppressing the cough centre in the medulla and are useful in the symptomatic relief of dry irritant cough.* They are only partially successful in suppressing cough due to carinal irritation. They are invaluable in the treatment of cough due to pleural diseases. Cough suppressants are particularly useful when complications of severe cough, such as rib fracture or cough syncope, produce discomfort. They should be avoided in patients with productive cough. *In general, cough suppressants do not impair voluntary coughing to clear secretions. They are not recommended in young children, particularly those younger than 2 years.*

CODEINE: This opium alkaloid, like morphine, depresses the cough centre but is less constipating. Its analgesic effect is useful if the cough is associated with pain. Similarly, the sedative effects are useful in apprehensive individuals having cough due to central stimuli.

A commonly employed preparation is linctus codeine which contains 15 mg of codeine phosphate in 5 mL (dose: 5 mL by mouth) and recommended doses are 15 mg-60 mg every 4-6 hours with the maximum of 300 mg/day.

It is a relatively safe drug, and its only bothersome adverse effect is constipation. But it can cause drowsiness, nausea and vomiting. *Codeine preparations are not recommended in children.*

Tolerance is not common, and drug dependence is rare at doses used for antitussive effects. However, codeine cough syrup abuse has been reported. Chronic administration at high doses or mixing cough syrup with alcohol can result in addiction.

Codeine is unlikely to be effective in the distressful cough of terminal lung cancer. In that condition, **diamorphine** linctus (3 mg/5 mL) in the dose of 2.5–10 mL every 4 h or **methadone** linctus (2 mg/5 mL) in the dose of 2.5–5 mL every 4 h is likely to be effective.

With several opioids, the dose required to suppress cough is lower than the analgesic dose.

DEXTROMETHORPHAN HYDROBROMIDE: It is the d-isomer of codeine analogue, methorphan. However, it does not act through the opioid receptors and has no analgesic or sedative property. *This has led to the belief that distinct receptors (other than the usual opioid receptors) mediate the antitussive action of opioids. It acts centrally to elevate the threshold for coughing.* It is as effective as codeine and is much safer; hence, it is commonly used in paediatric practice, though not for children below the age of 4 years. It does not depress respiration in the usual doses.

It can sometimes cause excitement, irritability and confusion (adult dose: 10–20 mg every 6–8 h (maximum 120 mg/day). The most important ADR is drug abuse. As it is readily available and relatively affordable, it can be misused for recreational purpose. Its active metabolite, dextrorphan is a noncompetitive NMDA receptor antagonist. Thus it will produce effects similar to ketamine and phencyclidine. Taken in a high dose it can induce psychotic state.

Laevopropoxyphene mesylate: This laevo-isomer of dextropropoxyphene, in the dose of 50–100 mg, appears to be as effective as an antitussive as 30 mg of dextropropoxyphene. It has no analgesic activity.

Pholcodeine, though related to opioids, has no opioid-like action. It is as effective as codeine as a cough suppressant, with a longer duration of action. It is nonsedating and nonaddicting. It is a common constituent of OTC cough mixtures.

NOSCAPINE: This opium alkaloid, belonging to the benzylisoquinoline group, is a **smooth muscle relaxant** such as papaverine. Its antitussive action is approximately equal to that of codeine. It does not produce constipation or drowsiness. Addiction does not occur. Sometimes it causes nausea. The antitussive dose is 15–30 mg 3–4 times a day. *Large doses can cause bronchospasm and hypotension due to histamine release.*

The **other synthetic compounds** used include oxeladine, pipezethate and piperidone. There is no convincing evidence about their superiority over codeine. *All cough suppressants are dangerous in the presence of excessive secretions, as failure to expel them may produce mechanical obstruction and atelectasis of the lung. They are also contraindicated in the presence of respiratory failure.*

PERIPHERAL COUGH SUPPRESSANTS

Benzonatate, chemically related to procaine, probably *acts on the stretch and cough receptors in the lungs. It also possesses some central action* and can cause sedation and headache. It is not recommended for those who are younger than 10 years.

Laevodropropizine and **moguisteine** are other nonopioid antitussives. The mechanism of action and uses of the former are similar to those of benzonatate; the mechanism of action of moguisteine remains to be elucidated.

Lignocaine, a local anaesthetic, in nebulised form is used for suppressing cough during pharyngeal examination, bronchoscopy and persistent cough in bronchial carcinoma.

OTHER ANTITUSSIVES

Cough may be the only symptom of bronchial hyperresponsiveness, including asthma. **Bronchodilators** are useful in these cases, as bronchospasm aggravates and may even initiate cough. The drugs commonly used are **salbutamol** and **orciprenaline**, usually given by inhalation (Chapter 27).

An **inhaled glucocorticoid** (Chapter 27) may be prescribed for *a short period* (2–3 weeks) for symptomatic treatment of persistent cough following a viral respiratory infection.

Therapeutic usefulness of **antihistaminics** as antitussives is limited to the cases where cough is due to conditions associated with postnasal drip. *They are of little value in allergic bronchospasm and may even have a deleterious effect because of their drying effect on the bronchial secretion.* Antihistaminics with a sedative action (e.g. diphenhyramine) may be useful in children who do not sleep because of cough provided no contraindication to their use (such as bronchial pathology) exists. *However, antihistaminics may occasionally cause paradoxical excitement.*

Sympathomimetic decongestants (Chapter 18) present in some cough mixtures can cause nervousness, insomnia, hallucinations, hypertension and dystonic reactions. *Some commercially available preparations promoted for cough and cold contain* **phenylpropanolamine** (PPA). *However, the use of PPA in cough mixtures has been banned as it may cause haemorrhagic stroke.*

LICORICE (*Glycyrrhiza glabra* L.), known as *Yashtimadhu* (or *Jeshtamadha* in Marathi) is widely used in traditional systems of medicine for treatment of cough and cold. The antitussive effects depend on both peripheral and central mechanisms.

The major active **phytoingredient** is **glycyrrhizin** (glycyrrhizic acid; glycyrrhizinate), which constitutes 10–25% of licorice root extract. *Glycyrrhizin is a triterpene glycoside with structural similarity to the adrenal steroids.* Excess consumption/ long term usage of licorice can lead to the classic symptoms of sodium and water retention with edema, potassium loss, hypertension, and muscular weakness. The deglycyrrhizinated form (DGL) is most often used to avoid these ADR. Licorice and DGL have a mild laxative effect and can protect the intestinal lining by increasing the production of mucus, thus alleviating heartburn and ulcers.

PHARMACOTHERAPY OF COUGH

Definitive treatment of cough depends on its cause which should be treated. *Mild acute cough generally does not need drugs.* The commonest cause of cough is common cold, which usually clears within 7 days and may not need active treatment. Only when cough serves no useful purpose and causes insomnia, or interferes with daily work and sleep, symptomatic treatment is indicated.

In case of productive cough, the patient should be encouraged to cough voluntarily in appropriate posture at regular intervals. Since inflamed trachea or bronchi are irritated by cold or dry air, a warm room with humid atmosphere is beneficial. Many patients with cough feel comfortable after a cup of warm tea or even warm water. Similarly, *simple steam inhalation with or without tincture benzoin, menthol or eucalyptus oil effectively liquefies tenacious respiratory tract secretions* (hydroponic therapy). Expectorants and mucolytics are prescribed for symptomatic management of productive cough.

Barking cough, stridor and chest wall withdrawal are characteristics of **croup**, which is common in children. Cough becomes worse at night. **Nebulised budesonide** or oral/IM **dexamethasone** (0.2–0.6 mg/kg, single dose) gives dramatic relief. Nebulised adrenaline gives immediate but short-lived relief. PH 1.33

It must be remembered that cough serves the useful purpose of clearing the respiratory tract. It should not be severely obtunded in patients with productive cough. Use of antitussives in sedated or debilitated patients may prove dangerous. They should be used cautiously in the acute phase of pertussis and bronchial asthma, as inspissation of mucus plugs may contribute to a fatal outcome. *Finally, cough suppressants, especially in a syrupy base, should be kept out of the reach of small children, as poisoning with them has been reported.*

Cough remedies: Most of the proprietary preparations available as 'cough remedies' generally contain a central cough suppressant, an expectorant, an antihistaminic, a bronchodilator and a decongestant in a pleasantly flavoured syrupy base. *Such drug combinations are considered irrational as they can dry up the secretions, prevent natural drainage, cause drowsiness and suppress cough, a protective reflex that helps to get rid of infective material. However, they have attractive colour and are pleasant to take. Moreover, they are heavily promoted,* which may distract a physician from thinking logically about their composition. Remember, they are expensive.

Chronic cough hypersensitivity syndrome is characterised by refractory cough not responding to conventional antitussives. It is believed to be due to cough hypersensitivity, abnormal laryngeal and pharyngeal sensations, allotussia and urge to cough. **Gabapentin** which inhibits central sensitisation has been claimed to help some patients with chronic cough syndrome.

DRUGS USED IN THE SYMPTOMATIC TREATMENT OF COUGH

Pharyngeal demulcents and local sialogogues

Syrups
Linctuses

Mucoactive drugs

Expectorants: Hypertonic saline, Guaifenesin, Potassium iodide, Vasicine

Mucolytics: N-acetylcysteine, Carbocysteine, Methylcysteine, Dornase alpha

Mucokinetics: Bromhexine, Ambroxol, Bronchodilators, Surfactants

Mucoregulators: Carbocysteine, Anticholinergics

Central cough suppressants

Opioids and related drugs

Codeine
Dextromethorphan
Pholcodeine
Levopropoxyphene
Noscapine

Nonopioids

Caramiphene
Pipezethate

Antihistaminics

Diphenhydramine
Chlorcyclizine

Peripherally acting compounds

Local anaesthetics

Benzonatate
Laevodropropizine
Lignocaine (nebulized)

CHAPTER 27

Pharmacotherapy of Bronchial Asthma, COPD and Rhinitis

Learning Objectives

This chapter will enable the reader:

1. To describe the pathophysiology of bronchial asthma, stating various clinical presentations of asthma.
2. To state the principles of therapy.
3. To classify drugs according to their mechanism of action.
4. To outline the pharmacotherapy of (a) acute attack of asthma, (b) prevention of acute attack, (c) chronic persistent asthma and (d) severe acute asthma (status asthmaticus) giving rationale for selected drug/s.
5. Describe ADR of the following drugs used in bronchial asthma: beta-2 agonists, methyl xanthines, glucocorticoids, anticholinergics, mast cell stabilisers, LT_1 receptor antagonists and omalizumab.
6. Enlist various inhalational steroids and state their advantages and limitations.
7. Outline the management of COPD.
8. Explain the rationale for use of surfactants in respiratory distress syndrome.
9. Explain the pharmacological basis for use of antibiotics, antihistaminics, nasal decongestants, anticholinergic drugs, topical glucocorticoids and immunotherapy in treatment of rhinitis.

KEY TERMS

bronchial hyper-responsiveness, p. 384
metered dose inhalation, p. 385
salbutamol, p. 386
long-acting beta agonists, p. 387
inhaled glucocorticoids, p. 389
bronchial asthma, clinical presentation, p. 392
asthma, step-wise management, p. 393
asthma exacerbation, therapy, p. 393
severe uncontrolled asthma, management, p. 393
biologicals in asthma, p. 394
COPD, treatment, p. 396
surfactants, p. 398
rhinitis, treatment, p. 398
allergic rhinitis, immunotherapy, p. 400

Bronchial asthma is a heterogenous group of conditions, which affects people worldwide, from infancy to old age. It is a clinical syndrome characterised by recurrent cough/paroxysmal dyspnoea, chest tightness and wheeze *due to increased resistance to air flow through the narrowed bronchi.* This narrowing is brought about by:

- *Bronchial hyper-reactivity and bronchospasm.*
- *Cellular infiltration and oedema of the bronchial mucosa.*
- *Blockage of the bronchial lumen by inspissated mucus.*

The symptoms of airway resistance vary over time and intensity. The diagnosis of asthma is made in a patient with reversible obstructive airway disease by objective evidence of:

1. Variability in ventilatory function over time.
2. Improvement following bronchodilator treatment.

Pathophysiology

The aetiology of bronchial asthma is multifactorial: genetic, developmental, environmental, inflammatory and immunological. Its pathogenesis is complex and involves:

- *Inflammation* due to infiltration of eosinophils, mast cells and CD4 lymphocytes.
- *Mucus cell hyperplasia.*
- *Remodelling of the airways* with fibrosis.

The major role of Th2 (T-helper type 2) cells in pathogenesis of asthma is now recognised.

Many patients have had well-defined allergen

exposures which are partly or substantially responsible for the asthmatic inflammation. These patients (even the asymptomatic ones, with normal lung function have inflamed airways and infiltration with mast cells, eosinophils, basophils, macrophages and activated helper T lymphocytes. *Lymphocyte-directed eosinophilic bronchitis is the hallmark of asthma.* Subacute mucosal inflammation and disruption of the protective epithelial barrier on the mucosal surface contribute to **bronchial hyper-responsiveness**, an exaggerated response to a variety of stimuli (asthmatic diathesis). *This inflammation is clinically silent with no apparent bronchoconstriction during the basal state of the disease.*

Exposure to an antigen causes cross-linking of IgE bound to the surface of mast cells and renders them more sensitive to reactivation (Fig. 27.1). A clinical acute attack is produced when the concerned antigen binds to the mast cell which gets activated and degranulated, with the release of histamine and various cytokines. This causes immediate bronchial

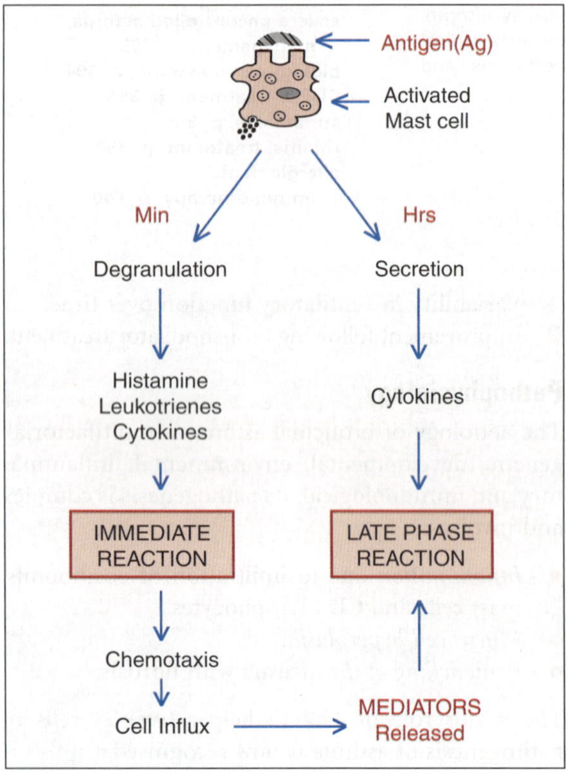

FIG. 27.1 Mast cell–dependent immediate and late phase reactions.

Box 27.1 Some Important Mediators Released by Mast Cells and Leucocytes

- ***From granules***
  Histamine, heparin
  Tryptase, chymotrypsin, proteases
- ***From membrane lipids***
  Sulfidopeptide leukotrienes,
  Prostaglandins, PAF
- ***Proinflammatory cytokines***
  TNF-α and interleukins 3, 4, 5 and 13

reactions (**early reaction**), leading to bronchospasm, local vasodilatation, increased capillary permeability, oedema and chemotaxis, with consequent influx of more inflammatory cells into the walls of the bronchi. The newly arrived cells release inflammatory mediators such as PG and LT which aggravate the airway inflammation and cause more sustained bronchoconstriction (**late phase reaction**). *The final common pathway for a clinical attack of asthma is the release of various mediators (Box 27.1) from a variety of inflammatory cells.*

An attack may also be triggered by factors like viral infection, irritants like dust, air pollutants, cold air, exercise, drugs and chemicals.

Majority of asthmatics (80%) are **atopic**, forming IgE antibody on exposure to common environmental allergens, house dust, mites, cockroaches, pets, pollen and so on. In such atopic subjects, challenge of the airways with allergens to which they are specifically sensitive triggers early and late phases of bronchoconstriction. *Mast cells are important in the acute airway response to an allergen and also contribute to their remodelling in chronic asthma.*

The **early reaction** is rapid in onset, reaching the maximum in 15–30 min after the challenge and recovering over the next 24 h.

Late-phase bronchoconstriction response begins 4–6 h after the challenge and lasts for up to 24 h. During this late (but not early) phase reaction, there occurs influx of neutrophils, eosinophils and macrophages into the airways, which suggests their role in the pathogenesis of this reaction. The acute inflammatory response usually resolves with the repair process, restoring the normal lung structure and function.

In **chronic asthma**, the recovery is incomplete, which leads to remodelling of the airway structure. Persistent epithelial damage exposes the deeper airway structures to further insults and promote persistent inflammation and cellular infiltration. Various mediators released cause angiogenesis, smooth muscle proliferation, fibrosis and airways thickening, causing a persistent obstruction to airflow.

Asthma is considered as:

- **Extrinsic**, when it is associated with history of atopy in the patient's childhood, a family history of allergies, illnesses such as hay fever, positive skin tests and raised serum IgE level. This is the commonest form.
- **Intrinsic**, when it occurs in middle-aged subjects with no family history of allergies, and clinically assumes a **'chronic form'**; there is a lack of identifiable allergen; serum IgE is not raised. However, an allergic factor may be involved in many cases of intrinsic asthma as well.

Currently, based on molecular phenotyping, asthma can also be classified as follows:

1. Th2 high phenotype (early-onset allergic asthma and late-onset eosinophilic asthma)
2. Th2 low phenotype (Obesity-related asthma and neutrophilic adult-onset asthma)

Irrespective of the type of asthma, persistent bronchial narrowing causes hyperinflation of the alveoli and disruption of alveolar walls with loss of elastic tissue (emphysema-like picture). PH 1.32, CT 2.16

Classification of Antiasthmatics

I. **Relievers:** These drugs are used to relieve the acute attack, as they produce **bronchodilatation**. They are:
   - **Selective beta-2 adrenergic receptor agonists:**
     i. *Short acting,* e.g. salbutamol, isoetharine, bitolterol (a prodrug), fenoterol, rimeterol
     ii. *Long acting,* e.g. formoterol, arformoterol
   - **Nonselective beta adrenergic agonists:** orciprenaline, adrenaline, ephedrine
   - **Phosphodiesterase inhibitors:** Theophylline derivatives – aminophylline.
   - **Anticholinergics:** Ipratropium bromide, tiotropium, aclidinium

II. **Controllers:** These drugs are used to control the inflammation (anti-inflammatory) and prevent the occurrence of acute attacks. They are further classified as:
   - **Glucocorticoids + Long-acting selective beta-2 adrenergic receptor agonists:** e.g., Budesonide + formoterol
   - **Glucocorticoids** e.g. inhaled corticosteroids (ICS)
   - **Leukotriene (LT) modifiers:**
     i. *LT receptor antagonists:* Montelukast and zafirlukast
     ii. *LT synthesis inhibitors:* Zileuton
   - **Mast cell stabilisers:** Sodium cromoglycate, nedocromil
   - **PAF antagonists:** Ketotifen
   - **Anti-IgE antibody:** Omalizumab

As the pathophysiology of asthma is restricted to the airways, direct, local delivery of drugs to the airways is the preferred method of administration. This route is convenient, rapid in onset, effective and reduces the systemic toxicity.

Inhalational Devices

These can be divided into four main groups:

- Pressurised metered dose inhalers (**MDIs**).
- Breath-activated inhalers including MDIs and dry powder inhalers.
- Inhalers with spacer devices.
- Nebulisers.

The **MDI** contains a canister which has pressurised inactive gas (drug). On pressing the canister a fixed dose of medicine is propelled out in each 'puff'. This type of inhaler is quick to use, small, and convenient to carry. It needs good co-ordination to press the canister and breathe in fully at the same time. The technique of using a MDI is described in Box 27.2.

Breath-activated inhalers are alternatives to the standard MDI. Some are still pressurised MDIs, but do not require the canister to be pressed. The other

Box 27.2 Technique of Using a Pressurised Inhaler-MDI

- Remove the cap. Hold the inhaler upright.
- Check whether the mouth piece is free of any foreign object
- Shake the inhaler.
- Instruct patient to tilt head back slightly, sit upright and breathe out normally away from the inhaler.
- Place the mouth piece into patient's mouth; tell him/her to close lips around it to form a good seal.
- Instruct the patient to press down on the canister firmly as he/she starts to breathe in slowly. (Press down until the medicine is released.)
- Tell the patient to breathe in slowly and deeply for a count of 3 to 5 seconds.
- Instruct the patient to hold his/her breath for 10 seconds or long as possible.
- While holding breath remove inhaler from the mouth.
- Breathe out gently away from inhaler.
- If more puffs are prescribed, repeat the next puff after 1-2 mins
- Replace the mouth piece cap.
- Advise the patient to rinse and gargle with water after using any steroid inhaler.

breath-activated inhalers include **dry powder inhalers** (e.g. rotahalers). By breathing in at the mouthpiece, the dose is triggered to get propelled. However, breathe in should be forceful to get the powder into the lungs. Need for co-ordination is lesser than for the standard MDI.

Spacer devices are used with pressurised MDIs. The spacer is placed between the inhaler and the mouth and holds the drug like a reservoir when the inhaler is pressed. A valve at the mouth end ensures that the medicine is kept within the spacer until the patient breathes in. Spacer devices do not require co-ordination between pressing the canister and inspiration by the patient. They are preferred in children, elderly and those who are breathless and find such synchronisation difficult.

Nebulisers are machines that turn the liquid form of short-acting bronchodilators into a fine mist, like an aerosol. The nebuliser is connected to a face mask and patient breathes in the drug. This does not require any co-ordination and large doses can be administered. Nebulisers are used mainly in hospital for severe attacks of asthma.

Non-adherence to regular inhaled therapy and *faulty inhalation technique are important causes of treatment failure.* Patients who find the inhalation route inconvenient or difficult to follow are given oral drug therapy which invariably causes more systemic adverse effects.

With all the methods of local administration, only about 10%–30% of the administered drug reaches the desired site, the distal bronchial tree. The rest is swallowed but undergoes first pass metabolism, thus minimising the systemic adverse effects.

PH 1.32, CT 2.16

I. BRONCHODILATORS (RELIEVERS)

Selective Short Acting β_2 agonists (SABA)

These drugs cause quick relief from an acute attack are called **reliever or rescue drugs**.

SABA are the rescue drugs par excellence as both, airway smooth muscle and mast cells have β_2 adrenergic receptors. They:

- **Relax the smooth muscle of all airways** from trachea to the terminal bronchi, irrespective of the spasmogen involved. Therefore, they serve as **physiological antagonists**.
- **Enhance mucociliary clearance** from the respiratory tract.
- **Suppress microvascular leakage in the airway.**
- **Inhibit mediator release** from the mast cells and the basophils, **and cytokine release** from the inflammatory cells in the airway.
- **May inhibit release of ACh** from the postganglionic cholinergic nerves in the respiratory tract.

These drugs, however, do not inhibit either the late response to allergens or the subsequent bronchial hyper-responsiveness.

There is no evidence that one β_2 agonist is superior to others, except with regard to the duration of action. The choice depends on the convenience and the cost. **Salbutamol** is usually preferred and is the prototype of this class (Chapter 18).

SALBUTAMOL (Albuterol): It is a selective β_2 adrenergic agonist related chemically to isoprenaline (Chapter 18).

- *It has a prominent bronchodilator action of rapid onset* (1–5 min after inhalation).
- *It has a poor cardiac* (β_1 *receptor*) *action.* Hence, it causes less palpitation or a rise of blood pressure.
- *It is resistant to inactivation by COMT and, therefore, has a longer duration of action.* The effect of a single inhalation or a single oral dose lasts for about 4–6 h.

Methods of administration: It is more rapidly effective by **MDI** (dose 100 mcg/puff) than orally (dose 2–4 mg) as it reaches smaller bronchi. The dose must be prescribed clearly as 'so many puffs at a time and the maximum number of puffs per day'.

Salbutamol may also be administered by a **nebuliser** or by a **dry powder inhaler.**

It may also be given subcutaneously or intramuscularly in the dose of 0.5 mg every 4 h and intravenously slowly, in the dose of 0.25 mg at the rate of 5–10 mcg/minute. It is generally well tolerated. Larger doses can cause dose-dependent ADR such as tachycardia, tremor and anxiety.

It must be kept in mind that all beta-adrenergic agonists may cause hypokalaemia which can be aggravated by the concurrent use of theophylline and its derivatives, diuretics and glucocorticoids, and by hypoxemia.

Salbutamol is used on an 'as needed' basis in acute attack of asthma. In an acute attack, it must be administered in adequate doses such as 10–12 puffs in 1 h. Inadequate dosage is the cause of apparent 'non responsiveness'.

Levosalbutamol: It is not clinically superior to salbutamol either in efficacy or ADR.

Terbutaline, fenoterol, bitolterol, pirbuterol, tolubuterol and **rimiterol** are other selective SABA with similar properties as those of salbutamol. However, *the use of more potent* β_2 *agonist than salbutamol, such as fenoterol, has been associated with greater cardiac toxicity in patients with acute asthma.*

Indications

SABA are very effective for:

- Treating acute attacks.
- Prevention of exercise-induced asthma.

They are less useful when taken regularly, and may increase allergic response and airway inflammation. Hence they should be used only as needed. They are safe during pregnancy. Excessive use of β_2 *agonists has been associated with an increased risk of severe exacerbations and asthma deaths.* **Hence SABA only treatment should not be preferred.** *Low-dose inhaled glucocorticoid (LICS) should be advocated with it.*

- Treating wheezing following upper respiratory tract viral infection. In infants and children younger than 5 years, they are used orally in **syrup** form or by a nebuliser.

They may be less effective in some patients who use a beta blocker concurrently.

Selective Long Acting β_2 Agonist (LABA)

SALMETEROL is a **long-acting** β_2 partial adrenergic agonist, weaker than salbutamol. It is used as the drug of choice in the prevention of nocturnal asthmatic attacks and those induced by exercise. Its onset of action is slow (10–15 min), and the duration of action is long (12 h). *It is not useful in relieving acute attacks.* It is available in pressurised MDI delivering 25 mcg/puff. The dose is 1–2 puffs every 12 h. It should not be used more than twice a day.

Formoterol, an analogue, has quicker onset (3–5 min.) than and similar duration of action as salmeterol. As a result, its combination with a glucocorticoid, budesonide is preferred for dual effect, reliever and controller. It is used as a reliever if the patient is already using budesonide-formoterol or beclomethasone dipropoionate-formoterol combinations as controller.

These drugs are usually well tolerated, however they are never administered alone as tolerance may develop during long-term therapy resulting in severe exacerbation. *They are always used in combination with an inhaled glucocorticoid to reduce the incidence of fatal asthmatic attacks.*

Nonselective Beta Adrenergic Agonists

Adrenaline, orciprenaline and ephedrine were used extensively earlier as bronchodilators but they are not recommended now due to availability of selective and safe bronchodilators.

Phosphodiesterase Inhibitors

AMINOPHYLLINE: This is a stable mixture of theophylline and ethylene diamine; the latter makes theophylline more water soluble (Chapter 12). It can be given orally or slowly intravenously. It:

- **Causes bronchodilatation** by its weak and nonselective inhibition of pulmonary enzyme PDE-4.
- **Inhibits adenosine receptors** in the airways.
- **Inhibits the late response to allergens** but does not inhibit the release of mediators.
- **Acts synergistically with beta adrenergic agonists.**

It is less effective orally because though it is absorbed, it undergoes first pass metabolism.

Adverse reactions: Given rapidly intravenously, it may cause nausea, vomiting, cardiac arrhythmias and collapse. *Deaths have been reported following rapid IV aminophylline, particularly in the presence of cardiac damage.* Rapid IV administration can also cause twitching of the facial muscles, and seizures. The repeated use of theophylline in children may cause learning difficulties and sleep disturbances. Hepatic enzyme inhibitors, e.g. ciprofloxacin, erythromycin and OC (pills), can increase the plasma concentration of theophylline.

It is safer in hypoxic subjects in status asthmaticus, and in patients with a concomitant cardiac disease. *It is especially helpful when one cannot decide whether a given attack is one of bronchial or cardiac asthma.*

Preparations and dosage: Aminophylline is available as 100 mg, 225 mg, and 350 mg tablets and as 25 mg/ml IV injection. Theophylline is available as immediate or controlled release tablets in varying strengths.

Indications:

- **Acute attack of asthma:** If treatment with inhaled selective SABA in adequate doses fails to relieve an acute attack in about 1/2 to 1 h, **aminophylline** is administered by IV infusion in 5% glucose in a dose of 5 mg/kg over 15−30 min, followed by 0.5−1 mg/kg/h for several hours not exceeding 25 mg/min. The infusion rate should be lowered in patients with cirrhosis, pneumonia, acute viral infection and congestive heart failure and in patients receiving drugs which interfere with its metabolic degradation.
- **Adjunct therapy of asthma: Aminophylline** or **theophylline** has weak efficacy in asthma. Moreover they may not be tolerated orally in therapeutically effective doses (1 g daily in divided doses) because of nausea. Their major drawback is the variability in bioavailability. Hence they are not recommended for the treatment of asthma. However, these drugs are cheaper. Slow release preparations of theophylline e.g. **Deriphylline** (containing etofylline with theophylline modified release tablets) in the dose of 150−450 mg given in the evening may be useful as adjuncts in preventing nocturnal attacks.

If an acute asthmatic attack is not terminated within 2 h by the above measures, the patient should be treated as a case of severe acute asthma (status asthmaticus).

Anticholinergics: As the airways have parasympathetic innervation, atropine-like drugs can induce bronchodilatation and have been used as a remedy for bronchial asthma.

IPRATROPIUM BROMIDE is a **short acting muscarinic antagonist (SAMA).** Administered by inhalation in the dose of 1−2 puffs (40−80 mcg) t.i.d., it relieves bronchospasm in patients with chronic bronchitis, and in prolonged bronchial hyper-responsiveness following viral respiratory infections. It is the preferred drug in patients with COPD (see section, Management of COPD).

It has a slow onset of action (30 min) and lower efficacy than β_2 agonists in the management of acute attacks. **Hence, it is not recommended for acute attacks.** It is, however, useful in patients with a concomitant heart disease and those intolerant to β_2 agonists. A combination of ipratropium and a beta adrenergic agonist by inhalation produces additive effects because ipratropium acts on large and medium-sized bronchi, whereas β_2 agonist acts predominantly on the smaller bronchi. *It is also useful in asthmatic attack induced by β blockers.*

Oxitropium bromide and **tiotropium** bromide are other analogues with similar properties; tiotropium has a longer duration of action (**long acting muscarinic antagonist; LAMA**).

II. ANTI-INFLAMMATORY (CONTROLLERS)

GLUCOCORTICOIDS

Detailed pharmacology of glucocorticoids is given in the Chapter 64.

Inhalational corticosteroids (**ICS**) are the **first-line therapy** for asthma since chronic inflammation is important in its pathogenesis. Glucocorticoids suppress the inflammatory response and improve lung function at multiple levels. They are promptly effective in small doses and their systemic toxicity, including suppression of HPA axis is low. They do not cure the asthmatic inflammation. They:

- **Inhibit phospholipase A_2** and thereby reduce the cellular histamine and SRS-A content.
- **Reduce the microvascular leakage** due to the mediators, thereby decreasing mucosal oedema.
- **Inhibit the influx of inflammatory cells** into the lungs after exposure to an allergen.
- **Stabilise the cellular lysosomal membranes.**
- **Inhibit the release of mediators from the macrophages and the eosinophils** in the lungs. *Therefore, they are useful in blocking the late response and the consequent bronchial hyperresponsiveness.*
- **Reduce bronchial hyperactivity by** blocking expression of COX-2 and cytokines.
- **Prevent and reverse the downregulation of the β adrenergic receptors,** and thus maintain/restore the responsiveness of the airway smooth muscle to β_2 agonists.
- **Reduce the immediate response to allergens** and **prevent exercise-induced asthma** when administered for long duration.

Clinically, they reduce the frequency of acute attacks as well as interval symptoms, and thus improve the quality of life. Effective, long-term suppression of airway inflammation reduces the need for bronchodilators. Hence ICS containing regiments should be started once asthma is diagnosed. Many patients can be maintained on low dose ICS. Concurrent use of glucocorticoids and a LABA is beneficial in preventing asthmatic attacks.

Limitations of inhaled glucocorticoids

- Locally, they may cause sore throat, coughing, hoarseness and rarely candidiasis.
- Higher doses produce limited additional benefits
- They may cause neutrophilia and even increase blood glucose levels. A physician should be aware of these effects of inhalational glucocorticoids.
- Long-term use of high doses may cause systemic adverse effects such as skin bruising, osteoporosis, cataract, glaucoma, HPA axis suppression and growth retardation in children (Chapter 64).

Hence, once good control is obtained, attempt should be made to taper down the dose.

The macrolide antibiotics (erythromycin and clarithromycin) increase the half-life of glucocorticoids and theophylline in the body.

BECLOMETHASONE DIPROPIONATE: This halogenated glucocorticoid ester is used in an MDI which delivers 50 mcg/puff of the drug. The usual dose recommended is two puffs (200 mcg) 3–4 times a day. Suppression of the hypothalamo−pituitary axis, is not significant and this is its major advantage (Chapter 64).

BUDESONIDE: This drug is more potent than beclomethasone. Its major advantage is that it is effective in the dose of 1−2 puffs b.i.d.; this improves patient compliance.

Fluticasone has properties similar to those of budesonide. It is expensive.

Mometasone furoate is another glucocorticoid used as a powder for inhalation.

Table 27.1 lists the doses of inhaled steroids.

Table 27.1 Doses of Inhaled Steroids

Drug (Formulation) HFA	mcg/puff	Low Dose, mcg	High Dose, mcg/day, in Divided Doses
Beclomethasone (MDI, HFA)	100, 200, 250	200–500	>1000
Beclomethasone (MDI, ultrafine, HFA)	100, 200	100–200	> 400
Budesonide[a] (DPI)	100, 200, 400	200–400	> 800
Fluticasone (MDI, DPI)	50, 125, 250	100–250	> 500
Ciclesonide (MDI)	80, 160	80–160	> 320
Mometasone furoate (DPI)	30, 60, 120	110–220	> 400
Flunisolide (MDI)	250	500–1000	> 2000
Triamcinolone (MDI)	100	400–1000	> 2000

[a]Solution for nebulisation is also available.

Clinically, all the inhaled steroids are equally effective. They can cause localised infection with *Candida albicans* in the throat. This can be prevented by rinsing the mouth after every dose. It may interfere with the growth of lungs and other organs in young children. A flare-up of allergic rhinitis and nasal polyps has been reported on stopping the treatment. *Steroid inhalation alone is of no value in treating acute attacks.*

Leukotriene modifiers

Leukotrienes liberated during inflammation are more potent and longer acting bronchoconstrictors than histamine (Chapter 25). They increase bronchial secretion, decrease mucociliary clearance, and increase vascular permeability. Drugs can modify the leukotriene system by

- **Acting as competitive antagonist** on type-1 cysteinyl LT receptors, e.g. montelukast.
- **Blocking the leukotriene synthesis,** e.g. zileuton.

MONTELUKAST: This is a competitive and selective LT_1 receptor antagonist (LTRA). Its oral bioavailability is 60%–70% and t½ 3–6 h. It is highly protein bound and metabolised by the liver. It is moderately effective in asthma with once to twice daily administration. It is expensive.

Adverse reactions: These are mild, self-limited and include dyspepsia, headache, eosinophilia and raised liver enzymes. Recently a risk of neuropsychiatric events has been reported. The drug may rarely cause systemic vasculitis.

Therapeutic uses:

- **Aspirin-induced bronchospasm**
- **Cold-air-induced airway obstruction**
- **Exercise-induced bronchospasm**
- **Add on therapy in asthma**
- **Allergic rhinitis**

Pranlukast and **zafirlukast** are the analogues of montelukast. The latter can cause severe hepatitis and can interact with warfarin to enhance its effect.

Zileuton, a 5-lipoxygenase inhibitor, is as effective as montelukast. It is available only as extended release formulation.

Leukotriene modifiers have no bronchodilator action and cannot be used as rescue drugs. For prophylaxis, they are less effective than low-dose inhaled glucocorticoids, particularly for exacerbations. Combined use of glucocorticoids and leukotriene modifiers may permit a reduction in steroid dose (**steroid sparing role**). They can be used as an alternative to low-dose inhaled glucocorticoid therapy in mild asthma, and in children. Their main advantage is that they are effective orally and hence can be used as substitute for cromolyn. *Their use mandates periodic monitoring of hepatic function. Their superiority over the older drugs is not established*, and they are expensive. They should be used only in selected cases.

Disodium chromoglycate (cromolyn sodium)

This is the sodium salt of 1,3-bis-(2-carboxychromon-5-yloxy)-2 hydroxy propane (Fig. 27.2). It is useful in preventing attacks of bronchial asthma in selected cases.

Mechanism of action: The drug prevents mast cell and eosinophil activation by altering the function of the delayed chloride channels in the cell membrane.

Pharmacological actions:

- It inhibits the release of spasmogenic autacoids after combination of the antigen and antibody. In this respect, like glucocorticoids, it acts as an anti-inflammatory agent.
- It also prevents the early response to allergens and exercise, and the subsequent bronchial hyper-responsiveness.

The drug relieves coughing due to asthma. It has a few other significant pharmacological actions.

Absorption, fate and excretion: It is absorbed poorly after oral administration (0.5%) but is absorbed better after inhalation (5%). The absorbed portion is rapidly eliminated unchanged in urine and bile.

Adverse reactions: Except some local irritation, no serious toxicity has been observed.

Preparation and dosage: Disodium cromoglycate 20 mg capsules. It is given by inhalation, 3–4 times daily using a **spinhaler**. Its effect is enhanced when the patient's ventilation is improved by *prior* (but not simultaneous) inhalation of a beta stimulant. It is available as powder for nasal insufflation and as 2% aqueous eye drops and ointment.

Indications:

- **Allergic bronchial asthma:** When inhaled during a symptom-free interval, it protects against an attack for several hours in most patients with extrinsic asthma. It is, however, ineffective when used after the beginning of an attack.

  It is more beneficial in patients with clear evidence of allergic factors and in those with **exercise-induced bronchospasm**. A single dose taken 15−30 min before exercise may prevent an acute attack for 1−2 h. It helps to reduce the requirement of glucocorticoids and bronchodilators. Some patients have to take the drug for 3–4 weeks before they notice its beneficial effects.
- **Other respiratory allergies:** It has been used in allergic alveolitis and in allergic rhinitis.
- **Miscellaneous:** It may also be useful in the treatment of allergic conjunctivitis, aphthous stomatitis, ulcerative colitis, food allergy and systemic mastocytosis with variable results.

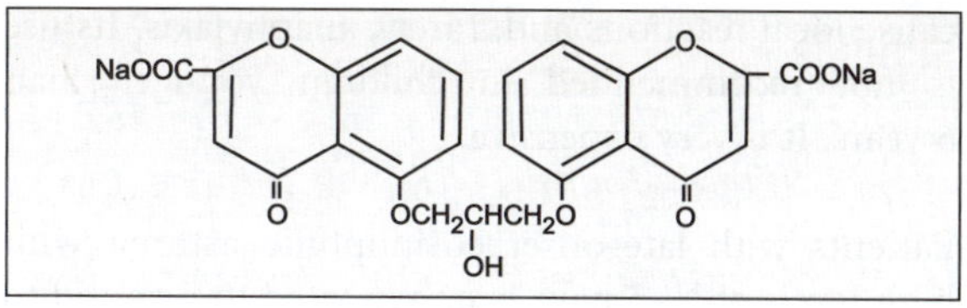

FIG. 27.2 Disodium cromoglycate.

Nedocromil sodium has properties similar to those of cromolyn but is effective orally. It also inhibits platelet activating factor (PAF). *Nedocromil and its analogues have now been largely superceded by low-dose inhaled glucocorticoids.*

PAF antagonist

KETOTIFEN, a H_1 receptor blocker, is claimed to be useful in asthma. It is believed to inhibit airway inflammation induced by PAF in primates. It can cause drowsiness. Its usefulness in asthma is equivocal.

Anti-IgE antibody

OMALIZUMAB: This is a recombinant, humanised anti-IgE monoclonal antibody (mAB). *It binds to IgE and prevents it from binding to IgE receptors on mast cells and basophils.* It thus prevents the allergic reaction at a very early step. It is administered as a single SC injection once in 2–4 weeks. The IgE−Ab complex is degraded in the liver; the elimination t½ is 26 days. *It is not a bronchodilator.*

In adults with allergic, moderate-to-severe persistent asthma, it reduces the dependence on glucocorticoids and decreases the frequency of asthma exacerbations. It may also be useful in seasonal allergic rhinitis and food allergy. It is generally well tolerated, but may cause local reactions and, rarely, anaphylaxis. Its use is not recommended in children younger than 6 years. It is very expensive.

Patients with late-onset eosinophilic asthma with high levels of IL-5 have been reported to respond to **mepolizumab,** a humanised mAB against IL-5. Other mAB for treatment of severe eosinophilic asthma are **reslizumab**, **benralizumab** (anti-L5 receptor antibody), and **dupilumab** (anti-IL-4 receptor antibody).

Other concurrent medications: Most chronic asthmatic patients have associated chronic bronchitis and lung damage. Such cases are treated by antibiotics whenever the sputum turns yellow or other signs of infection develop. Those prone to get repeated infections may need regular antimicrobial prophylaxis during winter or monsoon seasons.

> ***Antihistaminics** are not so useful in the treatment of asthma except in the presence of definite allergy.*

ASTHMA MANAGEMENT PH 1.1, CT 2.16

Earlier the asthma was classified as mild, moderate and severe asthma based on the presenting symptoms. Presently the terms 'mild, moderate and severe asthma' are redefined depending on the level of asthma control. *Asthma control is evaluated as ability of the prescribed drug/s to control symptoms and risk of adverse outcomes.* Thus, after starting the drug therapy, symptom control is reviewed after 4 weeks to check for presence of:

- Daytime asthma symptoms for more than a few minutes a day or more than once a week
- Activity limitation due to asthma
- SABA reliever medication needed more than once a week
- Night waking / coughing due to asthma

If drug/s can control all the above, then the asthma is considered as **well controlled.** If 1-2 of the above points are observed, then asthma is **partly controlled**, and if > 3 points persist, then asthma is labelled as **uncontrolled**.

Mild asthma is defined as asthma that is well controlled with as-needed ICS-formoterol, or with low dose ICS plus as-needed SABA.

Moderate asthma is defined as asthma that is well controlled with low or medium dose ICS-LABA.

Uncontrolled asthma includes one or more of the following:

- Poor symptom control (as evident from the above 4 points),
- Frequent exacerbations (≥2/year) requiring oral steroids,
- Serious exacerbations (≥1/year) requiring hospitalization.

Uncontrolled asthma can be classified as:

a. **Difficult-to-treat asthma:** When asthma is uncontrolled despite prescribing medium or high dose inhaled corticosteroids with a second controller (usually a LABA) or with maintenance oral steroids, or when asthma requires high dose treatment to maintain good symptom control and reduce the risk of exacerbations, one needs to check whether there are modifiable factors such as incorrect inhaler technique, poor adherence, smoking or comorbidities. If these factors are corrected, then the asthma gets controlled. This type of asthma is labelled as difficult to treat.
b. **Severe asthma** is defined as asthma that remains uncontrolled despite optimized treatment with high dose ICS-LABA. This implies that the inhaler technique / medication adherence / diagnosis of asthma / control of comorbidities (e.g. rhinosinusitis, GERD, obesity and obstructive sleep apnea) are all optimal, yet the patient is symptomatic. Also if the patient requires high dose ICS-LABA to prevent it from becoming uncontrolled, it is termed as severe asthma. *Thus the current definition of severe asthma is based on retrospective assessment, after at least 2–3 months of controller treatment received by the patient and not just by the clinical presentation as an acute exacerbation.*

Poor symptom control is burdensome to patients and increases the risk of exacerbations.

PHARMACOTHERAPY OF ASTHMA

It is directed to:

- Relieve bronchospasm
- Reduce bronchial inflammation and achieve good symptom control
- Prevent repeated attacks
- Minimize future risk of asthma-related mortality, persistent airflow limitation and adverse effects of treatment.

The medications for asthma are either:

- **Controller medications:** They usually have anti inflammatory / immunosuppressant action and are prescribed to all patients. They reduce airway inflammation, control symptoms, and reduce future risks such as exacerbations and related decline in lung function.
- **Reliever medications:** They are prescribed on an as-needed basis to relieve breakthrough symptoms, including worsening of asthma or exacerbations. They are also recommended for short-term prevention of exercise induced bronchoconstriction.

The initial choice of therapy depends on the clinical presentation of the patient as depicted in Table 27.2.

ICS + formoterol is the preferred drug regimen as patients have to use the same inhaler to relieve the acute attack and also as maintenance therapy, thus avoiding confusion (of using two different drug inhalers as controller and reliever) and ensuring better adherence. In addition, there is an evidence for reduction in risk of severe exacerbations, need for oral steroids, and hospitalizations with ICS + formoterol. The alternative treatment with **low dose ICS + SABA**, may be an option in countries where ICS-formoterol is not available / affordable. However, evidence for its efficacy and safety is weak. There may be difficulty of achieving good adherence, possibility of patient confusion and over-use of SABA alone.

Monitoring of therapy

Patient's response should be reviewed after 2–3 months, or earlier depending on clinical urgency to ensure that the patient uses the inhaler correctly and adheres to the treatment.

Depending on the worsening of symptoms, the drug treatment for the given patient will gradually be changed in a step-wise approach (Step 1-4 for treatment schedule as in Table 27.2).

As asthma symptom control is achieved and maintained for 2–3 months and lung function has reached a plateau, the drug treatment can be reduced without loss of asthma control (Step down from 4 to 1).

TREATMENT OF ACUTE EXACERBATION / ASTHMA FLARE

Exacerbations of asthma are episodes characterized by a progressive increase in symptoms of shortness of breath, cough, wheezing or chest tightness and progressive decrease in lung function, i.e. they represent a change from the patient's usual status that is sufficient to require a change in treatment. Exacerbations usually occur in response to exposure to a triggering factor (e.g. viral respiratory tract infection, allergen exposure, pollution, seasonal changes etc.) and/or poor adherence with controller medication.

If a patient who is prescribed as-needed combination of a low dose ICS+formoterol, experiences worsening of symptoms then doses of ICS+formoterol can be increased to a maximum of dose 72 mcg formoterol (for budesonide + formoterol). If there is no relief, then referral to a hospital is essential, wherein attempts are made to rapidly relieve airflow obstruction and hypoxemia, counteract the inflammatory pathophysiology, and prevent relapse. Refer Box 27.3 for management of the exacerbation in the hospital.

MANAGEMENT OF SEVERE UNCONTROLLED ASTHMA

There may be patients who despite taking regular and accurate treatment, may still worsen to severe uncontrolled asthma.

Table 27.2 Step-wise Management of Asthma

Step	Clinical Presentation	Description	Preferred Therapy	Alternate Therapy
1	**Infrequent asthma symptoms**	symptoms < twice a month and no risk factors for exacerbations, including no exacerbations in the last 12 months)	As-needed low dose ICS + formoterol combination MDI	Low dose ICS taken whenever SABA is taken, in combination or as separate inhalers
2)	**Presence of asthma symptoms**	Need for reliever ≥ twice a month	As-needed low dose ICS + formoterol combination MDI	Low dose ICS plus as-needed SABA. Before choosing this option, rule out non-adherence to daily ICS
3	**Troublesome asthma symptoms**	Symptoms on most days (4-5 days/week); or waking due to asthma once a week or more especially if risk factors exist	Low dose ICS-formoterol maintenance and reliever therapy (MART)	Low dose ICS-LABA with as-needed SABA OR Medium dose ICS plus as needed SABA. Consider likely adherence with daily maintenance treatment.
4	**Initial presentation is with severe uncontrolled asthma, or with an acute exacerbation**		Medium dose ICS-formoterol MART. A short course of oral glucocorticoids may be needed	Medium or high dose ICS-LABA with as-needed SABA. A short course of oral glucocorticoids may be needed. OR High dose ICS with as-needed SABA (Adherence is poor)

Adapted from GINA Guidelines 2023.

In these patients, in addition to Step 5 treatment, **LAMA** is added. If there is no improvement, then depending on the phenotypic assessment, **add-on biologic therapy** for severe asthma is indicated (Table 27.3).

Add-on azithromycin (500 mg three times a week for 6 months) can be considered after specialist referral (because of the potential for development of antibiotic resistance) for adult patients with persistent symptomatic asthma despite high dose ICS-LABA. Before prescribing azithromycin, sputum should be checked for atypical mycobacteria. ECG should be reviewed for QTc prolongation (and re-checked after 1 month on treatment). Patients may complain of diarrhoea and there is potential of developing antimicrobial resistance.

As a last resort, add-on low dose oral glucocorticoid (≤7.5 mg/day prednisone equivalent) therapy may be considered for some adults with severe asthma after exclusion of other contributory factors and when other add-on treatments including biologics are not available/ affordable. However the patient has to be counselled about the potential long term adverse effects of oral steroids.

Table 27.3 Biologicals in Severe Uncontrolled Asthma

Treatment Target	Drug	Recommended Route and Patients' age	Indications
Anti-IgE	Omalizumab	SC, ≥6 years	Allergic, moderate-to-severe persistent asthma
Anti-IL-5	Mepolizumab Reslizumab	SC, ≥6 years IV, ≥18 years	Severe eosinophilic asthma
Anti-IL-5 receptor blocker	Benralizumab	SC, ≥12 years	
Anti-IL-4 receptor α antagonist (binds to the IL-4 receptor α subunit)	Dupilumab	SC, ≥6 years	Severe eosinophilic/Type 2 asthma, or for adults or adolescents requiring treatment with maintenance oral steroids
Anti-thymic stromal lymphopoietin	Tezepelumab	SC, ≥12 years	Severe asthma

NON-PHARMACOLOGICAL THERAPY

Patient education focussing on inhaler technique and drug adherence are crucial in achieving asthma control, so also other non pharmacological strategies which supplement pharmacotherapy. These include:

- **Cessation of smoking** and avoiding environmental smoke exposure
- Performing **breathing** exercises.
- **Graded exercise training programme** to improve the sense of well-being and exercise tolerance. Patient must be counselled about prevention of breakthrough exercise-induced bronchoconstriction with use of SABA / low dose ICS-formoterol before exercise. Weight reduction is advisable for obese asthmatics.
- **Avoidance of medications that worsen asthma.** Refer Box 27.4. Beta blockers, which are used commonly to treat hypertension, angina, glaucoma, are contraindicated in patients with asthma. **Even the use of eye drops can cause fatal attacks.**
- Intake of healthy diet rich in fruits and vegetables.
- **Avoidance of indoor/outdoor allergens** (e.g.

Box 27.3 Treatment of acute exacerbation / asthma flare in hospital setting

- Correct dehydration and acidosis
- Humidified oxygen (50%–60%) by mask to maintain oxygen saturation at 93–95%
- Salbutamol (4–10 puffs every 20 minutes with MDI + spacer) for 1st hour. Thereafter, 4–10 puffs every 3–4 hours up to 6–10 puffs every 1–2 hours, or more often.
  - With moderate-severe exacerbations, initiate with both SABA and SAMA

  If no response,
  - IV Magnesium 2 g infusion over 20 minutes,
- High dose ICS within the first hour after presentation in patients not receiving systemic corticosteroids.

  Or

  Prednisolone 1 mg/kg/day orally (maximum 50 mg/day) for 5–7 days. IV hydrocortisone to those who are too dyspnoeic to swallow /vomiting/on non-invasive ventilation or intubation.
- Monitor serum K^+, arterial oxygen saturation
- Antibiotics for chest infection
- Exclude pneumothorax (X-ray chest)

If still poor response

- Shift to intensive care unit

On discharge

- Start controller medication on ICS+ LABA. If already on it prior to exacerbation, increase dose for the next 2–4 weeks. As-needed reliever medication continued.

Box 27.4 Some Drugs Known to Cause Bronchospasm

- Aspirin and other NSAIDs
- Beta adrenergic blockers
- Cholinergic drugs
- Quinine
- Morphine and other histamine liberators
- Sedatives
- Antihistaminics

house dust mite and/or pets especially for children or certain food products / chemicals. Allergen avoidance strategies are often complicated and expensive (see later section on hyposensitisation with immunotherapy), and there are no validated methods for identifying those who are likely to benefit.
- **Avoidance of occupational exposures, indoor / outdoor air pollution, emotional stress triggering factors and cold weather conditions.**

All these measures, when successful, enable the patient to live as normal a life as possible, including normal exercise tolerance, without experiencing severe adverse drug reactions. Box 27.5 depicts important points to remember about asthma management. PH 1.32, CT 2.16

Box 27.5 Points to Remember in Asthma

- Asthma is a heterogenous symptom complex.
- Each pattern with asthma should have a reliever inhaler along with ICS, even if the symptoms are infrequent to reduce the risk of serious exacerbation.
- Where symptoms of asthma persist in spite of low-dose inhaled glucocorticoids, add inhaled LABA instead of increasing the dose of inhaled glucocorticoids.
- High-dose inhaled glucocorticoids (more than 1500 mcg/day) increase the risk of its long-term toxicity.
- LABA are highly effective as prophylactics in exercise-induced and nocturnal asthma.
- Inhaled LABA should not be used as monotherapy but combined with inhaled glucocorticoids for long-term treatment.
- Oral aminophylline is much less effective than inhaled glucocorticoids.

CHRONIC OBSTRUCTIVE PULMONARY DISEASE (COPD)

COPD is a complex heterogeneous syndrome which results in a slow, albeit progressive loss of lung function due to chronic inflammation of the small airways and lung parenchymatous tissue. The risk factors are smoking, indoor air pollution, biomass fuel and occupational exposure. It is a major cause of mortality and morbidity all over the world. Often asthma coexists with COPD.

COPD is characterised by **'air flow resistance that is not reversible'.** It includes the following:

- **Emphysema,** an anatomically defined entity associated with enlarged and distorted lung alveoli.
- **Chronic bronchitis,** a clinical entity associated with diseases of small bronchioles with a chronic airflow obstruction, chronic cough and marked expectoration.

Chronic bronchitis without airflow obstruction is not COPD and hence spirometry is essential to confirm the diagnosis of COPD.

The main physiological abnormality in COPD is an accelerated rate of **decrease in the forced expiratory volume** (FEV_1) compared to normal individuals. There is hyperinflation which is present at rest and worsens on exercise, increasing the work of breathing. The **CO_2 diffusing capacity decreases** with the resultant hypoxemia. The situation becomes worse with comorbidities such as cardiovascular diseases.

An exacerbation of COPD can be defined as 'an event in the natural course of the chronic disease, characterised by increase in the baseline **dyspnoea, cough and mucopurulent sputum** beyond the normal variation'. It is usually triggered by bacteria, viruses and pollutants. The most common viruses are rhinovirus, coronavirus and influenza virus. In COPD, the lungs have lower airway bacterial colonisation, mainly by *Haemophilus influenzae, Moraxella catarrhalis, Streptococcus pneumoniae, Haemophilus parainfluenzae and Pseudomonas aeruginosa.* **Purulent sputum is a reliable marker for bacterial infection.**

PHARMACOTHERAPY OF COPD

The current therapy of COPD includes the following:

- **Inhaled bronchodilators** (β_2 agonists, anticholinergics)
- **Inhaled glucocorticoids**
- **Oxygen inhalation**
- **Prophylactic antibiotics**
- **Mucolytics**
- **Preventation of dehydration**

Table 27.4 Bronchodilator Regimens in COPD PH 1.32

Drug	Duration of Action (h)	Dose
Short Acting		
Salbutamol sulphate	4–6	2 puffs every 4 h (MDI 100 mcg/puff)
Ipratropium bromide	4–6	2 puffs every 4 h (MDI 20 mcg/puff)
Long acting		
Formoterol fumarate	8–12	One inhalation twice a day (DPI 12 mcg/inhalation)
Salmeterol xinafoate	8–12	One inhalation twice a day (DPI 50 mcg/inhalation)
Arformoterol	8–12	One nebulisation, 15 mcg twice a day
Aclidinium	12	One inhalation twice a day (DPI 400 mcg/inhalation)
Indacaterol	24	One inhalation once a day (DPI 75 mcg/inhalation)
Olodaterol	24	Two inhalations once a day (DPI 2.5 mcg/inhalation)
Umeclidinium	24	One inhalation once a day (DPI 62.5 mcg/inhalation)
Tiotropium bromide	>24	One inhalation once a day (DPI 18 mcg/inhalation)
Roflumilast	24	1 tablet per day (500 mcg) orally
Long-acting combinations: Steroids + beta-2 agonist		
Budesonide + formoterol	12	Two inhalations twice a day (MDI 160 mcg budesonide + 4.5 mcg formoterol/inhalation)
Fluticasone + salmeterol	12	Two inhalations twice a day (MDI 45, 115, 230 mcg fluticasone + 21 mcg salmeterol/inhalation)
Mometasone + formoterol	12	Two inhalations twice a day (MDI 100, 200 mcg mometasone + 5 mcg formoterol/inhalation)
Fluticasone + vilanterol	24	One inhalation once a day (DPI 100 mcg fluticasone + 25 mcg vilanterol/inhalation)
Long-acting combinations: Anticholinergic + beta-2 agonist		
Umeclidinium + vilanterol	24	One inhalation once a day (DPI 62.5 mcg umeclidirum + 25 mcg vilanterol/inhalation)
Tiotropium + olodaterol	24	Two inhalations once a day (DPI 2.5 mcg tiotropium + 2. 5 mcg olodaterol/inhalation)
Long acting Triple drug combinations: Steroids + Anticholinergic + beta-2 agonist		
Fluticasone + Umeclidinium + Vilanterol	24	One inhalation once a day (DPI 100 mcg fluticasone + 62.5 mcg umeclidinium + 25 mcg vilanterol)
Beclometasone + Glycopyrronium + Formoterol	12	Two inhalations once a day (MDI 100, 200 mcg beclometasone + 10 mcg glycopyrronium + 6 mcg eformoterol)
Budesonide + Glycopyrrolate + Formoterol	12	Two inhalations once a day (MDI 160 mcg budesonide + 9 mcg glycopyrrolate + 4.8 mcg formoterol)

Notes: MDI, metered dose inhaler; DPI, dry powder inhaler.

- **Physiotherapy, pulmonary rehabilitation and education**

Inhaled bronchodilators are the mainstay of therapy, and any one of the regimens given in Table 27.4 may be used. However, long-term use of combination therapy with an **inhaled glucocorticoid** (fluticasone, budesonide) and a **LABA** (salmeterol) gives better benefits with acceptable side effects. Inhaled glucocorticoids probably help to reduce the number of exacerbations, but they alone do not substantially modify airway obstruction. LAMA alone or LABA/LAMA combination can also be used. However triple combination, ICS+ LABA + LAMA has been shown to improve lung function, symptoms and reduce exacerbations compared to dual combinations or monotherapy. Addition of **theophylline** may be beneficial in some subjects.

Intermittently inhaled oxygen improves long-term survival in COPD, and home oxygen therapy (HOT) should be used along with pulmonary rehabilitation. Severe cases may need **oral glucocorticoid therapy**.

For patients with very **severe COPD** associated with chronic bronchitis, a selective and long acting PDE-4 inhibitor with anti-inflammatory activity, **roflumilast**, has shown to improve lung function and reduce exacerbations when added to LABA. These effects are also seen in patients not controlled on ICS + LABA combination.

Antibacterial prophylaxis: Patients with mucopurulent sputum should be treated promptly with antibiotics. Prophylactic use of erythromycin (250 mg twice a day)/**azithromycin** for 1year has been reported to be useful in preventing exacerbation in subjects with mucopurulent sputum. Acute exacerbation must be treated with antibiotics and oral glucocorticoids, administered after giving optimum combination inhaled therapy.

Mucolytic agents e.g. **N-acetylcysteine, carbocysteine** or **erdosteine**, (Chapter 26) given regularly may reduce exacerbations.

In order to reduce severe illness due to lower respiratory tract infections and death in COPD patients, especially the elderly, it is advisable that they receive influenza, pneumococcal, Tdap, varicella and COVID-19 vaccines.

Respiratory irritants such as smoke, chemicals and dust must be avoided. *Giving up smoking provides definite benefit.* Treatment of comorbid CVS conditions with statins, ACEI/ARB and selective β blockers may reduce the overall mortality. Patient education and pulmonary rehabilitation are equally important.

SURFACTANTS AND THE RESPIRATORY DISTRESS SYNDROME

Surfactant is secreted by type II pneumocytes within the alveolar epithelium of the lungs into the alveolar lumen. It is a complex mixture of phospholipids, proteins and carbohydrates. By its local action, it:

- **Reduces surface tension within the alveoli** and thereby facilitates their aeration at lower ventilatory pressures; this increases the lung compliance and reduces the work of breathing.
- **Aids in keeping the alveoli dry** (anti-oedema action).
- **Enhances oxygenation of blood at lower intra-alveolar, partial oxygen pressure.**
- **May play a role in the immune defense system** of the lungs.

  The secretion of the surfactant is stimulated by cortisol, adrenergic agonists, cholinergic agonists and prostaglandins.

Deficiency of surfactant action is observed in the following:

a. Neonatal respiratory distress syndrome (neonatal RDS).
b. Adult respiratory distress syndrome (ARDS).

Preparations

i. **Calfactant** and **beractant**, bovine-lung derived
ii. **Poractant alpha**, porcine-lung derived
iii. **Calfasceril**, recombinant

Adverse reactions: include bradycardia, hypotension and endotracheal tube blockage. Allergic reactions are rare.

Indications: Instillation of surfactant into the trachea of the newborns at risk of developing or already having RDS reduces the morbidity and mortality.

RHINITIS-DRUG THERAPY

Rhinitis, an inflammation of the nasal mucosa, can be

- **Noninfectious**, e.g. allergic rhinitis, which is frequently caused by seasonal allergy (e.g. hay fever, pollinosis) and leads to sneezing, nasal stuffiness, ocular pruritus, lacrimation and a postnasal drip. It can also be non allergic rhinitis without any infective origin due to pollution.
- **Infectious**, e.g. viral common cold and bacterial infection.

Chronic or nonseasonal rhinitis, often referred to as perennial rhinitis, results in daily episodes of rhinorrhoea, nasal congestion and sneezing that are present for several weeks during most months of the year.

It is caused by various allergic and nonallergic nasal disorders. It can be drug-induced. Long-term use of adrenergic blockers, cholinesterase inhibitors, estrogen preparations (including oral contraceptives) may cause chronic rhinitis. It can also be caused by the presence of a foreign body, nasal polyps, tumours and nasociliary disorders.

Non-pharmacological therapy: For all types of rhinitis is similar. Treat the cause if possible e.g. root cause of pollution should be investigated and dealt with. If not possible, them exposure to cigarette smoke, pollutants, allergens and other irritants should be avoided. In patients with pharyngitis, saline gargles, steam inhalation and warm mist therapy is helpful. Local instillation of hyperheated, humidified air directly into the nasal passages significantly relieves symptoms of allergic rhinitis. Nasal saline sprays and drops can be used to relieve nasal dryness and congestion. Nasal irrigation administered by squeeze bottle, or bulb syringe can help expel mucus and relieve congestion. The patient should drink plenty of fluids.

Drug therapy: No drug is likely to abolish the symptoms completely. In general,

- drugs are more effective in allergic rhinitis than in nonallergic forms and
- acute rhinitis responds more favourably than the chronic form.

The treatment is directed at preventing the release of inflammatory mediators such as histamine and leukotrienes, or blocking their effects. The drugs used are as follows:

- **Antihistaminics and antiallergic drugs (Chapter 23)**
- **Nasal decongestants (Chapter 18)**
- **Anticholinergic drugs (Chapter 20)**
- **Local corticosteroids (Chapter 64)**

The selection of drugs in individual patients depends upon whether it is noninfectious, allergic or infectious (common cold). The agents useful in the former, antihistaminics, cromolyn sodium and intranasal corticosteroids have little value in the latter. Nasal decongestants are beneficial in both. However, antibiotics should be reserved only for patients with bacterial infections.

Antihistaminics and antiallergic drugs: In allergic rhinitis, H_1 antihistaminics help to relieve rhinorrhoea, sneezing, nasal pruritus and conjunctivitis *but do not affect nasal congestion.* They are usually effective in seasonal allergic rhinitis when sneezing and rhinorrhoea predominate and oedema and congestion are minimal. A single daily dose of an antihistaminic with a long t½ taken at bedtime may relieve symptoms the following day. The nonsedating oral antihistaminics, such as cetirizine and loratadine, are preferred (Chapter 23) when sedation needs to be avoided.

Intranasal H_1 antihistaminics (e.g. azelastine, olopatadine) are equiefffficacious as their oral counterparts and they are more effective in relieving nasal congestion hence are recommended for initial treatment of intermittent allergic rhinitis symptoms. They have a more rapid onset of action than oral H_1 antihistaminics and intranasal corticosteroids.

Antiallergic drugs such as glucocorticoids and cromolyn sodium prevent the release of inflammatory mediators. Cromolyn sodium nasal spray is effective in preventing the symptoms of allergic rhinitis. It should be started 1-2 weeks before exposure to the allergen, and must be used 3-4 times daily. Intranasal cromolyn sodium is less effective than intranasal steroids.

Nasal decongestants: These synthetic alpha-adrenergic agonists (Chapter 18) when used locally by spray or as drops, constrict the dilated blood vessels in the mucosa of swollen turbinates and reduce oedema. The following drugs are commonly used:

- Ephedrine 0.5%
- Phenylephrine 0.25%
- Naphazoline 0.05%
- Oxymetazoline 0.05%
- Xylometazoline 0.05%

They provide temporary symptomatic relief in allergic rhinitis, common cold, acute rhinitis associated with other respiratory infections, nonallergic rhinitis with eosinophilic syndrome(NARES), sinusitis, and in acute otitis media with eustachian tube blockage. Addition of an intranasal decongestant for up to 4 weeks may be considered in patients with refractory nasal congestion that is unresponsive to an intranasal corticosteroid alone /intranasal antihistaminic+steroid combination. **Oral decongestants** (pseudophedrine) may be preferred when sinuses are involved (Chapter 18).

An oral decongestant can be used in combination with an oral H_1 -antihistaminic for acute relief of allergic rhinitis symptoms.

The most common adverse effects of the orally administered nasal decongestants (phenylephrine and pseudoephedrine) are insomnia and irritability. Topical decongestants sometimes cause local discomfort, stinging, burning, dryness of the mucosa. *Use of intranasal decongestants for more than 3-5 consecutive days is not recommended because of the risk of developing rhinitis medicamentosa (rebound nasal congestion). If rebound congestion develops then intranasal decongestant is replaced by intranasal steroids.*

Nasal decongestants are only palliative. Only a few drugs in very dilute solution are safe. *Ephedrine hydrochloride in isotonic saline, used as nasal drops, is also effective.* In infants and children, imidazole drugs such as naphazoline and tetrahydrozoline are known to cause disturbance of body temperature, CNS depression and even coma. *Hence, decongestants should be stored beyond the reach of children.*

Anticholinergic drugs: Rhinorrhoea occurs due to glandular hypersecretion, mediated by the cholinergic innervation of the nasal mucosa. Some patients with severe rhinorrhoea and congestion obtain more relief from topical antimuscarinic, **ipratropium bromide,** than from nasal decongestants. Intranasal ipratropium does not relieve sneezing or nasal itching or congestion. Addition of ipratropium may be beneficial in patients with rhinorrhea that is not completely controlled with intranasal corticosteroid treatment.

Topical glucocorticoids exert a marked anti-inflammatory effect on the nasal mucosa by inhibiting the release of inflammatory mediators from the mast cells and basophils, and by blocking the inflammatory effect of leucocytes in the nose. *Intranasal glucocorticoids are safe, and are the most effective agents available for the prophylaxis and treatment of seasonal and nonseasonal allergic rhinitis.* Topical glucocorticoids occasionally shrink nasal polyps and reduce nasal obstruction significantly. Small polyps may even disappear.

The efficacy of nasal spray preparation of beclomethasone dipropionate, flunisolide, budesonide, ciclesonide, fluocortil butyl and fluticasone is similar. They are modestly effective in reducing ocular symptoms. The onset of action of these intranasal glucocorticoids is 12 h and duration of action is 12-24 h. The adverse effects include dryness, irritation, burning, bleeding of nasal mucosa, sore throat, and headache. Occasionally, intranasal / oropharyngeal fungal infections and increased intraocular pressure have also been reported.

A short course (5-7 days) of an oral corticosteroid may be needed in patients with severe allergic rhinitis or rhinitis medicamentosa who cannot tolerate or do not respond to other drugs.

Injudicious use of commercially promoted combinations of decongestants with antihistaminics, glucocorticoids and antibiotics may be hazardous and not recommended.

The oral leukotriene receptor antagonist, montelukast is indicated for treatment of seasonal and perennial allergic rhinitis, but it can cause increased risk of suicidal behavior and other neuropsychiatric events. Hence it is used only when other treatments have been ineffective or intolerable.

Hyposensitisation with Immunotherapy: This comprises carrying out skin tests with several antigens individually, followed by serial injections of desensitising immunotherapy prepared from the 'offending' allergens. The use of such immunotherapy may benefit patients of moderate / severe allergic rhinitis *who have specific IgE antibodies to clinically relevant allergens (for e.g.* pollens causing seasonal hay fever, wasp and bee venom). However,

- Most atopic (allergic) patients are allergic to multiple allergens and are not likely to benefit from immunotherapy prepared from single allergen.
- Diagnostic tests are unreliable, if used by themselves.
- The allergen extract based immunotherapy can precipitate either severe asthma or anaphylaxis.

Immunotherapy can alter the natural history of allergic respiratory disease and induce long-term remission. **Subcutaneous immunotherapy (SCIT)** can be formulated to contain all relevant allergens for an individual patient. Similarly **sublingual immunotherapy (SLIT)** is also available for treatment of allergic rhinitis, induced by grass pollen, ragweed pollen, and dust mites. SCIT has been in use for many years and is generally considered more effective.

Local adverse effects of SCIT include pain, redness, and swelling at the injection sites. Anaphylaxis and, very rarely, death can occur, especially in patients with uncontrolled asthma. SLIT can cause local adverse effects such as mouth pruritus and edema, throat irritation and occasionally systemic adverse effects like nausea and mild abdominal pain. Anaphylaxis is rare.

Immunotherapy should be administered under medical supervision. After gradual dose increments over a few months, maintenance injections/doses are continued at 2-4-week intervals for 3-5 years. As SLIT is less likely to cause severe systemic reactions than SCIT, and can be self-administered, it may be better accepted for maintenance.

ANTIASTHMATICS

Relievers

- **Selective beta-2 adrenergic receptor agonists**
  - *Short acting*: Salbutamol, Isoetharine, Bitolterol, Fenoterol, Rimeterol
  - *Long acting*: Formoterol, Arformoterol
- **Nonselective beta adrenergic agonists**: Orciprenaline, Adrenaline, Ephedrine
- **Phosphodiesterase inhibitors**: Aminophylline, Choline theophyllinate
- **Anticholinergics**: Ipratropium bromide, Tiotropium, Aclidinium

Controllers

- **Glucocorticoids+Long-acting selective beta-2 adrenergic receptor agonists**: Budesonide + Formoterol
- **Glucocorticoids**: Inhaled corticosteroids (ICS): Beclomethasone, Budesonide, Fluticasone, Ciclesonide, Mometasone furoate, Flunisolide, Triamcinolone
- **Leukotriene (LT) modifiers**
  - *LT receptor antagonists*: Montelukast, Zafirlukast
  - *LT synthesis inhibitors*: Zileuton
- **Mast cell stabilisers**: Sodium cromoglycate, Nedocromil
- **PAF antagonists**: Ketotifen
- **Anti-IgE antibody**: Omalizumab

7

SECTION

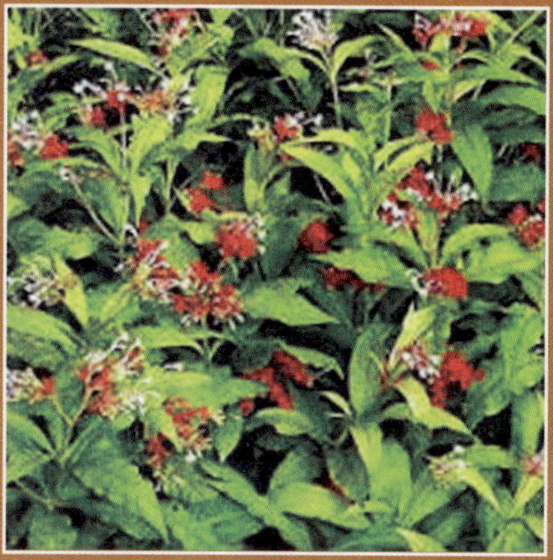
Rauwolfia serpentina

Cardiovascular Drugs

Section Outline

This section consists of the following chapters:

CHAPTER 28

Pharmacotherapy of Cardiac Arrhythmias

Learning Objectives

This chapter will enable the reader:

1. To be aware of electrophysiology of cardiac tissue.
2. To explain the mechanisms of cardiac arrhythmia.
3. To classify antiarrhythmic drugs based on mechanism of action giving examples of agents from each class.
4. To describe mechanism of action, pharmacological effects, ADR, indications and advantages of prototype drugs from each class.
5. To state the principles of therapy of arrhythmia.
6. To mention the appropriate drug/therapy of choice for
   a. sinus arrhythmia.
   b. premature beats.
   c. paroxysmal supraventricular tachycardia.
   d. paroxysmal ventricular tachycardia.
   e. ventricular fibrillation.
   f. digitalis induced arrhythmia.
   g. torsades de pointes.
7. To outline the management of atrial fibrillation.
8. To enumerate the agents which are used in the treatment of heart block giving rationale.

KEY TERMS

antifibrillatory and defibrillatory drugs, p. 405
automaticity, p. 407
excitability, p. 407
threshold potential, p. 407
conduction velocity, p. 407
disorders of impulse formation and conduction, p. 407
quinidine, p. 409
lignocaine, p. 412
propranolol, p. 414
amiodarone, p. 414
atrial fibrillation, treatment, p. 416
heart block, treatment, p. 418

Cardiac arrhythmia is defined as a disturbance of initiation or conduction of cardiac impulse. Most of us have occasional disturbances of cardiac rhythm which are transient and go unnoticed. Normal healthy heart, not genetically predisposed to arrhythmia, is resistant to such minor disturbances by triggers. However, sometimes arrhythmias can be symptomatic and even fatal.

Antiarrhythmic drugs are the drugs used to prevent or correct cardiac arrhythmias. The **antifibrillatory** drugs are compounds which prevent the development of atrial and/or ventricular fibrillation. The antifibrillatory drugs must be differentiated from the **defibrillatory drugs**, i.e. drugs capable of restoring normal sinus rhythm of the heart under atrial and/or ventricular fibrillation. Currently, no drug is available that can consistently restore normal rhythm to a fibrillating ventricle.

The cardiac cells (Fig. 28.1) are classified as follows:

1. **Excitable cells,** which include pacemakers such as sinoatrial node (SAN), conducting tissues such as atrioventricular node (AVN), bundle of His, bundle branches, Purkinje network and contractile myocytes. They constitute 30% of cardiac cells.
2. **Nonexcitable cells** (70%) form the extracellular matrix of collagen and elastin fibres; the latter decide the stretchability and stiffness of cardiac chambers, especially the left ventricular wall.

Electrophysiology of cardiac tissue: The excitable cardiac cell is bounded by a lipoprotein membrane which has *receptor channels* crossing it. These membrane channels permit passive movement of ions (Na^+, K^+, Ca^{++} and Cl^-)

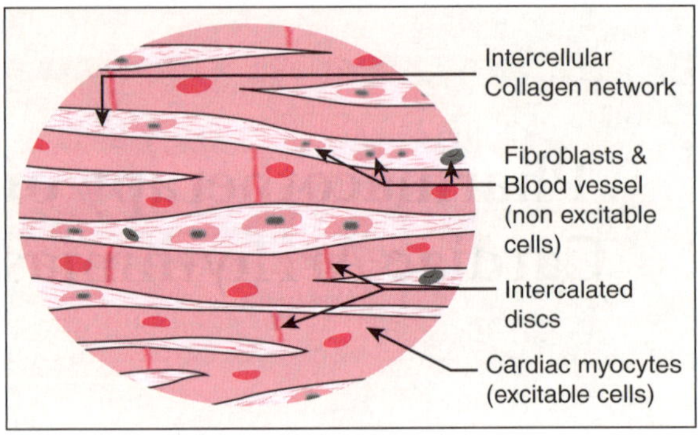

FIG. 28.1 Types of cardiac cells.

down their electrochemical gradients during the open, but not during the closed state. The ion channels in the gap junction connect myocyte to each other electrically. This allows the spread of the impulse rapidly and sequentially to all the cells of the heart (Fig. 28.1). **The Na^+ channels, known as 'fast' channels,** are present in the myocytes of the atria, ventricles and the His–Purkinje tissue; they are absent from the SAN and the AVN. The other ion channels are present in all the cardiac tissues. The *rapid depolarisation* (**phase 0**) is due to the influx of Na^+ into the cell, through the 'fast' channels with the late addition of Ca^{++}. The outward movement of K^+ is responsible for the *repolarisation* (**phases 1–3**) of all cardiac tissues (Fig. 28.2).

In addition to the above mentioned 'channels', there are two energy requiring **exchange pumps** in the cardiac myocyte cell membrane:

1. The adenosine triphosphate (ATP) energised Na^+-K^+ exchange pump which pumps Na^+ out of the cell and K^+ into the interior of the cell (see below).
2. The Na^+-Ca^{++} exchange pump, which mainly extrudes Ca^{++} from the cell to the exterior. Such extrusion is dependent on the activity of the Na^+-K^+ pump, and diminishes when the latter is made inoperative by digoxin (Chapter 31).

During the excitation of the cell, larger quantities of Na^+ and K^+ ions cross the cell membrane. These ion fluxes, are, in fact, responsible for the phenomenon of the continuously varying potential difference (**transmembrane electrical potential**) across the cell membrane. These variations in membrane potential can be graphically recorded as an **action potential** by inserting a microelectrode into the myocardiac cells. Fig. 28.2 shows the action potentials as recorded from the Ca^{++}-driven tissues, sinoatrial (SA) and atrioventricular (AV) nodes wherein the resting potential is 30–40 mV (Fig. 28.2A) and Na^+-driven tissues (others) of the heart (Fig. 28.2B), in which resting membrance potential is −60 to −90 mV.

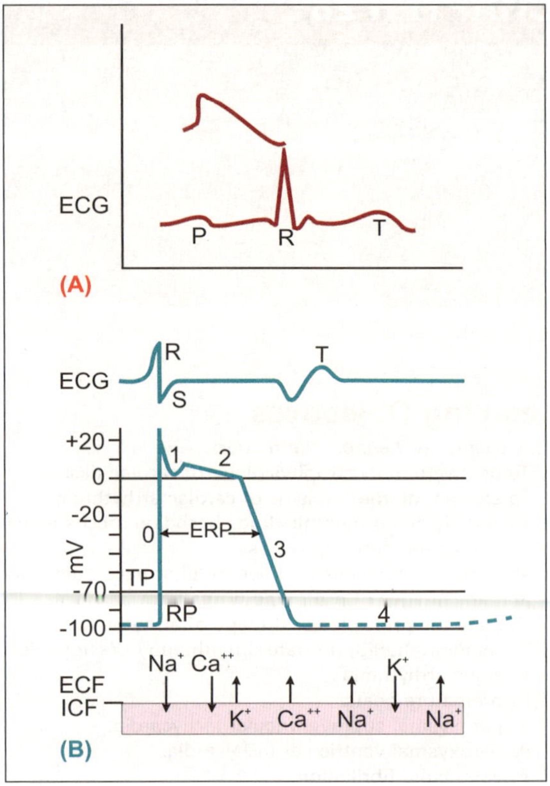

FIG. 28.2 Relationship between transmembrane cationic fluxes, ECG recording and transmembrane action potential recorded from mammalian (A) sinus node and (B) His–Purkinje fibre (ventricular). RP, resting potential; TP, threshold potential; (O), phase of depolarisation; (1, 2, 3), phases of repolarisation; (4), resting period.

In the normal heart, only the SAN and the AVN are capable of spontaneous depolarisation, i.e. generating an action potential without external stimulation. The other cardiac tissues merely respond by depolarisation to an action potential generated by the SAN. **The diseased heart may contain other sites capable of spontaneous depolarisation, giving rise to arrhythmias.**

When an atrial or a ventricular cell receives an action potential, it starts depolarising and Na^+ starts entering it. When such depolarisation reaches a **threshold potential** (TP in Fig. 28.2), the sodium channels open abruptly and a large amount of Na^+ enters the cell (potential becomes positive). **Phase '0' of the action potential** (Fig. 28.2) indicates **rapid depolarisation** of the cardiac cell membrane. During the latter part of phase 0, Na^+ channel gates close and cannot be reactivated. At this stage, Ca^{++} also enters the cell via the Ca^{++} channels. The entry of Ca^{++}

continues through **phases 1 and 2** via **the slow Ca^{++} channels**. The Ca^{++}, which enters the cell causes the release of Ca^{++} stored in the sarcoplasmic reticulum (SR) of the cardiac myocytes, raising the concentration of Ca^{++} within these cells. *The intracellular free calcium interacts with the* **troponin–actin–myosin system** *and causes contraction of the heart.* The P wave, the P–R interval and the QRS complex of the ECG are inscribed during phases 0 and 1 of the action potential propagation in the atria, the AV nodal tissue and the ventricles, respectively.

After depolarisation, the **repolarisation** occurs in several phases (Fig. 28.2):

- **Phase '1'** – A **short rapid repolarisation** due to the beginning of outward K^+ current and entry of Cl^- ions into the cells.
- **Phase '2'** – A **prolonged plateau phase** (delay in repolarisation) at the neutral level due to a balance between the Ca^{++} entering the cell (through slow calcium channel), small late but long-lasting Na^+ current and the K^+ leaving the cell. The ST segment of the ECG coincides with this phase of the action potential.
- **Phase '3'** – The **rapid repolarisation upto the resting potential** caused mainly by continued extrusion of K^+; it corresponds to the T wave.
- During phase 3, Ca^{++} is removed from the cytoplasm by an ATP-dependent active process, and by the extrusion from the cell via the Na^+/Ca^{++} exchange pump. The lowering of Ca^{++} concentration in the cytoplasm allows the cardiac muscle fibre to relax.
- **Phase '4'** – In this **resting phase,** the final ionic reconstitution of the cell is achieved by the Na^+-K^+ exchange pump which actively pushes Na^+ out of the cell and K^+ into the cell. The cycle is then repeated.

During the greater part of the action potential, the cardiac muscle is resistant to further stimulation (**refractoriness,** Fig. 28.3). This period is termed as the **effective** or **absolute refractory period** (**ERP** or **ARP**), and serves as normal physiological protective mechanism. During the ERP, a stimulus can evoke only a local, nonpropagated response. The **relative refractory period** extends from the end of ERP (second half of phase 3) to the end of phase 3. During this period, a stimulus of greater than the threshold strength is needed to evoke a response that is propagated, though slowly.

The above-mentioned concepts are important for understanding the mechanisms of action of antiarrhythmics in terms of Na^+-channel blocking, Ca-channel blocking and K^+-channel blocking.

Certain terms appear repeatedly during a discussion of cardioactive drugs; they are as follows:

- **Automaticity** is the capacity of a cell to undergo spontaneous diastolic depolarisation.
- **Excitability** is the ability of a cell to respond to an external stimulus by depolarisation.
- **Threshold potential** (TP) is the level of intracellular negativity at which abrupt and complete depolarisation occurs.
- **The conduction velocity of an impulse** is determined primarily by the slope of action potential and amplitude of phase 0 (Fig. 28.2) in that tissue.

Propagation of an impulse in the cardiac tissue depends on (a) the ERP of the tissue and (b) its conduction velocity.

The autonomic nervous system modulates the inotropic state of the myocardium by regulating the transmembrane ion movements, e.g. beta adrenergic stimulation allows the entry of larger amounts of Ca^{++} and exerts a positive inotropic effect. Beta adrenergic blockers counter this adrenergic influence and exert a negative inotropic effect.

Cardiac arrhythmias, mechanisms: According to the present concept, a triggering beat/s interacts with a predisposed cardiac tissue (substrate) to initiate and perpetuate cardiac arrhythmia. They could be due to the following:

1. **Disorders of impulse formation and/or**
2. **Disorders of impulse conduction**

- **Tachyarrhythmias** due to **disturbed impulse formation** are associated with spontaneous, irregular and rhythmic discharge from **ectopic pacemaker** activity from areas other than the SAN.

The differences among various atrial arrhythmias could be explained on the basis of the rate of discharge of the ectopic focus. Thus, an ectopic pacemaker with a rate 160–180/min causes **atrial tachycardia.** If the ectopic rate becomes more rapid, 220–300/min, it produces **atrial flutter**, while very rapid rates, more than 350/min, results in **atrial fibrillation** (AF).

- **Disorders of impulse conduction,** commonly referred to as **re-entry disturbances,** are the commoner of the two mechanisms of arrhythmias. According to this theory,

a. The affected myocardium has areas of depressed function with a prolonged refractory period.
b. Because of that, an impulse approaching such an area would be diverted to the adjacent excitable tissue.
c. The same impulse, after taking a circuitous route through normal tissue, will again reach the depressed area which by then becomes excitable.
d. Upon traversing it, the excitatory process is free to re-enter normal regions and restimulate the arrhythmia. Repetition of this cycle would produce an ectopic tachycardia.

In arrhythmias of the re-entrant type, conduction velocity and duration of RP are the two most critical electrophysiological properties which could be altered by drugs.

Clinically, it is usually not possible to determine whether an arrhythmia represents a disorder of impulse formation or impulse conduction. Identical arrhythmias on the ECG may result from disparate mechanisms. *Hence, except in a few cases, an antiarrhythmic drug cannot be selected simply on the basis of its effect on electrophysiological properties.*

Not all arrhythmias need the same aggressive drug therapy. If an arrhythmia is precipitated by hypotension, restitution of BP by vasopressor agents such as DA or NA may re-establish normal sinus rhythm. Furthermore, sinus tachycardia and sinus bradycardia generally need no treatment other than that of the underlying cause. *Only those which are lethal (VF), herald a more dangerous rhythm (ventricular premature beats in acute MI) or seriously compromise the cardiac output (AF with a fast ventricular rate) require rapid and effective therapy.*

In patients with arrhythmia any underlying cause such as a cardiovascular disorder, pulmonary disease, autonomic disorders, electrolyte disturbances, systemic disease and drug-induced toxicity must be evaluated before administering the antiarrhythmic drug. *In many situations, arrhythmias tend to be benign. Their treatment should be expectant, and potentially toxic drugs should be avoided.*

The basic electrophysiological actions of antiarrhythmic drugs (Fig. 28.3) are as follows:

- **Decreasing the slope of phase 4** (diastolic depolarisation) of the action potential in the excitable cardiac tissues. This action is possessed by all antiarrhythmic drugs and suppresses the enhanced automaticity of ectopic foci.
- **Shifting the threshold potential towards zero** (i.e. making it less negative). This again suppresses the automaticity of ectopic foci. Quinidine, procainamide, propranolol and potassium possess this action.

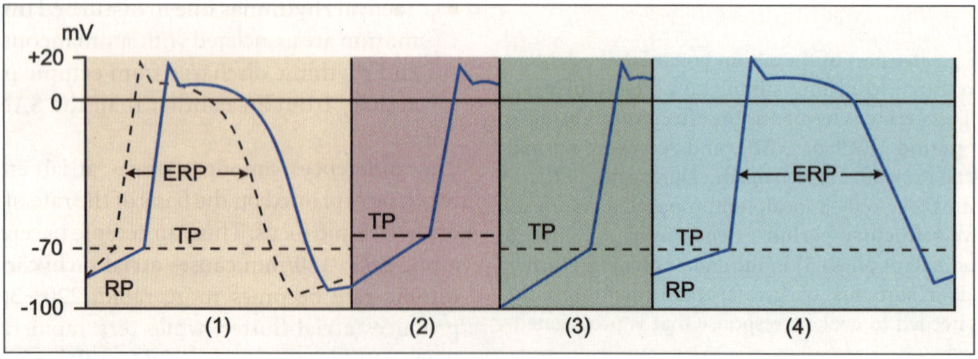

FIG. 28.3 **The normal pattern (dotted line) of the transmembrane action potential of a pacemaker cardiac cell and mechanisms of action of antiarrhythmic drugs: (1) delaying the spontaneous diastolic depolarisation from the resting potential (RP), thus decreasing the rate (all drugs); (2) increasing the excitation threshold potential (TP), e.g. quinidine, procainamide, propranolol; (3) prolonging the resting period in part by increasing the maximum diastolic intracellular negativity, e.g. phenytoin; and (4) increasing the effective refractory period (ERP), e.g. quinidine, procainamide.**

- **Shifting the resting potential away from zero** (i.e. making it more negative), which also slows the rate of diastolic depolarisation and suppressing automaticity. Lignocaine and phenytoin possess this action.
- **Increase in the action potential duration** (**APD**) thus increasing the effective refractory period (ERP) and blocking re-entrant impulses. Quinidine, procainamide, propranolol and potassium possess this action.
- **Shortening of the APD** by lignocaine and phenytoin, on the other hand, reduces the refractoriness of the AV junctional tissue.
- **Decreasing the slope of phase 0 of the action potential and slowing the conduction velocity of a propagated impulse.** This blocks the re-entrant impulses responsible for an arrhythmia. Quinidine, procainamide, disopyramide, lignocaine (in large doses) and verapamil possess this action. PH 1.30

Antiarrythmic Drugs - Classification

A. According to their mechanism of action (Vaughan Williams Classification):

Class I: Fast sodium channel blockers – They predominantly block sodium channels. In higher concentrations, they also block nerve conduction. With the usual doses, most drugs, have little effect on the normal conduction system. They impede the initial rapid depolarisation and slow the phase 0 depolarisation rate, without altering the resting potential. Hence they are called **membrane stabilisers** (Chapter 16). They are further subdivided into three groups:

Class IA: Those which cause moderate phase 0 depression and hence moderately suppress conduction. They *prolong repolarisation* (refractoriness) and *prolong the APD,* in addition to suppression of automaticity, e.g. quinidine, procainamide, disopyramide.

Class IB: Those which are weak phase 0 depressants (less potent Na^+ channel blockers) and **have little influence on conduction velocity**. They *shorten repolarisation* (refractoriness, phase 3) and *APD*. They suppress automaticity, e.g. lignocaine, phenytoin, mexiletine, tocainide.

Class IC: Those which cause marked phase 0 depression (most potent Na^+ channel blockers)**; they markedly slow conduction.** They have *no effect on repolarisation* but may prolong the APD, e.g. flecainide, propafenone.

Class II: Beta adrenergic blockers – They block the beta-1 cardiac receptors and mainly **suppress automaticity.**

Class III: Potassium channel blockers – They **markedly prolong repolarisation** (phase 3) and **increase the APD without affecting the conduction velocity.** They increase refractory period (RP), e.g. amiodarone, ibutilide, vernakalant, sotalol.

Class IV: Calcium channel blockers (CCB) – Their action is mostly limited to the SAN and AVN where they **suppress automaticity** in pacemaker cells and **slow the conduction** and increase the ERP. Duration of repolarisation is unchanged, e.g. verapamil, diltiazem (not nifedipine). They *shorten the APD* and depress the slow inward Ca^{++} current (phase 2)

Class V: Miscellaneous

- **Potassium channel openers** (e.g. adenosine): It does not cause prolongation of repolarisation.
- **Digitalis** (Chapter 31); potassium and magnesium.

Most of the antiarrhythmic drugs have multiple actions. Furthermore, the metabolites of some of these drugs contribute to or even are primarily responsible for the action.

B. According to their therapeutic use for the treatment of arrhythmia:

- **Supraventricular arrhythmias,** e.g. adenosine, CCB such as verapamil and diltiazem.
- **Both supraventricular and ventricular arrhythmias,** e.g. amiodarone, beta blockers, quinidine and procainamide.
- **Ventricular arrhythmias,** e.g. lignocaine.

All the antiarrhythmic drugs have both cardiac and noncardiac adverse effects.

CLASS I: FAST SODIUM CHANNEL BLOCKERS

Class IA Drugs

QUINIDINE: This first antiarrhythmic agent used to treat both atrial and ventricular arrhythmias is an isomer of the antimalarial drug quinine, one of the alkaloids occurring in the cinchona bark.

Pharmacological actions

These are as follows:

1. Cardiac actions
2. Extracardiac actions

Cardiac actions

It is a direct myocardiac depressant, and to a smaller extent vagolytic (antimuscarinic). It **blocks the sodium channels**. It also inhibits potassium channels in the cardiac cells.

- **Automaticity:** Quinidine **depresses automaticity** in all tissues, especially the ectopic pacemaker. This action helps to suppress the arrhythmias due to enhanced impulse formation. Quinidine does not suppress the automaticity of the normal SAN.
- **Excitability:** Quinidine **depresses the excitability of the cardiac tissue**, and hence a weak ectopic impulse becomes ineffective.
- **Conduction velocity:** Quinidine **slows the conduction** velocity in all the cardiac tissues. This property, along with the increased RP and decreased excitability, contributes to a decreased cardiac rate in arrhythmias due to the presence of an ectopic focus.
- **Refractory period:** It prolongs *(by a* **direct action***)* repolarisation and hence the RP. However, its vagolytic action (**indirect action**) increases the atrial RP and shortens that of the AVN while leaving that of the ventricles unaltered. The overall action of quinidine is:
  a. To prolong the RP markedly in the atria.
  b. To increase the RP in the ventricles to a smaller extent.
  c. To decrease the RP in the AVN.

Simple prolongation of RP prevents the heart from responding to premature or rapid stimulation. Re-entrant impulse finds the originally depolarised tissue still inexcitable. Quinidine thus abolishes the arrhythmias **due to re-entrant circuits**.

- **AV conduction:** Quinidine **depresses the conduction predominantly within the atria and the His–Purkinje system.** However, its vagolytic effect permits or even enhances the conduction in the AVN, causing tachycardia.
- **Contractility:** Quinidine exerts a **negative inotropic action on the heart**. This obviously is a disadvantage.
- **Effects on ECG:** Early changes comprise increase in the QT interval. A decrease in amplitude or inversion of the T wave and depression of the ST segment may also occur. Later changes include widening and frequent notching of the P wave, and a prolonged PR interval.

Widening of the QRS complex signifies a reduction of the conduction velocity, and if accompanied by a considerable increase in the RP of the ventricle might lead to the development of VT and to VF. **When, the QRS complex is widened by 25%–50% or more than 0.12–0.14 s, quinidine should be withheld.**

Extracardiac actions

- **Blood pressure:** Quinidine **lowers BP** in most patients.
- **Miscellaneous actions:** Quinidine depresses the skeletal muscle and like quinine shows antimalarial, antipyretic and weak oxytocic activities.

Absorption, fate and excretion: Quinidine is almost completely absorbed from the gut. Following a single oral dose, the peak effects are reached within 2–3 h and persist for 6–8 h. About 80% is bound to plasma albumin. It is primarily metabolised (75%) in the liver with a half-life of 4−8 h. One metabolite 3-hydroxyquinidine is as potent as quinidine. About 25% of the drug is excreted in the urine unchanged.

With the same quinidine regimen, there are wide differences in the serum quinidine levels in different persons.

Adverse reactions: Quinidine given intravenously could be very toxic.

- **Cardiac toxicity:** The drug causes bradycardia, conduction defects and heart failure, particularly in patients with marked cardiac damage. Two distinct, drug-induced ventricular arrhythmias may occur:
  a. *Torsades de pointes*
  b. *Incessant ventricular tachycardia*

All antiarrhythmics that prolong the QT interval markedly can precipitate a **polymorphic ventricular tachycardia** *known as torsades de pointes,*

Box 28.1 Some Drugs Causing the Prolongation of QTc

- **Antiarrhythmics (class IA):** Disopyramide, procainamide, quinidine
- **Antiarrhythmics (class III):** Amiodarone, dofetilide, ibutilide, dronedarone, sotalol
- **Antipsychotics:** Chlorpromazine, haloperidol, thioridazine, pimozide, ziprasidone, quetiapine
- **Antibiotics:** Erythromycin, clarithromycin, azithromycin, moxifloxacin
- **Miscellaneous:** Cisapride, quinine, methadone, pentamidine

which may result in syncope and sudden death. It is generally dose related. Drugs that cause similar prolongation of QTc (QT corrected) are listed in Box 28.1.

- **Hypotension:** Hypotension has been observed more commonly in older patients.
- **Embolic phenomena:** Sudden restoration of sinus rhythm by quinidine in a patient with chronic AF may dislodge the mural thrombi attached to auricular appendages. This might rarely precipitate embolic occlusion of the vessels of the vital organs.
- **Miscellaneous toxicity:**
  a. **Allergic Reactions:** The manifestations of intolerance include skin rashes, fever and thrombocytopenic purpura.
  b. **Gastrointestinal:** Nausea, vomiting and diarrhoea are common.
  c. **CNS:** Headache, dizziness and convulsions may result from a direct action of quinidine on the CNS.
  d. **Cinchonism:** It results from cumulative overdosage and includes impairment of hearing, ringing in ears, vertigo, blurred vision, light headedness, giddiness and tremor.

Drug interactions: Quinidine is metabolised by hepatic cytochrome P450 enzymes and hence induction or inhibition of these enzymes affects plasma concentration of quinidine (Chapter 3).

Preparations and dosage: Quinidine sulphate, 200 mg; dose 200–400 mg every 6 h. Extended-release formulation also available, dose 300 mg 8-12 h.

Indications: Quinidine, because of its toxicity, is now **rarely used to treat arrhythmias.**

- **Paroxysmal atrial, nodal and ventricular tachycardia: Adenosine is usually preferred.** Vasopressor agents and parasympathomimetic drugs may also help.
- **Atrial, nodal and ventricular premature beats:** Most supraventricular premature beats are benign, and the patient should be reassured about their harmless nature. Smoking and consumption of tea and coffee should be stopped. If these therapies are ineffective, a **beta blocker** or **amiodarone** may be used. *The development of ventricular premature beats during acute MI may herald the onset of ventricular tachycardia.* β Blockers and amiodarone are effective in many patients; quinidine may be used as the last resort.

PROCAINAMIDE: Procainamide, a derivative of procaine, a local anaesthetic (Chapter 16), is effective orally, intramuscularly and intravenously; it is not destroyed by esterase. **The cardiac and haemodynamic effects of procainamide are similar to those of quinidine. It is free from CNS toxicity.**

Absorption, fate and excretion: Procainamide is rapidly and almost completely absorbed from the gut. Given orally, the peak plasma level is reached within 1 h and declines by 4 h. It is minimally bound to plasma proteins, and about 60% is excreted unchanged in the urine. Impairment of renal function can produce cumulative toxicity.

Adverse reactions:

- **Allergic reactions** which include chills, fever, itching, skin rash and angioedema.
- **Cardiotoxicity** is similar to that of quinidine. Hypotension (or a shock-like state) occurs most often with the IV use.
- **Gastrointestinal ADR** such as anorexia, nausea and vomiting.
- **Blood:** Agranulocytosis and SLE are rare but serious manifestations.

Preparations and dosage:

i. Procainamide hydrochloride tablet 250 mg
ii. Procainamide hydrochloride injection, 100 mg per mL.

It is administered orally in the dose of 0.25–0.5 g every 4–6 h. In serious cases, 0.5–1 g may be given every 2–4 h. The maintenance dose is 0.25–0.5 g 6 hourly.

Indications: It may be used as a substitute for quinidine.

DISOPYRAMIDE PHOSPHATE: This drug has membrane depressant (quinidine-like) and anticholinergic properties. Its therapeutic effects and toxicity are similar to those of quinidine, but it is better tolerated.

Class IB Drugs

LIGNOCAINE (LIDOCAINE): This drug belonging to class IB is a local anaesthetic (Chapter 16). Given intravenously, it:

- **Selectively acts on diseased or ischemic myocardium** and depresses diastolic depolarisation and automaticity in **ventricular tissue.**
- Has a **rapid onset** and **short duration of action.**
- **Shortens the ventricular action potential.**
- Has **little influence on conduction velocity.**
- Does not significantly affect the electrophysiological function of the atria, SAN and AVN, and **causes hardly any change in the surface ECG.**
- **Has no haemodynamic adverse effects.**
- May produce **toxicity,** which is of a **short duration.**

Since the electrophysiological effects of lignocaine are primarily limited to ventricular myocardium, **it is most useful in abolishing ventricular arrhythmias.** Its lack of action on the AV nodal conduction velocity makes it a suitable drug in the treatment of digitalis-induced ventricular arrhythmia.

The drug is usually given intravenously, although it can also be given intramuscularly. It is not effective orally because of extensive hepatic first pass metabolism. Its plasma-protein-binding is 60%−80% with t½ of 15−30 min after a single injection.

Adverse reactions: In recommended dosage, lignocaine is a relatively safe drug. Adverse reactions include drowsiness, disorientation, muscle twitching, blurred vision and rarely convulsions. *An IV preparation of diazepam should be at hand while using IV lignocaine.* It diminishes the cardiac output and may cause hypotension, bradycardia and apnea. It should be avoided in the presence of liver damage and bradycardia.

Indications: It is the **drug of choice** for the following:

- Severe ventricular arrhythmias
- Emergency termination of ventricular tachycardia following recent MI and that occurring during cardiac surgery and cardiac catheterisation
- Digitalis-induced ventricular arrhythmias

Because of its immediate effect and short duration of action (10 min), lignocaine is given as a single large initial IV bolus, 1−2 mg/kg in 30 s, followed by a continuous IV infusion at the rate of 1−4 mg/min to maintain the effect. Smaller doses (50%) are used in patients with congestive heart failure, shock, hepatic dysfunction and in those more than 70 years.

TOCAINIDE: This is an amine analogue of lignocaine and can be given orally in the dose of 400−800 mg every 8 h. It can cause serious dose-related neurological adverse effects.

MEXILETINE: This drug resembles lignocaine, chemically as well as in its pharmacological actions. *It is, however, effective orally.* Adverse reactions are common and are dose related. They include vomiting, tremor, ataxia, blurred vision and hypotension. The dose is 400 mg followed by 200 mg t.i.d.

PHENYTOIN SODIUM (DIPHENYL HYDANTOIN): The hypothesis that the excitatory processes or substances initiating the discharge of impulses in cardiac arrhythmias may be similar to those responsible for epilepsy led to the use of phenytoin in the treatment of cardiac arrhythmias (Chapter 9).

Phenytoin, a **sodium channel inhibitor**, depresses the ventricular automaticity, but, like lignocaine, it does not decrease the conduction velocity between the ventricular fibres. Phenytoin has little effect on the surface electrocardiogram, although it may shorten the QT interval.

It is administered orally in the dose of 100−200 mg four times daily for the suppression of ectopic beats and for prophylaxis against recurrent paroxysmal tachycardia. Because of its long t½, the effect can be maintained by the administration of 1.0 g on the first day, 0.6 g on the second and third days and 0.4 g per day thereafter.

Indications: The main use of IV phenytoin is to **terminate digitalis-induced cardiac arrhythmias.**

Class IC Drugs

FLECAINIDE: This fluorinated analogue of procainamide (class 1C) is well absorbed on oral administration (t½ 14−20 h). It can also be given intravenously slowly. **It is highly effective in paroxysmal supraventricular tachycardia, tachycardia associated with the Wolff–Parkinson–White (WPW) syndrome and ventricular tachycardia.** It, however, causes prolongation of PR, QRS and QT intervals, and is liable to cause ventricular arrhythmias and unexplained sudden death. It has a negative inotropic effect. Less common toxicities include nausea, tremors and blurred vision. It is contraindicated in cases with heart failure and the sick sinus syndrome.

ENCAINIDE: It has properties and ADR similar to those of flecainide and is effective orally. *Both encainide and flecainide readily suppress ventricular premature beats after MI.*

PROPAFENONE: This class 1C antiarrhythmic drug also has mild beta blocker and calcium channel blocker activities. It has similar indications as flecainide but is relatively safe. At the onset of arrhythmia, 600 mg is administered orally, followed by 150−300 mg 8 hourly.

The adverse effects are dose related and include prolongation of the PR and QRS complex, conduction blocks, inhibition of sinus node and precipitation of CHF, dyspepsia and taste disturbances.

Moricizine: This phenothiazine derivative belongs to class IC and is used to treat supraventricular arrhythmias. Its active metabolites contribute to its long t½.

Class IC drugs, though potent antiarrhythmics, are also proarrhythmics and hence must be avoided in patients with structural damage to the heart.

Box 28.2 Cardiovascular Risks with Class I Antiarrhythmic Agents

- Bradycardia, heart block
- Heart failure
- New or worsened arrhythmias
  Torsades de pointes
  Increased frequency of ventricular tachycardia
- Increased mortality during long-term treatment

All drugs that block the sodium channels reduce the ventricular function and are potentially toxic. Box 28.2 lists the major risks with group I antiarrhythmics. **This propensity is highest with flecainide (class IC).**

Although the presence of ventricular premature beats and nonsustained ventricular tachycardia increase the risk in patients with recent MI, asymptomatic and mildly symptomatic patients with such arrhythmias may not benefit from antiarrhythmic drugs other than beta adrenergic blockers.

CLASS II: BETA-ADRENERGIC BLOCKERS

Myocardial β-receptor stimulation increases automaticity, enhances the A−V conduction velocity and shortens the refractory period especially in supraventricular tissues.

Beta-adrenergic blockers are useful because they:

- Antagonise the effects of beta-adrenoreceptor activation on the SAN and some ectopic foci.
- **Prolong the refractoriness of the AVN and slow down the ventricular rate.**
- Have a membrane stabilising property (propranolol, oxprenolol and acebutolol).
- **Reduce myocardial oxygen demand, particularly in the presence of IHD.**
- Are mainly useful in sinus tachycardia and supraventricular tachyarrhythmias, particularly those precipitated by exercise, emotions, thyrotoxicosis
- Are **generally well tolerated** and are **much safer than class I group of drugs. They reduce all-cause cardiovascular mortality** (see Chapter 18).

The broad spectrum of antiarrhythmic activity and established safety record make beta blockers agents of choice for general use as antiarrhythmic agents.

PROPRANOLOL: This beta blocker is well absorbed on oral administration, and it is used in the dose of 10–40 mg every 6–8 h. Its plasma t½ is 2–3 h following IV administration and 4–6 h after oral use. The drug is given slowly intravenously at the rate of 1 mg over 1 min, repeated at 2 min interval upto a total dose of 0.1 mg/kg. Other beta blockers, such as atenolol (25–100 mg/day), can also be used. Severe propranolol toxicity may result in progressive bradycardia and cardiac asystole.

Beta blockers prolong the PR interval, shorten QT_C and may potentiate the negative inotropic action of antiarrhythmic drugs, particularly verapamil, which can result in marked bradycardia and even asystole.

They are useful for the rate control in supraventicular tachycardia (SVT). **They exhibit synergistic effects when combined with other antiarrhythmic drugs from classes I and III** (see Chapter 31).

Esmolol is a rapidly acting cardioselective beta blocker with a t½ of 9 min because of rapid metabolism in RBC.

CLASS III: POTASSIUM CHANNEL BLOCKERS

SOTALOL: This class III drug is a noncardioselective beta blocker with potency similar to that of propranolol. However, **it has no membrane stabilising action.** It

- Prolongs the APD in the atria and the ventricles in a concentration-dependent fashion.
- Prolongs the ERP of all cardiac tissues, including the AVN and His–Purkinje system.
  These actions are unrelated to its beta-blocking action.
- Has no negative inotropic effect.
- Increases the ventricular fibrillation threshold in normal and ischemic myocardium, when given experimentally intravenously.

The surface ECG shows prolongation of PR and QT intervals.

Absorption, fate and excretion: Given orally, it is absorbed completely and does not undergo first pass metabolism in the liver. It is excreted unchanged (90%) in the urine. Its apparent plasma t½ is 7–18 h.

Adverse reactions: These are due to its beta-blocking properties, e.g. sinus bradycardia, conduction blocks and hypotension, and due to its property of prolonging the QT interval, e.g. *torsades de pointes* (similar to quinidine).

Preparations and dosage: Sotalol hydrochloride tablets (40, 80 and 160 mg) and a solution (10 mg/mL) for IV injection. It is important to avoid hypokalaemia during its use.

Indications: It has been found to be specifically useful in:

- **Unsustained ventricular arrhythmias** such as ventricular ectopic beats, even in patients with a reduced left ventricular function.
- **Sustained ventricular tachycardia.**
- **Recurrent atrioventricular nodal tachycardia.**
- **Prevention of ventricular tachycardia and fibrillation**

The main advantage of sotalol is that its use is associated with low incidence of adverse effects as compared to the class I antiarrhythmic agents. It is very expensive.

AMIODARONE: This class III drug exerts some class I as well as class II (noncompetitive beta blockade) and class IV actions. **It blocks Na^+, Ca^{++} and repolarising K^+ channels and thus has a broad spectrum of activity.** It:

- **Depresses the automaticity** of sinus, atria and the AVN.
- **Prolongs the ERP** of myocardial cells, the AVN and abnormal pathway.
- **Slows the conduction** in the AVN and specialised conducting tissues.

Thus, it reduces the cardiac rate, increases the cardiac output and causes a fall in the peripheral and coronary vascular resistance due to the direct effect on vascular smooth muscles.

It is used orally as well as intravenously. It has a large apparent volume of distribution and is stored in fat and tissues. **Its half-life is 18–60 days.** It is metabolised in the liver and excreted through the bile.

Adverse reactions: It causes various **dose-dependent** adverse effects. Photosensitivity is common. Other ADR include anorexia, nausea, abdominal pain, tremor, hallucinations, peripheral neuropathy, hepatic damage, hypotension and A−V block. Rarely, it can cause hypersensitivity, pneumonitis and pulmonary fibrosis. It contains iodine and can cause disorders of thyroid function (Chapter 62). *The drug is embryotoxic.*

It is also responsible for drug interactions. It inhibits warfarin metabolism. It enhances bradycardia and A−V block caused by beta blockers and Ca channel blockers.

Indications: Amiodarone is a **potent antiarrhythmic drug**, useful in preventing and treating both supraventricular and ventricular tachyarrhythmias. *Although its toxicity profile is wide, in the doses recommended, it appears to be well tolerated.*

It is particularly useful in patients with sustained ventricular tachycardia. It is now increasingly used to treat AF wherein it not only reduces the ventricular rate but can also restore sinus rhythm (**chemical cardioversion**).

Dronedarone: It is a structural analogue of amiodarone. It, however, does not cause thyroid dysfunction or pulmonary fibrosis, probably because of absence of iodine moieties in its structure. It is less effective than amiodarone.

Aprinidine, like amiodarone, is useful in controlling refractory ventricular tachyarrhythmias. Its electrophysiological effects resemble those of quinidine.

IBUTILIDE: This class III agent is used for chemical cardioversion of atrial flutter and fibrillation. It is as effective as amiodarone. It prolongs the atrial and ventricular RP with minimal effect on conduction. It has no negative ionotropic effect. Given intravenously, it acts within 1–2 h.

Dofetilide has similar properties as ibutilide but can be given orally.

VERNAKALANT: This new drug acts as antiarrhythmic by **blocking the ultrarapid delayed rectifier potassium current, mainly expressed in the atria.** It also blocks the sodium channel and muscarinic receptor-operated potassium channel. It is administered intravenously and has been used for rapid conversion of AF of a recent origin. It is contraindicated in patients with hypotension, bradycardia and severe heart disease.

CLASS IV: CALCIUM CHANNEL BLOCKERS

VERAPAMIL: This CCB is the *drug of choice for rapid conversion to sinus rhythm in cases of paroxysmal supraventricular tachycardia.* It is given intravenously in the dose of 5−10 mg injected over a period of 2−3 min and can be repeated, if necessary, after 30 min. It can also be given orally in the dose of 40−120 mg three times a day. It can also be used to reduce the ventricular rate in patients with AF and atrial flutter. *Verapamil IV is absolutely contraindicated in patients on beta blockers, quinidine or disopyramide* (see Chapter 29).

DILTIAZEM: Diltiazem has similar uses as verapamil in supraventricular arrhythmias. In fact, it may be the preferred drug because of its less marked negative inotropic effect. Like verapamil, it may be used orally or intravenously. *CCB are not likely to be useful in the prevention or suppression of most clinically important ventricular arrhythmias.*

CLASS V: MISCELLANEOUS

ADENOSINE: This is a naturally occurring purine nucleoside which is released during myocardial ischemia. **It has antiarrhythmic and potent vasodilator properties.**

Mechanism of action: It stimulates A_1 receptors on cardiac cells and increases the resting membrane potential. It suppresses automaticity and shortens APD, thereby slowing the sinus rate. Furthermore, it slows the A−V conduction. It dilates the coronaries and peripheral arteries.

It is rapidly metabolised by circulating adenosine deaminase and has a very short plasma t½ (4–8 s). Given as a rapid IV bolus, it can rapidly terminate narrow QRS complex paroxysmal, supraventricular tachycardia and is safer than verapamil as it lacks a negative inotropic action. *Unlike verapamil, adenosine an be used after a beta blocker.* It is contraindicated in the presence of asthma, sick sinus syndrome or A–V block.

Adverse reactions: They are not serious and usually short lasting. They include flushing, nausea, dyspnoea, bronchospasm, cough, headache, ventricular ectopy (proarrhythmic), bradycardia and A–V block.

DIGOXIN: It has a positive inotropic action, and hence it has been used in patients with AF susceptible to heart failure. It serves as a rate controlling agent slowing the A–V conduction in AF with an increased ventricular rate. Considering its ADR, its use as a stand-alone drug was on decline with the advent of beta blockers or CCB for the same purpose but it still served as an add on when rate control is inadequate with the other drugs. However, increased mortality with its use has been detected recently, which further declines its use.

POTASSIUM: The basic cardiac effects of potassium administration **without causing hyperkalaemia** are as follows:

- Diminution in the automaticity
- Reduction in conduction velocity
- Prolongation of the refractory period

These effects are most marked in the Purkinje fibres. In toxic doses, it is more likely to cause intraventricular conduction defects than A–V block (Chapter 31). *Correction of hypokalaemia, hypoxia and acid-base disturbances often restores sinus rhythm without the use of antiarrhythmic drugs.*

The administration of antiarrhythmic agents in the presence of hyperkalaemia can be disastrous.

MAGNESIUM, as magnesium sulphate 2–4 g by slow IV injection over 10–15 min, repeated once if necessary, is useful in the emergency treatment of ventricular tachycardia, including digoxin-induced and polymorphic ventricular tachycardia (especially *torsades de pointes*).

Cholinergic and anticholinergic drugs: Similar to vagal action, acetylcholine decreases the automaticity and slows the conduction through the AVN, increases its refractory period and may cause A–V block. **Edrophonium,** a short acting cholinesterase inhibitor, is sometimes useful in the treatment of supraventricular arrhythmia (Chapter 20).

ATROPINE: It blocks the effects of vagal stimulation (anticholinergic). It is useful for the diagnosis of sinus bradycardia, where it increases the heart rate, and in the treatment of heart block (see section, Drugs used in the treatment of heart block).

Table 28.1 illustrates electrophysiological, haemodynamic and ADR features of antiarrythmic agents from groups IA, IB, II and IV. Table 28.2 summarises the drug therapy of cardiac arrhythmias.

CHOICE OF ANTIARRHYTHMIC AGENT

It depends on the following:

- Correct diagnosis
- Urgency for treatment
- Route of administration
- Extent of cardiac damage
- The risk–benefit ratio of the drug concerned

ATRIAL FIBRILLATION: MANAGEMENT

The management of AF, perhaps the most common sustained cardiac rhythm disorder, has undergone considerable changes during the last decade. Many patients of AF are asymptomatic; often they present themselves with complications such as stroke as first manifestation.

The **medical management of AF** involves the following:

- Treatment of predisposing factors
- Control of heart rate
- Control of cardiac rhythm (conversion)
- Thromboprophylaxis

Paroxysmal AF is self-terminating usually within 48 h, while in **persistent AF**, the attack lasts for more than 7 days. When the arrhythmia persists in spite of therapy, it is diagnosed as **permanent.** The treatment of AF should be carried out **under the supervision of the specialist.**

Table 28.1 Principal Effects of Some Antiarrhythmic Drugs on the Heart

	Group IA (Quinidine, Procainamide, Disopyramide)	Group IB (Lignocaine, Phenytoin)	Group II (Propranolol)	Group IV (Verapamil)
Electrophysiological				
Automaticity	Decrease	Decrease	Decrease	Decrease
Excitability	Decrease	No change	Decrease	Decrease
Conduction velocity	Decrease	No change or increase	Decrease	Decrease
ERP	Increase	Decrease	Increase	Increase
Electrocardiogram				
PR duration	No change or increase	No change or decrease	No change or increase	No change or increase
QRS duration	Increase	No change	No change	No change
Q-T duration	Increase	No change or decrease	No change or decrease	No change
Haemodynamic				
Blood pressure	No change or decrease	No change or decrease	No change or decrease	No change or decrease
Cardiac output	Decrease	No change or decrease	Decrease	Decrease
Contractility	Decrease	No change or decrease	Decrease	Decrease
Left ventricular end diastolic pressure	May increase	No change or increase	May increase	May increase
Adverse effects	Proarrhythmic; negative inotropic effect; conduction block	Negative inotropic effect	Sinus bradycardia; conduction block; negative inotropic effect	Conduction block; negative inotropic effect

Table 28.2 Drug Treatment of Cardiac Arrhythmias

Arrhythmia	Emergency Treatment[a]: Preferred Treatment	Emergency Treatment[a]: Other Treatment	Chronic treatment prophylaxis
SA Node			
Sinus arrhythmia	Needs no treatment	–	–
Sinus tachycardia	Sedative, propranolol	Treat the cause	–
Sinus bradycardia	Atropine or temporary or transvenous pacing	Treat the cause	Permanent pacemaker
Atria			
Premature beats	Reassurance, propranolol	–	Radiofrequency ablation
Paroxysmal supraventricular tachycardia (PSVT)	DCC[a]/vagal maneuvers, adenosine IV, CCB: verapamil/diltiazem	Propranolol If LVEF <40%: digoxin[b]/amiodarone	Radiofrequency ablation, propranolol
Atrial fibrillation and atrial flutter	DCC[a] To control ventricular rate: verapamil, diltiazem, beta blockers	To terminate AF: (a) Elective DCC (b) Amiodarone/ibutilide/dofetilide (c) Procainamide	Rate controllers: diltiazem, beta blockers Rhythm controllers: amiodarone/dofetilide Stroke prevention: warfarin
Ventricles			
Premature beats	If symptomatic: beta blockers If LVF <40%: digoxin	–	Propranolol[c] Digoxin

Continued

Table 28.2 Drug Treatment of Cardiac Arrhythmias—cont'd

Arrhythmia	Emergency Treatment[a]		Chronic treatment prophylaxis
	Preferred Treatment	**Other Treatment**	
Paroxysmal ventricular tachycardia (PVT)	Amiodarone IV DCC[a]	Procainamide, lignocaine	Implantation of cardioverter defibrillator (ICD) ± amiodarone/beta blockers
Ventricular fibrillation	Defibrillation, epinephrine/vasopressin (if needed)	Amiodarone, lignocaine	ICD ± amiodarone/beta blockers
Digitalis-induced tachyarrhythmias	Lignocaine	Phenytoin	Procainamide
Torsades de pointes	DCC[a], magnesium, temporary pacing	Lignocaine, phenytoin isoprenaline	–
Second-/third-degree A–V block	Atropine temporary pacing	Isoprenaline	Permanent pacemaker

[a]DCC, direct current cardioversion (if haemodynamic unstability).
[b]If related to heart failure.
[c]Useful when ventricular tachyarrhythmias are associated with an increased sympathetic tone or circulating catecholamines. When using digoxin, verapamil or a beta blocker IV, drugs such as atropine and isoprenaline and cardiac pacemaker equipment should be at hand in the event of complete A–V block; for verapamil-induced complete A–V block, calcium gluconate 1 g IV is also effective.

1. **Treatment during an episode:** If the patient is severely symptomatic or haemodynamically unstable, and in urgent need of lowering of ventricular rate, he/she is best treated by DC cardioversion. For patients with the first episode of AF or rare recurrences of AF, particularly those that terminate spontaneously, no specific therapy to control the rhythm may be indicated.
2. **Cardiac rate control:** The immediate goal is to control symptoms due to an increased cardiac rate and or the underlying structural cardiac disease. The drugs used are given in Table 28.3. **For most patients, β blockers, or dihydropyridine CCB, are to be preferred for the initial treatment of the ventricular rate control.** In patients with decompensated CHF, digoxin may be used (See above Digoxin).
3. **Rhythm control:** Drugs used for control of cardiac rhythm are given in Table 28.3. For uncomplicated AF of <7 days, oral or IV administration of **class IC or III antiarrhythmic agents** can be used. **Propafenone** is a safe and effective therapy for conversion to sinus rhythm. For those who do not respond, electrical cardioversion can be considered.
4. **Thromboprophylaxis:** Warfarin used prophylactically reduces the incidence of ischaemic stroke but not that of haemorrhagic stroke. Aspirin–clopidogrel combination is less active than aspirin + warfarin for stroke prevention (see Chapter 33). *Anticoagulation, if started during an attack, has to be continued lifelong.*
5. **Maintenance therapy:** Patients with recurrent AF and minimal symptoms and those with persistent or permanent AF can be managed by long-term rate-control strategy. The commonly used drug for this purpose is oral amiodarone. Procainamide may be used in patients intolerant to amiodarone. *Flecainide, though effective, is proarrhythmic and is generally not preferred.*

DRUGS USED IN THE TREATMENT OF HEART BLOCK

ISOPRENALINE: Isoprenaline (Chapter 18) which enhances the rhythmicity of sinus as well as subsidiary nodal and ventricular pacemakers has proved invaluable in the treatment of advanced second degree and high grade A–V block. In emergency, the drug is administered intravenously slowly in the dose of 2 mg

Table 28.3 Drugs for Rate Control and Cardioversion in AF

Drug	Dose
For rate control	
• **Beta blockers**	
Propranolol	IV 1–3 mg, < 1mg/min; oral 80–240 mg t.i.d.
Metoprolol	IV 2.5–5 mg bolus every 5 min upto 15 mg; oral 25–200 mg o.d.
Esmolol	IV infusion loading dose: 0.5 mg/kg; maintenance: dose 0.05–0.12 mg/kg/min
• **Calcium channel blockers**	
Verapamil	IV 5–20 mg bolus; oral 140–180 mg t.i.d.
Diltiazem	IV 0.25 mg/kg bolus, then 5–20 mg/h; oral 30–60 mg t.i.d.
Amiodarone	IV 5mg/kg in the first hour, then 0.5–1 mg/min; oral 100–200 mg/day
For rhythm control	
• **Propafenone**	IV 2mg/kg; oral 450–600 mg
• **Amiodarone**[a]	IV 5mg/kg in the first hour, then 0.5–1 mg/per min
• **Ibutilide**	IV 1–2 mg
• **Flecainide**	IV 2 mg/kg; oral 200–300 mg
• **Vernakalant**	IV 3–5 mg

Source: Lip GYH, Tsc HF, Lane DA. Lancet 2012; 379: 648–61.

[a]Can also be used for AF more than a week. All others are used for AF less than a week.

in 500 mL of 5% dextrose under ECG control. In less urgent situations, it is generally given sublingually in the dose of 10–15 mg every 4–6 h. Isoprenaline is also effective in abolishing ventricular tachycardia in the presence of advanced AV block. It acts by:

- **Accelerating the basic sinoauricular pacemaker,** resulting in the suppression of ectopic ventricular activity.
- **Enhancing the A–V conduction.**
- **Increasing the cardiac output** as a result of the increased heart rate. This tends to augment the coronary flow.

The A–V conduction can also be improved during an emergency by **atropine 0.6 mg IV.**

Other drugs used are adrenaline, dopamine, aminophylline and glucagon, but they are less effective than isoprenaline.

Glucocorticoids are helpful when the heart block is due to an inflammatory disorder such as rheumatic fever.

No drug, however, is useful in the treatment of advanced heart block, and implantation of a permanent pacemaker is essential.

ANTIARRYTHMIC DRUGS

According to their mechanism of action (Vaughan Williams Classification)

Class I: Fast sodium channel blockers

Class IA: Those which cause moderate phase 0 depression

Quinidine
Procainamide
Disopyramide

Class IB: Those which are weak phase 0 depressants

Lignocaine
Phenytoin
Mexiletine
Tocainide

Class IC: Those which cause marked phase 0 depression

Flecainide
Propafenone

Class II: Beta adrenergic blockers

Propranolol
Atenolol
Metoprolol
Esmolol

Class III: Potassium channel blockers

Amiodarone
Sotalol
Ibutilide
Vernakalant

Class IV: Calcium channel blockers

Verapamil
Diltiazem

Class V: Miscellaneous

Adenosine
Digitalis
Potassium
Magnessium
Atropine

According to their therapeutic use for the treatment of arrhythmias

Supraventricular arrhythmias

Adenosine
Verapamil
Diltiazem

Both supraventricular and ventricular arrhythmias

Amiodarone
Beta blockers
Quinidine
Procainamide

Ventricular arrhythmias

Lignocaine

CHAPTER 29

Pharmacotherapy of Angina Pectoris, Acute MI and Peripheral Vascular Diseases

Learning Objectives

This chapter will enable the reader:

1. To state the clinical manifestations of IHD.
2. To be aware of physiology of coronary circulation and factors influencing it.
3. To be aware of physiological functions and pathological role of nitric oxide (NO).
4. To describe the clinical types of angina pectoris.
5. To classify antianginal drugs.
6. To describe pharmacological effects, salient pharmacokinetic features, ADR, drug interactions and indications for organic nitrates, beta adrenergic blocking drugs, calcium channel blockers and potassium channel activators giving suitable example of drugs from each group.
7. To discuss the importance of nonpharmacological treatment in management of IHD.
8. To enlist cytoprotectives used for treating angina.
9. To outline the management of (a) exertional angina, (b) variant angina and (c) unstable angina including therapy for chronic prophylaxis.
10. To compare and contrast verapamil, diltiazem, nifedipine and amlodipine
11. To outline the management of acute myocardial infarction.
12. To enumerate the drugs used in the treatment of peripheral vascular disorders stating the pharmacological basis for their use.

KEY TERMS

Angina pectoris occurs as a result of imbalance between the myocardial oxygen demand and supply. It is a common symptom of ischaemic heart disease (IHD). IHD can manifest in various ways:

1. Silent (asymptomatic) ischaemia
2. Stable angina of effort, microvascular angina and variant angina (vasospastic)
3. Acute coronary syndrome (ACS)
    a. Unstable angina (UA)
    b. Acute myocardial infarction (AMI)
        i. Non-ST-segment elevation MI (NSTEMI)
        ii. ST-segment elevation MI (STEMI)
4. Chronic heart failure (CHF)
5. Sudden cardiac death (SCD)

These clinical modalities are related to the:

- *Physiology of the coronary circulation*
- *Factors governing myocardial metabolism*
- *Mechanism regulating the genesis and appreciation of pain*

The design of the coronary circulation has three bad features:

- **The coronary arteries are functionally end arteries.** In health, there is little communication between the larger and smaller branches of coronary arteries, although collateral circulation does develop in patients who have had MI.
- **Unlike the skeletal muscle, the cardiac muscle shows almost maximum oxygen extraction at rest,** as shown by the comparative values of

oxygen saturation of coronary sinus blood (30%) and skeletal muscle venous blood (60%–70%). Hence, during exercise, the tissue demand for increased oxygen supply is met, at least partly, by increased oxygen extraction in the case of the skeletal muscle, but in the case of the cardiac muscle, it can only be met by increasing the coronary blood flow. Such increase can be severely limited by coronary artery disease.

- **The coronary blood flow is influenced by the inflow (aortic) pressure and the coronary vascular resistance.** The latter depends on (a) the state of dilatation of the coronary arterioles and (b) the pressure exerted upon the coronary vessels from the exterior by the contracting myocardium during systole. Thus, in contrast to other areas where the arterial blood flow is continuous, **coronary blood flow to the left ventricle is intermittent and occurs mainly during diastole**, whereas in the absence of pulmonary hypertension it is both systolic and diastolic in case of the right ventricle.

In spite of these limitations, the coronary circulation has a large reserve, and the coronary flow can increase up to 5 to 8 times the resting value in exercising healthy individuals.

Physiologically, **vascular endothelial cells control the vascular tone** by producing:

- **Vasodilators** such as **prostacyclin** (Chapter 25) and **NO/EDRF**
- **Vasoconstrictors** such as **endothelin** (Chapter 30) and **thromboxane A_2** produced by platelets

NITRIC OXIDE (ENDOTHELIUM-DERIVED RELAXING FACTOR – EDRF)

A labile factor that is released by endothelial cells, causing vascular relaxation was designated as EDRF. Later it was identified as nitric oxide (NO). It is synthesised by **nitric oxide synthases** (NOS). These enzymes utilise the amino acid l-arginine as the endogenous substrate for NO generation. Three NOS isoforms have been identified as follows:

1. **nNOS** (NOS-1) is found in high concentrations in central and peripheral neurons, endometrium and the skeletal muscle
2. **iNOS** (NOS-2) is found in vascular smooth muscle cells, macrophages, Kupffer cells, fibroblasts, neutrophils and endothelial cells
3. **eNOS** (NOS-3) is found in the vascular endothelium, brain and heart

Types 1 and 3 are **constitutive** *NOS* and their activities are regulated by intracellular calcium. These isoenzymes produce on demand short bursts of NO in small amounts. *Type 2, on the other hand, is the* **inducible NOS** *and is not expressed in resting cells.* When macrophages and other cells are activated, this enzyme triggers the production of large amounts of NO.

Actions of NO:

- **Direct,** partly mediated by the NO molecule itself and mainly by the interaction of NO with soluble guanylyl cyclase (which acts as the receptor for NO), resulting in the production of 3′5′-cyclic guanosine monophosphate (cGMP). It also inhibits calcium entry into the smooth muscle and inhibits K^+ channels.
- **Indirect,** mediated by the interaction of reactive nitrogen species (intermediates in NO synthesis) with oxygen and superoxide radicals, yielding **cytotoxic peroxynitrite anion.**

NO is a highly diffusible second messenger that produces effects far from its site of production. At low concentrations, the direct (physiological) effects of NO predominate while induced, high concentrations of NO cause indirect and often toxic effects.

Functions of NO:

- **Vasodilation:** NO causes vascular smooth muscle relaxation that helps to regulate blood flow and BP. NO is released from the endothelial cells following an influx of Ca^{++} into the endothelial cells. Thus, any agent or stimulus capable of eliciting an influx of Ca^{++} into these cells, such as acetylcholine, bradykinin or shear force, can activate NO biosynthesis.

Endothelial dysfunction (impaired NO production) is implicated in hypertension, cerebral and coronary vasospasm, atherosclerosis, ischaemic reperfusion injury and diabetes mellitus.

- **Platelet inhibition:** NO causes inhibition of platelet aggregation and adhesion.

- **Neurotransmission:** Nonadrenergic, noncholinergic (NANC) neurons innervate a variety of smooth muscles, such as those of the GI tract, the corpora cavernosa and the esophagus. **The exclusive neurotransmitter in the NANC is NO.** Thus NO is the physiological mediator of penile erection (Chapter 67) and gastric emptying.
- **Prevention of sickling of RBCs:** Its precursor l-arginine is used to treat pulmonary hypertension in sickle cell disease.
- **Immunostimulation:** Macrophages exposed to infective agents, increase the local production of NO. It probably serves as a cytotoxic agent.

Adverse effects of NO: It is an **important mediator of inflammation and neurodegenerative disorders**. Exposure to bacterial endotoxins can lead to *overproduction of NO, which can cause severe hypotension and/or endotoxic shock*. Excessive NO can be toxic to the host cells, including pancreatic islet cells.

ANGINA PECTORIS

Occurrence of angina pectoris depends on the balance between two factors:

(a) **Oxygen demand by the myocardium**. This may be compromised by either obstructive (atherosclerotic) or vasospastic disease of the coronary arteries.
(b) **Oxygen supply (coronary blood flow)**

Cardiac O_2 requirement increases with an increase in the following:

- *Heart size*
- *Heart rate*
- *Systemic blood pressure*
- *Myocardial contractility,* which is the rate at which the cardiac muscle fibre shortens

The last three are increased by heightened sympathetic activity. The myocardial oxygen consumption increases significantly during exercise and other states with increased sympathetic activity. If, the increase in coronary blood flow is unable to match this increased oxygen demand, angina develops. It is generally described by the patient as retrosternal pain, heaviness or discomfort, which may radiate to the neck, shoulder, back or the arm. In each patient, there exists at a given time a threshold (**angina index = heart rate × systolic BP**) at which angina occurs. **The angina index is a measure of the myocardial oxygen consumption.**

Clinically, angina can be:

- **Stable, exertional angina:** This commonest form is usually provoked by physical exertion or emotional stress and is relieved by rest and nitrates. The main pathophysiological factor appears to be an increased myocardial oxygen demand. The ECG shows ST depression during the attack.
- **Microvascular angina (cardiac syndrome X):** More common in women, this condition comprises (a) angina or angina-like chest pain on exercise, (b) ST segment depression on treadmill exercise testing and (c) **normal coronary angiography**. Endothelial or microvascular dysfunction is responsible for ischaemia, and hence it is also termed as microvascular angina. Therapeutic response to physical training and to beta blockers is better than to nitrates and calcium channel blockers (CCB).
- **Variant angina of Prinzmetal (vasospastic angina)**: It is characterised by **chest pain at rest**, and **ST elevation.** Spasm of large epicardial coronary arteries is responsible for this entity.

Unstable angina (UA) includes a variety of clinical syndromes such as new onset angina, angina occurring at rest or with minimal exertion, progressive angina with prolonged or more frequent attacks superimposed on chronic stable angina (*Crescendo angina*); it can progress to MI and sudden death (preinfarction angina). The ECG may show ST depression, and troponin test is *negative.* PH 1.28

DRUGS USED IN ANGINA PECTORIS

The drugs effective in the treatment of angina pectoris act by:

1. Dilating the coronary arteries and/or
2. Reducing the cardiac workload by reducing preload and afterload (Fig. 29.1)

Classification of Drugs Used in Angina

I. **Organic nitrates**
II. **Beta-adrenergic blocking agents**
III. **Calcium channel blockers**
IV. **Potassium channel activators**

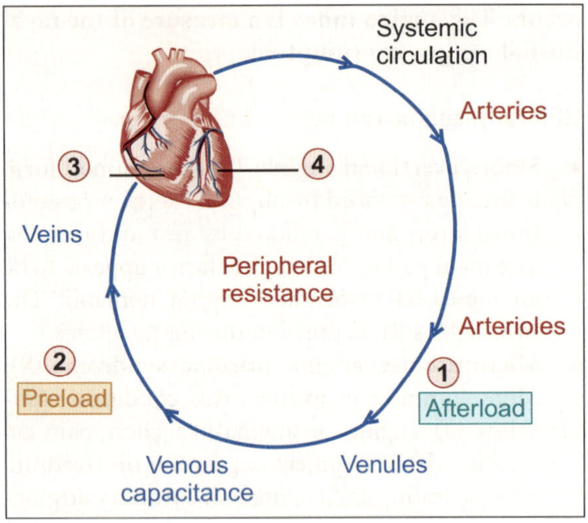

FIG. 29.1 **Antianginal drugs – mechanism of action. 1. *Reduce afterload* – CCB, beta blockers, nitrates. 2. *Reduce preload* – nitrates. 3. *Negative inotropic action* – beta blockers, CCB (verapamil and diltiazem). 4. *Coronary dilators* – nitrates and CCB.**

Additional beneficial effects can be obtained by using adjuncts such as

- **Cytoprotectives**
- **Antiplatelet drugs**
- **Antihyperlipidemic drugs**

ORGANIC NITRATES

Organic nitrates which are polyol esters of nitric acid are **potent vasodilators.**

Mechanism of action: Organic nitrates are reduced by reductases to organic nitrites, which are then **converted to NO** by mitochondrial aldehyde dehydrogenase. It acts as a direct vasodilator (Fig. 29.2). *Nitrates serve as exogenous sources of NO without involving endothelial cells, and are termed as NO donors.*

Pharmacological actions

Cardiovascular system

- **Hemodynamic actions:** Nitrates cause a **relaxation of the systemic venous and arteriolar bed. Venodilatation** causes peripheral pooling of blood and a reduction in venous return and in cardiac output. It thus reduces the preload (enddeastolic left ventricular pressure). **Arterial relaxation** is maximum in the large arteries (resulting in bounding pulse), followed by the arterioles, which reduces the **afterload** (resistance to left ventricular ejection) on the heart.
  The left ventricular workload and oxygen demand decrease. *The resultant improvement in the left ventricular function generally outlasts the measured pharmacological actions of individual doses of nitrates;* this is of great advantage in the therapy of angina pectoris.
  Sublingual nitroglycerine (NTG) is **predominantly a venodilator** causing reduction of ventricular preload.
- **Coronary circulation:** A transient decrease in the coronary resistance and an increase in the total

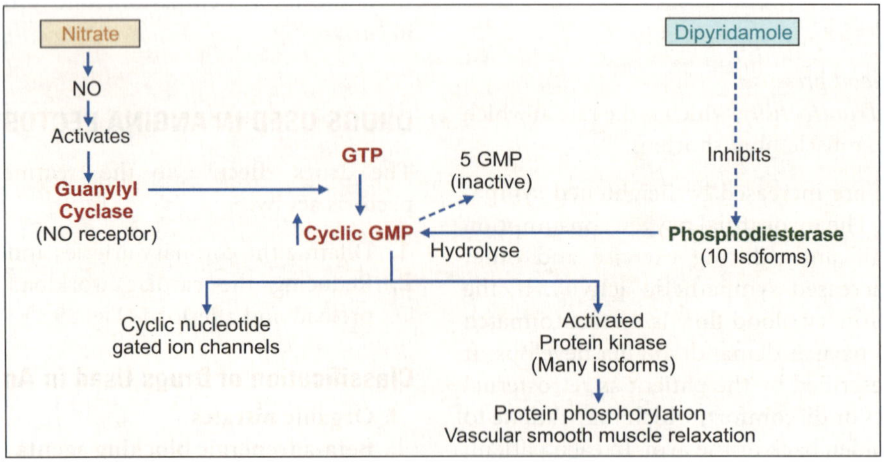

FIG. 29.2 **NO–cyclic GMP pathway and mechanism of action of nitrates and dipyridamole as vasodilators. GTP, guanosine triphosphate; Cyclic GMP, cyclic guanosine monophosphate.**

coronary flow occur in a normal subject. In patients with angina, nitrates:

i. *Dilate the large epicardial coronary arteries* without affecting the resistance of the arterioles.
ii. *Dilate collateral vessels.*
iii. *Cause selective redistribution of the coronary blood flow* with improved perfusion of ischaemic subendocardial areas.
Chronic administration promotes the development of interarterial anastomoses within the myocardium.

- **Effects in angina pectoris:** Nitrates help most patients with angina by increasing their exercise tolerance, but *without increasing their 'angina index'*. In such patients, they prevent the ECG changes of cardiac ischaemia during exercise. However, they do not increase the maximum aerobic capacity of the heart.

Other vascular beds: Nitrates cause dilatation of other vascular beds as well, e.g.:

1. Skin, giving rise to flushing
2. Meningeal vessels, resulting in throbbing headache
3. Pulmonary vessels, with fall in pulmonary arterial pressure
4. Kidneys, with a reduction in renal flow

Other smooth muscles: Nitrates relax the smooth muscles of the gall bladder, biliary ducts, sphincter of Oddi, bronchi, GI tract ureter and uterus.

Absorption, fate and excretion: Organic nitrates are readily absorbed from the sublingual mucosa, and cause more rapid and more predictable effects. This is because after sublingual administration, they bypass the liver where normally they are rapidly metabolised by denitration. With *relatively small sublingual doses,* the various organic nitrates have a similar duration of action, 10–45 min.

Large oral doses (30 mg of **isosorbide dinitrate** or 40–80 mg of **pentaerythritol tetranitrate**, every 4–6

Table 29.1 Nitrate and Nitrite Preparations for Clinical Use PH 1.28

Drug Preparations	Dose	Onset	Duration	Schedule	Remark
Glyceryl trinitrate (nitroglycerine)					
Tab. 0.3, 0.5 and 0.6 mg.	0.3–0.6 mg SL[a]	1–2 min	15–40 min	SOS	Volatile. Unstable in plastic containers. Store tablets in tightly closed amber coloured glass bottles, without cotton plugs, preferably in a fridge. Once a bottle is opened, it should be discarded after 8 weeks and fresh supply obtained. Sublingual tablets give immediate relief. Capsules, oral tablets and ointment for prophylaxis.
Sustained release cap. (2.5 and 6.5 mg) tablets: 2.6 and 6.4 mg	2.5 5.0 mg p.o.	60 min	8–12 h	8–12 hourly	
Sublingual spray	0.4 mg/metered dose	1–2 min	15–40 min for three doses	Every 5 min	
2% skin ointment (15 mg/inch)	½–2 inch applied without rubbing	20–60 min	4–6 h	4–6 hourly	
Transdermal patches (5,10, 15 mg)	5–15 mg	30–60 min	12 h	Once daily	
Isosorbide dinitrate					
Tab. 5, 10 mg	2.5–10 mg SL	10–30 min	1–2 h	3–4 hourly	Hepatic metabolism to isosorbide mononitrate. Useful in immediate relief and in prophylaxis
Buccal spray	1.25 mg/actuation	2–5 min	–	–	
Tab. oral 10, 20, 40 mg	10–40 mg p.o.	30–60 min	6–8 h	4 hourly	
Tab. sustained release	40–80 mg p.o.	60 min	12–18 h	12 hourly	
Isosorbide mononitrate					
Tab. 10, 20, 40 mg	10–20 mg p.o.	30–60 min	6–8 h	8–12 hourly	No first pass metabolism. Used in prophylaxis.
Pentaerythritol tetranitrate					
Tab. 30 mg	30 mg p.o.	15–30 min	4–6 h	8–12 hourly	Used in prophylaxis.

Notes: Tab., tablets; Cap., capsules; s.l., sublingually; p.o., orally.
[a]When the tablet, placed under the tongue, fails to produce local burning, flushing of the face and pounding in the head, it should be considered inert.

h) which exceed the metabolising capacity of the liver produce beneficial hemodynamic effects and are useful in prophylaxis. **NTG skin ointment and transdermal patches have a similar prolonged effect.**

Preparations and dosage: See Table 29.1. For IV use, NTG is diluted in 5% dextrose or 0.9% saline. It is administered in the dose of 5 mcg/min, increasing the rate every 3–5 min up to 80–100 mcg/min. It is useful in the treatment of refractory chest pain of myocardial ischaemia or MI, and refractory, variant angina.

Adverse reactions:

- **Headache:** Though common, it usually decreases gradually on repeated administration and can be controlled by aspirin.
- **Hypotension and syncope:** Transient episodes of giddiness, weakness and other signs of cerebral ischaemia associated with postural hypotension may develop. These are seen especially when the patient stands immobile. Hypoxemia may stimulate the central vagal nuclei and cold sweats, nausea, vomiting, involuntary passage of urine and faeces may accompany **postural hypotension**. Head-low position to augment the venous return quickly corrects the nitrite syncope. *Marked hypotension may occur when nitrates are used along with potent antihypertensives especially, vasodilators; it is also seen following the ingestion of alcoholic beverages or sildenafil* (Chapter 67) or aminophylline.
- **Tolerance** to nitrates can develop after repeated administration. **Cross-tolerance is common.** *Tolerance to the antianginal action develops commonly when the patient is exposed to nitrate for all the 24 h of the day.* Hence, **it is more common with long-acting nitrate preparations (SR tablets)** and **transdermal preparations.** *Tolerance is rare with sublingual nitrate because of the intermittent exposure.*
- **Withdrawal symptoms:** Sudden stoppage of nitrates during chronic administration may precipitate severe angina.

Indications:

- **All varieties of angina pectoris:** Discussed in the section, Treatment of angina pectoris.
- **At the onset of pain of acute MI** (see section, Acute myocardial infarction: management) except in those with inferior wall infarct (with the right ventricular involvement).
- **Paroxysmal nocturnal dyspnoea due to left ventricular failure (LVF) LVF:** NTG may give dramatic relief.
- **Acute LVF:** Nitroglycerine by IV infusion is useful in this condition.
- **Chronic heart failure:** Organic nitrates are sometimes used in the long-term management of a chronic heart failure due to IHD (Chapter 31).
- **Achalasia cardia.**
- **Acute anal fissure:** Local application (Chapter 40).
- **Cyanide poisoning:** Sodium nitrite IV is used to treat cyanide poisoning. Nitrites convert haemoglobin to methaemoglobin, which combines with cyanide ion and forms cyanmethemoglobin, a relatively nontoxic product (Chapter 75).

Contraindications to nitrates: These include cardiomyopathy, severe aortic or mitral stenosis, obstructive pericarditis and closed angle glaucoma.

BETA-ADRENERGIC BLOCKING AGENTS

These drugs are a cornerstone of the therapy of all stages of IHD, except Prinzmetal, vasospastic, variant angina. Only their actions relevant to angina are discussed below (also see Chapter 18).

Pharmacological actions: Increased sympathetic activity following exercise and emotional excitement increases heart rate, BP, myocardial contractility and oxidative metabolism and can precipitate an attack of angina in predisposed subjects. Beta blockers by blocking beta adrenergic activity prevent the angina attack. Moreover, they help to control BP in hypertensive patients. Like nitrates, beta blockers:

- **Increase the exercise tolerance without increasing the angina index.**
- **Prevent both subjective and ECG manifestations of cardiac ischaemia.**
- **Reduce ectopic activity and prevent arrhythmias** precipitated by exercise, emotion and conditions involving excessive sympathetic activity.
- **Decrease the NTG requirement.**

- Unlike nitrates, they **reduce heart rate and increase the diastolic relaxation time, which helps to improve coronary perfusion.** In most patients, the net effect is a beneficial reduction in cardiac workload and myocardial oxygen consumption. *However, they are not useful in acute attacks.*

Used prophylactically, they decrease the incidence of MI in such patients. For chronic prophylaxis, they are usually combined with nitrates. *Patients with cardiac decompensation should be stabilised before starting a beta blocker.*

Long-term use of beta blockers after MI and in patients with LV dysfunction reduces the rate of reinfarction and improves survival.

Clinically, all beta blockers are probably equally effective. Generally, the more selective beta blockers such as atenolol, metoprolol, bisoprolol and carvedilol are preferred.

Beta blockers are not useful in the therapy of variant angina of Prinzmetal.

Absorption, fate and excretion: Chapter 18.

Adverse reactions: The adverse reactions of relevance to antianginal therapy are:

- Precipitation or aggravation of CHF. Patients receiving both digoxin and a beta blocker should be watched for the development of heart block.
- Development of severe syncope on using NTG in patients on a beta blocker
- Bronchospasm
- Weight gain, glucose intolerance and erectile dysfunction can occur

Abrupt withdrawal of the beta-blocker can cause severe tachycardia, vasoconstiction, aggravation of angina and even precipitation of MI (Chapter 18).

Contraindications:

Presence of marked bradycardia, AV block, sick sinus syndrome, and severe heart failure are absolute contraindications for the use of beta blockers.

CALCIUM CHANNEL BLOCKERS (CCB)

In contrast to the contractile activity of the skeletal muscle, the contractility of the cardiac and vascular muscle is highly dependent on the extracellular calcium. Calcium transport in myocardial and vascular smooth muscle involves the following:

- **Voltage-dependent channel,** which is controlled by a gate that opens and closes in response to a voltage gradient.
- **Receptor operated channel,** which is normally activated by an alpha adrenergic agonist, such as NA, or angiotensin interacting with the alpha adrenergic receptors. They increase the degree of contraction of arterioles.
- **Sodium–calcium exchange,** which is an electrogenic mechanism. It operates bidirectionally to mediate the movement of calcium ions across the sarcolemma.
- **Calcium ATPase,** which extrudes calcium from the cell in an energy-dependent way.

Mechanism of action: CCB **bind to alpha-1 subunit of voltage-dependent L-channel,** and *inhibit the entry of calcium into the myocardial and vascular smooth muscles*, thus decreasing the availability of the intracellular calcium. They are **potent vasodilators.**

Classification of CCB

I. **Dihydropyridines** (DHP), e.g. nifedipine, amlodipine
II. **Non-DHP**
   - Phenylalkylamines, e.g. verapamil
   - Benzothiazepines, e.g. diltiazem

Pharmacological actions

Cardiovascular actions: Antianginal action of these drugs is due to:

1. **An improved coronary blood flow**
2. A **decrease in the oxygen demand of the heart** due to a reduction in the systemic vascular resistance. Verapamil, in addition, reduces the heart rate. *As a group, these drugs can be used in anginal patients with COPD in whom beta blockers are contraindicated.*
   - **Coronary artery dilatation:** These drugs are more potent than NTG as coronary artery dilators. CCBs dilate both, large epicardial as

well as the smaller intramyocardial coronary arterioles, even in the presence of coronary artery spasm. Furthermore, they can prevent the spasm even in diseased, atherosclerotic coronary arteries. This effect accounts for their efficacy in Prinzmetal angina.

- **Effect on peripheral blood vessels:** They lower the vascular resistance and the BP and are useful in the treatment of both systemic and pulmonary hypertension. The reduction in the afterload is also responsible for their beneficial effects in angina of effort. *The reduction in BP by nifedipine is accompanied by reflex tachycardia.*
- **Negative inotropic effect:** Non-DHP have a more pronounced effect on cardiac pacemaker, contractility and AV conduction which they depress. *Thus* **verapamil** *and* **diltiazem** *have negative inotropic actions and hence are not combined with beta blockers in the treatment of angina of effort.*
- **Antiarrhythmic effect:** Non-DHP:
    i. Decrease the rate of discharge of the SAN
    ii. Suppress ectopic pacemaker activity
    iii. Increase the refractory period of the AVN and slow the conduction (Chapter 28)

The slowing of the conduction prevents re-entrant excitation. This effect plus the improvement of cardiac ischaemia accounts for the potent (though selective) antiarrhythmic action. **Verapamil** and **diltiazem** are particularly potent in this respect. Both the drugs (but not nifedipine), however, can aggravate AV block.

Other actions: It also relaxes bronchial, ureteric and uterine smooth muscle.

Table 29.2 summarizes the properties of commonly used CCB.

VERAPAMIL: This drug is a synthetic papaverine derivative. It causes the following:

- **Suppression of SA and AV nodes which are Ca^{++} dependent**
- **Coronary and peripheral vasodilatation**
- **Potent antiarrhythmic effect**
- **Potent negative inotropic effect and may cause AV block**

It does not cause reflex sympathetic overactivity and tachycardia.

Given orally, it is absorbed completely but is substantially metabolised by first pass hepatic metabolism. It is highly protein bound. Adverse effects include constipation, vertigo, bradycardia, A–V block, CHF, hypotension and rarely cardiac asystole.

Table 29.2 Properties of Some Calcium Channel Blockers PH 1.28

	Verapamil	Diltiazem	Nifedipine	Amlodipine
Chemical class	Diphenylalkylamine	Benzothiazepine	Dihydropyridine	Dihydropyridine
Bioavailability	20%–35%	40%	40%–70%	40%–70%
Plasma half-life	6–12 h	3–6 h	2–5 h	35 h
Blocks AV conduction	+++	++	0	0
Antiarrthymic effect	+	+	0	0
Negative inotropic effect	++	+	±	±
Vasodilatation	++	+	+++	+++
Heart rate	□	N or □	□	N
Blocks reflex sympathetic effects	+	++	0	0
Dose (mg/day) in hypertension	120–240	60–120	30–60	2.5–10
Dose (mg/day) in angina	240–480	120–360	15–60	2.5–10
Dosage schedule	8 hourly	8 hourly	6–8 hourly	O.d.
Adverse effects	AV block, constipation	AV block	Palpitation, nausea, edema	Palpitation

Notes: 0, no effect; +/-, no or mild effect; +, Mild effect; ++, moderate effect; +++, potent effect; N, normal.

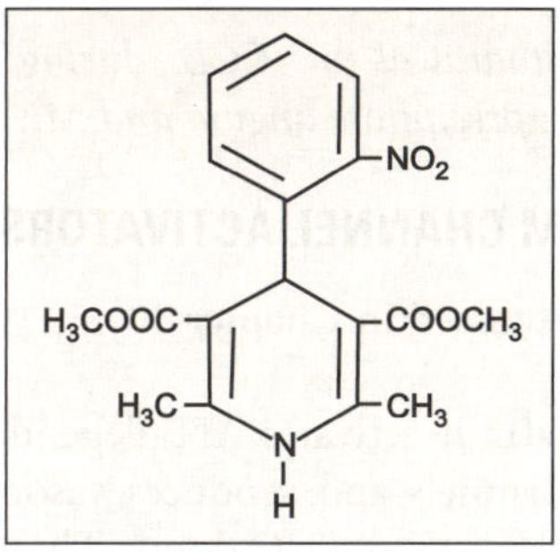

FIG. 29.3 **Nifedipine.**

It is used in the treatment of angina in the dose of 30–60 mg three times a day. For use in paroxysmal supraventricular tachycardia, see Chapter 28.

DILTIAZEM: This drug has properties intermediate between those of verapamil and nifedipine (see Table 29.2). It has less negative inotropic effect than verapamil and less vasodilating effect than nifedipine and verapamil. It can be combined with nitrates.

NIFEDIPINE: The pharmacological properties of this DHP derivative (Fig 29.3) are shown in Table 29.2.

Compared to verapamil, it:

- Has **negligible negative inotropic effect**
- Is a **more potent coronary and peripheral vasodilator**
- Causes **tachycardia**
- Is a **potent inhibitor of platelet aggregation**

It is admnistered either orally or (for a rapid effect) sublingually. *However, for long-term use, a sustained release formulation in the dose of 30–90 mg o.d. is preferred.*

Adverse reactions: These include headache, tachycardia, dizziness, fatigue, orthostatic hypotension, leg cramps, skin rashes and gingival hyperplasia. Occasionally, CHF may be precipitated.

Angina may worsen with nifedipine because of decrease in coronary perfusion pressure resulting from rapid fall in BP, increase in oxygen demand due to reflex sympathetic activation (tachycardia) and **coronary steal phenomenon.** In IHD, the narrowed coronary arteries are always maximally dilated to compensate for the decreased blood supply. **Nifedipine-induced arteriolar dilatation in the nonischaemic zone** *(there is no further dilatation of arterioles of the ischaemic zone) shunts oxygenated blood away from ischaemic zone to highly perfused nonischaemic zones of the heart. This stealing of coronary blood away from the ischaemic zone is termed as* **coronary steal phenomenon** *(Fig. 29.4), and may precipitate, angina. Hence nifedipine is not useful to treat agina. The slower-onset, longer-acting calcium blockers such as amlodipine do not cause this phenomenon.*

Indications:

Its main use is in the treatment of the following:

- **Hypertension** (Chapter 30)
- **Variant angina refractory to nitrate therapy**
- **Raynaud syndrome** (Chapter 30)

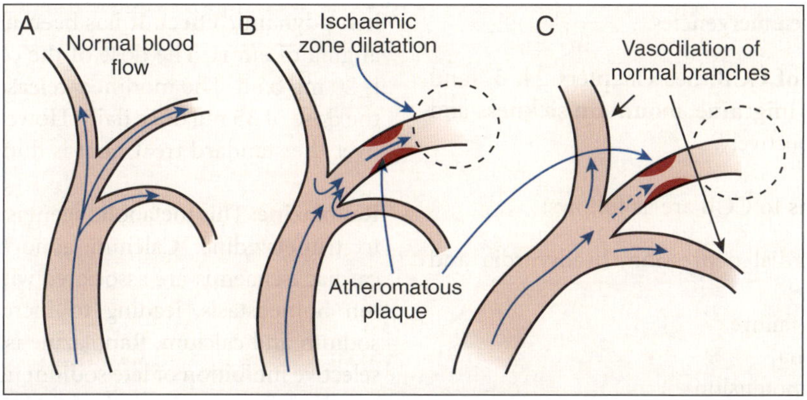

FIG. 29.4 **Coronary steal phenomena due to nifedipine. (A) Normal blood vessels: blood flow equally distributed to all branches. (B) Blood vessels in coronary disease: blood flow redistributed to ensure normal flow even to ischaemic myocardium. (C) Effect of nifedipine administration: blood flow diverted to normal myocardium due to vasodilatation leading to less blood supply to ischaemic myocardium.**

Nicardipine and **isradipine** are other DHP compounds with pharmacological properties and uses similar to those of nifedipine.

Amlodipine and **felodipine, with a long t½, are the second-generation DHP CCBs.** They are potent coronary and peripheral vasodilators; bradycardia and AV block are less liable to occur with their use (Table 29.2).

Nisoldipine: This dihydropyridine is available as SR tablets for prophylactic therapy for chronic stable angina and hypertension.

Nimodipine is related to nifedipine but is claimed to have a preferential vasodilating action on the cerebral arteries in animal studies. Its use is confined to the prevention of vascular spasm and subsequent ischaemic neurological damage following subarachnoid haemorrhage; its usefulness for this purpose is, however, uncertain. It is given in the dose of 60 mg every 4 h for the first few days.

Cilnidipine is a newer generation CCB, which blocks both, L- and N-type Ca^{++} channels. Blockade of N-type Ca^{++} channels attenuates NE release from sympathetic nerve endings, which in turn also inhibits renin-angiotensin system. Its efficacy as an antihypertensive is equal to amlodipidine but it causes lower incidence of ankle edema.

Clevidipine is a novel DHP compound with t½ of 2 min. It gets metabolised by plasma esterases. It has a rapid action and is used intravenously to control BP in hypertensive emergencies.

Noncardiac uses of CCB: See Chapters 24, 37 and 42 for their use in **migraine, mountain sickness** and as **tocolytics,** respectively.

Contraindications to CCB are as follows:

- Severe myocardial depression, bradycardia and heart block
- Clinical heart failure
- Unstable angina
- Preexisting hypotension
- Tight aortic stenosis

It is unwise to use them in patients on digoxin as they may exacerbate AV block or heart failure. They should be used in pregnancy only if absolutely necessary.

Abrupt withdrawal of CCB during long-term therapy can precipitate angina and MI.

POTASSIUM CHANNEL ACTIVATORS

These are discussed in Chapter 30.

NICORANDIL: It activates ATP-dependent myocyte potassium channels and produces vasodilatation. In addition, it also acts as a NO donor. Though it preferentially acts on the venous side and reduces the preload, it also acts on the arteriolar side and reduces the afterload. It is given orally in the dose of 10–20 mg b.i.d. Adverse effects are mostly due to vasodilator action and include headache, dizziness and dose-dependent hypotension.

Nicorandil is particularly useful as an alternative to nitrates when tolerance is a problem. It can be used in the presence of asthma or cardiac failure. It is expensive.

Pinacidil is similar to nicorandil in its properties, adverse reactions and uses. Its duration of action is about 6 h; the controlled release preparation (37.5 mg capsule) acts for about 12 h.

CYTOPROTECTIVES

Trimetazidine: This drug is a partial inhibitor of fatty acid oxidation (PFOX) pathway in the myocardium, thereby improving myocardial glucose metabolism in the presence of ischaemia. It is claimed to maintain normal LV function without exerting any hemodynamic effect. It has been used to treat stable angina of effort. The dose of the conventional tablet is 20 mg b.i.d. The modified-release tablet is given in the dose of 35 mg once daily. However, its superiority over the standard treatment is doubtful.

Ranolazine: This metabolic agent is chemically related to trimetazidine. Calcium abnormalities following cardiac ischaemia are associated with disregulation of ion homeostasis, leading to increased intracellular sodium and calcium. Ranolazine is claimed to act by selective inhibition of late sodium influx and thus prevents calcium overload via the Na^+–Ca^{++} exchanger. It also inhibits fatty acid oxidation. It has no effect on heart rate and BP. Its side effects are dizziness, nausea, asthenia and constipation. It is contra-indicated in hepatic impairment and in patients with pre-existing

Q–T prolongation. It is metabolised by CYP3A4 and can cause various drug interactions.

Perhexilene inhibits fatty acid oxidation. However, it causes hepatotoxicity and peripheral neuropathy.

Cytoprotective or metabolic drugs are much less effective and more expensive than the standard therapy. Their long-term safety profile is not known. They may be used as add-on drugs in resistant cases.

Ivabradine is a heart rate lowering agent which acts by selectively inhibiting the SAN. It has no other hemodynamic actions. It may be useful to treat high-resting heart rate in patients with CAD. *It is not useful in chronic stable angina.*

ANTIPLATELET DRUGS

ASPIRIN: Prophylactic aspirin reduces the incidence of MI in patients with chronic stable and unstable angina (Chapter 33).

Dipyridamole: This drug is a coronary dilator, but, unlike nitrates which dilate conductance vessels, it is claimed to dilate coronary resistance vessels (Fig. 29.2). It is a weak platelet inhibitor.

TREATMENT OF ANGINA PECTORIS

Exertional Angina (Angina of Effort)

The principles of treatment of angina of effort are outlined in Box 29.1.

Relief and prevention of individual attacks: NTG is the drug of choice in all types of angina. The patient is advised to carry the tablets and to put one **sublingually** as soon as premonitory symptoms develop. He/she should be advised to use NTG while sitting to avoid possible syncope. If symptoms are not relieved immediately, additional tablets may be used at 5 min intervals, **but not more than three tablets should be used in a 15 min** interval. Excessive absorption of the drug can cause hypotension.

NTG, or isosorbide dinitrate, used sublingually 10–15 min before a period of increased activity, such as walking, climbing or sexual intercourse, can frequently prevent the attack. This is the preferred method of using these drugs for prophylaxis.

Box 29.1 Principles of the Treatment of Angina of Effort PH 1.1

1. ***General***
   - **Reassurance**
   - **Measures to prevent progression**
     - i. Treatment of IHD risk factors, e.g. hypertension, hyperlipidaemia, diabetes and obesity
     - ii. Use of antiatherogenic agents, e.g. statins (Chapter 38)
     - iii. Advise about life style modification (control of emotional excitement, alcohol and smoking and weight control)
     - iv. Supervised, graded, physical exercises.
   - **Treatment of associated conditions** which increase oxygen demand, e.g. hyperthyroidism, anaemia, valvular heart disease, heart failure
   - **Avoidance of preparations containing sympathomimetic amines** (cold remedies, antiasthmatic and anorectic agents), atropine, aminophylline and antidepressants
2. ***Specific***
   - **Drugs for acute attack,** e.g. a nitrate (see Table 29.1)
   - **Chronic prophylaxis** (prevention of MI and improved survival) (see text)
     - i. Aspirin
     - ii. Use of nitrates, beta blockers, CCB
3. ***Surgical revascularisation***

Chronic prophylaxis: This comprises the following:

- **Nitrates:** Large oral doses of organic nitrates decrease the frequency of anginal attacks and increase the exercise tolerance. They, however, increase the risk of hypotension, tachycardia and tolerance. Nitrates can be combined with beta blockers or diltiazem which effectively counters the reflex tachycardia by nitrates.
- **Beta blockers:** All beta blockers seem to be equally effective and reasonably safe as antianginal drugs. **They are the drugs of choice for chronic prophylaxis of angina of effort (IHD).** They can be combined, if necessary with nitrates for this purpose. A selective beta blocker such as metoprolol (50–100 mg twice a day) or atenolol (50–100 mg once a day) may be preferred (Chapter 18).

Beta blockers are the drugs of choice in cardiac syndrome X but are not particularly effective against angina at rest. Their beneficial effect in the absence of sympathetic overactivity is small.

- **Calcium channel blockers:** In patients with angina of effort, these drugs appear to be as effective prophylactic as beta blockers, but they are less well tolerated.
  They are mainly used in patients not responding to a combination of beta blockers and nitrates, wherein DHP can be combined with beta blockers. They can be used in patients with COPD, asthma and AV conduction disturbances. *Verapamil can be used instead of a beta blocker to control tachycardia in thyrotoxic patients with asthma.*
- **Combination of a beta blocker and a CCB** is additive but not synergistic. *Verapamil should not be combined with beta blockers. Diltiazem may be combined with beta blockers only in patients with a normal cardiac function and without conduction defects.* The second-generation dihydropyridines (e.g. amlodipine) are particularly useful in patients with angina associated with hypertension.
  Box 29.2 outlines a step-wise approach to the drug treatment of angina.
- **Advice about the life style:** Excitement and emotional upset (stress) can precipitate anginal attacks. Rest, diet modification, choice of occupation not involving heavy manual work and mental relaxation are important. *In fact, the value of change in 'life style' and aggressive treatment of risk factors is far more important than that of any known drug.*
  The patient should avoid any type, amount or pace of activity known to precipitate anginal attack; if it is unavoidable, the prophylactic use of NTG or isosorbide dinitrate sublingually 10–15 min before commencing the activity is recommended.
  Alcohol should be avoided by patients with angina. It is not a coronary vasodilator. Alcohol has a negative inotropic action on the heart damaged by CAD.
- **Cessation of smoking:** Patients with angina *must be advised* to give up smoking, which increases the heart rate and oxygen consumption of the myocardium.

Box 29.2 Stepwise Approach to Drug Therapy of Angina

All patients are prescribed aspirin 75–150 mg/day orally and glyceryl trinitrate sublingually, whenever needed.

Control risk factors	Obesity, *hyperlipidaemia*, hypertension, diabetes and smoking. Consider using a statin.
Treat concomitant diseases	Anaemia, thyrotoxicosis, valvular disease and heart failure.
Mild to moderate symptoms	Beta blockers; if contraindicated, CCB. If both are not tolerated, use prophylactic isosorbide dinitrate/mononitrate, or nicorandil.
If symptoms persist	Combine beta blockers with a CCB. Cytoprotectives may be used.
If severe and not responding	Refer for revascularisation.

Variant Angina of Prinzmetal

The treatment of this condition comprises (a) NTG (SL) or (b) nifedipine, first chewed and then swallowed, for a rapid onset of action in acute attacks. Long-acting nitrates or DHP are used for prophylaxis. *Beta blockers are to be avoided.*

ACUTE CORONARY SYNDROME (ACS)

Unstable Angina — IM 2.15, PH 1.28

It requires aggressive treatment in an ICCU to prevent MI or sudden death. The patient is treated with aspirin (150–300 mg); sublingual NTG or IV isosorbide dinitrate/NTG. A beta blocker is administered to lower the heart rate to 50–60/min. Routine anticoagulation with heparin is helpful.

ACUTE MYOCARDIAL INFARCTION (MI): MANAGEMENT — IM 2.23, PH 1.28

Acute MI is a medical emergency and needs immediate attention. It is initiated by rupture or erosion of local atherosclerotic plaque leading to thrombus formation. The symptomatology varies from very mild (silent infarct) to severe presentation (with cardiogenic shock). **It is classified based on presence or absence of ST segment elevation as:**

- **STEMI**, which is usually precipitated by total occlusion by thrombus, and
- **NSTEMI**, which results due to partial occlusion.

Rise in **creatinine kinase–myocardial band** (CK-MB) and **troponin** indicates the degree of myocardial necrosis. These biochemical markers are always elevated in STEMI. In patients with NSTEMI, they are usually elevated but may be normal. In unstable angina, they are not elevated indicating the absence of necrosis. The pathology, ECG findings and management strategy for unstable angina, NSTEMI and STEMI is summarised in Table 29.3. Ideally patients with STEMI should be treated by Percutaneous Coronary Intervention (PCI) to achieve rapid reperfusion of coronary arteries but such facilities are often not available.

- **Relief of pain: In mild cases, sublingual nitroglycerine may suffice.** Transdermal or IV NTG therapy is helpful in relieving persistent pain. **In patients with severe pain,** the slow IV administration of 10 mg of **morphine** hydrochloride over 10 min ensures rapid relief from pain. **Morphine** may be repeated, if necessary, after 30 min. **Pethidine hydrochloride** (25–50 mg) may be given intravenously, particularly in the presence of bradycardia. Morphine may cause sinus bradycardia and respiratory depression. Alternatively **buprenorphine** 0.4 mg SC or 0.3–0.6 mg IM may be used and repeated, if necessary 6–8 hourly.
- **Oxygen and rest:** The patient should be confined to bed and made to breathe 100% oxygen by means of a face mask. **It is of not of much benefit in patients with normal oxygen levels.** Even a slight increase in activity could worsen the condition.
- **Thrombolytic therapy:** This is most useful in patients with STEMI (Chapter 33) and may be harmful in NSTEMI.
- **Antiplatelet therapy: Aspirin (100–300 mg) is chewed as soon as the diagnosis of MI is made.** It is continued once daily throughout convalescence and after recovery. It has shown to reduce the mortality significantly. For

Table 29.3 Pathology, ECG Findings and Management Strategy for STEMI, U NSTEMI and Unstable Angina IM 2.20

	STEMI	NSTEMI	Unstable Angina
Pathology	Fully occluding thrombus	Non-thrombotic plaque or partially occluding thrombus	Non-thrombotic plaque or partially occluding thrombus
ECG findings	ST segment elevation present	ST segment elevation absent	ST segment elevation absent
	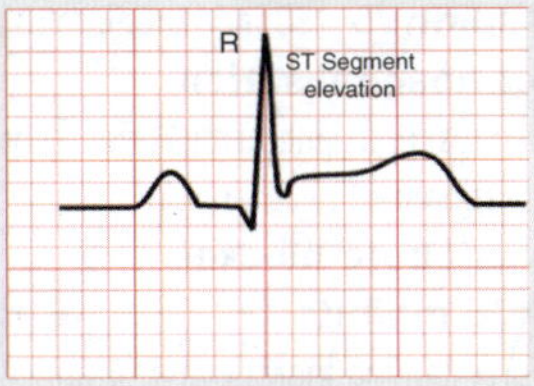	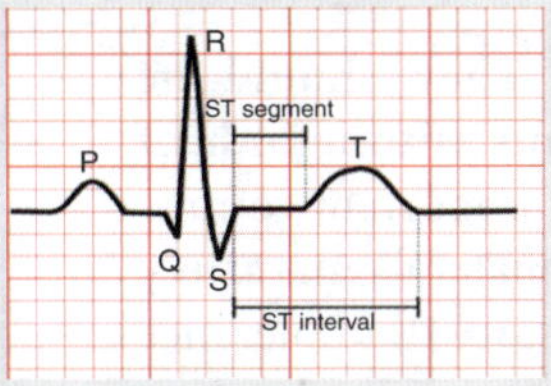	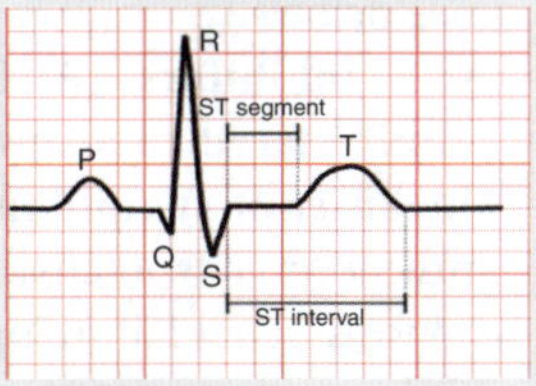
Biomarker levels(e.g. troponin)	Increased	Increased	Not increased
Immediate management	• Percutaneous coronary intervention within 120 mins, if facilities exist OR Thrombolytic therapy • Rest treatment same as for NSTEMI	• Oxygen • Morphine • Nitrates • beta blockers • Dual antiplatelet therapy • Anticoagulant	• Same as NSTEMI

patients intolerant to aspirin, clopidogrel can be used.

- **Maintenance of effective blood volume:** In the presence of cardiogenic shock, the effective circulating volume is reduced which should be corrected by the following:
  a. Elevating the lower limbs, and thus increasing the venous return to the heart
  b. Infusing 5% dextrose
- **Inotropic drugs: Dopamine and Dobutamine are the drugs of choice for regulating BP.** Dobutamine is less likely to cause arrhythmias and sinus tachycardia. If they are not available, NA may be used (Chapter 18).
- **Prevention and treatment of arrhythmias:** *Prophylactic therapy with class I antiarrhythmic drugs is not recommended in patients without an arrhythmia.* It is best not to give drugs empirically for a paroxysmal tachyarrhythmia or rapid irregularity of the pulse until an ECG is recorded.
  Digoxin may be given if CHF develops.
- **Beta blockers: Given within 4–6 h of the onset of symptoms, propranolol, atenolol and metoprolol may limit the infarct size and reduce early mortality.** The contraindications to the use of these drugs are: bronchospasm, resting bradycardia (less than 55/min), low systolic BP (less than 95 mm Hg) and heart block. *Currently, it is recommended that an oral beta blocker should be given to all patients who do not have a contraindication (Chapter 18).* Long-term use of beta blockers is beneficial (see below).
- **ACE inhibitors (ACEI): They should be administered to all patients within 24 h of the onset of symptoms,** if important contraindications (hypotension, bilateral renal artery stenosis, renal failure or history of intolerance to these drugs) are absent.
- **Anticoagulants:** Anticoagulants may be given to all patients with STEMI and NSTEMI. They prevent venous thrombosis, pulmonary embolism, and stroke in patients with severe LV dysfunction. Heparin, especially low molecular weight heparin (LMWH), given subcutaneously for 3–5 days is the preferred drug for this purpose (Chapter 33).
- **General measures:** Benzodiazepine to allay anxiety, soft low-calorie diet with no added salt, avoidance of caffeinated beverages, use of stool softener and life-style modifications are recommended.
- Lifelong continuation of low-dose (75–100 mg) aspirin is valuable to reduce the reinfarction rate.

Beta adrenergic blockers (atenolol, 50–100 mg o.d. or metoprolol 100 mg b.i.d.) have been shown to reduce mortality, sudden deaths and reinfarction after MI. This therapy should be used for at least 2–3 years after acute infarction.

ACE inhibitors reduce mortality, incidence of heart failure and reinfarction. They can be stopped after 1–2 years in many patients but must be continued lifelong in patients with left ventricular dysfunction, with or without symptoms and in patients of DM.

Box 29.3 summarises the medical treatment of acute MI.

Box 29.3 Principles of the Treatment of Acute Myocardial Infarction PH 1.1

Before hospitalisation
- For prompt relief of pain
  a. **Sublingual nitroglycerine** 0.4 mg every 5 min till pain is relieved (maximum three doses) in mild cases and in the absence of hypotension (systolic BP 90 mm).
  b. **IV morphine,** 1 mg per minute, titrated to a maximum total dose of 10 mg, together with IV metoclopramide 10 mg (antiemetic).
  c. Oxygen.
- **Aspirin** 75–150 mg (antiplatelet action).

After hospitalisation
- Bed rest and general measures (sedation, diet, bowel care, activity)
- Treatment of hypotension
- IV/oral **beta blocker**
- **ACE inhibitor**
- Thrombolytic therapy and/or anticoagulants (see text)
- Treatment of complications

Discharge and rehabilitation
- Graded increase in physical activity, including exercise therapy
- Aspirin
- ACE inhibitors
- Beta blockers
- Statin
- **Modification of cardiac risk factors:** smoking (including nicotine substitution), alcohol, hypertension, diabetes mellitus, hyperlipidaemia, obesity

Glucocorticoids and NSAID (except low-dose aspirin) should be avoided in patients with MI as they interfere with infarct healing.

DRUGS USED IN THE TREATMENT OF PERIPHERAL VASCULAR DISORDERS PH 1.28

Peripheral vascular disease (PVD) is many a times associated with CAD. It may be one of the following:

- **Obstructive:** Atherosclerosis or thromboangiitis obliterans (TAO) with large vessel involvement, or diabetes with small vessel involvement
- **Vasospastic:** Raynaud syndrome

Obstructive Peripheral Vascular Disease

In these patients, **vasodilator drugs are of little value** as they fail to increase the blood flow to ischaemic areas with blocked arteries/arterioles. Furthermore, the associated generalised vasodilatation can produce severe adverse reactions. Such patients may benefit from:

- **Correction of remediable underlying** factors such as CHF, anaemia or diabetes mellitus
- **Cessation of smoking**
- **Daily physical exercise** (such as walking) which can increase the walking distance
- **Foot care** (cleanliness, avoidance of any injury and prompt treatment of infection)
- **Drugs: Low-dose aspirin** (antiplatelet action), **statins** (cholesterol lowering action) and pentoxyphylline (hemorheologic action) have been used with variable success (Chapter 33)

All patients with PVD should be vaccinated against influenza.

Naftidofuryl oxalate 100 mg orally 2–3 times a day alleviates symptoms and increases pain-free walking distance in moderate peripheral obstructive vascular disease. It is not a direct vasodilator, and its mechanism of action is not clear. It is $5HT_2$ antagonist, and it inhibits 5HT induced vasoconstriction and platelet aggregation.

PENTOXIFYLLINE: This analogue of xanthines is claimed to decrease blood viscosity and maintain RBC flexibility during circulation and thus improve the microcirculation (**hemorheological action**). It has been claimed to be useful in patients with cerebrovascular disease, especially those getting transient ischaemic attacks and in those with intermittent claudication. The drug may reduce the plasma fibrinogen level and inhibit platelet aggregation. It causes mild GI upset and CNS adverse effects.

Cilostazol is a PDE3 inhibitor which inhibits platelets and dilates vessels. It improves symptoms of claudication, but the effect on cardiovascular mortality remains unclear. It may be useful in patients without rest pain and no peripheral tissue necrosis. It is contraindicated in patients with heart failure.

It is important to note that intermittent claudication can be of vascular origin (e.g. Burger's disease) or neurological origin. The former is only partially helped by vasodilators, while they are not at all useful in the latter group.

Vasospastic Diseases

Drugs useful in these conditions are as follows:

- **Calcium channel blockers,** e.g. nifedipine and diltiazem are preferred
- **Beta adrenergic stimulants:** nylidrin and isoxsuprine (Chapter 18)
- **Alpha adrenergic blockers:** tolazoline and prazosin (Chapter 18)
- **Anticoagulants:** heparin and warfarin, discussed in Chapter 33

In Raynaud syndrome, prazosin is used in the dose of 0.5 mg b.i.d. (first dose at bedtime); the maintenance dose is 1–2 mg b.i.d. Nifedipine is used in the dose of 5–20 mg t.i.d. NTG patch may be useful.

Other drugs claimed to be useful are nicotinic acid derivatives, cyclandelate, ketanserin and prostacyclin.

The drug therapy must always be combined with **nonpharmacological measures,** such as exercise, avoidance of exposure to cold and **cessation of smoking.** Sympathomimetics, e.g. decongestants, amphetamine and ephedrineas well as beta blockers should be avoided.

DRUGS USED IN THE TREATMENT OF ANGINA

Organic nitrates
- Glyceryl trinitrate
- Isosorbide dinitrate
- Isosorbide mononitrate
- Pentaerythritol tetranitrate

Beta-adrenergic blocking agents
- Propranolol
- Atenolol
- Metoprolol
- Bisoprolol

Potassium channel activators
- Nicorandil
- Pinacidil

Calcium channel blockers
- **Dihydropyridines (DHP)**
  - Nifedipine
  - Amlodipine
- **Non-DHP**
  - Phenylalkylamines
    - Verapamil
  - Benzothiazepines
    - Diltiazem

Cytoprotectives
- Trimetazidine
- Ranolazine

Other Agents
- Ivabradine
- Antiplatelet agents
- Antihyperlipidemic drugs

CHAPTER 30

Pharmacotherapy of Hypertension, Pulmonary Hypertension and Orthostatic Hypotension

Learning Objectives

This chapter will enable the reader:

1. To be aware of physiological factors and regulatory mechanisms involved in normal control of blood pressure (BP)
2. To classify antihypertensive drugs according to the site of action.
3. To explain the pharmacological basis for use of thiazides in hypertension.
4. To describe the mechanism of action, pharmacological effects, ADR and indications for angiotensin-converting enzyme inhibitors (ACEIs) and angiotensin receptor blockers.
5. To explain the rationale for use of following drugs to treat hypertension (highlighting their adverse reactions): calcium channel blockers, sympatholytics (centrally acting, ganglion-blocking drugs, adrenergic neuron–blocking drugs, beta-adrenergic antagonists, alpha-adrenergic antagonists and mixed adrenergic receptor blockers) and vasodilators.
6. To state the principles of antihypertensive drug therapy.
7. To describe the management of hypertension with emphasis on special populations, i.e. elderly, pregnant ladies and patients with other comorbid conditions.
8. To state the advantages and limitations of combining antihypertensives.
9. To outline the treatment of hypertensive crisis.
10. To enumerate the drugs used in the treatment of pulmonary hypertension stating the pharmacological basis for their use.
11. To outline the drug therapy for orthostatic hypertension.

KEY TERMS

Hypertension, which affects over 1 billion adults worldwide, is a major risk factor for cardiovascular and renal diseases. Clinically it can be divided into:

- **Primary or essential hypertension,** where the definite cause for the rise in blood pressure (BP) is not known
- **Secondary hypertension,** secondary to **renal** (e.g. chronic diffuse glomerulonephritis, pyelonephritis, polycystic kidneys), **endocrine** (e.g. Cushing syndrome, pheochromocytoma, primary hyperaldosteronism) and **vascular causes** (e.g. renal artery disease, coarctation of aorta)

Physiologically BP is a product of cardiac output (CO) and peripheral vascular resistance (**PVR**).

The syndrome of **essential hypertension** is characterised by elevation of the diastolic blood pressure (DBP) at rest, a normal CO (in most cases) and increased PVR, with documented natural history and with characteristic **pathological changes in the arterioles.**

Although, the 2017 guidelines (ACC-AHA) define high BP as a systolic BP ≥ 130 mm of Hg or diastolic BP ≥ 80 mm of Hg, currently clinic BP >140 systolic and/or > 90 mm of Hg or higher and daytime ambulatory BP monitoring average or home BP monitoring average of ≥135/85 mm Hg or higher *on several occasions qualifies as hypertension*, at all ages (NICE hypertension guideline, 2019; International Society of Hypertension, 2020; WHO, 2021). Systolic blood pressure (SBP) above 140 mm Hg plus DBP of below 90 mm Hg in the elderly is termed **isolated systolic hypertension.**

Hypertension, if untreated, leads to a variety of disabling cardiac, cerebrovascular and renal complications, with shortened life expectancy, regardless of its aetiology. Furthermore, *the risk of morbidity and mortality rises with BP. Control of BP with antihypertensives reduces this risk.*

Physiologically, the BP is controlled by two main types of systems (Fig. 30.1).

- **The adrenergic nervous system** which operates through the baroreceptors and is **mainly responsible for counteracting the acute changes in the BP**. Baroreceptor reflexes protect the circulation against stresses that alter arterial pressure acutely. When one stands up from the lying down position, the cardiac output tends to fall due to reduced venous return to the heart. This may lead to a fall in BP and fainting. Normally, it is prevented by a reflex increase in the heart rate and in the peripheral resistance through the baroreceptor mechanism.
- **The humoral renin–angiotensin–aldosterone system (RAAS),** which has a slow response, is **important in the long-term regulation of BP and operates through the kidneys** (Fig. 30.1).

Renin, a proteolytic enzyme, is produced and stored in the kidneys. It is released in response to:

- Reduction in the renal perfusion pressure
- Reduction in the sodium delivery to the macula densa
- Increase in the sympathetic activity
- Certain humoral factors

Renin cleaves the serum globulin **angiotensinogen** to an inactive decapeptide, 'angiotensin I'. The latter, during its passage through the lungs, is converted into an active octapeptide, **'angiotension II'** by the action of **angiotensin-converting enzyme** (ACE). Angiotensin II:

- **Is the most potent direct vasoconstrictor agent, effective in a dose as small as 0.1 mcg/kg body weight**
- Stimulates the synthesis and release of aldosterone from the adrenal cortex and thus regulates the ECF volume

In the circulation, angiotensin II is converted into a heptapeptide, angiotensin III, which is as potent as angiotensin II in its action on the adrenal cortex but is weaker in its other actions. '*The kidney thus plays an important role in determining the BP level, doing so via* **RAAS,** *which controls both vasoconstriction and volume, the two major determinants of BP and of tissue flow.*'

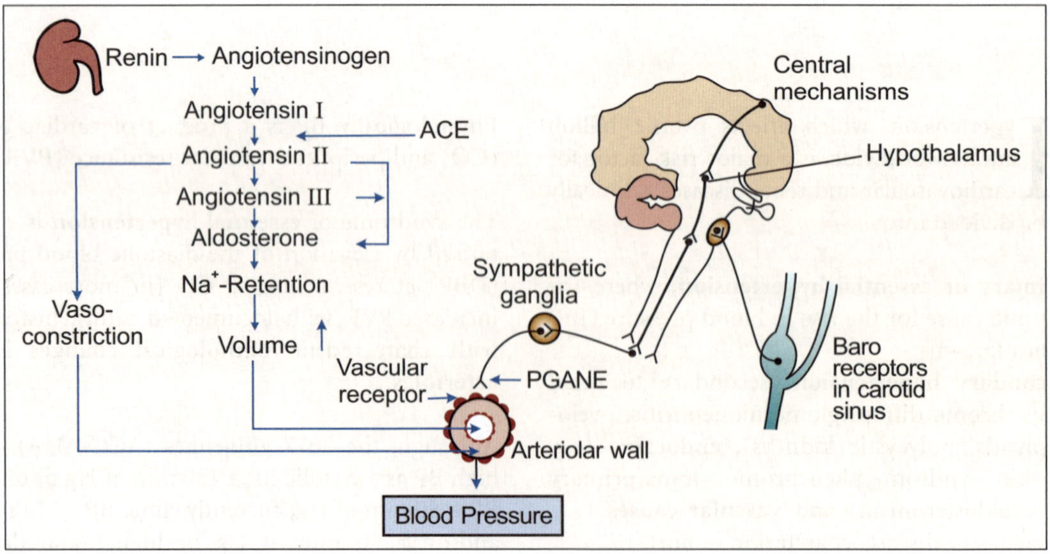

FIG. 30.1 **Physiology of BP control. PGANE, postganglionic adrenergic nerve ending.**

Renin and angiotensin are also produced locally in many tissues including blood vessels, brain, kidney, heart and adrenal glands. It is likely that these tissue angiotensin-generating systems are involved in the local control of cardiac, renal and vascular function, and cardiovascular damage.

The aetiology of primary hypertension is not clear. The factors implicated in its genesis are as follows:

- The chances of an individual developing hypertension increases with age and its prevalence is higher among individuals aged ≥60 years.
- There is a strong familial clustering of essential hypertension and *the inheritance is polygenic.*
- The arterial pressure is a function of the cardiac output and the peripheral resistance. Resistance to the blood flow resides chiefly in the arterioles. *Factors which tend to diminish their radius augment the total PVR and consequently, the BP.*
- The renin–angiotensin system is involved in the pathogenesis of some forms of secondary hypertension such as the renovascular hypertension. It is also believed to play a role in the pathogenesis of essential hypertension. On the basis of renin activity, patients with high BP can be divided into (1) those with high-renin activity or (2) those with **low-renin activity**.
- There is deficient vascular synthesis and release of nitric oxide (NO) in hypertensives.
- *There is a positive correlation between total body sodium and BP, and a negative one between total body potassium and BP in hypertensive patients.* Essential hypertension and age-related increase in BP are virtually absent in populations where less than 50 mmol of Na^+ (<3.00 g of salt) is consumed daily. **It appears that both excess of body sodium and deficit of body potassium contribute to the development of hypertension**. Increase in the intracellular Na^+ stimulates Na^+–Ca^{++} exchange pump, driving Ca^{++} into the cell. Increased cytosolic Ca^{++} triggers vascular smooth muscle contraction. Furthermore, sodium retention in the cell decreases NO synthesis by endothelial cells, whereas high-potassium diet causes endothelium-dependent vasodilatation. **Clinically, salt restriction reduces BP in many hypertensive patients.**

Classification of Antihypertensives PH 1.27

They can be classified according to site of action (Fig. 30.1).

I. **Diuretics:** Thiazides, chlorthalidone (thiazide-like)

II. **RAAS inhibitors:**
   - i. **Blockers of renin release:** Beta-adrenergic blockers
   - ii. **Direct renin inhibitors:** Aliskiren
   - iii. **ACE inhibitors (ACEIs):** Captopril, enalapril
   - iv. **Angiotensin receptor blockers (ARBs):** Losartan
   - v. **Aldosterone antagonists:** Spironolactone, eplererone

III. **Calcium channel blockers (CCBs):** Nifedipine, amlodipine, verapamil, diltiazem

IV. **Sympatholytic drugs**
   - i. **Drugs acting on adrenergic receptors:**
     - (a) *Alpha-adrenergic–blocking agents:* Phentolamine, phenoxybenzamine, prazosin, indoramin
     - (b) *Beta-adrenergic–blocking agents:* Propranolol, atenolol, metoprolol
     - (c) *Both alpha- and beta-adrenergic–blocking drugs:* Labetalol
   - ii. **Central sympatholytics:**
     - (a) *α_2-Adrenergic receptor stimulants:* Clonidine, alpha-methyldopa
     - (b) *Selective imidazole receptor (IR) stimulants:* Moxonidine
   - iii. **Adrenergic neuron blockers:** Guanethidine, reserpine
   - iv. **Ganglion-blocking agents:** Hexamethonium, trimethaphan

V. **Drugs acting directly on the vascular smooth muscle (vasodilators):**
   - (a) **Arteriolar vasodilators:** Hydralazine, diazoxide, minoxidil
   - (b) **Arteriolar-venular vasodilators:** Sodium nitroprusside

VI. **Potassium channel activators:** Diazoxide, minoxidil, pinacidil, nicorandil

VII. **Miscellaneous:** Metyrosine

All these drugs act by reducing the:

- cardiac output and/or
- the total PVR, without correcting the cause.

Various antihypertensives may ultimately reduce the BP by more than one mechanism. Furthermore, the haemodynamic alterations produced by a single parenteral dose of a drug may differ from those resulting from its prolonged oral use.

> *Currently, drugs used for the initial therapy of hypertension belong to any one of the three groups –* Thiazide or **thiazide-like diuretics, ACEI** or **ARB and CCB.**

THIAZIDES AS ANTIHYPERTENSIVES PH 1.24

The **thiazides** and related compounds **chlorthalidone** (Chapter 37) have proved extremely valuable in the treatment of mild-to-moderate hypertension. In addition, they enhance the effect of other antihypertensive agents. Chlorthalidone has a longer t½ of 40–60 h.

Mechanism of action: The thiazides probably reduce the BP by several mechanisms.

- The sodium depletion and consequent **reduction in plasma volume and cardiac output** produced by them are important in the initial days of therapy. Severe dietary restriction of sodium can produce a similar fall in BP.
  However, after a few weeks of thiazide therapy, the plasma volume and the cardiac output return to the pretreatment level.
- From then on, **decreased systemic vascular resistance, probably due to changes in the ionic composition** (Na^+–K^+) of the vascular wall, is important in maintaining the antihypertensive effect.
- **Activation of the K^+ channels** may also contribute to thiazide-induced vasodilatation.

Pharmacological actions: The antihypertensive effect is moderate and develops slowly. There is a reduction in both the SBP and the DBP. The maximum effect is obtained with 50 mg of **hydrochlorothiazide** or 12.5–25 mg of **chlorthalidone** once a day. *Increase in the dose does not enhance the hypotensive effect and there appears little difference in their antihypertensive action with equivalent doses of thiazides.* Differences do exist, however, in their duration of action (Chapter 37). The very potent diuretic furosemide is not recommended for the long-term management of hypertension because of its short duration of action and serious electrolyte disturbances. However, it can be valuable in patients with chronic kidney disease who do not respond to thiazides. **In patients with markedly decreased GFR (<50%), thiazides lose most of their diuretic and antihypertensive effects and are not useful.** Thiazides also increase the PRA which may contribute to the development of tolerance after prolonged use.

Adverse reactions: These include hypokalaemia, hyperuricaemia and hyperglycaemia (Chapter 37). *With the recommended low doses, hypokalaemia and other metabolic changes are generally not a problem.* Data indicate that:

- In the absence of digitalis and possibly overt heart disease, hypokalaemia is not associated with increased occurrence of ventricular arrhythmias.
- Although serum LDL-C levels do rise modestly after thiazide, the levels usually revert to the pretreatment levels during long-term use.

Routine potassium supplementation during thiazides use is not necessary. Those at high risk of developing hypokalaemia (patients with IHD, arrhythmias, diabetes, severe hepatic disease as well as those on digitalis or glucocorticoids) should receive prophylactic potassium supplements or potassium-sparing diuretics.

Advantages of low-dose thiazides and chlorthalidone:

- Their efficacy in mild-to-moderate hypertension is similar to other antihypertensive agents (see section choice of drug therapy)
- Postural hypotension is rare
- Blood flow to vital organs such as kidney and brain is not compromised
- They do not cause reflex tachycardia or reduce the cardiac output
- Unlike vasodilators, they do not cause compensatory volume overload and oedema
- They have substantial residual effects and BP rises slowly after discontinuation. Hence, missing a dose occasionally carries no risk of sudden rebound rise.
- With doses recommended, they are well tolerated, with minimal acceptable side effects. They

have been in use for several years and their long-term toxicity profile is well known. *They reduce calcium excretion and may prevent hip fractures and osteoporosis in postmenopausal women.*

- Clinically relevant drug interactions are few
- They can be combined with several other antihypertensives with synergistic effect
- They are convenient to take and remain effective for a long time

Oral thiazides and chlorthalidone still remain the most valuable, safe and highly cost-effective antihypertensive drugs.

That their use has been declining is not because they lack virtues, but is due to the 'absence of corporate promotion' and 'aggressive marketing' of newer but more expensive agents.

INDAPAMIDE: This indole derivative of chlorosulphonamide, is chemically related to chlorthalidone. Like chlorthalidone, it has a long duration of action ($t\frac{1}{2}$ of about 18 h). Given orally in the dose of 2.5 mg once daily, it reduces the BP in mild and moderate hypertension. Larger doses cause diuresis. It is available as 2.5 mg tablets. A sustained release (SR) preparation is available.

XIPAMIDE: This chlorosulphonamide diuretic has hypotensive effects as well as adverse effects similar to thiazides. It also resembles furosemide in that it is an effective diuretic in patients with renal failure. It is administered in a single daily dose of 20–40 mg.

LOOP DIURETICS: These drugs are not commonly used for treatment of hypertension (see Chapter 37) but **they are useful as antihypertensives in patients with moderate and severe renal impairment, wherein thiazides are ineffective**.

AMILORIDE and **TRIAMTERENE:** These are combined with loop or thiazide diuretics to prevent or correct hypokalaemia (Chapter 37).

RAAS INHIBITORS PH 1.26

Angiotensin-Converting Enzyme Inhibitors (ACEIs)

Introduction of this class of drugs distinctly improved the management of hypertension. Several ACEIs are now available. They have same pharmacodynamic properties and mainly differ in their pharmacokinetic properties (Table 30.1).

Mechanism of action: ACEIs competitively inhibit ACE and thus block the conversion of angiotensin I to angiotensin II (Fig. 30.1). **Thus they prevent:**

- The pressor effect of angiotensin II
- Aldosterone synthesis and release
- The metabolism of bradykinin (see Chapter 25). Inhibition of ACE raises the levels of bradykinin, a potent vasodilator, which may also contribute to its antihypertensive and cardioprotective effects.

Blockade of angiotensin II synthesis in the tissues (vascular, cardiac and renal) by ACEI may be responsible for their other beneficial effects. ACEIs cause a compensatory rise in the plasma levels of renin and angiotensin I.

Pharmacological actions: In healthy, sodium-replete humans, a single oral dose of ACEI lowers the systemic BP only slightly. By contrast, **a single dose of ACEI causes substantial lowering of BP in salt-depleted patients.**

In hypertensive patients:

- ACEIs cause vasodilation, lower systemic arterial resistance as well as both, SBP and DBP.
- There is no reflex tachycardia.
- The antihypertensive effect is seen in all types of hypertension, except that due to primary aldosteronism. **Concurrent use of a diuretic potentiates its action.**
- Renal, cerebral and coronary blood flow is increased.
- Baroreceptor function is reset; cardiovascular reflexes are not compromised and responses to posture and exercise are not impaired. **Postural hypotension is not a problem.**

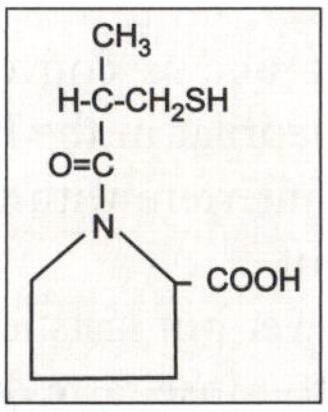

FIG. 30.2 **Captopril.**

- Secretion of aldosterone is reduced but adequate levels are maintained by other secretagogues, ACTH and potassium.

In patients with heart failure (HF): ACEIs produce several beneficial effects:

- They reduce the afterload and preload and increase cardiac output, and diminish the heart rate. BP is not much affected.
- There is a natriuretic (diuretic-sparing) effect following haemodynamic changes and reduction in aldosterone secretion. The venous return to the heart diminishes.
- Pulmonary arterial pressure, pulmonary capillary wedge pressure and left atrial and left ventricular filling pressure (preload) are reduced.
- They reduce cardiac remodelling and risk of coronary ischaemic events.
- Exercise tolerance increases.
- Survival is prolonged in chronic HF (CHF).

IM 11.18

In diabetic patients, ACEIs improve kidney function and reduce microalbuminuria **(renoprotection)**.

In patients with acute MI, early (within 24 h) administration of ACEI **reduces LV dysfunction and slows the progression of HF** (see Chapter 29).

Absorption, fate and excretion: The t½ of various ACEIs have been stated in Table 30.1. Captopril (Fig. 30.2) is rapidly absorbed from the gut with a bioavailability of about 65%. *Its absorption is reduced by food and so it is given 1 h before a meal*. It is cleared rapidly from the body by renal excretion (95%); about half is excreted as captopril and the other half as metabolites.

ENALAPRIL: This congener of captopril is without an SH group and is preferred to it. Enalapril differs from captopril in that:

- It is a prodrug and is converted to the active metabolite enalaprilat in the liver.
- Food does not interfere with its absorption.
- It is more potent.
- Its action is slower but lasts longer.
- It is less liable to cause taste disturbances, leucopenia and glomerulopathy.

Table 30.1 ACE Inhibitors in Current Use

Drug	t½[a] (h)	Usual Dosage (mg) in Hypertension[b]
Captopril	1.9	12.5–50 b.i.d.
Lisinopril	11–12	10–20 o.d.
Enalapril	11–12	5–20 o.d.
Ramipril	13–17	2.5–10 o.d.
Benazepril	10–11	10–40 o.d.
Fosinopril	12	10–40 o.d.
Quinapril	3	10–40 o.d.
Perindopril	2–10	4–16 o.d.
Trandolapril	6	2–8 o.d.
Moexipril	2–9	7.5–30 o.d./b.d.

Note: Drugs other than captopril and lisinopril are prodrugs.
[a]Of active drug/metabolite.
[b]Smaller doses in patients on diuretics, in CHF and with renal insufficiency.

Adverse reactions: ACEIs are generally well tolerated. Most adverse effects are the result of the specific inhibition of ACE. Relatively common adverse effect is **persistent dry cough.** It is believed to be due to raised levels of bradykinin. **A steep fall in BP may occur after the first dose in patients with severe hypertension who are on multidrug regimes including a diuretic, and generally in all salt-depleted patients.** *In such cases, ACEIs should be started in very small doses, preferably after stopping the diuretic.*

Aldosterone synthesis inhibition by ACEI causes **hyperkalaemia,** particularly in patients with renal insufficiency and in those taking a potassium-sparing diuretic. It should be used with caution in patients on an NSAID or a beta-blocker.

The other adverse effects are skin rashes, taste disturbances, vitiligo, headache, GI disturbances, muscle cramps and rarely leucopenia. **Proteinuria** (>1 g/day) has been described. Rarely, it causes serious angioedema. **The drug causes fetal toxicity in animals and should be avoided in pregnancy.**

Preparations and dosage: See Table 30.1. Because of reduced clearance, smaller doses are indicated in patients with impaired renal function.

In patients with HF, the starting dose of enalapril should be 2.5 mg/day in patients older than 60 years and 5 mg/day in patients younger than 60 years. Although it is used once daily in a few cases, its effect wanes off over 24 h and hence b.i.d. schedule is recommended. Usual maintenance dose is 10–20 mg per day.

Indications: In general, they are effective, reasonably safe with **flat dose–response curve** but more expensive drugs.

- **Hypertension:** These are useful in hypertension of all grades, including malignant hypertension. Combined with a thiazide they can reduce thiazide-induced hypokalaemia, hypercholesterolaemia, hyperglycaemia and hyperuricaemia. They can be used safely in asthma and diabetic patients. There is no rebound hypertension on stopping the drugs abruptly. They can be combined with an antihypertensive from any other class and are generally well tolerated by the elderly. Sexual function is not affected.
- **Heart failure:** ACEIs are indicated in all clinical manifestations of heart failure and in individuals with asymptomatic LV dysfunction (Chapter 31). Addition of ACEIs to conventional treatment in patients with severe HF can reduce mortality and improve symptoms.
- **Diabetic nephropathy:** ACEIs protect kidneys and decrease microalbuminuria in patients with insulin-dependent diabetes mellitus (DM) and nephropathy
- **Acute MI:** They reduce LV dysfunction and mortality (Chapter 29)

Contraindications for ACEI:

- Severe bilateral renal artery stenosis, as they reduce GFR and may cause renal failure
- Aortic stenosis
- Coarctation of the aorta
- Pregnancy
- Hypovolemia
- Severe hyperkalemia
- History of angioedema or hypersensitivity related to ACEI or hereditory angioedema
- Intake of angiotensin receptor/neprilysin inhibitor (ARNI) within the last 36 hours

Angiotensin Receptor Blockers (ARBs)

ACEIs inhibit ACE which is not a specific enzyme and has other substrates (bradykinin, substance P and neurokinins); inhibition of which may cause ADR such as cough and angioedema. Hence, specific ARBs have been developed (Table 30.2)

Table 30.2 Angiotensin Receptor Blockers

Drug	t½ (h)	Dosage (mg/day) in Hypertension
Losartan	2	25–100 o.d. or b.i.d.
Valsartan	6	40–320 o.d.
Candesartan	9	4–32 o.d.
Irbesartan	11–15	75–300 o.d.
Eprosartan	5	400–800 o.d. or b.i.d.
Telmisartan	24	20–80 o.d.
Olmesartan	14–16	10–40 o.d.
Azilsartan	11	40–80 mg o.d.

LOSARTAN: This phenyl tetrazole–substituted imidazole compound **acts as a selective, competitive blocker of angiotensin I receptor type 1 (AT_1)** and decreases PVR. However, AT_1 blockade can activate AT_2 and may increase the levels of bradykinin. Clinically, this effect is short lasting. It has some uricosuric action.

Given orally, it is well absorbed and undergoes hepatic first-pass metabolism, being partly converted to a more active metabolite. Its effect on the cardiovascular haemodynamics is similar to that of ACEI.

Adverse reactions: Like the ACEI, it can cause fetotoxicity and should not be used during pregnancy. It can precipitate renal failure in patients with bilateral renal artery stenosis and in those with low, fixed renal blood flow. It can cause skin rashes and neuropsychiatric disturbances such as insomnia, confusion, nightmares, agitation and depression. Even cough and angioedema can occur rarely.

Valsartan, Irbesartan, Eprosartan, Telmisartan, Candesartan, Olmesartan and **Azilsartan** are the other analogues of losartan.

Therapeutically, ACEI and ARB are equally effective for the treatment of hypertension, prevention of stroke and acute coronary syndromes. The choice between them depends upon familiarity and cost. ARBs have similar contraindications as ACEI.

Aldosterone Antagonists PH 1.24, PH 1.26

This class of drugs is discussed in Chapter 37.

SPIRONOLACTONE: This aldosterone antagonist by itself is not an antihypertensive agent. As an add-on drug, it may be particularly useful in hypertensive patients with significant hypokalaemia, hyperuricaemia, or glucose intolerance and also in resistant hypertension. It is the drug of choice in primary hyperaldosteronism. It is also recommended in small doses as an add-on drug in HF (Chapter 31).

Eplerenone: See Chapter 37.

Renin Inhibitors

This class of drugs inhibit renin which cleaves angiotensinogen from the liver to form angiotensin I, which is then converted to angiotensin II (Fig. 30.1). It thereby reduces both angiotensin I and II levels, and produces a fall in BP.

Aliskiren: This oral, nonpeptide, renin inhibitor, aliskiren, causes dose-dependent, direct inhibition of the PRA. It appears to have no special advantage over the other RAAS inhibitors. It should not be used along with ACEI /ARB or in pregnancy.

IM 11.18

CALCIUM CHANNEL BLOCKERS (CCBS)

Their properties and uses are discussed in detail in Chapter 29.

- CCBs are used in the long-term treatment of hypertension. Nifedipine has also been used in the management of hypertensive emergencies.
- They are often used as a monotherapy, particularly in moderately hypertensive patients with DM
- They are particularly preferred in patients with impaired renal function or asthma, and in acute hypertension during pregnancy
- They have no significant CNS effects. Oedema of feet may be observed.
- As these drugs are metabolised by liver, dose adjustment in patients with renal disease is less critical

There is some concern about the long-term safety of the short-acting dihydropyridines, like nifedipine, and are not recommended for long-term treatment of hypertension. **Diltiazem** *and* **amlodipine** *are as effective as diuretics, beta-blockers or their combination, in the long-term treatment of essential hypertension.*

Nitrates have a synergistic effect with CCB and can lead to sudden fall of BP and collapse.

SYMPATHOLYTIC DRUGS

Adrenergic Receptor Blockers

These include drugs which block either alpha- or beta- or both adrenergic receptors. Their detailed pharmacology is discussed in Chapter 18. Only their antihypertensive effects are discussed below.

I. Alpha-adrenergic–blocking agents: Peripheral vascular alpha-receptors are of two types (Chapter 18):

- **Postsynaptic α_1 receptors** which are **stimulatory in nature;** their activation causes vasoconstriction
- **Presynaptic α_2 receptors** (auto-receptors), which are **inhibitory in nature;** their activation inhibits NA release

Blockade of α_1 causes fall in BP. However, simultaneous blocking of α_2 results in enhanced output of NA that acts on cardiac beta receptors leading to tachycardia. Hence, nonselective alpha-adrenergic–blocking agents like phentolamine are not used in the treatment of essential hypertension (Chapter 18).

PHENTOLAMINE: It is a nonselective competitive blocker with a short duration of action. It can be administered intravenously in the dose of 2.5–10 mg *to prevent or treat severe hypertension due to release of catecholamines during removal of pheochromocytoma*.

PHENOXYBENZAMINE: This long-acting noncompetitive blocker is used in the preoperative management of pheochromocytoma (Chapter 18).

PRAZOSIN: This quinazoline derivative is a peripheral vasodilator (Chapter 18). **It acts by selective α_1-adrenergic receptor blockade**. Prazosin, thus, does not cause reflex tachycardia. Although it has a short plasma half-life (2.5–4 h), its effect lasts much longer (10 h).

- It controls both supine and standing BP with minimum of postural hypotension
- Tachycardia is minimal or absent
- It does not affect renal function, cardiac output or the RAAS
- It is effective in all grades of severity of hypertension but its main use is for the treatment of moderate-to-severe hypertension as an adjunct to diuretics and beta-blockers

Selective α_1 antagonists may decrease total and LDL cholesterol, and TG and increase HDL cholesterol levels.

Adverse reactions: It can cause giddiness, drowsiness, tiredness, nausea, diarrhoea and fluid retention. The first dose should be 0.5 mg or less and should be taken on retiring to bed at night, as some patients may have adverse reactions such as palpitation, postural hypotension and even collapse following the first dose (**first dose effect**). In females, it may cause urinary incontinence.

The therapy is started with 1–3 mg/day in divided doses. The maintenance dose is 3–7.5 mg/day. An SR preparation is also available.

Other uses: It is also used to treat CHF (Chapter 30), benign prostatic hyperplasia and prostatism with obstructive symptoms (Chapter 67). It is also used in the management of pulmonary edema due to scorpion sting (Chapter 7).

Terazosin, doxazosin and **alfuzosin** are the other analogues of prazosin.

INDORAMIN: This selective α_1-adrenergic blocker lowers the BP in a manner similar to that of prazosin.

For other uses of alpha-blockers, see Chapter 18.

II. Beta-Adrenergic–Blocking Agents: The exact **mechanism of their antihypertensive action** is not clear. However, the antihypertensive effect correlates best with their β_1-blocking action. Peripheral resistance is lowered during chronic administration. Reduction in cardiac output and lowering of plasma renin are variable during long-term therapy. They also increase the natriuretic peptide secretion 2–3 fold. The lipid-soluble agents (e.g. propranolol) have some central effect on catecholaminergic neurons, and reduce sympathetic outflow.

Pharmacological actions: The beta-blockers:

- Moderately lower the SBP and DBP, both in the supine and standing positions
- **Prevent the tachycardia caused by vasodilators**
- Protect against stress-induced hypertension
- Do not block baroreceptor mechanisms and **postural hypotension is not a problem**. Protective, alpha receptor constrictor mechanisms remain intact.
- **Are cardioprotective** and especially useful in patients with concurrent IHD (Chapter 29)
- Do not impair the kidney function
- Are generally safe and cost-effective

Absorption, fate and excretion: See Chapter 18 for details. The clinical hypotensive effect of a single dose lasts longer than the t½ (2–5 h) would suggest and hence, most of these drugs can be used twice daily. Longer acting drugs such as **atenolol can be used once daily**. The onset of antihypertensive effect is dose related but generally takes 5–7 days to become manifest. Highly lipid-soluble agents such as propranolol, metoprolol and oxprenolol are metabolised in the liver while highly water-soluble atenolol and nadolol are excreted by kidney.

Adverse reactions: Generally, these drugs are well tolerated and cause minimal ADR. Commonly they cause **bradycardia**. *Because beta receptor density increases during chronic administration, their abrupt withdrawal can result in potentially dangerous tachycardia, rebound rise in BP and angina pectoris.* **Cardiac enlargement is a relative contraindication to their use.** In some patients with established renal disease, deterioration of renal function may occur.

Most NSAIDs cause sodium retention probably because of the inhibition of formation of renal prostacyclin and reduce the antihypertensive effect of a beta-blocker. Highly lipid-soluble beta-blockers such as propranolol, metoprolol are likely to cause CNS adverse effects (Chapter 18).

Preparations and dose: See Chapter 18.

Indications: As a monotherapy, beta-blockers are used to treat mild-to-moderate hypertension, especially if the patient has another indication for beta blockers, e.g. migraine, IHD, HF or in young patients or those having palpitations, restlessness and anxiety. Relatively selective β_1-blockers (e.g. Atenolol) are preferred.

III. Alpha- and beta-adrenergic–blocking agents: By acting as competitive antagonists at both α_1 and β receptors, they cause a fall in the BP in patients with hypertension (Chapter 18).

LABETALOL: For details see Chapter 18. It is given orally in the dose of 100 mg twice daily and increased gradually up to 400–800 mg. However, it can be given intravenously to treat hypertensive emergencies (see under the section Treatment of hypertensive crises).

Carvedilol (6.25 mg b.i.d.) has similar actions as labetalol. It is also used in CHF (Chapter 31).

Central Sympatholytics

These drugs lower BP by stimulating the central α2-adrenergic receptors.

CLONIDINE: This imidazoline derivative (Fig. 30.3) has a potent antihypertensive action.

Mechanism of action: Clonidine activates the central postsynaptic adrenergic α_2 receptors in the vasomotor centre and the hypothalamus, and causes a decreased sympathetic outflow from the CNS leading to lowering of BP.

Larger doses stimulate the peripheral inhibitory presynaptic α_2 adrenoreceptors (autoreceptors). This reduces the peripheral NA release. Clonidine also reduces the PRA.

Pharmacological actions: *Given intravenously,* it produces a transient hypertensive response followed by a prolonged **fall in both, SBP and DBP** accompanied by bradycardia. *This initial hypertensive effect is not seen after its oral administration.*

Chronic administration of 0.3–1.5 mg/day:

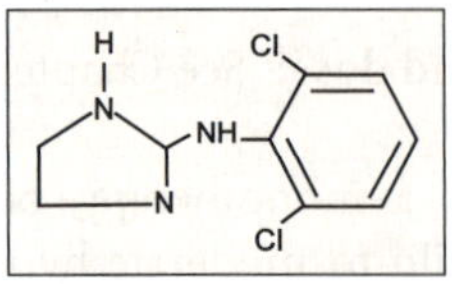

FIG. 30.3 Clonidine.

- Reduces both supine and standing BP without affecting the cardiovascular reflexes
- Diminishes the heart rate
- Does not cause postural hypotension
- Does not affect the renal blood flow and the GFR; hence, the drug is valuable in patients with compromised renal function
- Reduces the cardiac output, total PVR or both
- Results in tolerance to antihypertensive effect

Adverse reactions: It commonly causes sedation and dry mouth due to central effects. Vertigo, constipation, parotid pain, impotence, GI disturbances, allergic reactions and hallucinations may occur. Toxic doses cause marked bradycardia, miosis and hypotension.

Abrupt cessation of clonidine therapy can cause hyper-irritability and a dangerous and sometimes lethal rebound rise of BP. Therefore, when necessary, its withdrawal should be gradual.

Clonidine produces sodium and fluid retention and rapid development of tolerance to its antihypertensive effect. *Combination of clonidine and a beta-blocker can cause severe drowsiness.*

Preparations: Clonidine hydrochloride 0.025, 0.1, 0.15 mg tablets and 0.15 mg injection. A transdermal preparation releasing 0.1-0.3 mg/24 hr is also available; its effect lasts for 7 days.

Indications:

- **Hypertension:** It is now rarely used
- **Menopausal hot flushes** (Chapter 65)
- **Opiate, alcohol and nicotine withdrawal,** to control adrenergic symptoms

Guanfacine and **guanabenz** are related to clonidine and have actions similar to clonidine. Their duration of action, however, is prolonged.

ALPHA-METHYLDOPA: This isomer of methyldopa (Fig. 30.4), is a prodrug.

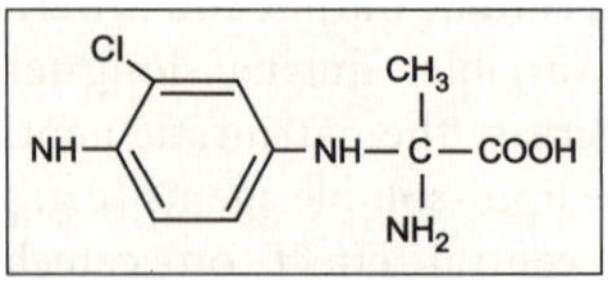

FIG. 30.4 Alpha-methyldopa.

Mechanism of Action: It is metabolised in the adrenergic neurons to an active metabolite, α-methylnoradrenaline and is stored in the vesicles of adrenergic neurons, instead of NA. When the adrenergic neuron discharges, α-methylnoradrenaline (a **false neurotransmitter**) is released instead of NA, which probably acts as an agonist at presynaptic α_2-adrenergic receptors in the brainstem and inhibits the central sympathetic outflow like clonidine. Methyldopa also inhibits renin release by the kidneys.

Pharmacological actions: After oral or IV administration, the hypotensive effect appears after a latent period of 3–6 h and 1–2 h, respectively. **Its pharmacological effects are similar to that of clonidine**.

Absorption, fate and excretion: Given orally, 50% of the drug is absorbed and is carried into the brain. As the drug metabolite gets stored in the neuronal endings the effect lasts longer (24 h), though its t½ is 1.5 h. The drug is almost completely excreted in urine in 12 h. In patients with severely impaired renal function, it may accumulate during chronic administration.

Adverse reactions: Commonly, it produces sedation. Other CNS effects are diminished intellectual drive, forgetfulness, nightmares, mental depression, Parkinsonism, hyperprolactinaemia and gynaecomastia. The drug may also cause retention of sodium and water, GI disturbances, constipation, failure to ejaculate, arthralgia and skin rashes. Tolerance to the antihypertensive effect may occur.

Alpha-methyldopa may produce cholestatic jaundice in a few cases and can rarely cause thrombocytopenia, leucopenia and systemic lupus erythematosus (SLE).

Preparations: Alpha-methyldopa hydrochloride 125, 250 and 500 mg tablets; injection 50 mg per mL.

Indications:

- **Hypertension during pregnancy:** It is a preferred drug based on its efficacy and safety in both the mother and fetus.

MOXONIDINE: This is claimed to be a **selective imidazole receptor (IR_1) agonist.** Moxonidine activates IR_1 in the medulla, thereby **reducing central sympathetic drive and PVR.** It has similar hypotensive action as clonidine and methyldopa with no special advantage.

Adrenergic Neuron Blockers

GUANETHIDINE: The drug is selectively taken up by adrenergic neuron ($Uptake_1$ process) where it replaces NA. It thus causes adrenergic neuron blockade by inhibition of the release of NA at the adrenergic nerve terminals. It blocks reuptake of NA, which may get released in the initial period. This allows its destruction by COMT. It also depletes vesicular NA stores at the adrenergic nerve endings in the heart and the aorta. The antihypertensive action of guanethidine is usually delayed for 48–72 h.

Adverse reaction: Marked sympathetic blockade causes postural hypotension, failure to ejaculate and fluid retention. Consequent predominance of cholinergic system results in diarrhoea and parotid pain. The use of adrenergic neuron blockers is now obsolete because of their toxicity.

RESERPINE: The root of the plant *Rauwolfia serpentina* has been in medicinal use in India since ancient times. Reserpine (Chapter 13), the alkaloid from its root is the most potent hypotensive agent whereas ajmaline has quinidine-like properties (Chapter 28).

Mechanism of action: Reserpine depletes the catecholamines, adrenaline, NA and DA from the various storage sites in the body. It also depletes 5-HT from the CNS.

Reserpine binds to storage vesicles in central and peripheral adrenergic neurons. This binding persists for a long time, and prevents the vesicles to concentrate and store biogenic amines, NA and DA. Thus, reserpine leads to depletion of the transmitter and consequently to peripheral sympathetic blockade. Its antihypertensive effects may be related to **both central and peripheral actions.**

Pharmacological actions: These are due to depletion of NA, 5-HT and DA. The effects of oral reserpine are established slowly (2–4 weeks) and maintained for a long time even after complete elimination of the drug, as it requires synthesis of new vesicles (**Hit and run drug**).

Hypotension is usually accompanied by **bradycardia.** Advantages are that there is no rebound hypertension on discontinuation of reserpine. Renal and muscle blood flow is not much affected.

It has sedative and antipsychotic actions (Chapter 13).

Adverse reactions: These usually develop as an extension of its pharmacological actions and **are dose dependent.**

Parasympathetic predominance due to peripheral sympathetic blockade causes adverse effects such as salivation, cutaneous vasodilatation, nasal congestion, increased motility of the gut and increased gastric acidity. The other adverse effects are orthostatic hypotension, mental depression, weight gain and with high doses, parkinsonism (depletion of DA), gynaecomastia and impotence in males and infertility in females.

Reserpine treatment causes upregulation of postsynaptic receptors and enhances the pressor response to sympathomimetic amines.

The above-mentioned **ADRs are not commonly observed with therapeutic doses (<0.25 mg/day).** The crude extract was used in India for many years and was well tolerated, relatively safe and cheap drug.

Preparations and dosage: Reserpine tablet 0.25 mg. Dose: 0.25 mg o.d. As little as 0.1 mg per day may be effective when combined with a diuretic.

Ganglionic Blockers

These drugs competitively block the nicotinic receptors (Nn) in both sympathetic and parasympathetic ganglia. The normal protective vasomotor reflexes mediated through the baroreceptors and the sympathetic nervous system are also blocked, which causes **marked postural hypotension** as their main ADR. Ganglionic blockers (e.g. hexamethonium, trimethaphan) once used to treat hypertension, are now obsolete because of the high incidence of serious ADR due to blockade of both the ganglia (Chapter 21).

VASODILATORS

Hydralazine: This drug (Fig. 30.5) was initially tested for antihistaminic activity and later evaluated as a hypotensive agent.

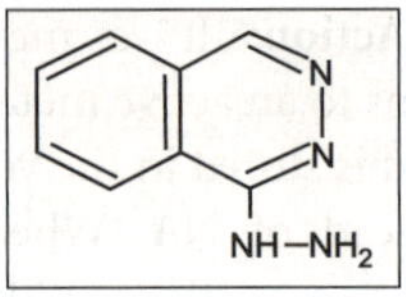

FIG. 30.5 Hydralazine.

Pharmacological actions:

- Hydralazine lowers the BP by causing a direct relaxation of the arteriolar wall
- The effect is slow in onset but prolonged. Even on its IV administration, the BP falls only after 15–20 min.
- The fall in BP is accompanied by a decrease in the total PVR, and by **a compensatory tachycardia, increase in stroke volume and in cardiac output.** Orthostatic hypotension is rare.
- The splanchnic, coronary, cerebral and renal blood flow may increase
- It causes increase in PRA and fluid retention

Absorption, fate and excretion: It is well absorbed after oral and parenteral administration. The drug is acetylated in the liver and there may be 'fast acetylators' and 'slow acetylators'. Elimination of the drug is almost complete within 24 h. Less than 5% of an oral dose is excreted unchanged in urine. **Hence, it can be used even in the presence of renal damage.**

Adverse reactions: The high incidence of ADR is the main drawback of hydralazine therapy. The manifestations are as follows:

- **Gastrointestinal irritation** producing nausea, vomiting, gastric hypersecretion, anorexia and diarrhoea
- **Cardiac effects:** These include palpitation, tachycardia and anginal attacks.
- **Others** like headache, nasal congestion, flushing, tremors, dizziness and salt and water retention
- **Intolerance:** The manifestations are fever, skin rash and polyneuritis. GI haemorrhage and pancytopenia are serious but rare manifestations.
- **Acute rheumatoid arthritis or SLE-like syndrome** may develop rarely with large doses.

Preparations and dose:

i. Hydralazine hydrochloride tablets 25 and 50 mg; maximum dose 100 mg daily

ii. Dihydralazine sulphate 25 mg table
iii. Injection 20 mg for IM/IV use

A combination of dihydralazine and reserpine with hydrochlorothiazide is also available.

SODIUM NITROPRUSSIDE: This drug, known since 1850, has been used as a colour indicator for acetone and aldehydes. It was regarded as a poison because of its cyanide group. Given by IV infusion, **it is metabolised to active compound NO which causes relaxation of arterioles and veins.** It:

- *Lowers the afterload and the preload* as a result of reduction in PVR and venous tone, respectively
- Reduces myocardial oxygen consumption with improvement in myocardial function in low output states
- Has rapid onset but very short duration
- Minimally affects heart rate and the regional blood flow
- Increases PRA
- Is rapidly metabolised to thiocyanate.

Adverse reactions: Hepatic dysfunction may result in excessive accumulation of toxic cyanide which may cause metabolic acidosis, arrhythmia and hypotension.

Prolonged administration of sodium nitroprusside either in high doses or in the presence of renal insufficiency may precipitate thiocyanate toxicity. This results in fatigue, anorexia, nausea, vomiting, sweating, disorientation, psychotic behaviour and muscle twitching. Larger doses may cause ataxia, rigidity, convulsions and metabolic acidosis.

Preparations and dose: Sodium nitroprusside is supplied as 50 mg powder to be dissolved in 500 mL of 5% dextrose in water, just prior to administration. When exposed to light, it is converted to cyanide; hence, a brown or black paper bag over the IV fluid container is necessary. Translucent plastic tubing may need taping. *Only freshly prepared solution should be used.*

Indications: It is mainly used to lower BP in hypertensive emergencies.

Nitrates have a synergistic effect with the vasodilator drugs and can lead to sudden fall of BP and collapse.

POTASSIUM CHANNEL ACTIVATORS

The group includes **minoxidil** and **diazoxide** used in hypertension; and **nicorandil** and **pinacidil** used in angina (Chapter 29).

Mechanism of action: Potassium channels play an important role in the regulation of membrane potential and excitability of cells. Potassium channel activators combine with ATP-modulated potassium channels; opening these channels causes potassium ions to leak out from the cell. This action hyperpolarises and stabilises the cell membrane of the vascular smooth muscle and reduces Ca^{++} entry, which prevents vasoconstriction, leading to relaxation. **Thus, they act as arterial vasodilators.** Nicorandil, in addition, also activates cGMP to produce NO.

These drugs reduce the excitability of the myocytes. They may have a role in the management of IHD because the ATP-modulated potassium channels are believed to be crucial in myocardial adaptation to ischaemic injury via 'preconditioning'.

MINOXIDIL: This prodrug (Fig. 30.6) is used orally as a peripheral vasodilator. Its active metabolite minoxidil N-O sulphate acts similar to hydralazine, but is more potent and more toxic. **It causes compensatory tachycardia, increased cardiac contractility, palpitation, angina and sodium retention.** It can also cause pulmonary hypertension (PH), hypertrichosis and headache. Because of its toxicity, the drug is reserved for resistant cases. See Chapter 69 for its use in alopecia.

DIAZOXIDE: It is a compound structurally related to the diuretic chlorothiazide but has **no diuretic activity. It is a potent, direct arteriolar vasodilator with t½ of 36 h.** As seen with hydralazine, compensatory reactions include tachycardia, increased cardiac contractility and sodium retention. It is highly

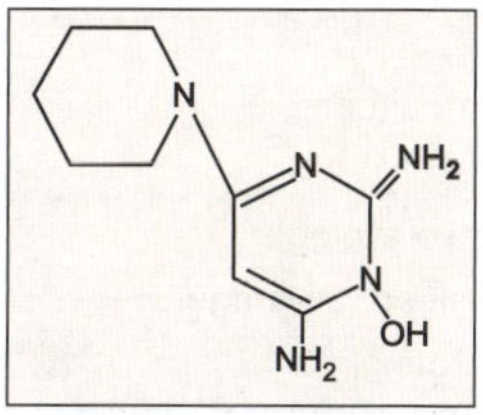

FIG. 30.6 Minoxidil.

protein bound. *When injected by IV bolus, it lowers the BP within 3–5 min, and is used in hypertensive emergencies.* **It also raises blood sugar levels** and is used to treat hypoglycaemia due to insulinoma (Chapter 63).

MISCELLANEOUS DRUGS

METYROSINE (Alpha-methyl tyrosine): This drug blocks the synthesis of catecholamines by inhibiting tyrosine hydroxylase. It is useful in the treatment of patients with pheochromocytoma.

HYPERTENSION – THERAPY IM 8.14

Effective treatment of hypertension is an important part of any programme to reduce the toll of cardiovascular disease, e.g. end-organ damage and mortality, in the society.

According to WHO for patients with a confirmed diagnosis of hypertension i.e. systolic blood pressure of ≥ 140 mmHg or diastolic blood pressure of ≥ 90 mmHg anti-hypertensive treatment should be initiated. For the individuals with cardiovascular disease the treatment should be initiated if systolic blood pressure is between 130-139 mmHg. Those who have high CVS risk, DM or chronic kidney disease (CKD) but no cardiovascular disease (CVD) should be treated if their systolic BP lies between 130-139mmHg.

Automated oscillometric devices are recommended for clinic BP measurements (AOBP). After a 5 min rest period, at least 3 readings are to be taken and averaged. Ambulatory BP monitoring (ABPM) and resting home BP monitoring (HBPM) allow detection of white coat hypertension and masked hypertension. In addition, ABPM allows daytime activity related BP and BP pattern (nocturnal hypertension, nocturnal BP dipping, early morning BP surge). The diagnostic BP levels for hypertension with these different measurements are depicted in Table 30.3.

Aims of treatment of hypertension

They are as follows:

a. Maintaining the BP, including the early morning BP, as near normal as possible (<140/90 mm Hg) without undue side effects
b. Maintaining/improving the quality of life, including the intellectual and sexual functions
c. Reduction in left ventricular mass
d. Prevention of cardiac arrhythmias, heart failure, stroke and other complications
e. Control of other CHD risk factors

To achieve all of the above, lifestyle management and pharmacological treatment should be adjusted to maximum tolerable effectiveness and should be adhered to on long-term basis in a cost-effective manner.

The drug treatment of essential hypertension is still 'empiric', as these drugs reduce the BP without correcting the cause. **However, the reduction of BP (even suboptimally) prevents or postpones renal, cardiac and cerebral complications and prolongs life. The control of hypertension in diabetic patients also helps to delay the onset of retinal and renal damage.**

Table 30.3 Diagnostic BP Levels based on Clinic, Ambulatory, and Home Blood Pressure Measurement

Type of Measurement	Systolic/Diastolic Blood Pressure (mmHg)
In Clinic	≥140 and/or ≥90
Ambulatory BP monitoring	
- 24-h average	≥130 and/or ≥80
- Daytime or awake average	≥135 and/or ≥85
- Night time or asleep aaverage	≥120 and/or ≥70
- Home BP monitoring	≥135 and/or ≥85

Adopted from: Asayama et al. *J Hum Hypertens* (2021). https://doi.org/10.1038/s41371-021-00486-8

It should be noted that:

- Every patient whose BP is elevated requires treatment, though not necessarily with antihypertensive drugs.
- Systolic hypertension is as damaging as diastolic hypertension.
- Treatment with antihypertensives, once started, will *generally* have to be continued for life. An occasional patient may be able to give up the treatment and may remain normotensive thereafter. How often this happens is not known, but it is rare.
- Success of the treatment depends upon the care and the time spent by the doctor upon educating and counselling the patient; and the patient's compliance.

Supportive treatment of hypertension

Reassurance by a physician and lifestyle modifications (Box 30.1) *are necessary in all hypertensive patients.* In addition, they are essential for normotensives with risk factors. In fact, these can prevent hypertension and may suffice in those with uncomplicated, mild hypertension; hence should be given a trial for 3-6 mths. These enhance the effect of antihypertensive medication, and reduce the number of drugs needed to control BP.

Although **sodium restriction** helps to reduce BP, rigid restriction of salt intake is rarely necessary, especially if diuretics are administered. Adequate rest, relaxation and sleep are desirable. Ambitions may have to be curbed or sacrificed for the reasons of health. Reassurance and a benzodiazepine could benefit the anxious patient. **The patient should be explained in detail what 'moderation in all things' actually means.** Yoga, meditation and stress control exercises are helpful. **Very strict restrictions are, however, often unnecessary**, as Page has aptly remarked, '*I firmly believe that those who follow directions minutely do better than the careless. But there are important areas of living in which we physicians know no more than others. Often when we don't know what to do, we proscribe instead of prescribing – we forbid this or that of the things people often most enjoy. I suppose this characteristic is a hangover from the days when anything that was pleasurable was sinful. Whether we forbid smoking, alcohol and such, may make a good deal of difference as to whether people will think life worth living. I should therefore remind you that smoke and alcohol were the oldest known preservatives and that Winston Churchill was 100% proof of this observation.*'

Box 30.1 Key Lifestyle Modification in Hypertensives

- Weight reduction in obese persons: About 1 mmHg reduction in SBP for every 1 kg weight loss
- Restriction of salt consumption to less than 5 g (about 2–3 g of sodium) a day[a]
- Increase in dietary potassium (fruits and vegetables) consumption[a]
- Healthy diet: Dietary Approaches to Stop Hypertension (DASH) include eating more fruits, vegetables, whole grains, low-fat dairy products, lean meat products and nuts and seeds. Saturated and total fat content should be reduced (Chapter 38) and trans fats should be eliminated.
- Physical exercise such as brisk walking (5–7 times a week; 30–60 min/session), and mental relaxation on a regular basis
- Reduction in alcohol (for those who drink ≤ 2 standard drinks in men and ≤1 standard drink in women), caffeine and cola beverages consumption
- Cessation of smoking
- Better adjustment at work and in family life

[a]Increased salt intake is a necessary but not sufficient cause for hypertension. One g reduction in salt intake reduces 1–3 mm Hg BP in individuals with or without hypertension. It may also prevent a recurrence in those who were previously normotensive on drugs. Salt restriction needs to be at least moderate (a reduction of salt intake to 4 g or less/day), sustained, and may take several weeks to be effective. Salt restriction also minimises the age-related rise in BP. Chloride is as important as sodium in elevating BP, and their effect is additive; other salts such as sodium citrate are less liable to elevate the BP. Liability for BP to be elevated by salt (*salt sensitivity*) is partly genetic. It is also seen in insulin resistance, hyperlipidaemia and microalbuminuria. It is alleviated by an increased potassium intake (optimal is 3.5-5 g potassium /day). *Extreme salt restriction, however, could be harmful.*

Aggressive reduction of BP is, however, likely to prove dangerous in the elderly, arteriosclerotic individuals with elevated SBP but normal DBP.

PRINCIPLES OF PHARMACOTHERAPY PH 1.1

- **Treatment initiation:** After the diagnosis of hypertension, treatment should be started within 4 weeks of diagnosis. However, if systolic BP ≥160 mmHg or diastolic ≥100 mmHg or if there is an end organ damage, no delay should be allowed.

- **Testing prior to treatment:** It is always better to do certain laboratory testing after clinical diagnosis of hypertension to identify 1. secondary hypertension, 2. comorbidities such as DM, hyperlipidaemia 3. end organ damage (e.g. CKD or left ventricular hypertrophy (LVH)), 4. cardiac risk stratification and to select certain antihypertensive drugs over others. These tests include serum electrolytes and creatinine, lipid panel, HbA1c or fasting glucose, urine dipstick, and electrocardiogram (ECG). However, the treatment should not be delayed just because of testing. These tests can be done after starting the treatment. Atherosclerotic CVD risk assessment is not needed to those having BP ≥ 140/90mm Hg. They are always at risk. It is mainly important for those with lower SBP (130–139 mmHg) as that would decide initiation of therapy.
- **Target BP goal:** Aim for at least a 20/10 mm Hg reduction within first 3 months. In the long run, aim should be to have **BP in the erect posture as near normal as possible – an SBP of < 140 mm Hg and a DBP of < 90 mm Hg in all patients of hypertension without comorbidity.** In hypertensive patients with either CVD or high risk for CVD, DM and/or CKD, the target systolic BP goal should be < 130 mmHg.

However, a higher level of BP may have to be accepted in elderly patients, in patients with impaired renal function and in those with IHD or cerebrovascular disease. This is done in order to avoid the possible complications (including myocardial and cerebral ischaemia or postural hypotension). However, the recent evidence shows that intensive BP control is not associated with increased hospitalization and does not increase the risk of orthostatic hypotension. Asymptomatic orthostatic hypotension in hypertensive adults is not associated with higher rates of CVD events, syncope, injurious falls, or acute renal failure and should not be a reason to withdraw or down-titrate treatment. **Lowering of DBP below 65 mm Hg must be avoided, as it increases the risk of stroke and CHD.**

- **Selection of antihypertensive:** The major factors in hypertension are as follows:
  - Peripheral vasoconstriction
  - Expansion of plasma volume
  - Hyperdynamic heart action, particularly in the young

With the availability of many effective and reasonably safe antihypertensives, greater flexibility can be exerted in choosing the initial drug. **What is most important is to reduce BP to the goal level. How that is done is less important.** Since the *majority of hypertensive patients will have BP reduction no matter what drug is used*, the initial choice of the drug should depend on the factors such as safety, cost, patient compliance and associated medical problems.

- **Commonly preferred anti-hypertensives: Drugs belonging to any one of the three groups – thiazide/thiazide-like diuretics, ACEIs/ ARBs, CCBs – can be used for the initial therapy of hypertension and also for subsequent add on therapy.** Their ADR are infrequent, usually mild, and can be managed or another agent can be substituted. They do not cause significant postural hypotension. Among these groups long-acting antihypertensives are preferred.

Long-term studies indicate that there are no important differences regarding efficacy, adverse effects or quality of life among the patients who receive thiazides, CCBs, ACEIs or ARBs. It is possible to **maintain both standing and supine BP normal or near normal in many patients**. *However, individual responses vary strikingly, even to the same drug. Hence, the drug therapy has to be* **'tailor-made' (patient-guided)** *for each patient.*

- **Factors guiding choice of therapy:** Generally **thiazides/CCBs (long-acting DHP)** are preferable for elderly (>65 years) and those of black ethnic origin at any age including those with DM. They are also the drugs of choice to prevent heart failure. Hydrochlorthiazide or **chlorthalidone** can be prescribed in nearly all cases. If the BP is not adequately controlled by thiazides, the therapy can be intensified with the addition of a **CCB (amlodipine)** or an **ACEI/ARB**.

If the patient is younger than 50 years and has evidence of tachycardia and hyperdynamic cardiac action, a beta-blocker (**Atenolol** 12.5–50 mg per day) may be the initial drug of choice. Beta blocker is generally not recommended as first line drug due to lesser benefit on stroke reduction compared to other three groups. Younger patients who have more responsive RAAS than older patients may be more benefited by ACEIs or ARBs.

Patients with special problems (Table 30.4) benefit from a nondiuretic as a first-line drug, e.g. a beta-blocker/CCB in a hypertensive patient with stable angina pectoris. Beta blockers are preferable if the patient has history of MI or heart failure. ACEIs/ARBs in patients with LV dysfunction or DM or severe proteinuria or kidney disease. *ACEI is the preferred drug in hypertensive patients with diabetic nephropathy* for several reasons:

- It does not alter or may even improve glucose tolerance
- It neither masks the symptoms and signs nor interferes with recovery from hypoglycaemia
- ACEIs protect the kidney in the long term

In the long run, at least half of the patients would need a minimum of two drugs to control their BP.

- **Use of drug combinations:** An appropriate combination of antihypertensive drugs can produce beneficial effects on:
  - BP
  - Adverse reactions
  - Haemodynamic effects

Combinations help to not only achieve better BP control but also reduce the incidence of ADR from individual drugs because of reduction in their doses as well as by their pharmacological actions. Fixed-dose combinations reduce pill burden and ensure better compliance to medication and therefore, better BP control. The Physician must have appropriate knowledge of clinical pharmacology of the drugs while prescribing these drug combinations. Fixed-dose combinations limit flexibility in dose adjustment of individual components, and pose difficulty in attributing ADR to a specific component.

It is rational to combine antihypertensive drugs with different pharmacodynamic actions or with different anatomical sites of action, e.g. a diuretic can be combined with a beta-blocker, or an ACEI/ARB. Extra care should be taken in patients who are at risk for postural hypotension.

An ACEI such as enalapril may be a good drug to add to thiazide, especially if the patient is suffering from heart failure.

In patients with repeated BP readings of more than 160/100 mm Hg (i.e. a baseline BP is 20/10 mmHg higher than the target BP), it is justifiable to start the therapy with two drugs, one of which preferably should be a thiazide/chlorthalidone.

- **Dose and frequency:** Start the **antihypertensive drug in small doses, increase gradually (start low, go slow) and infrequently every 4–6 weeks** (See below under the section, Management with Drugs) until the target BP goal is reached as the maximum effect of a drug or drug combination at a given dose level may take some days or weeks. Later on follow up can be done every 3-6 months.

Patients with very severe hypertension are at grave risk of developing 'hypertensive complications' such as cerebral haemorrhage, hypertensive encephalopathy, acute LVF, renal failure, etc. These patients and those with papilloedema (malignant hypertension) **need urgent and aggressive treatment** *with full doses of drugs, to achieve a rapid effect.*

- **Certain antihypertensive drugs need to be tapered.** This is because during chronic therapy, adjustments occur in homeostatic mechanisms including the reflex cardiovascular responses and in the end-organ receptor concentration; for example, during chronic beta blocker therapy, the number of beta-adrenergic receptors increases (upregulation). The reaction of the patient to the *abrupt cessation of drug therapy* depends upon 1. the dose and its duration of action, and 2. the readjustment time for the homeostatic mechanisms activated during drug therapy. If the former is much shorter than the latter (as is the case with propranolol and clonidine) *rebound rise in BP is likely to occur, with serious consequences* such as cerebral haemorrhage. If, on the other hand, the duration of action is prolonged (as is the case of reserpine), no such rebound occurs.

- In practice, it is wise to **be familiar with few preparations, use the preparations which one knows best,** and change them only if they are ineffective or adverse effects are troublesome.
- **Educate the patients about the drugs they are receiving and their possible adverse effects.** Impress upon the patient the hazards of uncontrolled or intermittently controlled hypertension and the rewards of keeping the BP under check continuously and lifelong.
- Give the patient a card bearing the names and doses of the drugs he/she is receiving.

MANAGEMENT WITH DRUGS IM 8.14

Generally, a stepped-care approach is recommended.

A. With monotherapy

- Start the therapy with **low dose** (usually half maximal dose) of an agent (**monotherapy**), appropriate for a given patient, depending upon the age, race and the comorbid conditions such as DM, angina and pregnancy (Table 30.4). So hydrochlorthiazide 12.5–25 mg or less/day, or **chlorthalidone** (12.5 mg) once daily can be used. Alternatives are long acting dihydropyridines, amlodipine (2.5-5 mg) once daily or enalapril (5-10 mg) or telmisartan (20-40 mg).
- If the BP is not controlled within 4-6 weeks of treatment, the dose should be increased in small increments (**start low, go slow**) till the desired BP level is achieved without undue ADRs or the maximum recommended dose is reached.

  The recommended maximum dose of a hydrochlorthiazide is 50 mg; chlorthalidone, 25 mg; amlopdipine, 10 mg; enalapril, 20 mg; and telmisartan 80 mg once daily. *Increasing the dose of hydrochlorothiazide beyond 50 mg o.d. usually does not produce any further therapeutic benefit.*
- If the BP is still not controlled, **another drug from a different class** may be added at half maximal dose which is likely to be well tolerated, as the compliance and the long-term efficacy of drugs depend on their long-term tolerability. The second drug can also be added without achieving maximum recommended dose of the initial drug.

  Of these two drugs, one should be preferably a diuretic in nearly all cases.

Table 30.4 Symptom Profiling of Antihypertensive Drugs IM 11.18

Associated	Recommended	Not Recommended
Migraine	BB	
Depression	Diuretics ACEI CCB Vasodilators α_1 blockers	Reserpine Clonidine Methyldopa BB
Bronchospasm	CCB Vasodilators	BB esp. propranolol
Palpitation	BB Diltiazem	Vasodilators
Angina pectoris	BB CCB	Vasodilators like hydralazine
Old MI	BB ACEI/ARB AA	CCB

Table 30.4 Symptom Profiling of Antihypertensive Drugs—cont'd

Associated	Recommended	Not Recommended
Heart failure	ACEI/ARB Diuretics, AA Vasodilators	CCB
Bradycardia		BB, Verapamil, Diltiazem
Left ventricular hypertrophy	ACE inhibitors	Direct-acting vasodilators
Raynaud's phenomenon	CCB α_1 blockers	BB
Fluid retention	Diuretics	Vasodilators Clonidine, BB
Thyrotoxicosis	BB	Drugs causing tachycardia
Recurrent TIA	ACEI/ARB, Diuretics, CCB	
Obesity	Low-dose thiazides, ACEI/ARB	BB
Hyperlipidaemia	Low-dose thiazides, α_1 blockers, ACEI, CCB	High-dose thiazides BB
Essential tremor	Propranolol	
Open-angle glaucoma	BB	
Diabetes mellitus	ACEI, ARB CCB	Potassium-sparing diuretics
Azotaemia	Loop diuretics Direct-acting vasodilators CCB, BB Alpha-methyldopa α_1 blockers	ACEI Potassium-sparing diuretics
History of sexual dysfunction	Gradual reduction of blood pressure (CCB, ACEI, and α_1 blockers are preferred)	Rapid reduction of blood pressure
Benign prostatic hyperplasia	α_1 blockers (relieve prostatism)	
Osteoporosis	Thiazides	Loop diuretics
Renal calculi	Thiazides	Loop diuretics
Chronic renal Disease	Loop diuretics ACEI/ARB+CCB	BB

Note: AA, aldosterone antagonist; BB, beta-blockers; CCB, calcium channel blockers.

The dose of the second agent is then titrated upwords every 4-6 weeks till the target BP level is achieved or its maximum dose is reached.

B. With combination therapy

- Another alternative is to use low-dose combination therapy as **initial therapy**. It can be used when baseline BP is ≥ 20/10 mmHg above target BP goal, and should be considered when baseline BP is ≥ 140/90 mmHg. This could be two single drug individual pills or fixed dose combination.

e.g. A thiazide (hydrochlorthiazide) with

a. a long-acting CCB (amlodipine) or
b. an ACEI or
c. an ARB.

In combination, both the are drugs at half the maximal doses. A CCB can be combined with an ACEI/ARB, but **an ACEI can never be combined with an ARB.**

- The BP is rechecked after 4-6 weeks and if the control is not achieved then the doses are increased gradually. Care should be taken in patients who have damaged target organs such as kidneys and heart. **A sudden reduction in BP may produce azotaemia or CAD.**

C. A two-drug combination will control BP in almost 90% of patients. If this is not achieved, it may be combined with reduction in salt intake to less than 4 g/day and increased intake of potassium in the form of fresh vegetables and fruits (the latter not in combination with an ACEI or ARB).

D. Patients in whom a two-drug combination does not achieve the desired target level of BP, a **third drug from another class** should be added from one the three drug classes mentioned earlier. This should be also added at half maximal doses and titrated to maximal level with BP checks at 4-6 weeks interval.

E. *Patients who do not reach the target BP using these strategies should be referred to a physician with expertise in treating hypertension. Such patients should be investigated in detail for a possible cause of secondary hypertension.* They may need combination with additional drugs such as an alpha-adrenergic blocker (**prazosin**), a centrally acting drug (**alpha-methyldopa**) or a direct-acting peripheral vasodilator such as **hydralazine.**

F. Once the BP is controlled then follow up can be done at 3-6 month interval. If it is maintained consistently, an attempt should be made to reduce the dose step-wise e.g. subsequently, smaller doses (12.5 mg o.d.) of chlorthalidone can be administered for maintenance therapy. Possibly omit one of the drugs, to determine the minimal therapeutic regimen that will maintain the BP less than 140/90 mm Hg, without any inconvenient, adverse effects.

HYPERTENSION IN THE ELDERLY

Both diastolic and isolated systolic high BP are cardiovascular risk factors in the elderly. **The beta-adrenergic responses of vascular smooth muscle and plasma renin levels decline with age.** The most consistent cardiovascular physiologic change in elderly patients is increased PVR.

Not all hypertensive old people need drug treatment. *Treatment should be considered for those elderly patients whose BP exceeds 150/90 mm Hg.*

Low-dose diuretic (thiazide <25 mg) or **chlorthalidone** (12.5–25 mg) **remain as the first choice for elderly patients as shown by several trials.** They also help against osteoporosis and dementia. Chlorthalidone is twice as potent as hydrochlorothiazide and has a longer duration of action. Chlorthalidone based therapy also has less incidence of CVS adverse events. However one should monitor electrolytes if thiazides are used. Even mild hypokalaemia needs to be treated.

Other agents used are amlodipine or ACEIs/ARBs, which may be used with or without thiazides. These are also well tolerated. They significantly lower the risk of stroke and coronary events. Amlodipine with its long t½ given in small doses of 2.5 mg on alternate days is also enough in some elderly patients.

It has been reported that lowering of BP results in a small but significant reduction in the risk of dementia or cognitive impairment in elderly.

*The **aim of therapy in the elderly** should be to lower the BP but the optimal BP target has remained unclear. Some propose the goal of 150/90 mmHg stating that no attempt should be made to make the BP 'normal' (<140 mm Hg) as it may cause* *increased risk of syncope and acute renal failure. On the other hand others have stated a BP goal of <140/90 mm Hg based on the recent evidence that "the lower the better".*

Considering that the elderly are vulnerable to develop complications from the antihypertensives such as orthostasis, falls and renal dysfunction due to their burden of comorbidities, advanced age and frailty, a personalized approach is needed focusing on chances of hypotension, presence of comorbidities, and adherence to medical prescriptions.

In case if an elderly attains BP <140/90 mm Hg and tolerates drug/s well with no adverse effects on health and quality of life, no adjustment should be made in doses. In patients older than 80 years the BP should not be lowered below 150/80 mm Hg. **In elderly with history of stroke, TIA or high risk for CVD, the target BP goal should be 130/80 mmHg.**

Isolated systolic hypertension (defined as SBP >160 mm Hg and DBP < 90 mm Hg) is often resistant to treatment; attempts to treat it aggressively lowers the DBP to such an extent (< 65mg mm Hg) as to compromise blood flow to vital organs such as brain and may precipitate cerebral or cardiac ischaemia. Furthermore, already existing orthostatic hypotension may be worsened.It may be treated with a low-dose thiazide or a beta-blocker, (or both) or with low dose of amlodipine alone.

Complex, multiple-drug regimes are best avoided in the elderly, as they may be confusing. Hypertension persisting after correction of heart failure, should be treated. An elderly patient with established stroke in old age does not benefit from such therapy.

HYPERTENSION IN PREGNANCY

In pregnancy haemodynamic state is of systemic vasodilation accompanied by an increase in cardiac output and decrease in total peripheral resistance. This results in a normal decrease in BP in the second trimester. Hypertension in pregnant women may be diagnosed when the SBP is ≥140 mm Hg and the DBP is ≥90 mm Hg on at least two occasions, at least six hours apart.

Hypertension during pregnancy may be:

- **Chronic hypertension,** either essential or secondary, dating from before the pregnancy. It may be diagnosed before 20 weeks of gestation.
- **Gestational hypertension** developing after mid pregnancy, after 20 weeks of gestation; this is usually mild and the BP returns to normal postpartum.
- **Pre-eclampsia** with moderate-to-severe hypertension, oedema and proteinuria.
- **Eclampsia**

Chronic hypertension especially *when secondary, long standing* and associated with organ damage, predisposes to pre-eclampsia. However, *more than 85% of women with mild pre-existing chronic, essential hypertension have uncomplicated pregnancies.* Hypertension during pregnancy needs treatment in order to possibly prevent pre-eclampsia; however, no treatment guarantees it.

Treatment is initiated when the SBP is ≥ 160 mmHg and/or the DBP is ≥105 mmHg. However, if target organ damage is present, then the treatment is initiated as DBP of ≥ 90 mmHg. Keeping a target BP goal of DBP as 85 mmHg prevents severe hypertension in pregnancy and does not pose risk to either mother or foetus.

Methyldopa is effective and is considered safe for the mother and the baby; it is the preferred drug in pregnant women. The alternative is **beta-blockers** (like atenolol); they are safe in the third trimester of pregnancy but may cause intrauterine growth retardation when prescribed earlier. However, beta-blockers mask an important index of fetal distress (i.e. bradycardia) because they themselves cause fetal bradycardia. **Labetol** has similar efficacy and safety profile as methyldopa.

CCBs (particularly nifedipine and, as an alternative, verapamil) and the direct-acting vasodilators (particularly hydralazine) can be used. If the patient is on thiazide diuretic, it may be continued especially if the patient has oedema. However, diuretics should not be used as first-line agents to treat hypertension in pregnancy, as they can deplete maternal intravascular volume, and may rarely cause neonatal thrombocytopenia.

ACEIs and ARBs are absolutely contraindicated during pregnancy, so also are direct renin inhibitors as they cause serious fetal toxicity, including renal and cardiac abnormalities and fetal death. Spironolactone should not be used due to fetal anti-androgen effects.

HYPERTENSION WITH COMORBID CONDITIONS

IM 8.14

- **Diabetes mellitus:** In around 80% patients with type2DM, hypertension coexists. The target BP goal is SBP <130 mm Hg and is to be achieved with lifestyle management and all recommended classes of drugs. Usually combination of 2-3 agents is required. In DM patients with heavy proteinuria or advanced kidney disease ACEI/ARB are indicated.
- **Renal disorder:** Control of BP halts the progress of renal failure and prolongs life. In CKD, the target BP to be achieved is SBP <130 mm Hg.
- **Recent MI or a stroke:** Antihypertensive drugs should be used cautiously in these as a rapid lowering of BP can worsen their condition.

Prevention of Cardiovascular Disease

Aspirin in daily dose of 75–150 mg can reduce major cardiovascular events in hypertensive patients. Hence, for primary prevention it is recommended in patients older than 50 years, only after BP is controlled.

In patients younger than 70 years, who have LDL cholesterol of >180 mg/dL, a **statin** may be used on long-term basis (Chapter 38). **Use of aspirin and statins should be considered in all high-risk patients irrespective of age.**

RESISTANT HYPERTENSION

In resistant hypertension the BP remains uncontrolled above goal despite the concurrent use of all 3 antihypertensive drugs of different classes administered at maximum or maximally tolerated doses and at the appropriate dosing interval. If the BP reaches the target goal but requires use of 4 or more antihypertensive agents of different classes then also it is classified as resistant hypertension.

It is necessary to rule out pseudo-resistance which is commonly due to faulty BP apparatus and/or faulty technique employed for measurement, error in BP measurement, the white coat effect, or suboptimal compliance to the prescribed regime. *The most common cause is noncompliance, probably present in 50%–70% of the patients.* The common causes of inadequate response to therapy are listed in Box 30.2.

Such patients are to be referred to a specialist for further treatment. Screening to rule out primary aldosteronism is essential. Usually optimization of the 3 drug regimen, with respect to agent, dose and timing, followed by substitution of a thiazide-like diuretic (chlorthalidone or indapamide) for hydrochlorothiazide helps. If still BP remains uncontrolled **spironolactone** or **eplerenone** can be added. Both have some disadvantages. Spironolactone has androgen -related adverse effects while eplerenone is less potent and has short half-life, requiring twice daily dosing. Both can cause hyperkalemia especially when ACEI/ARB are in the regimen and in patients with reduced GFR. Nonsteroidal mineralocorticoid receptor antagonists, such as **esaxerenone** and **finerenone**, are devoid of androgenic effect and can lower BP in resistant hypertension and reduce CVD in patients with DM and CKD. However, they are expensive. **Patiromer**, a K+-binding agent has shown to decrease spironolactone induced hyperkalemia in patients with resistant hypertension and CKD.

Box 30.2 Common Causes of Inadequate Response to Antihypertensive Treatment

- Visceral obesity
- Poor patient compliance
- Continued stress
- Inadequate drug therapy
- Concomitant use of certain drugs (Box 30.4)
- Excessive sodium intake (including that in medications)
- Smoking, too much of alcohol
- Secondary hypertension

IM 8.15

TREATMENT OF HYPERTENSIVE CRISES

High DBP (≥120 mm Hg) may sometimes be found in completely asymptomatic patients. Long-term treatment with *gradual reduction of BP* is sufficient in such cases to prevent severe organ damage.

On the other hand, **in hypertensive crises, BP must be reduced in several hours or even within 1 h to prevent death or severe damage to vital organ functions** (Box 30.3). They usually occur in patients with known hypertension, but may occur in previously normotensive persons.

- Hypertensive crises should be treated in a hospital ICU with **facilities for invasive BP monitoring. In its absence, IV antihypertensives should be avoided. The patients should be treated in a strictly supine position to avoid orthostatic complications.**
- Most hypertensive emergencies are characterised by vasoconstriction and normal or reduced plasma volume. If renal function is greatly impaired, even a small reduction in GFR may worsen it. Therefore, drugs which do not cause reduction in renal blood flow (sublingual nifedipine, fenoldopam and sodium nitroprusside) should be preferred.
- **Drastic lowering of BP in a few minutes is hazardous.** Such an immediate fall of BP below the autoregulatory range of cerebral blood flow (which in hypertensives can be as high as 120–160 mm Hg systolic) **can cause cerebral ischaemia and severe brain damage and may precipitate MI, blindness and stroke.** The initial reduction in DBP should be about 20%; further reduction of 10% every 2–4 h till the diastolic pressure reaches 90–100 mm Hg is desirable. *Drugs with long-plasma t½ may cause extended hypotension with its attendant complications. Close monitoring by frequent BP measurements is, therefore, mandatory.*

Box 30.3 Hypertensive Crises

A. **Hypertensive urgencies:** These may be defined as sudden or severe elevation of BP, usually with SBP > 180 mm Hg or DBP > 120 mm Hg or higher **with an impending complication**. Such patients need immediate treatment, preferably in an ICU. The DBP needs to be reduced to 100–110 mm Hg within 24–48 h without the use a loading dose. The BP may then be reduced further, gradually, over the next several days. Urgencies include the following:
   - Severe epistaxis
   - Severe perioperative hypertension
   - Unstable angina pectoris
   - Diabetic retinopathy
   - Pre-eclampsia
   - Tyramine ingestion during MAOI therapy
   - Amphetamine or cocaine intoxication
   - Hypertension with papilledema
   - Decrease in renal function
B. **Hypertensive emergencies:** These may be defined as severe elevation of BP to SBP >180 or DBP >120 mm Hg, **with evidence of target organ damage or dysfunction**. Such patients also require admission into an ICU and rapid, but not too rapid, lowering of BP to 150–160/100–110 *within 1 h;* the BP should be maintained at that level for a few days, before lowering it, slowly, still further. Examples of emergencies are as follows:
   - Hypertensive encephalopathy
   - Intracranial haemorrhage
   - Acute myocardial infarction
   - Acute LVF with pulmonary oedema
   - Eclampsia

The drugs used to reduce BP in hypertension crises are given in Table 30.5.

Nitroglycerine (NTG): It reduces BP in a few minutes. It is the preferred agent in advanced renal or hepatic insufficiency

Fenoldopam: This drug is a peripheral dopamine (D_1) receptor agonist with a short action. It causes peripheral and renal vasodilatation, and natriuresis. It is as effective as sodium nitroprusside.

Nifedipine: Sublingual nifedipine is effective in lowering the BP rapidly. Given in the dose of 10 mg, it acts within 2–3 min and the action lasts for 2–3 h. In less urgent cases, it is given orally in the dose of 10 mg 6 hourly. If a sublingual preparation is not available, the patient can chew a 10 mg tablet for immediate local absorption and should swallow a second 10 mg tablet at the same time. Nifedipine is the drug least liable to aggravate regional blood flow

Table 30.5 Some Parenteral/Oral Drugs in Hypertensive Emergencies

Drug	Dose	Onset	Duration	Remarks
Arteriolar and venous dilator				
Sodium nitroprusside	0.25–10 mcg/kg/min, IV infusion	Immediate	2–3 min	Thiocyanate toxicity
Nitroglycerine	Initial 5 mcg/min, then titrate by 5 mcg/min at 3–5-min intervals; if no response is seen at 20 mcg/min, incremental increases of 10–20 mcg/min may be used; maximum 100mcg/min	2–5 min	5–10 min	Preferred in patients with IHD
Arteriolar dilator				
Hydralazine	5–10 mg IV bolus every 30 min or 10–50 mg IM	10–20 min	2–4 h	May precipitate angina, MI, used in pregnancy
D_1 receptor agonist				
Fenoldopam	0.1–0.6 mcg/kg/min IV infusion	3–5 min	10–30 min	Maintains renal perfusion
Alpha- and beta-adrenergic blocker				
Labetalol	20-80 mg, IV bolus over 2 min, then 20-40 mg every10 min to max. total dose of 300 mg or 2 mg/min, IV infusion up to 300 mg	5–10 min	3–6 h	Avoid in patients with a cardiogenic shock or marked bradycardia
Nonseletive alpha blocker				
Phentolamine	5–15 mg IV bolus	1–2 min	3–10 min	For pheochromocytoma and MAOI interactions
Beta-adrenergic blocker				
Esmolol	80–500 mcg/kg IV for 1 min; then 50–300 mcg/kg/min for 4–5 min, may repeat loading dose or increase infusion up to 300 mcg/kg/min if necessary	3–5 min	10–20 min	For postoperative hypertension
CCB				
Nifedipine	SL 10 mg, then 10 mg p.o. 6 hourly.	2–3 min	2–3 h	May cause fluctuation in BP
Nicardipine	Initial 5 mg/h IV bolus, titrate by 2.5 mg/h every 5–15 min, max 15 mg/h	1–5 min	3–6 h	Can cause reflex tachycardia
ACE inhibitors				
Enalaprilat	0.625-1.25 mg IV over 5 min every 6–8 h; maximum 5 mg/dose	15–30 min	6 h	–

imbalances and to cause ischaemia of the brain, eyes or kidney, but it can cause undesirable fluctuations in BP. *Although not an ideal drug, given under supervision, it is the preferred drug when intensive care facilities are not available.* Nifedipine should be avoided in patients with CAD or with ECG evidence of LVH.

Diuretics should be used only to treat salt retention or acute LVF with pulmonary oedema. If diuretics are used, attention must be given for maintaining adequate hydration to avoid oligaemia.

DRUG-INDUCED HYPERTENSION

Some drugs used in therapeutics may cause a rise in BP as their adverse effect (Box 30.4).

Furthermore, some dietary supplements such as *bitter orange* have been reported to increase BP. It is

Box 30.4 Some Drugs Causing Hypertension

Hormones: Glucocorticoids, fludrocortisone, testosterone, ethinyl estradiol
Vasoconstrictors: Adrenergic agents, ergot alkaloids, anorexiants, decongestants
MAO inhibitors
Salt retaining drugs: NSAID, liquorice
Miscellaneous: Bromocriptine, alcohol, caffeine in excess, epoeitin alpha, cyclosporine

imperative, therefore, to enquire whether the patient is taking any such drug or herbal remedies while evaluating a hypertensive patient.

Many proprietary 'cold cures' and 'cough mixtures' contain adrenergic drugs, e.g. ephedrine, phenylephrine, phenteramine or phenylpropanolamine. Hence, *it is best to warn the patients on antihypertensives to avoid such preparations, as they may cause a sudden rise of BP. Their enquiry should form a part of history taking.*

PULMONARY HYPERTENSION

Pulmonary hypertension (PH) is an abnormal increase of BP in the lung vasculature arising from diverse aetiology – cardiac, pulmonary or intrinsic vascular disease. It is associated with shortness of breath, dizziness, oedema and markedly decreased exercise tolerance. It results in heart failure.

Increase in PH with normal pulmonary capillary wedge pressure is termed as *pulmonary arterial hypertension (PAH)*, which is a progressive disease. PAH is associated with abnormalities of pulmonary vascular endothelium and smooth muscle proliferation leading to increase pulmonary vascular resistance. PAH is also common in advanced cases of **idiopathic pulmonary fibrosis**.

Pulmonary perfusion is regulated by local production of **NO and prostacycline (which are vasodilators) and endothelin, (a vasoconstrictor in the lung)**. Their impaired release is reported in PAH. Although, there is no cure, drugs are now available which can prolong life and improve its quality.

ENDOTHELIN (ET): This 21-residue polypeptide, originally isolated from cultured vascular endothelium, is present in several tissues (brain, kidney, intestine, adrenal glands). It is a **potent endogenous vasoconstrictor that also has proliferative, profibrotic and proinflammatory effects.**

There are **two types of ET receptors, ETA and ETB.** ETA is expressed on vascular smooth muscles, heart, lung and kidney. ET-1 preferentially activates ETA which results in vasoconstriction, bronchoconstriction, aldosterone release and smooth muscle proliferation.

Classification of Endothelin Receptor Antagonists

I. **Nonselective:** Bosentan and macitentan
II. **Selective:** Ambrisentan

BOSENTAN: This substituted pyrimidine derivative acts as a **nonselective competitive antagonist** of ET1. In patients with PAH, it reduces the pulmonary vascular resistance and lowers the pulmonary arterial pressure.

The drug is well absorbed orally. It is highly (98%) protein bound and has a t½ of 3 h. It is metabolised in the liver, and the metabolites are excreted in the bile.

Adverse reactions: These include nausea, anaemia and liver damage. It is teratogenic and carcinogenic in animals, and is contraindicated during pregnancy.

Indications: It has been used to treat severe PAH, in the dose of 62.5–125 mg b.i.d.

Macitentan, a derivative of bosentan has similar properties. **Ambrisentan,** an analogue of bosentan, is a selective ETA antagonist.

Other drugs used in PAH are as follows:

1. **Prostacyclin analogues,** e.g. epoprostenol, beraprost, iloprost, treprostinil given by IV infusion (Chapter 25). The latter two can be given by inhalation.
2. **Prostacyclin (IP) receptor agonist e.g.** Selexipag, a selective nonprostanoid agent given orally
3. **Nitric oxide (NO)** by inhalation

4. **PDE5 inhibitors** such as sildenafil or tadalafil given orally (Chapter 67)
5. **Furosemide** given orally or intravenously

Pirfenidone, a pyridine immunosuppressant, is an **antifibrotic** drug for therapy of advanced *pulmonary fibrosis*. It reduces production of fibrosis-associated proteins and cytokines response to growth factors such as TGF-beta and platelet-derived growth factor (PDGF). It has shown some marginal benefits. ADRs include mild GI symptoms (nausea, vomiting, dyspepsia, anorexia), dizziness, photosensitivity, rashes and elevation of liver enzymes. The dose is three capsules (267 mg/capsule) three times a day.

Nintedanib is an intracellular inhibitor of tyrosine kinases and inhibits processes involved in the progression of lung fibrosis. The dose is 150 mg twice daily. The common ADR are diarrhoea, nausea, and vomiting.

Riociguat is an oral-soluble guanylate cyclase (sGC) stimulator for PAH. Riociguat acts directly by stimulating sGC and also indirectly by increasing sensitivity of sGC to NO.

Treatment of pulmonary hypertension, and pulmonary fibrosis is in general unsatisfactory.

ORTHOSTATIC HYPOTENSION

Orthostatic hypotension is defined as a reduction in the SBP of at least 20 mm Hg or in the DBP of at least 10 mm Hg within 3 min of standing from a supine or sitting position. It is often most troublesome on rising in the morning and after meals, especially breakfast. Severe orthostatic hypotension can be disabling and its management is unsatisfactory.

The first step is to establish that the condition is persistent and find out whether there is a remediable cause. Drug therapy (diuretics, nitrates, phenothiazines, anti-parkinsonian drugs, tricyclic antidepressants and antihypertensives) is by far the most common correctable cause. Often, **chronic orthostatic hypotension is due to autonomic failure, primary or secondary to diseases such as DM.**

It is important to treat the symptomatic orthostatic hypotension *and not just the BP reading alone.* Patients with starting SBP as low as 70 mm Hg may be completely symptom-free. It should be remembered that treatment of orthostatic hypotension may lead to supine hypertension.

In mild cases, nonpharmacological measures should be tried; advise to rise slowly, to take high-salt diet, to sleep with the head of the bed elevated 10 cm and to use 'support tights'.

Drug therapy is used for those who remain disabled, have severe syncopal episodes or are unable to stand. The patient is advised to drink two cups of coffee (250 mg of caffeine) before breakfast. **Midodrine,** an α_1 agonist, in a dose of 2.5 mg t.i.d. may be helpful. The dose may be increased gradually to the maximum of 10 mg t.i.d., if required. The last dose of the day is given at least 4 h before bedtime to reduce potential for supine hypertension. The alternatives are **pseudoephedrine** (30–60 mg t.i.d.) and **phenylephrine** (10 mg every 4 hourly).

In severe cases, fludrocortisone may be used despite its shortcomings (Chapter 64). **Droxidopa, a prodrug of noradrenaline,** has been recently approved for the oral treatment of adults with symptomatic neurogenic orthostatic hypotension caused by primary autonomic failure or nondiabetic autonomic neuropathy. Both these drugs cause supine hypertension.

ANTIHYPERTENSIVES

Diuretics

- *Thiazides*
  - Chlorothiazide
  - Hydrochlorothiazide
- *Thaizide-like*
  - Chlorthalidone
  - Indapamide
  - Metolazone
  - Xipamide

RAAS inhibitors

Blockers of renin release

- *Beta-adrenergic blockers*
  - Atenolol
  - Metoprolol

Direct renin inhibitors

- Aliskiren

ACE inhibitors (ACEIs)

- Captopril
- Enalapril
- Lisinopril
- Ramipril etc.

Angiotensin receptor blockers (ARBs)

- Losartan
- Valsartan
- Telmisartan
- Olmesartan etc.

Aldosterone antagonists

- Spironolactone
- Eplererone

Calcium channel blockers (CCBs)

- *DHP*
  - Amlodipine
  - Felodipine
  - Isradipine
  - Nifedipine extended release
- *Non DHP*
  - Verapamil
  - Diltiazem

Sympatholytic drugs

Drugs acting on adrenergic receptors

- *Alpha-adrenergic–blocking agents*
  - Prazosin
  - Terazosin
  - Alfuzosin
  - Doxazosin
  - Phentolamine
  - Phenoxybenzamine
- *Beta-adrenergic–blocking agents*
  - Propranolol
  - Atenolol
  - Metoprolol etc.
- *Both alpha- and beta-adrenergic–blocking drugs*
  - Labetalol
  - Carvedilol

Central sympatholytics

- *α_2-Adrenergic receptor stimulants*
  - Clonidine
  - Methyldopa
- *Selective imidazole receptor (IR) stimulants*
  - Moxonidine

Adrenergic neuron blockers

- Guanethidine
- Reserpine

Ganglion-blocking agents

- Hexamethonium
- Trimethaphan

Drugs acting directly on the vascular smooth muscle (vasodilators)

Arteriolar vasodilators

- Hydralazine
- Diazoxide
- Minoxidil

Arteriolar-venular vasodilators

- Sodium nitroprusside

Potassium channel activators

- Diazoxide
- Minoxidil
- Pinacidil
- Nicorandil

Miscellaneous

- Metyrosine

DRUGS USED IN THE TREATMENT OF PULMONARY ARTERIAL HYPERTENSION (PAH)

Endothelin receptor antagonists

Nonselective
- Bosentan
- Macitentan

Selective
- Ambrisentan

Prostacyclin analogues
- Epoprostenol
- Beraprost
- Iloprost
- Treprostinil

Prostacyclin (IP) receptor agonist
- Selexipag

PDE5 inhibitors
- Sildenafil
- Tadalafil

Nitric oxide (inhalation)

Soluble guanylate cyclase (sGC) stimulator
- Riociguat

Furosemide

Antifibrotic immunosuppressant (for fibosis)
- Pirfenidone
- Nintedanib

CHAPTER 31

Pharmacotherapy of Heart Failure

Learning Objectives

This chapter will enable the reader:

1. To be aware of physiology of cardiac contraction.
2. To be aware of pathophysiology of heart failure and its types.
3. To classify the drugs used in heart failure illustrating their sites of action.
4. To describe pharmacological basis for use of the following drugs in heart failure: ACE inhibitors, angiotensin receptor antagonists, ARNI, SGLT2 inhibitor, vasodilators (nitrovasodilators and hydralazine), vasopeptidase inhibitors, beta blockers, diuretics, aldosterone antagonists, digoxin, phosphodiesterase inhibitors, dopamine and dobutamine.
5. To describe pharmacological effects, ADR and indications for digitalis.
6. To state signs of overdigitalisation and outline management of digoxin toxicity.
7. To name newer agents used in HF with their pharmacological basis in brief.
8. To state nonpharmacological therapy for heart failure.
9. To outline management of heart failure and its complications.

KEY TERMS

heart failure, pathophysiology, p. 466
left ventricular ejection fraction, p. 467
ACEI in heart failure, p. 468
ARNI, p. 469
diuretics in heart failure, p. 470
metoprolol, p. 470
spironolactone, p. 471
SGLT2 inhibitors, p. 471
vericiguat, p. 471
digitalis, p. 471
digoxin toxicity, treatment, p. 473
digitalisation, p. 474
ionotropic agents, p. 474
omecamtiv mecarbil, p. 474
heart failure, nonpharmacological treatment, p. 475
chronic heart failure, therapy, p. 475
acute LVF with pulmonary oedema, management, p. 478

Heart failure (**HF**) is a serious condition with high morbidity and mortality. It is a complex clinical syndrome, which arises from abnormalities of cardiac structure, function or both that impair the ability of the heart to fill or eject blood. The pharmacotherapy of HF has made spectacular advances, in recent times leading to better prognosis.

The normal heart is capable of increasing the cardiac output (CO) up to 3–4 times the resting value during exercise and in other states of increased need. **HF may be defined as the inability of the heart to maintain the CO adequate to meet the metabolic demands of the body at all times.** It manifests as (1) **acute heart failure** *(as after MI)* or (2) **chronic heart failure** *(CHF)*.

Physiology of cardiac output: CO depends upon the rate of cardiac contraction (heart rate) and the stroke volume ejected by the ventricle with each beat. Thus,

$$\textbf{CO} = \textbf{Heart rate} \times \textbf{Stroke volume (SV)}$$

Heart rate is regulated by ANS, RAAS and thyroxine.

Stroke volume is regulated by

- **Preload,** the length of the ventricular muscle fibre at the onset of contraction, which reflects the ventricular end diastolic pressure
- **Afterload,** defined as the tension or stress developed in the ventricular wall during ejection of blood into the arteriolar system. It is dependent on the volume of the ventricular cavity, the thickness of the ventricular wall, the condition of the arterial wall, and the peripheral resistance.

- **Myocardial contractility,** the ability of the heart to contract in response to given preload and afterload

The principal mediator for the cardiac contractility is increased cytoplasmic Ca^{++}. Calcium ions activate myosin ATPase, which in turn breaks down ATP, the energy source for excitation-contraction coupling in cardiac muscle. This is mediated through two myofilaments, **actin** and **myosin**. Changes in the cytosolic Ca^{++} concentration is responsible for contraction and relaxation. Adrenergic system which acts via the neurotransmitter NA stimulates the cardiac β_1 receptors and modulates cardiac contractility.

Pathophysiology of HF

A failing heart is characterised by inability to provide a CO sufficient for the body's metabolic needs, initially during exercise, but later even at rest. **Basically, HF is failure of the heart as a pump.**

This can arise in several ways, as follows:

1. **Pressure overload** as in hypertension and stenosis of cardiac valves (mitral or aortic)
2. **Volume overload** as in congenital heart disease and in regurgitant lesions of the mitral and aortic valves
3. **Loss of cardiac muscle** due to infarction or chronic ischaemic damage
4. **Impaired cardiac contractility** due to causes such as myocarditis
5. **Restriction of cardiac filling** as in constrictive pericarditis (**diastolic HF**)

Thus when myocardial contractility is impaired and the ventricle dilates, the CO diminishes. To compensate for this, there is reflex peripheral vasoconstriction and increased afterload. However, the cardiac oxygen requirement also increases which tends to reduce the CO further, thus establishing a vicious cycle.

The diminished CO causes fatigue, diminution in exercise tolerance and a variety of compensatory circulatory changes. **The failing ventricle increases venous pressure. This results in:**

- **Pulmonary venous congestion,** pulmonary oedema and dyspnoea of left ventricular failure (LVF)
- **Systemic venous congestion,** liver enlargement and peripheral oedema of right ventricular failure

The important event in HF is the loss of functioning cardiac tissue. To compensate for this loss, both

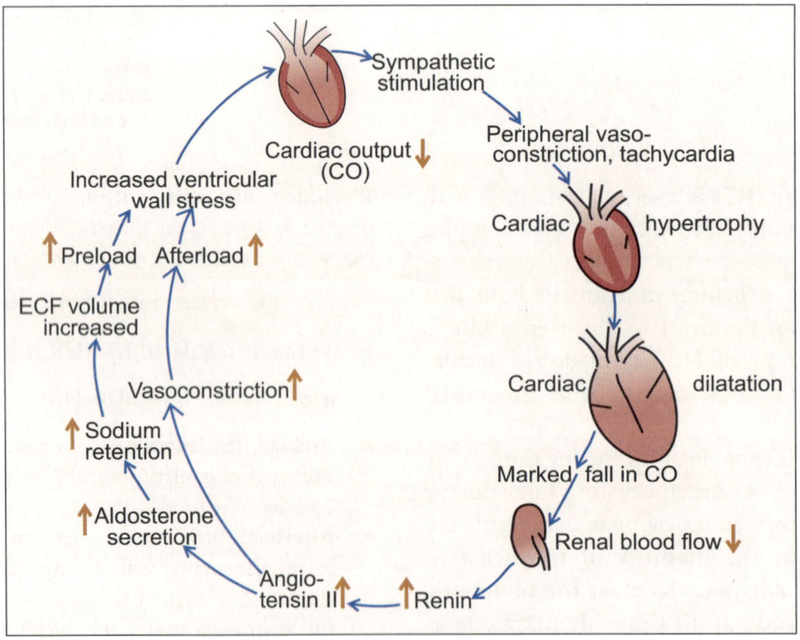

FIG. 31.1 Pathophysiology of CHF. Key events include (1) reduced myocardial contractility, (2) peripheral vasoconstriction due to activated adrenergic and renin–angiotensin–aldosterone systems and (3) increased ECF volume due to aldosterone secretion and sodium retention.

haemodynamic and neurohumoral adaptive mechanisms are activated to improve the force of ventricular contraction (Fig. 31.1). The compensatory mechanisms involved are as follows:

- **Increase in diastolic tension (preload),** which in early stages enhances the force of contraction according to Frank–Starling principle
- **Activation of adrenergic nervous system,** leading to increase in the circulating NA; chronic stimulation of the adrenergic system, however, causes increased afterload
- **Activation of RAAS**
- **Atrial stretch, stimulating secretion of atrial natriuretic peptide – ANP**
- **Release of endothelin, a vasoconstrictor**

In response to these mechanisms, ventricular remodelling occurs in which the ventricle hypertrophies; and in severe cases there is loss of myocytes with interstitial fibrosis. However, prolonged ventricular distension leads to progressive dilatation of the ventricles leading to **decompensated HF**. The failing heart is not able to maintain the CO. Further, activation of adrenergic system causes peripheral vasoconstriction, which increases the load on the ventricles (afterload).

When the CO falls, systemic perfusion pressure is maintained by two mechanisms:

1. **Peripheral vasoconstriction** caused by activation of adrenergic system early in the disease
2. **Sodium retention** caused by activation of RAAS which causes increase in aldosterone production

*The HF is not only a **disease** of the heart (a systolic dysfunction of the left ventricle) but is also a **disorder of the circulation**, involving both haemodynamic and neurohumoral factors.*

The major symptoms of HF, as explained earlier, are dyspnoea, decreased exercise tolerance, fatigue and fluid retention, which may result in pulmonary and/or systemic congestion. Some patients, however, do not show signs and symptoms of overload (congestion). *Hence, the term congestive HF is now replaced by the term HF.*

Among the techniques used to assess the global cardiac function, the most clinically convenient is the evaluation of **left ventricular ejection fraction** (LVEF), the ratio of the stroke volume to the end-diastolic volume of the left ventricle (**normal value is about 65%**).

Classification of HF on the basis on LVEF

1. **HF with preserved EF (HF_PEF)** with near normal heart size. These patients have near **normal LVEF** (>50%).
2. **HF with mildly reduced EF (HF_{mr}EF)** These patients have LVEF in range of 41%–49%.
   Both HF_PEF and HF_{mr}EF need confirmation from additional tests (apart from LVEF) such as spontaneous or provokable increased LV filling pressures (e.g. elevated natriuretic peptide, noninvasive and invasive hemodynamic measurement).
3. **HF with reduced EF (HF_REF)** with dilated heart. Patients with HF_REF have evidence of **abnormal LV systolic dysfunction and marked reduction in LVEF (<40%).**

Three important pathophysiological factors that contribute to the ventricular wall stress are as follows:

- Reduced cardiac contractility
- Peripheral vasoconstriction due to activation of sympathetic system and RAAS
- Sodium and water retention

PH 1.29

Classification of Drugs used in the Treatment of HF

I. **Vasodilators:** (Table 31.1)
   - **Arterial**, e.g. hydralazine. It reduces the afterload on the heart.
   - **Venous**, e.g. nitrates. They reduce the preload on the heart.
   - **Combined**, balanced arteriolar plus venous, e.g. ACEI, ARB, prazosin, sodium nitroprusside. They reduce both, preload and afterload.

II. **Angiotensin receptor neprilysin inhibitor (ARNI):** Valsartan + sacubitril combination

III. **Beta blockers:** Carvedilol, bisoprolol, metoprolol

Table 31.1 Beneficial Effects of Vasodilators in Heart Failure

Vasodilator Type	Preload	Afterload	VEDV	Stroke Volume
Arterial (hydralazine)	No change	Reduced	No change	Increased
Venous (nitrates)	Reduced	No change	Reduced	No change
Combined (ACEI)	Reduced	Reduced	Reduced	Increased

VEDV = ventricular end diastolic volume.

IV. **Diuretics:** Furosemide, aldosterone antagonists, thiazides

V. **Sodium Glucose cotransporter Type 2 (SGLT2) inhibitors:** Empagliflozin, dapagliflozin

VI. **Positive ionotropic agents:**
- **Sympathomimetics:** Dopamine, dobutamine
- **Phosphodiesterase (PDE) III inhibitors:** Amrinone, milrinone
- Omecamtiv mecarbil
- Digoxin

VIII. **Guanylate cyclase (GC) stimulator:** Vericiguat

IX. **Vasopeptidase inhibitors:** Omapatrilat

X. **Natriuretic peptides:** Nesiritide

ACEI (Box 31.1) PH 1.26, IM 1.24

Activation of the neurohumoral mechanisms in CHF increases, both **afterload** and **preload**, which in turn increase the cardiac work. *A reduction in either the afterload by arterial vasodilator or in the preload by venous vasodilators increases the CO.* ACEI, ARB, can reduce both preload and afterload. Table 31.1 depicts beneficial effects of ACEI/ nitrates and hydrallazine in heart failure. **ACEI, are considered the cornerstone of the therapy of patients with HF.**

ACEI has several advantages:

- They are **beneficial clinically and haemodynamically** *even in resistant HF.*
- They **control hypertension** which is an important risk factor.
- They **prolong survival** in CHF.
- **Tolerance is rare.**
- By blocking the local generation of angiotensin II, **they reduce its direct toxic effects** on the myocardium (*cardiac remodelling*) and reduce the risk of coronary ischaemic events.
- They **reduce the mortality rate** and the risk of haemodynamic and clinical progression in asymptomatic patient with left ventricular dysfunction following acute MI.

Box 31.1 Vasodilators Used in Chronic Heart Failure

- Captopril (6.25–50 mg t.i.d.), enalapril (10 -20 mg b.i.d.), lisinopril (2-40 mg o.d), Ramipril (10 mg o.d).
- Isosorbide dinitrate (20–40 mg orally or 2.5–10 mg sublingually, 6 hourly) or nitroglycerine ointment
- Hydralazine (50–75 mg 6 hourly)

All patients with asymptomatic or symptomatic LV dysfunction or LV enlargement are treated with ACEI as a first line therapy (Box 31.2). Patients who do not tolerate ACEI or remain symptomatic may be treated with **ARB or cardioselective beta blockers.**

Vasopeptidase inhibitors: These drugs **inhibit both ACE and neutral endopeptidase (NEP).** NEP is found mainly in the renal tubules but is also present in other tissues such as lungs, intestines, brain, heart and blood vessels.

- NEP catalyses the breakdown of ANP and some other peptide hormones including bradykinin.

Box 31.2 Use of ACEI in Heart Failure

- Start with small doses (captopril 6.25 mg, enalapril 2.5 mg, lisinopril 2.5 mg or ramipril 2.5 mg a day)
- Maximum doses are captopril 50 mg t.i.d., enalapril 10 mg b.i.d., lisinopril 30 mg o.d., or ramipril 5 mg b.i.d.
- Stop potassium supplements and potassium sparing diuretics before starting ACEI
- Stop other diuretics 24 h before the first dose of ACEI. They may be restarted the next day
- Patient should be sitting or lying down for 2–4 h, depending on the drug used, after the first dose of ACEI

- Its inhibition by vasopeptidase inhibitors prevents the breakdown of ANP and causes vasodilation and sodium excretion (Fig. 31.2).
- They also inhibit the production of angiotensin II. Thus, they may be useful in the treatment of HF and hypertension.

OMAPATRILAT: This vasopeptidase inhibitor given orally, is rapidly absorbed with plasma half-life of 14–19 h. It causes both arterial and venous dilatation and natriuresis. Toxicity reported includes dizziness, cough and angioedema.

NESIRITIDE: This, recombinant human B type natriuretic peptide (BNP), on i.v. administration binds to surface receptors on the vascular smooth muscle and endothelial cells and activates cGMP. It causes both arterial and venous vasodilatation and mild natriuresis. It also suppresses the RAAS. *However, it causes dose-dependent hypotension and hence should not be used routinely to treat severely decompensated HF.*

ANGIOTENSIN RECEPTOR NEPRILYSIN INHIBITOR (ARNI)

VALSARTAN + SACUBITRIL: This oral fixed dose combination is indicated for the treatment chronic heart failure.

Mechanism of action

The pathophysiology of heart failure involves an activated RAAS which leads to vasoconstriction, hypertension, increased aldosterone levels and sympathetic tone, eventually leading to cardiac remodelling, and worsening of HF. As compensatory mechanism the natriuretic peptides are increased leading to vasodilation, natriuresis, decreased BP, sympathetic tone, and aldosterone levels. Natriuretic peptides are broken down by an enzyme called neprilysin (an endogenous neutral endopeptidase). In addition neprilysin also metabolises bradykinin and angiotensin II.

Sacubitril is a pro-drug which on activation, acts as a neprilysin inhibitor, which prevents the breakdown of natriuretic peptides and prolongs their duration of action. When neprilysin is inhibited it will result in an accumulation of angiotensin II, hence a neprilysin inhibitor cannot be used alone; but must always be combined with an ARB to block the effect of the excess angiotensin II. Hence sacubitril is combined with valsartan, an ARB, as it antagonises the actions of angiotensin II.

This rational combination is recommended as first line drug in patients with chronic symptomatic HF to reduce morbidity and mortality. Neprilysin inhibitors also increase bradykinin levels hence, sacubitril cannot be used with an ACEI due to an increased risk of angioedema.

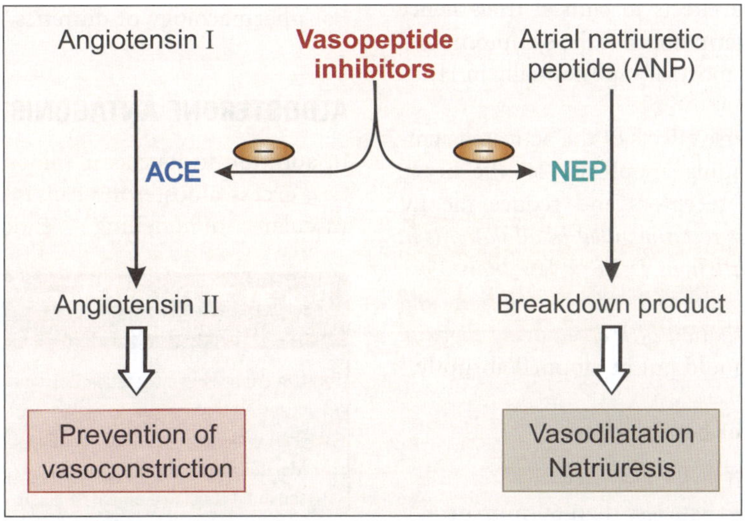

FIG. 31.2 Mechanism of action of vasopeptidase inhibitors. ACE, angiotensin converting enzyme; NEP, neutral endopeptidase.

Preparations and dosage: The formulation is available as an oral tablet containing a combination of valsartan + sacubitril in 3 dosage strengths i. 50 mg (26 + 24), ii. 100 mg (51+49) and iii. 200 mg (103 +97). Patients must be able to tolerate an ACEI or an ARB prior to being started on valsartan + sacubitril combination and at least a 36-hour washout period must be given before switching from an ACEI to valsartan + sacubitril. Patients on low-dose ACEI or ARB must receive 50 mg of combination mg twice per a day. The dose is doubled every 2 to 4 weeks as tolerated, upto 200 mg of combination orally twice a day. If patients were initially receiving a moderate to a high dose of ACEI / ARB, then 100 mg of valsartan + sacubitril combination twice a day is started.

Patients with GFR < 30 ml/ min or moderate hepatic impairment should start with 50 mg of combination twice a day.

Adverse reactions: These include hypotension, hyperkalemia, renal failure, cough, and angioedema.

BETA-ADRENERGIC BLOCKERS IM 1.24

Although the beta-adrenergic blockers can block the adverse cardiac effects of catecholamines, their use *in large doses* can worsen the HF owing to their negative inotropic action. However, the use of gradually increasing doses (*start low, go slow*) of **metoprolol/carvedilol/bisoprolol** (these three beta blockers have proven the beneficial effects in clinical trials hence preferred) over long term improve the symptoms and reduces the all-cause mortality substantially in HF.

They reduce the adverse effects of the activated sympathetic drive (including apoptosis) on the heart, upregulate the beta receptors and reduce the LV remodelling. *They are recommended in all patients in a stable condition, in whom LVEF is less than 35%, without substantial salt and water retention and without recent exacerbation of HF requiring digoxin.* Once started, they should not be stopped abruptly.

Contraindications for beta blockers

- HF after acute MI
- Patients with heart rate less than 60/min, or A-V block
- Patients with asthma or COPD
- Severe or unstable HF
- Those with HF and normal LVEF (i.e. diastolic HF)

Combination of an ACEI and a beta blocker is currently the cornerstone of the treatment of patients with left ventricular systolic dysfunction. As beta blockers and ACEI can worsen the fluid retention, it is necessary to optimise the diuretic drugs before starting beta blockers.

DIURETICS IM 1.24

Diuretics are used in HF to relieve sodium and water accumulation (**volume overload**) and thus reduce peripheral oedema, and dyspnoea due to pulmonary congestion. This gives quick symptomatic relief. But **if used alone, they have limitations:**

- They do not increase CO nor do they improve ventricular function
- With the excessive use of diuretics, CO and renal perfusion may diminish, with resultant fatigue, hypotension and impairment of renal function
- They do not improve the survival rate
- They can cause electrolyte disturbances

Therefore, diuretics alone are not recommended; they are combined with either ACEI or ARB. *Diuretics have no place in the absence of overt HF.* Box 31.3 outlines the principles of safe diuretic therapy of HF. For pharmacology of diuretics, see Chapter 37.

ALDOSTERONE ANTAGONISTS IM 1.24

In addition to its classic mineralocorticoid properties, excess aldosterone causes coronary and renovascular remodelling, endothelial cell and

Box 31.3 Diuretic Therapy of Chronic Heart Failure

- Use diuretics in moderation 2–3 times a week; avoid excessive doses
- Start with furosemide, add thiazide if needed
- Monitor blood chemistry, especially Na^+, K^+ and creatinine; serum K^+ should be at least 4 mEq/L
- Use diuretics in combination with an ACEI or ARB

baroreceptor dysfunction, potassium excretion and inhibition of myocardial NA uptake (Chapter 64). Morphological studies indicate that **chronic excess of aldosterone and salt loading cause fibrosis in the kidney** and other organs. It is known that ACEI in therapeutic doses do not completely abolish the secretion of aldosterone. The **aldosterone antagonist spironolactone** (Chapter 37) in the dose of 12.5–25 mg o.d. decreases the hospitalisation and mortality rates in patients with severe CHF who are already on the drugs discussed earlier. Further, the risk of hyperkalaemia is very low when such small doses of spironolactone are used. It also probably helps to conserve magnesium and thus prevent arrhythmias. *Monitoring of renal function and serum K^+ is mandatory*.

SODIUM-GLUCOSE CO-TRANSPORTER 2 (SGLT2) INHIBITORS

SGLT2 inhibitors were introduced as a new class of oral antidiabetic drugs (Chapter 63) that blocked SGLT2 transporters located in the proximal convoluted tubule of the nephron in the kidney. The SGLT2 are normally responsible for the resorption of filtered glucose (90%) along with sodium. **SGLT2 inhibition results in glycosuria and natriuresis, thus exerting antidiabetic effect.** This class of drugs opposed the adverse effects of diabetes, insulin resistance on cardiovascular metabolism and function, improved oxygen delivery and mitochondrial function.

The beneficial cardiovascular profile seen in diabetic patients led to evaluation of these drugs to be used in patients with HF. In addition, there are independent effects of SGLT2 inhibitors in HF such as:

- natriuresis
- preload and afterload reduction
- decreased BP
- regression of left ventricular hypertrophy
- renoprotective effect
- weight loss

SGLT2 inhibitors such as **empagliflozin** and **dapagliflozin** are added to the standard treatment of HF as they significantly reduce all-cause mortality, cardiovascular mortality, and hospitalizations associated with HF regardless of EF and diabetes status. Dose of both the drugs is 10 mg o.d.

The adverse effects include genital mycotic infections, volume depletion, hypotension, and ketoacidosis.

GUANYLATE CYCLASE (GC) STIMULATOR

Recently **vericiguat**, an oral soluble GC (sGC) stimulator, is approved as an add on therapy in patients with symptomatic chronic HF and LVEF <45%. Heart failure is associated with reduced synthesis and increased breakdown of NO and decreased soluble GC activity. Binding of NO to sGC increases production of cGMP, which leads to smooth muscle relaxation and vasodilatation. Vericiguat binds and stimulates sGC independently to cause vasodilatation and decrease in the cardiac load.

Vericiguat reduces the risk of hospitalization and CV death in patients with HF.

The adverse effects include anaemia and hypotension due to which it is not administered with PDE V inhibitors.

DIGITALIS AND OTHER INOTROPIC AGENTS

IM 1.24

Cardiac glycosides (digitalis) are plant derived, and have a steroid nucleus (CPP ring) and with an attached lactone ring (Fig. 31.3) in the chemical structure. Of the various cardiac glycosides only digoxin is used in clinical practice as a reserve drug in chronic HF.

Mechanism of Action: Digitalis acts as a potent positive inotropic agent by:

- **inhibiting the membrane bound Na^+–K^+ ATPase, which acts as a digitalis receptor (direct action).** This prevents extrusion of sodium and hastens the

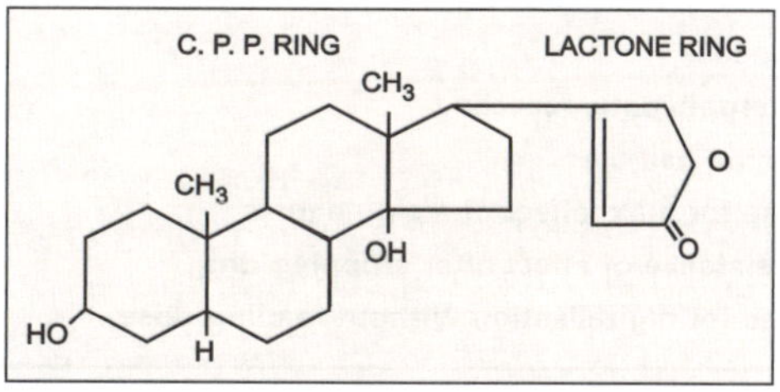

FIG. 31.3 **Structure of digitalis aglycone, digitoxigenin.**

entry of sodium into the cell during the resting phase (diastolic depolarisation). Along with sodium, some calcium also moves in and remains intracellularly because of the depressed function of the Na^{+}–Ca^{++} exchange pump. The accumulated intracellular sodium exchanges for the extracellular calcium, thus **increasing the cytoplasmic calcium, which results in increased contractility, automaticity and ectopic pacemaker activity in the heart.**

- **enhancing the vagal activity (indirect action)** and thus influencing the activity of the SA node, the atria and the AV node

Mechanism of action – digoxin.

Pharmacological actions: These can be divided into:

Cardiovascular actions: In the presence of CHF, digitalis:

- Increases the force of contraction, thus increasing the stroke output
- Shortens the duration of the systole, allowing greater time for both, ventricular filling and cardiac rest
- Reduces diastolic size of the heart. Reduction in cardiac size diminishes the oxygen consumption of the heart. **The digitalised heart, thus, can do the same work with less energy expenditure (oxygen utilisation).** Digitalis, therefore, is called a cardiotonic (and not merely a cardiac stimulant like adrenaline).

Digitalis, by improving the circulation, decreases the increased sympathetic tone in HF and thus, helps to reduce the heart rate and venous pressure. It also improves the coronary circulation and urinary output.

Digitalis exerts varying effects on the RP of different cardiac tissues. **Small doses** *shorten the atrial RP and* **larger doses** *prolong it. It prolongs the effective RP of AV node and depresses its conduction velocity.* **This action is of major importance in slowing the rapid ventricular rate in a patient with AF.** In contrast, *digitalis shortens the ventricular RP by direct action.* Large doses may produce extrasystoles, various degrees of A-V block and ventricular fibrillation as the terminal event.

Extracardiac actions:

Kidney: The urinary output is increased due to improved circulation and indirect inhibition of renin release.

Absorption, fate and excretion: Digoxin follows first order kinetics and its pharmacokinetics is summarised in Table 31.2. It is usually administered orally as IV can cause serious toxicity. IM 21.2

Adverse reactions: Digoxin can cause cardiac and extracardiac adverse effects, which are extension of its pharmacological actions:

- **Cardiac toxicity:** Digoxin produces all sorts of cardiac arrhythmias; the commonest are multifocal extrasystoles , bigeminy and even VF; followed by partial or complete A-V block. *Any arrhythmia occurring in a patient receiving digoxin should be*

Table 31.2 Pharmacokinetics of Oral Digoxin

	Digoxin
Absorption	70%–80%[a]
Plasma protein binding	25%
Disposal	Renal excretion of unchanged drug 50%–75%
Enterophepatic recycling	6%–8%
Plasma half-life	24–48 h
Time for max. effect of a single dose[c]	4–6 h
Persistence of effect after stopping drug	3–6 days
Time for digitalisation without loading dose	5–7 days

[a]Liquid-filled capsules of digoxin (Lanoxicaps) have higher bioavailability.
[b]Corresponding figures after IV dose is 1.5–3 h (digoxin).

assumed to be due to drug toxicity until proved otherwise.. Although anorexia, nausea and vomiting are the earliest signs of toxicity, cardiotoxicity can occur without them.

Digitalis toxicity is enhanced by excess of calcium ions. IV calcium salts should be avoided in individuals on digoxin.

- **Intracellular potassium depletion:** As inhibition of the sodium pump also prevents re-entry of potassium into the cell after repolarisation is complete, digitalis causes depletion of intracellular potassium. The serum potassium level, however, is not a reliable guide to the severity of K^+ depletion.

  Hypokalaemia enhances the cardiotoxicity of digitalis.
- **Gastrointestinal toxicity:** Digitalis, can produce nausea and vomiting due to stimulation of the CTZ . It also causes diarrhoea.
- **Opthalmological toxicity:** Visual disturbances including blurring, photophobia and disturbances of colour vision are fairly common.
- **Neurological toxicity:** Vertigo and headache can occur. Lassitude, confusion, disorientation, delirium, neuralgic pains and psychotic behaviour may appear.
- **Miscellaneous toxicity:** Includes skin rashes and gynaecomastia; the latter occurs as cardiac glycosides have a structural resemblance to estrogens.

Digoxin crosses the placental barrier, and may lead to premature delivery, and ECG abnormalities in the newborn.

Drug interactions: See Box 31.4. About 10% of patients convert large amounts of digoxin to inactive metabolites in the gut; in such patients oral antibiotics can cause a sudden increase in serum level.

Box 31.4 Drug Interactions of Digoxin

a. **Drugs which increase serum digoxin levels:** Quinidine; verapamil; methyldopa; indomethacin. Antibiotics (see text) and amiodarone
b. **Drugs which reduce serum digoxin levels:**
   - ***By induction of hepatic microsomal enzymes:*** Rifampicin
   - ***By reducing the bioavailability:*** Antacids; kaolin–pectin preparations; neomycin and cholestyramine
   - ***Drugs acting indirectly by interfering with serum K^+ and Ca^{++} levels,*** e.g. diuretics and IV calcium

Recognition of overdigitalisation: Overdigitalisation is to be suspected when the patient develops:

1. Anorexia, nausea and vomiting
2. Decrease in the pulse rate below 60 per minute, presence of extrasystoles, especially bigeminy or any other arrhythmia

A detailed analysis of the clinical situation, with special reference to past digitalisation, the patient's electrolyte and renal status, is necessary because the ECG alone may not be of help in diagnosing digoxin toxicity.

FM 10.1

Treatment of digoxin toxicity: See Box 31.5.

Preparations and dosages:

i. Digoxin tablet (Lanoxin) 0.125 or 0.25 mg
ii. Digoxin injection 0.25 mg/mL

Indications:

- **Heart Failure**

Digoxin is no more a drug of choice in HF because of its narrow therapeutic window and drug interactions.

Box 31.5 Principles of Treatment of Digoxin Toxicity FM 10.1

- Stop digoxin
- Stop diuretics
- Estimate serum potassium
- ***Bradycardia:*** atropine
- ***Mild toxicity (stable, VPBs):*** Potassium chloride 5-7.5g orally, daily in divided doses. For serious arrhythmia IV infusion is given (contraindicated in A-V block).
- ***Supraventricular tachyarrhythmias:*** Propranolol oral (10 – 40 mg every 6h) or IV (0.5-1 mg). Verapamil is contraindicated as it elevates serum digoxin concentration
- ***Ventricular tachycardia:*** Phenytoin IV (100 mg bolus every 5 -10 min upto a loading dose of 15mg /kg), or Lignocaine (loading dose 1-2 mg/ kg followed by a IV infusion at the rate of 1-4 mg/min
- ***Severe toxicity:*** antidigoxin antibodies (Digibind)
- Potassium is contraindicated in the presence of A-V block, hyperkalaemia or severe renal insufficiency

Moreover it does not alter the natural history of the disease nor does it substantially increase survival, in contrast to ACEI.

However, **low dose digoxin** (0.125–0.25 mg/day) **may be used as a reserve drug in patients with chronic heart failure if they do not respond /tolerate / afford other agents like ACEI, ARB, ARNI, aldosterone antagonists, diuretics and beta blockers.**

- **Atrial fibrillation:** Though digoxin was used for many years for this condition, its use is on decline (Chapter 28)

Digitalisation: is a process of administering digitalis to achieve steady state concentration by oral or IV route(Box 31.6). *Intravenous digitalisation is a potentially dangerous procedure, and is now rarely employed even in emergency. The therapeutic benefit, though proportionately smaller, comes even from partial digitalisation, because there is a linear dose–response relationship in the case of digoxin and there is no threshold for the positive inotropic effect of digoxin. Hence, except in special circumstances, the use of initial, large loading dose of digoxin should be avoided.*

OTHER INOTROPIC AGENTS

These agents stimulate the myocardium, but their mechanism of action differ from each other. Their usefulness is limited.

- Beta-adrenergic agonists, **dopamine** and **dobutamine** increase myocardial contractility, particularly in selected patients with severe HF. Although, these agents increase the velocity and force of contraction, they do not increase but often shorten the duration of systole (Chapter 32).
- **Phosphodiesterase (PDE) III inhibitors**

Box 31.6 Digoxin Dosage (mg) in Adults in Heart Failure

For routine, oral digitalisation: 0.25 mg once in 24 h; smaller doses (0.125 mg) in the elderly and in those in renal failure; digitalisation occurs in 5–7 days

For rapid, oral digitalisation: Loading dose of 0.75 mg in 24 h, followed by maintenance dose

For IV digitalisation: 0.5–1.0 mg

AMRINONE: It increases the force of contraction and rate of shortening of the cardiac muscle. It is a vasodilator and, reduces peripheral resistance (**ionodilator effect**). It has been used in patients with refractory HF. A common adverse effect is dose-related thrombocytopenia.

Milrinone has similar action as amrinone.

These drugs are not considered safe except for 48 h. They can cause serious arrhythmia on long-term use.

- **Omecamtiv mecarbil:** This new sarcomere directed drug, is a **selective cardiac myosin activator.** It increases myocardial contractility and stroke volume without increasing the calcium transit in myocytes and O2 consumption, thereby improving myocardial efficiency. The effect is dose dependent. The duration of left ventricular systole is increased. As the heart rate is decreased, the duration of diastole is not much altered. As a result, the coronary flow and left ventricular filling is not much altered. Thus, omecamtiv mecarbil may be an useful inotropic agent in the treatment of chronic HF caused by left ventricular dysfunction. It is under evaluation.

MANAGEMENT OF HEART FAILURE

The pharmacotherapy of HF has come a long way, since , William Withering , the master physician and botanist from Birmingham, in 1776, identified digitalis as the active ingredient from a mixture of twenty different herbs used by an old woman in Shropshire for the treatment of dropsy. Currently digitalis has taken a back seat due to availability of better and safe agents for HF.

The aim of pharmacotherapy for heart failure is

- Treatment of risk factors
- Provision of symptomatic relief
- Stabilisation of haemodynamics
- Reduction in the development of complications that result in hospitalization (acute LVF, cardiogenic shock)
- Prevention of disease progression.
- Improvement in quality of life and reduction in mortality

Patients with HF can present with ongoing symptoms as in **chronic HF** or as **acute complication**

(LVEF/ cardiogenic shock) warranting emergency hospitalisation. The New York Heart Association (NYHA) classification is used to characterize symptoms and functional capacity of patients with symptomatic HF (Box 31.7)

Box 31.7 The New York Heart Association (NYHA) Classification of Heart Failure

Class	Clinical Features
Class I	No symptoms and no limitation in ordinary physical activity, e.g. shortness of breath when walking, climbing stairs etc.
Class II	Mild symptoms (mild shortness of breath and/or angina) and slight limitation during ordinary activity
Class III	Marked limitation in activity due to symptoms, even during less-than-ordinary activity, e.g. walking short distances, comfortable only at rest.
Class IV	Severe limitations. Experiences symptoms even while at rest

NONPHARMACOLOGICAL TREATMENT OF HEART FAILURE

This is outlined in Box 31.8.

HF in many cases can be prevented by:

- **Controlling risk factors** such as hypertension, DM and correcting the structural anomalies like valve damage/stenosis
- **Controlling body weight and the sodium intake**

Box 31.8 Nonpharmacological Treatment of Heart Failure

- Salt and water restriction: advise *sodium* intake less than 2–3 g/day
- Weight reduction in the obese
- Cessation of smoking and alcohol consumption
- Limit physical activity in the acute phase of illness
- Stop any drug contributing to heart failure (Box 31.8)
- Influenza and pneumococcal vaccination has been recommended
- Supervised rehabilitation therapy including regular graded physical exercise which improves peak exercise capacity and the quality of life
- Surgical treatment, when appropriate

- **Use of ACEI after MI** and in patients with asymptomatic LV dysfunction
- **Avoidance of certain drugs.** Box 31.9 lists drugs to be avoided/used cautiously in CHF.

Box 31.9 Drugs to be Avoided in CHF

- Antiarrhythmics except beta blockers and amiodarone
- Calcium channel blockers
- NSAID
- Glucocorticoids
- Glitazones
- Metformin
- Cilostazol
- Sildenafil

Chronic HF (CHF)

The principles of rational therapy of CHF are outlined in Box 31.10.

Risk factors should be treated in all patients. **Restriction of sodium intake, (2.3 g/day) is beneficial to all.**

Box 31.10 Principles of Rational Therapy for Chronic Heart Failure

Reduction in ventricular wall stress and neurohumoral activation
- Bed rest
- ARNI/ACE inhibitors/ ARB
- Beta blockers
- **Aldosterone antagonist:** Spironolactones

Countering sodium and fluid retention by
- Restriction of sodium intake (<2.3 g/day)
- Restriction of fluid to <1.5 L/day
- Promotion of sodium excretion by using a diuretic, furosemide 20–40 mg
- SGLT2 inhibitors

Treatment of the cause, e.g. hypertension, arrhythmias, anaemia and thyrotoxicosis

Use of low dose aspirin, if evidence of ischaemic heart disease

PH 1.1

The standard treatment comprises of starting the initial drug as ARNI (valsartan + sacubitril combination) in all patients. ACEI or ARB can be used as initial drug in patients who are unable to tolerate/ afford an ARNI. Patients should also take a beta blocker (i.e., carvedilol, metoprolol, bisoprolol). In addition, aldosterone antagonist (i.e., spironolactone, eplerenone) and a SGLT2 inhibitor (i.e., dapagliflozin, empagliflozin) should be added in all the patients who do not have severe renal impairment. If patients have symptoms of congestion, a loop diuretic is added. Addition of a thiazide (eg, metolazone) to treatment with a loop diuretic should be reserved for patients who do not respond to moderate or high-dose loop diuretics to minimize electrolyte abnormalities.

All the above medications may be started simultaneously at initial (low) doses as recommended for HFrEF. Alternatively, these medications may be started sequentially, as guided by clinical or other factors, without need to achieve target dosing before initiating next medication. Finally, the drug doses should be increased to target level as tolerated.

In black patients with NYHA class III-IV symptoms, addition of hydralazine+isosorbide dinitrate may be considered who cannot tolerate the first line drugs or have renal insufficiency. Similarly in patients with symptomatic (NYHA class II to III) stable chronic HFrEF (LVEF ≤35%) who are receiving first line drugs, including a beta blocker at maximum tolerated dose, and who are in sinus rhythm with a heart rate of ≥70 bpm at rest, ivabradine (Chapter 28) may be added to the regimen as it can reduce HF hospitalizations and cardiovascular death.

Digoxin is a reserve drug and may be used in selected cases who do not benefit from the drugs mentioned above.

In selected high-risk patients with HFrEF not responding to optimal drug therapy vericiguat may be administered. In addition, patients with HF class II to IV symptoms, may receive omega-3 polyunsaturated fatty acid supplementation as adjunct therapy to reduce mortality and hospitalizations., It is continued even in patients who may become asymptomatic after treatment to prevent relapse of HF and LV dysfunction.

In patients with advanced HF refractory to optimal drug therapy can resort to device therapy such as implantable cardiac defibrillator, cardia resynchronization therapy. Patients who turn out to resistant even to device therapy are eligible for mechanical circulatory support or cardiac transplantation. Till these patients receive the device or mechanical circulatory support continuous intravenous inotropic support is offered as "bridge therapy".

Table 31.3 summarises the treatment of HF.

The treatment of patients with **current or previous symptomatic HFmrEF (LVEF, 41%–49%)**, is essentially the same as of HFrEF i.e use of ARNI, ACEI, / ARB, beta blockers, SGLT2 inhibitors and aldosterone antagonist to reduce the risk of hospitalization and deaths.

Patients with HFpEF and hypertension need antihypertensive drugs (titrated to attain optimum BP control) to prevent morbidity. SGLT2 inhibitors are recommended to these patients as they decrease/ prevent HF hospitalizations and cardiovascular mortality. In patients with HFpEF, management of atrial fibrillation can be useful to improve symptoms. In selected patients with HFpEF, aldosterone antagonist /ARNI/ ARB may be considered to decrease hospitalizations, particularly for patients with LVEF.

Box 31.11 lists important points to be remembered in the **management of chronic HF**.

Box 31.11 Points to Remember in Management of chronic HF

- ARNI /ACEI/ ARB are recommended in all patients
- Beta blockers in low doses substantially reduce morbidity and mortality and can be combined with ACEI
- SGLT2 inhibitors are recommended in all patients to prevent hospitalization and cardiovascular mortality
- Diuretics are needed for relief of pulmonary congestion and peripheral oedema
- Aldosterone antagonists are recommended for patients remaining symptomaic despite treatment with ACEI and beta blockers
- Digoxin has a limited role in patients with sinus rhythm. It improves symptoms and quality of life but does not reduce mortality
- Hydralazine + isosorbide dinitrate combination. ivabradine are indicated only in selected cases
- Patients with persistent angina may receive additional nitrate or a CCB such as amlodipine

Table 31.3 Stage-wise Management of Heart Failure

Stage[a]	Risk Factors for Heart Failure[b]	Symptoms of Heart Failure[c]	Structural Abnormalities in the Heart[d]	Treatment Recommended
A: Patients at high risk for HF	Present	Never	None	Treat risk factors;optimal treatment of HT, CVD, DM (add SGLT2 inhibitors in DM +CVD/ risk of CVD as they decrease hospitalization), Patient education.
B: Patients With Pre-HF	Evidence of any one of the following: • Risk factors • Structural heart disease • Increased filling LV pressures-increased natriuretic peptides/ cardiac troponin levels	Never	Detectable	In patients with LVEF ≤40%, ACEI / ARB + beta blockers started to prevent symptomatic HF and reduce mortality
C: Patients with symptomatic HF	Present	Currently present or H/O such symptoms	Detectable	ARNI in NYHA class II – III or ACEI /ARB in NYHA class II-IV+ beta blockers + Aldosterone antagonist + SGLT2inhibitors in all, ± Diuretics as needed, if congestion, present
D: Patients with advanced HF	Present	Refractory heart failure with marked symptoms at rest (EF <30%) resistant to maximal therapy, recurrent hospitalisations	Obvious	Difficult to treat; Resort to device therapy ICD-implantable cardioverter-defibrillator, CRT cardiac resynchronization therapy, mechanical circulatory support or cardiac transplantation

Note: Risk factor treatment and patient education is for all (A–D) groups.

[a]Stages as per the guidelines of the American College of Cardiology and The American Heart Association.

[b]Hypertension; diabetes mellitus; ischaemic heart disease; chronic lung disease; heavy smoking/alcohol consumption, H/O rheumatic fever, exposure to cardiotoxic agents, genetic variant / family H/O cardiomyopathy.

[c]Symptoms (current or past) of either left or right sided heart failure.

[d]Reduced left or right ventricular systolic function, reduced ejection fraction, reduced strain, ventricular hypertrophy, cardiac chamber enlargement, wall motion abnormalities,valvular heart disease, myocardial infarction.

The effectiveness of therapy can be monitored by observing the following:

Symptoms and signs of improvement:

- Increased urinary output
- Relief from fatigue, insomnia, orthopnoea and disappearance of basal rates
- Improved exercise tolerance
- Diminution in jugular venous pressure, hepato-jugular reflux and in liver size
- Disappearance of tachycardia and ventricular gallop
- Change of dry and paper like skin to normal, moist and elastic type

TREATMENT OF COMPLICATIONS OF HF

I Acute LVF

In **acute HF**, reduction of load (elevated LV filling pressure) and maintenance of CO as well as optimal blood pressure are the immediate aims of therapy. **Clinically, management of acute pulmonary oedema (see below) and cardiogenic shock is most urgent, and is preferably in ICU.**

Management of acute LVF

Acute LVF with pulmonary oedema is a medical emergency and is treated with IV **furosemide, and ACEI/ ARB** (Box 31.12). For patients hospitalized with HF, therapy with oral drugs which were used in chronic HF are continued and should be titrated with a goal to resolve congestion and rehospitalizations.

Management of acute HF has to be tailor-made guided by several factors such as concomitant diseases, left ventricular filling pressure and CO and hence is better left to specialist. In short,

- The patient without hypotension is made to lie in a **semiupright position** either by raising the head end of the bed or by using a back-rest, preferably with the legs hanging over the edge of the bed. Application of **tourniquets** to three limbs at a time, with rotation of the free limb every 15–20 min. **This helps to pool the blood in the limbs to reduce venous return and the preload.**
- **Oxygen** is administered at the rate of 6–8 L / minute
- **Furosemide** is injected intravenously in the dose of 40–60 mg, repeated every 30 min until diuresis sets in. *It acts by causing venodilatation, in addition to diuresis.* In patients hospitalized with HF when diuresis is inadequate to relieve congestion, the diuretic regimen is intensified using either: a) higher doses of intravenous loop diuretics. or b) addition of a second diuretic(aldosterone antagonist or thiazide)
- In patients who are admitted with decompensated HF, in the absence of systemic hypotension, intravenous nitroglycerin (5–10 mcg/min) or sodium nitroprusside may be considered as an adjuvant to diuretic therapy for relief of dyspnea
- If inotropic effect is desired, drugs such as **dopamine** or **dobutamine** may be added to the regimen

Box 31.12 Management of Acute LVF with Pulmonary Oedema

- Semiupright posture
- Tourniquets to three limbs in rotation
- Oxygen
- Furosemide 40–80 mg intravenously
- IV sodium nitroprusside or nitroglycerine
- Continued management of heart disease/heart failure, after resolution of acute heart failure

After resolution of acute HF, the patient should be investigated for possible cause of HF and treated accordingly.

II. Cardiogenic Shock

See Chapters 29 and 32. In patients with cardiogenic shock, temporary mechanical circulatory support is reasonable when end-organ function cannot be maintained by pharmacological measures to support cardiac function.

DRUGS USED IN THE TREATMENT OF HF

Vasodilators

Combined, balanced arteriolar plus venous

ACEI
- Enalapril
- Lisinopril
- Ramipril

ARB
- Losartan
- Candesartan
- Valsartan

Prazosin
Sodium nitroprusside

Arterial

Hydralazine

Venous

Nitrates
- Isosorbide dinitrate
- Nitroglycerin

Angiotensin receptor neprilysin inhibitor (ARNI)

Valsartan + Sacubitril

Beta blockers

Metoprolol
Carvedilol
Bisoprolol
Nebivolol

Diuretics

Furosemide
Aldosterone antagonists
(Spironolactone, Eplerenone)
Hydrochlorthiazide
Chlorthalidone

Sodium Glucose cotransporter Type 2 (SGLT2) inhibitors

Empagliflozin
Dapagliflozin

Positive ionotropic agents

Sympatho-mimetics
- Dopamine
- Dobutamine

Omecamtiv mecarbil

PDE Inhibitors
- Amrinone
- Milrinone
- Enoximone

Digoxin
Digitoxin

Guanylate cyclase (GC) stimulator

Vericiguat

Vasopeptidase inhibitors

Omapatrilat

Natriuretic peptides

Nesiritide

CHAPTER 32

Pharmacotherapy of Shock

Learning Objectives

This chapter will enable the reader:

1. To explain the pathophysiological mechanisms involved in different types of shock.
2. To be aware of clinical manifestations of shock.
3. To state the principles of management of circulatory failure.
4. To classify fluids used for volume replacement.
5. To state the uses of whole blood and its components, giving rationale.
6. To compare and contrast colloidal and crystalloid plasma expanders, giving suitable examples.
7. To explain the pharmacological basis for use of various cardiovascular drugs in shock.
8. To outline the management of hypovolemic shock, septic shock, cardiogenic shock, anaphylactic shock and neurogenic shock.
9. To comment on the use of vasodilators and steroids in shock.

KEY TERMS

Shock may be defined as complex acute systemic circulatory failure associated with hypoperfusion of tissues, which is incompatible with life if untreated and persisting for more than a short time. Hence prompt diagnosis and immediate resuscitation is essential.

Shock – Classification

Clinically, shock can be classified as:

I. **Hypovolemic or oligemic shock** due to
   a. Acute loss of plasma or blood (> 30% of blood volume in adults and 25% in children) as in burns and haemorrhage due to trauma, operation or obstetric emergencies like ectopic pregnancy or uterine rupture.
   b. Due to dehydration and sodium depletion as in excessive vomiting, diarrhoea, diabetic ketoacidosis and Addison disease.

II. **Bacteremic endotoxic or septic shock** produced as a result of severe infection usually with Gram-negative bacteria like *Escherichia coli*. Gram-positive organisms, particularly resistant staphylococci, can also produce shock by releasing an exotoxin called TSS toxin-1 (TSST-1) into the circulation. Deficiency of adrenal gland function and vasopressin production occurs in about half and one-third patients respectively. The mortality is still 40%–60%.

III. **Cardiogenic shock** due to acute heart failure, e.g. MI, acute myocarditis or severe paroxysmal tachycardia.

IV. **Anaphylactic shock** which is due to release of histamine and other mediators (Chapters 2 and 23).

V. **Neurogenic shock** due to pooling of blood in postcapillary capacitance blood vessels, e.g. shock encountered with spinal anaesthesia, spinal cord injury, abdominal and testicular trauma and perforation of a hollow viscus. In fact, it is a form of distributive shock.

VI. **Haemo-obstructive shock** produced as a result of obstruction of a main vascular channel, e.g. shock due to massive pulmonary embolism.

In all the above conditions, shock may be mediated by one or more of the following mechanisms; of these, *hypovolaemia is the most important*.

Mechanisms of Shock

Hypovolemic: This occurs due to a sudden reduction in the circulating blood volume, and can arise in many different ways. It evokes, through the baroreceptors, a generalised, compensatory sympatho-adrenal discharge and peripheral vasoconstriction. The latter is responsible for the clinical manifestations of shock. Though it helps to maintain the cardiac output and is important in short-term survival, it aggravates the hypovolaemia by making the microcirculation very sluggish, pooling the blood in the periphery which reduces effective intravascular volume.

Excessive vasoconstriction results in slowing of the blood flow, local haemoconcentration from loss of fluid from the capillaries into the tissues and in local formation of thrombi in the microcirculation. This causes tissue hypoxia leading to acidosis and to liberation of substances such as histamine, kinins, prostaglandins and cardiodepressant peptides into the circulation. Tissue hypoxia damages intracellular structures. Inadequate cerebral blood flow causes mental changes. Microcirculatory changes in the lungs lead to pulmonary oedema **(shock lung);** this is abetted by neurogenic and mechanical factors resulting in ventilatory failure and multiorgan dysfunction. Oligemic acute renal shut down completes the devastating picture.

Cardiogenic: This is due to failure of the heart as a pump as in acute myocardial infarction (MI). Rarely, in some cases, there is complete failure of the compensatory sympathoadrenal discharge.

Obstructive: Extracardiac obstructive diseases impair cardiac filling.

Distributive: In shock due to sepsis and burns, the peripheral resistance is initially low (warm shock); the cardiac output is elevated but is maldistributed as in shock with low cardiac output, with all the disastrous consequences. Later, the cardiac output falls and the peripheral resistance rises markedly.

The **septic shock** is initiated by the toxins released by the micro-organisms: exotoxins. These toxins cause the release of TNF-α and a variety of cytokines from the mononuclear phagocytes and the endothelial cells. They injure the vascular endothelium, increase its permeability, and cause fluid loss leading to hypovolaemia. They also depress the myocardium. Diffuse cell injury precipitates multiple organ failure. Many patients with septic shock have partial adrenocortical insufficiency.

Distributive shock may also occur following **anaphylaxis** and spinal cord or neurologic injury.

The **clinical picture** of shock is variable but generally consists of pallor, sweating, cold extremities, rapid and thready pulse and air hunger, all due to excessive sympatho-adrenal discharge. Cyanosis of the extremities may be present. Rarely, the extremities are warm (even in the absence of fever), whereas the circulation to the vital organs may be critically compromised. Oliguria (urine output less than 25 mL/h for 4 h or less than 500 mL/24 h in adults), mental changes (somnolence, confusion, restlessness) and acidosis are all indicators of reduced cardiac output and reduced tissue perfusion. *Central venous pressure (CVP) is the best guide to hypovolaemia.* If it is low to begin with and fails to rise during intravenous infusion of fluid at the rate of 10–20 mL/min for 10–15 min, hypovolaemia can be diagnosed. If during such infusion, the CVP exceeds 15 cm of water or rises more than 5 cm of water over the basal level, pump failure is a major component of the shock. In patients with chronic lung disease and after acute MI, CVP may not truthfully reflect left ventricular filling pressure.

By the time the BP falls, there is already a 25% deficit in the effective intravascular volume and hence an attempt should be made to diagnose and treat shock before the BP falls significantly. The femoral pulses are the best guide to the level of arterial pressure, since they are weak in hypotension but bounding in the presence of peripheral vasoconstriction with adequate arterial pressure. On the other hand, thready or absent radial or brachial pulses may be due to either severe hypotension or to reduction in extremity blood flow due to peripheral vasoconstriction.

Arterial hypoxaemia (reduced PaO_2), lactic acidosis and acidemia are the biochemical reflections of severe tissue hypoxia. PH 1.27

Management of Circulatory Failure: Aims

Successful management of circulatory failure aims at the following:

- **Early recognition of the shock state**
- **Correction of the initiating insult** (defibrillation, antibiotics, haemostasis, IV fluids, surgical removal of necrotic tissue)
- **Treatment of secondary consequences of shock** (e.g. acidosis, hypoxaemia)
- **Maintenance of function of vital organs** (e.g. cardiac output, B.P. and urine output)
- **Identification and treatment of aggravating factors**

Irrespective of type of shock, following is mandatory:

- The patient should be kept warm. Position the patient as lying flat with elevated legs (except in respiratory distress, acute pulmonary oedema).
- Venous access should be established through a peripheral IV line or central vein. Alternatively, intraosseous route may be used.
- Oxygen administration should be started to correct arterial hypoxaemia. Central venous O_2 saturation should be maintained at more than 70%.
- In case of respiratory distress, assisted ventilation is needed.
- Continuous monitoring is needed for consciousness, skin mottling and vital parameters like heart rate, BP, respiratory rate, hourly urinary output.

Restoration of blood volume: *Since increased blood flow to vital organs increases the likelihood of survival, therapy should augment cardiac output.* This is best achieved by restoring the intravascular blood volume as quickly as possible and may be the only treatment necessary, except in shock due to MI where the function of the heart itself is impaired. Fluid administration should be monitored by measurement of CVP and mean arterial BP. **Rise in CVP without a corresponding rise in arterial BP during IV fluid therapy denotes an overloading of the circulation.** To avoid it, CVP should be maintained <15 cm of water.

Fluids used for volume replacement are as follows:

1. **Whole blood and plasma**
2. **Colloidal plasma substitutes:** Dextran, hydroxyethyl starches, polyvinylpyrrolidone and oxypolygelatin
3. **Crystalloid plasma substitutes:** Normal saline (sodium chloride solution) and 5% dextrose

WHOLE BLOOD, PLASMA AND PLASMA FRACTIONS

BLOOD obtained from donors by aseptic technique, is preserved with either CPD (citrate–phosphate–dextrose) or CPDA (citrate–phosphate–dextrose–adenine) solution. Blood is stored at a constant temperature between 2°C and 6°C; storage below 2°C damages the RBC. It is vital to maintain the temperature constantly below 6°C to prevent the multiplication of bacterial contaminants. However, some bacilli can multiply even at a temperature below 6°C if they have previously been stimulated by exposure to a higher temperature. As the degree of haemolysis produced by such organisms is too insignificant for detection, **a bottle once taken out from the refrigerator and exposed to room temperature for 30 min or more should be discarded.**

The straw colour of the supernatant plasma serves as a convenient indicator to judge the suitability of blood sample for use. Pink or red stained plasma indicates haemolysis.

Blood should not be used after the stipulated period as the fragility of the erythrocytes increases after that period. Supernatant plasma, however, is stable and can be used. In the absence of an unusual haemolytic state or factor, the transfused erythrocytes have an average life of 4 months.

While transfusing **whole blood**, care must be taken to use only blood belonging to the *same* ABO blood group but preferably not from a genetically related donor (see GVHD below). **Rh- positive blood should not be given to Rh-negative individual, if it can be avoided;** at least it should not be repeated in an Rh-negative individual who has received Rh-positive blood transfusion previously.

Indications for Blood Transfusion

- **Acute haemorrhage:** Assessment of blood loss

is relatively easy in case of external injuries or gynaecological emergencies. Many times, however, one has to rely mainly on clinical signs such as pallor, tachycardia and hypotension to gauge the degree of blood loss.
An attempt should be made to maintain the following while treating acute blood loss:
a. Blood volume at 90% or more of normal
b. Haemoglobin level of at least 10 g/dL
c. Total serum proteins level of at least 60% of normal
d. Platelets above 50,000/mm^3
e. Plasma coagulation factors above 35% of normal

When the blood loss **is mild** (25% or less of the total blood volume) a crystalloid solution (see section, Crystalloid plasma expanders) should be infused in amounts 3–4 times the estimated blood loss. For **moderate blood loss** (26%–50% of the total blood volume), colloid plasma expanders may be adequate. For **larger estimated blood losses,** either packed blood cells or whole blood are needed to achieve adequate tissue oxygenation; *this may be in addition to crystalloid and colloid solutions.*
Adequacy of transfusion can be judged clinically from the reappearance of colour and warmth in the patient, filling of veins and the improvement in pulse and BP.
- **To provide leucocytes in cases of agranulocytosis:** Fresh blood is preferred as the leucocytes deteriorate on storage.
- **Severe anaemia:** With the availability of packed red blood cells, use of whole blood transfusion has become a rarity.
- **Intrauterine transfusion:** To reduce mortality in erythroblastosis fetalis.

Specific components like packed red cells, platelet concentrates or clotting factors obtained from plasma fractionation, are now available.

Complications of Blood Transfusion

- **Nonhaemolytic pyrexial reaction:** Rigor, a common manifestation, is mostly due to imperfect sterilisation of the apparatus. In such case, the transfusion should be stopped. The patient is covered with blankets. In severe cases aspirin, antihistaminics and glucocorticoids are employed. *Usually, it is due to pyrogens but may be caused by antibodies against antigens on donor leucocytes or platelets,* stimulated by a previous transfusion or pregnancy.
- **Allergy:** It is mandatory to enquire about previous history of urticaria in the donor to prevent this complication. Antihistaminics and adrenaline are used to treat this manifestation
- **Air embolism**
- **Heart failure** due to hypervolemia and circulatory overload
- **Transmission of disease:**
  1. ***Acute viral hepatitis B or C***
  2. ***Acquired immunodeficiency syndrome*** (AIDS) due to HIV
  3. ***Syphilis:*** *Treponema pallidum* does not survive refrigeration for more than three days; in an emergency, prophylactic use of penicillin can prevent this complication
  4. ***Malaria***

There is also the possibility of the recipient being harmed if the donor has received certain medications in recent or remote past.

- **Haemolytic reaction** due to mismatched transfusion is characterised by rigor, pain in loins, jaundice, haemoglobinuria, oliguria, bleeding and coma. The treatment of an acute haemolytic reaction is aimed at prevention of acute renal shut down. **Mannitol** 20 g (20%) should be administered rapidly, to initiate diuresis. If diuresis occurs, it should be maintained at 100 mL/h by giving normal saline, and IV **furosemide,** and by maintaining BP above 100 mm systolic. **Alkalinising the urine** with 40–50 mE moles of sodium bicarbonate, given intravenously, helps to hasten the excretion of free haemoglobin. If diuresis fails to occur, patient is treated for acute renal failure.
- **Hyperkalaemia:** Storing of blood at a temperature below 6°C causes an efflux of potassium from erythrocytes into the plasma. On restoration to room temperature, potassium re-enters the erythrocytes. *Failure to rewarm the blood to room temperature may lead to hyperkalaemia.*
- **Graft-versus-host disease (GVHD)** in which the donor lymphocytes attack and damage the host immune system. The mortality rate is high. It may be prevented either by avoiding transfusing blood from a genetically related donor or by irra-

diating such blood before transfusing it.

- **Iron overload** can occur in an adult after he/she has received 60–210 (mean, 120) units of blood. It is successfully treated by iron chelation (Chapter 34).
- **Citrate intoxication**, leading to cardiac irregularities and metabolic alkalosis due to metabolic conversion of citrate to bicarbonate, is a rare complication seen only after massive blood transfusions (more than 5 units of blood).
- Other complications after massive blood transfusion are hypocalcaemia; pulmonary insufficiency with adult respiratory distress syndrome; hypothermia (if blood is transfused without warming it to body temperature); and haemorrhagic diathesis.

Because of such complications of whole blood transfusion, when oxygen replacement is required, RBC replacement is to be preferred to whole blood.

PACKED RED CELLS can be transfused when it is desired to increase the oxygen carrying capacity of blood without increasing its volume. A packed red cell preparation is made by removal of 40% of the supernatant plasma. The red cell content of the remaining packed cells should be at least 5.5 million mm^3. **Concentrated red cells have to be infused within twelve hours of preparation**. There are less blood group antibodies in packed cells but still packed red cells are usually transfused in an ABO-identical manner (Box 32.1). If the patient's blood group is not known then it is permissible to transfuse packed red cells from an O group person (universal donor with Rh D negative) into a patient with any ABO group until the patient's blood group gets established. After that packed cells identical to the patient's own ABO blood group should be used. In addition, chances of anaphylactic reactions are less.

Box 32.1 Compatibility of Packed Red Cells

Patient's Blood Group	Compatible Packed Red Cells
A	A or O
B	B or O
AB	AB, A, B or O
O	O

Indications for Packed Red Cell Transfusion

Anaemia

1. Symptomatic acute or chronic anaemia: The decision for transfusion depends on both, Hb level (lower threshold for transfusion varies from 6 g/dL to 8 g/dL) and clinical symptomatology due to anaemia (resulting in tissue hypoxia) and co-morbidities
2. Aplastic and refractory anaemias
3. Thalassemia to reduce hemoglobin (Hb) S level to <30% of total Hb and other haemolytic anaemias
4. Cases of dyshaemopoiesis
5. As a preoperative measure
6. Acute blood loss refractory to crystalloid administration

One unit of packed red cells has haematocrit of 65%–70% which raises haematocrit of the recipient by approx. 3% and Hb by 1 g%. The amount of packed cells administered should not exceed 500 mL at a time.

In **chronic severe anaemia** and in sepsis, the myocardium is on the verge of ischaemia, and the rate of transfusion should not exceed 10–15 drops per minute. Failure to observe this precaution may result in heart failure. The amount administered in children under 25 kg is usually 15 mL/kg of body weight, whereas 10 mL/kg are administered in premature infants.

Adverse reactions:

Transfusion reactions to packed red cells are manifested as allergic reactions (erythema, urticaria, or flush), febrile non-hemolytic reactions, immediate or delayed hemolytic reactions. The most common reason for hemolytic reactions is ABO incompatibility and hence ABO testing is a must before every administration of packed red cells, even in emergencies!

PLASMA: **Fresh plasma** is prepared by separating a single unit (350 mL) of blood immediately after collection, for immediate infusion; and **fresh-frozen plasma** (FFP) is prepared by separating a single unit of blood (450 mL) within 6 h of collection and then storing the plasma at −30°C or lower. Blood derived FFP unit is 250 mL. Fresh plasma and FFP contain all the stable proteins (albumin, globulin) and the coagulation factors including **Factor VIII, factor IX**

and vWF; their main use is to treat/prevent bleeding due to deficiencies of coagulation factors e.g. patients with coagulopathy or those with liver diseases having abnormal coagulation tests before invasive procedures. For a patient with major bleeding following trauma, empirical transfusion of FFP along with red cells in a ratio of 1:1. Further administration is based on coagulation test results.

FFP is administered as 12–15 mL/kg. It should be transfused immediately after thawing or else it could be stored at 1–6°C after thawing but should be used within 24 h. Ideally, ABO compatibility of FFP should be matched with the recipient. However, Group AB plasma is a neutral plasma and hence is considered as universal for all the blood groups. Prothrombin time or partial thromboplastin time should be monitored and should not be allowed to go beyond 1.5 times the normal.

Plasma can also be prepared by separating stored blood within five days after its expiry date. Such plasma may then be freeze dried and stored. **The use of plasma merely to maintain blood volume is not recommended.**

NORMAL HUMAN SERUM ALBUMIN: This sterile preparation is obtained from human whole blood. It is used to raise the serum protein and reduce oedema level in hypoproteinemia, in hypovolemic shock, and as a vehicle for transfusing packed red cells. It is usually nontoxic and does not interfere with normal coagulation. The 5% solution is given undiluted usually at a rate of 2–4 mL/min. The 25% solution can be administered undiluted or diluted with sterile saline or 5% dextrose. Undiluted solution is used to treat the presence of oedema. In patients with low cardiac reserve, the rate of administration should be slow (1 mL/min).

PLASMA FRACTIONS: Plasma may also be used, by fractionating it, to prepare the following:

- *Individual coagulation factor concentrates,* such as prothrombin complex concentrate, Factor VIII concentrate (Chapter 33) to treat deficiencies of specific factors
- *Human immunoglobulin*
- *Fibrinogen*
- *Human and bovine thrombin*
- *Human fibrin*

These are discussed in Chapters 33 and 72.

- *Platelet concentrates* are discussed in Chapter 35

PLASMA EXPANDERS

PH 1.25

The plasma expanders are used to treat oligemic shock when blood and plasma are not available immediately.

Requirements of an Ideal Plasma Expander

1. It should have an oncotic pressure comparable to that of plasma
2. It should remain in the circulation for an adequate period and yet be eventually disposed of by metabolic degradation/excretion
3. It should not affect any visceral function adversely and should not have antigenic, allergenic or pyrogenic effects
4. It should not interfere with blood grouping or crossmatching
5. It should remain stable over a long period and at usual variations in environmental temperature. It should be easily sterilised and have a viscosity suitable for infusion.
6. It should be easily available

i. COLLOIDAL PLASMA EXPANDERS

Colloidal plasma expanders are substances of relatively high molecular weight, which, when infused, remain in circulation and augment the blood volume by increasing its oncotic pressure. They reduce capillary leak and thus decrease the amount of fluid requirement for resuscitation.

DEXTRAN: Dextran is isolated from beet root, where it is formed by the action of a contaminating bacterium *Leuconstoc mesenteroides.* Native dextran has a very high molecular weight (40 million) from which low molecular weight dextrans are prepared. Those used in therapeutics are **Dextran 70** (Macrodex, M.W. 70,000; 6% solution) and **Dextran 40** (Lomodex, MW 40,000; 10% solution). They are infused in the dose of 10 mL/kg body weight, in either isotonic saline or 5% dextrose.

- The oncotic pressure of dextrans is similar to that of plasma proteins and they persist in the plasma with an effective half-life of about 24 h.

- The dextrans also inhibit rouleaux formation by RBCs and have an antisludging effect on blood; they are claimed to improve the microcirculation independently of volume expansion.
- They may not interfere with typing, crossmatching or Rh determination.
- They can be stored without any special precautions for up to 10 years and thus can be stockpiled for emergency use.
  However, they coat the platelets and coagulation factors, and interfere with their function. In large doses, dextrans can cause widespread haemorrhages.

Dextran 70 tends to be retained in the body especially in the liver and the reticuloendo-thelial system. **Dextran 40** is rapidly excreted by the kidneys; as much as 50% is excreted in 24 h and the remainder in 4–7 days. Dextran molecules not excreted are slowly degraded enzymatically to glucose over a period of weeks. Allergic reactions including fatal shock are observed in about 10% of persons.

During its excretion through the renal tubules, dextran 40 can clog them and is known to precipitate acute oliguric renal failure which is gradual in onset (3–6 days) and hence may be missed initially. In order to guard against such possibility; dextran should not be used:

1. In quantities larger than 1 L (20 mL/kg) on day one and 10 mL/kg/day on subsequent days
2. If the urine output is less than 1500 mL per day or the blood urea is 60 mg/dL or higher
3. If the urine output drops further or the specific gravity of the urine rises above 1045 during its administration; in such cases, an attempt may be made to keep the urine output high with the use of diuretics and a high fluid intake
4. For more than 5 days

Dextrans can be easily sterilised by either filtration or autoclaving.

They are **contraindicated** in those who are known to be allergic to them; in HF; in existing or threatened acute oliguric renal failure; and in hypofibrinogenemia or marked thrombocytopenia.

HYDROXYETHYL STARCHES (HES): Addition of hydroxyethyl groups to starch molecules makes them resistant to hydrolysis by amylase and prolongs their intravascular half-life.

Though non-allergic, higher risk of death and a higher incidence of renal failure have been reported with HES in patients with septic shock, those with burns and in critically ill patients. HES induced coagulopathy increases risk of bleeding.

POLYVINYLPYRROLIDONE (PVP): This is a synthetic, water soluble, hydrophilic polymer of heterogeneous molecular sizes with a molecular weight between 35,000 and 40,000 and is given intravenously in buffered normal saline.

PVP may interfere with antibody formation. It can bind to drugs like penicillin and insulin and has a tendency to produce agglutination of erythrocytes. Hence, it interferes with blood grouping. *It is now rarely used.*

GELATIN POLYMERS: This polymer of degraded gelatin available commercially (**Haemaccel**) is a polypeptide with molecular weight of about 30,000–35,000. It is dissolved in an electrolyte solution with the final pH of the infusion 7.2–7.3. In this state, it can remain stable for 3 years at room temperature. Given intravenously, its t½-life is 4–5 h. Approximately 60%–80% of the gelatin is excreted unchanged by the kidneys. The preparation exerts osmotic activity similar to that of albumin.

It does not interfere with coagulation, blood grouping and crossmatching and is nonantigenic. Occasionally, it may cause flushing, urticaria and rigors. Bronchospasm and hypotension can occur. It is available as 3.5% gelatin polymer in 500 mL.

ii. CRYSTALLOID PLASMA EXPANDERS

PH 1.25

Crystalloids are solutions containing salts or other water-miscible agents. They can freely crossbiological barriers to enter interstitial tissue and hence, their effects are not restricted within vessels.

NORMAL SALINE, 0.9%, is the most widely used IV preparation. As its osmolality (308 mOsm/kg) matches that of serum, it is an excellent fluid for volume replacement. It distributes itself in the extracellular space, and infusion of 1 L of normal saline raises the blood volume by about 300 mL. It is mainly useful to replace lost sodium, chloride and water, particularly in cases of dehydration for emergency correction of hypovolaemia, e.g. haemorrhage, burns and diarrhoea. It is also used as a vehicle for giving IV drugs by drip. Though it is adequate to raise the effective blood volume and BP in emergencies, it leaves the blood rapidly and hence, has a short duration of effect. *Too rapid administration of large amounts can produce pulmonary oedema.* The febrile reaction that may occur with some products is usually due to the presence of pyrogens. Large volumes of normal saline may cause hyperchloremic metabolic acidosis, reduce renal cortical blood flow and induce acute kidney injury.

Its pH is 7.0 (i.e. neutral) when stored in a glass bottle but if packaged in polyvinyl chloride bags then it may range from 4.5 to 7.0. It is important to note that *noradrenaline is unstable at the neutral pH of normal saline but is stable at the acidic pH of dextrose solution.*

HYPERTONIC SALINE: In patients with acute severe sodium and water depletion, the amount of isotonic saline needed is so large that if injected quickly, it may overload the circulation. Serum sodium levels below 110 mmol/L may precipitate convulsions and coma. In such severe hyponatraemia, slow IV infusion of hypertonic saline (3%–5%) is used to relieve cerebral oedema temporarily and prevent neurological sequelae by restoring plasma volume and renal circulation. The injected hypertonic saline gets diluted by a shift of the water (which has entered into the ICF during severe sodium depletion) back to ECF. However, correction should be done slowly till serum Na^+ level of 125 mmol/L (no more) is reached over 24 h. Further rise in serum Na^+ to normal level should take several days. *Severe sodium depletion is generally associated with acidosis, which needs correction with sodium bicarbonate.* It is employed at times in critical care management to restore BP in haemorrhagic, shock or to reduce intracranial pressure in conditions causing acute intracranial hypertension but there is no evidence that it provides survival benefit.

HYPOTONIC SALINE: (0.45%): it is used to treat:

- Hypernatremia with extracellular volume depletion
- Hyperosmolar state with severe hyperglycaemia (0.45% saline with 5% dextrose)

BALANCED CRYSTALLOIDS

These are balanced electrolyte solutions containing a buffer such as lactate, acetate or gluconate. They are termed as "Balanced solutions" to indicate that they have ionic compositions similar to plasma. However, many of them have sodium concentrations lesser than ECF (hypotonic), and the buffers they contain differ from that found in plasma (bicarbonate and chloride). They include lactated Ringer solution, Ringer's acetate and multiple electrolyte solutions. The latter are marketed as Plasma-Lyte or Isolytes. Administration of large volumes of balanced crystalloids may cause hyperlactatemia, metabolic alkalosis, hypotonicity, and cardiotoxicity. The emerging evidence suggest that the chances of renal injury, need for renal replacement therapy, and mortality in critically ill patients are lesser with balanced crystalloids compared to normal saline. However, further confirmation is needed.

DEXTROSE 5% in water: When the glucose metabolism is normal, this solution is equivalent to administration of water alone. *As its osmolality is lower than that of serum, it is not optimum for volume replacement.* Water distributes itself in the total body water, and infusion of 1 L of dextrose in water raises the blood volume by about 100 mL only. *It is particularly useful when the kidney function is impaired.* It supplies nutrition. It can be used as a vehicle for drugs, especially noradrenaline. However, *phenytoin should not be infused in glucose-containing fluids.*

In general, colloids are considered superior to crystalloids in maintaining blood volume but the studies have failed to demonstrate their advantages. Moreover they are expensive and they may not always be available. Hence, 0.9% sodium chloride or Ringer-lactate is used commonly.

CARDIOVASCULAR DRUGS IN SHOCK

The major cardiovascular drugs used in shock are summarised in Table 32.1. For details see Chapter 18.

Table 32.1 Actions of Cardiovascular Drugs Used in Shock

Drug	Receptors			
	Dopamine	$Beta_1$	$Beta_2$	Alpha
Adrenaline[a]	–	+++	+++	++
Noradrenaline[b]	–	++ (small doses)	–	++ (large doses)
Dopamine[c]	++	+	–	+
Dobutamine	–	+++[d]	+	±
Phenylephrine	–	–	–	++
Isoprenaline	–	+++	+++	–
Glucagon: Positive inotropic and chronotropic action independent of beta-adrenergic receptors.				

[a]Low doses elevate systolic and decrease diastolic pressure; higher doses elevate both.
[b]Both systolic and diastolic pressures elevated.
[c]The action of dopamine varies with the dose. See Table 18.6.
[d]Dobutamine is a more potent ionotropic agent than isoprenaline.

Dopamine is indicated for reversing hypotension following MI, trauma, sepsis, kidney failure, overt heart failure and chronic CHF, when volume resuscitation is unsuccessful. When cardiogenic shock is identified or suspected, inotropic agent, such as **dobutamine,** (Chapter 18) is useful.

Noradrenaline is a preferred vasopressor. It is potent, has relatively low propensity to induce arrhythmias, and is associated with improved mortality compared to dopamine. The other drugs used are mephentermine, metaraminol and methoxamine (Chapter 18). **Mephentermine** acts chiefly by increasing the cardiac output. **Metaraminol** acts like NA but is less potent. **Methoxamine,** being a pure alpha adrenergic stimulant, is useful only in neurogenic shock. *Correction of acidosis restores sensitivity to the sympathomimetics.* To avoid infiltration into surrounding tissues the vasopressors are preferably infused through central venous or intraosseous catheters.

The main problem with sympathomimetics is the loss of responsiveness to them, apparently due to downregulation of adrenergic receptors, which may become evident within 8 h of continuous infusion. Therefore, their intermittent use is recommended in shock by some.

Except as a desperate resuscitative measure, the use of vasopressors should be preceded by expansion of intravascular volume. The systolic BP should be maintained around 90–100 mm Hg (or in previously hypertensive patients, 30 mm Hg below their usual pressure) during vasopressor infusion, as at infusion rates needed to raise the pressure higher, peripheral resistance rises disproportionately and compromises tissue perfusion. In severely ill patients, vasopressors may be used simultaneously with fluids, but their titration is needed with volume restoration.

Mechanical adjuncts such as venoarterial extracorporeal membrane oxygenation (VA-ECMO) and ventricular assist devices (VADs) aid circulation and may be employed.

MANAGEMENT OF VARIOUS TYPES OF SHOCK

PH 1.1

Table 32.2 illustrates the principles of management in various types of shock.

I. **Hypovolemic shock:**
- *Immediate treatment is directed towards restoration of effective blood volume by suitable fluids given intravenously.* Ringer lactate or 0.9% sodium chloride if used, the transfused volume should be 3 times the estimated losses. Plasma substitute amount will be 1.5 times the estimated losses. Hypovolemic shock is usually associated with metabolic acidosis as tissue hypoxia increases the production of lactic acid. This can be corrected by administration of

Table 32.2 Principles of Management of Shock PH 1.1

Treatment	Hypovolemic Shock	Endotoxic Shock	Cardiogenic Shock	Anaphylactic Shock
Volume replacement	Yes	Yes	Usually no	Possibly
Dopamine	Yes	Yes	Yes	Possibly
Dobutamine[a]	Possibly	Yes	Yes	No
Noradrenaline (only if severely hypotensive)	Yes	Yes	Yes	Yes
Adrenaline	No	No	No	Drug of choice
Vasodilators (sodium nitroprusside, nitroglycerine)	Possibly	No	Possibly	No
Phenylephrine[b]	No	Sometimes	No	Sometimes
Glucocorticoids	In Addison disease	Yes	No	Yes
Antihistaminics	No	No	No	Yes

Note: Isoprenaline is useful in toxicity due to beta blockers if bradycardia is the main problem (atropine may also be used for the same purpose); glucagon, dopamine and dobutamine are useful if hypotension is the main problem.
[a]May also be used along with dopamine.
[b]Also useful in spinal shock.

sodium bicarbonate. Associated diseases such as diabetes or Addison disease must be treated. As mentioned before packed red cells are administered after establishing the blood group.

- Correction of abnormalities of electrolyte balance.
- As soon as the clinical state of the patient permits, the causative factor should be corrected, if possible. If there is bleeding, control is achieved by compression, tourniquet or surgical haemostasis is used as the situation demands.
- **Morphine** is administered intravenously to relieve pain if shock is not associated with head injury or suspected acute abdomen.
- **Vasopressor agents** (DA or NA, see Table 32.2) may be employed to correct hypotension. However, *fluid deficit must be corrected before using vasopressors. Without such correction, the use of vasopressor agents may worsen the patient's condition* by reducing renal and cerebral blood flow and by increasing the oxygen consumption of the myocardium.

II. Bacteremic shock (Endotoxic shock): This is caused by severe infection and tissue hypoperfusion, leading to organ dysfunction. Emergency treatment comprises of prescribing appropriate antibiotic according to origin of infection, surgical intervention (if necessary), correction of acidosis, blood volume expansion (Ringer lactate or 0.9% sodium chloride or plasma substitute), and therapy for hypotension and for associated hypoglycaemia.

The initial antimicrobial drugs should be administered within first hour of recognition of sepsis after obtaining sample for antibiotic sensitivity and culture. Use of broad-spectrum, bactericidal multidrug regimens are preferred to cover all likely pathogens. In patients with high risk such as immunocompromisation, recent use of broad spectrum antibiotics, perforated abdominal organ, antifungal drugs are also considered. Once the organisms and sensitivity pattern is known, then rapid de-escalation to an appropriate antimicrobial agent is undertaken. A 7-10 days course suffices for most of the infections.

Noradrenaline is the first line vasopressor and is preferred over dopamine, which induces tachyarrhythmias and worsens the clinical outcome in sepsis. Vasopressin can be used as an adjunct as it has a sparing effect on norepinephrine, and reduces its dose. If there is inadequate cardiac output after fluid resuscitation, ionotrope like dobutamine is required. Adrenaline (in 1:10 000 dilution, 0.1 mcg/kg/minute) increases mean arterial pressure by increasing CO and vasomotor tone. It serves as a second line vasopressor or as an adjunct to decrease the dose of noradrenaline (especially if it is higher than 40-50 mcg/min) or as an ionotrope. However, adrenaline use is limited by risk of tachycardia, arrhythmia, and transient lactic acidosis.

As active lung injury often complicates severe sepsis, lung-protective ventilation, i.e. use of relatively low tidal volumes (6 mL/kg of ideal body weight), is reported to be beneficial in reducing mortality. Excessive tidal volume causes lung injury.

III. **Cardiogenic shock:** It is more common with STEMI than with non-STEMI. Approximately 80% patients with cardiogenic shock have LVF. The low cardiac output results in hypoperfusion and hypoxia of end organs which is life-threatening. The SBP remains <90 mmHg or mean arterial pressure <60-65 mmHg despite volume replacement and peripheral hypoperfusion is evident through raised lactate levels.

The treatment is focused on:

a. **Rapid revascularization of the infarct-related artery:** It forms the mainstay therapy for cardiogenic shock due to MI. Early revascularization is achieved with percutaneous coronary intervention (PCI) or coronary artery bypass graft (CABG) compared with initial medical therapy.

b. **Maintaining BP adequate to support renal and coronary perfusion:** This is done using vasopressors and adjusting volume status to ensure optimum LV filling pressure.

Noradrenaline is the first-line vasopressor compared to dopamine for the reasons mentioned earlier. Its infused at a rate of 2–4 µg/min and titrated upward based on BP. Dopamine should be avoided as first-line therapy for MI with cardiogenic shock based on hemodynamic and proarrhythmogenic effects. The former effects vary depending on dose, and there is an interpatient variability in responses (see Chapter 18). Dobutamine at a lower dose (2.5 µg/kg per min) has inotropic action with minimal positive chronotropic activity but with higher doses it causes moderate chronotropic activity. Its vasodilating activity prevents its use when a vasoconstrictor effect is required.

c. **Acute mechanical circulatory support:** It can offer better haemodynamic support.

In addition, hypoglycemia must be avoided. Any negative ionotropic agents like CCB should be discontinued.

IV. **Anaphylactic shock:** See Chapters 2 and 23

V. **Neurogenic shock:** This is treated like hypovolemic shock. Use of IV vasopressor (Tables 32.1 and 32.2) is indicated. Alternatively, ephedrine hydrochloride 0.5–1 mL of 45 mg/mL solution may be injected intramuscularly prophylactically.

VI. **Haemo-obstructive shock:** This is treated like cardiogenic shock.

Vasodilators in shock: Their use is restricted to the treatment of continued ischaemic pain or cardiogenic shock in acute MI. *Nitroglycerin IV infusion, along with dobutamine infusion is the preferred regimen.* They are not used in the presence of marked hypotension.

Glucocorticoids in shock: Glucocorticoids are of definite value in shock due to **adrenocortical insufficiency** and **anaphylaxis.** In septic shock they downregulate the maladaptive inflammatory response. Many patients in septic shock may have partial, adrenocortical insufficiency caused by adrenal suppression or glucocorticoid tissue resistance. Steroids have vasopressor-sparing role and have shown to reduce the duration of shock, ventilator use, and ICU stay. However, there is no conclusive evidence that use of glucocorticoids improve survival. Hence they are used as an adjunct for those requiring higher doses of vasopressors or in refractory septic shock. Longer course of low doses of a glucocorticoid (200 mg hydrocortisone per 24 h by continuous IV infusion drip, or 50 mg bolus in 4 divided doses or equivalent doses administered intramuscularly of methylprednisolone, betamethasone, or dexamethasone) for at least 3 days may be helpful in reducing mortality. Glucocorticoids are of no value in cardiogenic, hypovolemic and traumatic shock.

8

SECTION

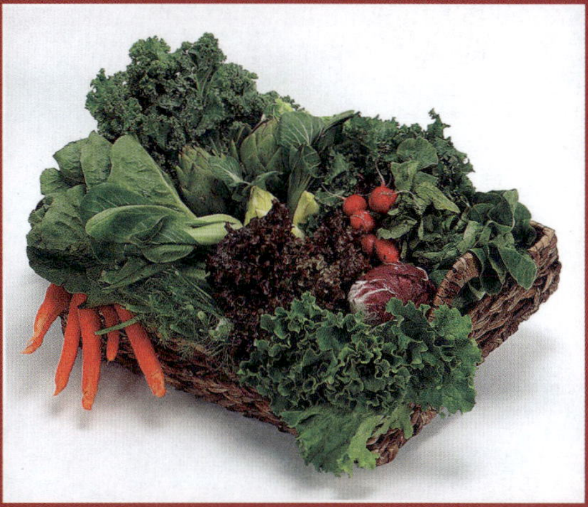

Carrot and green leafy vegetables

Drugs Acting on Blood and Blood Forming Organs

Section Outline

This section consists of the following chapters:

CHAPTER 33

Drugs and Blood Coagulation

Learning Objectives

This chapter will enable the reader:

1. To be aware of physiology of haemostasis.
2. To state the role of platelets in haemostasis and classify antiplatelet drugs.
3. To compare mechanism of action, indications, ADR of antiplatelet agents of various classes.
4. To classify anticoagulants on the basis of mechanism of action.
5. To describe mechanism of action, pharmacological effects, salient pharmacokinetic features, ADR, drug interactions, indications and monitoring strategy for heparin, warfarin and direct thrombin inhibitors.
6. To compare and contrast unfractionated heparin and low molecular weight heparins (LMWH).
7. To state advantages and disadvantages of different classes of oral anticoagulants.
8. To enlist fibrinolytics and state their mechanism of action, ADR and indications.
9. To classify haemostatic agents and state their mechanism of action, ADR and indications.
10. To outline the management of acute variceal bleeding.
11. To enlist sclerosing agents.

KEY TERMS

platelet aggregation, p. 493
coagulation, p. 494
aspirin, p. 496
clopidogrel, p. 496
heparin, p. 498
fondaparinux, p. 501
rivaroxaban, p. 501
warfarin sodium, p. 502
international normalised ratio, p. 502
anticoagulant therapy, contraindications, p. 506
fibrinolytic agents, p. 506
thrombolytic therapy, contraindications, p. 508
prothrombin complex concentrate p. 510
vitamin K, p. 510

Drugs are often used in therapeutics to prevent blood coagulation for thrombolysis and to arrest blood loss. They do that by acting on various stages of coagulation:

- Platelet aggregation
- Clot or fibrin formation
- Fibrinolysis

Haemostasis is the spontaneous arrest of bleeding from damaged blood vessels. When cut, the precapillary vessels constrict, following which:

1. Platelets adhere (**platelet adhesion**) to the exposed collagen fibrils of the injured vessel via a specific, platelet-collagen receptor, **glycoprotein Ib-IX-V complex**. Exposed collagen captures von Willebrand factor (VWF) from circulating blood, which provides binding site for platelets. It allows platelets to slow down, allowing interaction of other platelet receptors with matrix proteins leading to stable platelet adhesion.
2. This causes platelet intracellular signaling and triggers **platelet activation**. The activated platelets change shape and release preformed platelet granule constituents (5HT) and newly synthesized mediators of coagulation including adenosine diphosphate (**ADP**). **Activated platelets also generate thromboxane** A_2, a potent platelet agonist that recruits additional platelets at the site and aids vasoconstriction.
3. While changing the shape, platelet fibrinogen receptors (GPIIb/IIIa) get activated, and initiate platelet aggregation, which is reversible. It is strengthened by thromboxane A2 and ADP (irreversible aggregation). ADP promotes **platelet aggregation**, by interacting with ADP receptors (P2Y1 and P2Y12) on the platelet surface. P2Y1

receptors assist platelets to lose their individual membranes, form a viscous mass and aggregate. P2Y12 receptors complete the aggregation process, thus forming a **primary haemostatic plug.**

Platelet and coagulation activation are interconnected processes. During activation, the platelet membrane phospholipids become negatively charged, which facilitates binding of coagulation factors. This initiates coagulation cascade as described under Coagulation Physiology. Activated platelets also release thrombin, which activates the platelets further and cause conformational change in **glycoprotein IIb/IIIa**.

Coagulation Physiology

Coagulation involves a series of interactions among various clotting factors and other substances (kallekrein, calcium, platelet factor) present in the plasma. *The clotting factors* are synthesised by the liver. Factors II or prothrombin, VII, IX and X are *vitamin K dependent* for their synthesis. During the process of clotting, each factor undergoes partial proteolysis to form an enzyme (activated factor labelled by the subscript 'a' e.g. Xa). The activated factor then brings about similar proteolysis of the next factor in the cascade of coagulation.

The coagulation is initiated *in vitro* by the **intrinsic pathway** whereas it is initiated *in vivo* by the **extrinsic pathway** (Fig. 33.1). These pathways merge with the generation of factor Xa.

The initial event in the **intrinsic pathway** appears to be the activation of factor XII to factor XIIa following a contact with a foreign surface such as glass. The initiators of the **extrinsic pathway** are not normally present in the blood; they are added following tissue injury; in their presence, factor VII converts factors IX and X to active factors IXa and Xa, respectively. **The two pathways have the common objective of generating factor Xa from factor X.**

The activated factor Xa converts prothrombin (II) to thrombin (IIa). Thrombin ultimately converts fibrinogen attached to the activated platelet receptor, glycoprotein IIb/IIIa into soluble fibrin (**friable clot**). It also activates factor XIII, which then stabilises soluble fibrin strands as insoluble fibrin (**firm clot**)(Fig. 33.1). Normally, the blood is kept fluid by:

- **The rapid flow of blood**, which keeps the local concentration of clotting factors low.
- **Antithrombin III**, which inactivates all the clotting factors in the blood as well as any thrombin formed in the circulation.
- **Removal by fibrinolysis of traces of fibrin formed in the circulation.**

Disturbances in haemostasis include **hypercoagulability** and **excessive bleeding**. The latter may be due to deficiency of platelets or clotting factors.

Hypercoagulability is due to:

- Stasis within the venous system.

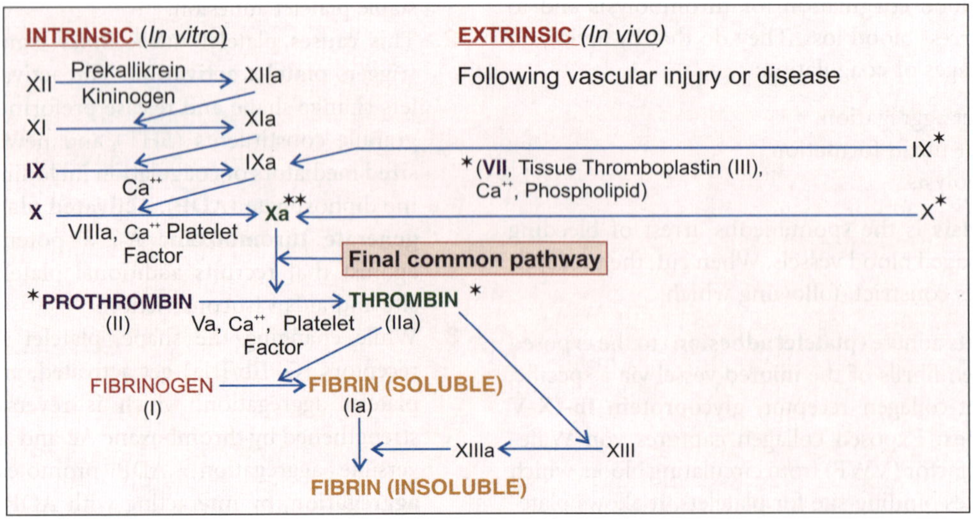

FIG. 33.1 Clotting factors and blood clotting. *Inhibited by warfarin; **inhibited by heparin.

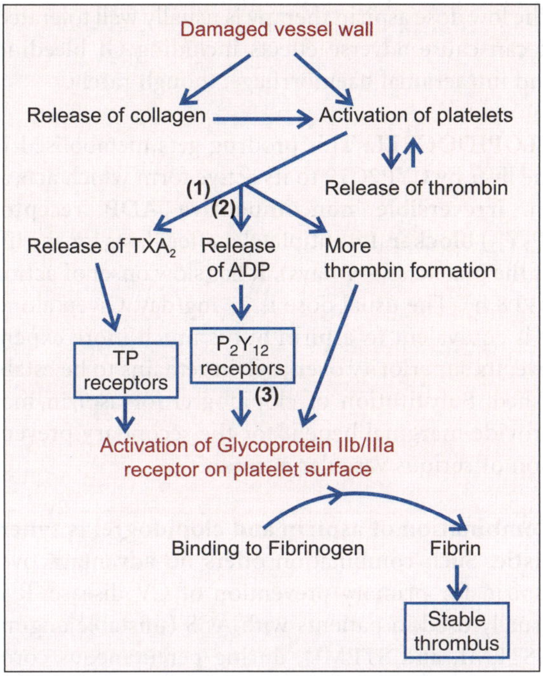

FIG. 33.2 Mechanism of thrombosis and its inhibition by drugs (1) aspirin; (2) clopidogrel and (3) glycoprotein IIb/IIIa antagonists. Prostacyclin is a physiological inhibitor (see text).

- Injury to or disease of the vessel wall.
- A hypercoagulable state of blood.

Thrombogenesis is a pathological process, leading to an intravascular thrombus formation. It is normally prevented by several regulatory mechanisms such as normal vascular endothelium, PGI_2, antithrombin, protein C and heparan sulphate proteoglycans synthesised by the vascular endothelium.

There are **two types of thrombi:**

1. **Arterial** (white thrombus)
2. **Venous** (red thrombus)

The process of formation of an **arterial thrombus** is an extension of the processes of platelet adhesion, granule release and platelet aggregation. It is predominantly made up of aggregated platelets and contains little thrombin. The arterial thrombus may occlude the artery or gets disintegrated to embolise the distal arterial tree. It may lead to ischaemic necrosis of the tissue such as heart. By contrast, a **venous thrombus** forms in an area of venous stasis. It is largely a mass of fibrin with RBCs entangled in its mesh and has few platelets.

Fig. 33.2 depicts the steps in thrombosis and their inhibitors. **Drugs used in the prevention and treatment of thrombosis** are as follows: PH 1.25

- **Antiplatelet agents**
- **Anticoagulants**
- **Fibrinolytic agents**
- **Haemorrheological agents** (Chapter 28)

ANTIPLATELET AGENTS

A balance between platelet TXA_2 and vascular PGI_2 regulates the platelet aggregability. TXA_2, is a potent vasoconstrictor, and promotes platelet aggregation by inhibiting adenylyl cyclase and lowering cAMP. Unlike TXA_2, PGI_2 is formed by the vascular endothelium. It stimulates adenylyl cyclase and the formation of cAMP, which prevents adhesion of circulating platelets to the healthy endothelium and their aggregation.

Platelet adhesion and thrombosis in atheromatous plaques are due to failure of local generation of PGI_2 by the vascular endothelial cells (**endothelial dysfunction**).

Apart from PGI_2, the endothelial cells also produce NO which increases the platelet cAMP resulting in inhibition of platelet aggregation. Prevention of platelet aggregation can prevent thrombosis.

Antiplatelet Agents Classification PH 1.25

I. **Prostacyclin PGI_2 analogue**, e.g. epoprostanol
II. **TXA_2 synthesis inhibitor**, e.g. aspirin.
III. **ADP receptor (P_2Y_{12}) antagonists**, e.g. clopidogrel, prasugrel, ticagrelor
IV. **Phosphodiesterase inhibitors**, e.g. dipyridamole
V. **Glycoprotein IIb/IIIa antagonists**, e.g. abciximab
VI. **Protease activated receptor (PAR-1) antagonist**, e.g. vorapaxar

PROSTACYCLIN (PGI_2) is naturally produced by the endothelial cells. It is also present in other tissues such as the brain, the gut and the kidney. It is formed from PG-endoperoxide (Chapter 25). Prostacyclin is very unstable with a short half-life of 3 min. Hence **epoprostanol**, an analogue of PGI_2, is used for preventing platelet aggregation during haemodialysis and to treat primary pulmonary hypertension (Chapter 25). It causes vasodilatation, resulting in hypotension, tachycardia, headache and intense facial flushing. It also causes nausea, vomiting, diarrhoea, dizziness, jaw pain and musculoskeletal pain.

ASPIRIN: Aspirin selectively acetylates platelet cyclooxygenase irreversibly (Chapter 11). The enzyme of vessel walls is less sensitive to aspirin than is that of platelets. **Hence, small doses of aspirin selectively inhibit the synthesis of TXA_2 by platelets (Fig. 33.1) whereas higher doses also inhibit PGI_2 formation in the vessel.** Aspirin in the oral dose of 75–150 mg daily is useful in:

- Preventing MI in patients with angina and reinfarction in patients with MI. IM 2.23
- Acute coronary syndromes (ACS) such as unstable angina. For immediate platelet inhibition, it is used in the dose of 150–300 mg.
- Patients undergoing revascularisation.
- Preventing stroke in patients with cerebrovascular disease in the dose of 150–300 mg.
- Preventing ischaemic limb complications in patients with atherosclerotic peripheral vascular disease.
- Pregnant women at high risk of developing preeclampsia; for this purpose, it is started between the 12th and 16th weeks of pregnancy and continued daily until delivery. *Its routine use in all pregnant women to prevent preeclampsia is, however, not recommended.*

In hypertensive patients, aspirin therapy should not be initiated until the BP is controlled.

Based on the results of current clinical trials, low-dose aspirin (75–100 mg orally daily) is not shown to offer major benefit for decreasing the incidence of CHD in adults with high risk factors (primary prevention). Hence aspirin use for the primary prevention of ASCVD may be considered among select adults 40 - 70 years of age who are at higher ASCVD risk but not at increased bleeding risk. **It should not be administered on routine basis for adults > 70 years of age.**

The low dose aspirin therapy is usually well tolerated. It can cause adverse effects including GI bleeding, and intracranial haemorrhage, though rarely.

CLOPIDOGREL: This prodrug gets metabolised in the liver by CYP2C19 to its active form which acts as an **irreversible noncompetitive ADP receptor (P_2Y_{12}) blocker.** Its antiplatelet effect lasts for the life of the platelets (5–7 days). It has slow onset of action (t½ 8 h). The usual dose is 75 mg/day. Given alone, it is equivalent to aspirin but is much more expensive. Its superiority over aspirin remains to be established. Substitution of clopidogrel for aspirin may provide marginal benefit for the secondary prevention of serious vascular events.

Combination of aspirin and clopidogrel is synergistic. Such combination offers no advantage over aspirin for primary prevention of CV disease. It is usually used in patients with ACS (unstable angina, NSTEMI, and STEMI), during percutaneous coronary intervention (PCI) and other vascularisation procedures.

Clopidogrel has several drawbacks such as delayed onset of action, large interindividual variability in platelet response, irreversibility of its inhibitory effect on platelets, genetic polymorphisms (CYP2C19) and drug–drug interactions with CYP3A4 inhibitors like atorvastatin.

Hence, low dose aspirin still remains the relatively safe, efficacious and cost-effective antiplatelet regimen for routine use.

PRASUGREL, a theinopyridine, is also a **prodrug** with an **irreversible antagonistic** action like clopidogrel at P_2Y_{12} receptor. It undergoes hepatic metabolism by cytochrome P450 to active metabolites, which are eliminated by both, renal and fecal routes. Its t½ is 7 hours.

Adverse reactions: As compared to clopidogrel, prasugrel is associated with higher rates of fatal and life-threatening bleeding. It is contraindicated in patients with a history of stroke or TIA or in patients over 75 years of age since such patients are at a higher risk of intracranial bleed. It has been reported to cause thrombotic thrombocytopenic purpura.

Preparation and dosages: It is available as tablets to be administered initially as a loading dose of 60 mg, followed by 10 mg once daily. For patients weighing less than 60 kg, the daily dose needs to be reduced to 5 mg.

It is used after coronary intervention for acute coronary syndrome to reduce thrombotic cardiovascular events.

TICAGRELOR: This cyclopentine triazolopyrimidine **reversibly inhibits P_2Y_{12} ADP receptors.** It does not require hepatic activation and hence its **action is more rapid and more complete**. The recovery after stoppage is rapid. The drug is metabolised by CYP3A4. It is effective in patients not responding to clopidogrel. Adverse effects include dyspnoea, bradyarrhythmia and increase serum uric acid and creatinine level.

Combinations of newer antiplatelet agents with aspirin are more effective than that with clopidogrel. However, they may have higher risk of bleeding.

DIPYRIDAMOLE: This vasodilator **reversibly inhibits platelet phosphodiesterase enzyme** (Fig. 33.3) and thus, increases cAMP. It has a weak therapeutic effect. Its main use is as an adjunct to warfarin in patients with artificial heart valves. It is used orally in the dose of 100 mg q.i.d. By itself, it is hardly of any benefit.

Cilostazol is a phosphodiesterase inhibitor (see Chapter 29). IM 2.23

Glycoprotein IIb/IIIa antagonists: These agents compete with fibrinogen to occupy the glycoprotein IIb/IIIa receptors (Fig. 33.3). **They inhibit the final common pathway of platelet aggregation. Thus, they are effective against any platelet aggregating agent** and are more potent than other antiplatelet drugs. Their onset of action is rapid. They include:

1. **Monoclonal antibody against the platelet receptor**, e.g. abciximab
2. **Synthetic inhibitors of glycoprotein IIb/IIIa**, e.g. tirofiban – *a nonpeptide*; eptifibatide – *a cyclic heptapeptide*

ABCIXIMAB: This monoclonal antibody blocks platelet receptors and inhibits platelet aggregation. Given as IV bolus, followed by infusion for 12 h, it produces an immediate effect **which lasts for 18–24 h** after stopping the infusion. Small amounts of the drug can be detected on circulating platelets for 7–14 days. It is an effective antithrombotic agent in ACS that requires

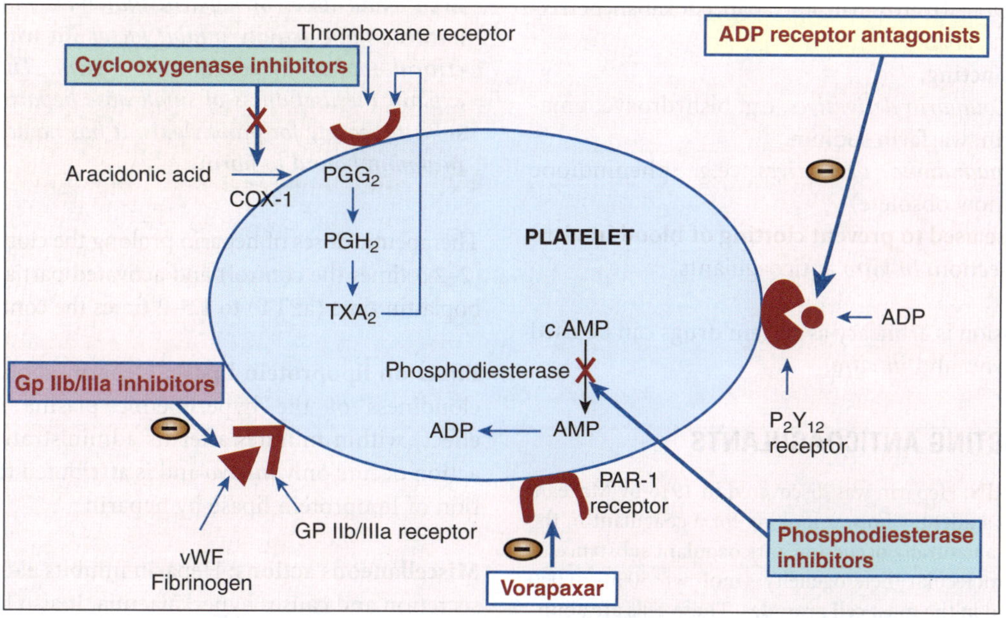

FIG. 33.3 Target sites for antiplatelet drugs.

percutaneous coronary intervention. It acts synergistically with aspirin and heparin. The drug is effective in refractory unstable angina and has also been used in ischaemic stroke. The major adverse effect is thrombocytopenia, which is reversed by platelet transfusion; monitoring of platelet count is necessary.

Tirofiban and **eptifibatide** are competitive inhibitors of the GpIIb/IIIa complex, with a plasma t½ of 2–2.5 h. Their effect disappears within 4–6 h after stopping the infusion.

Vorapaxar: Thrombin activates the platelets by acting on protease activated receptors (PAR-1) on platelets. Vorapaxar selectively inhibits PAR-1 and thus blocks the cellular action of thrombin and serves as a modestly effective antiplatelet agent.

Classification of Anticoagulants PH 1.25

A. Those used for preventing clotting of blood inside the intact vasculature.

Fast acting:

I. *Heparin, LMWHs*

II. *Direct thrombin inhibitors*

Parenteral: Lepirudin, bivalirudin, Argatroban,

Oral: Dabigatran

III. *Factor Xa inhibitors*

Parenteral: Fondaparinux, danaparoid

Oral: Rivaroxaban, apixaban, edoxaban, betrixaban

Slow acting:

I. *Coumarin derivatives,* e.g. bishydroxycoumarin, warfarin sodium.

II. *Indandione derivatives,* e.g. phenindione (now obsolete)

B. Those used to prevent clotting of blood in vitro

See section, *In vitro* anticoagulants.

The division is arbitrary as certain drugs can be used both *in vivo* and *in vitro.*

FAST-ACTING ANTICOAGULANTS

I. HEPARIN: Heparin was discovered in 1916 by McLean, a medical student, who was looking for a coagulant in the liver. It is a naturally occurring anticoagulant substance of marked molecular heterogeneity (mol wt 5000–30,000 Da), found in the **mast cell granules**. These cells are abundant in the liver (hence the name heparin), and in the lung. When released, it is rapidly degraded by macrophages and cannot be detected in normal plasma.

Purified, *unfractionated (native)* heparin (UFH) preparations are obtained from the lung and the intestinal mucosa of pigs and cattle.

Heparin is a mucopolysaccharide composed of a number of sulphated D-glucosamine and D-glucuronic acid units linked through an oxygen bridge (glucosaminoglycans) with more than 40–45 saccharides per chain. **Very high content of esterified sulphuric acid makes heparin a strongly electronegative compound, which is responsible for its anticoagulant activity.** It is *the strongest organic acid occurring in the body.*

Pharmacological actions:

As an anticoagulant: Heparin prevents the clotting of blood both, *in vivo* and *in vitro.*

Heparin binds to and **activates antithrombin III** which then inactivates factor IXa, Xa and thrombin. The heparin-antithrombin complex becomes almost 1000 fold more active inhibitor than antithrombin alone, producing instantaneous action.

> *Even small doses of heparin that have much less antithrombin activity inhibit factor Xa which is a critical moiety in coagulation system. This may explain the usefulness of small dose heparin given subcutaneously for prophylaxis. It has no action on thrombin bound to fibrin.*

Therapeutic doses of heparin prolong the clotting time (2–2.5 times the control) and activated partial thromboplastin time (aPTT) to 1.5–2 times the control.

Effect on lipoprotein lipase: Heparin abolishes the cloudiness of the hyperlipemic plasma (Tyndall effect) within minutes after its administration. This action occurs only *in vivo* and is attributed to activation of lipoprotein lipase by heparin.

Miscellaneous actions: Heparin inhibits aldosterone secretion and causes hyperkalaemia. It also has some anti-inflammatory action.

Absorption, fate and excretion: Heparin is poorly absorbed orally. It is well-absorbed after SC injection. Usually, it is given intravenously. It circulates bound to plasma proteins. The mast cells take up heparin in their granules and act as a storage depot for exogenously administered heparin. It is also taken up by the endothelial cells. *Heparin does not cross the placental barrier and is not secreted in the milk.*

The onset of anticoagulant action with an IV dose is almost immediate and reaches peak within 5–10 min; whereas after SC administration, it is delayed up to 1 h. The clotting time returns to normal within 2–4 h with a t½ of about 60 min. *The aqueous preparation is, therefore, administered at 2–4 hourly interval.*

Heparin is metabolised mainly in the liver by an enzyme, *heparinase*. Following IV administration, 25%–50% of a single dose may appear in the urine in active form. Its elimination from plasma involves both, first and zero order kinetics. *Thus clinically, the dose–response relation is not linear; instead, the anticoagulant response increases disproportionately in intensity and duration with increasing doses.*

Adverse reactions:

- **Allergic and anaphylactoid reactions** are rare and include asthma, urticaria, rhinitis and fever. It is advisable to give a trial dose of 1000 U of heparin.
- **Bleeding:** Excessive or injudicious use of heparin may produce haemorrhage from various sites such as peptic ulcer, kidneys and haemorrhoids. It is advisable to avoid aspirin and other drugs which interfere with platelet function during heparin therapy.
- **Thrombocytopenia:** UFH causes transient, mild thrombocytopenia in 25% of patients and severe thrombocytopenia in a few. The mild reaction results from heparin induced platelet aggregation. The severe form, which occurs on 8th to 12th day of treatment, is due to the formation of heparin dependent antiplatelet antibodies; this can result in tolerance to its anticoagulant action. The incidence is less with low molecular weight (LMW) heparins. *It is recommended that a platelet count should be obtained before starting the therapy and frequently during the therapy.*
- **Alopecia:** Transient alopecia may occur after prolonged heparin therapy.
- **Osteoporosis:** Use of heparin in the dose of 15,000 U daily for a period of 6 months or more has been reported to cause osteoporosis.
- **Miscellaneous:** SGOT and SGPT levels may rise during therapy with heparin.

Preparations and dosage: UFH is available as solution for injection either as **heparin sodium** 1000 U/ml, 5000 U/ml and 25000 U/ml or **heparin calcium** as 25000 U/ml or as IV flush available in a dose of 10 U/ml and 100 U/ml. Also available as **heparin sodium gel/cream/ointment** containing 50, 200, 1000 U/gm. Since the commercial preparations of heparin vary in their potency (as U/mg), the dosage of heparin must be prescribed in units.

Small fixed doses of heparin are given deep subcutaneously to prevent venous thromboembolism. Larger doses are needed to prevent the propagation of an established thrombus; still larger doses may be necessary in acute pulmonary embolism. *When large doses are used, they must be adjusted according to the clotting time and aPTT* (see below).

Heparin is not injected intramuscularly as it can cause a haematoma.

i. **Low fixed dose, SC regimen** (prophylactic): 5000 U given every 8–12 h, starting 1–2 h before the operation and continuing till the patient is discharged. *Determination of aPTT is not needed.*
ii. **Dose-adjusted SC regimen** (therapeutic): This regimen employs either 8000–10,000 U hourly or 15,000–20,000 U 12 hourly, the actual dose being adjusted in either instance according to the results of aPTT.
iii. **IV intermittent regimen** (therapeutic): 60-100 U/kg every 4-6 h or **IV infusion** in isotonic saline (0.5 U/kg/min).

Advantages of UFH:

- Its anticoagulant effect can be *completely and rapidly reversed by prothrombin*
- It has a *shorter t½*
- There is no renal elimination; hence it is *safer in patients with renal impairment*

- *It directly inhibits the contact activation pathway* that is important in the formation of thrombi in stent, catheter etc.
- It is cheaper than LMW heparin.

LOW MOLECULAR WEIGHT HEPARINS (LMWH): These are prepared by fractionation of native heparin; they are more homogeneous molecularly with molecular weight between 4000 and 6500. Given subcutaneously once or twice daily, these compounds have at least as much antithrombotic activity as UFH. Their **advantages** are that, they:

- *Are absorbed more uniformly* than the UFH after SC administration.
- *Have a longer duration of action* (t½ 4 h).
- *Inactivate factor Xa selectively*; their action against thrombin is minimal.
- *Have a predictable anticoagulant effect because they bind less avidly to cells and to heparin binding proteins.*
- *Interact relatively less with platelets* and lead to fewer bleeding episodes.
- *Are less antigenic.*
- *Cause thrombocytopenia and osteoporosis infrequently.*

These properties make their use attractive for outpatient and domiciliary use. However, they are more expensive.

Examples of LMW heparins are **enoxaparin, dalteparin** sodium, **tinzaparin, pamaparin** and **reviparin**. They vary in their pharmacokinetic properties and dose. Their uses are similar to those of native heparin (Table 33.1). *However, native heparin still remains the parenteral anticoagulant of choice in cardiopulmonary bypass and DIC.*

Box 33.1 Monitoring Heparin Therapy

- ***Whole blood clotting time*** (Lee-White), which should be kept at 2–3 times the normal
- ***Activated partial thromboplastin time (aPTT)*** which should be kept at 1½–2 times the normal

Box 33.1 lists the methods of monitoring heparin therapy. *Small doses of heparin subcutaneously, for prophylaxis and LMWH do not generally require monitoring.*

Heparin antagonists: The anticoagulant effects of heparin can be arrested by the administration of **strongly basic compounds which react with the strongly acidic groups of heparin,** thereby abolishing its activity, e.g. protamine sulphate.

PROTAMINE SULPHATE: It is a mixture of simple, low molecular weight polypeptides, found in the sperms of certain fish. It binds firmly to heparin and inactivates it. Protamine sulphate as 1% solution, is administered slowly intravenously, not more than 50 mg over a 10-min period. One milligram of protamine sulphate neutralises the anticoagulant effect of 100 U of heparin. If more than 30 min have elapsed after heparin administration half of this dose is required. A patient given protamine should be observed for recurrence of bleeding as protamine sulphate itself has

Table 33.1 Doses of Commonly Used LMWH

Preparation	For Prophylaxis of Deep Vein Thrombosis (DVT)	For Treatment of DVT and Pulmonary Embolism
Enoxaparin	3000 U subcutaneously 2 h before surgery; then 3000 U (30 mg) SC twice daily for 7–10 days In high risk patients, 4,000 IU (40 mg) SC injection 12 hours before surgery and resumed 12 hours post- surgery once/day	100 U/kg (1mg/kg) subcutaneously twice daily or 150 U/kg (1.5mg/kg) once daily for 5 days
Dalteparin	2500 U subcutaneously 1–2 h before surgery; then 2500 U every 24 h for 5–7 days	100 U/kg subcutaneously twice daily for 5 days
Tinzaparin	3500 U subcutaneously 2 h before surgery; then 3500 U every 24 h for 7–10 days	175 U/kg subcutaneously once daily for 6 days

anticoagulant activity. Moreover, the action of heparin lasts longer than that of protamine.

Protamine IV injection may cause a sudden fall in BP, bradycardia, dyspnoea and transitory flushing. It only partially neutralises LMWH and has no effect on the anticoagulant activity of fondaparinux.

II. DIRECT THROMBIN INHIBITORS

Parenteral

HIRUDIN: This is a polypeptide obtained from the leech *Hirudo medicinalis*. It is synthesised by recombinant DNA technique **(lepirudin).**

- *It binds directly to thrombin without requiring antithrombin or cofactors and inactivates free as well as fibrin-bound thrombin irreversibly.*
- It not only prevents conversion of fibrinogen to fibrin, but also blocks thrombin-catalysed platelet aggregation, and activation of other clotting factors.
- It has a short duration of action and hence it is given by IV infusion.
- There is no antidote.
- Its activity is monitored by the same tests as that of heparin.

Bivalirudin, a synthetic analogue of hirudin, has rapid onset and offset of action (due to reversible binding; t½ 25 min). **Desirudin** is also an analogue of hirudin.

Argatroban: is a **reversible direct thrombin inhibitor** with t½ of 45 min. It is given as an IV infusion. It can be used as an alternative to lepirudin.

Oral

DABIGATRAN: Dabigatran etexilate is a prodrug. Given **orally**, it is converted to the active agent dabigatran which is a **direct inhibitor of thrombin**. Given once daily, it is claimed to be as effective as enoxaparin for the treatment and prevention of venous thromboembolism. The drug appears to have an ADR profile similar to that of enoxaparin. **It does not need coagulation monitoring.**

Idarucizumab is the first specific antidote for controlling life threatening bleeding due to dabigatran but not due to factor Xa inhibitors. Hemodialysis can be used to eliminate dabigatran from the body.

All the direct thrombin inhibitors are used in patients with or at risk of developing heparin induced thrombocytopenia.

III. FACTOR Xa INHIBITORS

Parenteral

FONDAPARINUX is a synthetic pentasaccharide unit of heparin that binds to antithrombin and enhances inactivation of factor Xa. Its t½ is 17 h. It is excreted by the kidney. It does not cause thrombocytopenia. It is not neutralised by protamine. It is given as 2.5 mg subcutaneously once daily.

DANAPAROID: This heparinoid, obtained from porcine intestinal mucosa, is a mixture of glucosaminoglycans. It inhibits factor Xa. It is given subcutaneously twice a day, for prophylaxis.

Oral

RIVAROXABAN: It is an **orally acting, direct, reversible selective factor Xa inhibitor** used for prevention and treatment of arterial and venous thromboembolism. It does not require monitoring. (Table 33.2). Others are **apixaban**, **edoxaban** and **betrixaban**.

Andexanet alfa (genetically modified variant of human factor Xa) acts as an antidote for urgent reversal of the anticoagulant effect of rivaroxaban, edoxaban and apixaban. It acts as a decoy receptor and binds to direct oral anticoagulants (DOAC), which frees up the natural factor Xa for haemostasis. It is very expensive.

SLOW-ACTING ORAL ANTICOAGULANTS

COUMARIN DERIVATIVES: Bishydroxycoumarin or dicoumarol, the first coumarin compound (Fig. 33.4), isolated from spoilt sweet clover, and was proved to be the causative factor in a cattle disease termed 'Sweet Clover Disease', characterised by a severe haemorrhagic tendency. The various coumarin drugs exert qualitatively similar pharmacological actions. The most commonly used drug is **warfarin sodium**.

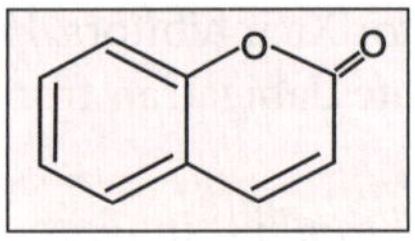

FIG. 33.4 **Coumarin ring.**

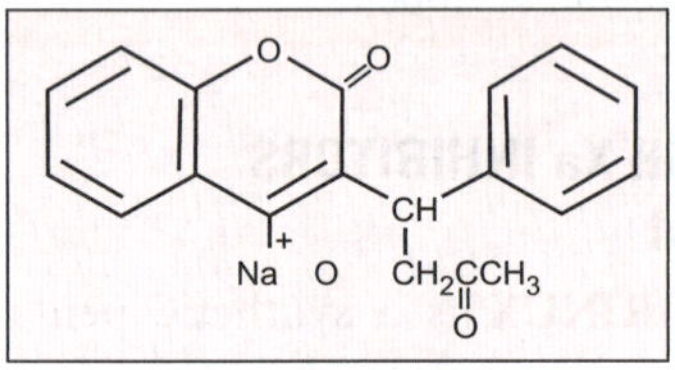

FIG. 33.5 **Warfarin.**

WARFARIN SODIUM: This coumarin (Fig. 33.5), originally employed as a rodent poison, is **the most widely used coumarin anticoagulant**. It is a racemic mixture of two isomers, S (t½ 35 h) and R (t½ 50 h), in almost equal proportions.

Mechanism of anticoagulant action:
Coagulation factors II (prothrombin), VII, IX and X are synthesised in the liver but are biologically inactive until they are carboxylated. Carboxylation is directly coupled to the oxidation of vitamin K to its epoxide. To sustain the carboxylation, the epoxide is converted back to the reduced form of vitamin K by the enzymes vitamin K epoxide reductase and vitamin K reductase (Fig. 33.6). **Warfarin being structurally similar to vitamin K, competitively inhibits vitamin K epoxide reductase.** This prevents regeneration of reduced form of vitamin K and therefore to inhibition of carboxylation. **Coumarins, Thus it inhibits vitamin K–dependent synthesis of coagulation factors.**

It has a slow onset of action. After initiating therapy with the maintenance dose 5–10 mg/day (*no loading dose*), therapeutic INR level is achieved in 36 h but clinical effect is seen within 4–5 days. This is because it *prevents* the formation of active essential clotting factors by the liver but *does not destroy* the circulating ones. It takes 3–7 days for prothrombin time to return to normal after cessation of therapy.

Therapy with warfarin is monitored by **estimating prothrombin time,** which is expressed as *International Normalised Ratio (INR)*. It does not alter the bleeding time.

Absorption, fate and excretion: The intestinal absorption of warfarin is slow and incomplete. It is extensively bound to plasma proteins. **It can cross the placenta but is not secreted in the milk.** It is mainly metabolised in the liver. There is a considerable individual variation (as much as 14 fold) in the rate of detoxification.

Adverse reactions:

- **Bleeding:** The incidence of haemorrhage is 5%–6%. There is no correlation between the onset and degree of haemorrhage and the dose, or the prothrombin levels. Bleeding is considered as major if it occurs at a critical site or the patient is hemodynamically unstable or the clinically overt bleeding is associated with lowering of Hb by ≥2 g/dl or need of > 2 units of packed RBC transfusion.
  If INR is above therapeutic range, then warfarin is withheld and after INR reaches back in the range, warfarin is started at a lower dose. However, if INR is 10 or higher then 2-5 mg of vitamin K_1 is given orally, which enables the liver to synthesize active clotting factors. However, the IV administration of vitamin K is associated with a latent period of several hours. *Therefore, in the immediate treatment of severe haemorrhage, prompt administration of fresh whole blood,* recombinant factor VIIa *or prothrombin complex concentrate is necessary as they act more rapidly than vitamin K.*

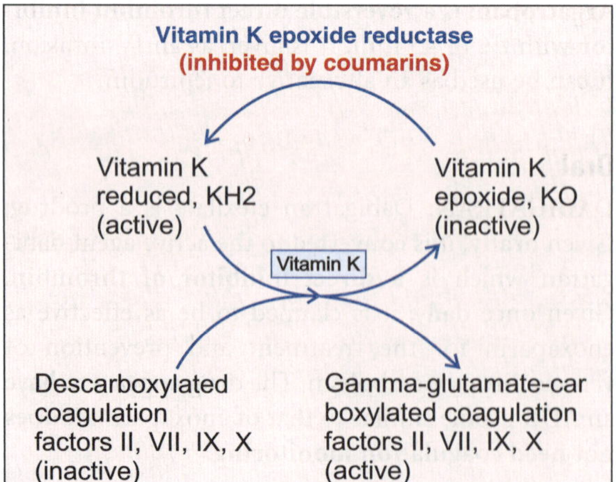

FIG. 33.6 **Vitamin K cycle and site of action of coumarin anticoagulants.**

Menadione (synthetic vitamin K, vitamin K_3) is ineffective in countering the bleeding caused by warfarin.

For management of bleeding also see section, Hemostatic agents.

- **Fetal toxicity:** Warfarin may cause fatal haemorrhage in the fetus. It is teratogenic (Chapter 78) **and is contraindicated during pregnancy.** Women on long-term warfarin therapy should avoid pregnancy.
- **Cutaneous gangrene:** Petechiae that coalesce to painful ecchymoses, haemorrhagic bullae and finally to necrosis/gangrene occur occasionally within 3–8 days after starting treatment with large doses of warfarin. The lesions affect women more often than men and involve the adipose tissue of breasts, buttocks, thighs and the distal lower extremities.
- **Miscellaneous:** Warfarin may rarely cause alopecia, urticaria, anorexia, vomiting and diarrhoea.

Drug interactions: The major drawback of warfarin is the possibility of multiple drug interactions Box 33.2. It can cause drug interactions by:

- **Inhibiting the platelet function** (aspirin, NSAID).
- **Stimulating hepatic microsomal catabolism of warfarin** (barbiturates, rifampicin, griseofulvin, carbamazepine).
- **Displacing warfarin from protein binding** (sulphonamides, phenylbutazone, chlorpropamide)
- **Inhibiting the metabolic clearance of warfarin** (cimetidine, omeprazole, amiodarone).

Drugs like tolbutamide and phenytoin may accumulate in the body following coumarins and hence, doses of these drugs must be reduced.

Box 33.2 Drug Interactions of Coumarin Anticoagulants

- **Drugs which prolong prothrombin time and may cause bleeding:** Aspirin, phenylbutazone, other NSAID, heparin, clofibrate, thyroxine, amiodarone, anabolic steroids, cimetidine, omeprazole, metronidazole, cotrimoxazole, high doses of penicillins, erythromycin, some cephalosporins, moxalactam
- **Drugs which shorten prothrombin time:** Barbiturates, chloral hydrate, meprobamate, rifampicin, griseofulvin, cholestyramine, carbamazepine. When these drugs are stopped, bleeding may occur in a patient on oral anticoagulants

Preparation and dosage: Warfarin sodium available as 0.5, 1, 2, 3 and 5 mg tablets and as 1 mg/ml oral suspension. It is used once a day in the dose of 2.5–10 mg. It has a cumulative action and the maintenance dose (usually in the range of 3-9 mg) may have to be gradually decreased after the first week or so. *No loading dose is used to initiate therapy. Its haemostatic effect varies within individuals depending upon the vitamin K intake and polymorphism of vitamin K reductase and liver CYP2C9.* The dose of warfarin is adjusted by measuring INR, which is generally maintained between 2.0 and 3.5.

Its **advantages** are as follows:

- *It is almost 99% absorbed* and gives more steady plasma levels; approximately 97% of the drug is bound to plasma albumin.
- *It has a rapid onset and predictable duration of action;* therefore, the therapy is easier to regulate.
- *It is water soluble and can be given parenterally.* Parenteral administration, however, does not accelerate the speed of anticoagulation.

If warfarin is employed for long-term anticoagulant therapy, it takes about 3 days for the prothrombin time to return to normal after drug discontinuation.

Factors affecting the dosage and activity of the oral anticoagulants: See Box 33.3.

Advantages and disadvantages of different classes of oral anticoagulants is presented in Table 33.2.

Box 33.4 summarises the main actions of anticoagulant drugs.

Box 33.3 Factors Affecting the Dosage of Oral Anticoagulants

- Genetic differences in the rate of drug metabolism
- Age and sex
- Vitamin K deficiency caused by poor diet, bowel disease or biliary disease enhances the response to oral anticoagulants
- Chronic alcoholism, liver disease, kidney disease and vitamin C deficiency enhance the response
- Hypermetabolic states

Table 33.2 Advantages and Disadvantages of Different Classes of Oral Anticoagulants

Drug Class	Advantages	Disadvantages
Vit. K antagonists (Warfarin)	• Large data on therapeutic utility and adverse effects • Once daily dosing • Antidote available • Cost effective	• Marked variability in dose requirements • Dietary restrictions • INR monitoring required • Numerous drug interactions
Factor Xa inhibitors (Rivaroxaban)	• INR monitoring not required • Once daily dosing • Appears to have less incidence of intracranial and fatal bleeding • No dietary restrictions	• No specific antidote • Missing a dose can predispose to thrombotic risk. • No method to evaluate extent of anticoagulant effect • Dose adjustment required in renal impairment • Non dialyzable
Thrombin inhibitors (Dabigatran)	• INR monitoring not required • Dialyzable • Appears to have less incidence of intracranial and fatal bleeding	• No specific antidote • No method to evaluate extent of anticoagulant effect • Dose adjustment required in renal impairment • Twice daily dosing and must be stored in original container

Anticoagulant Therapy

Arterial and venous thrombosis differ in their causes, pathologic effects and management. *In case of arterial thrombus (White thrombus) platelet aggregation is the important event in its initiation.* In contrast, a typical clot (red thrombus) has red cells entangled in fibrin and a much smaller platelet- leucocyte element. In venous 'thrombosis' and pulmonary embolism, the structure responsible for the clinical state is usually a clot, and not a 'thrombus'. *The drugs which interfere with the clotting mechanism may not necessarily modify the arterial thrombus formation unless they affect the platelet behaviour.* Although such drugs may satisfy the conventional definition of an 'anticoagulant' they are not 'antithrombotic' agents.

- Extension of an existing venous thrombus
- Development of emboli (venous thromboembolism).

Box 33.4 Main Actions of Anticoagulant Drugs

- ***Heparin*** accelerates inactivation of thrombin by antithrombin III
- ***LMWHs,*** mainly, inactivate factor Xa (activated factor X)
- ***Rivaroxaban*** inhibits factor Xa
- ***Hirudin, lepirudin*** and ***dabigatran*** inactivate thrombin
- ***Warfarin*** inhibits the vitamin K–dependent synthesis of several active coagulation factors, including prothrombin

Conventional anticoagulants do not influence the established arterial thrombus, nor can it reverse ischaemic tissue damage.

Heparin is the drug of choice when rapid induction of anticoagulation is desired. It can be used safely during late pregnancy. The disadvantages of heparin are its narrow therapeutic window, high cost and the need for parenteral administration.

The disadvantages of oral anticoagulants are as follows:

1. Delayed onset of action
2. Variable therapeutic effect
3. Need for an elaborate laboratory control

The maximum therapeutic response to oral warfarin is achieved 3–5 days after the initial dose. Hence, in order to obtain immediate therapeutic response, heparin is given intravenously, intermittently at 4–8 h interval. Combined IV heparin and oral warfarin therapy gives the patients the advantage of immediate and prolonged anticoagulation.

Indications for anticoagulant therapy:

- **Prevention of deep venous thrombosis (DVT) and pulmonary embolism (PE):** Anticoagulants

Table 33.3 Drugs for Thromboprophylaxis

Drug (Dose)	Mechanism of Action	Antidote
Warfarin (2–10 mg orally o.d.)[a]	Vit-K dependent clotting factors synthesis inhibitor	Vitamin K
Enoxaparin (40 mg subcutaneously o.d.)	Antithrombin mediated inhibitor of factor Xa	Protamine sulphate
Fondaparinux (2.5 mg subcutaneously o.d.)[b]	Antithrombin mediated inhibition of factor Xa	None
Desirudin (15 mg subcutaneously 12 hourly)[c]	Direct inhibitor of thrombin	Antibodies
Dabigatran exilate (oral 110 mg once, then 220 mg once/daily)	Direct inhibitor of thrombin	Idarucizumab
Rivaroxaban (10 mg orally o.d.)[b]	Direct inhibitor of factor Xa	Andexanet alfa
Apixaban (orally 2.5 mg bid)	Direct inhibitor of factor Xa	Andexanet alfa
Betrixaban (orally 160 mg once, then 80 mg once/day)	Direct inhibitor of factor Xa	None
Aspirin/Clopidogrel	Antiplatelet action	None

[a]Needs monitoring.
[b]Is avoided, if creatinine clearance is <30 mL/min.
[c]Only in presence of heparin induced thrombocytopenia.

are most useful in this condition and are used prophylactically. They prevent:

a. Extension of an existing venous thrombus
b. Development of emboli (venous thromboembolism)

LMWH is recommended for prevention of DVT/PE in most orthopedic and nonorthopedic surgical patients, for whom postoperative prophylaxis is indicated.

Low fixed dose heparin considerably **reduces the incidence of pulmonary embolism,** if used **prophylactically** in postoperative therapy and in patients with acute MI. Dalteparin is given subcutaneously in doses of 5000 U every 8–12 h; the first dose being given 2 h before surgery. *Laboratory monitoring is not necessary* and risk of haemorrhage is minimal. Pressure over the injection site minimises local bleeding into the tissues.

It is also used for prevention of DVT in patients confined to prolonged bed rest. Other agents currently used for **thromboprophylaxis** are listed in Table 33.3.

- **Treatment of DVT and PE:** LMWH (dalteparin −200 IU/kg SC once daily or enoxaparin 1 mg/kg SC bid or 1.5 mg/kg SC once daily) or fondaparinux (5–10 mg SC once daily), with or without warfarin (2–10 mg once daily), has generally been recommended for initial treatment (5–10 days) of DVT or PE. Oral alternatives apixaban and rivaroxaban can be used. Following initial parenteral therapy, warfarin is used for maintenance therapy. Direct oral anticoagulants (DOAC) like apixaban/rivaroxaban/dabigatran or edoxaban can be other effective and safer alternatives to warfarin. But they are expensive. Warfarin or UFH is recommended for treatment of patients having creatinine clearance <30 mL/min. In pregnancy LMWH is recommended.

Duration of therapy of patients with VTE or PE should be minimum for 3 months.

- **Myocardial infarction:** Chapter 29.
- **Mitral valve disease with AF:** Chapter 28.
- **Miscellaneous:** They are also used in case of artificial heart valves in order to prevent emboli and during cardiac bypass surgery.

As a rule, anticoagulants are not indicated in cerebrovascular disease for fear of causing cerebral haemorrhage.

Contraindications to anticoagulants are summarised in Box 33.5.

Box 33.5 Contraindications to Anticoagulant Therapy

- Haemorrhagic tendency and blood dyscrasias
- Benign or malignant ulcers, such as in the gut, colitis, diverticulitis, recent operation upon the CNS, eye or prostate gland
- In subacute bacterial endocarditis, anticoagulants may cause detachment of the bacterial vegetations from the damaged valves into general circulation
- Threatened abortion, injury to the brain the spinal cord and stroke
- Regional and lumbar block anaesthesia
- Prothrombin deficiency, severe hepatic, renal impairment and severe uncontrolled hypertension
- An uncooperative patient, inadequate laboratory facility and uninformed or casual medical supervision
- Pregnancy

IN VITRO ANTICOAGULANTS

Physical methods: Clotting can be delayed by cooling the blood or by collecting it in coated vessels so that platelets are not broken up. The coating used is paraffin, collodion or silicone.

Oxalates and citrates: These act by removal of calcium ions. Potassium oxalate 0.1% precipitates serum calcium as calcium oxalate. Sodium citrate combines with calcium and forms calcium sodium citrate. The anticoagulant solution (B.P.) contains 2.5% of sodium citrate in 0.9% saline. Citrate is usually employed as an anticoagulant for blood to be transfused. The final strength of citrate is 3.8%. Potassium oxalate produces convulsions and hence is not employed in vivo.

EDTA (ethylenediamine tetraacetic acid) a chelating agent, has a great affinity for calcium and its sodium salt has been used as an anticoagulant (see also Chapter 74).

Heparin: discussed earlier.

FIBRINOLYTIC AGENTS PH 1.25

The process of fibrinolysis or dissolution of blood clot is schematically represented in Fig. 33.7.

Mechanism of action:

All fibrinolytic agents in use act directly or indirectly as plasminogen activators. Plasminogen is an inactive precursor. An activator substance (tPA, urokinase), present in tissues, converts plasminogen to **fibrinolytic enzyme plasmin**. The plasmin breaks down fibrin clots. It is relatively nonspecific in action and it can also act on proteins and clotting factors.

During the formation of a thrombus, plasminogen binds to fibrin. The fibrin-bound plasminogen is more susceptible to the activation than the plasminogen in circulation.

Fibrinolytics–Classification

Indirect Plasminogen Activator

- **Streptokinase**

Direct Plasminogen Activator

- **Recombinant tissue-type plasminogen activators**, alteplase reteplase, tenecteplase
- **Urokinase**
- **Acylated plasminogen-streptokinase activator (APSAC) complex** (anistreplase)

STREPTOKINASE: It is used in the treatment of DVT in the dose of 250,000 U intravenously in 30 min, followed by 100,000 U every hour for 24–72 h (Chapter 76). A loading dose is given to neutralise the antibodies following any previous dose.

ALTEPLASE, tPA (tissue-type plasminogen activator), a natural protein in man, is now prepared by recombinant DNA technology. **It preferentially activates plasminogen bound to fibrin clot and avoids systemic activation of plasminogen.**

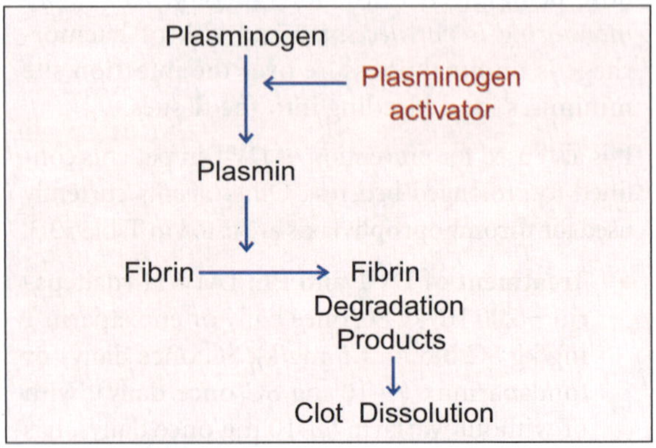

FIG. 33.7 Mechanism of fibrinolysis.

Fibrinogen depletion and bleeding is thus minimised. It is as effective as streptokinase. It has a short t½ of 8 min. It is metabolised by the liver. Patients weighing <67 kg should receive a total dose of 1.5 mg/kg Heparin 5000 U is given IV bolus prior to administration of tPA.

Reteplase (t½ 1.6 h) and **tenecteplase** (t½ 2 h) are the other recombinant analogues of human tPA. They have long plasma half-lives and can be given as bolus injection.

UROKINASE: This enzyme, originally isolated from human urine, is now obtained from cultured human renal cells. It is a **potent direct plasminogen activator**. It is *nonantigenic, nonpyrogenic and does not cause allergic reactions.* However, it lacks fibrin specificity and is very expensive. It is also used to lyse fibrin or blood deposits in the anterior chamber of the eye. It is not used for coronary thrombolysis.

FIBRINOLYTIC THERAPY

Choice of Fibrinolytics

Alteplase, reteplase and **tenecteplase** are more **fibrin-specific**. They bind strongly to fibrin and are capable of dissolving resistant thrombi **better than fibrin-non-specific agents, streptokinase, anistreplase and urokinase. With the doses used in the treatment of acute MI, the lytic activity is greatest with streptokinase, intermediate with urokinase and least with tPA.**

The therapeutic goal is to reestablish the blood flow through the occluded vessel within a short time, so as to prevent organ damage.

Therapeutically, when treatment is begun within the first 6 h of the onset of chest pain in MI, a similar incidence of reperfusion is provided by all the agents. *Rethrombosis, after reperfusion, occurs in roughly inverse proportion to the length of the plasma half-life of the drug used, with the lowest incidence with streptokinase, and the highest with tPA. Hence, heparin is administered simultaneously with tPA, primarily to enhance reperfusion and decrease the rate of rethrombosis.* Since streptokinase produces more prolonged and extensive anticoagulant effect, simultaneous administration of heparin is not required (Table 33.4).

Adverse reactions:

- **Bleeding** is the commonest adverse effect with all these agents. *Vascular injury rather than changes in blood coagulation is the main cause of bleeding.* In case of bleeding the drug should be stopped and fresh frozen plasma may be given.

Table 33.4 Properties of Fibrinolytic Agents IM 2.23

Characteristic	Streptokinase	Alteplase (tPA)[a]	Tenecteplase[a]
Plasma half-life (t½ min)	15–25	<5	20
Fibrin specificity	+	+++	+++
Plasminogen binding	Indirect	Direct	Direct
Potential for allergy/ hypotension	Yes	No	No
Total dose	1.5 million units	100 mg	50 mg
Administration for MI	1.5 million units in 100 mL saline over 30–60 min	1. **Accelerated infusion:** 15 mg IV bolus, then 50 mg infused over 30 min, then 35 mg over 1 h OR 2. **As 3-h infusion:** 60 mg over the first hour (of which 6–10 mg as a bolus), 20 mg over the second hour, and 20 mg over the third hour	Single IV bolus 0.5 mg/kg administered over 5–10 seconds
Early heparinisation	Not required	Yes	Yes

[a]Appears to result in a higher rate of early coronary reperfusion compared to streptokinase.

Box 33.6 Contraindications to Thrombolytic Therapy

- Active bleeding, bleeding tendency
- Recent major trauma (within 3 months)
- Invasive or surgical procedure in the past 10 days
- GI or genitourinary bleeding in the past 2-4 weeks
- Prolonged cardiopulmonary resuscitation (within 3 weeks)
- Neurosurgical procedure in the past 2 months
- Stroke or transient cerebral ischaemic attack in the past 3 months
- History of cerebral tumour, aneurysm or arteriovenous malformation
- Active peptic ulcer disease
- Hypertension (severe, uncontrolled)
- Diabetes mellitus with proliferative retinopathy
- Pregnancy
- INR > 1.7 with current warfarin therapy

- **Multiple microemboli** can occur following disintegration of existing thrombus.
- **Allergic reactions:** Streptokinase, being a bacterial protein, is antigenic. Hence, it may cause allergic and febrile reactions and rarely (0.1%) anaphylactoid reaction; therapy with urokinase and other tPAs does not provoke allergic reaction.
- **Hypotension** may occur more often with rapid administration of streptokinase.
- **Haemorrhagic stroke** is a dreaded complication of thrombolytic therapy.

Intramuscular injections are contraindicated during thrombolytic therapy.

The important contraindications to fibrinolytic therapy are listed in Box 33.6.

Probably 10%–20% of reperfused arteries undergo rethrombosis. Heparin in the dose of 5000 U (IV bolus) followed by 1000 U hourly (by IV infusion) for 3–5 days and aspirin (150 mg/day) have been recommended. Rethrombosis of veins is probably most often related to incomplete lysis of the original thrombus, and the present management emphasises adequate anticoagulation with heparin as the best approach to preventing rethrombosis.

Indications: Fibrinolytic agent by accelerating the rate of vascular reperfusion, improves rapidly the manifestations of vessel occlusion.

- **Myocardial infarction (MI):** IM 2.15, 2.23

Fibrinolytic therapy is most useful in patients with STEMI (Chapter 29).

As progression of ischemia and infarction from the subendocardium to the epicardium occurs in about 6 h, fibrinolytic therapy, begun within 6 h of the onset of MI reduces mortality and preserves LV function.

Among various fibrinolytic agents, streptokinase and tPA (alteplase) are commonly used. There appears to be little difference in left ventricular function or predischarge patency rates between the use of either drugs.

The dosage regimens for streptokinase, alteplase and tenecteplase are presented in Table 33.4. Fibrinolytic therapy is followed by 75–150 mg of **aspirin** daily, for 4 weeks. *Patients are not routinely treated with fibrinolytics later than 6 h after infarction unless they are at high risk; they can, however, be given aspirin.*

- **Ischaemic stroke:** Because of the risk of conversion of a nonhaemorrhagic stroke into a haemorrhagic one, such therapy is highly controversial in ischaemic strokes. *In such cases occlusion by clot must be demonstrated by MRI. Reteplase and tenecteplase are given by IV bolus.*
- **Pulmonary embolism:** Heparin is the mainstay of treatment of pulmonary embolism. A thrombolytic therapy is useful adjunct in patients with severe (massive) pulmonary embolism and right ventricular dysfunction.
- **Acute peripheral arterial occlusion:** It is used especially for dissolving occlusion of small arteries that cannot be surgically treated. Thrombolytic therapy for arterial thrombi in locations other than the limbs or the coronary arteries has been reported for virtually all organs.
- **Deep venous thrombosis (DVT):** Anticoagulation is the treatment of choice (see earlier). Fibrinolytic therapy may be used to treat those with high risk of pulmonary embolism and those with axillary vein thrombosis.

  Clinically, no large differences are seen between streptokinase and tPA. Streptokinase is more cost-effective than tPA. *If the patient has received streptokinase even 4 days earlier, tPA is preferred.*

Administration of heparin and aspirin remains the mainstay of treatment in unstable angina. Thrombolytics are not useful and are not recommended.

ARVIN: Arvin is a purified enzyme obtained from the venom of the Malayan pit viper, *Agkistroden rhodostoma*. The enzyme:

- **Converts fibrinogen to an imperfect fibrin polymer** that breaks up easily in the circulation and is lysed
- **Produces fibrinogen depletion** independently of the coagulation.

The therapy is controlled by measuring plasma fibrinogen.

The enzyme has been used to treat venous thrombosis. Administered intravenously, it reduces the fibrinogen levels, with peak anticoagulant activity at 8–12 h after its administration. Fibrinogen levels return to normal within 3 weeks after cessation of therapy. It can also be used intramuscularly/subcutaneously.

Unlike the conventional anticoagulants, it does not cause a haemorrhagic tendency. Haemolytic anaemia, urticaria and unilateral impairment of vision have been reported. Specific antivenom antidote is available to treat the toxicity.

HAEMOSTATIC AGENTS

Bleeding can be controlled by physical methods such as application of direct pressure, tourniquet, cold and use of cautery. Drugs like **desmopressin** (Chapter 37) and **adrenaline** (Chapter 18) can be used to produce vasoconstriction. Adrenaline is used in the form of nasal pack to control epistaxis after ruling out any systemic cause such as hypertension.

When bleeding is the consequence of a specific defect in haemostasis such as haemophilia, the ideal treatment is to correct the defect. Major blood loss commonly occurs during surgery, trauma and some medical conditions. In such cases **nonspecific haemostatic therapy** has to be employed.

Classification of Haemostatic Drugs:

i. **Agents acting locally**
ii. **Transfusional agents** such as specific coagulation factors
iii. **Nontransfusional agents,** e.g. Vtamin K and antifibrinolytic agents, e.g. Epsilon aminocaproic acid and Tranexamic acid.

I. **Agents acting locally:** These agents control oozing of blood from minute vessels but are not effective in controlling bleeding from large vessels. They are as follows:

THROMBIN: Thrombin is obtained from bovine/human plasma. It is stable as a dry powder stored between 2°C and 8°C. Thrombin therapy is restricted to local application in oozing of blood. It has also been used, mixed with plasma, to anchor skin grafts.

THROMBOPLASTIN: Thromboplastin is a powder prepared from the acetone extracts of brain and/or lung tissue of freshly killed rabbits. It is used for determination of prothrombin time and as a local haemostatic in surgery.

FIBRIN: Fibrin obtained from human plasma is used in the dehydrated form as sheets to cover bleeding surfaces. When used in combination with a thrombin solution, it also acts as a mechanical barrier and holds thrombin in position over the bleeding area.

GEL FOAM: Gel foam is a porous, pressed form of gelatin sponge used in conjunction with thrombin to control oozing of blood from surface wounds. Gel foam is moistened with isotonic saline before use. It is completely absorbed within 4–6 weeks and hence, may be left in place after suturing of a wound. It is available as cones, packs, sponges and powder.

OXIDISED CELLULOSE (Oxycel): It is a surgical gauze treated with nitrogen dioxide. It promotes clotting by a reaction between haemoglobin and cellulosic acid. Oxycel, when wet with tissue fluid, becomes sticky and gummy and exerts its haemostatic effect by mechanical blockage. Oxycel is usually absorbed completely within 2–10 days.

MICROFIBRILLAR COLLAGEN: This haemostatic material is prepared from purified, bovine corium collagen. When applied to a bleeding surface, it attracts platelets to initiate formation of a platelet plug followed by a natural clot. Used along with manual pressure, it is effective in controlling capillary bleeding, even in patients on heparin or oral anticoagulants, and in haemophiliacs. It is nonallergenic but can promote local infection. As it is inactivated by autoclaving, it should not be sterilised.

II. **Transfusional agents** (such as specific coagulation factors):

HUMAN FIBRINOGEN: Fibrinogen, a sterile fraction from human plasma, is used for restoring normal fibrinogen levels in haemorrhagic complications caused by acute afibrinogenemia. Fibrinogen and thrombin may be employed together for local haemostasis.

ANTIHAEMOPHILIC GLOBULIN (AHG): Haemophilia A and Christmas disease (haemophilia B) are the two commonest hereditary haemorrhagic states, due to deficiency of specific clotting factors VIII and IX respectively. *Antihaemophilic globulin or concentrate of factor VIII (AHG) is highly effective in the treatment of classical haemophilia-A.* High potency human AHG is now prepared by recombinant DNA technique. Simultaneous use of fibrinolytic inhibitors like EACA can reduce the dose of AHG required. The half-life of injected factor VIII in a haemophiliac, is about 12 h. In case of nonavailability of AHG, fresh plasma or blood transfusion is used. **Desmopressin** (Chapter 37), which causes release of AHG from its stores, transiently increases its blood level and may be helpful in mild-moderate haemophilic bleeding.

Pure recombinant factor VIII, factor IX and activated factor VII ($rFVII_a$) are available. They are very expensive.

PROTHROMBIN COMPLEX CONCENTRATE (4F- PCC): This contains four coagulation factors II, VII, IX and X as well as the inhibitor protein C and its cofactor protein S. *It causes complete and rapid reversal of warfarin.* As it is a concentrated product, risk of volume overload is lesser than plasma or whole blood. As compared to plasma or blood, its infusion time is less, shelf life is longer and safety profile is better. It also lacks blood group specificity. However, it is very expensive.

It is indicated when urgent hemostasis is needed as in case of major bleeding due to warfarin, deficiency of prothrombin complex coagulation factors, haemophilia B (factor IX deficiency) or intracerebral haemorrhage or bleeding during CABG.

FRESH FROZEN PLASMA: is suitable for the treatment of most coagulation disorders, since it provides all the clotting factors. For **blood,** See Chapter 32.

III. **Nontransfusional agents** e.g. **vitamin K** and antifibrinolytic agents, (**epsilon aminocaproic acid** and **tranexamic acid**):

VITAMIN K: Vitamin K comprises three distinct fat soluble, naphthoquinone compounds which participate in the biosynthesis of several clotting factors:

a. **Vitamin K_1** (phytonadione) is found in several foods and also prepared synthetically.
b. **Vitamin K_2**, produced by the bacteria in the GI tract and supplies almost 50% of the human requirements.
c. **Vitamin K_3** (menadione) a **synthetic compound** used for therapeutic purposes. The diphosphate salt of menadione is water soluble.

Pharmacological actions: Vitamin K in its reduced form participates in the carboxylation of the biologically inactive coagulation factors, e.g. II, VII, IX and X (Fig. 33.5). Vitamin K is also shown to be involved in electron transport (coenzyme) and oxidative phosphorylation.

Absorption, fate and excretion: Vitamin K is produced by the flora of the human intestine. The fat soluble vitamins K_1 and K_2 are absorbed in the presence of bile salts, whereas the water soluble synthetic menadione can be absorbed even in their absence. The exact daily requirement of vitamin K is not known. Both the lipid and water soluble preparations are satisfactorily absorbed on parenteral administration (either SC, or IM or IV).

Adverse reactions: These are rare after oral administration. However, serious anaphylactoid reactions can occur after IV use. Large doses of synthetic menadione have produced haemolytic anaemia, hyperbilirubinemia and kernicterus in newborn, especially in premature infants. Menadione competes with bile salts for glucuronide detoxification mechanism causing the accumulation of bile salts in the blood and this results in jaundice. Haemolysis with menadione is usually seen in infants, whose RBC lack the enzyme G6PD.

Indications:

- **Adult vitamin K deficiency** which may be produced by (1) malabsorption syndrome or obstructive jaundice, (2) long-term intravenous feeding (prophylactic use) and (3) prolonged periods of malnutrition. Menadione may be used in
- **Vitamin K deficiency in infants** during acute diarrhoea.
- **Neonatal vitamin K deficiency**, for prevention and treatment.
- **Bleeding state during coumarin anticoagulant (warfarin) therapy.** In case of major bleeding event, 5-10 mg IV vitamin K is given. For rapid hemostasis, prothrombin complex concentrate may be given concurrently. For other events that require hospitalization, 2-5 mg of oral or intravenous vitamin K can be used.

> *Menadione preparations are **NOT** useful in treating oral anticoagulant induced bleeding, and may cause adverse reactions in neonates with vitamin K deficiency. They should not be used in the last weeks of pregnancy.*

Preparations:

i. Vitamin K_1 tablets (1 mg and 10 mg), drops (200 mcg/ml) and injection (10 mg/ml) for IV use. Dose: 2.5–25 mg orally; 5–10 mg intravenously over 30 min to reduce the risk of anaphylactoid reaction.
ii. Menadione 10 mg tablets. Dose 2.5–10 mg daily.
iii. Menadione sodium diphosphate injection, 5 and 10 mg/mL. Dose 5–15 mg once or twice daily, subcutaneously, intramuscularly or intravenously. Menadione sodium bisulphite injection 10 mg/ml and 1 mg/0.5 ml.

EPSILON AMINOCAPROIC ACID (EACA): This is a water soluble analogue of the amino acid lysine (Fig. 33.8).

Mechanism of action: Lysine analogue reversibly binds to plasminogen and inhibits fibrin binding to plasminogen. It thus inhibits the activation of plasminogen to plasmin. This impairs fibrinolysis with consequent stabilisation of clot.

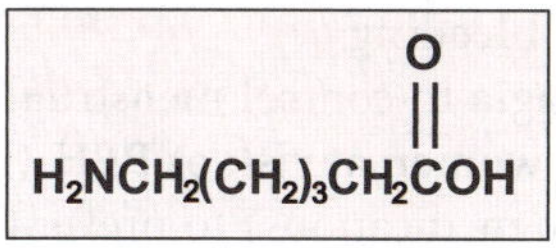

FIG. 33.8 Aminocaproic acid.

Orally, it is rapidly absorbed; the peak level after a single dose is achieved in about 2 h. About 60%–90% of the dose is excreted in the urine within 24 h. A blood level of 13 mg per 100 mL is required for plasminogen inhibition, whereas 130 mg per 100 mL inhibits plasmin activity.

Adverse reactions: Mild ADRs include nasal stuffiness, abdominal discomfort, dyspepsia, hypotension, conjunctival erythema, nausea, vomiting, diarrhoea and skin rash. A rare, lethal complication is disseminated intravascular thrombosis.

Preparation and dosage: It is available as 500 mg tablet and 250 mg/ml injection.

Indications: The drug has been found to be useful in preventing the hyperplasminaemic bleeding state following the damage to tissues rich in plasminogen activator. Tranexemic acid which is more potent with longer t½ is now preferred to EACA for therapeutic use.

TRANEXAMIC ACID (TA), also a derivative of lysine, is about **10 times more potent than EACA and has a longer duration of action.** It is clinically preferred and is used in the dose of 1–1.5 g 3–4 times daily. Adverse reactions are mild and include nausea, diarrhoea and hypotension.

Indications:

- **Patients undergoing elective surgery** prophylactically, to prevent clot breakdown (fibrinolysis) and reduce perioperative blood loss. Although the drug has been employed to control bleeding during prostatectomy, it is contraindicated in the event of haematuria because of the risk of ureteral occlusion by unlysed clot.
- **Bleeding trauma patients** to reduce mortality.

- **Upper GI bleeding**
- **Menorrhagia** to control menstrual blood loss.
- **Pregnant women at risk of PPH** (in addition to uterotonic medications) to prevent PPH.
- **Bleeding associated with PPH:** It has been reported that administration of 1 g of IV **TA to women with PPH reduces mortality considerably, especially if given soon after bleeding onset (within 3 h of birth).**

Both EACA and TA are contraindicated in patients with subarachnoid haemorrhage because they may induce vasospasm and ischaemic stroke.

Ethamsylate is used for similar indications as EACA and TA. It probably acts by correcting abnormal platelet adhesion. It does not stabilise fibrin. The oral dose is 500 mg q.i.d.

Ecallantide, a kallikrein inhibitor has been used in cardiothoracic surgery to prevent blood loss but was found to be less effective than TA (Chapter 25).

Aprotinin: See Chapter 25.

DESMOPRESSIN: This analogue of arginine vasopressin (Chapter 37), given intravenously or subcutaneously, increases for a short time the plasma concentration of factor VIII in haemophiliacs, and of von Willebrand factor, the adhesive protein that is deficient or defective, in patients with von Willebrand disease. *Demopressin is considered a treatment of choice for patients with mild hemophillia-A or type I von Willebrand disease.* It shortens or normalises the bleeding time in patients with congenital defects of platelet function. Desmopressin is also used for acute variceal bleeding (see below). Adverse effects are mild and include headache, water retention and hyponatremia.

The major risk involved in using agents that potentiate haemostasis is thrombotic complications.

CONJUGATED ESTROGENS (Refer Chapter 65 for menorrhagia): Given intravenously in the dose of 0.6 mg/kg, daily, they improve platelet function, shorten the prolonged bleeding time and reduce or stop bleeding in uremic patients. Compared to desmopressin, they have a delayed onset but much longer duration of action on bleeding time. They can be combined with desmopressin for synergistic effect. They have been used daily for 5–7 days with hardly any adverse reaction.

Vitamin C: Vitamin C (50–100 mg t.i.d.) specifically controls bleeding due to scurvy.

MANAGEMENT OF ACUTE VARICEAL BLEEDING

Bleeding from oesophageal varices is a common complication of advanced cirrhosis of the liver. Oesophageal varices are dilated anastomoses between systemic veins and portal venous system, which help to decompress the increased portal venous pressure. In cirrhosis, increased cardiac output and splanchnic vasodilatation causes increased blood flow to the liver. This along with increased portal venous resistance leads to dilation of oesophageal/gastric varices, which tend to rupture and cause haematemesis. IM 15.14

Acute bleeding can be controlled by reducing the portal pressure by using:

- **l-Arginine vasopressin, desmopressin** or long-acting analogue **terlipressin** (triglycyl-lysine-vasopressin) which constrict the splanchnic blood vessels and decrease the blood flow in portal venous system. Vasopressin is given as 20 U IV infusion. Terlipressin is given intravenously as bolus, 4 hourly usually for 48–72 h.
- **Somatostatin/octreotide** also decreases splanchnic blood flow (Chapter 60).
- **Prophylactically, nonselective beta-adrenergic blockers such as propranolol or nadolol may be useful.** Because of the β_1 receptor antagonism, they reduce the cardiac output, whereas the β_2 antagonism allows unopposed α adrenergic vasoconstriction. In practice, their dose can be regulated by monitoring the reduction (20%) in pulse, although direct measurement of the portal/systemic venous pressure gradient is ideal.

SCLEROSING AGENTS

Sclerosing agents are irritating substances employed to obliterate varicose veins and uncomplicated piles.

They act locally. The important preparations are as follows:

- **Sodium tetradecyl sulphate** is an anionic detergent, marketed as 0.5%–3.0% solution: given intravenously as 0.5–1.0 mL at up to 4 sites.
- **Ethoxy scleral** (3%) in 5% aqueous ethanol (polidocanol), a nonionic detergent.
- **Phenol**, 5% in vegetable oil, 2–3 mL, injected into the submucosal layer at the base of each pile; maximum total dose 10 mL at any one time.
- **Sodium linoleate** given intravenously/locally as 0.5–5 mL.
- **Ethanolamine oleate** 5%. Dose: 2–5 mL divided between 3 and 4 sites.
- **Sodium morrhuate** 1–2 mL of 5% solution per site. Total 15–25 mL at one sitting.

ANTIPLATELET AGENTS

Prostacyclin (PGI_2)
- Epoprostanol

TXA_2 synthesis inhibitor
- Aspirin

ADP receptor (P_2Y_{12}) antagonists
- Clopidogrel
- Prasugrel
- Ticagrelor

Phosphodiesterase inhibitors
- Dipyridamole
- Cilostazol

Glycoprotein IIb/IIIa antagonists
- Abciximab
- Eptifibatide
- Tirofiban

Protease activated receptor (PAR-1) antagonist
- Vorapaxar

ANTICOAGULANTS

Those used for preventing clotting of blood inside the intact vasculature (*in vivo*)

Fast acting

Heparin
Low molecular weight heparins (LMWHs)
- Enoxaparin
- Dalteparin
- Tinzaparin

Direct thrombin inhibitors
Parenteral:
- Lepirudin
- Bivalirudin
- Argatroban

Oral:
- Dabigatran

Factor Xa inhibitors
Parenteral:
- Fondaparinux
- Danaparoid

Oral:
- Rivaroxaban
- Apixaban
- Edoxaban
- Betrixaban

Slow acting

Coumarin derivatives
- Bishydroxycoumarin
- Warfarin sodium

Indandione derivatives:
- Phenindione (now obsolete)

ANTICOAGULANTS

Those used to prevent clotting of blood *in vitro*

- Potassium oxalate
- Sodium citrate
- EDTA (Ethylenediamine tetraacetic acid) disodium salt
- Heparin

FIBRINOLYTICS

Indirect Plasminogen Activator

Streptokinase

Direct Plasminogen Activator

Recombinant tissue-type plasminogen activators

- Alteplase, Reteplase
- Tenecteplase

Urokinase

Acylated plasminogen-streptokinase activator (APSAC) complex

- Anistreplase

HAEMOSTATIC DRUGS

Agents acting locally

- Thrombin
- Thromboplastin
- Fibrin
- Gel foam
- Oxidized cellulose
- microfibrillar collagen

Transfusional agents

Specific coagulation Factors

- Human fibrinogen
- Antihaemophilic globulin (AHG)
- Recombinant factor VIII, factor IX,
- Activated factor VII
- Prothrombin complex concentrate (4F-PCC)
- Fresh frozen plasma

Nontransfusional agents

- Vitamin K (Menadione)
- Epsilon aminocaproic acid (EACA)
- Tranexamic acid

CHAPTER 34

Drugs Effective in Iron Deficiency and Other Related Anaemias

Learning Objectives

This chapter will enable the reader:

1. To be aware of physiology of erythropoiesis and factors affecting the same.
2. To classify types of anaemia.
3. To explain ferrokinetics in normal person and in patient with iron deficiency anaemia giving daily requirements in both the groups.
4. To enumerate iron formulations giving their elemental iron content and state importance of elemental iron content.
5. To discuss ADR and indications of oral and parenteral iron therapy.
6. To outline the management of iron-deficiency anaemia.
7. To discuss the pharmacotherapy of iron poisoning.
8. To describe pharmacological effects, ADR and indications for erythropoietin.

KEY TERMS

ferrokinetics, p. 516
factors affecting iron absorption, p. 516
daily dietary iron requirements, p. 518
iron preparations, oral, p. 518
iron dextran, p. 519
erythropoietin, p. 522
iron poisoning, treatment, p. 523
desferrioxamine mesylate, p. 523

Anaemia is one of the most common disorders in clinical practice. It is characterised by a decrease in the oxygen carrying capacity of the blood which is determined by the haemoglobin content of the erythrocytes (RBC). *Reduction in the blood haemoglobin level and in the number of circulating erythrocytes are the hallmarks of anaemia.*

Erythropoiesis: The erythrocytes are produced in the bone marrow from the precursor cells, proerythroblasts which subsequently differentiate to normoblast and then reticulocyte. It takes the reticulocyte approximately 4 days to mature into a normal erythrocyte. The normal life span of a human erythrocyte is roughly 110–120 days and it is destroyed by the reticuloendothelial system.

Various factors such as lack of oxygen, vitamin C, growth hormone and thyroxine stimulate erythropoiesis. Kidneys also play an important role in erythropoiesis through the glycoprotein hormone, **erythropoietin** (EPO). EPO serves as an oxygen sensor and stimulates production of erythrocytes which are oxygen carriers. Deficiency of dietary factors such as iron, folic acid and vitamin B12, and of EPO disturbs the normal erythropoiesis resulting in anaemia.

Anaemias may be classified according to their aetiology as anaemias due to:

1. **Increased requirement of essential nutrients**, e.g. in pregnancy, growing children, lactating women
2. **Nutritional deficiency or malabsorption of factors essential for blood formation**, e.g. iron, folic acid, vitamin B_{12}, vitamin C and pyridoxine
3. **Blood loss** such as menorrhagia, GI loss and hookworm infestation
4. **Excessive haemolysis**, e.g. thalassemia, sickle cell anaemia, malaria and autoimmune haemolytic anaemia
5. **Aplasia or hypoplasia of the bone marrow**, such as idiopathic or following certain drugs such as anticancer drugs and chloramphenicol
6. **Deficiencies of erythropoietin** as in chronic renal disease
7. **Anaemias of impaired release and/or utilization of iron despite normal storage**, e.g. due to chronic infections, rheumatoid arthritis, liver disease and cancer

FERROKINETICS

Every cell in the body contains iron. The total iron content of the body varies between 2–3 g depending upon the body weight and haemoglobin level. In adult males the iron content is estimated to be about 50 mg/kg while in adult females it is 35 mg/kg.

Iron absorption: The amount of iron available from food depends upon its iron content as well as the bioavailability of iron from different foods.

Absorption of inorganic iron salts can occur from any part of the GI tract; however, there exists an absorption gradient, decreasing from the duodenum to colon. *Maximum iron absorption occurs in the duodenum.*

Thus absorption of iron is limited to 1–2 mg; most of the iron needed is provided through recycling of body iron.

Mechanism of iron absorption: The iron is absorbed via the brush borders of the intestinal lining cells. The absorption depends as much on its form as on its absolute amount. **Two mechanisms** for iron absorption exist, as follows:

1. **An active transport process** whereby *ferrous iron from intestinal lumen gets transported into the mucosal cells with the help of a carrier protein.* The absorbed iron combines with **apoferritin** to form ferritin and is stored. Iron is actively released into blood as Fe^{+++} from basolateral side by ferroproteins as per body needs. **When apoferritin gets fully saturated to ferritin, no more iron is absorbed.** Thus, in normal individuals the body is protected from possible iron overload. In iron deficiency, the amount of apoferritin is reduced and iron passes through the cells into the blood.
   Within the mucosal cells, iron exists as follows:
   a. Mobile iron – Fe^{+++}
   b. Storage iron – ferritin.
   This intracellular ferritin is eventually excreted during desquamation of the epithelial cells, as a part of the regular shedding of the intestinal mucosa.
2. **A passive transport process,** by which iron diffuses across the intestinal villi, perhaps in combination with amino acids such as glycine and serine. This mechanism probably operates primarily at doses of iron exceeding the amounts in a normal diet.

Factors affecting iron absorption:

- **Type of dietary iron:** Food iron is ionised in the stomach under the influence of gastric acid. Hypochlorhydria may thus reduce the amount of iron absorbed from the food.
  Iron from animal foods is better absorbed than that from vegetable foods; **heme iron** is by far the most available (20%–40%), and its absorption is independent of the food composition. It gets absorbed intact. However, **nonheme fraction** represents by far the largest amount in a vegetarian diet. *This form needs reduction to ferrous iron (Fe^{++}) prior to absorption.*
  The mean absorption of iron from vegetable foods ranges from 1% for rice, 5% for wheat to 6% for soyabeans, whereas for animal foods it ranges from 11% for fish, 12% for meat haemoglobin to 13% for liver. Ferric hydroxide iron complexes present in the vegetarian foods are absorbed poorly. *Milk and milk products are a poor source of iron.*
- **Reducing agents present in the diet**, such as ascorbate, succinate and the SH groups of amino acids like cysteine, and proteins **convert ferric iron to ferrous form and help the iron absorption.**
- **A diet poor in phosphorus** enhances iron absorption, whereas **phytates and organic phosphates (as in vegetarian foods) reduce iron absorption** by forming insoluble and unabsorbable complexes. A cereal based diet decreases iron bioavailabity. Wheat is rich in phytates; only about 5% of wheat iron is absorbed. Egg iron is strongly complexed to the phosphate of yolk phosphoproteins and is poorly absorbed.
- **Drugs: Antacids** such as calcium carbonate, aluminium hydroxide and magnesium hydroxide reduce iron absorption. Other drugs like tetracycline, levodopa, fluroquinolones, captopril, bisphosphonates, PPI and thyroxine interfere with iron absorption.
- **Administration of iron along with or after food reduces its absorption.** However, in practice, ferrous salts are usually administered after food to minimise gastric irritation.
- **Pancreatic secretion has an inhibitory effect on iron absorption** and prevents iron overload. In severe chronic pancreatitis and liver cirrhosis, iron absorption is greatly increased. **Pyridoxine**

deficiency also enhances iron absorption despite elevated plasma iron levels.

- **Iron deficiency accelerates iron absorption.** Individuals with iron deficiency absorb 20%–30% of the food iron (compared to 5%–10% in normals), whereas the absorption of iron in organic form (vegetables and meat) is approximately doubled, and that of inorganic iron is increased five to six fold.
- **Pica:** Iron deficiency can promote appetite for bizarre foods (pica). If clay is consumed (geophagia), there occurs chelation of iron in the gut, worsening the iron deficiency.
- **GI disorders:** Partial gastrectomy and extensive bowel surgery reduce absorption of food iron. Absorption of inorganic iron salts, however, is less impaired. Cachexia, infectious diseases, (*H. pylori* infection), gluten sensitivity and malabsorption syndrome reduce iron absorption.
- **Chronic inflammatory diseases: Hepcidin,** a peptide hormone of liver, is an acute phase reactant induced by inflammatory cytokines as observed in chronic diseases such as RA, IBD, tuberculosis and cancer. It decreases iron absorption from GIT, reduces its transport and blocks its release from the stored sites. It is thus responsible for iron deficiency anaemia in above conditions. *Such patients are unresponsive to oral iron and might need intravenous iron.*

Iron transport and utilisation: Iron circulates in the blood bound to a beta globulin fraction, **transferrin** (also termed as siderophilin) to reach the sites of its intracellular utilisation. In iron deficiency, increased number of transferrin receptors increases the cellular iron uptake. *The liver parenchymal cells are the major site of transferrin synthesis. Normally, transferrin is one-third saturated with iron.*

The body iron is present as:

- **Heme.** About two-thirds of the total body iron is in the form of haemoglobin. Remaining heme is present in myoglobin (heme protein of skeletal and cardiac muscle) and parenchymal iron. The latter exists in cytochrome oxidase and other cellular enzymes involved in tissue respiration or cellular metabolism.
- **Iron bound to protein**, without heme formation, as the storage compounds (30% of the total body iron). These include water soluble **ferritin** and insoluble **haemosiderin** present in bone marrow, liver, spleen and other areas with prominent reticuloendothelial components. Both ferritin and haemosiderin are available for heme synthesis. **Iron deficiency anaemia does not manifest until the stores are largely depleted.**
  The concentration of serum ferritin is normally in equilibrium with body iron stores. **Serum ferritin is the most sensitive index of iron status and is used to diagnose iron deficiency** (if levels are< 30 mcg/L). Serum ferritin level of 1 mcg/L corresponds to 8 mg of storage iron.
- **Transport iron** bound to transferrin

Plasma iron is normally in equilibrium with iron stores. The normal plasma iron level varies from 66 - 146 mcg/100 mL. The plasma iron level and plasma unsaturated binding capacity are modified by:

1. Iron deficiency which is associated with a reduction in serum iron levels and an increase in iron binding capacity.
2. Haemochromatosis which is associated with high serum iron levels and reduced binding capacity. A similar picture is seen in pernicious and aplastic anaemias.
3. Acute and chronic infections which are generally associated with reduced serum iron due to sequestration and decreased binding capacity.

The daily iron turnover has been estimated to be approximately 35 mg. The major contribution to this, 21 mg, comes from the normal red cell destruction; iron thus released is reutilised. About 11 mg of iron is contributed by that fraction which is not used for haemoglobin production during its stay in the marrow, whereas the remaining 2–3 mg comes from the storage sites, intestinal absorption and the ECF.

From these 35 mg of iron, about 32 mg enter the 'erythropoietic labile pool', a poorly defined compartment, primarily in the bone, for erythropoiesis. Approximately, 1 mg of iron goes for storage and into the ECF each, and about 1 mg is excreted.

The **labile iron pool** is that part of body iron which is readily available for utilisation for haemoglobin synthesis. Iron quickly enters this pool either after absorption from the intestine, after release from the RBC breakdown or following an iron injection. If the amount entering this labile pool is in excess of needs, then, it is transferred into **storage pool**.

Iron transfer to maturing erythrocytes occurs mainly by binding transferrin to specific receptor sites present on the membrane of the erythrocyte precursors. The iron released and inserted into the porphyrin ring to form heme is controlled by mitochondrial enzymes. Failure of this process causes **sideroachrestic anemias**. The anaemias of lead poisoning and of thalassemia are of this type. In such cases iron granules are seen in the cytoplasm of erythroblasts.

Iron excretion: Iron is tenaciously conserved. The body iron is regulated mostly by regulation of iron absorption by the gut. The total iron excreted daily is 0.5–1 mg via:

- **Intestine:** Iron is excreted in the faeces with the exfoliation of the villous cells, and in trace amounts in bile.
- **Skin:** Traces of iron are lost by desquamation of the skin and hair and through sweat.
- **Urine:** Urinary iron excretion is 0.1 mg daily.
- **Menstrual blood:** One ml of blood contains 0.5 mg of iron and the iron loss due to menstruation in a 28 days cycle is 0.3–0.6 mg/day.
- **Milk:** Up to 1.5 mg appears in milk daily, during lactation.

Iron requirements and sources: Box 34.1 gives the daily iron requirements. Vegetable foods rich in iron (containing 10 mg of iron per 100 g) include cereals like bajra, rice bran, whole wheat flour, pulses like Bengal gram, many leafy vegetables like spinach, peas and beans, condiments like turmeric and tamarind pulp, bananas and jaggery. The iron content of milk is so poor (0.2 mg%) that an infant fed on cow's milk alone would need 10 L daily to get its daily requirement of iron! Among the nonvegetarian foods, egg yolk, crab muscle, meat, liver and heart are rich in iron.

Box 34.1 Daily Dietary Iron Requirements[a]

- Children, 8–18 mg
- Adult men, 10–15 mg
- Menstruating women, 15–20 mg[b]
- Pregnant and lactating women, 20–25 mg[c]

[a]Based on 5%–10% absorption of food iron.
[b]Based on the monthly loss of 50 mL of blood (=25 mg of iron).
[c]Based on the fetal accumulation of 200–400 mg of iron and loss during child birth.

IRON FORMULATIONS

Iron formulations are available for oral and parenteral use.

Preparations and dosage of oral iron formulations

Table 34.1 lists the commonly used oral iron salts:

i. Dried ferrous sulphate tablet 200 mg. Modified-release tablets 325 mg and spansules 150 mg are also available
ii. Ferrous sulphate syrup. 60 mg of ferrous sulphate (12 mg of iron) in 5 mL.
iii. Ferrous sulphate paediatric drops for infants contain 125 mg of ferrous sulphate (25 mg of iron) in each mL.
iv. Ferrous gluconate 300 mg tablets. Elixir of ferrous gluconate 36 mg of iron per 5 mL.
v. Ferrous fumarate: 200 mg tablets. 305 mg capsules, oral solution ferrous fumarate 28 mg/ml and 140mg/5ml are also available
vi. Iron and ammonium citrate is a scaly ferric preparation soluble in water and is administered in the form of a mixture in the dose of 2 g t.i.d.
viii. Ferric hydroxide polymaltose complex (100 mg of elemental iron per tablet). This is an expensive preparation which offers hardly any advantage. Therapeutic failures have been reported with this preparation.
ix. Ferrous ascorbate

Adverse reactions to oral iron: All iron preparations are probably equally toxic per unit mass of soluble iron. They produce mild **GI disturbances** characterised by colicky pain, nausea, vomiting, diarrhoea or constipation, and gastric distress in about 6%–12% of individuals. These disturbances can be minimised by giving iron with food and by a gradual increase in the dosage.

The daily dose should not exceed six 200 mg tablets of exsiccated ferrous sulphate (180 mg of elementary iron). Iron administered in liquid form may combine with sulphide ions in the mouth forming black iron sulphide which causes blackening of teeth; this can be avoided by using a straw for drinking. *Oral iron invariably makes the faeces black due to iron sulphide.*

Acute iron poisoning is rare in adults but is not uncommon in children and infants. Doses of 1 g or

Table 34.1 Iron Preparations for Oral Therapy

Preparation	Therapeutic Dose[b] (mg/day)	Total iron Content (mg)	Percent of Elemental Iron
Exsiccated ferrous sulphate	600	180	32
Ferrous gluconate	900	108	12
Ferrous fumarate	600	198	33
Iron and ammonium citrate[a]	6000	1200	18
Ferrous succinate	300	105	35
Ferrous ascorbate	750	100	13

[a]Given only in liquid form; the rest either as tablets or in liquid form.
[b]Prophylactic dose 1/3rd or less.

more of ferrous sulphate are considered toxic in children. Toxicity is associated with severe GI irritation, haematemesis, vomiting, diarrhoea, cardiovascular collapse and shock. Death may occur within 12–48 h. Some may develop jaundice, hypoglycaemia and convulsions. Even if recovery occurs, sequelae such as GI obstruction may prove troublesome (for treatment see later). *Every patient should be warned to keep the tablets away from children who may mistake them for sweets.*

Preparations and dosage of parenteral iron formulations:

Parenteral iron releases inorganic ferric iron.

For IM use:

i. Iron–dextran: 15 mL vial, 50 mg of elemental iron/mL
ii. Iron–sorbitol–citric acid complex: 1.5 mL vial, 50 mg of iron/mL

For IV use:

i. High molecular weight iron dextran, 1–2 mL vial, 50 mg iron/mL
ii. Low molecular iron dextran 2 mL vial, 50 mg of iron/mL
iii. Iron sucrose (ferric hydroxide complexed with sucrose), 5 mL vial, 20 mg of iron/mL
iv. Ferric gluconate, 5 mL vial, 12.5 mg iron/mL
v. Ferric carboxymaltose, 15 mL single use vial, 50 mg iron/mL, given as 2 doses separated by at least 7 days
vi. Iron isomaltoside (IIM) 50 mg iron/ml and 100 mg iron/ml
vii. Ferumoxytol, 17 mL single use vial, 30 mg iron/mL, given as 2 doses separated by 2–8 days

Iron sorbitol is rapidly absorbed into the blood, and saturates transferrin. It is mostly stored in the liver and bone marrow. Mobilisation of iron dextran from IM injection site varies from 50% to 90%. Iron dextran, unlike iron sorbitol citric acid, does not saturate transferrin rapidly. It is absorbed from the muscle via the lymphatics and is converted by hepatic parenchymal cells into ferritin which in turn releases iron. **Iron isomaltoside** has iron tightly bound to carbohydrate in matrix structure This prevents the release of labile iron and reduces chances of iron toxicity.

IV iron can be administered by infusion either as a total single dose or repeated bolus of multiple doses. Utilisation of IV iron is 70%–100%. The initial dose of IV iron preparations is usually 20–30 mg of iron (1–1.5 mL). It is gradually increased to 100–200 mg (5–10 mL) and repeated daily, till the total dose is given.

Parenteral and oral iron preparations should not be administered concomitantly.

Adverse reactions to parenteral iron:

- **Intramuscular preparations** may cause local pain, permanent skin discoloration and local inflammation and regional lymphadenopathy. The systemic toxicity which may develop within

10 min of injection includes headache, fever, myalgia, arthralgia, backache, tachycardia, flushing, haemolysis and circulatory collapse. These effects are probably due to excessive amounts of free iron in the plasma. Iron sorbitol, in addition, may cause disorientation and temporary loss of taste.

- **With IV therapy**, the systemic reactions are similar to those observed following IM iron. Anaphylactoid reactions can occur within the first few minutes of administration. Severe chest pain, respiratory distress and circulatory collapse have been reported. Extravasation into the subcutaneous tissue can cause abscess.
- The urine of a person on iron sorbitol therapy turns black on standing, probably due to conversion of excreted iron into iron sulphide and the patient should be warned about this effect.

PHARMACOTHERAPY OF IRON DEFICIENCY ANAEMIA PH 1.35, IM 9.14, PE 13.5

Iron deficiency anaemia can occur due to the following:

1. Absolute iron deficiency
2. Functional iron deficiency as in erythropoeitin stimulated erythropoeisis
3. Sequestration of iron by hepcidine (see earlier).

As iron deficiency develops, iron stores diminish, as reflected by reduced and later absent stainable iron, haemosiderin. The most sensitive diagnostic test for detection of early or mild iron deficiency is the iron staining of the bone marrow. *In fact, prelatent iron deficiency is characterised by the absence of stainable iron in the bone marrow, increased iron absorption but no decrease in either serum iron or haemoglobin concentration.*

The iron deficiency anaemia is characterised by the presence of small erythrocytes (**microcytosis**) poorly filled with haemoglobin (**hypochromia**) and many cells of bizarre shapes (**poikilocytosis**) and variable sizes (**anisocytosis**). **All hypochromic anaemias, however, are not due to iron deficiency.** Evidence indicates that the metabolic importance of iron extends far beyond the red blood cell. *Even in the absence of anaemia, iron deficiency can produce adverse effects on brain function and abnormalities in behaviour; and can delay mental and motor development in children. Rule out thalassemia trait before starting long-term iron therapy unless the cause of iron deficiency (e.g. bleeding) is obvious.*

Indications for iron therapy are summarised in Box 34.2.

The aims of treatment of iron deficiency anaemia are as follows:

- **Correction of haemoglobin**
- **Correction of the underlying cause**
- **Building up body iron stores**

Both, correction of haemoglobin and replenishment of body stores can be achieved by oral iron supplements. It is an effective, convenient and well tolerated therapy. Many oral iron formulations are marketed but **routinely any cost effective preparation such as ferrous sulphate, ferrous fumerate or ferrous gluconate is preferred.** The fluid preparations, however, are preferred in children and in the presence of dysphagia and peptic ulcer. Sustained release and enteric coated iron preparations are generally poorly dissolved in the gastric and intestinal secretions, and may be lost in the faeces.

Absorption of ferrous sulphate in the usual therapeutic dose varies from 20% to 50% in iron deficient patients. Thus the recommended doses of oral iron deliver 40–60 mg of iron per day to the erythroid marrow, which is adequate to stimulate haemoglobin production 2-3 times the normal.

Box 34.2 Indications for Iron Therapy

Prophylactic: Pregnancy; infancy; rapidly growing children; menstruating women; elderly, professional blood donors; following partial gastrectomy

Therapeutic: i.e. to treat existing iron deficiency anaemia

- ***Nutritional deficiency*** due to deficient intake or decreased absorption
- ***Anaemia of pregnancy, infancy, prematurity and prolonged breast feeding***
- ***Anaemia due to acute or chronic blood loss*** as in menorrhagia, peptic ulcer and hook-worm infestation. (Blood loss of 100 mL corresponds to a loss of 50 mg of iron)
- ***Chronic kidney disease***
- ***Chronic inflammatory disease***

While prescribing it is essential to note the elemental iron in the preparation and calculate the dose. The dose ranges from 100 to 200 mg of elemental iron (2-3 mg/kg) per day but lower doses may be as effective and better tolerated (15–30 mg daily) and should be considered in patients not tolerating recommended doses. Dose should be increased at weekly intervals to reduce GI disturbances. If it is not tolerated, other preparations such as ferrous gluconate or ferrous fumarate may be substituted.

Ideally, iron should be given on an empty stomach, but it is better tolerated after food so initially therapy should be started with food and then gradually paced out the timings so that by 2 weeks, it can be taken either at least 1 hour before or 2 hours after a meal. However, iron should not be co-administered with milk, curd, cheese, calcium syrup/ tablets and drugs interfering its absorption.

It is necessary to warn the patient that the colour of stool may change to black or there may be temporary staining of the teeth and that he/she may experience either constipation or loose motions.

Patient should be advised regarding intake of iron rich food (green leafy vegetables like spinach, beans like soyabeans and rajma, nuts, raisins, jiggery, eggs (especially egg yolks), fish and meat). Foods rich in vitamin C such as citrus fruits, strawberries, tomatoes, and even potatoes also increase iron absorption.

Though the response to oral iron therapy depends on the severity of anaemia, ability to tolerate oral iron, and presence of co-morbidities, it is quite predictable. The **reticulocyte count** in the peripheral blood begins to rise within a week, reaches a peak at 10–14 days and returns to normal after about 3 weeks. Reticulocyte response is more striking in children than in adults; however, in children with haemoglobin, more than 7.5 g% and in adults, the rise in haemoglobin level may be the only indication of response to iron therapy.

The response is considered satisfactory when the haemoglobin level increases by about 1.5 g/100 mL of blood within 3 weeks. Most patients respond to oral therapy satisfactorily if iron is taken regularly and it is absorbed. Normal haemoglobin level is usually attained within 1–3 months, depending mainly on the initial haemoglobin level. *It is important, however, to continue with the therapy for 12–20 weeks after the haemoglobin level has returned to normal, in order to replenish the depleted iron stores.* Box 34.3 lists the causes of failure to oral iron therapy.

Indications for parenteral iron: *Response to oral or parenteral iron preparations is essentially similar, with average daily haemoglobin rise of about 0.2 g%.* Hence, parenteral therapy is used only under special circumstances (Box 34.4).

The parenteral dose is calculated on the basis that 25 mg of elemental iron is needed to correct 1% deficit of haemoglobin. The total dose needed is calculated by formula:

[Body weight (kg) × 2.3 × Hb deficit (Expected Hb − Patient Hb)] + 500 − 1000 mg iron for repletion of stores.

Iron dextran and iron sorbitol citric acid complex are the commonly used preparations. They are injected deep intramuscularly into the upper and outer quadrant of the buttock. The injection is made by 'Z' technique, pulling the skin and subcutaneous tissue to one side before entering the muscle to avoid leakage and skin staining. After an initial test dose of 25 mg, 100 mg are given daily or every

Box 34.3 Causes of Failure of Oral Iron Therapy

- Incorrect diagnosis
- Noncompliance
- Continued loss of blood
- Defective iron absorption
- Gluten sensitivity
- *H. pylori* infection or chronic inflammation
- Severe protein deficiency
- Underlying CKD or malignancy

Box 34.4 Indications for Parenteral Iron Therapy

- Inability to tolerate oral iron
- Failure to absorb adequate amounts of oral iron, e.g. malabsorption or extensive bowel resection
- Ulcerative colitis, colostomy and intestinal shunts
- Depleted iron stores as in patients with chronic bleeding, in whom the average daily iron loss equals or exceeds absorption of iron from oral iron preparations
- When the patient cannot be relied upon to take oral iron medication
- Patients with advanced kidney disease requiring erythropoietin
- Chronic inflammatory diseases

few days till the total calculated dose is administered. A single dose should not exceed 25 mg for infants, 50 mg for children and 100 mg for adults.

Intravenous infusion of total dose of low molecular weight iron dextran in 500 mL 5% glucose or normal saline can be given over 3–4 h. The drug concentration in the infusion must not exceed 5%. The initial infusion rate is 10 drops per minute. If no ill effects are seen over 30 min, it may be increased to 30–40 drops. Prednisolone IV before and after the infusion decreases the incidence of myalgias and arthralgias. *The merit of this therapy is that it circumvents the problems of oral iron absorption and the patient gets the required iron in one dose* and the iron stores may be rapidly restored, which would take months to achieve by the oral route.

IV iron dextran *is contraindicated in early pregnancy* but seems to be safe during late pregnancy.

Alternatively, **ferric gluconate** or **iron sucrose** is used **in repeated IV boluses** in the dose of 100–200 mg of elemental iron. Doses larger than 100 mg may be diluted in normal saline and infused over 30 min. Lower doses can be injected slowly over 2–3 min. *Prior test dose or medication is not needed.*

Prophylactic iron therapy

Women in the reproductive age should receive 100 mg of oral iron weekly (or 15 to 30 mg of iron per day). During pregnancy oral iron supplements (equivalent to 100 mg of elemental iron daily) should be administered from 14-16 weeks onwards, till 100 days postpartum.

Prophylactic iron therapy is also advocated for infants and children, more so in those with low birth weights. Biannual deworming with albendazole is also recommended.

Professional blood donors should receive routinely 300 mg of ferrous sulphate daily for 1 month after each donation of 500 mL.

ADJUVANTS TO IRON THERAPY

Various substances claimed to enhance the efficacy of iron are vitamin C, cobalt, copper, zinc and manganese. Vitamin C may increase the iron absorption but it is not necessary to use costly iron preparations incorporating vitamin C to achieve this effect. The therapeutic value of these supplements in the treatment of iron deficiency anaemia is doubtful. However, *nutritional iron deficiency is commonly associated with folate deficiency and folic acid is combined with iron with beneficial effects. The use of expensive pills containing several minerals and vitamins along with iron is unnecessary and wasteful.*

ERYTHROPOIETIN (EPO) AND ANEMIA PH 1.35

Anaemia is an almost invariable feature of chronic renal failure. The critical defect is inadequate secretion of erythropoietin, the major hormonal regulator of RBC production, produced by the kidney.

ERYTHROPOIETIN (epoetin α and β) has molecular weight about 36,000. It is a glycoprotein hormone mainly synthesised by the kidney in response to hypoxemia. Some amount is also produced by the liver, which is its important source to maintain erythropoiesis in patients with degenerated kidneys.

Thyroxine, growth hormone, prolactin, testosterone, $beta_2$ adrenergic agonists, PGs and angiotensin II stimulate erythropoietin production, while alkylating agents, estrogens and beta-adrenergic blocking drugs inhibit it.

Commercial **recombinant rHuEPO, epoetin alfa,** has the same amino acid sequence as the natural human erythropoietin. Given intravenously, it has a plasma t½ of 6–8 h. The target cell for erythropoietin is the early erythroid colony forming unit. It is metabolised in the liver.

Adverse reactions: are aggravation of hypertension, associated with a too-rapid rise in haematocrit, increased viscosity, higher rate of thrombosis and stroke. It is nonimmunogenic.

Indications:

- **Anaemia of end stage renal failure:** It is a normochromic, normocytic, hypoproliferative anaemia. The IV or SC administration of erythropoietin causes dose dependent rise in the haematocrit and eliminates the need for transfusions. Most patients respond to a dose of 35–80 IU/kg three times a week. Correction of coexisting iron deficiency should be done before erythropoietin therapy.
- **Anaemia in premature babies.**
- **To permit the autologous blood transfusion:** Injection of 600 IU/kg of erythropoietin thrice a week makes it possible both to donate more blood and to maintain higher haematocrit at the time of elective surgery in an individual.

EPO is sometimes misused by athletes to increase Hb and thus O_2 supply to tissues.

Darbepoetin alfa is a long acting, synthetic analogue of epoietin. Its properties and uses are similar to those of epoietin. It can be injected *once a week*. **Methoxy polyethylene glycol epoetin beta** is an isoform of EPO which is longer acting and given intravenously/subcutaneously at 2–4 weeks interval.

TREATMENT OF IRON POISONING FM 9.3

Acute Oral Iron Poisoning:

1. Milk and egg yolk mixture is administered to bind the iron.
2. **Desferrioxamine** 1–2 g intramuscularly is administered.
3. Gastric lavage with water containing desferrioxamine is given initially, followed by 5–10 g of the same in 100 mL of water being left in the stomach to adsorb any more iron. If desferrioxamine is not available, **calcium disodium edetate** 35–40 mg/kg may be used.
4. An IV infusion of desferrioxamine (see below).
5. Early replacement of body fluids and electrolytes using isotonic saline, correction of metabolic acidosis and hypotension by using ringer lactate and vasopressor agents, respectively, are indicated.
6. Diazepam to control convulsions.

DESFERRIOXAMINE MESYLATE: This compound, obtained from *Streptomyces pilosus*, is a potent and **specific chelator of iron.** It readily binds ferric iron to form ferrioxamine, a stable and water soluble chelate. Ferrioxamine is excreted two-thirds in the urine and one-third in the bile. It colours the urine reddish brown. Desferrioxamine also removes iron from haemosiderin except that in the bone marrow; **desferrioxamine 100 mg binds 8.5 mg of iron.**

It is administered by IV infusion or intramuscularly. It is generally well tolerated. Rapid IV injection can produce hypotension, tachycardia and anaphylactoid reactions and urticaria. Allergic reactions and cataract formation are known to occur during its *chronic administration* for iron storage diseases. It is contraindicated in patients with severe renal disease or anuria, and in pregnant women.

Indications:

- **Acute iron intoxication:** In severe cases (in shock), the drug is administered by IV infusion: 10–15 mg/kg/h to a maximum of 80 mg/kg in 24 h. In less severe cases (without shock), it is given in the dose of 1–2 g every 3–12 h; maximum dose 6 g in 24 h. In less severe cases (without shock), it is given intramuscularly in the dose of 40 mg/kg every 4–12 h.
- **Haemochromatosis:** Desferrioxamine is useful in the *prevention and treatment* of iron overload in patients with chronic anaemia such as in thalassemia major treated with multiple transfusions.

Deferiprone: This is an orally effective iron chelator. It is less effective than desferrioxamine. It causes nausea, vomiting abdominal pain, arthralgia and nutropenia. It is excreted mainly in urine as metabolite. The dose is 25–30 mg/kg t.i.d.

Deferasirox: This oral, selective iron chelator is given once daily. The drug-iron complex is excreted in the feces. Its uses are similar to those of desferrioxime. The dose is 20–30 mg/kg once a day.

CHAPTER 35

Drugs Effective in Megaloblastic Anaemias, Neutropenia and Thrombocytopenia

Learning Objectives

This chapter will enable the reader:

1. To be aware of the pathophysiology of megaloblastic anaemia.
2. To be aware of the physiological functions of vitamin B_{12} and folic acid and their daily requirements.
3. To enumerate the formulations of vitamin B_{12} and folic acid and their indications.
4. To outline the management of megaloblastic anaemia.
5. To give the pharmacological basis of use of folinic acid.
6. To enumerate the drugs used in neutropenia, their ADR and indications.
7. To enlist the drugs used in thrombocytopenia.

KEY TERMS

vitamin B_{12} and folic acid, physiological role, p. 525
vitamin B_{12}, absorption, p. 525
vitamin B_{12}, metabolic actions, p. 526
vitamin B_{12} and folate actions, interrelation between, p. 526
megaloblastic anemia, p. 529
folic acid, metabolic actions, p. 529
folic acid, absorption, p. 529
folinic acid, p. 531
neutropenia, drugs used, p. 531
thrombocytopenia, drugs used, p. 531

Megaloblastic anaemias are characterised by the presence of abnormally large, nucleated, red cell precursors, known as megaloblasts, in the bone marrow. A megaloblast is viewed as an example of the unbalanced growth between the cytoplasm and the nucleus due to defective synthesis of nucleoproteins. **In almost 95% of the cases with megaloblastic bone marrow, vitamin B_{12} and/or folic acid deficiency is present.**

Although folic acid and vitamin B_{12} influence different metabolic pathways in the synthesis of nucleoproteins, the final result of deficiency of either of these is defective DNA (deoxyribonucleic acid) synthesis. Since DNA is present in every cell, the basic abnormality affects all proliferating cells such as those in buccal cavity, tongue and GI tract, leading to glossitis, stomatitis and intestinal malabsorption. Other organs affected include the cervical and vaginal squamous epithelium, the ovary and testes. The precursors of white cells (giant metamyelocytes) and those of platelets show abnormal mitotic activity. These abnormally large cells give rise to abnormally large offsprings that appear in the peripheral blood, which shows fully haemoglobinised (**hyperchromic**), large, red cells called macrocytes, polymorphonuclear leucocytes with hypersegmented nuclei and giant platelets. The anaemia is thus described as **macrocytic hyperchromic**. Such abnormal cells have a shortened life span and may undergo early haemolysis, which sometimes gives rise to associated jaundice. The anaemia is also associated with pancytopenia (leucopenia, neutropenia and thrombocytopenia). *Vitamin B_{12} deficiency causes damage to myelin in peripheral nerves, spinal cord and brain. With folate deficiency, the loss of body weight is much more marked and nervous instability may be present;* but, the damage to the myelin is doubtful.

All the macrocytic anaemias, however, are not megaloblastic. Thus, the macrocytic anaemias due to liver disease, myxoedema, following certain haemolytic states, and leukaemias usually have normoblastic bone marrow.

Physiological Role of Vitamin B_{12} and Folic Acid

Physiologically, both these vitamins play an important role in the synthesis of DNA and RNA. The deficiency picture produced by both is clinically indistinguishable except that the neurological disturbances are commoner with vitamin B_{12} deficiency than with folic acid deficiency; the peripheral blood picture and bone marrow changes are also similar and only certain special tests give the correct clue about the precise diagnosis.

Small 'physiological' doses of either folic acid or vitamin B_{12} will selectively improve the blood picture only in those persons suffering from a deficiency of the particular vitamin being administered; large 'pharmacologic' doses of either vitamin, however, will cause a haematological response irrespective of the type of deficiency, vitamin B_{12} or folic acid or both.

COBALAMINS: Chemically, vitamin B_{12} belongs to the family of cobalamins which are *cobalt containing carrinoid compounds.*

Of these, cyanocobalamin and hydroxocobalamin are commonly used therapeutically. They are discussed below under the general heading 'Vitamin B_{12}'.

VITAMIN B_{12}: Vitamin B_{12} is synthesised solely by micro-organisms in soil, water and animal intestine or rumen. **It is almost absent in plant products. In man, as in animals, it is synthesised in the colon by micro-organisms;** however, it is hardly absorbed from this site and hence, is excreted (about 3–5 mcg daily) in faeces. Some of the animals like rabbits and rats eat their own faeces (coprophagy), and hence they have very high serum levels of vitamin B_{12}. Nonvegetarian foods like muscle, liver, kidney, oysters, fish and egg yolk are rich in vitamin B_{12}; dairy food contains smaller amounts. The vitamin B_{12} content of cow's milk is considerably more than that of human milk.

The daily dietary intake of vitamin B_{12} varies considerably and is high in nonvegetarians and likely to be very low in vegetarians, some of whom may not even consume sufficient amount of milk or milk products; however, vegetarians may obtain enough vitamin B_{12} from contaminated water and in the form of coenzyme B_{12} by ingesting legumes and nodules of root vegetable in which vitamin B_{12} is synthesised by micro-organisms.

The minimum daily requirement of vitamin B_{12} in adults is not exactly known but is believed to be extremely small, about 1 mcg per day. Taking into consideration the incomplete absorption of B_{12} present in food, the recommended daily dietary intake is 2 mcg for adults, 3 mcg in pregnancy and lactation and 0.3 mcg for infants.

Absorption of vitamin B_{12}: The cobalamins in food exist in a bound form and are metabolically inactive until they are released by heat (cooking) and by proteolysis in the stomach. The gastric juice contains cobalamin binding protein, called R-type protein (cobalophilin and haptocoin). This protein binds cobalamin with higher affinity than does IF. Thus, at acidic pH, the dietary cobalamin enters the duodenum bound to R-type protein.

Pancreatic proteases degrade this complex in the jejunum, and cobalamin is presented to the IF, a glycoprotein, produced by the parietal cells of the fundus and the body of the stomach. IF-cobalamin complex binds specifically to cubulin receptors on terminal ileum with high affinity. Vitamin B_{12} enters the cells and stored in lysosomes. Finally, it is released for transportation into the blood.

Thus, very little or none of the dietary cobalamin is absorbed in cases with pernicious anaemia, gastric diseases and after gastrectomy as the IF is absent. IF is antigenic and antibodies against IF are known.

The maximum absorption of vitamin B_{12} occurs within 8–12 h following a physiological dose (1–5 mcg), uninfluenced by vitamin B_{12} concentration.

Given subcutaneously or intramuscularly, cyanocobalamin is rapidly absorbed and the plasma level reaches the peak in 1 h. Cyanocobalamin can also get absorbed without the help of IF, but the dose needed is much higher **(500–1000 mcg)**.

Vitamin B_{12} transport and storage: Almost 80% of absorbed vitamin B_{12} is transported in the plasma, bound to beta$_2$ globulin called **transcobalamin II.** Only <10% circulates as a free fraction. The transcobalamin II is taken up by cells by endocytosis. During the process, it is degraded and the released cobalamin is converted to two coenzymes, **methylcobalamin** and **adenosyl cobalamin.**

The major form of vitamin B_{12} in the serum is methylcobalamin attached to a globulin. The total body stores of cobalamin in normal adult are estimated at about 3–5 mg, of which a large portion is present in the liver. Not all of this, however, is available for haemopoesis.

Turnover of vitamin B_{12} is very slow and only 0.2%–0.3% of the total B_{12} contained in the body is excreted per day. Vitamin B_{12} is excreted in the bile but most of it is reabsorbed, so that there is a closed **enterohepatic circulation.** *This is how the body conserves vitamin B_{12} and this would explain partly why even strict vegans with a very low intake of this vitamin rarely develop clinical vitamin B_{12}–deficiency syndrome.*

Excretion: The daily urinary loss of vitamin B_{12} is very small, less than 0.25 mcg. Only the cobalamin not bound to proteins is capable of being excreted by glomerular filtration. *Conservation of the vitamin by enterohepatic circulation and its very slow excretion explain why it takes a long time, perhaps 10 years, for deficiency to develop in the presence of deficient intake or absorption.* The half-life of a tracer dose of radioactive vitamin B_{12} in the liver is about 12 months.

If vitamin B_{12} is injected, only the amount necessary for the saturation of the binding sites is retained; the remaining excess is excreted in the urine. It is calculated that 80%–95% of a 50 mcg dose of injected vitamin B_{12} is retained. As the dose exceeds 100 mcg, large proportions (90%) of the injected dose appear in the urine within 48 h.

Vitamin B_{12} crosses the placental barrier and the cord blood level of vitamin B_{12} is significantly higher than the maternal blood levels. PH 1.35

Metabolic actions of vitamin B_{12}: Cyanocobalamin itself is inactive in man. After absorption it is converted to active forms, **methyl cobalamin and 5-deoxyadenosylcobalamin.**

1. On entry into the cell, methyl group from N_5-methyl tetrahydrofolic acid ($MeFH_4$) is transferred to cobalamin to form methyl cobalamin. The methyl group from methyl cobalamin is transferred to homocysteine to form **methyl-homocysteine** also called **methionine** (Fig. 35.1). In the absence of vitamin B_{12}, the conversion of dietary and stored

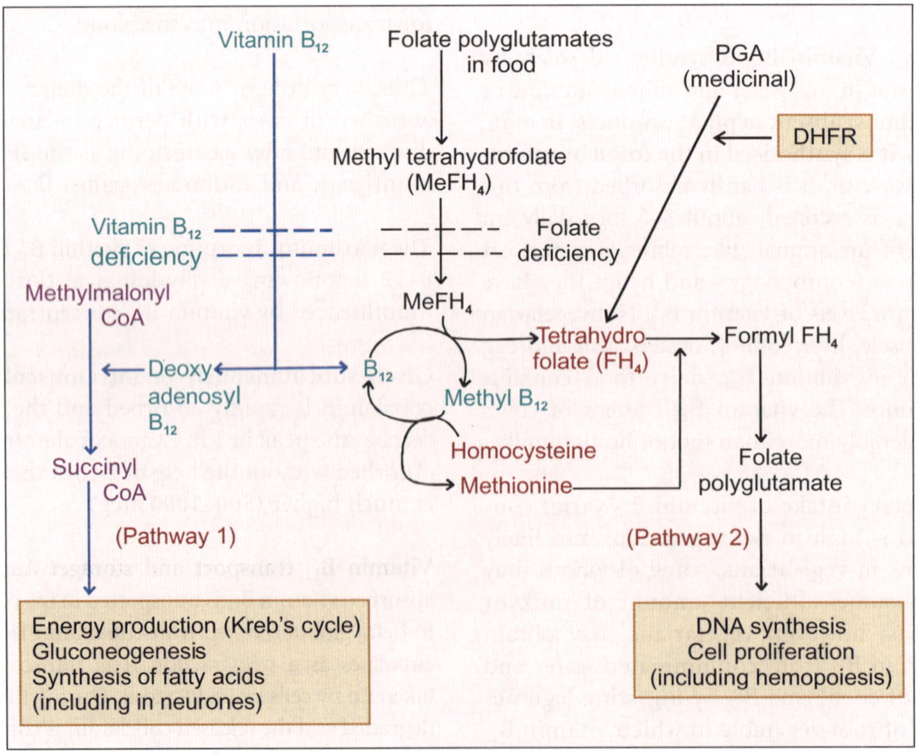

FIG. 35.1 **Interrelation between vitamin B_{12} and folate actions. PGA, pteroyl glutamic acid; DHFR, dihydrofolate reductase.**

folate ($MeFH_4$) to FH_4 is blocked (Fig. 35.1), resulting in deficiency of essential folate cofactors and accumulation of $MeFH_4$ ('methyltetrahydrofolate trap'). As a result biochemical reactions requiring folate cofactors will suffer. This may explain the similarity of GI lesions and peripheral blood picture seen in megaloblastic anaemia due to deficiency of either vitamin B_{12} or folic acid.

2. Vitamin B_{12} is needed for the development and myelination of CNS and its function. Because the neurons do not divide, impaired DNA synthesis cannot explain the demyelination that occurs in vitamin B_{12} deficiency. It is suggested that tissue deficiency of deoxyadenosyl cobalamin and failure of transmethylation reactions are important in causing deficiency of myelin synthesis. Deoxyadenosyl cobalamin is necessary for the conversion of methyl malonyl CoA to succinyl CoA (Fig. 35.1). Lack of adenosyl cobalamin causes accumulation of methylmalonyl CoA. **Deficiency of vitamin B_{12} thus interferes with the production of lipoprotein in myelin tissue and may explain the neurological complications** such as peripheral neuritis, optic atrophy, subacute combined degeneration of the spinal cord and brain atrophy.
3. Purine biosynthesis is reduced in cobalamin deficiency and this abnormality may also contribute to defective DNA synthesis. Both methyl tetrahydrofolate trapping and lack of deoxyadenosyl B_{12} contribute to impairment of purine synthesis.
Vitamin B_{12} plays some role in folate uptake and storage.

Vitamin B_{12} does not seem to have any other significant pharmacological actions, even in large doses.

Serum vitamin B_{12} levels: The serum level in normals consuming nonvegetarian food varies between 140 and 750 pg/mL (means 205 pg/mL). *The levels in healthy subjects consuming lacto vegetarian food are considerably lower, some of them even below 100 pg/mL without any clinical or haematological evidence of deficiency.* Although vitamin B_{12}–deficiency anaemia is accompanied by low serum levels, *it is doubtful whether a low serum level of vitamin B_{12} by itself signifies tissue deficiency in otherwise healthy vegetarians.*

Only characteristic peripheral blood picture and estimation of serum methylmalonic acid and total homocysteine (both of which are markedly increased) will help in correct diagnosis. With currently employed automeasured assays for vitamin B_{12}, both false-positive and false-negative results are common up to 50%. Furthermore, the results obtained differ from laboratory to laboratory and hence could be unreliable.

Preparations and dosage: PH 1.35

i. Cyanocobalamin, pink-coloured injection, contains 100 mcg/mL. *It should be administered either intramuscularly or subcutaneously.* It is also available as 50 mcg and 1 mg tablets and 7 mcg/ml oral solution.
ii. Hydroxocobalamin injection, 100, 500 or 1000 mcg/mL
iii. Vitamin B_{12} for oral administration is available as a part of multivitamin formulations. Such preparations may be helpful in treating *dietary* deficiency of vitamin B_{12} but are ineffective in patients with deficiency.

Oral formulations of vitamin B_{12} are not recommended to treat established vitamin B_{12} deficiency in the initial period; however, after parenteral therapy, 1–2 mg/day of oral hydroxocobalamin can be given as maintenance doses. Large oral doses get absorbed using another transport system which does not require IF or functional terminal ileum but has a lower efficiency.

Adverse reactions: Vitamin B_{12} given orally is very safe. *Cyanocobalamin should never be injected intravenously, as it has been reported to cause anaphylactoid reactions very rarely. The use of hydroxocobalamin can lead to the development of antibodies to the transcobalamin–vitamin B_{12} complex*. Hence, IM or SC cyanocobalamin, is the treatment of choice in vitamin B_{12} deficiency.

Indications: IM 9.14

1. **Megaloblastic anaemia due to vitamin B_{12} deficiency:**
   - **Deficient intake** in nutritional megaloblastic anaemia is often seen in *strict vegans.* Majority of the nutritional megaloblastic anaemias observed in India are mainly due to folate deficiency. The nutritional B_{12}

deficiency can be corrected by parenteral administration of vitamin B_{12}. Exclusively breast fed infants of mothers with the vitamin B_{12} deficiency, could develop vitamin B_{12} deficiency.

- **Impaired absorption** of Vitamin B_{12} is observed in pernicious anaemia (due to lack of IF), after gastrectomy or resection of small bowel, in malabsorption syndromes and in GI diseases involving stomach and intestine such as malignancy, and chronic pancreatitis. Long-term use of biguanides, antacids, H_2 receptors blockers and proton pump inhibitors can impair vitamin B_{12} absorption and cause vitamin B_{12} deficiency. In all these cases, vitamin B_{12} should be given *parenterally*.

  Cyanocobalamin *is the drug of choice for pernicious anaemia.* Initially, it is given in the dose of 1000 mcg intramuscularly or deep subcutaneously daily for 1–2 weeks to replenish the body stores. Then, a similar dose may be given intramuscularly every week for 4 weeks and then monthly. The reticulocyte response occurs on the 3rd to 4th day and reaches the peak by the 5th to 8th day. In patients with pernicious anaemia and in cases with incurable GI lesions, the treatment has to be continued lifelong.
- **Infestation with the fish tapeworm** also causes megaloblastic anaemia due to preferential uptake of dietary vitamin B_{12} by the worm. This is not common in India but heavy worm infestation may contribute to such a deficiency.
- **Inadequate utilisation** of vitamin B_{12} which may occur in infants who inherit the deficiency of certain enzymes necessary for conversion of vitamin B_{12} to its coenzyme forms. Hereditary deficiency of transcobalamine II may also cause cobalamin deficiency.

2. **Vitamin B_{12}–deficiency neuropathies** such as tropical neuropathy, subacute combined degeneration, tobacco and tropical amblyopia, which sometimes occur without clearcut megaloblastic anaemia, respond to parenteral vitamin B_{12} therapy. The sensory component improves much less than the motor component. There is some evidence to suggest that certain well defined neurological and ophthalmic syndrome (tobacco amblyopia) may represent the chronic neurotoxic effects of cyanide, and that hydroxocobalamin may help in the detoxication of cyanide by binding to it (see Chapter 75).

Vitamin B_{12}, given in massive doses, has been claimed to be useful in such varied conditions as infective hepatitis, infertility, herpes zoster, toxic amblyopia and trigeminal neuralgia; *there is no evidence to suggest that this vitamin is of any value in such conditions. Nor there is any conclusive evidence to suggest its usefulness in patients with mental disorders. Its use as general 'tonic' is irrational.*

HYDROXOCOBALAMIN: It is absorbed slowly on injection and is more protein bound than cyanocobalamin. It is excreted slowly and hence, higher blood levels are maintained over a longer period than with cyanocobalamin. It is given initially as 1 mg intramuscularly every 2–3 days for five doses. Maintenance dose is 1 mg every 3 months.

Methylcobalamin: *There is no evidence for superiority of this expensive analogue over cyanocobalamin and hydroxocobalamin, which are cost-effective.*

FOLIC ACID (PTEROYLMONO-GLUTAMIC ACID): It is named folic acid because it is commonly present in green leaves. The term 'folate' is used in the generic sense and includes other chemical forms, dihydro and tetrahyro folic acid.

Folate is present in abundance in green vegetables, liver and yeast. Moderate amounts are present in eggs, meat, fish and dairy foods. Most of the folic acid in vegetables is in conjugated form, usually as triglutamic and heptaglutamic acid conjugates. **Prolonged boiling during cooking destroys most of the folate in the food.**

Vitamin C protects the reduced product, tetrahydrofolic acid, from oxidative destruction. It also protects the folate in the food. Hence, food poor in vitamin C content is generally low in folate content.

Many microorganisms including those in the colon synthesise folic acid. It is doubtful, however, whether it is available for utilisation in man.

Absorption: Folic acid conjugates are hydrolysed to **pteroylmonoglutamic acid** by conjugases found throughout the GI mucosa. Pteroylmonoglutamic acid is absorbed almost completely in the small intestine, particularly in the jejunum. *Physiological doses (1 mg) are absorbed by an active process by binding to folate receptors, whereas large doses get absorbed by diffusion.* Absorption of food folate, however, is incomplete. Inhibition of conjugase by certain drugs (e.g. phenytoin) or its decreased concentration due to intestinal pathology may cause malabsorption of polyglutamates in the diet.

Transport, storage and fate: Given orally, folic acid appears in the blood within 30 min. It circulates in the plasma mainly as ***N*-methyl tetrahydrofolate ($MeFH_4$)**. The majority is loosely bound to albumin, from which it is readily taken up by the cells. **Inside the cells, it is converted to tetrahydrofolate (FH_4)** by the cobalamine dependent enzyme, methionine synthetase.

The amount of folic acid excreted in the urine is dependent on the dose. Only a small amount appears in the urine following ingestion of 0.1 mg of folic acid, whereas **almost 90% is excreted** after 15 mg dose. Folate appears in the urine within 6 h after ingestion, and excretion is complete within 24 h.

The total body stores of folate are in the range of 5–10 mg, of which almost one-third is present in the liver mostly as methylfolate. **Unlike vitamin B_{12}, folate gets selectively concentrated in the spinal fluid.**

Folate is incorporated in red cells during erythropoiesis and the amount decreases only slightly during their life span. **Red cell folate is, therefore, a useful indicator of body folate status.**

The exact daily requirement of folate in man is not known; but it appears to be 200 mcg in adults, 100 mcg for children and 300–400 mcg in pregnancy and lactation. The folate losses from the body are about 50% of the amount ingested, **the recommended daily intake is 400 mcg for adults, 200 mcg for children and 600–800 mcg in pregnancy.** PH 1.35

Metabolic actions of folate: Folic acid by itself is inactive. Folate transfers one carbon units such as methyl and formyl groups to various substrates in enzymatic reactions. Its coenzymes are involved in various metabolic reactions (Fig. 35.1).

- Biosynthesis of purine and pyrimidine nucleotides
- FH_4 is able to accept one carbon fragment such as methyl, formyl and methylene groups; the folate coenzymes participate in reactions in which one carbon fragment is transferred from one molecule to another. **The important reactions of this type are conversion of homocysteine to methionine** (Refer to metabolic actions of vitamin B_{12}) and of serine to glycine.

These reactions are necessary for the biosynthesis of DNA and RNA and hence, for cell division. **In folate deficiency, homocysteine accumulates in the blood due to lack of 5-methyl tetrahydrofolate.** Fig. 35.1 depicts the interrelation between actions of vitamin B_{12} and folic acid.

Diagnosis of folic acid deficiency: Low blood level of folic acid, in itself, cannot be considered as a definite indication of folic acid deficiency. Various other tests (e.g. serum homocysteine level) have been proposed for diagnosing folic acid deficiency, but none of these is without fallacies.

Adverse reactions: Folic acid is nontoxic in man, and no adverse effects have been reported.

Preparations and dosage: Folic acid tablet contains 5 mg of the drug. It is also available as 0.4 mg tablets and 0.5 mcg/ml oral solution. Dose 1–5 mg. It can be increased upto 15 mg in malabsorption states, while 0.2–0.5 mg is the prophylactic dose for megaloblastic anemia.

It can also be given parenterally. IM 9.14

Indications: Folic acid is used in the treatment of megaloblastic anaemia due to folate deficiency. These are as follows:

- **Dietary deficiency:** Nutritional megaloblastic anaemia is the commonest type of megaloblastic anaemia occurring due to undernutrition. Megaloblastic anaemia of protein caloric undernutrition of infancy and childhood is mostly due to folic acid deficiency. Cooking habits involving prolonged boiling of food with spices, which destroys folic acid, and possibly loss of folate in sweat further contribute to its deficiency. Whenever there is deficiency of folate there is also a lack of other nutrients and the ideal treatment lies in correcting the diet. Supplementation with folic acid orally can, however, avoid and correct this deficiency.

- **Anaemia due to increased requirements:** The commonest type of megaloblastic anaemia **in pregnancy** is due to folate deficiency caused by the increased requirement both by the fetus and the mother. *Folate deficiency during pregnancy is so common that prophylactic use of folic acid along with iron from conception till the end of lactation is justified.* Daily prophylactic dose of 600–800 mcg of folic acid with about 100–200 mg of elemental iron is all that is needed. In the treatment of established anaemia, folic acid is given orally, 5 mg daily. Increased demand for folic acid also occurs in various pathological states like hyperthyroidism, rheumatoid arthritis, leukaemia, haemolytic anaemia, chronic infections, exfoliative skin disease, myelofibrosis and in cancer; this is probably due to rapid cell synthesis.
- **Anaemia due to impaired absorption:** This is observed in malabsorption syndrome associated with tropical sprue, extensive organic disease of the jejunum, etc.
  In other types of malabsorptive states such as idiopathic steatorrhoea, adult celiac disease and nontropical sprue, sensitivity to the gluten fraction of wheat protein is often the offending cause. In such cases and in gluten enteropathy in children, administration of gluten-free diet gives dramatic results; many patients in this group, however, also suffer from folic acid deficiency. In such conditions, folic acid is given intramuscularly in a dose of 5 mg daily, followed by oral therapy as soon as the diarrhoea ceases.
- **Anaemia due to drug-induced folate deficiency:** Certain antiepileptic drugs like phenobarbitone, phenytoin and primidone may cause folic acid–deficiency anaemia by impairing its absorption and/or its utilisation. Drugs like methotrexate, the antimalarial pyrimethamine and the antibacterial drug trimethoprim can also cause folate deficiency by blocking the conversion of folic acid to tetrahydrofolate. A supplement of folic acid, 1 mg daily, orally, can correct this deficiency. **The antiepileptic treatment need not be stopped.**
- **Certain other megaloblastic anaemias as** in liver disease, chronic alcoholism and scurvy are usually associated with folate deficiency
- **Prevention of neural tube defects** (NTD): Any woman who can become pregnant should be prescribed 400 mcg of folic acid daily, as otherwise the conceptus might develop NTD which are liable to occur during the first week of gestation, even before the subject knows that she is pregnant. Furthermore, if the woman is at high risk for NTD (has past/family history of NTD, or is taking carbamazepine or valproate), she should be prescribed 5 mg of a folic acid daily at least 1 month before planned conception. *However, as many pregnancies may be unplanned, it is recommended for all women with childbearing potential.*
- **Folate deficiency of ageing** may be associated with elevated serum homocysteine levels and degenerating vascular disease in the elderly. Folate supplementation (400–1000 mcg/day) given prophylactically, may be useful.

Folate deficiency is also observed in those who are exposed to excessive UV light, e.g. after skin tanning. The UV rays penetrate the skin and destroy folates in the cutaneous circulation and can cause deficiency.

Folate deficiency as a cause of neuropathy is not universally accepted, although cases of encephalopathy giving rise to a confusional state, usually diagnosed as senile dementia and/or myelopathy, responding to folic acid have been reported. Hence, folic acid may be tried empirically in obscure chronic neurological disorder not responding to vitamin B_{12} therapy.

Administration of folic acid alone is contraindicated in pernicious anaemia as, although it may correct the haematological abnormality, it can precipitate or worsen the neurological complications. It has been postulated that folic acid accelerates the utilisation of the meagre vitamin B_{12} stores (Pathway 2 in Fig. 35.1) in an already deficient subject and may aggravate deficiency of vitamin B_{12}.

Subjective improvement such as feeling of well-being and decrease in the soreness in the mouth occur early after the start of therapy. Megaloblasts disappear from the peripheral blood within 48 h, and reticulocyte peak within 7 days. Rise in haemoglobin is observed in 10–15 days.

FOLINIC ACID (citrovorum factor): This is N5 formyl tetrahydrofolinic acid. It was originally found in the liver and was demonstrated to have a growth promoting effect on the organism *Leuconostoc citrovorum*. It is available in 1-mL ampoules for injection. Its only use is in the treatment of toxicity due to folic acid antagonists like methotrexate.

DRUGS USED IN NEUTROPENIA PH 1.35

Recombinant preparations of human granulocyte colony stimulating factor (G-CSF) and granulocyte/macrophage colony stimulating factor (GM-CSF) are used in the treatment of neutropenia.

FILGRASTIM is a glycoprotein which is not glycosylated unlike the natural G-CSF. It stimulates neutrophil progenitors to produce mature neutrophils, stimulates their release from bone marrow storage pool and also increases their phagocytic and cytotoxic capacity. Filgrastim has t½ of 3.5 h. **Lenograstim** is the glycosylated analogue of filgrastim.

Pegfilgrastim is filgrastim conjugated to polyethyleneglycol (PEG), which minimises its glomerular filtration. Its t½ is 5–8 h. It is given as a single injection (6 mg subcutaneously) per chemotherapy cycle.

Forms of GM-CSF available worldwide are **sargramostim** (from yeast) and **molgramostim** (from *E. coli*). They stimulate proliferation and differentiation of partially committed haemopoietic progenitor cells to produce end cells of granulocyte and monocyte/macrophage lineages. They also activate some of the functions of the fully differentiated cells. Their administration stimulates myelopoiesis. Their t½ is 2–3 h.

These agents are given subcutaneously or slow IV infusion. Dosages are adjusted based on the blood counts and duration. Therapy duration is 7–14 days.

Adverse reactions: These agents are well tolerated but can cause bone pain, fever, myalgia, lethargy and pain at the injection site. Hypersensitivity reactions including skin rashes can occur with higher doses. Hypotension, flushing, nausea, vomiting and dyspnoea (especially after first IV infusion) have also been reported. Prolonged administration can lead to capillary leak syndrome with peripheral oedema and pleural and pericardial effusion. Supraventricular arrhythmias, and elevation of serum creatinine and hepatic enzymes are also reported. These agents stimulate growth of tumour cells with myeloid characters.

Indications:

- To reduce the severity and duration of neutropenia induced by cytotoxic cancer chemotherapy
- To shorten the duration of neutropenia in patients undergoing bone marrow transplantation
- To stimulate the release of progenitor cells in circulation and to reduce number of collections of peripheral blood stem cells (PBSC) necessary for transplant in patient undergoing PBSC transplantation
- To expand the number of harvested progenitor cells *ex vivo* before infusing them
- To increase the peripheral blood neutrophils in prospective donors
- For persistent neutropenia in patients with AIDS

They may be used in patients with aplastic anaemia and myelodysplasia.

See Chapter 36 for drugs causing neutropenia.

DRUGS USED IN THROMBOCYTOPENIA

OPRELVEKIN: It is a **recombinant human IL-11** available for cancer-chemotherapy-induced severe thrombocytopenia. This thrombopoietic growth factor stimulates the hematopoietic stem cells and megakaryocyte progenitor cells to proliferate and mature as platelets. Given subcutaneously, thrombopoietic response occurs within 5–9 days. Two forms of **r-thrombopoietin** are also available. However, **platelet transfusions are commonly used to treat thrombocytopenia.** Considering the immunogenicity of recombinant preparations, smaller molecular weight thrombopoeitin-mimetics such as

Romiplostim (for SC use) and **Eltrombopag** (for oral use) have been developed. These agents promote megakaryocyte growth and maturation by binding to thrombopoietin receptors. They are used in the treatment of idiopathic thrombocytopenia (ITP) and thrombocytopenia that may occur in hepatitis C, viral infections, cancer chemotherapy and myelodysplastic syndromes.

CHAPTER 36

Drug-Induced Blood Dyscrasias

Learning Objectives

This chapter will enable the reader:

1. To classify drug-induced blood dyscrasias.
2. To enlist drugs causing megaloblastic anaemia.
3. To enumerate drugs causing aplastic anaemia and present key points in its treatment.
4. To enlist drugs causing haemolytic anaemia.
5. To explain the basis of drug-induced haemolytic reactions in G-6-PD-deficient individuals.
6. To mention drugs causing methaemoglobinaemia and state its treatment.
7. To enumerate drugs causing neutropenia and present key points in its treatment.
8. To enlist drugs causing thrombocytopenia and present key points in its treatment.

KEY TERMS

drugs causing aplastic anaemia, p. 534
aplastic anaemia, treatment, p. 534
drugs causing haemolysis in G-6-PD deficiency, p. 534
drugs causing methaemoglobinaemia, p. 534
drugs causing neutropenia, p. 535
drugs causing thrombocytopenia, p. 535

Various types of blood dyscrasias may occur following the use of certain drugs in toxic doses or sometimes even in therapeutic doses (e.g. bleeding due to NSAIDs and anticoagulants). These reactions can be grouped into the following:

- **Those due to impaired production of blood cells,** e.g. aplastic anaemia
- **Those due to increased destruction of blood cells,** e.g. haemolytic anaemias
- **Those due to derangement of blood cell functions,** e.g. methaemoglobinaemia

The important drug-induced blood dyscrasias are as follows:

Drug-induced anaemias: Megaloblastic anaemia following certain drugs has already been discussed in Chapter 35. Drugs responsible for this can be grouped as follows:

I. **Folic acid inhibitors:**
   - **DHF reductase inhibitors or folic acid antagonists:** Methotrexate, pyrimethamine, triamterene, trimethoprim
   - **Associated with impaired absorption and/or utilisation of folic acid:** Phenytoin, primidone, barbiturates, cycloserine, alcohol and probably oral contraceptive agents

II. **Those which cause vitamin B_{12} malabsorption:** PAS, colchicine, neomycin

III. **Antiinflammatory drugs and anticoagulants** can cause iron-deficiency anaemia secondary to blood loss

IV. **Isoniazid (INH)** causes pyridoxine responsive anaemia which is a hypochromic microcytic anaemia with normal serum iron. The anaemia is probably due to inability of iron to get incorporated into haemoglobin. It responds to the oral administration of pyridoxine.

Aplastic anaemia: This is the most severe type of blood dyscrasia; fortunately, it is rare. The evidence that a given drug is responsible for aplastic anaemia in a given patient is largely circumstantial and in many cases toxicity may occur 2 weeks to 6 months after cessation of therapy. It is associated with

Box 36.1 Drugs Causing Aplastic Anaemia

NSAIDs: Indomethacin, phenylbutazone, oxyphenbutazone
Anticancer drugs: Cytotoxic drugs, vinca alkaloids
Antimicrobials: Chloramphenicol, sulphonamides
Insecticides: DDT, gamma benzene hydrochloride
Antithyroid drugs: Propylthiouracil, perchlorate
Oral antidiabetic drugs: Sulphonylureas
Anti-epileptics: Carbamazepine, phenytoin
Miscellaneous: Gold salts, acetazolamide, penicillamine

PH 1.35

pancytopenia and hypocellular bone marrow. The mortality is very high (more than 50%) and recovery, if it takes place, occurs only after illness for many months. Drugs that are commonly known to produce aplastic anaemia are listed in Box 36.1.

The treatment of aplastic anaemia is outlined in Box 36.2.

Haemolytic anaemia (haemolytic reaction)occurs generally with drugs which can oxidise haemoglobin. Normally, the RBCs contain the enzyme, glucose 6-phosphate dehydrogenase (G-6-PD). Normal functioning of G-6-PD is necessary for maintaining glutathione in its reduced form, which in turn protects the red blood cells from the damage by oxidising agents. The drug- damaged red cells show precipitated denatured haemoglobin, identified as Heinz bodies in an appropriate blood smear preparation.

Box 36.2 Treatment of Aplastic Anaemia

- **Withdrawal of offending agent**
- **Blood transfusions** to control bleeding and relieve anemia symptoms: red blood cell and platelet transfusions
- **Bone marrow transplantation**
- **Immunosuppressants:** Horse antithymocyte globulin (ATG), rabbit antilymphocyte globulin, cyclosporine, steroids (prednisolone 20-40 mg/day). Immunosuppression may be effective in 70%–80% of the patients and is usually recommended in subjects for whom bone marrow transplantation is not available
- **Bone marrow stimulants:** sargramostim, filgrastim/pegfilgrastim, and epoetin alfa - help stimulate the bone marrow to produce new blood cells
- **Prophylactic antimicrobials**

Individuals, in whom RBCs are deficient in G-6-PD, reduced glutathione (GSH) or glutathione reductase are more susceptible to drug-induced haemolysis. Such a deficiency is hereditary. It is known to occur predominantly in Negros and is relatively rare in white population. Its presence has also been noted in Indians.

A haemolytic reaction with oxidant drugs can occur even in normal individuals without G-6-PD deficiency, if the concentration of the oxidant drug is sufficiently high. Drugs which are known to cause haemolytic reactions in G-6-PD deficiency are listed in Box 36.3. Similar reactions can also occur due to improper functioning of phosphogluconate dehydrogenase and glutathione reductase. *In a patient with persistent jaundice (non-obstructive) possibility of G-6-PD deficiency should be ruled out.*

Drugs can also cause haemolysis by an immune mechanism, where the RBC destruction is caused by circulating antibodies. Drugs which can cause immune haemolytic anaemia are methyldopa, quinine, quinidine, stibophen and phenacetin. Patients with abnormal haemoglobins may develop haemolysis if they are given sulphonamides or 8-aminoquinoline drugs. The treatment of haemolytic reactions is essentially symptomatic. Glucocorticoids such as hydrocortisone may produce some beneficial effects in blood dyscrasias caused by immune mechanisms.

Methaemoglobinaemia: The oxygen carrying capacity of red cell haemoglobin is dependent on the availability of haemoglobin iron in the ferrous form. Drugs such as phenacetin, sulphonamides, bismuth subnitrate, ammonium nitrate and nitrites are known to oxidise the haemoglobin iron from ferrous

Box 36.3 Drugs Causing Haemolysis in G-6-PD Deficiency

Antibacterial agents: Sulphonamides, furazolidone, nitrofurantoin, chloramphenicol, fluoroquinolones
Antileprosy drugs (sulphones): Dapsone
Antimalarials: Primaquine, quinine
Miscellaneous agents: Salicylates, doxorubicin, rasburicase, water soluble analogues of vitamin K, niridazole, methylene blue, phenazopyridine

to ferric state and thus cause methaemoglobinaemia. Infants below 6 months are more susceptible to this reaction, probably on account of a low concentration of the erythrocyte enzyme nicotinamide adenine dinucleotide hydrogen (NADH) which normally reduces methaemoglobin to haemoglobin. This enzyme is also genetically deficient in certain individuals who are more prone to develop drug-induced methaemoglobinaemia.

Treatment consists of stoppage of the offending drug and the administration of methylene blue, an effective antidote. 50 mL of 1% solution is administered intravenously.

Neutropenia: In this condition, specific depression of leucocytes, particularly granulocytes, occurs. Drugs known to produce this condition do so relatively frequently, in 1 in 1000 to 1 in 100 of patients. Certain drugs like amidopyrine and dipyrone produce neutropenia by an immune mechanism. However, with drugs like phenothiazines and antithyroid compounds the exact mechanism is not known. Drugs that are commonly known to produce neutropenia are listed in Box 36.4.

Box 36.4 Drugs Causing Neutropenia and Agranulocytosis

Antipsychotics: Chlorpromazine and related drugs, clozapine
Antidepressants: TCA (imipramine)
Analgesics: NSAIDs (phenylbutazone, analgin, indomethacin)
Antiepileptics: Carbamazepine, phenytoin, valproic acid, ethosuximide
Diuretics: Thiazides, furosemide, acetazolamide
Antihypertensives: Propranolol, ACEI (enalapril, captopril)
Antibacterial agents: Chloramphenicol, sulphonamides, dapsone, streptomycin, cotrimoxazole, macrolides, penicillins, cephalosporins, vancomycin
Antifungal agents: Amphotericin B, flucytosine
Antimalarial agents: Chloroquine, quinine, amodiaquine
Antithyroid drugs: Propylthiouracil, methimazole
Miscellaneous: Tocainide, thiacetazone, deferiprone, H_2 blockers, isotretinoin, sulphasalazine, gold preparations

Periodic blood counts may not necessarily predict impending neutropenia. **Patients taking such drugs, therefore, should be warned about unexplained fever, or sore throat with ulceration, and should be instructed to report immediately.** The mortality rate is more than 20%, mainly as a result of infection, which needs prompt treatment. Blood transfusion may be necessary. Treatment with human GCSF is discussed in Chapter 35.

Thrombocytopenia: This is a less frequent complication and in most cases is due to immune mechanisms. Drugs known to cause thrombocytopenia are listed in Box 36.5. Quinidine is most commonly involved in causing this reaction. In addition, all drugs causing aplastic anaemia also cause thrombocytopenia.

Box 36.5 Drugs Causing Thrombocytopenia

Immune mediated
Antiarrhythmics: Quinidine, procainamide, amiodarone
Antimicrobials: Sulphonamides, penicillins, cephalosporins, rifampicin, ethambutol, linezolid, daptomycin, levofloxacin, valacyclovir, vancomycin
Antiepileptics: Phenytoin, carbamazepine, valproic acid
Analgesics: NSAIDs
Antiplatelets: Eptifibatide, tirofiban, abciximab
Diuretics: Thiazides, furosemide, acetazolamide
H_2 receptor antagonists: Cimetidine, ranitidine
Miscellaneous: Alpha methyldopa, gold compounds, danazol, heparin, quinine, mirtazepine
Nonimmune mediated
Anticancer drugs: Bleomycin, vincristine, carboplatin, cytosine arabinoside, irinotecan, alkylating agents

9
SECTION

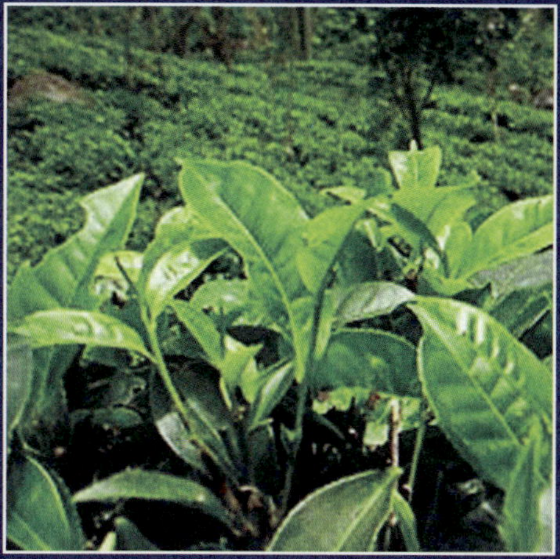
Camellia sinensis

Drugs Affecting Renal Functions

Section Outline

This section consists of the following chapter:

CHAPTER 37

Diuretic and Antidiuretic Drugs, and Drug-Induced Nephrotoxicity

Learning Objectives

This chapter will enable the reader:

1. To be aware of the physiology of urine formation.
2. To classify diuretics according to efficacy giving examples of agents from each class.
3. To explain the site and mechanism of action, pharmacological effects, adverse effects and indications for osmotic diuretics, carbonic anhydrase inhibitors, thiazides, loop diuretics and potassium-sparing diuretics.
4. To state the nondiuretic uses of diuretics.
5. To outline the management of various types of oedema, i.e. cardiac oedema, cirrhotic oedema, pulmonary oedema, cerebral oedema and nutritional oedema.
6. To explain the mechanisms of diuretic resistance.
7. To explain the complications of diuretic therapy.
8. To outline the management of acute renal failure.
9. To be aware of the physiological functions of vasopressin.
10. To mention the mechanism of action, pharmacological effects, ADR, indications of vasopressin and its analogues as well as vasopressin receptor agonists.
11. To explain the pharmacological basis for use of thiazides, chlorpropamide and carbamazepine in treatment of diabetes insipidus.
12. To enlist different types of drug induced nephrotoxicity with suitable examples.

KEY TERMS

The kidneys play an important role in regulating the volume and the maintaining the electrolyte composition of the body fluids. They also secrete erythropoietin and thus serve as an endocrine organ. They have a rich blood supply; almost 25% of cardiac output is received by the kidneys. Hence, several drugs and their metabolites during their passage through the kidneys can cause either beneficial or adverse effects.

The functional unit of the kidney is termed as the **nephron** (Fig. 37.1). Drugs can modify the renal functions:

- **Indirectly by modifying its blood supply**
- **Directly by affecting the nephron function.** Most of the therapeutically useful agents act mainly by modifying various functions of the nephron.

Physiology of Urine Formation

The volume and composition of urine are essentially determined by **glomerular filtration, tubular reabsorption** and **active tubular secretion**.

Urine formation begins in the glomerular capillary tufts by the process of ultrafiltration of the plasma. Both the renal plasma flow and glomerular filtration can be affected by factors which may cause sodium retention and oedema, e.g. chronic heart failure and renal vascular disease. **The GFR is directly related to the cortical blood flow** since 90%–95% of the renal blood flow passes through the cortex. **The medullary blood flow is an important factor contributing to the concentrating ability of the kidney.**

PGE_2 synthesised in the renal medulla participates in the autoregulation of renal blood flow and glomerular filtration.

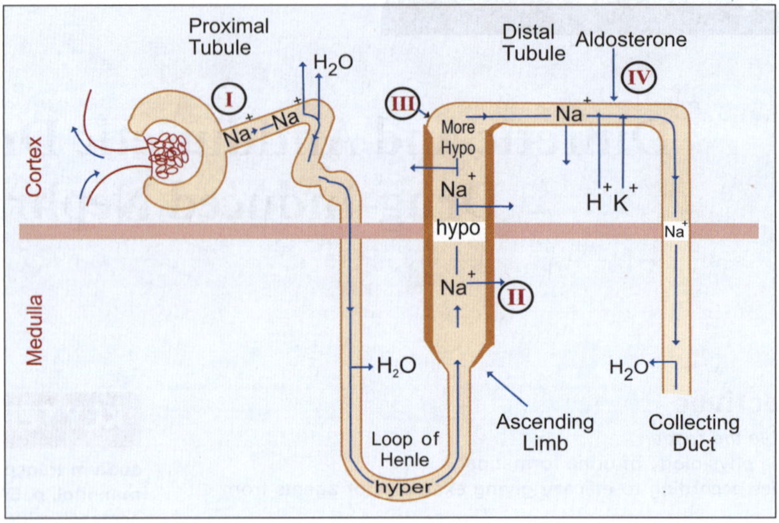

FIG 37.1 The simplified schematic diagram showing functional subdivisions of a mammalian nephron and sites of diuretic action on sodium reabsorption: (I) proximal tubule, (II) ascending limb of Henle's loop, (III) early distal tubule and (IV) distal tubular Na^+/K^+ exchange site.

The transport of sodium and other solutes across the tubular epithelial cells involves several mechanisms: (1) solute movement with bulk water flow; (2) simple diffusion; (3) channel-mediated diffusion; (4) carrier-mediated or facilitated diffusion (**uniport**); (5) primary ATP-mediated transport and (6) secondary ATP-mediated transport which is either in the same direction (cotransport or **symport**) or in opposite directions (counter transport or **antiport**). Sodium is actively transported from the basolateral surface of tubular epithelial cells, involving Na^+–K^+–ATPase pump.

Nearly, 60%–70% of the filtered sodium is reabsorbed in the **proximal tubule** along with water (*obligatory reabsorption*), so that the tubular fluid remains isotonic with plasma. The sodium reabsorption in the proximal tubule varies with changes in ECF and GFR; it is enhanced markedly in response to contraction of ECF volume and acute reduction in GFR from any cause, whereas it is depressed following ECF expansion which causes the release of a natriuretic hormone. *Reabsorption of sodium is the event of primary importance in tubular reabsorption of chloride, water and urea.* Bicarbonates are absorbed with the help of carbonic anhydrase enzyme.

Quantitatively less (25%) of filtered sodium is absorbed from the **loop of Henle** (Fig. 37.1). Juxtaglomerular apparatus (JG) is located at the vascular pole of the glomerulus and contains the myoepithelial cells, which secrete renin. **The JG apparatus is responsible for tubulo-glomerular feedback which regulates the glomerular haemodynamics by altering the renin secretion.**

The loop of Henle acts as a **counter-current multiplier**. According to the counter-current concept, the descending and the ascending limbs of the loop (Fig. 37.1) have relatively different permeabilities to water and sodium:

1. In the **thick segment of the ascending limb**, sodium and chloride are actively transported (**symport**) from the tubular lumen to the interstitium. The tubular epithelium at this site is impermeable to water and hence, the tubular fluid becomes dilute (hypotonic) and the interstitium becomes hypertonic.
2. In contrast, the **descending limb** is permeable to water, which is absorbed readily into the hypertonic interstitium

Hence, the tubular fluid, which is isotonic with plasma at its entry into the descending limb of the loop of Henle, becomes progressively more hypertonic as it approaches the tip of the loop. From then on, its osmolality diminishes progressively because of passive reabsorption of Na^+ from the ascending thin limb and active extrusion of chloride (accompanied by sodium) from the ascending thick limb of the loop. Thus, the fluid entering the distal convoluted tubule (site III) is hypotonic to plasma. This circular and repetitive transfer of sodium across the loop is called the **hairpin counter-current multiplier system.** It is largely responsible for creating a hypertonic medullary interstitium. **Preferential transport of sodium by the ascending limb with its low water permeability is important in the process of concentration of the urine.**

The active reabsorption of sodium along with chloride through specific sodium channels continues in the **late distal convoluted tubule and the collecting tubule.**

Most of the potassium filtered by the glomeruli (80%) is reabsorbed in the proximal tubules and the fluid presented to the distal tubule probably does not contain any potassium. **The potassium that appears in the urine is, therefore, secreted by the distal tubule in exchange for sodium which is reabsorbed.** The exchange of potassium is largely under the influence of aldosterone. Excess of aldosterone causes sodium retention and potassium depletion.

Most of the *filtered calcium (70%) is reabsorbed in the proximal tubule. About 25% of the filtered magnesium is reabsorbed in the proximal tubule, whereas 70% is reabsorbed in the thick ascending limb.*

The final volume and composition of the urine to be excreted is regulated by the **collecting duct.** The urine entering the collecting tubule is isotonic with plasma. *Under the influence of arginine Vasopressin (AVP), collecting ducts are relatively permeable to water which passes freely to hyperosmotic renal medulla, thus concentrating the urine further.* Collecting ducts in addition, also reabsorb sodium actively under the influence of aldosterone and secrete H^+ and ammonium ions.

Since tubules normally absorb over 99% of the glomerular filtrate, marked diuresis can be achieved by interfering with the tubular reabsorption of sodium. However, a diuretic acting on the proximal tubule alone is not so potent since its effect is counterbalanced by increased distal reabsorption.

DIURETICS

Diuretic are the drugs which increase the rate of urine formation together with natriuresis.

Only a few drugs produce diuresis by increasing the GFR; **most of the diuretics used therapeutically act by interfering with sodium reabsorption by the tubules.**

Classification of Diuretics PH 1.24

I. **Weakly efficacious diuretics**
   - **Osmotic diuretics** such as mannitol, isosorbide, sucrose and glycerol
   - **Carbonic anhydrase inhibitors** such as acetazolamide
   - **Potassium-sparing diuretics**
     1. **Aldosterone antagonists:** Spironolactone, potassium canreonate and eplerenone
     2. **Renal epithelial sodium channel inhibitors:** Triamterene and amiloride

II. **Moderately efficacious diuretics**
   - **Benzothiadiazines (thiazides) and related compounds** such as chlorthalidone, chlorexolone, and indapamide.

III. **Highly efficacious diuretics (high ceiling-loop diuretics),** e.g. furosemide, mefruside, bumetanide and ethacrynic acid.

Classification of diuretics according to the site of action is given in Table 37.1.

Water, when given in excess, acts as a physiological diuretic. During water diuresis, the antidiuretic hormone (ADH) remains inhibited. The urine consists of water that is excreted along with the electrolytes (**osmolar clearance**) as well as the solute free portion (**free water clearance**). In oedema, the basic problem is sodium retention, followed by secondary water retention. In such cases, water does not act as a diuretic. **Water diuresis** is used to wash out drugs which irritate the urinary tract or possess limited solubility in the urine, e.g. salicylates or sulphonamides. It is also useful in urinary tract infection (UTI).

WEAKLY EFFICACIOUS DIURETICS

These diuretics have a weak action and cause excretion of less than 5% the filtered NaCl.

OSMOTIC DIURETICS

Osmotic diuretics are solutes with the following properties. They are:

- **Pharmacologically inert**
- **Generally nonmetabolisable**
- **Increase osmolality of the plasma and tubular fluid**
- **Freely filtered at the glomerulus**

Table 37.1 Site of Action of Diuretics and Their Effects

Site of Action	Drug Group	Mechanism of Action	Effect on Ions
Proximal tubule	Carbonic anhydrase inhibitors	Inhibition of carbonic anhydrase	Inhibition of Na^+–H^+ exchange indirectly
Loop of Henle and proximal tubule	Osmotic diuretics	Osmotic effect reduces medullary tonicity	Limits passive reabsorption of Na^+
Thick ascending limb of loop of Henle	Loop diuretics	Inhibition of Na^+–K^+–2 Cl^- symport	Inhibition of reabsorption of Na^+ and Cl^- and increased excretion of K^+
Site in distal tubule before Na^+/H^+ exchange	Thiazides	Inhibition of Na^+–Cl^- symport	Inhibition of reabsorption of Na^+ and Cl^- and increased excretion of K^+
Late segment of distal tubule (site of Na^+/H^+ exchange) and collecting duct	Aldosterone antagonist	Blockade of mineralocorticoid receptors	Inhibition of Na^+ reabsorption and reduced excretion of K^+
	Triamterene, amiloride	Inhibition of renal epithelial sodium channels	

- **Not significantly reabsorbed by the renal tubules**

Mechanism of action: In the proximal tubule, sodium is actively absorbed from tubular lumen, dragging water passively along with it. In the presence of a nonabsorbable solute such as mannitol, diffusion of water is reduced relative to that of sodium. As a consequence the net absorption of sodium diminishes. *There is an enhanced urine flow with a relatively smaller increase in the sodium excretion.* However, this action is of secondary importance; the main site of action of the osmotic diuretics is the loop of Henle. They expand the ECF and increase the renal blood flow, thereby reducing the medullary tonicity, which inhibits water extraction from the descending limb. This limits the passive reabsorption of sodium from the thick ascending limb of the loop.

The **other osmotically active solutes** are urea, glucose and isosorbide. *In case of glucose, this mechanism becomes operative when the tubular maximum limit for reabsorption of glucose is exceeded because of hyperglycaemia, as in DM.*

The osmotic diuretics retain their effectiveness even when GFR is acutely reduced (as in hypotension or dehydration). Although the GFR is reduced, a substance like mannitol is filtered at the glomerulus and is excreted in the voided urine, dragging water (and sodium) with it, causing diuresis.

MANNITOL: It is a sugar (polyhydroxy aliphatic alcohol) which, when injected intravenously, is not metabolised and is rapidly filtered by the glomeruli causing osmotic diuresis. It increases excretion of all the electrolytes including magnesium and calcium.

To be effective, mannitol has to be administered in sufficiently large doses. It is not a suitable diuretic to treat cardiac oedema, because it increases the ECF volume by extracting water from the cells, thus increasing further the load on the heart. When the renal tubules are damaged, in addition to reduction in GFR (as happens with nephrotoxic agents or with prolonged, severe, renal ischemia), they become permeable to mannitol, which then loses its capacity to induce diuresis.

Adverse reactions: It can cause headache, nausea, chills, polydipsia, confusion and pain in the chest. Excessive amounts or rapid infusion of mannitol can cause cellular dehydration; pulmonary oedema in patients with HF and hyponatraemia. Extravasation of mannitol may cause thrombophlebitis.

It is supplied as 25% solution in ampoules of 50 mL for IV use. Contraindications to mannitol are given in Box 37.1.

Indications:

- **Barbiturate poisoning:** It is useful in *barbiturate poisoning* to increase the urinary elimination of barbiturate. In such cases, it is infused as a 5%–25% solution. However, the loop diuretic furosemide is preferred.
- **Threatened acute renal failure:** It is also useful in any condition of threatened acute oliguric renal failure from prerenal causes (e.g. severe gastroenteritis) which result in hypovolaemia and hypotension. In such cases, after initial correction of hypovolaemia, mannitol is given to maintain the high urine flow rate. This may prevent the establishment of acute renal failure (ARF).
  Mannitol is also used preoperatively during aortic surgery or surgery in a deeply jaundiced patient, which are known to increase the risk of ARF. It is also useful in preventing acute oliguric renal failure after severe trauma and haemolytic transfusion reactions.
- **Raised intraocular pressure (IOP):** Mannitol infusion is used in the dose of 1.5–2 g/kg (in 30–60 min) to reduce IOP **in acute congestive glaucoma** (see Chapter 70)
- **Cerebral oedema:** See Box 37.5
- **During rapid dialysis,** to maintain osmolality of ECF

GLYCEROL: Glycerol is used orally in the dose of 1–1.5 g/kg (maximum dose 120 g per day), as a 50%–75% solution, prior to ophthalmological procedures. Glycerol has been claimed to avoid the 'rebound oedema', which may occur after mannitol. It can be used in the presence of dehydration and cardiac failure where mannitol cannot be used. It has been used in the treatment of acute cerebral infarction, given IV daily 10% in 500 mL saline for 6 days. Rapid infusion of high concentrations (30%) can cause haemolysis. It also causes hyperglycaemia.

Box 37.1 Contraindications to Mannitol

- Pulmonary congestion/oedema
- Intracranial bleeding, except during craniotomy
- Heart failure
- Metabolic oedema with abnormal capillary fragility
- Established acute renal failure with anuria

CARBONIC ANHYDRASE INHIBITORS

ACETAZOLAMIDE: This drug (Fig. 37.2), a **weak diuretic,** is unique because of its mechanism of action.

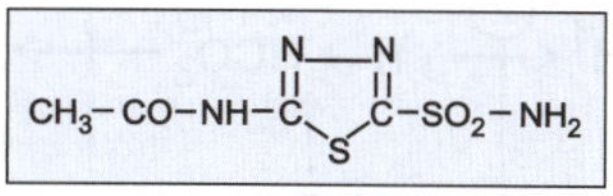

Fig. 37.2 Acetazolamide.

Mechanism of action: In the proximal tubule, H^+ ion is transported from the tubular cell cytoplasm to the tubular lumen in exchange for the Na^+ ion which is absorbed into the tubular cell (antiport) and is pushed out into the interstitium by Na^+–K^+–ATPase pump (Fig. 37.3). In the lumen, H^+ reacts with the filtered HCO_3 to form H_2CO_3 which splits into CO_2 and water.

$$H^+ + HCO_3^- \rightarrow H_2CO_3$$
$$H_2CO_3 \rightarrow H_2O + CO_2$$

The CO_2 diffuses across the luminal membrane into the tubular epithelial cell where it forms H_2CO_3, a reaction that is catalysed by **cytoplasmic carbonic anhydrase**. Within the cytoplasm, H_2CO_3 splits into HCO_3 and H^+. The hydrogen ion then repeats the above cycle and exchanges with luminal Na+ which is reabsorbed into the tubular cell. The HCO_3 in the tubular cell cytoplasm gets transferred into the interstitium, where it combines with Na^+ to form $NaHCO_3$. $NaHCO_3$ thus formed is reabsorbed into the systemic circulation.

Thus the enzyme carbonic anhydrase plays an important role in the tubular reabsorption of sodium and bicarbonate (Fig. 37.3). The enzyme carbonic anhydrase is also present in the gastric mucosa, pancreas, eyes, CNS and RBC.

Acetazolamide inhibits carbonic anhydrase so that:

a. carbonic acid (H_2CO_3) is not formed
b. hydrogen ion is not made available for sodium exchange, leading to excretion of luminal sodium along with water
c. *bicarbonate remains in the poorly diffusible form and hence excreted in large amounts with sodium*

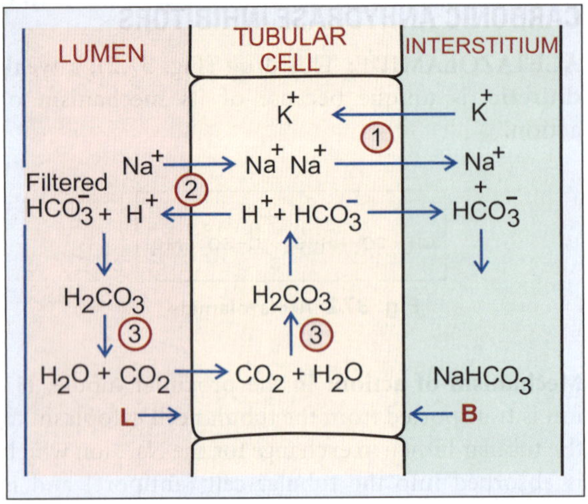

Fig. 37.3 **Carbonic anhydrase action in renal tubules. 1, Na^+K^+ ATPase; 2, Na^+/H^+ exchanger; 3, carbonic anhydrase, L, luminal cell membrane; B, basolateral cell membrane. L, B and cytoplasm are rich in carbonic anhydrase.**

Pharmacological actions:

Kidney and electrolytes: As acetazolamide is a carbonic anhydrase inhibitor, it causes loss of sodium, potassium, bicarbonate and phosphate ions in the urine. The urine becomes alkaline. Since exchange of potassium and hydrogen ions with sodium occurs in the distal tubule, the decrease in available hydrogen ion may promote more loss of potassium. The resulting decrease in the ECF base may cause metabolic acidosis which ends the diuretic action. Acetazolamide is thus a self-limiting diuretic.

Eye: Carbonic anhydrase present in the ciliary processes is important in the production of aqueous humour, which has a high bicarbonate content. Acetazolamide reduces the intraocular pressure by inhibiting this enzyme (Chapter 70).

CNS: Acetazolamide decreases the CSF formation. For its antiepileptic action, see Chapter 9.

Absorption, fate and excretion: Acetazolamide, given orally, is well absorbed. It is not metabolised but is actively secreted into the urine by the proximal tubular cells through the organic acid pathway.

Adverse reactions: It can cause excessive potassium loss (hypokalemia) and metabolic acidosis. Occasionally, it may cause drowsiness and paraesthesiae. It can lead to renal calcium and phosphorus calculi formation. Rarely, it causes skin rashes, blood dyscrasias, and kidney damage. Salicylates enhance its toxicity by inhibiting its plasma protein binding and by interfering with its renal tubular secretion.

Preparation and dosage: Acetazolamide 0.25 g tablet; dose: 1–2 tablets daily in divided doses. Sodium acetazolamide can be given parenterally.

Indications: *It is no more used as a diuretic.* Its use is restricted to the following:

- **Prophylaxis and treatment of high altitude illness:** This term is used to describe the cerebral and pulmonary syndromes that can develop in unacclimatised persons after rapid ascent to high altitude. At these heights, the low partial pressure of atmospheric oxygen causes marked hypoxemia, resulting in tissue hypoxia. Resulting neurohumoral and haemodynamic responses lead to hyperperfusion of microvascular beds, capillary leakage and consequent local oedema.

The **cerebral syndrome** comprises acute mountain sickness and cerebral oedema. Early symptoms of the cerebral syndrome are headache, and impairment of memory, judgement and ability to perform complex calculations. Other manifestations are anorexia, malaise and insomnia. The **pulmonary syndrome** is due to high altitude noncardiogenic pulmonary oedema. The early symptoms are decreased performance and dry cough. Later manifestations are respiratory distress, resting tachycardia, tachypnoea, fever and pink or frank bloody sputum and later noncardiogenic pulmonary oedema with pulmonary arterial hypertension and retinal haemorrhages. Coma and death can occur.

Thus respiratory alkalosis caused by hyperventilation further limits the rise in ventilation and leads to symptoms of acute mountain sickness. Acetazolamide counteracts this respiratory alkalosis, allows chemoreceptors to respond more effectively to hypoxic stimuli at high altitude, improves ventilation and hastens acclimatization. The principles of prevention and treatment of these conditions are presented in Box 37.2.

- **Treatment of glaucoma** (Chapter 70)
- **Treatment of resistant epilepsy** (Chapter 9)
- **Prevention of attacks of periodic paralysis**

METHAZOLAMIDE, another carbonic anhydrase inhibitor, related to acetazolamide, is used orally in the treatment of glaucoma (Chapter 70).

POTASSIUM-SPARING DIURETICS

These agents **inhibit Na^+ absorption** in the distal tubule, collecting ducts and concomitantly, indirectly **suppress the secretion of K^+ and H^+**, thus preventing potassium loss. They are as follows:

- **Aldosterone antagonist:** spironolactone
- **Direct inhibitors of renal epithelial sodium channels:** triamterene and amiloride

Both drugs can cause hyperkalaemic, hyperchloraemic and metabolic acidosis. However, they do not affect renal haemodynamics.

SPIRONOLACTONE: Spironolactone, with structural similarity to aldosterone (Fig. 37.4), is a commonly employed **aldosterone antagonist.**

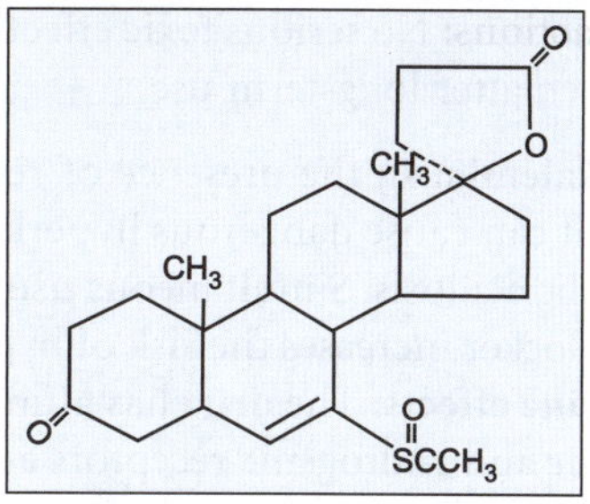

Fig. 37.4 Spironolactone.

Mechanism of action: It enters the tubular cells from basolateral surface and competitively antagonises aldosterone, in the distal part of the nephron, (**late distal diuretic**). It thus prevents potassium secretion (loss) and decreases sodium reabsorption. By itself, it does not produce significant natriuresis in normal individuals. Even in oedema associated with an excess of aldosterone, its natriuretic action is weak.

Given orally, its full response is observed after 3–5 days. It has a short t½ of 1.6 h. Its major action is due to an **active metabolite, canrenone** (t½ 17 h). *In combination with thiazide or loop diuretics, it prevents loss of potassium*. It is metabolised to several inactive compounds.

Box 37.2 Prevention and Treatment of High Altitude Sickness

I. **For acute mountain sickness and cerebral oedema:**
   a. Gradual ascent to high altitude to promote acclimatisation
   b. Avoidance of overexertion
   c. Descent to lower altitude at the first appearance of symptoms. Descent may be simulated by stay in a portable hyperbaric oxygen chamber (Chapter 75).
   d. Supplementary oxygen
   e. **Drugs:**
      (i) Prophylactic **acetazolamide** 250 mg 12 hourly, the day before, during and for 5 days after the ascent. It causes mild metabolic acidosis, which increases the respiratory drive, prevents hypoxemia and produces a pharmacological response resembling an acclimatisation response. *Acetazolamide ameliorates symptoms but does not reduce the risk of cerebral oedema, pulmonary oedema or retinal haemorrhages.* Hence, it *is no substitute for slow ascent.*
      (ii) **Dexamethasone**, 4 mg every 8–12 h, begun on the day of the ascent, continued for 3 days at high altitude, and then tapered quickly, may be useful in reducing the incidence and early symptoms of acute mountain sickness. *Acetazolamide and dexamethasone are useful for both prevention and treatment.*
      (iii) Adjunct drugs used are **NSAID** and **antiemetics,** when necessary

II. **For pulmonary syndrome:** The nonpharmacological measures are the same as above.
   (i) **Nifedipine** is the preferred drug. It probably lowers pulmonary arterial pressure, which is critical in the development of pulmonary oedema
   (ii) **Beta adrenergic agonists:** They clear the fluid from the alveolar space and may lower pulmonary arterial pressure
   (iii) **Dexamethasone** if cerebral symptoms develop

Prophylactic nifedipine should be considered before a future ascent in a person with a history of high altitude pulmonary oedema.

Adverse reactions: No serious toxic effects have been reported even after long-term use.

- **Hyperkalemia:** In the presence of renal insufficiency, it can cause dangerous hyperkalemia and metabolic acidosis. Simultaneous use of ACEI or a beta blocker increases the risk of hyperkalemia.
- **Endocrine effects:** The drug has affinity for progesterone and androgenic receptors and has been shown to block gonadal and adrenal steroidogenesis. This may cause decreased libido, gynecomastia, impotence and menstrual irregularity.
- **Miscellaneous effects:** Spironolactone may cause lethargy and drowsiness. It may increase blood urea nitrogen and serum uric acid levels. It can cause gastritis and is avoided in patients with acid-peptic disease. NSAIDS may inhibit the excretion of this drug.

Preparation and dosage: Spironolactone (micro crystalline), 25, 50, 100 mg tablet. Dose: 100–200 mg per day (maximum 400 mg) in divided doses.

Indications: It is used in

- The **treatment of oedema** particularly cirrhotic oedema (see section on management of edema-cirrhotic edema and ascites)
- **Severe chronic heart failure** (Chapter 31)
- The **treatment of hypertension,** as an adjunct to thiazide diuretics (Chapter 30)
- **Patients with hirsutism due to polycystic ovarian disease** (Chapter 67)
- The **treatment of primary hyperaldosteronism** (Conn syndrome): It corrects the electrolyte abnormalities and lowers the BP

POTASSIUM CANREONATE: This prodrug gets converted to canrenone in the body, and has similar uses as spironolactone but it can be given parenterally. It is given intravenously, slowly, up to 400 mg per day, in divided doses.

EPLERENONE blocks the mineralocorticoid receptors in the kidney, heart, blood vessels and brain more selectively than spironolactone; it has lower affinity for the androgen and progesterone receptors.

It is metabolised by the liver and has a t½ of 4–6 h. The ADR include GI intolerance, dizziness, hyperkalemia and hypertriglyceridemia. Its probable advantage over spironolactone is the lower incidence of endocrine side effects. It is used to treat:

- **Hypertension,** in the dose of 50 mg o.d., increased to 100 mg o.d. (maximum dose) within 4 weeks, as required
- **Post-MI heart failure,** in one half of the above dosage

Recently oral nonsteroidal mineralocorticoid receptor antagonist **Finerenone** has been approved as an add on therapy to slow the progression of chronic kidney disease (CKD) and reduce the risk of cardiovascular events in patients with advanced CKD and type 2 diabetes. It appears to cause less hyperkalemia.

TRIAMTERENE: This drug (Fig. 37.5) increases the excretion of water, sodium, chloride and bicarbonate but it **depresses the excretion of potassium.** In this respect, it resembles the aldosterone antagonist spironolactone.

Mechanism of action: It acts on the late distal tubule and collecting duct and blocks renal epithelial Na^+ channels competitively, thus prevents K^+ loss. It also spares magnesium loss. *Triamterene has no antihypertensive action.*

It is administered orally in the dose of 100–200 mg. It is secreted by proximal tubules. Its peak effect is reached in about 2 h, and the action lasts for 10 h because of an active metabolite.

Adverse reactions: No serious toxic effects have been noted. Besides causing hyperkalemia, the drug may cause troublesome diarrhoea. Occasionally, skin rash and dryness of mouth have been noted. It may cause a decrease in glucose tolerance and a rise in blood urea level. Chronic administration decreases the uric acid excretion and may cause renal calculi.

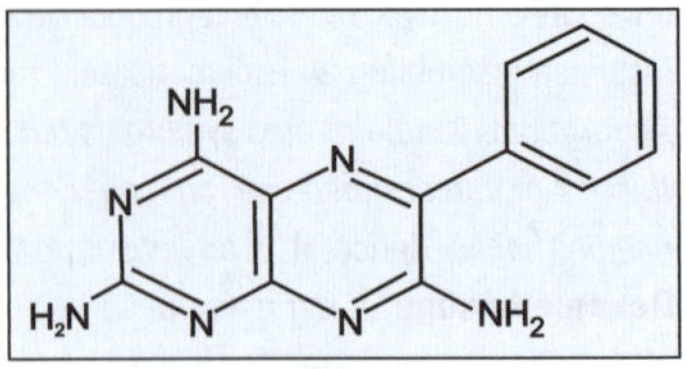

Fig. 37.5 Triamterene.

Indications:

- **Potassium-sparing diuretic:** Triamterene itself is a weak diuretic. However, it is usually combined with a thiazide or loop diuretic to prevent the potassium loss.
- **Pseudo-aldosteronism:** The drug has also been used in 'pseudo-aldosteronism', a familial renal disorder characterised by hypertension, and hypokalemia but without increased aldosterone secretion. In such patients, spironolactone is not of much use as the aldosterone secretion is subnormal.

AMILORIDE HYDROCHLORIDE: This compound, a guanidine derivative, has a weak diuretic activity, and is given orally. Its action is similar to that of triamterene. It prevents potassium loss. It has t½ of 6 h and is excreted unchanged in the urine. It is reported to cause photosensitivity. It is used:

- **As a diuretic,** in combination with other diuretics. On weight basis, it is more potent than triamterene.
- **In lithium-induced diabetes insipidus** as it blocks lithium reabsorption from the collecting tubules.
- **In cystic fibrosis:** An aerosolised preparation facilitates mucociliary clearance by blocking bronchial epithelial sodium channels. Reduced reabsorption of Na^+ increases the hydration of bronchial secretions.

MODERATELY EFFICACIOUS DIURETICS

They:

i. Inhibit Na^+–$C1^-$ symport
ii. Have a moderate action and cause excretion of 5%–10% of the filtered NaCl
iii. Have a wide spectrum of duration of action (8–72 h)
iv. Are ineffective with GFR<30 mL/min

BENZOTHIADIAZINES (THIAZIDES)

Introduction of **thiazide diuretics** (Fig. 37.6) revolutionised the oral diuretic therapy.

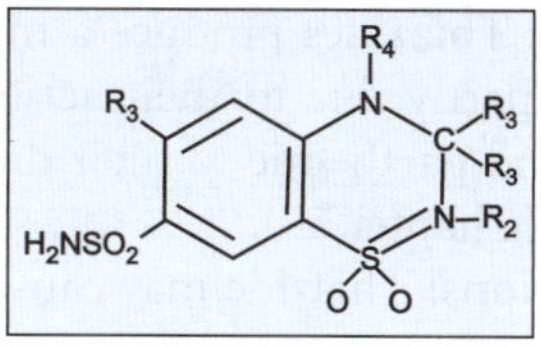

Fig. 37.6 Benzothiadiazine nucleus.

Mechanism of action: Like acetazolamide, these drugs are secreted into the tubular fluid and block the electroneutral Na^+–$C1^-$ symport in the distal convoluted tubule by competing with Na^+ and Cl^- for the binding sites and increase their excretion. **Thiazides primarily act on the site proximal to the sodium and potassium exchange region in the distal tubule** (site III, Fig. 37.1). Hence, they are sometimes known as *early distal diuretics.* The GFR is not affected.

Pharmacological actions:

Kidneys

- Thiazides increase Na^+ and Cl^- excretion but as almost 90% of the filtered load of sodium is reabsorbed before reaching the distal tubules, **they exert only a moderate diuretic effect.**
- Chlorothiazide has a weak carbonic anhydrase inhibitory activity and it causes some loss of bicarbonate. The newer thiazides, however, do not significantly increase the bicarbonate loss.
- Because of the marked inhibitory action on sodium reabsorption, a large amount of sodium is made available to the distal segment where exchange of K^+ with Na^+ takes place. *This may cause increased potassium loss.*
- Excessive renal loss of sodium and chloride may cause hyponatraemia and hypochloraemia; excessive potassium loss can cause hypokalemia, thus leading to *hypokalaemic hypochloraemic alkalosis.* Long-term use causes hypomagnesaemia.
- Initially, the drug causes a diminution in sodium reabsorption in the distal tubule and a gradual reduction in the ECF volume. When the ECF volume falls to slightly below normal, the reabsorption of sodium from the proximal tubule is stimulated, resulting in diminished amount of sodium delivered into the distal tubule. This may explain its decrease diuretic activity and resistance.
- Thiazides are less effective when GFR falls below 30–40 mL/min.

Blood vessels: Thiazides produce a mild antihypertensive effect partly due to their action on sodium metabolism and partly due to their direct action on blood vessels (Chapter 30).

Metabolic actions: Thiazide may cause.

- **Hyperglycaemia:** The mechanism by which thiazides cause hyperglycaemia is not known. These drugs can unmask or aggravate the pre-existing diabetes mellitus. Diazoxide, a thiazide derivative with potent hyperglycaemic action, has been used in the treatment of hypoglycaemia.
  However, during long-term therapy of hypertension, thiazides do not significantly increase the incidence of diabetes mellitus.
- **Hyperuricaemia:** Thiazides also decrease the reabsorption of uric acid from proximal tubule, thus raising plasma uric acid level. In addition, they compete with uric acid for urate transporter causing uric acid retention. Usually, this is asymptomatic but, occasionally, it can precipitate gout.
- **Hypercalcaemia:** Unlike loop diuretics (see section, Loop diuretics), *thiazides reduce urinary calcium loss by acting on distal convoluted tubules* and **promote calcium retention; they are useful in treating idiopathic hypercalciuria.**
- **Hyperlipidaemia:** *Serum cholesterol and triglycerides may increase slightly; however, this has hardly any significance as the elevation is not persistent beyond 6–12 months of treatment.*

Other action: In patients with nephrogenic type diabetes insipidus, thiazides decrease urinary volume (see section, Antidiuretic agents).

Absorption, fate and excretion: Thiazides are well absorbed from the intestine and the effect starts within 1 h. They are distributed throughout the ECF and are relatively concentrated in the kidney. They can cross the placental barrier. Like other organic acids, thiazides are secreted into the tubules and excreted in urine.

The long acting thiazides are long acting because of greater plasma protein binding and greater lipid solubility. Bendroflumethiazide, polythiazide and indapamide are primarily metabolised in the liver; whereas chlorothiazide, hydrochlorothiazide, hydroflumethiazide and chlorthalidone are excreted in the urine. **Plasma half-life of thiazides is sufficient to permit their use once or twice daily.**

Adverse reactions: These are as follows:

- Eelectrolyte disturbances resulting in **hypokalaemic and hypochloraemic alkalosis**. Hypokalemia increases the risk of fatal toxicity of certain arrhythmias (Chapter 28) and drugs like digoxin (Chapter 31). They may cause dilutional hyponatraemia
- Because of structural similarity to sulphonamides, allergic reactions such as dermatitis and thrombocytopenia may rarely occur
- In the presence of renal and hepatic insufficiency, these drugs may precipitate renal failure or hepatic coma

Preparations and dosage: Table 37.2.

Indications:

- **As diuretics:** Thiazides produce effective diuresis in most of the patients with sodium retention and oedema. **There is no special advantage in using any particular preparation;** hydrochlorothiazide is usually preferred. Occasionally, patients may develop resistance to these drugs. In majority of such cases, hypokalemia may be present which needs correction. Excessive potassium loss can be prevented by combining thiazide drugs with spironolactone or triameterene (see section, Potassium sparing diuretics).
- **As antihypertensives:** See Chapter 30.
- **In the prevention of recurrent renal calculi:** In patients with idiopathic hypercalciuria, hydrochlorothiazide (50 mg twice a day) reduces the frequency of stone formation.
- **In nephrogenic diabetes insipidus:** See section, Antidiuretic agents.

Thiazide-like diuretics: These drugs, structurally similar to thiazides, have similar mechanism but longer duration of action. As diuretics, they offer limited advantage over thiazides. These are as follows:

CHLORTHALIDONE: This phthalimidine derivative is absorbed slowly, and is not significantly metabolised.

Table 37.2 Commonly Used Benzothiadiazine and Related Diuretics

Name	Tablet (mg)	Daily Dose as Antihypertensive (mg)	Daily Dose as Diuretic (mg)	Duration of Diuretic Action (h)
Hydrochlorothiazide	12.5, 25, 50	12.5–25	25–200; children: 2 mg/kg	12 or more
Hydroflumethiazide	25, 50	12.5–25	25–200	18–24
Benzthiazide	25	12.5–25	50–200	12–18
Cyclopenthiazide	0.5	0.25–0.5	0.5–1	18–24
Bendroflumethiazide	2.5, 5	1.25–2.5	2.5–5	18–24
Chlorthalidone	6.25, 12.5, 100	12.5–25	50–200	48–72
Metolazone	5	1.25–2.5	5–10	18–24

It remains preferentially bound to renal tissue for prolonged periods. Hence, **its duration of action is longer,** up to 48 h. *It may be preferred in the treatment of hypertension and can be given on alternate days.* It is more liable to cause hypokalemia than the thiazides. It has been reported to be useful in the treatment of hypoparathyroidism where it corrects hypocalcaemia without the danger of causing hypercalcaemia which is inherent in vitamin D therapy of this condition.

Indapamide and **xipamide** are used in the treatment of hypertension (Chapter 30).

Clopamide is administered in a single daily dose of 20–60 mg in the morning, on alternate days. It has longer duration of action (18–24 h).

QUINAZOLINONES: **Quinethazone** and **metolazone** belong to this group. These compounds have diuretic characteristics similar to those of thiazides. Metolazone has the advantage of being effective even when GFR < 30 ml/min.

HIGHLY EFFICACIOUS DIURETICS

They:

- Inhibit Na^+–K^+–$2Cl^-$ symport
- Have a rapid onset and short duration of action
- Cause excretion of 15%–20% of the filtered NaCl
- Are effective even in the presence of markedly reduced GFR
- Tend to be effective when drugs from group II (thiazides), given in maximum doses, fail to act

LOOP DIURETICS

FUROSEMIDE (Frusemide): It is a potent, oral, diuretic, possessing a halogenated sulphamoyl benzene ring common to thiazide diuretics (Fig. 37.7).

Mechanism of action: Like thiazides, furosemide is secreted into the tubular fluid via the organic acid pathway. **The drug acts along the entire nephron (sites II and III in** Fig. 37.1), primarily on the thick ascending limb of the loop of Henle with the exception only of the distal site where Na^+ is exchanged for K^+ and H^+.

- It blocks the Na^+–K^+–$2Cl^-$ symport. It is far more efficacious than thiazides.
- Unlike thiazides, urinary excretion of Na^+ may continue uninterruptedly even when the patient's ECF volume has been severely depleted
- It also inhibits the reabsorption of Ca^{++} and Mg^{++} and causes their loss
- Given IV bolus, it is a venodilator and increases the renal blood flow
- It increases PGE_2 synthesis in the kidneys, which has a locally protective, vasodilator effects

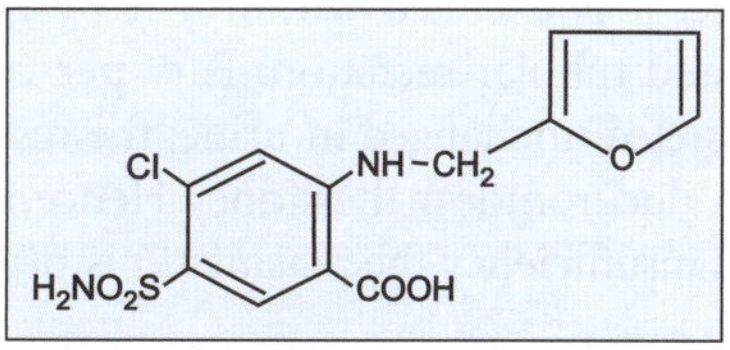

Fig. 37.7 Furosemide. Note the sulphamoyl benzene ring.

Pharmacological actions:

Kidneys:

- Intense diuretic action starts within an hour of oral administration and is completed in 4–6 h. **It has a steep dose–response curve without a ceiling effect.** Because of its short duration of action, furosemide is administered twice a day when sustained diuresis is desired.
- It causes marked sodium, potassium, chloride and phosphate loss. The bicarbonate loss is less marked.
- Excessive chloride loss can cause hypochloraemic alkalosis. The associated potassium loss leads to hypokalemia.
- Furosemide causes little change in the urinary pH and its diuretic action is less affected by the prevailing state of electrolyte or acid–base balance
- GFR is not affected
- Loop diuretics are potent renin releasers

Blood vessels and blood pressure: *Intravenous furosemide dilates the peripheral vasculature, lowers the arterial BP, and causes rapid venous pooling of blood, thus reducing the cardiac preload and afterload*. This action of bringing about a redistribution of blood from the congested pulmonary circulation into the systemic, capacitance vessels is more rapid than its diuretic effect and is perhaps more important in the treatment of acute LVF with pulmonary oedema.

Its effects on the BP on oral administration are comparable to those of thiazide diuretics.

Metabolic actions: Like thiazides, furosemide can cause hyperglycaemia, hyperuricaemia and rise in blood urea. *Calcium and magnesium excretion is increased.*

Absorption, fate and excretion: The drug is rapidly absorbed (60%–100%) from the GI tract. Food reduces its bioavailability. It has rapid onset and short duration of action. Given intravenously, the diuresis begins within 2 min and lasts for 2–3 h. It is best given in a single dose. It is excreted within 4 h by glomerular filtration and tubular secretion. Fifty per cent of the dose is excreted unchanged in urine; the rest is conjugated with glucuronide in the kidney. Hence, in patients with renal insufficiency the plasma t½ is prolonged.

Adverse reactions: Generally, it is well tolerated.

- Being a potent diuretic, it causes excessive loss of sodium, potassium and chloride and can precipitate serious hypovolaemia.
- It can cause fatigue, dizziness, cramps and orthostatic hypotension.
- Rapid diuresis with excessive K^+ loss can precipitate hepatic coma in the presence of liver disease
- Less common reactions include skin rashes, nausea, diarrhoea and rarely acute pancreatitis, thrombocytopenia and neutropenia.
- It can unmask latent diabetes mellitus.
- It increases plasma triglycerides, total and LDL cholesterol.
- **Hearing loss,** usually transient, with or without tinnitus, has been reported following *very large doses* in patients with renal failure.
- Furosemide can enhance the toxicity of lithium, aminoglycosides and cephalosporins. Its action is inhibited by NSAID such as indomethacin.

It should be avoided in pregnancy.

Preparations and dosage: Furosemide tablet 20, 40, 500 mg. Furosemide injection, 20 mg in 2 mL. Dose: 40–100 mg daily.

Indications:

- **As a diuretic:** Furosemide is a very effective, potent and usually safe diuretic. However, it has no distinct advantage over thiazides, in the treatment of moderate oedema. **It is more useful in severe oedema.**
- **Pulmonary oedema:** *Given intravenously, it can be life-saving in patients with pulmonary oedema*
- **Acute renal failure:** See section, Acute renal failure
- **Chronic renal failure:** The dose–response curve with furosemide shows a steep rise due to its high ceiling effect. This makes it possible to use increasing doses of furosemide (unlike thiazide) to cause diuresis in patients with advanced renal failure with marked decrease in GFR (as low as 2 mL/min). *Since the drug continues to act even in the presence of electrolyte and acid–base disturbances, close monitoring of the therapeutic response and blood chemistry is very essential.*
- **Barbiturate poisoning:** It is used to induce forced diuresis (Chapter 6).
- **Hypercalcaemia:** Intravenous furosemide, together with normal saline infusion, is valuable

in the emergency management of hypercalcaemia (Chapter 68).

- **As an antihypertensive:** Furosemide is not recommended for long-term antihypertensive therapy because of high dose requirements, short duration of action and its high diuretic potential.

Torsemide, bumetanide, axosemide, tripamide and **piretanide** are the other diuretics belonging to the furosemide group.

ETHACRYNIC ACID: Ethacrynic acid, an unsaturated ketone derivative of phenoxyacetic acid, is a potent oral diuretic like furosemide. Chemically, it is unrelated to other diuretics.

The diuretic and metabolic effects of ethacrynic acid are similar to those of furosemide. Like furosemide, it can be used in oedematous states, especially in patients allergic to sulphonamides. However, it is more prone to cause adverse effects particularly, nausea and deafness.

The **electrolyte excretion pattern** following the administration of various diuretics is presented in Table 37.3.

Indications for diuretic therapy are given in Box 37.3. The **nondiuretic uses of diuretic drugs** are given in Box 37.4. These are discussed in the respective chapters.

MANAGEMENT OF OEDEMA PH 1.1

Increase in extracellular sodium and fluid volume leads to the development of **'pitting' oedema.** The oedematous states observed in practice are mostly due to decreased rate of renal excretion of sodium and water.

Factors involved in promoting excessive sodium retention are as follows:

1. **Decreased cardiac output** and GFR as in HF
2. **Increased levels of aldosterone** as in oedema due to hepatic cirrhosis
3. **Intrinsic renal disease** such as acute nephritis

Oedema can also occur due to **hypoalbuminaemia** (serum albumin < 2.5 g%) as observed in hypoproteinaemic states, nutritional oedema, cirrhosis and nephrotic syndrome).

Although the treatment of underlying pathology is important in all such cases, great relief can be obtained by using proper diuretics.

Oedema due to sodium retention can be treated by:

- **Restricting sodium intake**
- **Ensuring adequate renal perfusion,** by improving cardiac efficiency, as in cardiac oedema
- **Promoting sodium and water excretion** by using diuretics and aldosterone antagonists

Usually, these approaches are combined. *Some pitting oedemas that are idiopathic, postural and drug induced (see Box 37.6) do not need drug treatment.*

Cardiac Oedema

Diuretics are not the first choice in the treatment of chronic HF and their routine use in all cases of HF

Table 37.3 Electrolyte Excretion Pattern Following Diuretics

Drug	Urinary Electrolytes				Urine pH
	Na^+	K^+	Cl^-	HCO_3^-	
Acetazolamide	++	+	−	++	8.2
Thiazides	+++	++	+	±	7.4
Furosemide	++++	++	++++	±	6.0
Spironolactone	+	a	+	±	7.2
Triamterene	++	a	++	+	7.2
Mannitol	+++	+	++	+	6.5

[a]Denotes potassium retention.
[−]Denotes no change.

Box 37.3 Indications for Diuretic Therapy

- Oedema associated with sodium retention such as cardiac, hepatic and renal oedema
- Pulmonary and cerebral oedema
- Drug poisoning such as due to barbiturates or salicylates
- Acute oliguric renal failure
- Oedema of pregnancy and idiopathic oedema

Box 37.4 Nondiuretic Uses of Diuretic Drugs

- Hypertension (hydrochlorothiazide)
- Idiopathic calcium urolithiasis (hydrochlorothiazide)
- Diabetes insipidus (hydrochlorothiazide, amiloride)
- Hypercalcaemia (furosemide)
- Hyponatraemic states due to water retention (furosemide)
- Glaucoma (acetazolamide, mannitol)
- Mountain sickness (acetazolamide)
- Cystic fibrosis (amiloride)
- Acute LVF (furosemide)

from the beginning is not recommended (Chapter 31). Hence, it is important to improve cardiac function and to restore adequate renal perfusion. Adequate GFR is ensured by the following:

- **Complete rest**
- **Improving the cardiac output**
- **Treating the underlying cause** such as anaemia, hypertension or hyperthyroidism

In addition, restriction of sodium intake is needed.

In mild HF, one should aim at diuresis which causes a weight reduction of less than 1 kg per day. A moderate efficacy diuretic such as thiazide is preferred to a loop diuretic. When planning continuous diuretic therapy, ACEI ± spironolactone is combined with the primary diuretic right from the beginning to prevent the development of diuretic resistance due to secondary hyperaldosteronism.

As the disease progresses, the use of furosemide is inevitable. With a **single-daily-dose of furosemide,** intense sodium retention post-diuresis can limit the efficacy of the drug. This can be overcome by increasing the daily dose of furosemide, administered in 2–3 divided doses per day. Patients with severe HF may need larger oral/parenteral dose of furosemide.

Cirrhotic Oedema and Ascites IM 5.16

This is due to the following:

- **Increased portal venous pressure**
- **Decreased plasma colloid osmotic pressure following hypoalbuminaemia**
- **Secondary rise in aldosterone secretion**

The treatment therefore would be, bed rest, salt restriction (to 20 mEq/day) and use of spironolactone. **Diuretics like furosemide (40-80 mg/day) are used only in severe cases.**

The danger of precipitating hypokalemia and azotaemia (volume contraction) with diuretic therapy is higher in cirrhotic oedema; the chances of precipitating hepatic encephalopathy are also high. Hence, the diuretic therapy should be undertaken under supervision with checks on serum electrolytes. *The dose used should be the smallest possible one and oral potassium supplements should be given.*

Seriously ill cirrhotic patients with ascites should not be treated too vigorously, as this may precipitate hepatic coma, azotaemia and death.

Renal Oedema

Diuretics are ineffective in treating oedema due to acute glomerulonephritis.

The treatment of **nephrotic syndrome** depends upon the underlying cause; in patients with diabetic nephrotic syndrome, furosemide is the diuretic of choice. In 'idiopathic' nephrotic syndrome due to 'minimal change disease' in children, the treatment comprises of:

a. Salt restriction
b. Dietary protein supplementation, unless concurrent renal insufficiency is present

c. Prednisolone (a glucocorticoid) in adequate doses (2 mg/kg/day)
d. Judicious use of diuretics; furosemide is the drug of choice, but increasingly large doses and sometimes IV bolus (100-200 mg) are required

It must be remembered that the concurrent use of large doses of furosemide and a glucocorticoid in a nephrotic child who has secondary hyperaldosteronism may cause severe hypokalemia. In such circumstances spironolactone is added

Pulmonary Oedema

It is a medical emergency and needs immediate treatment. The treatment depends upon aetiology (Chapter 31). Attention is paid to circulation, gas exchange and lung mechanics. Infection, acidaemia, anaemia and renal failure, when present, must be treated.

Cerebral Oedema

See Box 37.5.

Nutritional Oedema

This is due to hypoalbuminaemia, and it responds to increased protein intake. **Diuretics are usually not indicated.** In severe cases, weak diuretics may be used to obtain temporary relief from the oedema; **vigorous diuretic therapy is, however, dangerous and should be avoided.**

Box 37.6 lists **the drugs that can cause fluid retention** and oedema. In majority of the cases, it is mild, dose-related and reversible without requiring any drug therapy.

Choice of a diuretic: The choice of a diuretic in the treatment of oedema would depend on:

- Nature of the disease
- Potency of the drug
- Electrolyte changes associated with its use
- Possibility of development of tolerance
- Convenience of administration

Majority of the patients with oedema respond satisfactorily to relatively small doses of a moderately effective diuretic, like thiazides, which is often preferred for routine use as they are safe and cheap.

Box 37.5 Treatment of Cerebral Oedema

- **Mannitol** 25–50 g IV every 3–5 h to a maximum of 2 g/kg/day
- **Furosemide** 20–80 mg IV every 4–12 h to supplement the effect of mannitol
- **Replacement of fluids** to maintain serum osmolality
- **Glucocorticoids** (Dexamethasone 8 mg IV every 6–8 h) in intracranial neoplasms. Also see Chapter 64
- **Mechanical hyperventilation** to achieve a CO_2 partial pressure of 25–30 mm Hg
- **Oral glycerine** 30 mL t.i.d.
- **Magnesium sulphate**, saturated solution, 50–200 mL rectally
- **Surgical decompression** if all above measures fail

Box 37.6 Drugs Causing Fluid Retention

- NSAIDs
- Vasodilators: CCB, hydralazine
- Steroids: Cortisone, hydrocortisone, fludrocortisone, testosterone, estrogen, danazol
- Thiazolidinediones

Only when quick and vigorous response is needed, loop diuretic like furosemide is employed. *Vigorous treatment with potent diuretics, coupled with strict restriction of sodium intake to clear the oedema, may lead to rapid development of serious electrolyte disturbances, volume depletion and even death* (see below).

Combination of diuretics: *Sequential nephron blocking* may be needed sometimes. For example,

a. A potassium-sparing diuretic added to a thiazide or to furosemide, prevents hypokalemia
b. Addition of a thiazide may promote diuresis in patients resistant to furosemide
c. The concurrent use of furosemide and mannitol, minimises the dose of furosemide in patients with acute oliguric renal failure

COMPLICATIONS OF DIURETIC THERAPY

Diuretic therapy, no doubt, is very effective and many times life-saving. However, it can produce various complications. These are as follows:

a. **Allergic reactions:** These include various types of skin eruptions, urticaria, occasional blood dyscrasias and rarely interstitial nephritis. Such reactions are usually confined to a single drug or class of drugs. In such circumstances, a drug from another group may be substituted.

b. **Disturbances of electrolyte balance**: These occur more commonly and are usually predictable. These include the following:
   - **Acute sodium depletion and hypovolaemia:** This is a relatively common complication especially following the loop diuretics particularly, in patients on sodium restriction and in those with undetected renal disease. The patient who improves dramatically initially, suddenly becomes lethargic and sleepy. Signs of dehydration are present. Increasing the sodium intake reverses this condition. In severe cases, IV sodium chloride may be necessary.
   - **Chronic sodium depletion:** This is less common and is characterised by lethargy, weakness and disorientation. Absence of demonstrable oedema along with a low serum sodium is the cardinal requirement for its diagnosis.
   - **Potassium depletion and hypokalemia:** This occurs during long-term use of thiazides and loop diuretics. It is especially liable to occur when these drugs are used in large doses continuously rather than in small doses, intermittently and in states (such as cirrhosis of liver) with high circulating levels of aldosterone (secondary hyperaldosteronism) to begin with. It can be seen in patients who are diabetic, elderly and on glucocorticoids.

     By itself hypokalemia can impair renal function and can cause arrhythmias in patients receiving digitalis and those drugs which prolong QT interval.

Hypokalemia can be prevented/corrected by the following:

i. **Increased dietary intake of potassium or potassium chloride supplement:** However, routine administration of supplemental potassium is not necessary when thiazides are used to treat hypertension and in young patients with good appetite

ii. **Potassium-sparing diuretics:** They are valuable but *when they are given, potassium supplements should be omitted except in cirrhotic patients* to avoid hyperkalemia

   - **Hyperkalemia:** This is less common and occurs in cases with uraemia and with drugs like triamterene
   - **Hypochloraemic alkalosis:** This occurs following thiazides and loop diuretics
   - **Metabolic acidosis:** This is seen following carbonic anhydrase inhibition (acetazolamide), and is discussed earlier
   - **Chronic dilutional hyponatraemia:** This state is sometimes seen in patients with HF **where serum sodium is persistently low in spite of severe oedema.** This is because there is relatively more water retention than sodium retention by the kidneys resulting in extreme dilution of ECF; its mechanism is not clear. It may be aggravated following diuretics. The treatment is difficult. Rigid restriction of water intake (less than 700–800 mL daily) is recommended. Glucocorticoids may be helpful in some cases.

c. **Selective adverse effects:** These are discussed under each individual drug. Thiazides and loop diuretics can cause magnesium deficiency which can give rise to ventricular arrhythmias.

DIURETIC RESISTANCE

In practice, diuretic resistance can be due to:

- **Drug-related factors** such as the choice of the diuretic; its dose; or interfering drugs such as NSAID, lithium or probenecid
- **Patient-related factors** such as noncompliance with instructions about bed rest or salt and fluid intake
- **Disease-related factors** such as markedly low GFR; severe hypokalemia, hyponatraemia, hypovolaemia, or hypomagnesaemia; or severe HF

Correction of the underlying factors often restores the response. With proper use of diuretics, there would be only a few patients who show refractoriness. In many such cases, correction of underlying electrolyte disturbances restores the responsiveness. Treatment of extrarenal factors such as pulmonary infection, adequate bed rest and appropriate use of other drugs like steroids/NSAIDs may help in some patients.

IM 10.25

ACUTE RENAL FAILURE (ARF)

ARF may be defined as a state in which the kidney's ability to maintain homeostasis has declined suddenly, with resultant retention of metabolic waste products as well as electrolyte, acid–base and volume disturbances.

The aims of therapy are:

i. to treat the cause (if possible);
ii. to maintain the urine output at 30–50 mL/h in adults without causing fluid overload;
iii. to maintain the BP normal; nutritional care and
iv. prevention and treatment of infection, hyperkalemia, metabolic acidosis, hyperphosphatemia and other complications; all this while awaiting spontaneous recovery of renal function.

Principles of management of established ARF are presented in Box 37.7 but ideally the management should be left to the specialist.

ANTIDIURETIC AGENTS

PH 1.24

VASOPRESSIN: It is an antidiuretic hormone (ADH). This polypeptide hormone is released from the posterior lobe of the pituitary along with oxytocin. Given in pharmacological doses, it has a vasopressor action and hence, is called **vasopressin.** Human vasopressin is **arginine vasopressin (AVP).**

Its rate of secretion is mainly determined by the plasma osmolality. Thus, dehydration stimulates whereas hydration inhibits AVP secretion. An increase or a decrease in the circulating blood volume may also influence the secretion. Angiotensin is a potent stimulator of AVP release. In addition, pain, nausea, hypoxia and some hormones and neurotransmitters can modify its secretion. Some drugs can also stimulate or inhibit its release (Table 37.4).

Box 37.7 Principles of Management of Established ARF PH 1.1

- Isolation and barrier nursing to prevent infection
- Clinical monitoring (weight; BP; urine output and signs of dehydration or over hydration)
- Laboratory monitoring for anaemia; electrolyte and acid base balance
- Ensure an intake of 30–50 kcal/kg/day
- Restrict protein intake
- Restrict fluid intake to 300 mL (urine output + insensible losses from the skin and the lungs + visible losses such as sweat, vomit, stool)
- Restrict sodium chloride intake to 2–4 g/day
- Restrict K^+ intake to 40 mEq/day
- Restrict phosphorus intake to 800 mg/day
- Administer phosphorous-binding antacids such as aluminium hydroxide
- Avoid magnesium containing drugs
- Adjust doses of drugs to renal status
- Maintain blood pressure
- Detection and treatment of acidosis, hyperkalemia and hypo- or hypernatremia
- Treatment of infection, anaemia and GI bleeding
- Haemodialysis

Mechanism of action: AVP acts on two G-protein-coupled receptors, **V_1** (**V_{1a}** and **V_{1b}**) and **V_2**.

V_1 receptors are located in the vascular smooth muscle, bladder and uterine smooth muscle, liver, platelets and in the CNS.

Activation of V_{1a} increases intracellular calcium and causes vasoconstriction, including that of the coronary vessels. AVP acts directly on the cardiac myocytes which hypertrophy. It may also potentiate the synthesis of endothelin. In patients with HF plasma AVP may rise early during the disease. **V_{1b} receptors are involved in vasopressin-stimulated secretion of ACTH.**

V_2 receptors are found predominantly in the renal collecting duct. Their stimulation increases water permeability of the apical membrane promoting water reabsorption (**anti-diuretic action**).

In addition, V_2 receptor activation greatly increases the permeability of urea in the terminal portions of the collecting duct and Na^+ transport in thick ascending limb and collecting duct.

Table 37.4 Drugs and AVP Release

Stimulants	Inhibitors
Tricyclic antidepressants	Alcohol phenytoin
Nicotine	Chlorpromazine
Adrenaline	Haloperidol
Morphine(high doses)	Promethazine
Barbiturates	Morphine (low dose)
Cyclophosphamide	Butorphanol
Vincristine	Glucocorticoids

Physiological and pharmacological actions:

Kidney: Under the influence of AVP, the distal tubule and the collecting duct reabsorbs water and reduces urine volume. Hence it is called as **antidiuretic hormone**. In addition, V_1, receptor activation reduces the renal medullary blood flow. **Production of PGE_2 is stimulated.** Absence of AVP causes pituitary (central) diabetes insipidus.

The antidiuretic response to AVP is enhanced by NSAID, chlorpropamide and carbamazepine; it is inhibited by lithium and demeclocycline.

Cardiovascular system: In large doses, it directly stimulates the vascular smooth muscle and raises BP. It also constricts the coronary and cerebral blood vessels. The hormone causes an initial tachycardia, probably secondary to coronary insufficiency and resultant hypotension, followed by bradycardia.

Other smooth muscles: AVP stimulates the GI smooth muscle.

Miscellaneous: Stimulation of $\mathbf{V_2}$ receptors increases the level of coagulation factor VII and von Willebrand factor. AVP, stored in the platelets, plays a role in platelet aggregation.

Absorption, fate and excretion: When administered subcutaneously or intramuscularly, the drug remains in the body for a few hours; given intravenously, it is rapidly metabolised. However, vasopressin tannate in oil, administered subcutaneously or intramuscularly, produces an effect lasting for 24–48 h.

AVP is rapidly metabolised in the body, largely during passage through the liver and the kidney. Its plasma t½ is 20 min or less.

Adverse reactions: It may produce nausea, biliary colic and abdominal cramps due to increased peristaltic activity. Hypotension and shock are serious but rare adverse effects.

Preparations and dosage:

i. Vasopressin injection 20 U per mL; dose 5–10 U every 4–6 h subcutaneously or intramuscularly
ii. Synthetic vasopressin analogue, DDAVP (1-deamino-8-d-arginine-vasopressin, Desmopressin), *administered intranasally* (5-10 mcg b.i.d.) has greater antidiuretic and lesser pressor activity. Its action lasts for 13–22 h. It can also be given subcutaneously or intravenously (dose 1–4 mcg/day), orally (100–600 mcg/day) and sublingually.
iii. Lysine-8-vasopressin is more stable and is used *intranasally* by spray (2 units/spray; 1–4 sprays 3–7 times a day)

Indications:

I. **Those related to vascular and smooth muscle (V_1 receptor) actions,** where **AVP** is used:
   - **Postoperative ileus and abdominal distension**
   - **Oesophageal varices due to portal hypertension:** Triglycyl lysine vasopressin (glypressin), an analogue, releases slowly the active hormone *in vivo*, that causes marked splanchnic vasoconstriction. The effect lasts for 10 h after a single bolus injection (Chapter 33).
   - **Acute haemorrhagic gastritis**
   - **Vasopressin IV has been found effective in the treatment of asystolic cardiac arrest. It may be given in a single dose of 40 IU, IM**

II. **Those related to antidiuretic action and release of blood coagulation factors (V_2 receptors),** where **desmopressin** is useful
   - **Diabetes insipidus:** Desmopressin is the treatment of choice. It is administered intranasally or by SC/IM injection. If desmopressin is not available, AVP may be used. As this is replacement therapy, it is lifelong in most cases. **It is effective in central (pituitary) but not in nephrogenic diabetes insipidus.**

- **Nocturnal enuresis:** Desmopressin intranasally or orally (as tablet) at bedtime has been used for its short-term treatment.
- **Bleeding disorders:** Haemophilia A (factor VIII deficiency) and von Willebrand disease (Chapter 33)

BENZOTHIADIAZINES: Surprisingly, benzothiadiazines are **effective in controlling central as well as nephrogenic diabetes insipidus**. The mechanism of action is not known. Various possibilities have been suggested; they probably act by causing a negative sodium balance and reducing the GFR. This leads to a decrease in volume and an increase in concentration of urine. A long acting drug such as **polythiazide** is usually preferred. Since symptomless hypokalemia is commonly associated with this therapy, a potassium-sparing diuretic may be added to this regimen.

In nephrogenic diabetes insipidus, where there is renal unresponsiveness to the action of desmopressin, thiazides are the most effective form of therapy.

In both idiopathic and nephrogenic diabetes insipidus, the beneficial effect of benzothiadiazines is reduced by liberal salt intake.

CHLORPROPAMIDE: This drug, used in the treatment of diabetes mellitus (Chapter 63), is effective in the treatment of diabetes insipidus. It probably acts by increasing the sensitivity of renal tubules to low and otherwise ineffective concentrations of AVP. Unlike thiazide diuretics, the response to chlorpropamide is not reduced by high sodium intake or steroid administration. **It is not useful in nephrogenic diabetes insipidus.** It is usually given in the dose of 250–500 mg once daily orally.

Carbamazepine (400–600 mg/day) is effective in patients with partial diabetes insipidus. It probably acts by stimulating vasopressin release from the neurohypophysis. Action of carbamazepine and chlorpropamide is overcome by ethanol, which inhibits the release of AVP.

VASOPRESSIN RECEPTOR ANTAGONISTS

PH 1.24

CONIVAPTAN: This competitive, nonselective vasopressin – **V_1/V_2 receptor antagonist** causes decreased permeability of the renal collecting ducts to water, leading to excretion of free water (**aquaresis**). It is 99% protein bound and is metabolised in the liver by CYP3A4. *It is administered parenterally for short-term treatment of euvolemic hyponatraemia, usually caused by SIADH, hypothyroidism and adrenocortical insufficiency.* In general, the drug is well tolerated but may cause headache, thirst, dry mouth, hypokalemia, hypotension and vomiting. Excessive correction of hyponatraemia increases the risk of osmotic demyelination syndrome.

Tolvaptan, another benzazepine derivative, has more **selective V_2 antagonistic action**. It is effective orally and has been used to treat euvolemic and hypervolemic hyponatraemia in patients with HF, cirrhosis and SIADH. Adverse effects reported are similar to those of conivaptan. These antagonists are generally not useful in the treatment of patients with hyponatraemia, who suffer from severe CNS symptoms due to cerebral oedema. In such patients, the cerebral oedema is best treated with hypertonic saline.

DRUGS AND NEPHROTOXICITY

Kidney has a rich blood supply and further, it can concentrate the drugs and their metabolites locally. This exposes the renal tubules to very high concentrations of the drugs, which may cause renal damage.

Drugs can cause nephrotoxicity:

- **Directly**, e.g. NSAID, aminoglycosides, heavy metals, chemicals such as ethylene glycol
- **Indirectly**, e.g. vitamin D causing hypercalcaemia, leading to the formation of renal calculi; diuretics causing hypokalemia may cause renal tubular damage and cytotoxic drugs causing hyperuricaemia
- **By immunological mechanisms.** Many drugs can produce variety of damages such as glomerulitis, interstitial nephritis, vasculitis and SLE. Examples are sulphonamides, INH, rifampicin, gold, phenytoin, hydralazine and procainamide

Nephrotoxicity can be 'acute' leading to ARF or may be 'chronic' and responsible for chronic renal

Table 37.5 Drugs Causing Nephrotoxicity

Site of Action	Drugs	Nature of Toxicity
Extrarenal	Tetracyclines, corticosteroids	Aggravation of azotaemia probably via increased protein breakdown
Arteries and arterioles	Heavy metals, e.g. arsenic, bismuth and gold salts, long acting sulphonamides, iodides, thiazides and bevacizumab	Vasculitis, thrombotic microangiopathy
Glomeruli	Hydralazine, long acting sulphonamides. Interferons	Nephrotic syndrome, podocytopathy, glomerulopathy
Convoluted tubules	Aminoglycoside antibiotics, e.g. kanamycin, gentamicin, colistin, amphotericin B, polymyxin B, vancomycin and cephaloridine cisplatin	Necrosis of proximal and/or distal tubular epithelium
Interstitium	NSAIDs, phenytoin, sulphonamides and cyclosporine	Interstitial nephritis with papillary necrosis. May cause acute renal failure or chronic nephropathy
Collecting ducts	Acetazolamide, sulphonamides and antineoplastic drugs – methotrexate	Crystalluria, calculi and hyperuricaemia
Ureters	Methysergide	Obstruction due to retroperitoneal fibrosis

disease. Drugs can damage the kidney at various sites from renal arteries to the ureters. They can also cause the renal damage by crystal or calculi formation. From among the many compounds incriminated in producing such damage, only some of the better known nephrotoxic agents are included in Table 37.5.

Chronic nephropathy due to prolonged ingestion of NSAID has received considerable attention. Patients suffering from this syndrome may present with haematuria, renal colic, urinary infection and finally hypertension and renal failure. The lesions are reversible if the syndrome is detected early and the offending drug stopped (see Chapter 11). Hence always enquire about chronic use of NSAID when patients present with such signs and symptoms.

Drug-induced nephrotic syndrome has been observed following therapeutic use of drugs like tolbutamide, probenecid, penicillamine, and gold salts. It is characterised by marked proteinuria.

Compounds like antiepileptic drugs, sulphonamides, phenylbutazone, tetracyclines, antihypertensive agents like hydralazine; and methyldopa can induce systemic lupus erythematosus (SLE) and affect the kidney. The damage may be reversible on discontinuation of the drug.

Apart from the therapeutic agents, **many chemicals** also cause nephrotoxicity. These include such compounds as aniline, carbon tetrachloride, phenol, ethylene glycol, phosphorus, arsenic, cadmium and mercuric chloride.

In the presence of kidney damage, the t½ of drugs that are mainly excreted by kidney is prolonged, e.g. beta lactams, fluroquinolones, aminoglycosides, atenolol, ACEI and digoxin. In such patients, it is necessary to reduce the doses of such drugs to avoid toxicity.

In general, the serum creatinine is a useful rough guide to the severity of impairment of renal function. In mild failure, with a GFR of 25–50 mL/min, it is 1.8–2.8 mg%. With GFR of 10–25 mL/min, it is 2.9–7.9 mg%, whereas in severe renal failure (GFR $<$10 mL/min), serum creatinine is $\geq$8 mg%.

Renal function deteriorates with age but this reduction, until marked, is not reflected in the serum creatinine level. *It should be noted that many apparently healthy elderly subjects also may have a GFR of less than 50 mL/min, and therefore, caution is needed in prescribing certain drugs in the elderly and those with DM.*

DIURETICS

Weak diuretics

Osmotic diuretics
- Sodium
- Potassium salts

Xanthine derivatives
- Aminophylline

Carbonic anhydrase inhibitors
- Acetazolamide

Moderately efficacious diuretics

Osmotic diuretics
- Mannitol
- Isosorbide
- Sucrose
- Glycerol

Benzothiadiazines (thiazides)
- Hydrochlorothiazide
- Hydroflumethiazide
- Benzthiazide

Thiazide-like diuretics
- Chlorthalidone
- Chlorexolone
- Indapamide
- Metolazone

Highly efficacious diuretics (high ceiling or loop diuretics)

- Furosemide
- Torsemide
- Bumetanide
- Ethacrynic acid

Potassium-sparing diuretics

Aldosterone antagonists
- Spironolactone
- Potassium canreonate
- Eplerenone

Renal epithelial sodium channel inhibitors
- Triamterene
- Amiloride

VASOPRESSIN RECEPTOR MODULATORS

Vasopressin receptor agonists

- Vasopressin
- Lysine-8-vasopressin
- Desmopressin (V_2 selective)

Vasopressin receptor antagonists

- Conivaptan
- Tolvaptan (V_2 selective)

10

SECTION

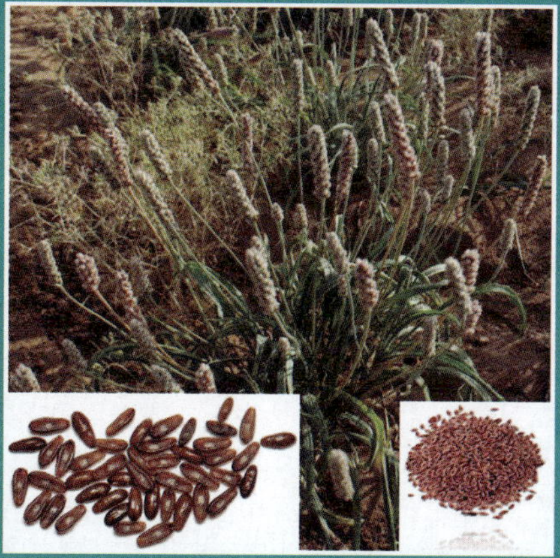

Plantago psyllium

Drugs Used in Disorders of the Gastrointestinal Tract

Section Outline

This section consists of the following chapters:

CHAPTER 38

Appetite Stimulants, Digestants, Antiflatulents, Appetite Suppressants and Antihyperlipidemic Agents

Learning Objectives

This chapter will enable the reader:

1. To enlist appetite stimulants.
2. To enumerate digestants with their mechanism of action and indications.
3. To enlist antiflatulents and carminatives with their mechanism of action and indications.
4. To be aware of the physiology of energy balance.
5. To classify anorexiants on the basis of their mechanism of action.
6. To outline the treatment of obesity.
7. To explain the key mechanisms that can lead to atherosclerosis.
8. To explain the principles of diet therapy in hyperlipoproteinemia.
9. To classify antihyperlipdemic drugs on basis of their mechanism of action.
10. To describe pharmacological effects, salient pharmacokinetic features, ADR, indications and drug interactions of statins, ezetimibe, bile acid sequestrants, fibrates and nicotinic acid.
11. To justify the therapeutic utility of fish oil.
12. To state the choice of lipid-lowering drugs in the treatment of hypercholesterolemia, combined hyperlipidaemia and hypertriglyceridemia.

KEY TERMS

Appetite, a desire to eat or drink, is a complex phenomenon influenced by several neurohormonal factors. Dopamine- and 5-HT-mediated processes in the CNS and ghrelin, a gut-brain peptide, probably play an important role in appetite regulation.

Loss of appetite (**anorexia**) is a common complaint in clinical practice. Its aetiology varies from prolonged, debilitating illnesses such as tuberculosis, heart failure, cancer to psychiatric diseases such as depression. It is imperative, therefore, to investigate thoroughly an individual complaining of **persistent anorexia and weight loss** for the underlying cause and treat the same.

Temporary anorexia due to short illnesses usually needs no treatment. However, appetite stimulants may be prescribed for a short time.

APPETITE STIMULANTS

There is no safe and reliable appetite stimulant. Symptomatically, appetite can often be improved by varying the diet and by use of such simple preparations as lemon pickles, bitters such as bitter orange peel and soups. The aromatic bitter appetite stimulants combine the property of bitterness with that of an aromatic volatile oil, e.g. orange, ginger and cardamom. *Use of costly appetite stimulants and 'tonics' for this purpose is unnecessary.*

Vitamin B_{12} and **anabolic steroids** may stimulate appetite but whether that is their primary action or secondary to their metabolic effects remains to be established. The 5-HT antagonist **cyproheptadine** has also some appetite stimulating property; however, used in large doses, it inhibits the release of ACTH and depresses the circulating cortisol level (Chapter 24).

Megestrol acetate and **glucocorticoids** may be useful in increasing the appetite but not necessarily to gain weight in patients with cancer-induced cachexia.

Alcohol (10%), in small quantities, given before a meal it can augment the gastric secretion both reflexly by stimulation of the taste buds and by a direct action (Chapter 6). It is a major constituent of popular 'tonics'. Many tonics dispensed in fancy bottles contain 10%–15% of alcohol. *Repeated ingestion of alcohol, however, causes chronic gastritis and a diminution in appetite. The use of alcohol containing 'tonics' in children is to be condemned.* **Prolonged use of alcohol in any form is to be discouraged.**

DIGESTANTS

PH 1.34, PH 1.61

The digestants are the drugs that are claimed to aid digestion in the gastrointestinal tract. The commonly used digestants are as follows:

Pepsin: This is a proteolytic enzyme, obtained from the glandular layer of the fresh stomach of the hog. It is administered orally in the dose of 0.5–1 g. It is of doubtful value except perhaps in patients with gastric achylia, a condition characterised by defective acid and pepsin secretion.

Enzyme, **papain**, obtained from vegetable source (papaya), also has proteolytic properties.

PANCREATIN: This contains the **enzymes amylase, trypsin and lipase** and is obtained from hog or ox pancreas. It has been employed as a replacement therapy in chronic pancreatitis, obstruction caused by the cancer of the head of pancreas, cystic fibrosis and after total gastrectomy. It is not useful in GI disorders unrelated to pancreatic enzyme insufficiency. It is administered orally as enteric coated capsules, to prevent its gastric inactivation. However, this preparation contains very small amounts of enzymatic activity per tablet or capsule, compared to quantities necessary for efficient digestion. Hence, even with large doses, total correction of steatorrhoea may not occur. Prolonged use of pancreatin may cause fibrosing colonopathy.

BILE ACIDS AND BILE SALTS: Bile acids are important in emulsifying the fats in the intestine. Along with bile salts they increase the flow as well as the concentration of bile and are termed **choleretics**. They are used in liver cirrhosis and functional hepatic insufficiency. Their benefits however are doubtful.

PH 1.34

URSODEOXYCHOLIC ACID (ursodiol), is formed from chenodeoxycholic acid by colonic bacteria. It is the commonly used bile acid therapeutically. It decreases hepatic cholesterol secretion and improves solubility of cholesterol in bile but it does not increase the secretion of bile acids into bile. Given orally, it is absorbed rapidly and taken up by the liver.

It is usually well tolerated but some patients may experience diarrhoea, nausea, vomiting, dyspepsia, abdominal pain, rash, itching and hair loss.

Indications

- **Primary biliary cirrhosis:** Ursodiol, given orally in the dose of 8–12 mg/kg/day, in divided doses, has been reported to cause clinical, biochemical and histological improvement. It acts by modifying the composition of bile acids in the liver, thereby hindering the progression of the pathological process. It lowers the serum cholesterol levels in these patients.
- **Gallstones:** Ursodeoxycholic acid, 8-10 mg/kg/day is indicated **for radiolucent cholesterol stones**, 5 mm or less in diameter,as alternative option for surgical removal. It needs to be administered for a prolonged time, sometimes up to 2 years. Gall stones are very common and asymptomatic gallstones are often an incidental finding on ultrasonography. In most cases, they need no treatment. True symptoms of gallstone disease include acute cholecystitis, biliary colic, jaundice and acute pancreatitis, and if severe symptoms, cholecystectomy is the best treatment. However, this may not guarantee improvement in all digestive symptoms of the patient. Therapy with ursodiol, however, is unsuitable in patients with (1) noncholesterol stones; (2) nonfunctioning gall bladder or (3) severe recurrent symptoms. *Gallstones in the bile duct are more serious and need surgical treatment.*

ANTIFLATULENTS AND CARMINATIVES

PH 1.34

These are the drugs used to expel gas from the stomach or the intestines in the treatment of *flatulence and colics*. Most of these drugs are **aromatic volatile oils**. *They act by mild stimulation thereby increasing the GI motility and causing relaxation of sphincters.* They produce a feeling of warmth in the stomach. They do not affect the gastric acid secretion significantly. Indian food contains enough carminatives in the form of various spices and condiments. The common ones are cardamom seeds, ginger, fennel seeds, asafoetida, cinnamon bark, cloves, coriander and anise. Along with sodium bicarbonate, they form important constituents of various **'gripe water'** mixtures commonly used in infants to relieve colicky pain.

Although carminatives may afford some quick symptomatic relief and audible satisfaction, *it must be remembered that flatulent dyspepsia may be associated with disorders such as peptic ulcer, biliary tract disease, the irritable bowel syndrome, alimentary tumours and even IHD.*

DIMETHYLPOLYSILOXANE: This silicone derivative has been advocated in symptomatic treatment of postprandial and postoperative flatulence and abdominal distension. It is believed to act as a defoaming agent, allowing the gas to escape from the GI tract, providing comfort to the patient with 'gases'. It is available as 40 mg tablets. **Simethicone** is a mixture of dimethylpolysiloxane and silicagel.

IM 14.13

ANOREXIANTS AND TREATMENT OF OBESITY

Obesity is defined as 'a condition of abnormal or excessive accumulation of adipose tissue, to the extent that health may be impaired'. People with abdominal fat distribution or **android** obesity are at greater risk to its consequences than those with the less serious **gynoid** fat distribution where fat is more evenly and peripherally distributed around the body.

Sedentary lifestyle of modern living, combined with the abundant availability of tempting, high-fat (junk) foods has caused almost an epidemic of obesity. However, not everyone who partakes of such foods becomes obese. *The tendency to become obese is definitely inherited. The mortality rises exponentially with increasing body weight and the incidence of heart disease, hypertension, diabetes, sleep apnoea, osteoarthritis and bowel cancer is higher in the obese than in the nonobese.*

Regulation of energy balance: *Obesity is a disorder of energy balance.* Hypothalamus is a major centre that regulates food consumption by modulating hunger and satiety. Hypothalamus also controls the energy expenditure via the adrenergic nervous system and the pituitary hormones.

The central control of the bodyweight is a complex phenomenon, not well understood, regulated by multiple brain nuclei and many NTs (Box 38.1). Of these, **neuropeptide Y is the most potent appetite stimulant** and is abundantly present in the hypothalamus. It also suppresses the sympathetic activity and thus reduces energy expenditure.

Ghrelin, a 28 amino acid, gut-brain peptide which is **a potent inducer of growth hormone release** has also powerful **appetite stimulating** (**orexigenic**) properties. It is produced mainly by neuroendocrine cells in the gastric fundus and acts on the hypothalamus. Given in human volunteers, it stimulates appetite, induces hunger and increases food consumption. Reduction in ghrelin secretion is one of the mechanisms of appetite reduction after gastric surgery for weight reduction.

Leptin is another peptide hormone synthesised in the fat cells. It acts on the hypothalamus to signal adequacy of body fat stores, **suppress food intake and increase the calorie expenditure through inhibition of neuropeptide Y.** Deficiency of leptin stimulates appetite.

It also facilitates puberty in adolescents, and fertility in adults. It is not a trigger but a **permissive factor for LHRH release** in both the situations. Leptin has been used

Box 38.1 Neuropeptides Affecting Energy Balance

- ***Increase food intake:***
  Noradrenaline, GHRH
  Neuropeptide Y, ghrelin, opioids
  Endogenous cannabinoids
- ***Inhibit food intake:***
  5-HT, dopamine
  Cholecystokinin (CCK), CRH
  neurotensin, bombesin
  Glucagon-like peptide, α MSH

successfully in overcoming amenorrhoea in females with anorexia nervosa and those participating in vigorous sports.

Normally, body weight is tightly regulated and a small excess of food consumption over burning of calories is all that is required to cause weight gain. *Daily excess of 100 kcal (a small chocolate bar or one chapati) would result in 4–5 kg weight gain in 1 year! Even modest weight loss of 10% improves physical performance and glucose tolerance. What is most important, however, is maintenance of the reduced weight for long-term benefit.*

Clinically, overweight and obesity are assessed in terms of **body mass index** (BMI = body weight in kg/height in m^2) and waist circumferences. The normal value in adults is 18.5–24.9; overweight is BMI of 25–29.9; and obesity is 30 or higher. BMI of 35 or more means severe obesity. According to the new Asian criteria, a person with a BMI > 23 is considered as obese. *The perils of obesity, diabetes, hypertension and hyperlipidaemia increase from a BMI of 23.*

Alternatively, obesity is diagnosed even with normal BMI if the waist circumference exceeds 102 cm in men and 88 cm in women in the western countries; for Asians, the corresponding figures are 90 and 80 cm, respectively.

Many of the comorbidities of obesity present themselves in the form of the so-called **metabolic syndrome**. The latter is related to an excess of intra-abdominal rather than subcutaneous fat (Chapter 63).

Some obese individuals show psychological disturbances and a compulsive desire to eat, though such individuals may not derive satisfaction from the act of eating.

Treatment of obesity is essentially medical. Surgical treatment (on the GI tract) may be useful only in severe, resistant cases. The **general principles of** treatment are outlined in Box 38.2.

In an obese individual, if an organic cause such as an endocrine disease is present, it should be treated. **Commonly, obesity is due to excessive eating and lack of adequate exercise.** The patient must be made to appreciate this at the beginning of the treatment and explained that *diet is the mainstay of the treatment of obesity*; he/she must be adequately motivated by the concept of 'positive health'. It must also be emphasised that dietary treatment of obesity consists of a lifelong reorientation of his/her eating habits (and often those of his/her family) and not merely of a 'course' of dieting.

Box 38.2 Principles of Treatment of Obesity PH 1.1

- Change in lifestyle; regular exercise
- Nutritionally adequate, low-calorie diet, containing at least 1 g of protein/kg of desirable body weight
- Fat intake below 25% of total calories prescribed
- Liberal use of fibre-containing foods
- Behavioural intervention
- Restriction of alcohol and smoking
- Pharmacotherapy as adjunct

Diet in obesity: There are many diets for obesity and there is no ideal diet for the weight loss. It has, however, been established that **nothing about the diet matters except its calorie content.**

- The best diet is one which is **low in calorie content** (1000–1500 kcal/ day), contains all the essential nutrients, provides a variety and is simple for the patient to follow for prolonged periods. It is better to reduce the daily calorie intake progressively in steps of 500 cal. *The diet should also conform to the patient's pocket.* 'It is prudent to avoid well-advertised, fancy and expensive nutritional supplements'.
- *Diet rich in fruits, vegetables and whole grain, especially pulses and nuts, is to be preferred.* Excessive intake of fat (butter, eggs, oil), sweets (chocolate, pastries) and red meat should be avoided. Proprietary slimming foods are expensive and ineffective. The age-old Indian religious custom of fasting on certain days of the month has, much to recommend it, as it can atone for the minor sins of the palate indulged in at other times and thus, help to keep good health.
- Apart from the caloric restriction for obesity, the individuals having co-morbidities such as hypertension, gout, diabetes mellitus, etc.

need additional dietary modifications.
- Sodium content in diet should be reduced and extra salt or salt rich items like pickles, papads, processed foods need to be avoided.

If the patient realises the importance of dieting and exercise and if he/she has the necessary will, then the treatment of obesity is not that difficult and can easily be carried out at home without the help of expensive 'obesity clinics', and fashionable 'health clubs'!

The most simple and cost-effective moderate exercise recommended is 'brisk' walking (during which an individual finds speaking difficult but not impossible). Other exercises recommended are stair climbing, cycling, jogging or swimming. Physical activity should be carried out for 30–60 min/day.

The results of therapy are likely to be more satisfactory in **hypertrophic** obesity (enlarged, distended fat cells, with usual onset in adult life) than in the **hyperplastic** variety (more numerous fat cells, with usual onset in childhood).

The patient should be told at the onset of therapy that an average weekly loss of 0.5–0.8 kg is adequate and would result in annual loss of about 25 kg. This can be achieved by consuming 500–1000 fewer calories per day.

Use of **appetite suppressants (anorexiants)** may help the patient to adjust to the prescribed diet. *However,* **these drugs only supplement and are not a substitute for the dietary restrictions.**

Classification of Drugs Used for Obesity

I. **Centrally acting, appetite suppressants (anorexiants)**
   - **Adrenergic agents**, e.g. benzamphetamine, phentermine, mazindol, phendimetrazine
   - **5-HT agonists**, e.g. fluoxetine, lorcaserin

II. **Drugs acting in the GI tract**
   - **Bulk anorexiants**, e.g. dietary fibre, methylcellulose, guar gum
   - **Nonabsorbable fat substitutes**, e.g. olestra
   - **Lipase inhibitors**, e.g. orlistat

III. **Drug combinations,** e.g. phenteramine + topiramate, bupropion + naltrexone

IV. **Miscellaneous,** e.g. metformin, liraglutide (GLP-1 agonist)

Salient Pharmacological Features of Antiobesity Drugs

I. **Anorexiants**

Amphetamine and related compounds: *They* (Chapter 18) *are not recommended because of* drug dependence and sympathomimetic ADR like hypertension, tachycardia, insomnia and nervousness. **Methylamphetamine is highly addictive and is extensively abused.**

Other related drugs are phenteramine, phendimetrazine, mazindol and diethylpropion. Of these, the first two are suspected to produce dependence and could be abused.

Fluoxetine: This 5-HT reuptake inhibitor antidepressant (Chapter 14), in the dose of 60 mg/day, is associated with weight loss; but its long-term use should be avoided in view of the experience with fenfluramine, which was found to cause cardiac valvular injury and primary pulmonary hypertension.

Lorcaserin: This is a **selective central $5HT_{2C}$ receptor agonist.** It suppresses the appetite. It has a t½ of 11 h and is extensively metabolised by the liver. Headache, nausea, dizziness and euphoria (at doses >40 mg) are the frequently reported adverse effects. Lorcaserin inhibits CYP2D6 and hence increases the concentration of other drugs metabolised by this enzyme (e.g. dextromethorphan). Its long-term toxicity is not yet known.

The limitations of the centrally acting anorexiants are summarised in Box 38.3. **None of these**

Box 38.3 Limitations of Centrally Acting Anorexiants

- Short-term efficacy
- Relapse of weight gain
- Possible toxicity during long-term therapy
- Weight cycling as a result of drug holiday, leading to adverse outcomes such as coronary heart disease
- Inability to prevent obesity-related illnesses and to prolong life
- Poor compliance

drugs are effective and safe for long-term therapy.

II. Drugs acting in the GI tract

Bulk anorexiants:

Methylcellulose, a nondigestible polysaccharide, when ingested, swells and adds to the bulk in the diet. Though used as an agent to promote satiety, it is no more effective than a high residue low caloric diet for the obvious reason that an obese person is interested in eating good food and not something that would merely distend the stomach. It forms an important, cheap constituent of many 'costly', commercially promoted preparations for the treatment of obesity. **Guar gum, karaya gum** (sterculia gum, kanormal) and **glucomannan** are the other bulking agents.

Digestion inhibitors:

OLESTRA: This is a mixture of sucrose-fatty-acid esters that is **neither digested nor absorbed from the GI tract.** When used as a component of diet, it increases the bowel function and stool bulk. It is recommended as a fat substitute in cooking. Long-term effects on the health are yet not fully known. It is expensive.

ORLISTAT: Orlistat (tetrahydrolipostatin) is **related to a lipase inhibitor, lipostatin** produced by the mould, *Streptomyces toxytricini.*

- It acts by inhibiting pancreatic and other lipases including phospholipase A_2.
- It is not absorbed and the effects are confined to the GI tract, where it prevents the lipase-catalysed breakdown (GI lipase inhibition) of triglycerides (TG) and subsequent absorption.
- It causes a modest reduction in the plasma levels of total cholesterol and LDL cholesterol but not of TG.
- It causes modest weight loss over 1–4 years.
- It is almost completely excreted unchanged in faeces.

The common ADRs are abdominal pain, flatulence, increased defecation of oily/fatty stools with anal leaking, which can be inconvenient and socially embarrassing. Rarely hepatotoxicity has been reported. It is used in the dose of 120 mg 2–3 times daily, with meals, for a maximum of 2 years.

Isn't it better to eat less fat, rather than eating it and then preventing its absorption by a 'pill'?

III. Drug combinations

a. **Phenteramine** in combination with **topiramate,** an antiepileptic (Chapter 9), given once daily causes dose dependent weight loss. However, because of ADR, the discontinuation rate is nearly 40%. Topiramate is also a carbonic anhydrase inhibitor and can cause metabolic acidosis.

b. **Bupropion,** a weak antidepressant, also stimulates hypothalamic neurons to produce anorexigenic effects. However, these neurons also secrete beta endorphin, an endogenous opioid, which counters this action. Hence, **bupropion is combined with naltrexone,** an opioid antagonist. The combination is reported to cause weight loss but the effect is not sustained. Moreover, its neuropsychiatric toxicity limits its usefulness (Chapter 14).

IV. Miscellaneous

The antidiabetic, **metformin,** induces weight loss in diabetic and some nondiabetic obese individuals GLP analogues such as **Liraglutide (3mg SC once daily) and semaglutide (2.4 mg SC per week)** are approved in the treatment of obesity. (Chapter 63).

Experts recommend that drugs may be considered in adults with a BMI of over 27 in the presence of an obesity-related complication and in those with a BMI of over 30 even in the absence of such a complication. Most effective drugs are phentermine+ topiramate combination and semaglutide SC. There are intragastric balloon devices also available which are placed endoscopically for 6 months and then deflated. In addition, recently nonsystemic oral superabsorbent hydrogel formulation of cellulose and citric acid has been approved. These capsules when taken before meals with water create a sense of satiety and hence reduce food intake. For persons with a BMI of over 40, bariatric surgery may be considered. As obesity is a chronic disease and as relapse is common after cessation of drug therapy, prolonged, lifelong, drug therapy may be desirable. **However, none of the available drugs is safe enough for prolonged use.** They also fail to maintain weight loss over 10% in a year. *Irrespective of the drugs used, if significant weight loss does not occur within 4–6 months of therapy, the drug is discontinued.*

Thus, currently the treatment of obesity mainly depends on **permanent lifestyle modifications** *such as change in eating habits and regular physical exercise, supported by behavioural therapy.*

Box 38.4 presents examples of drugs that can cause anorexia and Box 38.5 lists the drugs which may cause weight gain.

ATHEROSCLEROSIS AND HYPERLIPIDEMIA

The plasma lipids are water insoluble and transported in several classes of lipoproteins. These classes are as follows:

- Chylomicrons
- Chylomicron remnants
- Very low density lipoproteins (VLDL)
- Intermediate density lipoproteins (IDL)
- Low density lipoproteins (LDL)
- High density lipoproteins (HDL)
- Lipoprotein (a)

The lipoproteins contain a nonpolar core of TG and cholesterol esters, surrounded by a polar coat made up of phospholipids, unesterified cholesterol and apoproteins. The lipid in the chylomicrons and VLDL is mostly TG whereas that in the LDL is mostly cholesterol. *High serum LDL and VLDL levels are considered as atherogenic, whereas high HDL* (over 60 mg/dL) *has a protective effect.* Asians commonly have low HDL levels (<35 mg/dL), probably because of high carbohydrate diet.

Box 38.4 Some Drugs Causing Anorexia

- Aminophylline
- Amphetamines and related drugs
- Antimicrobials: Metronidazole, fluoroquinolones, erythromycin, nitrofurantoin, tetracycline
- Antimalarials
- Metformin
- Digitalis
- Levodopa

Box 38.5 Drugs Which May Cause Weight Gain

- **Antipsychotics**, especially Olanzapine
- **Antidepressants:** Tricyclics, SSRI, MAOI, mirtazapine
- **Hormones:** Glucocorticoids, insulin, progestogens, oral contraceptives and danazol
- **Beta blockers**
- **Oral antidiabetic drugs:** Sulphonylureas, glitazones
- **Anticonvulsants:** Phenytoin, sodium valproate
- **Antihistaminics,** especially the first generation agents
- **Pizotifen**

The normal fasting plasma is clear and contains about 700 mg of total lipids, comprising TG, cholesterol and phospholipids. About 70% of cholesterol is in ester form. Body derives cholesterol from:

1. Diet absorbed from the intestine.
2. Large amount by de novo synthesis by the liver and peripheral tissues.

In health the plasma cholesterol and TG levels are regulated by several factors such as age, sex, race, genetics, diet, exercise and stress.

Atherosclerosis, a disease which affects *large and medium-sized arteries*, is now a leading cause of death in many developed countries. Its etiology is not known. The atherosclerotic lesion is a localised plaque in the intima and is composed of cholesterol esters, proliferation of smooth muscle, deposition of fibrous proteins (predominantly collagen) and calcification. Such plaques

- *Narrow the arterial lumen causing distal ischaemia and even thrombosis.*
- *Weaken the arterial wall, leading to formation of aneurysms.*

The coronary and the cerebral vessels are common sites of atherosclerosis.

Experimental and epidemiological evidence suggests a relationship between atherosclerosis and elevated levels of plasma lipids (cholesterol and TG). Although there is no diagnostic abnormal pattern of the plasma lipids in atherosclerotic patients, they have an **increase**

Table 38.1 Serum Lipid Levels (mg/dL) and the Risk of IHD[a]

Lipid	Desirable Level (Low Risk)	Borderline Level (Moderate Risk)	Abnormal Level (High Risk)
Total cholesterol	<200	200–240	>240
LDL cholesterol	<130	130–160	>160
HDL cholesterol	>60	40–60	<40
Triglycerides	<200	200–400	>400

[a]The risk increases further with other risk factors such as smoking, diabetes and hypertension.

in plasma LDL cholesterol and TG. The risk of IHD in such subjects is about thrice that in those with normal plasma cholesterol. A reduction of plasma lipids helps to prevent the progression of atherosclerosis. *Studies have confirmed that a reduction in elevated plasma LDL cholesterol does reduce the risk of MI.*

Table 38.1 shows the risk of IHD associated with different levels of serum lipids.

Hyperlipoproteinaemias which are incriminated in the pathogenesis of atherosclerosis are divided into five Fredrickson's types (I–V) depending on the class of lipoprotein(s) elevated. Determination of the total TG, total cholesterol and HDL cholesterol levels also allows to diagnose (a) hyperlipidaemia and (b) hyperlipoproteinaemia type. Type I hyperlipoproteinaemia is due to a defect in lipoprotein lipase and is induced by dietary fat. Type II is hereditary. Type III is due to hereditary dysbetalipoproteinaemia. Types IV and V are carbohydrate induced and are associated with insulin resistance as well.

The commonest hyperlipidaemias are secondary to dietary excess, uncontrolled DM, hypothyroidism, alcoholism, nephrotic syndrome, chronic renal failure and drugs such as etretinate, glucocorticoids used for prolonged periods and protease inhibitors. Therefore, every patient with hyperlipidaemia (defined as elevation of cholesterol and/or TG) should be investigated for such factors before starting lipid-lowering therapy.

Elevation of plasma LDL cholesterol, especially when combined with reduced HDL, is associated with increased risk of atherosclerotic arterial disease. Raised concentration of TG and VLDL may also contribute. Extreme elevation of plasma TG can lead to pancreatitis.

ANTIHYPERLIPIDEMIC/DYSLIPIDEMIC DRUGS PH 1.31, IM 2.18, IM 11.18

Classification of anti-hyperlipidemic drugs based on target lipoprotein:

I. Elevated LDL-C
   - **HMG-CoA reductase inhibitors** (statins)
   - **Intestinal Mucosal transporter inhibitor-NPC1L1**, e.g. ezetimibe
   - **PCSK-9 inhibitors**, e.g. alirocumab, evolocumab
   - **Cholestyramine resins**, e.g. colestipol, colesevalam

II. Elevated TG e.g. fibric acid derivatives (fibrates), fish oil

III. Elevated LDL-C and TG e.g. nicotinic acid

STATINS **(HMG-CoA-reductase inhibitors):** Drugs belonging to this class are structural analogues of HMG-CoA. They are listed in Table 38.2.

Table 38.2 Recommended Statin Doses

Statins	High-Intensity Statin Therapy (mg/day)	Moderate-Intensity Statin Therapy (mg/day)
Atorvastatin	40–80	10–20
Rosuvastatin	20–40	5–10
Simvastatin	–	20–40
Pravastatin	–	40–80
Lovastatin	–	40
Fluvastatin	–	Extended-release: 80 40 twice a day
Pitavastatin	–	2–4

Mechanism of action: Normally, about 70%–75% of plasma LDL is extracted by hepatocytes. Cholesterol esters from LDL molecules are hydrolysed in the liver to free cholesterol. The liver also produces cholesterol by *de novosynthesis* by a pathway involving formation of mevalonic acid by the *enzyme, Hydroxy methyl glutaryl coenzyme A reductase (HMG-CoA reductase)* (Fig. 38.1). **Statins inhibit this rate-limiting enzyme.** The decreased hepatic cholesterol synthesis causes increased synthesis of high affinity **LDL receptors (upregulation)** on the surface of hepatocytes. This results into increased clearance (uptake) of cholesterol-rich plasma LDL with subsequent reduction in plasma LDL cholesterol (Fig. 38.2). This action is dose dependent and maximum effect is generally seen within 6 weeks. Effect of statins on HDL-C is variable.

Statins also possess other **lipid-independent effects.** These are as follows:

- Decrease in platelet aggregation and in fibrinogen levels.
- Improvement in endothelial function and increase in local NO production.
- Decrease in macrophage infiltration into the vessel wall.
- Decrease in the arterial muscle proliferation.

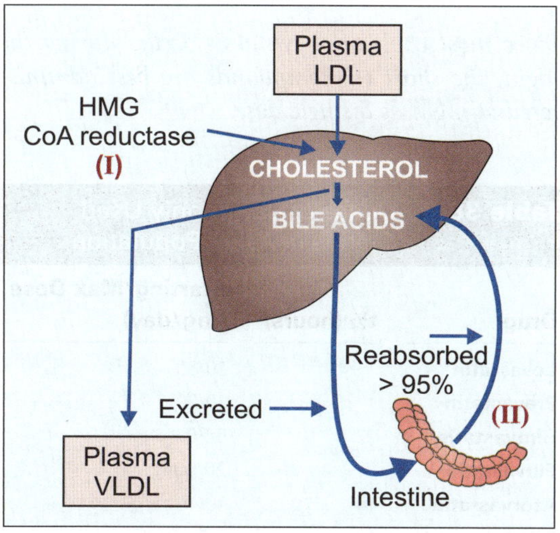

Fig. 38.1 Hepatic regulation of synthesis of cholesterol and bile acids. (I) Site of action of statins; (II) site of action of resins and ezetimibe.

- Retardation of the progression of hypertrophy of the vessel wall
- Decrease LDL oxidation in the vessel wall

These **pleiotropic effects** contribute to anti-inflammatory potential of statins. However, their precise contribution to the overall beneficial effects in the patients is not clear.

Absorption, fate and excretion: Oral absorption of all the statins (except fluvastatin) varies from 40%–90%. Fluvastatin is absorbed almost completely. Lovastatin and simvastatin are prodrugs and are hydrolysed in the GIT to the active metabolites. *Atorvastatin, fluvastatin and rosuvastatin are fluorinated compounds that are active as such.* All undergo first-pass metabolism and most of the dose is excreted in the bile; only about 5%–20%is excreted in the urine.

Adverse reactions: Generally statins are well tolerated and appear to be reasonably safe. ADRs are mostly mild and dose dependent. They may cause reversible rise in hepatic aminotransferase levels. Small rise in the plasma creatinephosphokinase (CPK) level is not uncommon. Rarely, it may be marked, and accompanied by muscular pains (myositis) and even myopathy. Rhabdomyolysis is rare.

Rarely, statins may cause impotence, gynaecomastia, peripheral neuropathy, memory loss, insomnia, mood changes and depression.

Clinical trials demonstrate that statins may increase the risk of new-onset diabetes but incidence is not as much as they reduce the cardiovascular risk.

Statins are contraindicated in pregnancy and in a woman planning to become pregnant, during breast-feeding, in children and in patients with severe liver disease.

Drug interactions: Combination of a statin with a fibric acid derivative and nicotinic acid potentiates the rise in plasma CPK level.

Lovastatin, simvastatin and **atorvastatin** undergo extensive first-pass metabolism by CYP3A4 and their toxicity can be increased by the concurrent use of

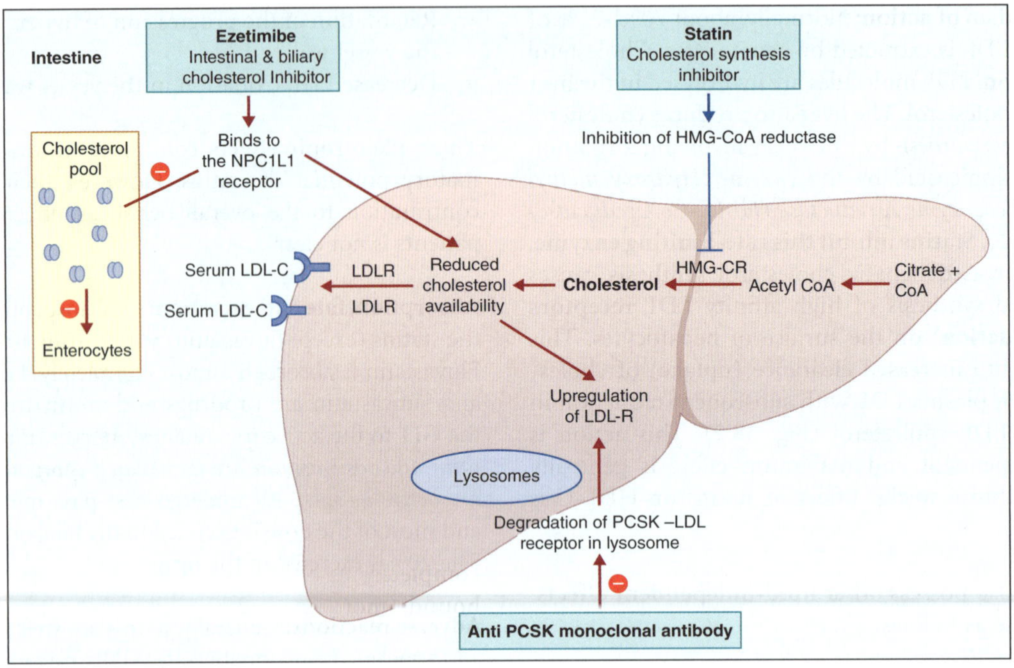

Fig. 38.2 Target sites for statin, ezetimibe and PCSK–9 inhibitors.

hepatic microsomal enzyme inhibitors such as ketoconazole, isoniazid, erythromycin, cyclosporine and HIV protease inhibitors. **Fluvastatin** and **rosuvastatin** are metabolised by hepatic CYP2C9. Inhibitors of this enzyme such as ketoconazole, metronidazole and cimetidine can increase their plasma levels.

Indications: Statins, used alone in maximum doses, can lower LDL level by 30%–50% (Table 38.4). Statin therapy can reduce the 5-year incidence of major coronary events, and stroke significantly, largely irrespective of the initial lipid level. *In general, statins are more effective in patients with high risk factors irrespective of the LDL cholesterol level. They retard the atherosclerotic process.* Statins are useful in:

- **Familial hypercholesterolemia.**
- **Atherosclerotic cardiovascular disease (ASCVD) for treatment and prevention:** See section on Management of hyperlipidemia

Choice of statin: Therapeutically, there are no clear differences among various statins. Hence the choice of the statin depends upon the degree of LDL-C elevation, drug pharmacokinetics, drug interactions, presence of hepatic/renal disease and cost. *Atorvastatin, simvastatin and rosuvastatin are more potent than other statins.* Atorvastatin and fluvastatin need no dose adjustment in patients with renal impairment. Pravastatin and fluvastatin are not metabolised by CYP3A4 and are likely to cause few drug interactions. *Atorvastatin and rosuvastatin have long t½ (see Table 38.3) and can be taken at any time of the day.*

Since most cholesterol synthesis occurs during the night, the short t½ compounds are best administered at night as a single dose.

Table 38.3 Doses of Commonly Used Statins in Asian Population

Drug	t½ (hours)	Starting/Max Dose (mg/day)
Lovastatin	1–4	10/80
Pravastatin	1	10/20
Simvastatin	12	5/20
Fluvastatin	6	20/60
Atorvastatin	14	10/40
Rosuvastatin	19	2.5/20

Notes: Atorvastatin may be given at any time of the day; pravastatin and fluvastatin at bedtime; others with evening meal.

EZETIMIBE: The prodrug, 2-azetidinone, is converted in intestine to an active metabolite ezetimibe glucuronide (t½– 22 h). It acts by inhibiting the intestinal mucosal transporter NPC1L1, and reduces the *absorption of cholesterol by the small intestine (Fig. 38.1 and Fig. 38.2). This in turn decreases the delivery of dietary and biliary cholesterol to the liver. Reduction of hepatic cholesterol stores causes an increase in the LDL receptors on the hepatocytes (upregulation) and an increased LDL cholesterol clearance from the circulation*. The plasma total and LDL cholesterol decreases with minimal increase in HDL-C (See Table 38.4). It also interrupts the entero-hepatic cycling of cholesterol. It is 90% bound to plasma proteins and is largely excreted in the faeces.

Adverse reactions are fatigue, dizziness, headache, abdominal discomfort, diarrhoea, arthralgia and hypersensitivity reactions.

Indications: It is used as an add-on drug in the dose of 5–10 mg/day. It acts synergistically when combined with statins. It should be avoided in children and in pregnant/lactating women.

PCSK-9 inhibitors: Proprotein convertase subtilisinkexin type 9 (PCSK-9) binds to LDL receptors on liver cells and promote receptor degradation. Thus LDL cholesterol clearance from blood is prevented (Fig 38.2). Human monoclonal antibodies **alirocumab** and **evolocumab** given subcutaneously prevent PCSK-9 binding to hepatocyte LDL-C receptors and increase hepatic uptake of LDL-C leading to fall in blood LDL-C levels. They have been used to treat heterozygous familial hypercholesterolemia and statin resistant patients. They may cause neurocognitive toxicity. They need further evaluation. They are prohibitively expensive.

FIBRATES are the derivatives of fibric (isobutyric) acid (Fig. 38.3) and include **gemfibrozil**, **bezafibrate** and **fenofibrate**.

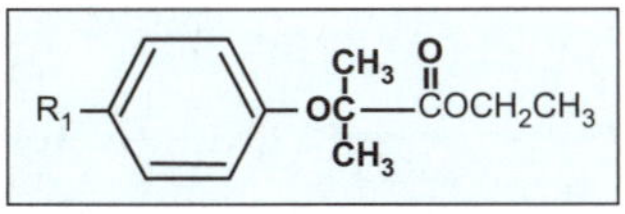

Fig. 38.3 **Fibrate nucleus. R differs with the analogue.**

Mechanism of action: These drugs **stimulate** the nuclear transcription receptor, **Peroxisome Proliferator Activated Receptor-alpha (PPAR-α)** that controls the expression of genes, which mediate TG metabolism. They:

a. Increase lipoprotein lipase (lpL) activity and the hydrolysis of TG
b. Promote HDL production
c. Reduce the incorporation of fatty acids into VLDL in the liver, thus inhibiting its synthesis and secretion

The plasma TG declines by 50% and cholesterol by 10%–15%. HDL increases by 20% (Table 38.4). They reduce plasma fibrinogen levels, to increase fibrinolysis and to reduce platelet aggregation.

Absorption, fate and excretion: They are almost completely absorbed from the gut, are highly protein bound (more than 90%). *They are largely excreted unchanged in the urine.*

Adverse reactions: Fibrates are generally well tolerated although, they occasionally produce allergic reactions, nausea and diarrhoea. *Though rare, potentially serious effects on the skeletal (myositis) and cardiac muscle have been reported.* Fibrates should be avoided in patients with renal or hepatic damage and in alcoholics (with hypertriglyceridemia) who are predisposed to myositis. Long-term therapy is associated with an increase in gallstone formation. *The combination of a fibrate and a statin increases the chance of rhabdomyolysis and myopathy.* These drugs displace acidic drugs from their plasma protein binding and may enhance the action of warfarin and sulphonylureas.

Preparations and dosage:

i. Fenofibrate: 145 and 160 mg tablets and 45, 67, 134, 160, 200 and 267 mg single dose capsules. Dose: One tablet/capsule o.d. with a meal.
ii. Gemfibrozil 300 and 600 mg capsules. Dose: 600 mg twice a day 30 minutes before meals.
iii. Bezafibrate: 200 mg tablets and 400 mg modified release tablets. Doses: 200 mg three times a day with meals. For modified release tablet, 400 mg once daily.

Indications: They are mainly useful in reducing plasma TG. Fenofibrate is preferred to gemfibrozil.

NICOTINIC ACID: This vitamin in large doses effectively and rapidly reduces plasma TG by lowering VLDL levels; LDL levels diminish more slowly, whereas HDL levels rise during therapy. *Nicotinamide lacks these actions.*

Mechanism of action: In the adipose tissue, nicotinic acid inhibits adenylyl cyclase and prevents lipolysis. This reduces the transport of fatty acids to the liver. In the liver, it reduces both synthesis and esterification of fatty acids. The end result is reduction in the hepatic production of VLDL and in plasma TG, VLDL cholesterol and LDL cholesterol (Table 38.4).

Adverse reactions: In pharmacological doses, nicotinic acid produces intense cutaneous flushing and pruritus by increasing the local prostaglandin levels. This can be minimised by starting with a small dose and gradually building it up to the full dose, and by taking the drug with meals; further, one tablet of aspirin, taken 30 min earlier, markedly reduces the flush. Other adverse reactions are nausea, vomiting, diarrhoea; abnormalities of liver function, clinical jaundice; hyperuricaemia, hyperglycaemia and potentiation of hypotension caused by antihypertensives.

Indications: *Nicotinic acid is useful in all forms of hyperlipoproteinaemias except type I.* The starting dose is 250 mg once daily (with meal); dose/ frequency increased every 4 to 7 days to reach 1.5 to 2 g daily in 2 to 3 divided doses with maximum dose as 6 g daily in 3 divided doses. With sustained release formulations dose is 250 -750 mg t.i.d, and extended release formulations 500 mg at bedtime for 4 weeks, then 1 g at bedtime.

Fish oil: Epidemiological evidence suggests that fatty-fish-eating communities have a lower incidence of IHD than non–fish eaters. **Omega-3 PUFA** *in the fish oil decreases hepatic production of TG and increases its clearance.* Thus, they reduce plasma TG but have little effect on HDL and LDL cholesterol and can sometimes increase total cholesterol up to 50%. They also lead to synthesis of leukotrienes and prostaglandins of series 1 and 3, which are less proinflammatory than those of series 2 (Chapter 25). Unlike gemfibrozil and niacin, omega-3 PUFAs do not interact with statins to enhance the incidence of myositis. They may decrease the risk of cardiac death in recent MI. *But, in chronic IHD there is a possibility of a proarrhythmic effect.*

Adverse effects: These include eructations, dyspepsia and unpleasant after taste. Large doses of Omega-3 PUFA can inhibit platelet aggregation and may worsen glycaemic control in diabetes.

CHOLESTYRAMINE RESIN: This insoluble chloride salt of a basic anion exchange resin has a strong affinity for bile salts (cholates) in the intestine (Fig. 38.1). It binds the cholates into an insoluble complex which is excreted in faeces. The result is decreased absorption of exogenous cholesterol and increased metabolism of endogenous cholesterol into bile acids in the liver. This leads to increased LDL receptors on liver cells and increased removal of LDL from the circulation. The dose is 12–24 g per day in a single or divided doses.

Adverse reactions: These include nausea, vomiting, bloating and constipation. Large doses may interfere with absorption of fats and fat-soluble vitamins, causing steatorrhoea. It also interferes with the absorption of thyroid hormones, tetracyclines, warfarin andphenobarbitone.

Indications: It is usedin combination with antihyperlipidemic drugs to treat hyperlipidaemia, but it is not a drug of choice. It may be useful in hyperlipidemic pregnant women and for relieving pruritus associated with biliary cirrhosis and cholestatic jaundice.

Table 38.4 Effects of Lipid-Lowering Agents on Lipid Fractions

Drug	Total Cholesterol	LDL Cholesterol	HDL Cholesterol	Triglycerides (TG)
Statins	↓	↓↓	↑	↓
Ezetimibe	↓	↓	–	–
Fibrates	↓	↑	↑	↓↓
Nicotinic acid (NA)	↓	↓	↑↑	↓

Notes: ↑/↑↑, increases; ↓/↓↓, decreases.

Colestipol and **colesevalam,** like cholestyramine, are bile acid sequestrants.

GUGULIPID: This is the steroidal fraction derived from the plant *Commiphoramukul* and has moderate and variable hypocholesterolemic activity. It is well tolerated. It is available as 25 mg tablets.

FIBRE: Soluble fibres (pectins in citrus fruits, mucilages in psyllium husk and seeds, gums in oat products and in beans) have a modest effect in lowering serum cholesterol. Psyllium husk (isapgol) is administered in the dose of 2.5–5 g twice a day; oat bran is used in the dose of 50–150 g a day. Insoluble fibre such as is present in wheat bran is not effective in lowering serum cholesterol (Chapter 40).

NEWER ANTIHYPERLIPIDEMIC DRUGS

1. **Inhibitor of microsomal triglyceride transfer: Lomitapide** inhibits the intracellular transfer of TG into triglyceride-rich lipoproteins. It thus prevents the formation of VLDLs and chylomicrons in hepatocytes and intestinal epithelial cells respectively. Lomitapide is co-administered with statin if patients are not responding to maximally tolerated dose of statin.
2. **ATP-citrate lyase inhibitor: Bempedoic acid** acts by inhibiting *de novo* hepatocyte cholesterol biosynthesis by reducing the flow of acetyl-CoA to HMG-CoA reductase. It acts synergistic with statins and reduces LDL-C by 65%. However, it increases the risk of myopathy and should not be given with simvastatin or rosuvastatin. It can be combined with ezetimibe.
3. **Inhibitor of angiopoietin-like protein 3: Evinacumab-dgnb** is a recombinant human monoclonal antibody that binds to and inhibits angiopoietin-like protein 3. This causes reduction in LDL-C and TG. It is given intravenously for patients with homozygous familial hypercholesterolemia.

MANAGEMENT OF HYPERLIPIDEMIA

Stress reduction, weight reduction, modification of diet, abstinence from alcohol and smoking and treatment of the causative disease, if any, such as hypothyroidism and DM are more important than lipid-lowering drugs. The cornerstone of the current therapy is improvement in the lifestylefor the primary and secondary prevention of coronary artery diseases (CAD). It is claimed that existing CAD can be reversed by appropriate nonsurgical and even nonpharmacological regimens (such that of 'Dean Ornish'), which comprises the following:

- **Dietary modification**
- **Increased physical activity**
- **Reduction in the body weight to the ideal level**
- **Elimination of associated risk factors,** e.g. smoking, alcohol
- **Stress control**

Dietary modification (Box 38.6) implies:

- *Decrease in the consumption of foods rich in saturated fats (restricted up 10% of total calories). The dietary cholesterol appears to contribute relatively insignificantly to serum cholesterol level. However, processed products rich in cholesterol may be harmful as they contain transfat.*
- *Reduction in the intake of salt, sugars and sugar containing products and beverages.*
- *Avoidance of red meat and processed meat products.*
- *Increase the consumption of poultry, low-fat fish and skimmed milk, together with large helpings of vegetables, legumes, fruits and mixed nuts.*

In fact, the traditional Indian vegetarian diet, which contains grains, nuts, curd, low fat dairy products, less of salt and sugar, lot of fibres, pulses, legumes and nuts, has much to recommend in this respect. It has

Box 38.6 Principles of Diet Therapy in Hyperlipidemia PH 1.1

- Restriction of fat calories to less than 20% of total calories
- Saturated, monounsaturated and polyunsaturated fats should form one-third each of the total dietary fat. Avoid trans-fatty acids
- Increased consumption of vegetables, fresh fruit, cereals, nuts especially walnuts and almonds (in moderation) and whole grain products
- Avoid refined carbohydrates
- Increased consumption of fish, where possible/permitted
- Drastic reduction in alcohol consumption and smoking

The above principles may need to be modified in case of children, pregnant women and old people.

similarities to Mediterranean diet, which contains olive oil and is claimed to prevent cardiovascular diseases.

- *Decrease the consumption of total fats to 15%–20% of the daily caloric intake.* Only one-third of these fat calories should be supplied by saturated fats (fats of animal origin and coconut oil), one-third by mono-unsaturated fats (olive oil, mustard oil, til oil and groundnut oil), and the rest one-third by polyunsaturated fats (sunflower, corn and safflower oils).

Saturated fatty acids (SFA) are straight chained and vary in the chain length. Unsaturated fatty acids (UFA), on the other hand, also vary in the number and the position of their double bonds. In natural products, the double bonds are in cisform; whereas **in the case of commercial products, they are converted into trans form (TFA)** following partial hydrogenation. The **trans forms:**

a. Are more stable and have higher melting points.
b. Though unsaturated, **they decrease HDL cholesterol and increase LDL cholesterol, TG and lipoproteins.**
c. Can also cause endothelial dysfunction.
d. Promote abdominal fat accumulation, and insulin resistance in animals.
e. Their consumption is associated with increased risk of IHD in humans.

As deep-fried and bakery food products are the major dietary sources of TFA, these should be avoided.

Hydrogenated fats and prolonged heating of fats also have deleterious effects similar to those of saturated fats and should be avoided.

- *Use of complex carbohydrates*: With the reduction in the total fat content of the diet, carbohydrates become a major source of calories. Use of complex carbohydrates such as starchy foods (cereals, beans, pulses) should be encouraged.
- *Consumption of omega 3 fatty acids*: Traditional approaches to prophylaxis of atherosclerosis have focused on one aspect of its pathogenesis, i.e. platelet function or blood lipids. Coastal eskimos who eat a traditional diet of fish and seals have a low incidence of cardiovascular diseases, chronic inflammatory diseases such as psoriasis and asthma. This is believed to be due to consumption of **fatty fish rich in two omega-3-fatty acids – eicosapentaenoic acidand docosahexaenoic acid, as against omega-6 fatty acids** (linoleic acid), present in vegetable oils, which is converted to arachidonic acid (Chapter 25).

Studies indicate that:

a. The administration of omega-3-polyunsaturated fatty acids in the form of salmon or cod liver oil results in reduction in platelet responsiveness, lowering of blood lipids and improvement of blood flow.
b. Long-term intake of cod liver oil promotes the formation of the PGI_2.
c. Exogenous eicosapentaenoic acid dose-dependently suppresses formation of leukotriene-B4.

Vegetarians get omega-3 fatty acids from nuts (especially walnuts), dark green leafy vegetables, flaxseed, pumpkin seeds, soya beans, hemp seeds and linseed,canola and sunflower oil, but to a smaller extent. These fatty acids may play a role in the prophylaxis of atherosclerosis (Chapter 25).

Finally while prescribing the diet, we should focus more on the dietary pattern and not so much on the individual components of the diet.

Drug therapy is indicated in those:

- **In whom the dietary measures are not successful or who find the dietary restrictions irksome.**
- **Who are at a risk of pancreatitis** because of very high TG levels (1000 mg%).

Drug therapy should be started with the understanding that it will have to be continued **life-long**. *The drugs do not cure the basic disorder of lipoprotein metabolism but symptomatically control only one aspect of the disease process.*

Choice of lipid-lowering drugs: The current evidence indicates that the **statins are the lipid-lowering drugs of choice for most patients at risk of atherosclerotic cardiovascular disease (ASCVD). They are indicated for both treatment and prevention in individuals:**

- With **clinical evidence of ASCVD** e.g. IHD, MI.
- With **primary elevation of LDL cholesterol > 190 mg%**

Table 38.5 Choice of Lipid-Lowering Drugs

Drug	Hypercholesterolemia (Elevated LDL-C + TG < 200 mg/dL)	Combined Hyperlipidaemia (Elevated LDL-C + TG 200–400 mg/dL)	Hypertriglyceridemia (TG > 400 mg/dL)
Statins	Drugs of choice	Effective	–
Fibrates	–	Effective in high doses	Drugs of choice
Nicotinic acid	Effective; usefulness limited by adverse effects	Drug of choice	Effective but poorly tolerated

Notes: Statins can be combined with nicotinic acid or a fibrate or ezetimibe in resistant cases.

- **Aged 40–75 years with DM and LDL cholesterol between 70–189 mg%without clinical evidence of ASCVD**
- Aged 40–75 years, having LDL cholesterol between 70–189 mg%with no evidence of DM or ASCVD but **having estimated 10-years ASCVD risk of 7.5%or higher**. This risk is calculated based on the presence of risk factors.

Patients with clinical evidence of ASCVD and those with LDL-cholesterol >190 mg%are treated with **high intensity statin therapy**, which reduces LDL-cholesterol by >50%. Others are treated with **moderate intensity**, wherein a decrease by 30% to <50% is expected (Table 38.2). *Considering that low doses are required in Asian populations (Table 38.3), studies in Indians to establish dose range are needed.*

There is no unanimity about what can be considered as an 'ideal'level of serum cholesterol and hence, currently importance is given to the clinically relevant risk factors rather than chasing a particular target level for LDL cholesterol. Routine use of statin in subject with >75 years and without evidence of ASCVD and those with HF (see Chapter 31) do not seem to be beneficial.

Though statins are used for all types of hyperlipidemias, the choice of drugs for combined hypercholesterolemia and for hypertriglyceridemia are outlined in Table 38.5.

Hyperlipidemia is associated with homocysteinaemia, hence **folic acid** supplements are used to prevent homocysteinaemia (Chapter 35).

DRUGS USED IN THE TREATMENT OF OBESITY

Centrally acting, appetite suppressants (anorexiants)

Adrenergic agents
- Benzamphetamine
- Phentermine
- Mazindol
- Phendimetrazine

5-HT agonists
- Fluoxetine
- Lorcaserin

Drugs acting in the GI tract

Bulk anorexiants
- Dietary fibre
- Methylcellulose
- Guar gum

Nonabsorbable fat substitutes
- Olestra

Lipase inhibitors
- Orlistat

Drug combinations
- Phenteramine + Topiramate
- Bupropion + Naltrexone

Miscellaneous
- Metformin
- Liraglutide (GLP-1 agonist)

ANTIHYPERLIPIDEMIC DRUGS BASED ON TARGET LIPOPROTEIN

Elevated LDL-C

HMG-CoA reductase inhibitors
- Atorvastatin
- Rosuvastatin
- Simvastatin
- Pravastatin
- Lovastatin

Intestinal mucosal transporter NPC1L1 inhibitor
- Ezetimibe

PCSK-9 inhibitors
- Alirocumab
- Evolocumab

Cholestyramine resins
- Colestipol
- Colesevelam

Elevated TG
- Fibric acid derivatives (fibrates)
- Fish oil

Elevated LDL-C and TG
- Nicotinic acid

CHAPTER 39

Emetics, Drug Therapy of Vomiting, Vertigo and Diarrhoea

Learning Objectives

This chapter will enable the reader:

1. To classify emetics and state their indications and contraindications.
2. To enlist drugs that cause vomiting as ADR.
3. To classify antiemetics based on their mechanism of action giving suitable examples from each class.
4. To explain the pharmacological effects, ADR and indications for antihistaminics, phenothiazines, prokinetic drugs, anti-$5HT_3$ drugs, cannabinoid class of antiemetic drugs.
5. To outline the therapy of vomiting during pregnancy and motion sickness.
6. To outline the treatment of vertigo.
7. To explain the key features in the pathophysiology of diarrhoea, which are targeted during treatment.
8. To outline the therapy of infective diarrhoea.
9. To explain the management of dehydration and electrolyte disturbances associated with diarrhoea.
10. To describe the mechanism of action, indications, contraindications and adverse effects of GI protectives, adsorbents, opioids, racecadroteil, atropine substitutes, PG inhibitors, chloride channel inhibitor and probiotics.
11. To outline the pharmacotherapy of irritable bowel syndrome (IBS).
12. To outline the management of inflammatory bowel disease (IBD).
13. To enlist the drugs causing diarrhoea as adverse effect.

KEY TERMS

emetics, p. 580
antiemetics, p. 581
motion sickness, p. 584
vertigo, p. 584
prokinetics, p. 585
diarrhoea, mechanisms, p. 586
travellers' diarrhoea, p. 587
oral rehydration therapy, p. 588
racecadotril, p. 591
irritable bowel syndrome, p. 592
ulcerative colitis, p. 593
sulphasalazine, p. 593

Vomiting, though unpleasant, is a protective reflex which helps the stomach to get rid of noxious material. Vomiting also occurs in physiological situations such as pregnancy but often it is an indication of ill health and needs to be treated.

Physiology of vomiting: The act of vomiting is accompanied by a complex series of movements, controlled by the vomiting centre. It receives afferent impulses from

- Higher centres in the brain
- Chemoreceptor trigger zone (CTZ)
- Vestibular apparatus
- Peripheral structures including the GI tract and nucleus tractus solitarius

Fig. 39.1 shows the mechanism of vomiting and the receptors involved.

A major sensory relay station in the afferent vomiting pathway is the **CTZ**, situated in the lateral border of the area postrema of the medulla oblongata. *Histologically, CTZ resembles the carotid body and is not a part of the brain. It is in direct contact with the circulating blood and is outside the BBB.* A variety of drugs like morphine, apomorphine, alkylating agents and digitalis stimulate the CTZ, whereas the phenothiazines and certain antihistaminics depress it. However, the CTZ, being a purely sensory relay station, is incapable of initiating vomiting in the absence of vomiting centre, whereas direct stimulation of the latter evokes vomiting. Irritation or overdistension of the GI tract and delayed gastric emptying cause vomiting by direct stimulation of the vomiting centre via visceral vagal afferents. Similarly, it is likely that vomiting of central origin due to emotions, nauseous odours, and similar factors is due to impulses directly reaching the vomiting centre. On the other hand, **vomiting of vestibular origin** is mediated by the pathway – vestibular nuclei, cerebellum, CTZ and the vomiting centre.

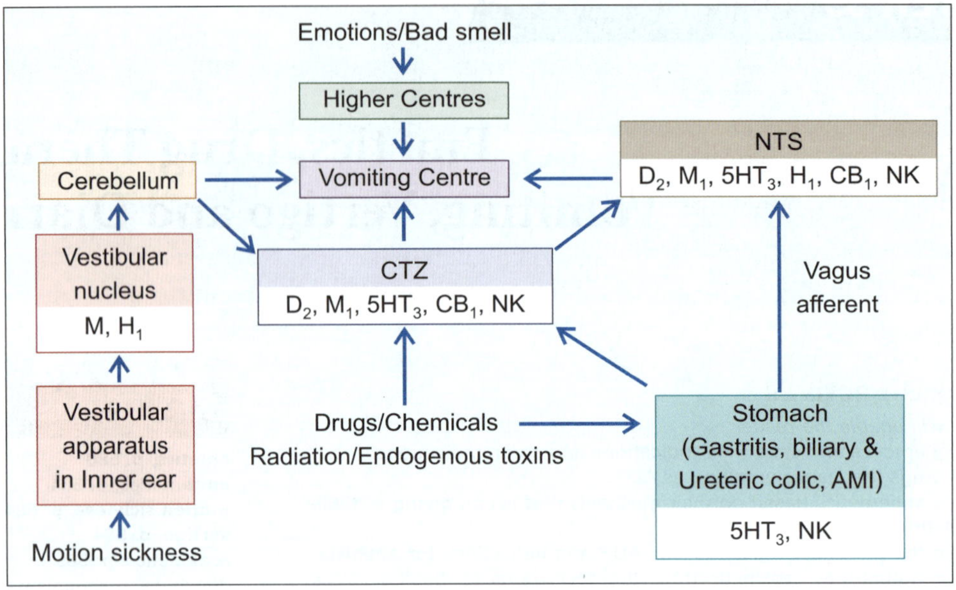

FIG. 39.1 **Mechanism of vomiting. AMI, acute myocardial infarction; CTZ, chemoreceptor trigger zone; H, histamine receptors; M, muscarinic receptors; NK, neurokinin receptor; NTS, nucleus tractus solitarius.**

Gastroesophageal reflux (GER) is not true vomiting; it occurs as a result of failed normal oesophageal function. GER is effortless and generally *not associated with autonomic symptoms.*

Apart from 5-HT, other NT such as DA, neurokinins (NK) and histamine probably play an important role in the process of vomiting. Three different NKs have been identified: substance P, neurokinin A and neurokinin B which are believed to act as neurotransmitters/neuromodulators. **Substance P** has been identified in the nucleus tractus solitarius and the area postrema of the brainstem, and also with 5-HT within the enterochromaffin cells of the GI tract. It is excitatory in nature and can induce vomiting.

Vomiting is usually preceded by the feeling of nausea and increased secretion of saliva, bronchial fluid and sweat. The muscles involved in the act of coughing also take part in the act of vomiting, and the vagal, vomiting and cough centres have a close functional relationship. Vomiting can also be induced voluntarily.

EMETICS

The drugs that are administered to induce vomiting are termed emetics.

Classification of Emetics

I. **Centrally acting emetics,** e.g. apomorphine, morphine.
II. **Peripherally acting emetics,** e.g. mustard, antimony-potassium tartrate [tartar emetic], hypertonic sodium chloride
III. **Both peripherally and centrally acting emetics,** e.g. ipecacuanha.

Salient Pharmacological Features of Emetics

I. **Centrally acting emetics**

APOMORPHINE: This drug (Chapters 10 and 15), given subcutaneously, causes vomiting within 15 min by stimulating CTZ. Vomiting is often accompanied by sedation. Apomorphine-induced vomiting is effectively suppressed by chlorpromazine. The drug can cause severe vomiting, hypotension, syncope, convulsions, coma and respiratory depression.

Although apomorphine is a highly effective emetic, it is not used as an emetic.

II. **Peripherally acting emetics:** These cause vomiting reflexly by irritating the gastric mucosa. The drugs are as follows:

MUSTARD: This acts by virtue of its volatile oil in the presence of water. It is uncertain in action, but it is safe and easily available common household remedy. Dose: 1 teaspoonful in 300 mL water.

SODIUM CHLORIDE (hypertonic): Given orally, it withdraws fluid from the gastric cell lining. This causes irritation with reflex emesis.

III. **Both peripherally and centrally acting emetics**
IPECACUANHA SYRUP: It contains, an alkaloid emetine which can evoke emesis in poisoning with drugs that depress the CTZ, e.g. chlorpromazine. The usual adult dose is 15 mL by mouth and may be repeated after 20 min if the individual fails to vomit. It should be avoided in infants.

Indications: The therapeutic use of emetics is limited to certain cases of poisoning, *especially where facilities for gastric lavage are not available.*

Emetics should generally be **avoided in**

- Children and the elderly
- Pregnant women
- Patients with cardiac decompensation, hypertension, hernia, peptic ulcer and pulmonary tuberculosis
- Poisoning caused by caustic agents

DRUG THERAPY OF VOMITING

ANTIEMETICS are drugs which specifically prevent or relieve nausea and vomiting.

Classification of Antiemetics: PH 1.34

I. **Antihistaminics,** e.g. cyclizine, meclizine, promethazine, dimenhydrinate (Chapter 23)
II. **Antidopaminergics** (D_2 receptors), e.g. chlorpromazine and related drugs (Chapter 13) metoclopramide, domperidone
III. **$5HT_3$ antagonists,** e.g. ondansetron, granisetron, dolasetron and palonosetron (Chapter 24); and ginger
IV. **Antimuscarinics,** e.g. scopolamine
V. **Antagonists of the NK_1 receptors for substance P,** e.g. aprepitant, netupitant
VI. **Miscellaneous** e.g. nabilone (a cannabinoid), trimethobenzamide, benzquinamide

Clinically, the antiemetics are grouped according to their potency as follows:

- **Highly efficacious:** Ondansetron, granisetron and high-dose metoclopramide.
- **Moderately efficacious:** Low-dose metoclopramide, phenothiazines (prochlorperazine), butyrophenones (droperidol) and cannabinoids.
- **Weakly efficacious:** Anticholinergics, antihistaminics and benzodiazepines (lorazepam).

ANTIHISTAMINIC–ANTIEMETIC DRUGS

Antihistaminics: H_1 receptor antagonists used include the **phenothiazine antihistaminics**, promethazine and its chlorotheophyllinate, dimenhydrinate and the **piperazine antihistaminics**, cyclizine, buclizine, meclizine and cinnarizine (Chapter 23). Some of these have antimuscarinic action. Antihistaminics act on the vomiting centre and also have mild sedative effect. They are effective in motion sickness, in vomiting due to labyrinthine disorders (vestibular neuronitis, Meniere disease) and in vomiting during pregnancy. *Vomiting due to gastroenteritis does not respond well to antihistaminic antiemetics.*

ANTIDOPAMINERGIC ANTIEMETICS

Phenothiazines (Chapter 13) like chlorpromazine, prochlorperazine are dopamine D_2 antagonists. *They selectively depress the CTZ but have no action on the vomiting centre.* **Hence, they are ineffective in motion sickness.** They are, however, the drugs of choice in nausea and vomiting due to uraemia, carcinomatosis, radiation sickness and that due to drugs. Among the phenothiazines, **triflupromazine and the piperazine phenothiazines are more effective** than others. However, they can cause extrapyramidal adverse effects.

In general, the phenothiazines are preferred when vomiting is severe and hazardous but is of short duration, e.g. postoperative vomiting. On the other hand, the antihistaminic antiemetics, though less effective than the phenothiazines, are safer and preferred for long-term use.

PH 1.34

METOCLOPRAMIDE: This antiemetic, chemically related to procainamide, acts predominantly as a **dopamine antagonist.** It also has **$5\text{-}HT_4$** agonist properties. Its antiemetic effect has two components:

- *Peripherally, it promotes the forward propulsion of the contents of the upper GI tract* **(prokinetic action)** *due to its agonist action on the 5-HT_4 receptors present on the myentric plexus.* It enhances the action of ACh at the muscarinic receptors, which are restricted to the proximal gut.
- *Central inhibition of vomiting* due to the blockade of DA receptors in the CTZ.

Pharmacological actions: The drug increases the resting tone of the gastroesophageal sphincter and stimulates coordinated gastric motility. An injection of 20 mg produces gastric emptying within 90 min in most patients. It also increases the activity of the pyloric antrum and duodenal peristalsis, and accelerates transit along the small bowel. It has no significant action on the biliary tract and the large bowel motility.

By its central action, metoclopramide reduces postoperative vomiting and vomiting due to morphine and pethidine.

The drug stimulates prolactin secretion.

Adverse reactions: It is a relatively safe drug. It can cause drowsiness, dystonic or extrapyramidal reactions and diarrhoea. The others include lassitude, skin rash, hyperprolactenaemia, gynaecomastia and galactorrhoea. It may aggravate sodium retention and hypokalaemia in patients with oedema. Extrapyramidal (EP) reactions and malignant neuroleptic syndrome following metoclopramide are dose related; and *the daily intake of this drug should not exceed 0.5 mg/kg*.

Preparations and dosage: 10-mg tablets; dose 5–10 mg t.i.d., as syrup (1mg/ml) and as an IM/IV injection (5mg/ml); 10–20 mg.

Indications:

- **As an antiemetic,** especially in postoperative vomiting, *in low doses* (10 mg i.m. or i.v. three times a day).
- **Before and during cancer chemotherapy** to prevent nausea and vomiting, in high doses (0.5–3 mg/kg i.v. over 15 min).
- **To accelerate gastric emptying** (prokinetic) before induction of general anaesthesia for emergency surgery; *prior administration of atropine can, however, block this effect.*
- **To assist the passage of tubes** *(including an endoscope)* **into the duodenum.**
- **To treat gastroparesis and gastroesophageal reflux disease (GERD)** with retention from a variety of causes, e.g. vagotomy, diabetes, gastritis and gastric ulcers.

DOMPERIDONE: This agent acts as a **selective D_2 receptor antagonist at CTZ.** It does not have ACh like effect. As it does not cross the BBB easily, unlike metoclopramide, it causes fewer EP reactions and rarely, hyperprolactinemia and galactorrhoea. The drug is effective orally as well as parenterally. The oral dose is 10–20 mg 3–4 times a day.

Selective 5-HT_3 antagonists, e.g. ondansetron, palanosetron are used to prevent and treat chemotherapy-induced vomiting, postoperative and postradiation vomiting (see Chapter 24).

ANTIMUSCARINIC ANTIEMETICS

SCOPOLAMINE: The belladonna alkaloid, scopolamine is among the first drugs to be used in the treatment of motion sickness. *A central muscarinic antagonism of ACh may be the basis of its therapeutic efficacy.* Scopolamine is more effective when used prophylactically than during an attack. The drug may cause drowsiness, dizziness, blurring of vision, dry mouth and urinary retention. *Scopolamine is also available in transdermal delivery system,* as an adhesive unit, for placement behind the ear.

Substance P/NK_1 receptor antagonists, e.g. **aprepitant, netupitant, rolapitant** selectively inhibit effects of substance P, a neuropeptide that binds to NK_1 receptors and thus, exert antiemetic actions. Adverse effects include headache, dyspepsia, and constipation. Usually these antagonists are given in combination with $5HT_3$ receptor antagonists in the treatment of highly emetogenic chemotherapy-induced vomiting.

NABILONE: This synthetic cannabinoid is used to treat nausea and vomiting caused by cancer chemotherapy, unresponsive to conventional antiemetics. The adverse reactions are mainly neurological and comprise drowsiness, vertigo, visual disturbances, headache, dysphoria, confusion, hallucinations and psychosis. Hypotension, tachycardia and abdominal pain may occur. Its use is contraindicated in severe hepatic impairment, pregnancy and breast-feeding. The adult dose is 1–2 mg t.i.d.

DRONABINOL: This Δ-9 tetrahydrocannobinol (Δ-9 THC), a natural ingredient of cannabis, is prepared synthetically. It acts on CB_1 receptors and is used orally to prevent and treat cancer-chemotherapy-induced nausea and vomiting. The ADR are wider than those of nabilone and include drug abuse.

Glucocorticoids such as dexamethasone given parenterally in large doses are used as *adjuncts* in the management of resistant nausea and vomiting induced by cancer chemotherapeutic agents.

PHARMACOTHERAPY OF VOMITING

Vomiting may be psychic in origin and initiated by sights or bad smells or may arise reflexly following GI irritation, MI, biliary and renal colic. Similarly excessive stimulation of vestibular apparatus as in motion sickness can cause vomiting. Certain drugs (Box 39.1), metabolites (as in uraemia) and raised intracranial tension act on the CTZ to produce vomiting. Finally, any severe pain may make a person prone for vomiting.

Similar stimuli in progressively increasing intensity produce successively anorexia, nausea and vomiting. There appear to be wide differences in individual susceptibility to stimuli that can trigger vomiting , e.g. infants are less susceptible to motion sickness than older children and adults (among whom again there are wide individual differences); women are more susceptible than men and the elderly are less susceptible than young adults to postanaesthetic vomiting. Estrogens are believed to lower the threshold of the CTZ, thus possibly explaining the vomiting of pregnancy and the nausea following the administration of combination OC therapy.

Box 39.1 Some Drugs which Cause Vomiting

- Antimicrobials: Erythromycin, tetracyclines, fluoroquinolones, metronidazole
- Anticancer drugs
- Amiodarone
- Opioids
- Chloroquine; quinine
- Diltiazem
- Emetine
- Ergot alkaloids

The treatment of vomiting consists of

- **Treatment of the cause,** e.g. relief of pain, treatment of GI infection, correction of metabolic acidosis
- **Symptomatic treatment** with antiemetics
- **Supportive therapy,** e.g. correction of dehydration

Therapy of Vomiting During Pregnancy

The aetiology of vomiting of early pregnancy is not established. It is usually mild. It reaches peak by 10th week and usually resolves by 14th week.

The patient is advised to take frequent small meals and more fluids. Psychotherapy including reassurance and placebo therapy are often helpful. Though it is ideal to avoid drugs in the first trimester, some women are severely nauseated and need drug therapy.

Drugs employed are **vitamin B_6 (pyridoxine)**, **antiemetic antihistaminics** (dimenhydrinate, doxylamine, cyclizine, meclizine) and **metoclopramide.** Usually, **doxylamine** 40 mg + **pyridoxine** 40 mg combination b.i.d. is considered safe and effective. **Dimenhydrinate** (50–100 mg) is safe and rapid in onset, and can be used as a suppository. **Prochlorperazine,** a phenothiazine, 5–10 mg is reported to be safe and can be given intravenously in severe cases (Chapter 23). **Ginger,** along with sugar, is safe and effective home remedy in mild cases. Its active components have 5-HT_3 antagonistic action. *Finally, vomiting due to an unrelated but associated condition such as peptic ulcer, hepatitis, drug reaction or gall bladder disease should be ruled out.*

Therapy of Motion Sickness

Motion sickness is a syndrome characterised by vertigo and nausea resulting from body motion. The word 'nausea' is derived from Greek word 'nautical' as it usually occurs at sea.

The receptors for motion sickness are located in the vestibular apparatus. Other stimuli such as visual, proprioceptive and emotional, may facilitate or enhance motion sickness. Children are more susceptible to motion sickness and the vulnerability diminishes with advancing age.

The susceptibility to motion sickness is determined by the balance of activation between the ACh and NA sensitive neurons in the reticular activating system adjacent to the vestibular nuclei. Drugs (a) that block ACh in the CNS, e.g. scopolamine, and (b) those which activate the central sympathetic areas, are highly effective in its treatment. It is easier to prevent motion sickness than to treat it.

SCOPOLAMINE: Scopolamine is more effective when used prophylactically than during an attack. A single oral dose of 0.3–0.6 mg in an adult, 15 min before food and 30 min before a journey, gives satisfactory protection. The drug action persists for 2–3 h.

Scopolamine transdermal patch is also available and placed behind the ear to prevent vomiting for 72 h.

The piperazine **antihistaminics** (cyclizine, buclizine, meclizine) have a prolonged action, a single dose providing relief for 6–12 h and are hence preferred. The action of meclizine is claimed to persist for 24 h. They are administered orally, 30 min before the journey.

Box 39.2 lists the applications of antiemetics in vomiting from different causes. For anti-5-HT_3 antiemetics see Chapter 24.

Box 39.2 Antiemetics in Various Types of Vomiting

GI irritation: Anticholinergics; in severe cases, a phenothiazine
Motion sickness: Scopolamine; dimenhydrinate; cyclizine, meclizine
Pregnancy: Doxylamine, pyridoxine, dimenhydrinate
Uraemia, cancer, radiation sickness, anticancer chemotherapy: Phenothiazine and butyrophenone antipsychotics; metoclopramide; ondansetron; nabilone; dexamethasone (as adjunctive drugs during cancer chemotherapy)
Gastroparesis: Prokinetic drugs
Postoperative: Prokinetic drugs, antihistaminics

THERAPY OF VERTIGO AND DIZZINESS

Vertigo is a hallucination of movement, generally spinning, caused by a disturbance of the orientation-detecting system of a person.

Orientation in space is achieved by integrating information mainly from:

- *Vestibular system*
- *Vision*
- *The proprioceptors in the muscles and joints* (somatosensory)

The collected information is processed in the sensory integrating areas of the reticular formation. When the information contains a new or an unusual element, vertigo can occur, e.g. it can occur in normal subjects following a spin or even unfamiliar head movement.

Vertigo can occur due to physiological stimulation or pathological dysfunction in any of the above systems. Phobic postural vertigo is observed in patients with panic attacks.

In all cases of vertigo, complete neurological examination is a must. If a cause for vertigo can be established, it may be amenable to specific treatment.

Dizziness is less specific than *vertigo* and comprises all symptoms of disequilibration including lightheadedness, giddiness, swimminess, floating, etc.; its pathogenesis is similar to that of vertigo. Individual patients may not be able to differentiate between vertigo and dizziness. **Both are caused by different pathological processes in CNS, CVS and metabolic disease.** Impaired sensation from the feet, poor vision in the elderly subject may cause lightheadedness or dizziness mostly during walking. **This is not vertigo.**

Drug therapy of vertigo: Box 39.3 lists the drugs used for the symptomatic therapy.

An acute attack of vertigo is best treated with bed rest for couple of days and vestibular support drugs such as antihistaminics, benzodiazepines and phenothiazines. Chronic persisting vertigo due to central or peripheral causes may be treated symptomatically by small doses of antihistaminics.

Antihistaminics suppress the vestibular end organ receptors and thus *inhibit the activation of the central muscarinic receptors.* Of the antihistaminics, **cinnarizine** 15 mg three times a day is highly effective antivertigo agent. The other antihistaminics used include **cyclizine, meclizine, dimenhydrinate** and **promethazine** (Chapter 23).

Phenothiazines (prochlorperazine) and central anticholinergics (**scopolamine**) suppress the central vestibular nuclei and pathways. Chronic use of central sedatives (and even their withdrawal after prolonged use) can be associated with dizziness. However, benzodiazepines are likely to be helpful when anxiety is a prominent feature. When depression is a major response, amitriptyline may be useful (Chapter 14).

Betahistine, a vasodilator, may be useful in some cases of **Meniere disease** (Chapter 23). Meniere disease is initially treated with low salt diet (1 g/day) and a thiazide diuretic. If this is not effective, an antihistaminic or betahistine should be used.

Glucocorticoids (methylprednisolone 40–80 mg/day for 4–5 days, followed by 20 mg/day for 4 days) have been used to suppress intralabyrinthine oedema due to virus infection.

Box 39.3 Drugs Used in Vertigo

- ***Vestibular suppressants,*** e.g. phenothiazine antihistaminics (prochlorperazine)
- ***Central sedatives,*** e.g. scopolamine, benzodiazepines
- ***Betahistine***
- ***Diuretics***
- ***Glucocorticoids***

PROKINETICS

Prokinetic agents are drugs that enhance coordinated GI motility and transit of material in the GI tract. These drugs either enhance the release of excitatory neurotransmitter at the nerve-muscle junction without interfering with the normal physiological pattern and rhythm of motility, or antagonise dopamine which is present peripherally in the upper GI tract and has inhibitory effect on the GI motility and intragastric pressure. These effects are believed to be due to the suppression of ACh release from the primary motor neurons in the myenteric plexus, the activity of which is modulated by inhibitory D2 neurons. The conventional cholinergic drugs are not termed as prokinetics as they increase GI motility in an uncoordinated manner that produces little or no net propulsive motor activity.

Prokinetic drugs include:

- **D_2 antagonists**, e.g. **metoclopramide** and **domperidone** (Table 39.1). By acting as dopamine antagonists in the CTZ, they also act as central antiemetics.
- **5HT receptor agonists:** Since 5-HT plays an important role in GI motility and is present in the neurons of the myenteric plexus, prokinetic action can also be achieved by the action of **5-HT_4 receptor agonists**, e.g. **cisapride** and **metoclopramide** (Chapter 24).

CISAPRIDE: This **prokinetic** drug stimulates GI motility by acting as a **5-HT_4 receptor agonist**. It modulates the activity of the primary motor neurons in the myenteric plexus. It also has an action on the colon. *It has no direct antiemetic action.*

Adverse reactions include increased urinary frequency, abdominal cramps and diarrhoea. It prolongs the QT interval and *serious cardiac arrhythmias and sudden death have been reported*, because of which it has been withdrawn from the market in some countries including India.

Mosapride is a selective **5-HT_4** agonist claimed to have fewer side effects. **Itopride** has actions similar to those of metoclopramide. Another analogue, Prucalopride is approved for use in adults with

Table 39.1 Actions of Prokinetic Drugs PH 1.34

Action	Metoclopramide	Domperidone	Cisapride
5-HT4 agonist	+++	–	+++
Antidopaminergic (D2)	++	+++	–
CNS	++	+	–
Hyperprolactinemia	++	+++	–
Antiemetic	++	++	–
Prokinetic	Upper GI tract	Upper GI tract	Upper GI tract and colon

chronic constipation in whom laxatives fail to provide adequate relief. Tegaserod, a **5-HT$_4$** agonist is also approved for IBS-C in women.

- **Motilin receptor agonists: Erythromycin,** a macrolide antibiotic, causes diarrhoea as a major side effect due to **activation of motilin** receptors. Motilin is a peptide hormone, found in the GI tract; it increases the smooth muscle contractibility. Erythromycin has been used as a prokinetic drug in patients with diabetic gastroparesis.

DRUG THERAPY OF DIARRHOEA IM 6.13

Diarrhoea is a common problem in clinical practice and, like vomiting, it can be caused by a variety of conditions varying from infections and allergy to emotional disturbances. **It is defined as the frequent passage of liquid or unformed stools with or without blood or mucus;** in the case of former, it is usually due to a known cause such as amoebic or bacillary dysentery.

Box 39.4 outlines the pathophysiology of diarrhoea.

Box 39.4 Pathophysiology of Diarrhoea

Osmotic diarrhoea due to poorly absorbable, osmotically active substances as after ingestion of osmotic laxatives, in lactase deficiency and in malabsorption syndromes
Secretory diarrhoea due to active ion secretion by the small intestinal epithelium as in cholera, enterotoxigenic *E. coli* diarrhoea and carcinoid syndrome
Deranged intestinal motility as in irritable bowel syndrome, thyrotoxicosis and diabetic neuropathy
Altered mucosal morphology as in viral gastroenteritis, bacterial infection with tissue invasion, GI cancers and radiation enteritis
Allergic diarrhoea as in food allergy
Drug-induced diarrhoea (see Box 39.5)
Miscellaneous such as in neurological and endocrine disease

Most diarrhoeal diseases act through multiple mechanisms and affect many types of cells in the intestinal tract, including neurons, endocrine cells, inflammatory cells and epithelial cells. **The mechanisms include:**

- *Increase in the adenylate cyclase and cAMP content of the intestinal epithelial cells*, resulting in a decrease in sodium absorption and stimulation of chloride secretion.
- *Stimulation of enteric nerves and 5-HT-containing neuroendocrine cells.*
- *Initiation of intestinal metabolism of arachidonic acid by the cyclo-oxygenase pathway with the formation of PGs.*

In nearly all forms of acute infectious diarrhoeas, the abnormally formed stools indicate small bowel hypersecretion of fluid and electrolytes and not increased intestinal motility.

Not all diarrhoeas need drug treatment. For example, irritant diarrhoea can be self-limited.

PH 1.34, IM 6.13, PE 24.5, PE 24.8

Treatment of diarrhoea consists of the following:

I. **Specific treatment:** This depends upon the cause. The common pathogens responsible for acute diarrhoea and drugs used in their treatment are listed in Table 39.2.
The initial clinical evaluation of the patient with acute diarrhoea should include assessment of its severity, the need for rehydration and the likely cause, based on history, clinical findings and stool examination. Specific therapy of diarrhoea would be easy if the responsible pathogen could be identified quickly.

Table 39.2 Clinical Features and Drugs Recommended in Acute Infective Diarrhoeas IM 6.13

	Organism	Blood in Stool	Polymorphs in Stool	Vomiting	Drugs Recommended
I	**Bacterial**				
	Shigella	+	+++	+++	Ciprofloxacin; norfloxacin; ampicillin; cotrimoxazole; nitazoxanide
	Salmonella (non-typhi species)	+	+++	+	Cotrimoxazole; fluoroquinolone or ceftriaxone in severe cases
	E. coli	++	++	+	Fluoroquinolone; cotrimoxazole; Avoid antimotility drugs
	E. coli (Shiga toxin producing)	+++	±	+	
	Vibrio	±	±	±	Doxycycline; fluoroquinolone
	Campylobacter	+	++	+	Azithromycin
	C. difficile	+	+++	–	Metronidazole
II	**Protozoal**				
	E. histolytica	±	±	±	Metronidazole
	Giardia	–	–	±	Metronidazole
	Cryptosporidium	–	–	–	Azithromycin; nitazoxanide
	Cyclospora	–	–	+	Cotrimoxazole
III	**Viral**	–	–	++	No antimicrobial

IM 16.14

IM 16.13

Many patients suffer from **simple diarrhoea** manifested by watery stools, low grade fever, malaise, nausea and sometimes vomiting. *In the developed countries*, it is usually of viral origin, whereas in developing countries, it is more often due to a bacterial pathogen. The pathogen commonly involved is enterotoxigenic *Escherichia coli*, which is a major cause of infant diarrhoea. The other pathogens involved are the enteropathogenic *E. coli*; enteroinvasive *E. coli*; shigatoxin producing *E. coli*; shigella; salmonella; campylobacter; *Entamoeba histolytica*; cyclosporidium and others. Such patients tend to have more severe diarrhoea, fever and blood in stools (**dysentery**) (Table 39.2). Cotrimoxaozole, which was earlier effective against all the strains of *E. coli*, has now been replaced by **ampicillin (500 mg q.i.d.) or a fluoroquinolone (e.g. norfloxacin 400 mg b.i.d. or ciprofloxacin 500 mg b.i.d. for 5-7 days), which are now considered as the drugs of choice in patients with bacterial dysentery.** Most patients show a rapid response except for those infected with *C. jejuni*. Such patients are best treated with **azithromycin,** 1 g as a single dose or 500 mg/day for 3 days.

Travellers' diarrhoea has been treated with **rifaximin,** a new nonabsorbable rifampin derivative in the dose of 200 mg t.i.d. for 3 days, as an alternative to fluoroquinolones. It is well tolerated *but is ineffective in patients with fever or blood in stool* and in those infected by *C. jejuni*. It should be avoided in pregnancy.

Neonates with acute bacillary dysentery should be treated with parenteral antibiotics.

Patients with cholera or **cholera-like gastroenteritis** should be treated with **doxycycline** in a single dose of 300 mg (Chapter 47). It is effective within 48 h. **Antimicrobials are ineffective in viral diarrhoea.**

If diarrhoea persists for more than 5–7 days despite treatment, the causative organism is likely to be a protozoon. Lack of evidence of a pathogen should arouse the suspicion of IgA deficiency or irritable bowel syndrome.

II. Correction of dehydration and electrolyte

disturbances: *This is the most important aspect of treatment of diarrhoea* and in many cases, it may be the only treatment needed. *In all cases the* **initial therapy should always include rehydration and nutritional support.**

Massive diarrhoea with watery stools causes marked depletion of sodium, potassium and bicarbonate and metabolic acidosis resulting in high mortality. Hence, **immediate replacement of the fluid and electrolyte losses is life saving.** It is ideal to tailor-make the fluid and electrolyte therapy in a seriously ill patient by monitoring the blood chemistry. This, however, may not always be possible.

The extent of dehydration in severe diarrhoea can be estimated by noting the quality of pulse, BP, condition of the neck veins and skin turgor. The plasma protein concentration and plasma specific gravity can be reliable guides, in judging the degree of dehydration. Normal plasma specific gravity is 1.025. It has been estimated that for each 0.001 increase in the plasma specific gravity, an adult patient requires about 4 mL of fluid per kg body weight.

In an emergency, isotonic saline along with isotonic sodium bicarbonate, should be used in the proportion of 2:1. This would correct sodium loss and acidosis. If i.v. sodium bicarbonate is not available, 5% solution of sodium bicarbonate may be given orally *ad lib.* Potassium should be given, preferably orally. About 15 mmol of potassium is needed to **correct the potassium loss** in a litre of stools. The quantity of stools passed should, therefore, be noted. Potassium can be conveniently administered as 200 mL of tender coconut water for each litre of stools passed. Alternatively, potassium salts such as potassium chloride may be given orally or by i.v. infusion under medical supervision.

Coma and convulsions during diarrhoea often indicate hypoglycaemia and need for i.v. glucose.

In a collapsed patient, i.v. fluids are given rapidly initially, at the rate of at least 100 mL/min, to correct hypovolaemia and to avoid irreversible shock. Later on, the infusion may be adjusted according to the loss of fluids in stools and sweat. In practice, i.v. therapy is monitored by noting the state of the neck veins and the urine output. Usually i.v. fluid therapy is continued until the shock state is corrected and the patient is strong enough to drink the *oral glucose-electrolyte solution.*

Oral Rehydration Therapy (ORT) PH 2.2

The sodium and water absorption by the small bowel is enhanced by the addition of glucose to the oral fluid. This is because sodium is absorbed in the small intestine via sodium glucose transporter type 1 present along the brush border of the intestinal cells. Physiologically the ratio of sodium: glucose absorption is 2:1 . This implies that for efficient sodium absorption presence of glucose is essential. Hence, once the initial hypovolaemia is corrected dehydration can be successfully treated with oral fluids containing glucose. Mild to *moderate dehydration and acidosis due to diarrhoea can be corrected in 3–6 h by* **oral rehydration therapy alone**. *The treatment should continue even when diarrhoea is not controlled.*

Advantages of ORT:

- It is far less expensive than i.v. fluids.
- No expertise is needed to administer the fluid.
- The solution can be prepared on the spot with drinking water.
- It can be given by family members and non-professionals as well as by health workers.

Patients strong enough to drink, generally take the solution avidly. They may continue to vomit and in some cases the stool volume may increase. In spite of this, there is a net absorption of water and electrolytes. Moreover, vomiting which is probably caused by acidosis and volume depletion, is likely to be corrected by the oral therapy itself. *One teaspoonful given to a child every minute can provide 200–300* mL/h. *'A conscientious mother can work wonders'.* Adults can take 750–1000 mL/h for several hours until signs of dehydration disappear and abundant pale urine is produced. If the patient needs rest, the same fluid may be given by a nasogastric tube.

- **WHO-recommended, modified ORS:** Its composition is shown in Table 39.3. ORS that contains less sodium and glucose than the WHO recommended ORS should be avoided. ORS can also be prepared at home (Table 39.3).
  Children under five years should be given plain

Table 39.3 Composition of ORS

Substance	WHO		Homemade (Measure)
	Weight (g)	Components (mmol/L)	
Sodium chloride	2.6	Na^+ 75	¾ teaspoon (table salt)
Potassium chloride	1.5	K^+ 20	½ teaspoon
Trisodium dihydrate citrate[a]	2.9	HCO^-_3 equivalent 10	¾ teaspoon
Glucose (anhydrous)[b]	13.5	Glucose75	1½ tbsp
Water	1000	Total osmolarity 245	1 L

[a]Citrate in ORS diminishes stool output in high output diarrhoeas.
[b]Glucose 20 g can be replaced by 40 g of sucrose. Alternatively, it can be replaced by 50 g of cooked rice powder. Cl^- content is 65 mmol/L.

water in addition to above solution in quantities approximately one-third of the total volume administered.

- **Cereal-based oral rehydration solution (CORS):** The correct concentration of Na^+ and glucose in the ORS and its osmolality are critical for optimal effect and safety. ORS in which rice and other food sources of starch are substituted for glucose effectively replace lost fluids, decrease vomiting, and reduce the severity of diarrhoea. *The cereal (rice)-based solutions, may also shorten the duration of illness.* Rice contains a low molecular weight fraction, which has a direct effect on the chloride channel. It inhibits the response of the crypt cell chloride channel to cAMP. Thus, rice-based ORS in cholera, inhibits chloride channel, the target of toxigenic secretory states. Addition of sodium bicarbonate and potassium chloride is not critical to the success of cereal-based ORS. *Interestingly, the use of rice conjee in diarrhoea is traditional in India for ages!* Physiologically, cereal-based ORS are identical to their glucose-based counterparts. The dominant component in the cereals is starch from rice, corn, wheat, potato, sorghum, millet or even plantain. Starch is a large polymer of glucose that is converted into glucose at the intestinal brush border by enzymes. This digestive process supplies a larger number of glucose molecules for transfer of sodium ions from lumen into the blood. The cereal proteins also provide small peptides and amino acids which also facilitate the absorption of additional sodium ions. Of course, **the presence of sufficient digestive enzyme is essential for the success of such solutions.** In the vast majority, this is not the problem, except perhaps in infants in whom intestinal glucoamylase is not fully developed.
- **Zinc supplemented ORS:** Zinc maintains the GI mucosal integrity. It also imparts local immunity. Deficiency of zinc has been shown to worsen diarrhoea. Moreover diarrhoea itself leads to zinc deficiency. Hence, UNICEF-WHO has proposed zinc-supplemented ORS. Such ORS has also shown to reduce the duration of diarrhoea and the stool frequency. In children less than 6 month, 10 mg/day of zinc and for older children 20 mg/day of zinc is advocated.

If there is severe dehydration, urgent restoration of circulating volume is undertaken with IV administration of **Ringer lactate**. In adults and children ≥ 5 years of age, 30ml/kg is infused over 30 min and if required it is repeated once. Thereafter 70ml/kg is administered over 3 hours. For children under 5 years 20 ml/kg is administered over 15 min and this amount can be repeated twice if required. Thereafter 70ml/kg is administered over 3 hours. Close monitoring is needed to prevent fluid overload in young children and elderly.

Usually the patient is able to drink orally within 2 hours and can be shifted on ORS.

III. **Symptomatic and supportive treatment:** Drugs used for symptomatic treatment may act by various mechanisms

They can be classified as

- GI protectives and adsorbents
- Antimotility and antisecretory agents

1. **GI protectives and adsorbents:** These agents may be useful predominantly because of their ability to adsorb noxious substances such as gases, bacteria and bacterial toxins. In addition, some of these possess an astringent action, whereas others protect the GI mucous membrane from the irritants by coating it physically. They are cheap, and reasonably safe but *their usefulness is limited to the treatment of mild diarrhoea*. However, they may adsorb simultaneously administered anti-infective agents and anticholinergics. The drugs are as follows:

   BISMUTH SALTS: The commonly used bismuth salts are **bismuth subcarbonate** and **bismuth subsalicylate**. They have astringent, adsorbent and antimicrobial actions. They also act against *Helicobater pylori* (Chapter 41).
   Bismuth subsalicylate binds toxins produced by *V. cholerae* and *E. coli*. In case of subsalicylate salt, it is possible that the liberated salicylic acid may inhibit the PG synthesis responsible for intestinal inflammation and hypermotility. Salicylate may also exert an antisecretory action.
   They are devoid of serious toxicity. Other bismuth salts used are bismuth subgallate and bismuth subnitrate.

   PECTIN: It is a purified carbohydrate obtained from the extract of the inner portion of citrus fruits or from apple pomace. It consists chiefly of partially methoxylated polygalacturonic acids. Its mechanism of action is not clear. When ingested, it passes into the intestinal tract where it probably acts by physically coating the mucosa. **It helps to produce formed stools.**
   It forms a viscous, colloidal solution with 20 parts of water. The solution is tasteless; it is administered either as a colloidal suspension alone or with kaolin. Pectin can also be given in the form of cooked apple or overripe banana.

   ACTIVATED WOOD CHARCOAL: This preparation is the residue from the destructive distillation of vegetable matter such as saw dust, cellulose residue and coconut shells, treated with zinc chloride to increase its adsorptive power. It is employed in the treatment of flatulence, nonulcer dyspepsia and various types of diarrhoeas. As a suspension in water, it is used for gastric lavage and for the emergency treatment of poisoning with alkaloids like morphine, strychnine and atropine (see Chapter 2).

   Other preparations: These are **prepared chalk,** a native form of calcium carbonate (often used as an antacid); and **light kaolin**, which is hydrated aluminium silicate. Both these agents are insoluble in water and form a protective coating on the intestinal mucosa. They may also have some adsorbent properties. They are administered as suspension, and form an important constituent of 'over-the-counter' (OTC) antidiarrhoeal remedies. *There is no rigorous demonstration that these GI protectives and adsorbents help in diarrhoea, although their administration may result in more formed stools.*

2. **Antimotility and antisecretory agents**

   Antimotility drugs may be used in simple diarrhoea but should be avoided in infective diarrhoea and in children.

- **Opioids:** Morphine-like compounds **inhibit** the first phase of the peristaltic reflex, the **acetylcholine dependent contraction of the longitudinal muscle,** followed by a **depression of rapid PG sensitive phase**. In addition, they also produce antisecretory effect by acting on intestinal opiate receptors. Thus they provide symptomatic relief. However, their routine use is not advocated. In the presence of acute inflammatory bowel disease, they can precipitate *paralytic ileus in children and in the elderly. Opioids, diphenoxylate and loperamide are not recommended for use in children under 2 years as they can cause respiratory depression. They should be avoided in infective diarrhoeas at all ages.*

The **preparations** used are as follows:

i. Codeine phosphate, 15–60 mg at 8–12 hourly.
ii. Diphenoxylate, a pethidine substitute in the dose of 2.5 mg mg along with 0.025 mg of atropine 3–4 times a day. *Atropine in such a low dose induces only dryness of mouth without exerting any antidiarrhoeal effect.* The purpose is to discourage excessive intake of the formulation and thus prevent addiction.

LOPERAMIDE: It has a structural resemblance to pethidine. It acts directly on intestinal opioid (μ) receptors. In addition, loperamide has antisecretory activity against cholera toxin and some forms of E. coli toxin, presumably by acting on Gi -linked receptors and blocks the toxin induced stimulation of adenylyl cyclase activity. The action is prompt and prolonged. It has a characteristic tissue distribution; almost 85% of the drug is recovered from the gut. It has high antidiarrhoeal specificity. It does not easily cross the BBB and is devoid of CNS toxicity. It is not used in children <2 years. Overdosing can result in cardiac events including torsades de pointes, cardiac arrest, and death hence.

RACECADOTRIL: Given orally, this **antisecretory prodrug** is hydrolysed to the active compound thiorphan. In the peripheral tissues, including the intestines, membrane-bound encephalinase enzymes degrade endogenous opioids/encephalins. Thiorphan inhibits encephalinase, thus increasing the availability of local encephalins which acts on the opioid delta receptors in the GI tract. Its efficacy is claimed to be as much as that of loperamide. It may be used to treat acute diarrhoea in children below the age of 2 years.

- **Atropine and its substitutes** such as hyoscine butylbromide (10–20 mg) or propantheline, are useful to relieve colic associated with diarrhoea (Chapter 20).
- **PG inhibitors:** Prostaglandins are known to stimulate intestinal fluid secretion and intestinal motility, thus causing diarrhoea. It is possible that $PGF_2\alpha$ release is involved in the genesis of certain diarrhoeas. PG inhibitors such as **aspirin** and **indomethacin** have been shown to be effective in diarrhoeas induced by bacterial toxins in animals, and in certain diarrhoeas in humans (Chapter 11).
- **Chloride channel inhibitor: Crofelemer,** a natural product derived from the red sap of the South American plant *Croton lechleri* **inhibits the secretion of chloride ions into the intestinal lumen.** The common ADRs include URTI, bronchitis, cough, flatulence and increased bilirubin. It is indicated for symptomatic relief of noninfectious diarrhoea in patients with HIV on antiretrioviral drug therapy.
  Nutmeg, in combination with ginger, jaggery and ghee, is an age-old Indian household remedy for diarrhoea. **PG inhibition is believed to be the mechanism of its antidiarrhoeal effect.** Nutmeg often works where other drugs have failed.

3. **Supportive treatment** includes (1) probiotics and (2) nutrient intake. These are as follows: PE 24.5

- **Probiotics:** These are live, nonpathogenic bacteria or yeasts which have been used for centuries in the form of cheap and easily available home-made curd (yogurt), whey and buttermilk for health benefits. Probiotics contain variable lactobacillus species and *Saccharomyces boulardi*, an yeast. Acetic, lactic and propionic acids produced by these bacilli lower the intestinal pH and inhibit the growth of certain pathogenic intestinal bacteria, e.g. *E. coli* and clostradium spp. Probiotics may also act physically to prevent adhesion and colonisation by pathogenic organisms and may also enhance immune responses. Clinically, they may be beneficial in infectious (rotavirus-induced) or antibiotic associated diarrhoea, irritable bowel syndrome (IBS) and inflammatory bowel diseases. *Considering this, Indian dietary habits of having curd or buttermilk with meal are commendable!*
  Probiotics may occasionally produce mild and transient flatulence. Antibiotics may inactivate bacteria derived probiotics. Commercially, they are available as powders, liquids and capsules.
- **Energy and nutrient intake** is impaired during acute diarrhoea and in the catabolic state that

may persist afterwards. Adults and children should be discouraged from fasting. Fluid-electrolyte balance is maintained by drinking boiled water, fruit juice and buttermilk and by eating salted biscuits. Intake of starchy foods (**rice conjee**) reduces diarrhoeal fluid output and is cost-effective (see earlier). The diet should be nonirritant, nonoily, easily digestable and palatable such as soft rice, ripe bananas and cooked apple. *Continued feeding improves the outcome in children.* Milk and milk products should be avoided since transient lactase deficiency may occur. Temporary reduction in the intake of foods rich in fibre (unrefined cereals, fruits and vegetables) is desirable in acute diarrhoea.

CHRONIC DIARRHOEA

Chronic diarrhoea, lasting for more than 3–4 weeks, is due to various causes and needs detailed evaluation. The drug therapy would depend on its cause. In many cases, it is noninfectious, e.g. irritable bowel syndrome, osmotic diarrhoea, steatorrhoea (gluten sensitivity), inflammatory bowel disease such as ulcerative colitis, and drug-induced diarrhoea (Box 39.5).

Irritable Bowel Syndrome (IBS) PH 1.34

As per Western criteria, IBS is diagnosed when the subject complains of recurrent abdominal pain or discomfort (bloating) at least 3 days a month in the past three months, associated with the following: (a) relief after defecation and (b) onset associated with change in frequency of stools or with change in the form of the stools. The disorder can be subdivided into:

Box 39.5 Drugs Causing Diarrhoea

- Magnesium antacids
- Antibiotics: Erythromycin, ampicillin, tetracyclines
- GI prokinetic drugs, e.g. cisapride
- Quinidine
- Prostaglandin analogues
- Anticholinesterases
- Colchicine
- Emetine
- Cytotoxic drugs
- Lithium

1. IBS with constipation (IBS-C)
2. IBS with diarrhoea (IBD-D)
3. The mixed type with both hard and soft stools

In India, IBS is more common in middle aged men. Majority of patients (90%) have combination of upper abdominal discomfort and lower abdominal fullness, relieved by defecation. Nearly 70% have feeling of inadequate evacuation. *Diarrhoea or constipation diagnosed as per Western criteria is uncommon and stool frequency is usually within normal limits (1–2/day) for most of the patients.*

The exact cause of IBS is not known. General examination is usually normal. IBS is often associated with emotional stress, anxiety or depression. *The treatment is symptomatic.* **Education of the patient about the benign nature of the ailment is essential.** Avoidance of fried spicy and pungent food is likely to be helpful; so is avoidance of stress. *Patients with predominant diarrhoea should be tested for gluten (wheat) sensitivity and milk intolerance.*

Drug Therapy of IBS: Pain in these patients is considered to be due to visceral hypersensitivity to physiological and noxious stimuli. Serotonin appears to be involved in this **syndrome of visceral hyperalgaesia.**

- **Smooth-muscle relaxants** provide moderate degree of relief to patients who complain of postprandial **abdominal pain,** distension and disturbed defecation. These include:
  1. **Antimuscarinics** like **dicyclomine,** propantheline, isopropamide and cimetropium.
  2. **Direct smooth muscle relaxants** like **mebeverine, alverine** and **doloverine.** This group is devoid of anticholinergic side effects and is particularly useful when colonic hypermotility is suspected.
  3. **Miscellaneous: Trimebutine** exerts antimuscarinic and weak mu opioid agonistic effects; **pinaverium** is a GI L-type CCB and **otilonium bromide,** NK_2 receptor blocker, is a weak antimuscarinic and a CCB. They are more expensive.
- **Alosetron** is a potent and selective $5\text{-}HT_3$ receptor antagonist. Given in the dose of 1 mg

b.i.d., it decreases intestinal motility and secretion, thereby relieving abdominal pain and discomfort and may control diarrhoea. Commonly, it causes constipation; rarely it can cause dangerous ischemia of the bowel. It is recommended only in women with IBS not responding to other therapy.

- **Eluxadoline,** an opioid which is a mixed MOR agonist and KOR agonist, acts locally to reduce abdominal pain and approved for the treatment of diarrhea-predominant IBS in adults.

The patients with predominant constipation benefit from bulk forming agents such as isapgol; whereas those in whom 'gas' is the major symptom are likely to benefit from a reduction in consumption of unrefined fibre products such as bran.

Tricyclic antidepressants (chapter 14) such as amitriptyline (10-25 mg), nortriptyline, imipramine, or desipramine (12.5 -25 mg) in doses lower than antidepressant dose are used in IBS-D. SSRIs have fewer side effects and have been advocated particularly for patients with IBS- C because SSRIs can increase bowel movements. However, they probably are not as effective as tricyclic antidepressants in the management of visceral pain. Relaxation and cognitive behavioural therapy may be helpful.

Inflammatory Bowel Disease (IBD) PH 1.34

Both **ulcerative colitis** *(UC)* and **Crohn's disease** are IBD; their exact cause of inflammation is not known.

Ulcerative colitis affects mainly the rectum and the colon causing proctitis, left sided colitis and pancolitis. Clinically, it causes diarrhoea with blood in the stools, urgency, tenesmus, weight loss and may cause systemic symptoms. Generally, it is mild but sometimes it can develop into toxic colitis with severely ulcerated mucosa.

UC seems to result from a breakdown of the homeostatic balance between the host's mucosal immunity and the enteric microflora, which results in an aberrant immune response against nonpathogenic gut commensals. The main abnormality driving inflammation in UC involves an exaggerated T-cell response, which causes mucosal hyper-responsiveness to commensals in genetically predisposed host. TNF-α is elevated in the blood, stool samples and intestinal mucosa of patients.

Crohn's disease affects the small intestine and the colon. The lesions in ulcerative colitis are superficial whereas those in Crohn's disease are transmural.

In both the conditions, proper nutrition and electrolyte balance must be maintained. **Antidiarrhoeal drugs are not recommended in severe colitis as they can precipitate toxic dilatation of the colon and perforation.** IM 16.16

Treatment of IBD: The mainstay of drug therapy for UC is **sulphasalazine** or **mesalazine** (5-aminosalicylates) and **glucocorticoids** (Table 39.4). They can induce and maintain a remission in UC in about 20% cases but their beneficial effect in Crohn's disease is less predictable. *Mesalazine and glucocorticoids can be used during pregnancy and are generally safe.*

SULPHASALAZINE is sulphapyridine linked to 5-aminosalicylic acid, **mesalazine** (mesalamine) by an azo bond. Given orally, it reaches the colon unaltered and is split by the colonic bacteria into its constituents. Sulphapyridine is absorbed, is acetylated in the liver and excreted in the urine. It has no therapeutic action in UC. **Mesalazine which is poorly absorbed induces remission in UC as well as Crohn's disease.**

Mechanism of action: This is not known. However, its anti-inflammatory (not mediated through COX) and free radical scavenging properties are believed to be responsible for its beneficial effects. It has variable effects on PG production. *It modulates inflammatory mediators derived from both the COX and lipoxygenase pathways and interferes with the production of inflammatory cytokines.* 5-Aminosalicylic acid inhibits the activity of nuclear factor-β (NF-β), an important transcription factor for producing proinflammatory cytokines. Mucosal secretion is reduced. It also inhibits cellular functions

Table 39.4 Drugs Used in IBD

Drugs	Doses/Day (in Divided Doses)
Anti-inflammatory	
Oral[a]	
Sulphasalazine	2–4 g
Olsalazine	1–2 g
Mesalazine	1.5–4.8 g
Prednisolone	40–60 mg
Budesonide	9 mg
Methylprednisolone	60 mg
Topical	
Mesalazine enema	1 g
Hydrocortisone enema	100–200 mg/60 ml
Beclomethasone enema	3 mg
Budesonide foam	4 mg
Parenteral	
Hydrocortisone	300 mg
Antimicrobials[b]	
Metronidazole; ciprofloxacin; rifaximin; cotrimoxazole; clarithromycin: in severe cases	
Immunosuppressants	
Azathioprine	50–150 mg
Mercaptopurine	60–90 mg
Methotrexate[c]	15–25 mg
Cyclosporine	2–4 mg/kg
TNF-α inhibitors	
Adalimumab	
Cetrolizumab	
Golimumab	
Infliximab	
Integrin receptor antagonists	
Natalizumab	
Vedolizumab	
Interleukin-12 and -23 antagonists	
Ustekinumab	
Janus kinase inhibitor	
Tofacitinib	

[a]Used for maintenance.
[b]More useful in Crohn's disease.
[c]Parenterally once a week.

of NK cells, mucosal lymphocytes, and macrophages including migration of inflammatory cells.

Adverse reactions to sulphasalazine include nausea, malena, headache, myalgias and sulpha-induced allergic reactions. Folate deficiency can occur, and folic acid 1 mg/day orally is recommended during long-term treatment. The drug may reduce sperm motility and cause reversible oligospermia.

Sulphasalazine is also used in the treatment of rheumatoid arthritis (Chapter 73).

MESALAZINE is rapidly absorbed from the jejunum, and hence is marketed as delayed release forms (Table 39.5). The drug may cause nausea, abdominal pain, diarrhoea. Rarely interstitial nephritis, pancreatitis, hepatotoxicity, pericarditis and SLE like syndrome can occur.

GLUCOCORTICOIDS: They are used only as short-term treatment in acute UC and Crohn's disease. They are not used for maintenance therapy. See Chapter 64.

Patients suffering from **mild-to-moderate UC** may respond to **mesalazine suppositories** (1 g/day) or enemas (2–4 g/day). The response is seen within 2 weeks. In 40–50% patients remission is induced. If this fails, additional **mesalazine oral therapy** can be instituted. **Glucocorticoid enemas** (hydrocortisone 100 mg/day) are also used. Patients not responding to rectal glucocorticoids (**Table 39.4**) are given oral glucocorticoids. *Topical enema is less likely to be effective in Crohn's disease, because of patchy distribution of lesions.*

Patients not responding or having **moderate and severe acute exacerbations of UC or Crohn's disease** respond to **additional oral or i.v. glucocorticoid therapy** (prednisolone 60 mg/d).

Severe cases should receive **IV glucocorticoid** for 5–7 days. The patients with IBD may be classified as: **glucocorticoid responsive** (40%), **glucocorticoid dependent** and **glucocorticoid unresponsive** (20%). The therapeutic response is generally observed in 1–2 weeks. **The unresponsive patients do not improve even with prolonged, high dose therapy.**

Glucocorticoid therapy may sometimes lead to intercurrent, opportunistic infections, sepsis and osteoporosis. Reactivation of pulmonary

Table 39.5 Mesalazine (MS) Preparations

Preparation	Chemical/Pharmaceutical Form	Delivery of MS	Distribution of MS	Dose
Sulphasalazine	MS linked to sulphapyridine	Bacterial cleavage	Colon doses	2–6 g/day in divided
Balsalazine	MS linked to an inert molecule	Bacterial cleavage	Colon	2.25 g (three 750 mg capsules) t.i.d.
Olsalazine	MS linked to MS	Bacterial cleavage	Colon	1.5–3.g/day in divided doses
MS	Time release preparation	Time release pH independent	Ileum and colon	3–4 g/day in divided doses
MS	pH-sensitive coated MS[a]	Release at pH > 7	Ileum and colon	2.4–4.8 g/day in divided doses
MS suppository	MS	Direct	Rectum	0.5–1 g o.d./b.i.d.
MS enema	MS	Direct	Left colon	4 g in 60 mL

Preparation without a sulphonamide are better tolerated than sulphasalazine and therefore are preferred.
[a]Should not be coadministered with antacids, PPI and H_2 blockers.

tuberculosis is another dreaded complication (Chapter 64).

ANTIMICROBIALS: These (Table 39.4) are used:

1. as adjuncts to the above drugs in active IBD
2. as treatment for a specific complication of Crohn's disease such as an intra-abdominal or perianal abscess

Many patients with Crohn disease benefit from **oral metronidazole** given for long-term (3 months). It is also beneficial in maintaining remission in Crohn's disease. Its efficacy in UC is doubtful.

IMMUNOSUPPRESSANTS: Patients with **glucocorticoid dependent UC and those who relapse** after adequate mesalazine can be treated with **azathioprine** (2–2.5 mg/kg orally once daily) or **mercaptopurine** (Maintenance dose 1–1.5 mg/kg orally once daily; Chapter 72). *When given with mesalazine, their toxicity increases because mesalazine inhibits their metabolising enzyme, thiopurine methyltransferase.*

Those who do not respond (**resistant cases**) and all those with severe, extensive disease may need **TNF-α antagonist** with or without azathioprine or Janus kinase inhibitor, **tofacitinib** and anti-integrin antibodies, **natalizumab** and **vedolizumab. Etrolizumab** is reserved for resistant Crohn's disease. **Ustekinumab**, a monoclonal antibody that blocks IL-12 and -23, is used as a last resort (Chapter 72). All these drugs may cause severe and sometimes fatal infection.

Recently **ozanimod**, a sphingosine-1-phosphate (S1P) receptor modulator (used in multiple sclerosis) is approved for the treatment of moderate-to-severe ulcerative colitis in patients who have failed biological.

After remission, oral or rectal **mesalazine** is used for long term in the dose of 1.6–3 g/day for maintenance of remission. Long-term follow-up of the patients is necessary due to the probability of occurence of colorectal cancer.

Table 39.6 illustrates preferred drugs in remission induction and maintenance phases of UC and Crohn's disease.

Intestinal Malabsorption

Some of the diarrhoeas associated with fat malabsorption improve with substitution of medium chain triglycerides in place of long chain fatty acids. Bile

Table 39.6 Drugs in Remission Induction and Maintenance Phases of UC and Crohn's Disease

Ulcerative Colitis		Crohn's Disease	
Induction	**Maintenance of Remission**	**Induction**	**Maintenance of Remission**
Mild-Moderate		**Mild-Moderate**	
Mesalazine (oral/topical)	Mesalazine (oral/topical)	Budesonide	Azathioprine
Olsalazine	Olsalazine		Mercaptopurine
Hydrocortisone (topical)			
Budesonide (topical)			
Moderate-Severe		**Moderate-Severe**	
Prednisone	Azathioprine	Prednisone	TNF α inhibitors
Hydrocortisone	Mercaptopurine	Methylprednisolone	Azathioprine
Methylprednisolone	TNF α inhibitors	TNF α inhibitors	Mercaptopurine
Pouchitis		**Perianal and Fistulising Disease**	
Ciprofloxacin	Ciprofloxacin	Metronidazole ±	Azathioprine
Metronidazole	Metronidazole	Ciprofloxacin	Mercaptopurine
	Rifaximin	Infliximab	Infliximab
	Probiotics		

salt binding resin like cholestyramine, colestipol or colesevelam are also used 1–3 times daily before meals. **Osmotic diarrhoea** due to intestinal lactase deficiency (seen in infants) improves on reducing consumption of milk and dairy products which contains lactose. Diarrhoea due to **carcinoid syndrome** responds to 5-HT antagonists or octreotide (Chapter 61), whereas that due to blind loop syndrome responds to antibacterial therapy.

Drug-Induced Diarrhoea

Many drugs (Box 39.5) including self-administered OTC remedies promoted for a variety of ailments, including hyperacidity, flatulence and alleged constipation, may contain laxatives, e.g. magnesium salts and herbal products. *This awareness will help to reduce the need for extensive and expensive evaluation of patients with chronic diarrhoea, whose initial evaluation is unrevealing.*

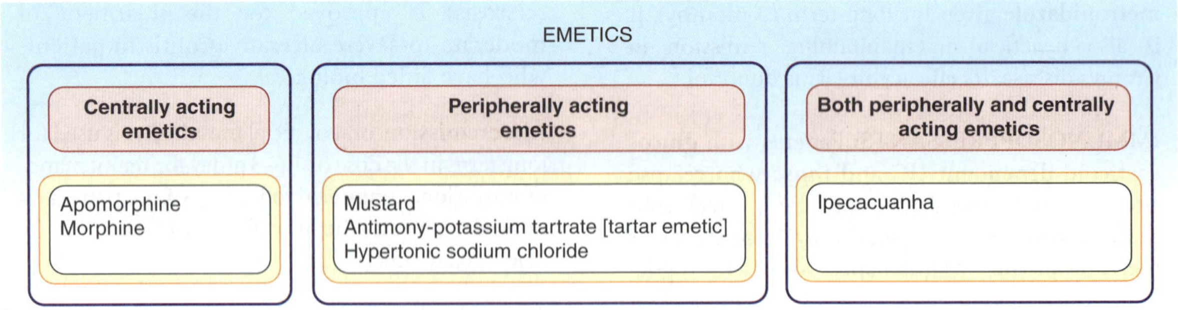

ANTIEMETICS

Antihistaminics
- Cyclizine
- Meclizine
- Promethazine
- Dimenhydrinate
- Doxylamine

Antidopaminergics
- Chlorpromazine
- Prochlorperazine
- Haloperidol
- Droperidol
- Metoclopramide
- Domperidone

$5HT_3$ antagonists
- Ondansetron
- Granisetron
- Dolasetron
- Palonosetron

Antimuscarinics
- Scopolamine

Antagonists of the NK_1 receptors for substance P
- Aprepitant
- Netupitant
- Fosaprepitant
- Rolapitant

Miscellaneous
- Nabilone and Dronabinol (cannabinoid receptor antagonists)
- Dexamethasone
- Diazepam
- Lorazepam
- Trimethobenzamide
- Benzquinamide

CLINICAL CLASSIFICATION OF ANTIEMETICS

Highly efficacious
- Ondansetron
- Granisetron
- High-dose metoclopramide

Moderately efficacious
- Low-dose metoclopramide
- Phenothiazines (prochlorperazine)
- Butyrophenones (droperidol)
- Cannabinoids

Weakly efficacious
- Anticholinergics
- Antihistaminics
- Benzodiazepines (lorazepam)

ANTIVERTIGO DRUGS

Vestibular suppressants
- Phenothiazine antihistaminics (prochlorperazine)

Central sedatives
- Scopolamine
- Benzodiazepines

Betahistine

Diuretics

Glucocorticoids

DRUGS USED IN THE TREATMENT OF IBD

Anti-inflammatory

Oral
- Sulphasalazine
- Mesalazine
- Steroids (prednisolone)

Topical
- Mesalazine enema
- Hydrocortisone enema

Parenteral
- Hydrocortisone

Antimicrobials
- Metronidazole
- Ciprofloxacin
- Rifaximin
- Cotrimoxazole

Immunosuppressants
- Azathioprine
- Methotrexate

TNF-α inhibitors
- Adalimumab
- Cetrolizumab

Integrin receptor antagonists
- Natalizumab
- Vedolizumab

Janus kinase inhibitor
- Tofacitinib

Interleukin-12 and -23 antagonists
- Ustekinumab

Sphingosine-1-phosphate (S1P) receptor modulator
- Ozanimod

CHAPTER 40

Pharmacotherapy of Constipation

Learning Objectives

This chapter will enable the reader:

1. To be aware of the regulation of GI motility and physiology of defecation.
2. To classify laxatives giving suitable examples.
3. To explain the mechanism of action, indications, contraindications and ADR of anthraquinones, irritant oils, stimulant laxatives, osmotic laxatives, bulk laxatives, emollient laxatives and chloride channel activators.
4. To outline the management of constipation.
5. To enlist drugs causing constipation as an adverse effect.
6. To enumerate the treatment of anal fissures and haemorrhoids.

KEY TERMS

People have been very particular about the 'regular bowel habit' from the earliest times and purgation, believed to be the panacea for many diseases, formed an important part of medieval therapeutics. Even today, many people have wrong notions about the quantity, consistency and frequency of stools in health and 'ritual purgation of children and the obsessional catharsis of adults' is still not uncommon. Drugs used for the treatment of constipation are widely advertised and are extensively used by lay people as they are easily available over-the-counter without a prescription. Almost half of the patients suffering from digestive tract disorders complain of 'constipation' and often drugs are self-prescribed.

Drugs which are used to promote defecation are called **laxatives**.

Regulation of GI motility: Orderly movement of ingested material through the gut is essential for adequate absorption of fluids, electrolytes and nutrients.

The CNS (via the sympathetic and the parasympathetic nerves), local neuronal reflexes and the circulating, enteric peptide hormones play an important role in regulating the neurohumoral control of the GI smooth muscles.

The enteric nervous system (ENS) integrates information from the periphery and the CNS and modulates the effector function. The various NTs released from the enteric neurons as well as the enteric peptide hormones are both, excitatory and inhibitory (Table 40.1). The complex interactions among them coordinate the GI movements. However, unlike the enteric NTs, which affect the GI function immediately, the peptide hormones have a delayed action. Since the CNS plays an important role in controlling the activity of the GI smooth muscle, **psychological disturbances also cause GI motility disorders.**

Physiology of defaecation: Intestinal movements are mainly of three types:

- **Pendular**, due to annular contraction of longitudinal muscles
- **Segmental**, due to contraction of circular muscles
- **Peristaltic**

Table 40.1 Some Enteric Neurotransmitters and Peptide Hormones which Control GI Motility

Excitatory	Inhibitory
Acetylcholine	Vasoactive inhibitory
Gastrin	Polypeptide (VIP)
Neurokinins	Noradrenaline
Cholecystokinin	Nitric oxide
5-Hydroxytryptamine	ATP
Somatostatin (in small doses)	Somatostatin (in large doses)
Motilin	Peptide YY
Enkephalin	Enteroglucagon

The first two are responsible for mixing of the food, whereas peristalsis helps in propulsion. The peristaltic waves occur frequently up to the ileum but are infrequent in the transverse, descending and pelvic colon, except during the gastrocolic reflex. Normally, food leaves the stomach in about ½–2½ h and its residue reaches the caecum by about 5–6 h. It takes approximately 18–24 h before the process of evacuation starts and the total time necessary for complete clearance of the ingested material is approximately 5–6 days. The global transit time (the time after ingestion to complete clearance from the GI tract) of a radio-opaque marker, such as barium sulphate, is about 5 days. If it is normal, the patient is probably not constipated.

The Asians have relatively shorter colonic transit time (CTT) of 15–24 h than the mean CTT of 30.7 h in the Americans. The normal frequency of stools (1–2/day) among Indians is higher than that (3 or more times a week) in the Western populations. These differences could be due to differences in the diet, especially its fibre content.

Most of the ingested water (2 L) and fluids secreted (9 L) by the various gastroinstestinal glands are reabsorbed by the ileum. About 1–1.5 L is absorbed by the colon and only 100–200 mL of water is excreted into the stools. Hence, laxatives which act mainly in the small intestine are likely to produce considerable loss of fluids and electrolytes and interfere with absorption of food. On the other hand, laxatives which act only on the colon produce relatively less fluid loss and do not interfere with the absorption of food.

The rate of intestinal passage of food depends on the nature of the diet and its fluidity. The greater the indigestible residue and water content, the more rapidly it reaches the rectum and produces its distension which initiates the act of defaecation. If this sensation is ignored habitually, it may lead to the development of constipation. *A diminished intake of both water and indigestible residue can also lead to constipation.* Furthermore, constipation, though commonly due to a lax, atonic colon, may also be associated with a hypersegmenting, high pressure bowel. Emotional stress and physical exercise can also modulate the GI transit.

Laxation *suggests the elimination of soft, formed stool without griping and without much loss of water. In large doses, many laxatives promote* **catharsis** *which means purgation, the passage of fluid stools and griping.* Laxatives act through multiple mechanisms affecting the epithelial transfer, directly or indirectly, leading to decreased sodium absorption and increase in chloride secretion by intestinal epithelial cells. Similarly, increase in faecal concentration of PGs has been observed following some laxatives.

Table 40.2 lists the effects of other drugs on GI motility.

Classification of Laxatives PH 1.34

Laxatives can also be classified according to their mechanism of action as follows:

Table 40.2 Drugs and GI Motility

Drugs	Stomach	Small Intestine	Colon
Cholinergics: Carbachol and neostigmine	E	E	E
Dopamine antagonists: Metoclopramide and domperidone	E	E	–
5-HT$_4$ agonist: Cisapride	E	E	E
Antimuscarinic: Atropine	I	I	I
CCB: Verapamil and nifedipine	I	I	I
Macrolide antibiotic[a]: Erythromycin	E	E	?
Opioids	I	I	I
Nitrates	?	I	I
Peppermint oil	?	I	I

Note: E, excitatory; I, inhibitory; ?, not clear.
[a]Probably act on the motilin receptors.

I. **Stimulant or irritant laxatives:**
   - **Anthraquinones,** e.g. *Cascara sagrada* and senna
   - **Irritant oils,** e.g. castor oil
   - **Miscellaneous,** e.g. phenolphthalein, bisacodyl and sodium picosulphate

II. **Osmotic laxatives,** e.g. magnesium sulphate, milk of magnesia, magnesium citrate, potassium sodium tartrate, lactulose and polyethylene glycol (PEG)

III. **Bulk laxatives,** e.g. methyl cellulose, agar agar, plantago seeds and bran.

IV. **Emollient laxatives (faecal emollient),** e.g. liquid paraffin and dioctyl sodium sulphosuccinate

V. **Chloride channel activators,** e.g. lubiprostone and linaclotide

VI. **Mu Opioid Receptor Antagonists:** e.g. methylnaltrexon and naloxegol

VII. **Prokinetic agents,** such as 5-HT4 receptor agonist, e.g. tegaserod

Clinical Classification according to the onset of laxative effect following the therapeutic doses:

- **Slow onset** which soften the stool after 1–3 days of daily use: Bulk laxatives, mineral oil, dioctyl sodium sulphosuccinate and lactulose
- **Intermediate onset** which cause soft or semifluid stool in 6–12 h of a single dose: Saline laxatives (low dose), bisacodyl (oral) and anthraquinone group
- **Rapid onset** which produce watery evacuation in 2–6 h of a single dose: Saline laxatives (high dose), castor oil, bisacodyl and glycerin suppository (rectal)

ANTHRAQUINONES

The two most commonly used agents are ***Cascara sagrada*** and **senna**. Cascara sagrada is obtained from the bark of a tree *Rhamnus purshiana*. The dried **senna** fruits (senna pods) and leaves are obtained from the plants *Cassia acutifolia and Cassia angustifolia*, respectively.

The active constituent anthraquinone is present as an inactive precursor glycoside in the leaves, pods and roots of these plants. On oral administration, the active anthraquinone derivatives, mainly oxymethylanthraquinones, are liberated in the small intestine, where they are partly absorbed. These agents do not act on the small intestine, probably because the release of the active principle is too slow. However, sufficient quantity reaches the large intestine, via the blood as well as by intestinal propulsion of the unabsorbed portion.

Anthraquinone acts by stimulation of the large bowel, and also probably by inhibiting NaCl and water absorption in the colon.

Pharmacological actions: As these drugs act mainly on the large bowel, evacuation occurs 6–8 h after their ingestion. Stools are usually semisolid and the incidence of griping is low. There are no other important actions of the absorbed anthraquinone derivatives and excreted in urine. However, they are excreted in milk and may cause diarrhoea in breast-fed infants.

Adverse reactions: They are relatively safe and the only important toxicity is excessive purgation and griping. Cascara is more bitter in taste, whereas senna produces more griping.

The urinary excretion of some of the constituents impart yellowish brown color to the acidic urine, and reddish violet colour to alkaline urine, hence the patient has to be counselled regarding this.

Chronic use may lead to benign melanotic pigmentation of the colonic mucosa.

They are employed as cold water decoction as home remedies in India for their laxative effect. The dose in each case is 0.6–2 g at bedtime. Other preparations include senna fluid extract, dose 2 mL and senna syrup, dose 8 mL. Laxative preparations containing standardised, purified concentrates and those containing purified senna glycosides are also available.

Aloe and **rhubarb,** used as vegetable foodstuffs, also have a mild laxative effect.

IRRITANT OILS

CASTOR OIL: It is a fixed oil obtained from the seeds of *Ricinus communis* Linn. Chemically, it is a triglyceride of ricinoleic acid, an unsaturated hydroxy fatty acid. Castor oil itself is nonirritant and is used as hair oil or applied to skin as emollient. *When ingested, it is hydrolysed in the intestine by pancreatic lipase to glycerol and ricinoleic acid, which acts as an intestinal irritant and produces purgation.*

Pharmacological actions: *As ricinoleic acid acts on the small intestine*, it produces copious, liquid stools, with associated fluid loss. Colonic emptying may be so complete that the patient may not pass a stool for next few days. The action is evident within 2–3 h. It causes griping. Ricinoleic acid that is absorbed is metabolised like any other fatty acid.

It is not recommended as a laxative.

MISCELLANEOUS STIMULANT LAXATIVES

BISACODYL: This drug, structurally related to phenolphthalein, is used orally and as rectal suppository. It is rapidly converted by intestinal enzymes and bacteria to *its active desacetyl metabolite which directly stimulates the large bowel.* It is not absorbed from the gut and is less toxic. It is supplied as 5 mg enteric coated tablets for oral use and as 10 mg rectal suppositories. Prolonged use (more than 10 days) may cause local irritation.

SODIUM PICOSULPHATE: Like bisacodyl, this drug is hydrolysed by colonic bacteria. *It acts on the large bowel* and produces a soft, formed stool in 10–14 h. It is well tolerated. The oral, adult dose is 5–15 mg as a single bedtime dose. A low volume oral solution is also available for bowel cleansing prior to colonoscopy.

Phenolphthalein, though used as a laxative earlier, is no more recommended because of its potential carcinogenicity. This agent undergoes **enterohepatic circulation** and the faeces and urine may get a reddish colour.

OSMOTIC LAXATIVES

Certain salts (magnesium, sodium and potassium salts called as saline laxatives), nonabsorbable disaccharides and higher alcohols, given orally, are not much absorbed and are retained in the GI tract. Such preparations exert an osmotic effect and hold considerable amounts of water, thus increasing the intestinal bulk. This acts as a mechanical stimulus causing an increase in the intestinal motor activity and evacuation. Release of cholecystokinin-pancreozymin with consequent stimulation of intestinal secretory and motor activity has been proposed as an additional mechanism of action of the magnesium salts.

Pharmacological actions: *These compounds act in the small as well as the large intestines* and, therefore, produce a *watery evacuation within 3–6 h*. They have a quick onset of action, and hence are given early in the morning before breakfast. They do not cause irritation and there is very little griping. Patients should be instructed to take plenty of water along with these drugs since administration of a hypertonic solution may produce dehydration.

Small amounts of these drugs may get absorbed into the circulation and may rarely cause toxicity, in the presence of kidney damage. Thus, the absorption of magnesium may cause CNS depression, whereas that of sodium may worsen the existing CHF. This is most unlikely in normal subjects, as the small amount absorbed is rapidly excreted by the kidneys.

Preparations and dosage:

i. Magnesium sulphate, $MgSO_4{\cdot}7H_2O$ (Epsom salt) – bitter salt, soluble in water. Dose 5–10 g. Hypertonic solution is sometimes used rectally to reduce increased intracranial tension.
ii. Milk of magnesia is a 7.0%–8.5% aqueous suspension of magnesium hydroxide (83 mg/ml). Dose: 2.4–4.8 g daily.
iii. Magnesium carbonate, heavy or light. Dose: 2–4 g. As a suspension, it can be given in a dose of 10 ml thrice daily.
iv. Magnesium citrate is pleasant to take but expensive.
v. Magnesium oxide. Dose: 2–4 g.
vi. Sodium potassium tartrate (Rochelle salt) is administered in the dose of 8–16 g. Tartrate ion, not being absorbed from the GI tract, does not produce systemic toxicity.
vii. Seidlitz powder is a mixture, in which 2.5 g of sodium bicarbonate and 7.5 g of Rochelle salt are dispensed together in a blue paper, whereas

2.5 g of tartaric acid is dispensed in a white paper. The user dissolves the contents of two papers separately in 30 mL of water and drinks the mixture after the effervescence begins to subside. *The powders must not be taken separately.* Carbon dioxide evolved acts as a carminative and masks the unpleasant saline taste.

IM 5.16

LACTULOSE: This is a synthetic nonabsorbable disaccharide which is metabolised by bacterial action in the distal ileum and colon to lactate and other organic acids and exerts an osmotic effect. The lactic acid can also bind to ammonia. Because of this property as well as its laxative effect, lactulose is used in the dose of 30–50 mL of the solution (3.5 g of lactulose per 5 mL) with plenty of water, three times a day in the treatment of hepatic coma; the dose is adjusted to produce 2–3 soft stools per day.

Lactitol: This synthetic disaccharide is more palatable than lactulose.

GLYCERIN: Glycerin is used in the form of **rectal suppositories** (3 g for adults and 1–1.5 g for children). It acts by its osmotic effect to soften and lubricate the dried up faeces. It may also stimulate rectal contractions. Glycerin is also used as a glycerin-edible oil (30–50 mL of each) **enema,** introduced into the rectum with a syringe. Other indications for glycerin are as follows:

Oral glycerin:

- Treatment of **acute congestive glaucoma** (Chapter 70) and **cerebral oedema** (Chapter 37)
- **As a sweetening/flavouring agent**

Topical glycerin:

- **As a hygroscopic agent** along with magnesium sulphate as dressing for wounds, ulcers and abscesses (Chapter 69)
- **As an emollient**

***In vitro* uses:**

- **As a vehicle for drugs**

Polyethylene glycol (PEG)-electrolytes: is supplied as a powder or as a ready-to-use electrolyte solution. Since the solution is isotonic, dehydration does not occur. It can be used for bowel cleansing before bowel surgery, colonoscopy, radiological examination, and to treat acute poisoning. It is administered orally in the dose of 250 mL every 15–20 min, over a period of 4 h (4 L). It can also be given by nasogastric tube at the rate of 25 mL/min. The dose to treat constipation is 17 gms in 125–250 ml of water orally once a day. After reconstitution, the solution should be stored in a fridge, and used within 24 h. It is not recommended in patients weighing less than 20 kg.

BULK LAXATIVES

These are natural or semisynthetic polysaccharides and cellulose derivatives.

Pharmacological actions: *They are not absorbed and increase the indigestible residue. They absorb water and swell up, thus providing the stimulus of mechanical distension for evacuation.* Their action is mild and is usually seen 12–36 h after ingestion.

- They produce evacuation of solid or semisolid stools without irritation or griping.
- Some of these agents also have lubricating properties.
- Usually, these drugs are administered at bed time, with plenty of water.
- Safe and do not have any systemic toxicity

Intestinal obstruction has been reported but very rarely.

Because these agents help to produce formed stools, they are also recommended in the treatment of diarrhoea. As many of these agents, when administered in a palatable form, can increase the bulk of indigestible material in the diet, they have also been used in the treatment of obesity for satisfying appetite.

AGAR: It is a mucilagenous substance extracted from marine algae. It contains indigestible hemicellulose. With water, it forms a gel which has emollient or lubricating properties. The dose is 4 g; occasionally, however, a large dose 40 g may be required.

ISAPGOL: consists of dried seeds of *Plantago ovata Forsk.* The seeds, which are hard and pinkish-grey to brown in colour, contain a large amount of natural mucilage. They are used as household remedy. Many OTC preparations contain Psyllium husk derived from plantago seeds. Dose: 5–15 g.

SABZA: This consists of the dried seeds of *Ocimum basilicum* Linn, a plant belonging to the tulasi family. The seeds are rich in mucilage and can be used as a substitute for isapgol.

HALIV: Seeds of *Lepidium sativum* (Garden cress) are used traditionally for relieving constipation. They have shown to possess prokinetic and laxative activities. The seeds also have rich amount of proteins (25%), fats (16%), calcium, iron, folic acid and vitamin A and C. The dietary fibre content of its bran is high. Used along with milk, ghee, sugar/jaggery, they have therapeutic and nutritional value. *Haliv* is a tastier and pleasant laxative than others. However, it should be avoided in pregnancy due to its possible teratogenic effects.

BRAN: It is the byproduct of the milling of wheat and contains almost 40% of fibre. Processed bran is palatable as such and it may be mixed with flour for preparing chapatis/bread. Dose: 12–24 g daily, in divided doses.

METHYL CELLULOSE AND SODIUM CARBOXYMETHYL CELLULOSE are hydrophilic, semisynthetic derivatives of cellulose. Methylcellulose (available as 500 mg tablets) is administered in the dose of 1 g, 1–4 times daily, whereas sodium carboxymethyl cellulose is administered in the dose of 1.5 g, 1–4 times a day. The preparations should be taken with 30–40 mL of water to minimise the risk of oesophageal obstruction.

Bulk forming laxatives are especially useful in patients with:

- **Irritable bowel syndrome**
- **Haemorrhoids and anal fissures**
- **Chronic diarrhoea** associated with diverticular disease and ulcerative colitis
- **Colostomy or ileostomy**

Dietary fibre and bowel disorders: Unrefined plant products (fruits, vegetables, pulses, nuts and especially wholegrain products such as 100% whole-wheat flour and unpolished rice) are rich in indigestible cell wall materials. This material, known in the past as 'roughage' or 'residue' is now called 'fibre'. *Chemically, this consists mainly of cellulose, hemicelluloses, pectins and lignin*. Following ingestion, they hold water, form gels, exchange cations and bind bile acids. *In the colon, they are mainly broken down to short-chain fatty acids, which may influence the colonic function favourably*. Thus, the stool becomes bulkier and softer so that the need for straining is decreased. Occasionally, frequency of defaecation is increased. Increased intake of such fibre has been found useful not only in simple constipation but also in spastic colon, irritable bowel syndrome, colonic diverticular disease, and in anal fissures and piles. Higher consumption of fibre rich food (vegetables and fruits) may decrease the duration of contact of locally (in the colon) formed carcinogens with the colonic wall and may be helpful in preventing colonic cancer.

The best way of increasing the fibre-intake is to include fibre-rich foods in the diet. In persons who cannot or will not consume sufficient fibre-rich food, **wheat bran** may be added to food or taken with water. Eating of raw fruits and certain raw vegetables may however, often cause abdominal discomfort, bloating, griping and diarrhoea and should be avoided. A daily intake of 20–60 g of dietary fibre would appear to be sufficient for easy bowel movements.

EMOLLIENT LAXATIVES

LIQUID PARAFFIN: This mineral oil is the most widely used emollient laxative. It consists of a mixture of hydrocarbons obtained from petroleum. It is not significantly absorbed on oral administration and exerts a softening and lubricating effect on faeces.

Pharmacological actions: *It is a mild lubricant and by itself does not initiate peristalsis. Because of its lubricant action, the straining during defaecation can be avoided.* It is usually given at bed time, but can be taken at any time of the day.

It is almost nontoxic but used repeatedly, it may interfere with the absorption of essential fat soluble substances and may cause a deficiency of vitamins A,

D and K. The small amount which is absorbed from the intestinal tract may get deposited in the intestinal mucosa, liver and spleen. Its chronic use can cause granulomatous fibrosis in the intestinal wall and more diffusely in the reticuloendothelial system. Rarely, it can cause lipoid pneumonitis, if it gets into the lungs during its administration in bedridden patient and in old people. *It should not be used in children under three years of age.*

Preparation and dosage: Liquid paraffin is a colourless, oily liquid (1mg/ml). Dose: 10–30 mL. It is also available in emulsified form.

Edible oils like coconut oil, groundnut oil, cotton seed oil and corn oil are employed as lubricant laxatives. However, they are digested and hence, fairly large doses are needed for lubricant effect. The usual dose is 30 mL.

DIOCTYL SODIUM SULFOSUCCINATE: This drug, which is used in pharmaceutical industry as a dispersing agent, *acts by its physical property of lowering surface tension.* It does not stimulate peristalsis but promotes softening of faeces. It is slow acting and takes 1–2 days to act. It should not be combined with liquid paraffin as it may enhance the absorption of the latter.

Dose: 100–200 mg three times a day.

5-HT$_4$ RECEPTOR AGONISTS

Tegaserod: This prokinetic drug acts as a 5-HT$_4$ agonist in the entire GI tract and was used in women with IBS with predominant constipation (IBS-C). It has been withdrawn from the market for possible risk of cardiac events. However, it has been reintroduced in 2019 for IBS-C in women under 65 years.

CHLORIDE CHANNEL ACTIVATORS

LUBIPROSTONE: *This drug acts locally in the GI tract by opening chloride channels, resulting in secretion of chloride-rich intestinal fluid. This accelerates small intestinal and colonic transit.* It also delays gastric emptying. The adverse effects are nausea (31%), headache, diarrhoea and occasionally dyspnoea. It is contraindicated during pregnancy and should be avoided during child bearing age. High dose (24 mcg b.i.d.) is used in opioid induced constipation chronic idiopathic constipation, whereas low dose (8 mcg b.i.d.) is used for women with IBS having predominant constipation. It is of limited value and is expensive.

Linaclotide, a 14-amino acid synthetic peptide, given orally activates guanylate cyclase-C receptors on the luminal surface of the intestinal epithelium increasing intracellular cGMP. This results in activation of the chloride channel. Its common adverse effects are diarrhoea, abdominal pain, flatulence, and abdominal distension. Linaclotide has been used to treat chronic idiopathic constipation or IBS with constipation.

Plecanatide, another guanylate cyclase-C activator is approved for the treatment of chronic idiopathic constipation in adults at a dose of 3 mg daily.

Recently, a new drug **Tenapanor**, an inhibitor of isoform 3 of the Na^+–H^+ exchanger present in the GI tract. **Tenapanor** reduces the absorption of Na^+ and enhances intestinal fluid volume and transit. It is approved for the treatment of IBS-C in adults at a dose of 50 mg orally twice daily.

MU OPOID RECEPTOR ANTAGONISTS

Naloxegol, derived from naloxone, acts as an antagonist of peripheral gut opioid receptors (Chapter 10). It reverses the opioid induced effects on the GI muscle contractility, water and electrolyte secretion and rectal sphincter tone and relieves constipation. Adverse effects are dose related and include nausea, flatulence and abdominal pain. It is claimed to be more effective than lubiprostone in the **treatment of opioid induced resistant constipation**. It can precipitate opioid withdrawal in cancer patients taking opioids.

Other peripherally acting mu opoid receptor antagonists include **methylnaltrexone** and **naldemedine**. Recently fixed drug combination of oxycodone +naloxone(ratio 2:1) is available as an oral formulation to relieve opioid induced constipation when opioid pain relief is still required. Naloxone displaces oxycodone from the mu opioid receptors in the GIT without interfering with the analgesic effect of oxycodone.

Indications for laxatives:

- **In food or drug poisoning** to flush the intestinal tract. Saline laxatives are generally preferred.
- **To provide a fresh stool sample** for parasitic examination.
- **Following anthelmintic therapy,** to eliminate the parasites; saline laxatives are preferred.
- **Preoperatively in abdominal surgery or prior to radiological examination of the abdomen** (bowel cleansing action).
- **In drug induced constipation** such as that during the use of opioids or drugs with antimuscarinic property.
- **In constipation** due to diminished intestinal tone as in old age and pregnancy.
- **In patients with painful anal conditions** (fissure, thrombosed piles), **cardiac disease** (acute MI) and typhoid fever in order to spare the patient from straining during defecation. In these conditions, a lubricating laxative such as liquid paraffin is preferred.
- **In patients with severe neuromuscular disease** who have poor muscle strength.
- **In patients with hepatic encephalopathy,** to reduce the colonic absorption of ammonia and other unknown toxins e.g. lactulose.
- **In children with encopresis** (passage of normal stools in socially unacceptable places; it is normal in the first 3 years of life) and **in congenital/ acquired megacolon.**

In general, laxatives are more often misused than used properly. Such misuse can cause serious harm (see section constipation and laxatives).

Contraindications:

Laxatives are absolutely contraindicated in patients with undiagnosed acute abdomen and in cases with intestinal obstruction and inflammatory bowel disease as violent contractions may lead to intestinal perforation and peritonitis.

Irritant laxatives should be avoided during pregnancy as these may cause pelvic congestion, although abortion following therapeutic doses of laxatives is most unlikely. Similarly, these drugs should also be avoided in case of typhoid fever and in very ill cardiac patients.

ENEMAS: See Chapter 1 for general information on enemas. Their use for bowel evacuation is discussed here; the use of retention enemas for other purposes is discussed in appropriate chapters.

Evacuant enemas cause fragmentation, liquefaction or lubrication of the faeces. Fluid distention of the bowel wall causes reflex evacuation. They act locally and may be preferred to laxatives in some situations. As an enema, one may introduce into the rectum plain tap water (this should be used only in adults, but not in infants or children); soapsuds (only neutral and not alkaline); isotonic sodium chloride (one level-teaspoon common salt per half litre of water); mineral or vegetable oil; glycerine; a surfactant (docusate sodium) or a stimulant laxative (bisacodyl).

The enema should be administered very gently to prevent local injury to the bowel. Tap water enema may cause water intoxication, especially in infants and children. *Irritant substances such as hot water, household detergents and strongly hypertonic salt solutions should not be used.*

The **indications for evacuant enema** are as follows:

- **Faecal impaction:** This may have to be treated initially by introducing a mineral or vegetable oil, followed by enema and digital evacuation, if required
- To empty the colon and the rectum **before radiologic or endoscopic examination**
- To cleanse the large bowel **prior to surgery or childbirth**
- In patients with **incontinence or colostomies**
- **As substitutes for glycerin suppositories and oral laxatives** to re-establish the rectal reflex in constipated patients

MANAGEMENT OF CONSTIPATION PH 1.1

Constipation may be defined as 'functional impairment in the inherent capacity of the colon to produce normally formed stools at regular intervals'. Individuals are known to differ widely in the 'normal' habits concerning the frequency, quantity and consistency of stools, and **missing a bowel movement does not necessarily affect the health adversely.** Failure to realise this may lead to self-medication and to laxative habit. In most cases, 'chronic constipation' is functional and can be corrected by simple measures such as increasing the roughage and water intake, exercise and by treatment of emotional factors, if any. The proper 'habit time' (conditioned effect) should be developed and the natural reflex, when it occurs, should not be ignored habitually. **Presence of any local organic cause such as painful fissure should be ruled out.**

The bulk residue can be increased and stools can be softened by simple measures such as increasing bran or leafy vegetables in the diet or by using bulk laxatives like isapgol, methyl cellulose or agar agar. **Food fibre is more effective as a laxative than synthetic fibre.** Cereal fibre (bran) is more effective in this respect than fruits and vegetables. Such measures are particularly useful in patients with irritable bowel syndrome, who may complain of constant or intermittent symptoms with the passage of small, round 'rabbit' or 'sheep' stools and abdominal pain aggravated by fatigue, smoking and mental tension. The pain could be related to the ingestion of certain foods such as coffee, spices, fried foods, certain vegetables and fruits and even milk. *Only in a few cases of chronic constipation, mild stimulant laxatives from the vegetable group may be necessary in initial stages.*

In old or obese individuals and in convalescing patients who find it difficult to strain, **lubricant drugs** or suppositories are useful, whereas in those in whom spastic colon is suspected, use of antimuscarinic preparations may be beneficial. Constipation associated with diseases like vitamin B deficiency or hypothyroidism will be corrected following vitamin B or thyroxine therapy. For the elderly, drinking of plenty of water and abdominal muscle exercises are recommended. Retraining of bowel habits is important. *Use of lubricants along with a bulk laxative is safer, effective and economical in such patients.*

In pregnant ladies presenting with constipation lubricant laxatives like liquid paraffin and lactulose are used. If satisfactory evacuation fails to occur following lubricant laxatives, simple enema or a suppository may be employed.

Constipation in infants and children sometimes poses a problem. In many cases, however, it is exaggerated by the anxious parents who believe that a daily good evacuation is necessary for good health. It is essential, therefore, that parents, particularly mothers, should know that the dire consequences of constipation are mostly imaginary. **Breast fed babies may have infrequent stools, sometimes once every four days, without any abnormal symptoms.** This obviously needs no treatment. In artificially fed babies, hard stools are often produced because of under-feeding or deficient intake of water and sugar in the feeds; the water requirement in warm countries like India is usually more than that in the temperate zones. In such cases, increasing the water intake and adding sugar to feeds corrects the constipation. Daily consumption of a few black raisins or a fig is known to help children with constipation. Occasionally, however, one has to prescribe a laxative particularly in those children in whom passing of hard stools is associated with considerable discomfort. The drug usually advocated is **magnesium hydroxide mixture** (milk of magnesia). **Suppositories containing glycerine** may be prescribed when other methods are not helpful. It acts by its hygroscopic action within 10–20 min. It is reliable, safe and cheap. In some cases with really formidable constipation, enemas are necessary to clear the bowel.

Disadvantages of Laxatives

They on repeated administration may cause:

- **GI disturbances** like dyspepsia, anorexia, nausea and spastic colitis
- **Nutritional deficiency** of calories, vitamins, and minerals due to interference with their absorption
- **Loss of fluid and electrolytes,** particularly potassium and calcium, giving rise to hypokalaemia and osteomalacia
- **Dependence on drugs** and later even resistance to all the mild laxatives, due to the development of spastic colon
- **Drug toxicity**

Box 40.1 Drugs Causing Constipation PH 3.4

- Drugs with antimuscarinic action (atropine and its derivatives antihistaminics, antiparkinsonian agents, tricyclic antidepressants and phenothiazines)
- Prostaglandin inhibitors (NSAIDs)
- Opioids
- Calcium carbonate and aluminium hydroxide used as antacids
- Sympathomimetic amines
- Antidiarrhoeal agents
- Miscellaneous: Clonidine, iron, MAO inhibitors, verapamil and phenytoin

After a thorough evacuation following a laxative, it may take some days to normalise the bowel movement and individuals should be told about this. Otherwise, they may feel that the constipation is continuing and continue to take the purgative.

It is important that family physicians should counter the false notions created in the minds of lay people, many times by commercial advertisements, and must emphasise the limitations of laxatives rather than prescribe them readily, whenever the patient complains of 'constipation'.

In the clinical management of **persistent constipation,** *it is very essential to carry out an abdominal and rectal examination to exclude any local rectal or anal lesion to exclude possible local organic disease.* In the elderly irregular bowel movements with constipation may be the only warning symptom of possible colorectal cancer.

Box 40.1 gives the commonly used drugs which may cause constipation.

TREATMENT OF HAEMORRHOIDS AND ANAL FISSURE

Perianal pruritus, soreness and excoriations are common symptoms in addition to bleeding in haemorrhoids; and acute anal pain due to spasm of the anal sphincter occurs in anal fissure. These patients can be helped by:

- Avoidance of hard stools by the use of **bulk laxatives** and/or **liquid paraffin** and a **high fibre diet**
- **Local application of a bland, zinc salt containing ointment**.
- Application of an ointment containing a local anaesthetic such as **lignocaine** before passing a stool.
- **Nitro-glycerine ointment** (0.2%) or **isosorbide dinitrate** 1% ointment is used for local application in cases of anal fissure(Chapter 29), with relief of spasm and pain, and healing of the fissure. While prescribing the nitrate preparations, the patient should be warned that headache might follow their application,
- Local injection of **botulinum toxin** (Chapter 22) into the anal sphincter has been used in resistant cases. It acts by preventing the release of acetylcholine locally.

Preparations for local application containing antibiotics and corticosteroids have little rationale and may even be harmful. **For sclerosant therapy of bleeding haemorrhoids see Chapter 33.**

LAXATIVES

Stimulant or irritant laxatives

Anthraquinone group
- Cascara sagrada
- Senna

Irritant oils
- Castor oil

Miscellaneous
- Phenolphthalein
- Bisacodyl
- Sodium picosulphate

Osmotic laxatives

- Magnesium sulphate
- Milk of magnesia
- Magnesium citrate
- Potassium sodium tartrate
- Lactulose
- Polyethylene glycol (PEG)

Bulk laxatives

- Methyl cellulose
- Agar agar
- Plantago seeds (Psyllium)
- Bran

Emollient laxatives

- Liquid paraffin
- Dioctyl sodium sulphosuccinate (Docusate sodium)

Chloride channel activators

- Lubiprostone
- Linaclotide (Guanylate cyclase-C agonist)

Mu Opioid Receptor Antagonists (for opioid induced constipation)

- Methylnaltrexon
- Naloxegol
- Naldemedine

Prokinetic agents

- Tegaserod

Clinical classification of laxatives

Slow onset
- Bulk laxatives
- Mineral oil
- Dioctyl sodium sulphosuccinate
- Lactulose

Intermediate onset
- Saline laxatives (low dose)
- Bisacodyl (oral)
- Anthraquinone group

Rapid onset
- Saline laxatives (high dose)
- Castor oil
- Bisacodyl (rectal)
- Glycerin suppository (rectal)

CHAPTER 41

Pharmacotherapy of Peptic Ulcer Disease

Learning Objectives

This chapter will enable the reader:

1. To be aware of the pathophysiology of peptic ulcer.
2. To classify drugs used for treatment of peptic ulcer.
3. To explain the mechanism of action, salient pharmacokinetic features, ADR, drug interactions and indications of proton pump inhibitors, H_2 receptor antagonists, anticholinergic agents and mucosal protective agents.
4. To outline the management of peptic ulcer.
5. To enlist the various drugs and regimens used for eradication of *H. pylori*, giving rationale for the same.
6. To outline the management of gastro-oesophageal reflux disease.
7. To state the treatment of NSAID-induced ulcers.

KEY TERMS

regulation of gastric acid secretion, p. 610
omeprazole, p. 613
H_2 receptor antagonists, p. 614
antacids, p. 616
peptic ulcer, management, p. 619
***H. pylori* infection, p. 620**
gastroesophageal reflux disease, p. 622
NSAID induced ulcers, therapy, p. 623
Prescribing PPI with NSAID, guidance, p. 623

Peptic ulcer disease is one of the common GI disorders in clinical practice. The common forms of peptic ulcer are as follows:

- **Duodenal ulcer** (DU)
- **Gastric ulcer** (GU)
- **Stress ulcer**(s)
- **NSAID-induced ulcer**

Of these, the DU is largely a disease of adult males. It occurs commonly in younger individuals and is evenly distributed among various socioeconomic groups. Gastric ulcer (GU), on the other hand, occurs most frequently in the older age group and in the lower socioeconomic class of individuals.

Peptic ulceration occurs mostly in areas which are bathed by the acid juice. Although the exact aetiology of ulceration is not known, a high association between *Helicobacter pylori* infection of the stomach and duodenum and peptic ulcer disease has now been established.

Physiology of gastric acid secretion: The gastric juice is a mixture containing hydrochloric acid, pepsin, rennin (in children), neutral chlorides, mucus, intrinsic factor and traces of potassium, ammonium and calcium which is screted by gastric glands. The gastric glands are of two types:

1. The **oxyntic glands** (80% of gastric glands) – body and fundus
2. **Pyloric glands** (20% of gastric glands) – antrum region

The **oxyntic glands** contain parietal or oxyntic cells (which secrete HCl and intrinsic factor), chief cells (which secrete pepsinogen), mucous neck cells and surface epithelial cells (which secrete mucus), G cells (which secrete gastrin), enterochromaffin-like-cells (ECL-which secrete histamine).

Gastric acid secretion is regulated by intricate central and peripheral mechanisms. (a) Central mechanism acts through the vagus nerve. (b) Peripherally, ACh liberated from the post-ganglionic nerve fibres directly stimulates the parietal cells.

Three distinct but interdependent pathways deliver chemical messengers that stimulate acid secretion by parietal cells (Fig. 41.1):

- **The neurocrine pathway**, that acts through the vagal efferent transmitter **acetylcholine**
- **The endocrine pathway**, which delivers hormone **gastrin from antral G cells**
- **The paracrine pathway**, which delivers tissue factors, such as **histamine from ECL cells**

The parietal cells possess a specific hydrogen–potassium–ATPase enzyme (**proton pump**), which is activated by protein kinases, histamine, acetylcholine and gastrin. It serves as a common final pathway for gastric acid secretion. When stimulated, it causes the transport of H^+ ions across the parietal cells in exchange of K^+ ions. Hydrogen ions combine with Cl^- ions to form HCl (Fig. 41.1).

ACh may enhance the acid secretion not only by stimulating the parietal cell directly, but also by reducing the somatostatin, a potent inhibitor of acid secretion.

Prostaglandin E (PGE) is produced by cells throughout the GI tract. **PGE, inhibits the secretion of gastric acid in humans, particularly, that stimulated by food and NSAIDs.**

The **pyloric glands**, present in pyloric antrum, secrete:

- *Gastrin, directly into the blood*
- *An alkaline, viscid, mucus-rich juice, into the stomach*

The rate and the composition of the secretion from the gastric glands is dependent on various factors and varies considerably as discussed below.

Phases of gastric secretion: Gastric acid secretion is generally divided into three phases:

- *Basal or interdigestive*
- *Neurogenic (or Cephalic)*
- *Hormonal (Gastric and Intestinal)*

Basal secretion: This follows a circadian rhythm, reaching its peak around midnight and its nadir at approximately 7 a.m. measured as nocturnal acid secretion, it is high in some patients with DU.

Gastric secretion in response to food may be divided into two phases, neurogenic and hormonal.

Neurogenic phase: The secretion occurs as a result of sight, smell, taste or even simple thought of food. The juice secreted is highly acidic and rich in pepsin. It is **mediated**

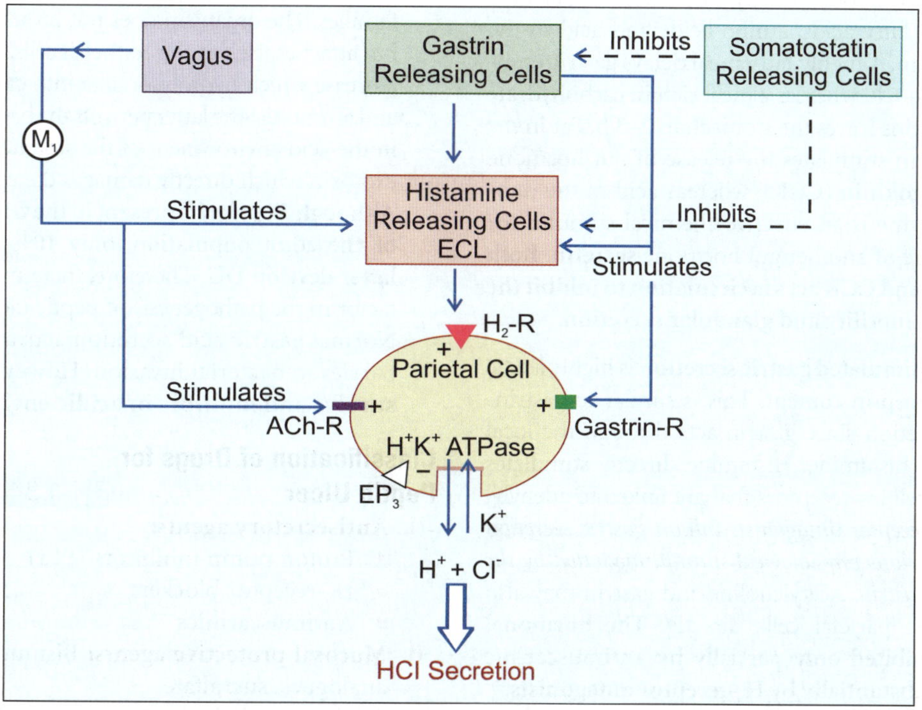

FIG. 41.1 Mechanisms involved in regulation of gastric acid secretion by the parietal cells. R, receptors; ECL, enterochromaffin like (cells). Gastrin acts mostly indirectly by releasing histamine; EP_3–R, PG receptor for PGE_2; M_1, muscarinic; H_2, histaminic.

by the vagus and is abolished by vagotomy and antimuscarinic drugs. In man, depression and fear result in a suppression of gastric secretion, whereas anger and resentment result in increased production.

Hormonal phase: Stimulation of the parietal cells by **gastrin** increases gastric secretion. Gastrin-containing cells are stimulated by food in the stomach and by neuronal input. Gastrin stimulates the ECL cells to release histamine, which activates the H_2-receptors in the parietal cells (Fig. 41.1). In addition, acid secretion is stimulated chemically, specifically by an increase in intraluminal pH and by certain foods, principally proteins and individual amino acids.

After a meal, the secretion of acid is modulated by a *negative-feedback* mechanism:

- Antral acidification inhibits the further release of gastrin. As the luminal pH approaches 3.5–3.0, inhibition of gastrin becomes apparent and is almost complete at pH 1.5.
- **Somatostatin** and its analogue **octreotide** inhibit the antral release of gastrin and also decrease acid secretion directly.
- Gastric secretion is also inhibited by reflexes initiated in the duodenum by distension, hypertonic contents, fatty acids, amino acids and acid in the duodenum. A highly fatty meal delays gastric emptying to 4–6 h, whereas a meal rich in carbohydrate and proteins leaves the stomach in 2–3 h. Fat in the duodenum stimulates the release of gut hormone **cholecystokinin** (CCK), whereas acid in the duodenal chyme is an effective chemical stimulus for the release of another gut hormone **secretin. Both secretin and CCK act via circulation to inhibit the stomach motility and glandular secretion.**

Histamine-stimulated gastric secretion is highly acidic but poor in pepsin content. This is similar to gastrin-induced secretion since gastrin acts through the local liberation of histamine. Histamine directly stimulates the parietal cell H_2-receptors that are linked to adenylyl cyclase. *H_2-receptor antagonists inhibit gastric secretion elicited by various physiological stimuli, mediated by the vagus or by gastrin.* Acetylcholine and gastrin may also stimulate the parietal cells directly. **The hormonal phase is inhibited only partially by antimuscarinic drugs but substantially by H_2-receptor antagonists.**

Factors which are postulated to protect the gastric and duodenal mucosa against the effects of the 'aggressive factors' are summarised in Box 41.1.

Box 41.1 Factors Protecting the Gastric and Duodenal Mucosa

- ***Mucus*** produced by the cells of the gastric mucous glands
- ***Bicarbonate*** secreted by the surface epithelial cells
- ***Rich mucosal blood flow*** which removes the acid that might diffuse through the mucosa
- ***Prostaglandins E*** which enhance all the normal gastroduodenal protective mechanisms
- ***Various growth factors*** *such as epidermal growth factor, and transforming growth factor*
- ***A competent pyloric sphincter*** which prevents the regurgitation of the aggressive factors (bile acids and pancreatic enzymes) into the stomach

- **Role of *H. pylori*:** Nearly all patients with DU and almost 80% of patients with GU show colonisation of the stomach by *H. pylori*. Those with infection of the gastric antrum have hyperacidity and develop DU; those with infection of the body of the stomach develop low acidity and GU. It is also strongly implicated in the pathogenesis of gastric carcinoma and gastric lymphoma.
  The infection is acquired by faecal–oral route in early childhood and is mainly transmitted within families. The organism does not invade the mucosa but attaches itself to the epithelial cells. It secretes (a) a urease which hydrolyses urea into carbon dioxide and ammonia; the latter permits the bacilli to survive in the acid environment of the stomach and (b) an exotoxin which directly damages the epithelial cells. **Although *H. pylori* is present in the GI tract of 50% of the adult population, only 10%–20% of the latter develop DU.** Therefore, there must be a host factor in the pathogenesis of peptic ulcer disease.
  Normal gastric acid secretion acts as a chemical barrier to bacterial invasion. **However, *H. pylori* survive and multiply in acidic environment.**

Classification of Drugs for Peptic Ulcer

PH 1.34, IM 15.15

I. **Antisecretory agents:**
   - Proton pump inhibitors (PPI)
   - H_2-receptor blockers
   - Antimuscarinics

II. **Mucosal protective agents:** Bismuth salts, PGE analogues, sucralfate

III. **Acid neutralising agents:** Systemic and non-systemic antacids

IV. **Antihelicobacter antimicrobials** given in combination

- Amoxicillin, clarithromycin, tetracycline, metronidazole
- Bismuth subsalicylate

ANTISECRETORY AGENTS

These drugs reduce the gastric acidity by acting on the target sites of parietal cells (Fig. 41.1).

Proton Pump Inhibitors (PPIs)

All PPIs are prodrugs and require activation at an acid pH.

Mechanism of action: After absorption from the intestine, PPI diffuse from the blood into the parietal cells, and get ionised at the acid pH and **irreversibly inactivate the enzyme H^+–K^+-ATPase (proton pump)**, which is the final common pathway for acid secretion in response to all stimuli (Fig. 41.1).This causes marked inhibition of gastric acid secretion. They have negligible effect on pepsin content. The effect lasts till the enzyme is regenerated following stoppage of the drug. There is less rebound increase in acidity following the drug withdrawal.

Mechanism of action – PPIs.

All PPI have short plasma t½, 0.5–2 h but the action lasts much longer. *They are acid labile and the tablet should be swallowed unbroken/uncrushed; or the drug should be given as enteric coated formulations or delayed release formulations. Film coated formulations wherein coating containing bicarbonate and oral suspensions of powdered omeoprazole with sodium bicarbonate are also available. Sodium bicarbonate neutralises acid and improves bioavailability of acid-labile omeoprazole.*

OMEPRAZOLE: This is a substituted benzimidazole (Fig. 41.2) with potent and prolonged action. As the concentration of the proton pump molecules in the parietal cells is highest after a prolonged fast at night, the *PPIs act best when taken about ½ h before the breakfast.* A second dose may be administered ½ h before the dinner. As only a fraction of the PP molecules are activated at a given time, a single daily dose takes 4–5 days to achieve the maximum reduction of acid secretion (65%–90%). It also selectively inhibits gastric mucosal carbonic anhydrase.

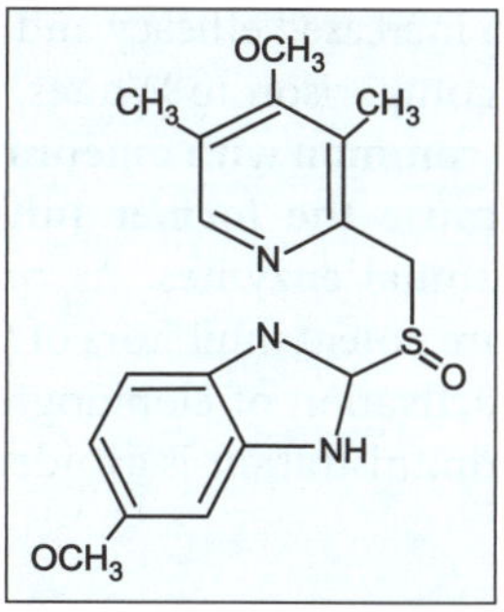

FIG. 41.2 Omeprazole.

Lansoprazole, pantoprazole, esomeprazole and **rabeprazole** are the other analogues of omeprazole (Table 41.1). Pantoprazole, esomeprazole and rabeprazole are available for IV use.

Adverse reactions: PPI are generally well tolerated. GI disturbances, dizziness and drowsiness may occur. Gynecomastia,hepatic failure, subacute myopathy, arthralgia, severe rash, and acute interstitial nephritis can also occur rarely. *They cause marked hypergastrinaemia due to prolonged achlorhydria.* Long-term use of PPI may cause malabsorption of iron, magnesium and vitamin B_{12}. Use of PPI for more than 5 years may be associated with increased incidence of osteoporotic fractures. Experimental studies have shown that omeprazole and other PPI cause alteration in gut microflora (dysbiosis) and may increase susceptibility to infection with *Clostridium difficile*.

Drug interactions: PPI are metabolised by hepatic CYPs, especially by CYP2C19 and CYP3A4. Asians are more likely to possess CYP2C19 genotype variant that correlates with slow metabolism of PPI, hence

Table 41.1 Proton Pump Inhibitors

Drug	Bioavailability (%)	Dose[a] (mg/day)
Omeprazole	40–65	20–40
Pantoprazole	77	40
Lansoprazole	80–90	15–30
Rabeprazole	52	20–40
Esomeprazole	50–89	20–40
Dexlansoprazole	80	30–60

[a]For peptic ulcer and GERD, in single or two divided doses.

contributing to increased efficacy and toxicity in this population in comparison to Whites. **Drug interactions are more common with omeprazole than with other PPI because the former inhibits multiple hepatic microsomal enzymes.** As omeprazole and esomeprazole are potent inhibitors of CYP2C19, they interfere with activation of clopidogrel. Hence their concomitant administration is avoided.

Indications:

- **Duodenal and gastric ulcers:** They are used in the treatment of DU. They appear to be less effective in promoting the healing of GU (see section, Management of peptic ulcer). With once a day (20–40 mg) regimen, 90% DU heal in 2 weeks and almost all heal in 4 weeks. Gastric ulcers require larger doses for 8 weeks. For patients with **bleeding ulcers, high dose IV PPI** may reduce need for endoscopic haemostasis. They also reduce chances of rebleeding. **Oral doses (40 mg 12 hourly)** of omeprazole is another alternative. DU resistant to H_2 blockers also respond to PPI.
- **Zolinger–Ellison syndrome:** They are used to treat multiple peptic ulcers due to gastric hypersecretion from excessive circulating gastrin.
- **Gastroesophageal reflux disease (GERD):** See Box 41.8
- **Prevention of acute erosive gastritis in acutely stressed patients:** In this condition, prophylaxis with intensive antacid regimens and/or PPI/H_2 blockers is recommended during the period of risk.
- **NSAID-induced ulcers.**

Recently similar to PPI, a new class of drugs called **potassium-competitive acid blockers** have been introduced. The drugs are weak bases that bind competitively and reversibly to the potassium binding site of the H^+/ K^+–ATPase. As these drugs have large molecular size they prevent the access of K^+ to their binding site, thus blocking activation of the H^+/K^+–ATPase. In comparison to PPI, they do not require acid-catalyzed activation, have early onset of action, can bind to both the active and inactive forms of the H^+/K^+–ATPase, resulting in a faster and longer duration of acid suppression. Drugs in this class include, **revaprazan**, **tegoprazan**, and **vonoprazan**. The reported adverse effects are diarrhea, nasopharyngitis, dyspepsia, headache, and abdominal pain.

H_2-Receptor Antagonists

Because of their structural similarity to histamine (Fig. 41.3), these **drugs act selectively by competitive blockade of parietal cell H_2-receptors.** They are highly effective. However, they can cause tolerance probably due to down regulation of receptors. A rebound increase in acid secretion may occur after their withdrawal.

CIMETIDINE: Cimetidine inhibits markedly (80%–90%) histamine, pentagastrin, caffeine and vagus (ACh) stimulated gastric acid secretion. It also inhibits the basal and meal-stimulated gastric secretion. Given orally, it reduces the acid secretion to about 20% within an hour. *Pepsin secretion is less affected. Food does not interfere with its action.* It has no significant action on gastric emptying.

Absorption, fate and excretion: It is well absorbed (60%–80%) orally, but its bioavailability is reduced to one-third when it is given with sucralfate or large doses of antacids; these should not be given within 2 h of H_2-receptor antagonists. Therapeutic effect of a single dose lasts for 5–8 h. It is largely excreted unchanged in the urine within 24 h. It can cross the placenta and is secreted in milk.

Adverse reactions: The drug is generally well tolerated. The adverse effects include rashes, diarrhoea,

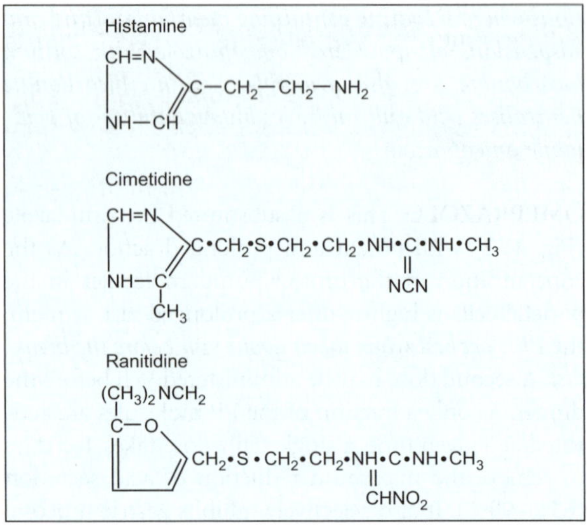

FIG. 41.3 Histamine and H_2-receptor antagonists.

muscle pain, fatigue and bradycardia. It must be noted that histamine and H_2-receptors are widely distributed in various areas such as brain, heart, blood vessels and bone marrow (Chapter 23). Blockade of cerebral H_2-receptors can cause drowsiness, mental confusion, delirium and hallucinations in the elderly and in those with hepatic or renal failure. It is a weak antiandrogen and may rarely cause gynaecomastia, hyperprolactinaemia and sexual dysfunction.

Drug interactions: It is a CYP1A2, CYP2C19, CYP3A4 and CYP2D6 inhibitor and reduces the clearance of drugs which are metabolised by oxidation, e.g. phenobarbitone, phenytoin, propranolol, warfarin, theophylline and diazepam; the hepatotoxicity of INH and paracetamol is enhanced.

Preparations and dosage: Cimetidine 200 mg tablet and as injection 100 mg/mL for IM or slow IV use.

In cases with DU, it is usually given in the dose of 400 mg twice or thrice daily after meals, or 800 mg at bedtime. **Because of its adverse effect profile and propensity to cause drug interactions it is not the preferred H2 blocker.**

RANITIDINE: It is a nitroethane derivative of furan. It:

a. Is 5–10 times more potent than cimetidine.
b. Is more selective and longer lasting than cimetidine, with plasma t½ of 1.6–2.4 h
c. Is adequately absorbed and 50% gets metabolised in the liver
d. Can control gastric acid secretion for up to 8–12 h when administered as a single oral dose of 150 mg
e. **Does not inhibit hepatic drug metabolism and hence there is a lesser possibility to cause drug interactions**
f. Has less antiandrogenic effects
g. Causes little, if any, central effects

Adverse reactions: It may cause skin rash, constipation and faecal concretions.

Preparations and dosage: The dose is 150 mg 12 hourly or 300 mg once daily preferably at bed time. It is also available as IV preparation.

FAMOTIDINE: Unlike cimetidine and ranitidine it has a thiazole ring. It has properties similar to ranitidine but is long acting. Only 25% is metabolised in the liver. Its plasma t½ is 3–4 h, and therapeutic effect lasts for 24 h.

- Famotidine is 30 times more potent than cimetidine and 7.5 times more potent than ranitidine.
- A single oral dose of 40 mg at night for 8 weeks produces healing of DU in most cases, while a dose of 20 mg reduces the relapse considerably. Preparations for IM or IV use are also available.
- It is well tolerated but may cause headache, dizziness and GI symptoms.
- *It does not interfere with drug metabolising enzymes in the liver.*
- *It is most cost effective and is to be preferred.*

Nizatidine and **roxatidine** are other drugs with similar properties, and have no significant advantages over ranitidine and famotidine.

Indications for H_2 blockers:

- Short-term therapy for gastritis.
- **Duodenal and gastric ulcers:** H_2 blockers have a faster onset of action than PPIs, but they are less effective than PPIs in relieving heartburn and healing of ulcers. Tolerance can develop quickly with their continuous use.
- **Zollinger–Ellison syndrome:** PPI are more effective than H_2 blockers.
- **Gastroesophageal reflux disease (GERD):** H_2 blockers are effective but less so than PPI (Box 41.8).
- **Prevention of acute erosive gastritis in acutely stressed patients**
- **NSAID-induced ulcers.**

Antimuscarinic Drugs

Experimentally, antimuscarinic drugs like atropine and its derivatives inhibit the basal and maximum gastric acid secretion by up to 40%. Clinical evidence indicates that tension type of ulcer pain which is relatively uncommon may be relieved but the commoner pain related to the food ingestion is little affected. Further, these drugs cause various anticholinergic side effects (Chapter 20). In the absence of antacids, they would prolong the contact of the acid secretion with the ulcer; this may aggravate the symptoms.

In the presence of pyloric stenosis, these drugs may cause gastric retention. They are no more recommended in DU.

PIRENZEPINE: This drug has selective antimuscarinic action on M_1 muscarinic receptors in the stomach and has been shown to reduce gastric acidity.

MUCOSAL PROTECTIVE DRUGS

BISMUTH SALTS: The preparations commonly used are: **colloidal bismuth subcitrate and bismuth subsalicylate.** They are not absorbed and the white precipitate (Bismuth chelate) formed in the gastric acid (pH < 3.5) coats the ulcer crater with bismuth-glycoprotein complex; the latter is relatively impermeable to the H^+ ion and acts as a diffusion barrier to gastric acid. **It is** also **toxic to *H. pylori*.** They are used as tablets before each of the three main meals and at bed time. The drugs may commonly cause constipation, black stools and rarely neurotoxicity.

SUCRALFATE: This drug is a complex of sulphated sucrose and aluminium hydroxide. In the acid environment of the stomach, it forms a gel which coats the ulcer crater for more than 6 h, thus forming a physicochemical defence barrier. The coating is not disturbed by food and is relatively impermeable to the H^+ ions. It also binds pepsin and bile acids. It is well tolerated. It promotes healing of peptic ulcers. It may be used as maintenance treatment to prevent recurrence. It is given as 1 g tablets, taken 1 h before a meal and at bed time (four times daily) for 4–8 weeks. *An antacid should not be taken ½ h before or after sucralfate.* By 4 weeks 70%–80% ulcers heal. The drug may cause constipation, dryness of mouth and abdominal discomfort. Rarely, it may cause aluminium toxicity and hypophosphatemia. It interferes with the absorption of ciprofloxacin, phenytoin, digoxin and aminophylline.

PROSTAGLANDIN E: Both the gastric and intestinal mucosa synthesise prostaglandins (PG). **PGE and PGI reduce the secretion of gastric acid and at lower concentrations may promote cytoprotection** by acting on EP3 receptors. Analogues of PGE_1 (**Misoprostol,** 15-deoxy-16-hydroxy-16 methyl PGE_1) and of PGE_2 (**enprostil, arbaprostil, rioprostil**), given orally, produce similar effects. The protective effect lasts for hours. These drugs may cause dose-related diarrhoea and oxytocic effects (Chapter 42). **They are inferior to H_2-receptor antagonists in the treatment of DU.** They are useful to prevent ulceration and bleeding from the gastric mucosa in patients who take large doses of aspirin or NSAID. *They should not be used in pregnant women and those contemplating pregnancy. They are very expensive.*

Rebapimide, a quinolone derivative, is claimed to act as a gastric mucosal cytoprotectant. It probably acts by stimulation of gastric PG generation. It has used to treat gastric ulcers and acute gastritis. It needs further evaluation.

ANTACIDS

Antacids are substances which, on ingestion, react chemically with gastric acid and lower the acidity of gastric contents. They produce symptomatic relief of pain, mainly by reducing the acidity and partly by the consequent relief of muscle spasm. Reduction in acidity inhibits the action of pepsin. It also increases the tone of the oesophagogastric sphincter and reduces the reflux of the acid, gastric contents into the oesophagus.

If adequate relief of symptoms in DU is to be brought about without seriously interfering with peptic digestion of food, the gastric pH must be raised from the usual level of 1–2 to between 3.5 and 4.5. Although this is possible with antacids, it is difficult to maintain it continuously. *Hence, to achieve even a reasonable control of gastric acidity regular and frequent administration of an antacid round the clock would be necessary,* which is its main disadvantage.

In spite of their limitations, antacids are valuable as they produce immediate, symptomatic relief in patients with gastritis, reflux oesophagitis and DU. As OTC drugs, they are often used for the symptomatic treatment of dyspepsia.

Antacids – Classification

I. **Nonsystemic antacids:** Such as aluminium hydroxide gel, magnesium trisilicate, magnesium hydroxide, calcium carbonate.

II. **Systemic antacids:** Sodium bicarbonate

Sodium bicarbonate is absorbed and may cause alkalosis; hence, it is called 'systemic antacid'.

Mechanism of action: These drugs acting as weak bases neutralise the gastric HCl. They act rapidly and raise the gastric pH to above 4.

The activity of various antacids is compared on the basis of their acid neutralising capacity which is defined as 'the mEq of 1 N HCL of acid neutralised per g or ml of the antacid to bring the pH to 3.5 in 15 minutes'

Nonsystemic Antacids

These are water insoluble and largely unabsorbable basic agents. The base may be hydroxide or carbonate or trisilicate, combined with cation such as Mg^{++}, Al^{+++} or Ca^{++}. In the stomach, during neutralisation of the acid, the cation, e.g. Mg^{++} forms a chloride. In the alkaline pH of the small intestine, the chloride salt reacts with the bicarbonate from the intestinal juices to regenerate the original salt (hydroxide or carbonate). **There is, thus, no net gain or loss of H or HCO_3 ions to the body. Hence, systemic alkalosis is avoided.**

Nonsystemic antacids are insoluble till they come into contact with the gastric acid. The antacid which escapes this reaction remains in the stomach and reacts with the acid subsequently secreted. **Hence, their duration of action is, longer than that of soluble antacids.**

ALUMINIUM HYDROXIDE GEL: This is available either as a white, colloidal, viscous suspension or as dried gel in the form of powder or tablets. It reacts with gastric acid to form aluminium chloride.

Each millilitre of 4% gel suspension neutralises 1.2–2.5 mEq of acid. The neutralising action is slow. The gastric pH is raised to 4. The acid neutralising capacity differs according to the process of manufacture and age of the product and to vary from batch to batch. Pepsin activity is not significantly inhibited. It has, however, astringent and demulcent properties by which it forms a protective coating over the ulcer crater. It may also adsorb toxins, gases and bacteria.

In the intestines, $Al(OH)_3$, is regenerated from $AlCl_3$ and chloride liberated is reabsorbed.

Adverse reactions: Constipation is the common ADR. This can be countered by combining it with magnesium trisilicate. Aluminium hydroxide may prevent the absorption of phosphate from the intestines. This may rarely cause osteomalacia. In patients with chronic renal failure, high plasma aluminium may rarely cause encephalopathy and deposition of aluminium in the bone with resultant osteodystrophy.

Preparations and dosage:

i. Aluminium hydroxide gel 4–8 mL every 2–4 h.
ii. Aluminium hydroxide 0.5 g tablets; 1–2 tablets to be chewed q.i.d.

ALUMINIUM PHOSPHATE GEL: It is sometimes preferred to aluminium hydroxide gel, as it does not interfere with phosphate absorption.

MAGNESIUM TRISILICATE: It is a fine, white, tasteless powder, insoluble in water. In the stomach, it reacts with acid to form hydrated silicon dioxide. As it becomes gelatinous in consistency, it provides a protective coating to the ulcer crater.

The neutralising action of magnesium trisilicate is slow in onset but prolonged. In the intestines, magnesium chloride reacts with the bicarbonate to form magnesium carbonate, which is excreted in faeces; about 7% is absorbed and excreted in the urine.

Hydrated silica gel has adsorbent properties similar to those of aluminium hydroxide gel.

One gram of magnesium trisilicate neutralises about 9–11 mEq of gastric acid.

Adverse reactions: It may cause mild diarrhoea which can be countered by combining it with aluminium hydroxide. A small amount of magnesium absorbed may produce CNS depression in the presence of impaired renal function.

Dose: 2–4 g every 1–4 h. **The tablet should be chewed before it is swallowed.** The drug can also be used in powder form.

MAGNESIUM OXIDE AND HYDROXIDE: Magnesium oxide, on contact with water, is converted to magnesium hydroxide which combines with gastric acid. It is a quick acting antacid with prolonged action. In small intestine, $Mg(OH)_2$ is regenerated and excreted in faeces. One gram of magnesium oxide neutralises 50 mEq of the acid. The dose is rather bulky.

Magnesium hydroxide is available as **'Milk of magnesia'** containing 7%–8.5% of magnesium hydroxide. It is more palatable than other formulations of magnesium salts.

Adverse reactions: These are similar to those of other magnesium salts.

Dose: Milk of magnesia as an antacid 4 mL; as a laxative 15 mL.

MAGNESIUM CARBONATE: This antacid has properties similar to those of magnesium hydroxide except that carbon dioxide is liberated during neutralisation of the acid.

CALCIUM CARBONATE: It occurs as a white, powder with a chalky taste. In the stomach, it reacts with gastric acid to form calcium chloride. In the intestine, $CaCl_2$ reacts with bicarbonate to regenerate $CaCO_3$ which is excreted in faeces. **Calcium carbonate acts quickly and has a high acid neutralising capacity.** One gram neutralises 21 mEq of the acid. Its action is prolonged and it is inexpensive.

Calcium carbonate increases serum gastrin level and gastric acid secretion above the basal level. Prolonged therapy may cause hypercalcaemia, hyperphosphatemia and renal calcinosis.

Dose: Powdered precipitated chalk or tablet containing 1 g of calcium carbonate. Dose: 2–4 g.

Systemic Antacids

SODIUM BICARBONATE: Sodium bicarbonate is a white, water soluble and completely absorbable antacid. It reacts with the gastric acid to form sodium chloride, water and carbon dioxide. One gram of the drug neutralises 12 mEq of acid. In the intestine, sodium chloride remains unchanged.

Excess of bicarbonate of the intestinal contents is absorbed, and may cause systemic alkalosis. **It is an effective and rapidly acting antacid. Its duration of action, however, is short.** Eructation of the carbon dioxide liberated during the process of acid neutralisation often gives the patient a sense of relief from abdominal discomfort. This is the basis of its reputed carminative action. *During its repeated administration in sufficient quantities, the output of the gastric juice and acid far exceeds the basal secretion.* This is probably because the continuous maintenance of raised pH in pyloric antrum stimulates gastrin secretion.

Adverse reactions: The release of carbon dioxide with resultant belching, flatulence, feeling of fullness, nausea and exacerbation of oesophageal reflux are the common side-effects. Systemic alkalosis and oedema due to sodium retention are rarely encountered.

Indications:

- **As an antacid:** For quick action, a dose 1–5 g in water, repeated as required.
- **Metabolic acidosis:** In severe cases (pH 7.1 or less, or HCO_3 less than 10 mmol/L) acidosis can be corrected by a slow IV infusion of 7.5% sodium bicarbonate in quantities sufficient (1 mmol/kg over 20–30 min) to raise the plasma bicarbonate concentration to about 15–20 mmol/L. No attempts should be made to correct the acidosis rapidly or fully.
- **Alkalinisation of urine:** To render urine alkaline in the treatment of certain urinary tract infections and to prevent precipitation of substances such as sulphonamide and uric acid.
- **Topical use:** Sodium bicarbonate solution is used as an antipruritic lotion, as an eye wash, mouth wash, douche and to loosen ear wax.

ANTACID THERAPY

Antacids are among the most abused drugs. Their indiscriminate use without an attempt to establish the cause of 'dyspepsia' can sometimes lead to masking of the warning symptoms of a serious condition like cancer of the stomach. When used properly, they promptly relieve the pain of gastritis and duodenal ulcer and promote healing. They are relatively cheap.

While using antacids, it is necessary to remember that:

- *They should be prescribed in optimal dose at 1 and 3 h after each meal, at bed time and as needed for pain.* In the fasting state antacids have only a transient intragastric buffering effect, about 15–30 min. When ingested 1 h after meal, however, they have a much longer effect, about 3–4 h.
- *The in vitro buffering effect of an antacid may not necessarily correlate with its* in vivo effect.
- *The quantity of an antacid required to produce optimal buffering varies from one patient to another.*
- *Antacid tablets, though more convenient than liquids, are less effective buffers,* unless they are chewed; hence, liquid formulations are to be preferred.
- *Antacids may interfere with absorption of other drugs* (Table 41.2).
- *Persistent reduction in gastric acidity by antacids may rarely increase susceptibility to intestinal pathogens.*

Choice of an antacid: Adequate dosage and frequency of administration are more important than the actual antacid chosen. Cost is also a major consideration. In general, systemic antacids should be avoided. **Magnesium trisilicate, is more effective than aluminium hydroxide.**

Table 41.2 Drug Interactions of Antacids

Antacids	Decrease in Bioavailability of
Aluminium compounds	Phosphate, iron salts, tetracyclines, antimuscarinic drugs, phenothiazines, digoxin, indomethacin (but not aspirin), prednisolone, ranitidine, sulphadiazine and fat-soluble vitamins
Calcium carbonate	Antimuscarinic agents, iron, phenothiazines, quinidine and tetracyclines
Magnesium salts	Digoxin and tetracyclines

Note: Although the clinical significance of the above drug interactions is uncertain, it is prudent to avoid simultaneous administration of antacids and drugs intended for systemic absorption.

Antacid combinations do not necessarily produce better results than individual antacids, but may counter the mutual adverse reactions.

MANAGEMENT OF PEPTIC ULCER IM 15.15

The management of peptic ulcer is essentially medical. It has undergone a major change with the discovery of the association of DU with *H. pylori* infection.

Therapeutic objectives:

- **To control gastric acidity, hypermotility and promote ulcer healing** (Box 41.2)
- **To treat H. pylori infection**
- **To prevent the complications and recurrence**

Exogenous factors such as smoking, NSAID, glucocorticoids and alcohol have been strongly associated with ulcerogenesis, and nonhealing of peptic ulcers.

The principles of medical treatment of peptic ulcer are outlined in Box 41.3.

Box 41.2 Measures to Control Gastric Acidity

- Neutralising gastric acid using antacids
- Inhibiting the gastric acid secretion and protecting the gastric mucosa
  a. **H_2-receptor antagonists**
  b. **Proton pump inhibitors**
  c. **Mucosal protectives**
- Cessation of smoking
- Withdrawal of gastric acid secretion stimulants such as alcohol, caffeine and soft cola drinks
- Avoiding acid-inducing drugs

Box 41.3 Principles of Medical Treatment of Peptic Ulcer Disease PH 1.1

- Withdrawal of offending agents such as NSAID, smoking, alcohol and caffeine
- Dietary modification
- Antisecretory drugs (PPI)
- Treatment of *H. pylori* infection (See text).
- Antacids (routine use is not recommended)
- Rest and sedatives in acute stage as poor sleep quality can cause recurrence.

- **Withdrawal of the offending agents:** For example, tobacco, NSAID, alcohol and caffeine-containing beverages.
- **Diet:** Peptic ulcer disease can be effectively treated with the usual 3–4 meals a day. Night feeds should be avoided. Irritants such as chilly, other spices and fried food should be avoided. Edible vegetable oils, ghee and butter taken as such may be helpful, as these have an inhibitory effect on gastric acid secretion.
- **Antisecretory drugs and antacids:** The mean diurnal gastric pH is about 1.4–2.0; **low pH is mainly found at night.** For the treatment of DU, the pH has to be elevated to a level higher than 3.0 for about 16–18 h a day. For the treatment of reflux oesophagitis, it must be raised to at least 4.0 for 16–18 h per day. This can be achieved by 8–12 weeks' course of therapy with an H_2-receptor blocker or a PPI.

PPIs are the most potent antisecretory drugs available; all of them are equally effective. They may be prescribed twice daily for 3–5 days; after that a single prebreakfast dose may be prescribed for 8–12 weeks. If the ulcer recurs, another course of full therapy is indicated.

H_2-receptor antagonists, *as a class, are remarkably free from adverse reactions.* **The total daily dose of these drugs is usually given after the evening meal.** Cimetidine 800 mg is equivalent to 300 mg of ranitidine, 40 mg of famotidine and 300 mg of nizatidine. Famotidine is perhaps the most cost-effective with a longer duration of action. However, it takes longer time for ulcer healing as compared to PPI. An H_2 blocker can be used as needed for patients who have breakthrough nocturnal symptoms while taking a PPI. Antacids can be used as adjuncts for quick pain relief. Patients with Zollinger–Ellison syndrome who are resistant to H_2-receptor blockers should be treated with PPI.

Although antisecretory drugs alone can cause ulcer healing, they do not cure the disease and recurrence can occur after stoppage of therapy. Hence, they are now always combined with anti *H. pylori* therapy. MI 3.6

- **Treatment of *H. pylori* infection:** *Eradication of documented H. pylori infection is now considered the mainstay of treatment of documented DU and GU.* Antibiotics are used in combination regimens using triple or quadruple therapy. Recommended regimens are shown in Box 41.4. **Bismuth-containing quadruple therapy** (a PPI, bismuth, tetracycline, and metronidazole/ tinidazole) and **concomitant quadruple therapy** (a PPI, clarithromycin, amoxicillin, and metronidazole/ tinidazole) are currently recommended as first line treatment of *H. pylori* infection. *The concurrent administration of a PPI or an H_2-receptor antagonist enhances the eradication of H. pylori.* PPIs are superior in this respect. The organism may develop resistance to metronidazole in 20%–30% of cases.

To ensure complete cure, antisecretory and antimicrobial therapy is usually given together for the first 10–14 days, followed by antisecretory therapy (PPI or an H_2 blocker) alone for 6–8 weeks to ensure complete cure. Efficacy of the antimicrobial therapy is assessed by a negative urea breath test. Patients

Box 41.4 Suggested Antimicrobial Regimens for *H. pylori* Infection

1. Clarithromycin 500 mg b.i.d. + amoxicillin 1 g b.i.d. + metronidazole 400mg b.i.d + PPI b.i.d.
2. Tetracycline 500 mg q.i.d. + metronidazole 200 mg q.i.d. + bismuth subsalicylate 2 tablets q.i.d. + omeprazole 20 mg b.i.d. or ranitidine 150 mg b.i.d.
3. Clarithromycin 500 mg b.i.d. + metronidazole 400 mg b.i.d. + omeprazole 20 mg b.i.d.
4. Clarithromycin 500 mg b.i.d. + amoxicillin 1 g b.i.d. + omeprazole 20 mg b.i.d.

Clarithromycin is very expensive. Tetracycline can be substituted for metronidazole or amoxicillin.
Other PPI or H_2 blocker can be used instead of omeprazole.
Duration: 10–14 days.
Sequential therapy: PPI + amoxicillin 1 g b.i.d for 5 days followed by PPI + clarithromycin 500 mg and tinidazole/ metronidazole 500 mg bi.d for 5 days

who are still infected should be treated with a different regimen, not used initially. *Once H. pylori infection is eradicated, long-term maintenance antisecretory therapy is not needed.*

Some experts feel that a course of antimicrobial therapy is justified in all patients with documented DU even without demonstrating *H. pylori* infection. However, it is not indicated in reflux oesophagitis and nonulcer dyspepsia. In patients with GU, malignancy should be ruled out.

Box 41.5 summarises the current guidelines for treatment of *H. pylori* infection.

- **Adjuvant therapy:** A sympathetic discussion of the patient's problems may be useful in relieving the anxiety and tension. An antianxiety or an antidepressant drug may be needed in some cases. Tricyclic antidepressants also possess antimuscarinic action (Chapter 14).
- **Prevention of recurrence:** In the absence of documented *H. pylori* infection (which is curable) no treatment, available at present, can permanently prevent a recurrence of the peptic ulcer. However, ranitidine (150 mg daily), used prophylactically reduce ulcer recurrence and prevent complications in resistant cases. Patients should be advised to avoid smoking, alcohol and **certain drugs** (Box 41.6). Many elderly persons with osteoarthritis often receive potent *anti-inflammatory* drugs (NSAIDs) **in high doses,** whereas all that they require is an analgesic such as paracetamol or low dose ibuprofen (200 mg). *Up to four-fifths of gastric ulcers have been attributed to smoking and use of NSAID.*

Failure to respond to medical treatment indicates chronicity or the presence of some complication. A gastric ulcer may undergo malignant change.

Box 41.5 Current Guidelines for Treatment of *H. pylori* Infection

1. **Strongly recommended in**
   - ***Duodenal and gastric ulcer*** (whether active or not, including complicated peptic ulcer disease)
   - ***Gastric lymphoma***
   - ***Atrophic gastritis***
   - ***Recent resection for gastric cancer***
2. **May be useful in**
   - ***Functional dyspepsia***
   - ***First degree relatives of patients with gastric cancer (prophylaxis)***

Acute Erosive Gastritis (Box 41.7)

Acute erosive gastritis with bleeding occurs as a complication of a serious medical or surgical illness and is common in intensive care units. Compromise in the gastric mucosal blood supply appears to be an important aetiological factor. Patients at risk must be given prophylactic treatment; and any patient who has begun to bleed deserves aggressive management. The incidence of bleeding is reduced if the gastric pH is maintained above 5.0.

Box 41.6 Drugs to be Avoided in Peptic Ulcer Disease

- Salicylates and other NSAID
- Clopidogrel
- Caffeine, theophylline
- Glucocorticoids in pharmacological (but not in replacement) doses
- Some iron salts
- Bisphosphonates
- Mycophenolate mofetil
- Potassium chloride

Box 41.7 Prevention and Treatment of Acute Erosive Gastritis

- Prevention of hypovolaemia, systemic acidosis, sepsis and hypoalbuminemia
- Maintenance of intragastric pH above 5.0 with the use of antacids, an H_2-receptor blocking agent or PPI; the latter is more convenient
- Ranitidine: 50 mg IM or IV every 6–8 h; or 6.25 mg/h by IV infusion, Famotidine: 20 mg every 6–12 h IM or IV Pantoprazole repeated as bolus or by continuous infusion over 24 h
- Antacid in liquid form: 15–30 mL/h by a nasogastric drip

Table 41.3 Prescribing PPI with NSAID based on Gastrointestinal Risk Factors

Cardiovascular risk	Gastrointestinal risk*		
	Low (No risk fator)	**Moderate (1-2 risk factors)**	**High (> 2 risk factors; history of previously complicated ulcer)**
Low	NSAID alone (the least ulcerogenic NSAID at the lowest effective dose is to be prescribed)	NSAID+PPI	Alternative therapy if possible OR COX-2 Inhibitor + PPI
High (those who require low- dose aspirin)	Naproxen + PPI	Naproxen + PPI	Avoid NSAIDs or COX-2 inhibitors and use alternative therapy

Gastrointestinal Risk factors: 1. Age >65 years; 2. High dose NSAID therapy; 3. Previous history of uncomplicated ulcer; 4. Evidence of *H. pylori* infection; 5. Concurrent use of aspirin (including low dose), corticosteroids or anticoagulants

Gastroesophageal Reflux Disease (GERD) PH 1.34

This is a chronic, unremitting, essentially incurable disease that relapses on cessation of drug therapy. It is characterised by 'the reflux of gastric acid contents into the oesophagus, leading to oesophagitis and reflux symptoms sufficient to impair the quality of life'. It is subdivided into **nonerosive** GERD and **erosive** GERD. The commonest symptom is heartburn followed by cough; about half the patients have erosive oesophagitis. Incompetence of the lower oesophageal sphincter (LES), its transient, repeated relaxation not associated with swallowing, and delayed gastric emptying seem to be the important factors in its pathogenesis.

The **current guidelines for the treatment of** GERD are outlined in Box 41.8. *Acid suppression is the key measure in both acute and long-term therapy of GERD.* It is advisable to start the therapy with **PPI** given b.i.d. (20–60 min before breakfast and dinner) and once the symptoms are relieved, substitute it with **H_2-receptor blockers/antacids** in nonerosive but not in erosive GERD.

Patients with infrequent heart–burn and dyspepsia (less than 3–4 times a week) and mild GERD can be managed with an H_2 antagonist alone such as famotidine 20 mg o.d. or b.i.d. as needed.

Box 41.8 Current Guidelines for Treatment of GERD

- ***Nonpharmacological measures:*** Reassurance and advice about lifestyle; elevation of the head of the bed by 15–20 cm; weight reduction in obese patients; avoidance of tight garments, large meals and lying down for 2–3 h after a meal; cessation of smoking; avoidance of reflux-inducing foods (such as spicy or fatty foods, citrus fruits, chocolates and coffee), carbonated drinks, alcohol, NSAID, CCBs, theophylline and antimuscarinics
- ***Antacids*** help to relieve mild reflux symptoms promptly
- ***PPI (high dose)*** are the most effective drugs for promotion of healing of the erosive oesophageal lesions. Maintenance therapy up to 1 year may be needed
- ***H_2-receptor antagonists*** are less effective than PPIs in erosive oesophagitis but may be cost-effective in long-term maintenance therapy. *In nonerosive GERD, they are almost as effective as PPIs and much less expensive*
- ***Prokinetic drugs*** are not recommended for routine use. However, they may be used as add-on drugs in refractory cases
- ***On demand therapy*** is a cost-effective alternative to continuous maintenance therapy in case of mild, nonerosive GERD
- When symptoms have resolved, an attempt should be made to stop therapy. However, sometimes long-term treatment is needed in a few cases
- ***Routine anti-H. pylori therapy is not indicated in GERD***

NSAID-Induced Ulcers

Aspirin and other NSAIDs are known to cause dyspepsia and symptomatic gastric ulcers, particularly when given in **large doses and for long periods** as in rheumatoid arthritis (RA) (Chapter 11).

The drugs used for prophylaxis are:

(1) **PPI** which are more effective.
(2) **H_2-receptor antagonists**
(3) **Misoprostol**, a PG analogue, given concurrently (400 mcg b.i.d.) with NSAIDs.

They are not needed in patients receiving small doses of NSAIDs for a short period.

However, for those who have gastrointestinal risk factors, co-prescribing a PPI with NSAID is essential (Table 41.3).

PPI are being marketed as a fixed dose combination (FDC) with nonselective NSAIDs. *There is no convincing evidence that such a combination prevents GI complications in the long term.* Such FDCs are not recommended because the dosage regimens of individual drugs in the FDC are not compatible (Chapter 11).

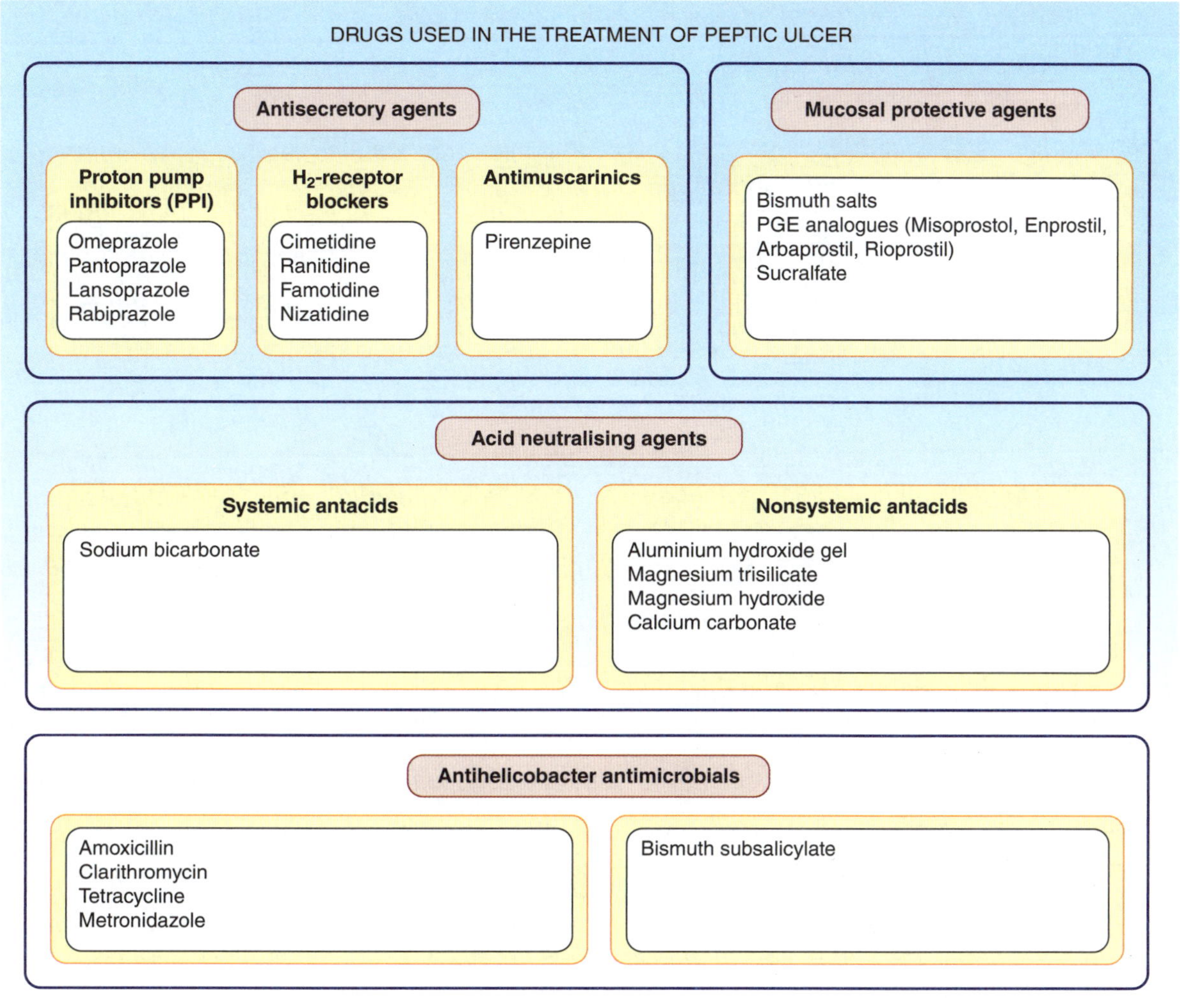

11

SECTION

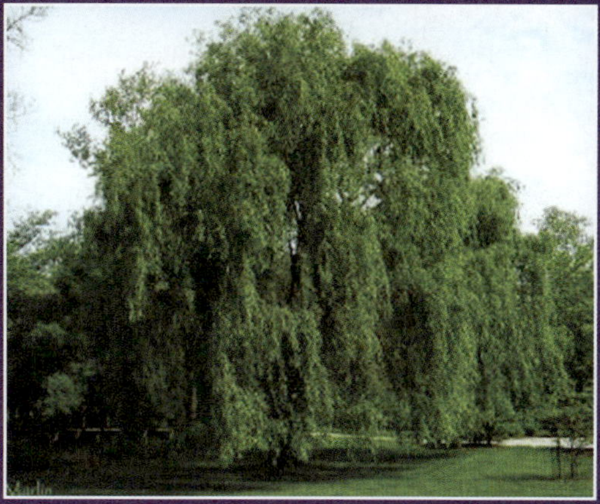

Salix alba

Oxytocics and Uterine Relaxants

Section Outline

This section consists of the following chapters:

CHAPTER 42

Pharmacology of Ergot Alkaloids, Oxytocics and Tocolytics

Learning Objectives

This chapter will enable reader:

1. To compare pharmacological effects of ergotamine, ergometrine and dihydroergotamine.
2. To state adverse effects of ergot alkaloids.
3. To define the term, 'oxytocics' and enlist them.
4. To explain the mechanism of action, salient pharmacokinetic features, adverse effects, indications and contraindications of oxytocin, methylergometrine and prostaglandins.
5. To classify tocolytics.
6. To explain the pharmacological effects, ADR, indications and contraindications of calcium channel blockers, COX inhibitors and β_2 agonists.

KEY TERMS

PH 1.41

Ergot has been termed a treasure house of pharmacological constituents and many drugs have been developed for various therapeutic indications. Ergot is obtained from a fungus *Claviceps purpurea,* which grows mainly on rye and occasionally on other grains. Ergot spores, carried by insects or wind, are deposited on the ovaries of young rye where they germinate. Their hyphal filaments penetrate deep into the rye, and destroy the entire grain substance with formation of a hardened, black purple body termed the sclerotium, which serves as the commercial source of ergot.

Chemistry of ergot: Ergot contains ergot alkaloids, of which levorotatory forms are active. In addition, histamine, tyramine, acetylcholine and several other constituents are present.

Classification of Ergot Alkaloids

I. **Amino acid alkaloids:** Ergotamine, ergosine and ergotoxin(e.g.ergocornine, ergocristine and ergocryptine), of which only ergotamine is used therapeutically.
II. **Semisynthetic dihydrogenated amino acid alkaloids:** Dihydroergotamine (DHE).
III. **Amine alkaloid:** Ergometrine (ergonovine).
IV. **Semisynthetic amine alkaloids:** Methylergometrine, methysergide

Pharmacological actions (Table 42.1):

All the ergot alkaloids and their dihydrogenated derivatives:

- Block the α adrenergic receptors (Chapter 18) and
- Directly stimulate the vascular and uterine muscle.

Cardiovascular system: The stimulant activity on the vascular smooth muscle is higher among the natural amino acid alkaloids (ergotamine being the most potent vasoconstrictor) while their dihydrogenated derivatives cause increased α adrenergic blockade with minimal direct vasoconstrictor effect. *Thus, the natural amino acid alkaloids usually raise the BP and may constrict coronary vessels.* Peripheral vasoconstriction is accompanied by damage to the capillary endothelium.

Table 42.1 Pharmacological Actions of Ergot Preparations

Preparation	Uterus (Contraction)	Alpha Adrenergic Blocking Action	Vasoconstriction	5-HT[a] Antagonism
Ergotamine	+++ (delayed)	+++	++++	+++
Ergometrine	++++	±	+	+++
DHE	++ (on pregnant uterus)	++++	++	+

[a]All are also partial 5-HT agonists.

Dihydroergotamine (DHE) also retains the vasoconstrictor effect in addition to adrenergic blocking activity.

The amine ergot alkaloid, **ergometrine**, is devoid of adrenergic blocking activity and causes minimal vasoconstriction (Table 42.1).

Ergot alkaloids also depress the vasomotor centre, induce bradycardia by central vagal stimulation and direct myocardial depression.

CTZ: Ergot alkaloids may cause vomiting by stimulation of the CTZ and emetic centre through 5 HT Receptors. They are also antagonists of 5-HT_2.

Uterus: See under section Oxytocics.

Gastrointestinal tract: Ergotamine increases peristaltic activity and can potentiate the action of neostigmine on the gut.

Miscellaneous: Ergotamine and ergometrine are partial 5-HT agonists on certain blood vessels and selective antagonists on various smooth muscles.

Absorption, fate and excretion: Ergotamine and DHE are erratically absorbed from the gut, and have poor bioavailability. *Ergometrine and methylergometrine, on the other hand, are rapidly and completely absorbed.* They are metabolised in the liver and the degradation products eliminated in urine. Liver damage enhances the toxicity.

Adverse reactions:
Ergotamine and DHE often produce nausea, vomiting, miosis and postural hypotension. Toxicity of ergotamine and DHE is mainly due to direct vascular actions; ergotamine is more toxic than DHE.They may cause angina due to coronary constriction. On prolonged administration, they may also induce paraesthesiae, tingling, numbness and occasionally thrombosis and gangrene (Chapter 18).

For adverse effects of ergometrine and methylergometrine, see section Oxytocics.

Preparations and dosage:

i. Preparations of ergotamine and DHE (Chapter 18)
ii. Preparations of ergometrine and methylergometrine (section Oxytocics)

Indications:

- **Migraine:** Ergotamine is used to treat acute attacks of migraine (Chapter 24).
- **Postpartum haemorrhage (PPH)** – see section under Oxytocics
- **Uterine involution** - see section under Oxytocics

BROMOERGOCRIPTINE: This synthetic ergot derivative is not an oxytocic. It is discussed in Chapter 66.

OXYTOCICS

PH 1.41

Oxytocics are the drugs which stimulate uterine contractions (oxytocin, prostaglandins and ergot alkaloids), and are used to:

- **Minimise the placental blood loss**
- **Induce or augment labour**
- **Induce abortion**

OXYTOCIN

The posterior pituitary extract has two distinct pharmacologically active principles:

- **Vasopressin** which acts on the kidney and the

blood vessels (Chapter 37)

- **Oxytocin**, which has a dominant action on the uterus and the myoepithelium of the mammary gland

Oxytocin and vasopressin are **synthesised in hypothalamic nuclei**. They travel along the hypothalamo-hypophyseal tract to the posterior lobe of the pituitary where they are stored. They are released under a variety of stimuli, such as dehydration, haemorrhage, dilatation of the cervix and uterus and emotional stimuli. **Oxytocin is a bonding hormone**; increased levels are observed during 'love making'and on the battlefield. As both oxytocin and vasopressin are bound to a common protein, such stimuli cause simultaneous release of both.

Oxytocin is a nonapeptide usually represented in the simplified form given in Fig. 42.1. The polypeptide is freely water soluble and acid stable. Oxytocin used in therapy is a synthetic preparation whose structure is identical to natural oxytocin.

Pharmacological actions:

Uterus: The oxytocic activity of oxytocin varies according to the dose, the species, the stage of oestrous cycle, and the stage of gestation. These effects are highly dependent on the presence of estrogen. In the early period of pregnancy only very high doses are effective. However, as the pregnancy advances, from 5th to 6th month onwards, the sensitivity of pregnant uterus to oxytocin increases rapidly.

- **Small doses**, *given by IV infusion, exert a physiological action on the pregnant uterus. The upper uterine segment, consisting of the fundus and body, is contracted, whereas the lower uterine segment, consisting of the cervical portion, is dilated.* This results in an expulsion of the fetus from the uterine cavity. The contractions also squeeze the maternal blood out of the placenta into the maternal inferior vena cava. The periods of relaxation which intervene between the two successive contractions allow refilling of the placental blood vessels by the maternal arterial blood and thus prevent asphyxial injury to the fetus. *Oxytocin, therefore, can be used by slow IV infusion for inducing labour at term* in contrast to ergot preparations which are contraindicated prepartum.
- **With high doses,** the uterine tone increases, the contractions become more powerful and frequent, and asphyxial injury to the fetus may develop due to direct compression and ischemia caused by inadequate filling of the placental blood vessels.

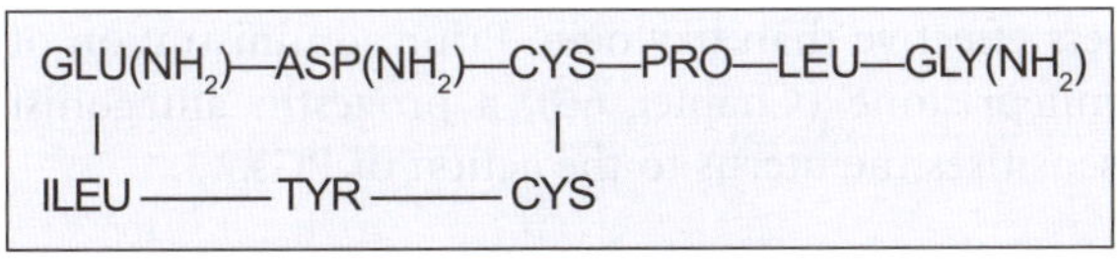

FIG. 42.1 Oxytocin.

Mammary gland: It stimulates the myoepithelium, a modified smooth muscle, which surrounds the alveolar ramifications of the mammary gland and causes expulsion of milk from the alveolar lumen and ducts into large cisterns and sinuses. This is termed milk ejection or milk 'letdown'. The milk ejection reflex is initiated by the stimulus of suckling, which results in the release of oxytocin.

Cardiovascular system: In small doses, it produces a vasodilator effect by direct vascular muscle relaxation. Transient hypotension and flushing accompanied by tachycardia are usually observed. *The usual infusion rates employed in obstetrics do not modify the BP.* The hypotensive phase is followed by a rise in BP, probably due to an increase in the cardiac output.

Kidney: *Synthetic oxytocin possesses antidiuretic activity in man* and a dose of 100 mU causes a definite antidiuresis in postpartum women; this is associated with a diminution in the renal plasma flow and the GFR. The renal effects of oxytocin may be due to constriction of renal cortical vessels.

Absorption, fate and excretion: Given orally, it is inactivated by trypsin. On IM administration, it is absorbed rapidly. The t½ *in nonpregnant women* is about 10–15 min. The removal from the circulation is mainly by kidneys and the liver. Plasma from men and nonpregnant women does not inactivate oxytocin but the plasma, the uterine tissue and the placenta in pregnant women contain an enzyme termed 'oxytocinase' which inactivates oxytocin. Thus, *t½ of oxytocin in pregnant women at term is approximately 3 min.*

Oxytocin is also absorbed from the nasal and buccal mucous membranes. Absorption from these routes, however, is erratic.

Adverse reactions: Oxytocin given by IV infusion may occasionally cause water retention leading to water intoxication. It is characterised by nausea, vomiting, anorexia, weight gain and lethargy. Injudicious use of oxytocin during labour may result in premature birth, fetal death, too rapid a delivery or uterine rupture.

Preparation and dosage:

i. Oxytocin injection contains 5U, 10 U/ml; 5 U/0.5 ml is also available.

Indications:

- **Induction and augmentation of labour at term:** For the induction of labour, oxytocin is administered by IV infusion, 5 U in 500 mL of 5% dextrose solution. *The uterine response must be closely monitored and the dose be regulated by monitoring of fetal heart rate.*
  Before using oxytocin, following points must be ruled out:
  i. Cephalopelvic disproportion
  ii. Multiparous women (para 4 and over),
  iii. Malpresentation of the fetus,
  iv. Complete placenta previa,
  v. Uterine scars
  vi. Fetal distress
- **Hypotonic uterine dysfunction** (Uterine inertia): Oxytocin is occasionally employed to initiate uterine contractions in cases of prolonged, stubborn and hypotonic uterine inertia.
- **Postpartum haemorrhage (PPH):** Oxytocin can be routinely administered 5–10 U intravenously *after the delivery of placenta* to produce a firm contraction of the uterus and thus prevent PPH. The drug may also be administered in the same dose after delivery of the anterior shoulder of the fetus to produce a prompt expulsion of the placenta and to prevent PPH. The same dose may also be injected directly into the uterus, after delivering the fetus by caesarean section. **For treatment of PPH,** a dose of 20–40 U in 1 L of 5% dextrose is preferred. Alternatively, it can be given intramuscularly.
- **Miscellaneous:** Oxytocin may be given intranasally in the dose of 40 U 2–5 min before breast feeding to promote milk ejection when this component of lactation appears to be deficient in nursing mothers.

It is often used in veterinary practice to increase the milk yield.

Oxytocin is no more employed to induce therapeutic abortion.

PROSTAGLANDINS (PG, Prostin)

Prostaglandins are C20 fatty acids containing a cyclopentane ring, and are described in Chapter 25; only the actions on uterus are discussed below.

Apart from human seminal fluid, PGs are found in the ovary, myometrium and menstrual fluid. Their physiological significance, however, is not well understood. Majority of PGs in varying doses inhibit the spontaneous activity of isolated non-pregnant human myometrium. However, *PGF_2 and PGE in low doses stimulate both, the tone and amplitude of the uterine contractions.* Four PGs have been isolated from human amniotic fluid, obtained during normal labour and during spontaneous abortion. Experimentally, they are shown to sensitise the uterus to oxytocin as well as causing oxytocin release. **Since PGF_2 has smooth muscle stimulating action, it is possible that it participates in the process of labour.**

During pregnancy PGs act in at least three different ways:

- **As uterine smooth muscle stimulants,** causing uterus to contract.
- **As cervical primers,** thus hastening the process of softening and dilation of the cervix, sometimes referred to as 'cervical ripening'. Unlike oxytocin, $PGF_2\alpha$ and PGE_2 actually decrease cervical stiffness.
- **As luteolytic agents,** inhibiting the secretion of progesterone by corpus luteum. This effect has not been observed in humans.

PGs are most effective in the second trimester (13th–20th weeks), whereas in the third trimester, PGs are less effective than oxytocin. Prior administration of mifepristone (Chapter 66), a progestin antagonist sensitises the uterus to the action of PGs.

Adverse reactions: These are not troublesome with

smaller doses but could be **severe with larger doses**. They include nausea, vomiting, abdominal cramps, diarrhoea, headache, fever and vasodilatation. PGs should be used cautiously in the presence of raised intraocular pressure, hypertension, diabetes, angina or epilepsy. They are contraindicated in the presence of cardiac, renal, pulmonary or hepatic disease. Smoking and alcohol should be avoided during their use and for 48 h afterwards.

Preparations and dosage:

i. Dinoprost (Prostin $F_2\alpha$) 5 mg/mL for intraamniotic use to induce abortion. Dose: 40 mg slowly injected into the amniotic sac; further dose of 10-40 mg may be repeated after 24 h, if the membranes are still intact.
ii. Dinoprostone (Prostin E_2) Available as injection- 1 mg/ml; pessary- 3 mg; vaginal gel- 1 mg, 2 mg; vaginal device-10 mg; oral tablet -3 mg for induction of labor. Prefilled syringes containing Dinoprostone 0.5 mg to be administered as endocervical injection for cervical ripening is also available.
iii. Carboprost (Prostin/15 m) is 15-15 dimethyl $PGF_2\alpha$ analogue with a longer duration of action. Dose: 250 mcg/mL deep intramuscularly.
iv. Misoprostol, PGE_1 (Chapter 66) has been used orally/intravaginally to bring about medical abortion. The intravaginal administration is also used to cause cervical dilatation.
v. Gemeprost, PGE_1, as vaginal pessary in the dose of 1mg every 3 hourly (maximum upto 5 mg) is used for cervical dilatation.

Indications:

- **Therapeutic abortion:** *PGs are not used for terminating early, first trimester pregnancies* because of the high incidence of incomplete abortions and consequent need for surgical procedures. The dose needed usually causes pain and adverse GI reactions. Many clinicians, therefore, prefer suction evacuation to PGs (Chapter 66).
  PGs are now widely used to terminate the pregnancy in the second trimester. Gemeprost, administered vaginally as pessaries, is the preferred PG for this purpose. Alternatively, oral or intravaginal misoprostol may be used. They are combined with mifeprostone (Chapter 66).
  All methods of abortion using PGs alone cause a high incidence of adverse effects and there is a possibility of delivering a live fetus. Some of them may also cause bronchospasm. There is no absolutely safe method of terminating pregnancy in the second trimester.
- **Cervical priming:** Dinoprostone has been used extra-amniotically for cervical priming. Endocervical gels, suppositories and oral tablets containing PGs may also be useful.
- **Postpartum haemorrhage:** The PG analogue, carboprost, given intramuscularly, is effective in managing PPH due to uterine atony. However, the *less expensive ergometrine is preferred.*
- **Induction and augmentation of labour at term:** Dinoprostone may be preferred to oxytocin for this purpose in the presence of chronic renal failure or pre-eclampsia because of its diuretic action. The PGs can cause hyperstimulation of the uterus which compromises uteroplacental blood flow, and they have a longer duration of action than oxytocin. *Signs of uterine hypertonus and fetal distress should therefore be watched for.*

As the obstetric regimens of PGs are complicated, the manufacturer's literature should be read before using these drugs.

ERGOT ALKALOIDS AS OXYTOCICS

All the natural ergot alkaloids possess *oxytocic action*. The magnitude of response depends upon the alkaloid employed, the dose used, the degree of uterine maturity and stage of gestation. **Ergotamine** elicits a delayed but powerful response; DHE, however, is active only on pregnant uterus at term. **Ergometrine** and **methylergometrine** are therapeutically used as uterine stimulants, as they elicit an immediate and powerful response:

- **Small doses** produce an increase in the force of contraction, with **normal relaxation in between consecutive contractions**.
- **Larger doses** cause more powerful, tetanic, and frequent contractions and the resting muscle tone increases markedly.
- **Very large doses** cause a sustained contracture.

Their oxytocic effect is seen within 10–15 min of oral, 3–5 min of SC and 1–2 min of IV administration.

Both ergotamine and ergometrine are capable of stimulating the uterus during any phase of oestrous cycle or gestation. In general, the uterus at full term and immediately after delivery is highly sensitive.

Ergometrine has several advantages over ergotamine. It is:

- Effective orally and elicits a prompt and marked contractile response, even in small doses.
- Devoid of significant adrenergic blocking, vasoconstrictor and emetic activity.
- Less toxic.

Compared to oxytocin, ergometrine increases the tone of the cervix. Oxytocin decreases it. Further, the frequency of contractions is increased more with ergot alkaloids than with oxytocin.

Adverse reactions: Ergometrine and methylergometrine may produce nausea and vomiting but serious toxic effects are rare. If administered in higher doses can cause hypertension, seizures, headache and sometimes hypotension.*Their use during I and II stages of labour may, result in the death of the fetus in utero or rupture of the uterus.*

Preparations and dosage:

i. Ergometrine tablet. Dose: 0.2–0.4 mg. In PPH and post-abortion bleeding, doses can be doubled.
ii. Ergometrine maleate injection contains 0.5 mg/mL. Dose: 0.2–0.5 mg intramuscularly and 0.2–0.4 mg intravenously. Doses may be doubled/quadrupled if needed.
iii. Methylergometrine maleate tablet 0.125 mg. Dose: 0.125 mg t.i.d.
iv. Methylergometrine injection 0.2 mg/mL. Dose: 0.2 mg subcutaneously, intramuscularly or intravenously.

Indications:

- **Postpartum haemorrhage (PPH):** Ergometrine and methylergometrine are extremely useful in both prophylaxis and treatment of PPH. For prophylaxis, *they are administered after the expulsion of the placenta*, in the IM dose of 0.2–0.3 mg. If immediate action is desired, an IV dose of 0.2 mg is given. However, IV administration may result in dangerous hypertension.
- **Uterine involution:** Ergometrine, 0.2 mg orally t.i.d., is employed for 7 days after child birth to hasten the uterine involution, although its beneficial effect on the normal process of involution is not established. It is, however, useful in the same dose in cases of delayed involution where it hastens involution, prevents bleeding and checks the spread of infection.

TOCOLYTICS (Uterine relaxants) PH 1.41

Tocolytics are the drugs which inhibit myometrial contractions. Although they are uterine relaxants, not all uterine relaxants are effective tocolytics, e.g. ephedrine and atropine. Tocolytics are used to prevent spontaneous preterm birth (before completion of 37 weeks of gestation). The major goal in preventing preterm birth is to eliminate the risk of neonatal complications and death. Since the contracting uterus is the most commonly recognised mechanism, stopping the contractions by using the tocolytics constitutes the major therapeutic approach.

Tocolytics – Classification

I. **Calcium channel blockers** e.g. Nifedipine
II. **COX (cycloxygenase) inhibitors** e.g. Indomethacin
III. **Beta-2 adrenergic agonists** e.g. Ritodrine and Salbutamol
IV. **Nitric oxide (NO) donors** e.g. Nitroglycerine
V. **Oxytocin receptors antagonist** e.g. atosiban
VI. **Magnesium sulphate**

Before starting tocolytic therapy, accurate estimation of gestational age, including clinical and laboratory evaluation for the possible cause of preterm labour should be done.

Calcium channel blockers: Nifedipine (Chapter 29) may be administered sublingually/orally in the loading dose of 10 mg, and the dose repeated every 20 min for 3 doses. Maintenance dose of 10 mg may be given orally every 4–6 h. It is effective in reducing neonatal complications and is relatively safe. It can be used at any gestational age.

COX inhibitors: Human decidua, myometrium and fetal membranes express COX-1 enzyme. During labour, there is a dramatic increase in COX-2 in the decidua and the myometrium. **Indomethacin** (Chapter 11), given early, inhibits COX nonselectively and hence PG synthesis, and thus acts as a tocolytic. *It is avoided in more than 32 weeks of gestation to prevent in utero closure/narrowing of the ductus arteriorus.*

Beta-2 adrenergic agonists: Salbutamol, terbutaline and **ritodrine** (selective beta-2 agonists, Chapters 18, 27) as IV infusion have been used previously to delay preterm delivery in uncomplicated labour. They are contraindicated in pre-eclampsia. Although they delay preterm delivery for 24–72 h and reduce the immediate risk, a significant reduction in perinatal morbidity and mortality has not been convincingly demonstrated. Further, their adverse effect profile is less favourable than that of CCB.

Nitric oxide (NO) donor: Nitroglycerine intravenously (Chapter 29) can delay preterm labour for 48 h. Transdermal NTG can prolong gestation to 37 weeks.

Magnesium sulphate: Magnesium sulphate is used for neuroprotection of fetus in preterm labour and has been found to reduce the risk of cerebral palsy in surviving infants. However, it has not demonstrated pregnancy prolongation and clinically it showed no benefit as tocolytic over placebo.

Thus, there is no first line ideal tocolytic. Tocolytics may not always prevent preterm birth. However, these drugs offer certain benefits. A delay of 24–48 h in labour can be utilised (a) for administering a glucocorticoid (betamethasone, dexamethasone) to bring about maturation of the fetal lungs and thus decrease the occurrence of neonatal respiratory distress syndrome (Chapter 64) and (b) to transfer the patient to a centre where neonatal ICU is available. *Ideally, tocolytics should not be given for more than 48 h, and the treatment should be individualised.*

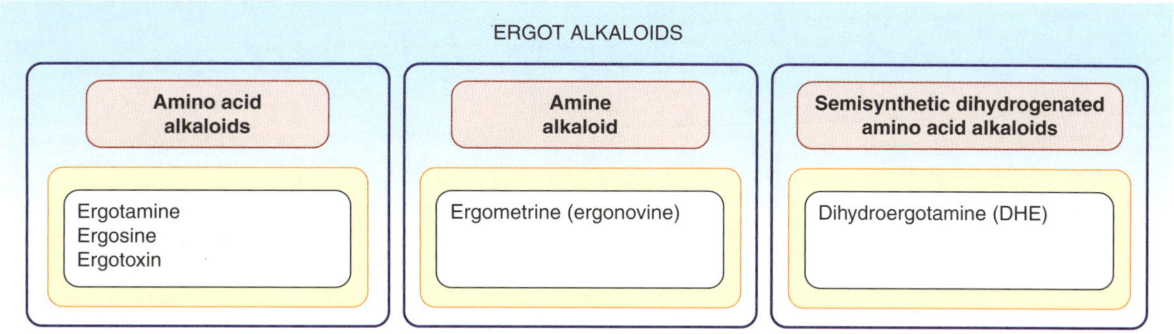

TOCOLYTICS

Calcium channel blockers
- Nifedipine

COX (cycloxygenase) inhibitors
- Indomethacin

Beta-2 adrenergic agonists
- Ritodrine
- Salbutamol

Nitric oxide (NO) donors
- Nitroglycerine

Oxytocin receptors antagonist
- atosiban

Magnesium sulphate

SECTION 12

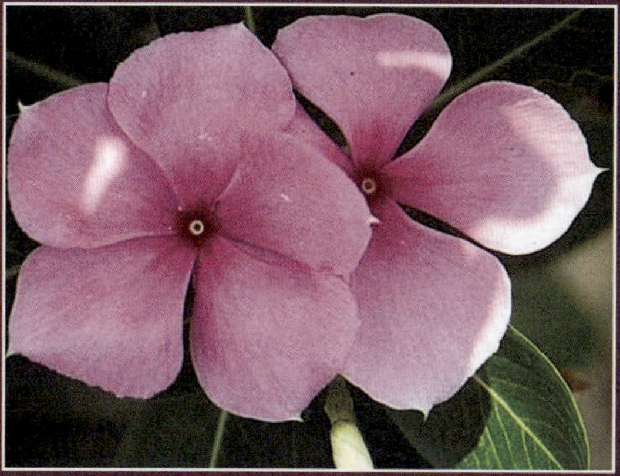

Vinca rosea

Chemotherapy

Section Outline

This section consists of the following chapters:

SECTION 12

Chemotherapy

CHAPTER 43

Sulphonamides, Trimethoprim, Cotrimoxazole, Nitrofurans and Quinolones

Learning Objectives

This chapter will enable reader:

1. To classify antimicrobial agents, depending on mechanism of action and antimicrobial spectrum.
2. To enumerate factors determining the efficacy of chemotherapeutic agents.
3. To explain concentration/time dependent killing and postantibiotic effect.
4. To explain mechanism of action of sulphonamides.
5. To explain reasons for reduced use of sulphonamides in clinical practice and state conditions wherein they have retained their place.
6. To state the mechanism of action, salient pharmacokinetic features, ADR and uses of cotrimoxazole.
7. To classify fluoroquinolones (FQ) based on their spectrum of antimicrobial activity and clinical use.
8. To state the mechanism of action, salient pharmacokinetic features, ADR and indications for FQ.

KEY TERMS

chemotherapy, p. 637
bactericidal, bacteriostatic definition, p. 638
concentration- or time-dependent antibiotic effect, p. 639
antimicrobial agents, targets, p. 639
cotrimoxazole, p. 643
nitrofurantoin, p. 645
sulfonamides, current indications, p. 642
fluoroquinolones, p. 645
fluoroquinolones, differences amongst generations, p. 647

The word **Chemotherapy** can be defined as the use of chemical compounds in the treatment of infectious diseases, so as to destroy offending organisms and parasites without damaging the host tissues. The evolution of chemotherapy can be traced through three distinct periods:

1. **A pre-Ehrlich era before 1891**
2. **The period of Paul Ehrlich**
3. **The period after 1935, highlighted by the discovery of sulphonamides and antibiotics**

In the long *pre-Ehrlich era*, many compounds were employed in therapeutics empirically, occasionally with beneficial and often with disastrous consequences. Thus, the usefulness of Cinchona bark in the treatment of malaria and of mercury in syphilis was known for many years.

Paul Ehrlich (1854–1915), an organic chemist, was struck by the fact that certain vital dyes like methylene blue specifically killed and stained certain bacterial cells and he reasoned that chemical substances might be produced that could unite with and destroy the parasitic agents of disease without in any way injuring the host cells. He demonstrated the efficacy of methylene blue in the treatment of human malaria. He also synthesised a series of arsenical compounds effective against spirochaetal infections.

A drug could exert either a curative or a toxic effect depending upon its affinity for the parasite or the host. Thus, a compound with a high affinity for the host tissue, an *organotropic* compound, could be toxic, whereas one with high affinity for parasites, a *parasitotropic* compound, might be curative. Based on this hypothesis, Ehrlich introduced arsephenamine, the first effective chemotherapeutic agent in man, in the treatment of syphilis.

Ehrlich is aptly called '**the Father of Modern Chemotherapy**' (Nobel Prize in 1908).

Gerhard Domagk, Fritz Mietsch and their colleagues in 1935 demonstrated that 'Prontosil', an azo dye with a sulphonamide side chain, inhibits the growth of Streptococci *in vivo*. Later Nitti, Bovet and Fuller proved that prontosil owed its therapeutic efficacy to its conversion into sulphanilamide. Since then several sulphonamides were synthesised. Domagk was awarded a Nobel Prize in 1939.

In 1928, Sir Alexander Fleming discovered penicillin, which inhibited the growth of a number of Gram-positive organisms. The work of Chain, Abraham and Florey in 1941 during the 2nd World War established penicillin as the first most potent anti-infective agent. In 1945, Fleming, Chain and Florey were awarded the Nobel Prize. The isolation of 6-aminopenicillanic acid nucleus of penicillin led to the development of various semisynthetic penicillins.

In 1944, after more than 10,000 microorganisms had been screened, Schatz, Bugie and Waksman reported the isolation of streptomycin from *Streptomyces griseus*. Selman Waksman also defined an **antibiotic** as '*a chemical substance produced by microorganisms having the property of inhibiting the growth of or destroying other microorganisms in high dilution*'. **Streptomycin,** unlike penicillin, was found to be **effective against Gram-negative organisms, and against *Mycobacterium tuberculosis*.**

Majority of antibiotics are obtained from fungi but some like bacitracin, colistin and polymyxin B are obtained from bacteria. Some are now synthesised, e.g. chloramphenicol, imipenem. The important factors in determining the efficacy of chemotherapeutic agents are outlined in Box 43.1.

Box 43.1 Factors Determining the Efficacy of Chemotherapeutic Agents

- Host defence
- Source of infection
- Tissue(s) affected
- Margin of safety
- Bacterial susceptibility/resistance to the agent being used

Of these, the **host defence plays an important part in the curative action of most of the specific remedies.** PH 1.42

Mechanism of action: *An antimicrobial agent may act by killing the organism* **(bactericidal)** *or by inhibiting its growth* **(bacteriostatic).** Bactericidal drugs, in general are most effective against rapidly multiplying bacteria. Often, a bacteriostatic drug in higher concentration may act as bactericidal.

The selective toxic action on the infecting organism is the key to beneficial actions of antibiotics. These drugs act at multiple targets in bacterial cell (Fig. 43.1):

- *The cell wall*
- *The cytoplasmic membrane*
- *The ribosomes*
- *The RNA molecules involved in transcription of genetic information*

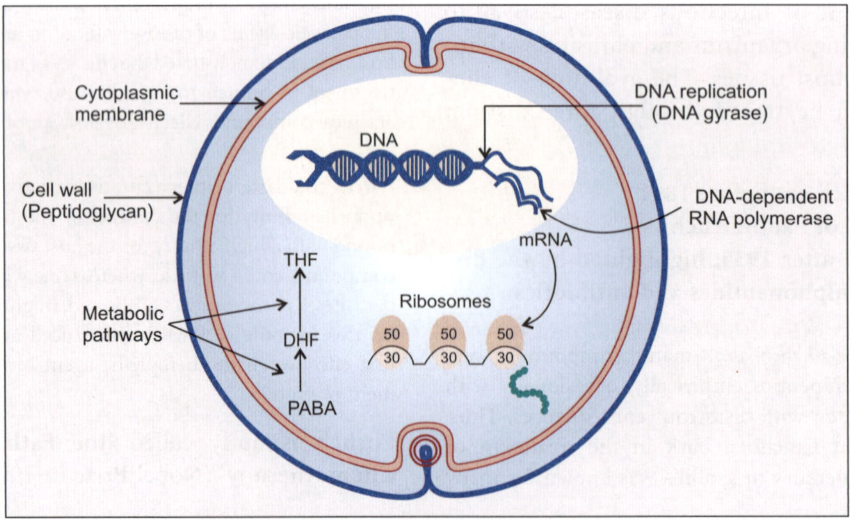

FIG. 43.1 Targets for antimicrobial agents.

- *Enzymes required for DNA synthesis/replication*
- *Metabolic pathways*

The cell wall of bacteria is a thick rigid envelope, mainly composed of sugar and peptides called **mucopeptide** or **murein**. It is much thicker in Gram-positive cells than in Gram-negative cells. Underneath the rigid cell wall is a cytoplasmic membrane which encloses the cytoplasm. This membrane has lipoprotein structural elements, which account for selective permeability to water, ions and nutrients. *Antimicrobials attacking this membrane may alter the permeability of the cell or may disorganise the lipoproteins leading to cell death.*

Inside the cytoplasm are ribosomes, spherical particles, which are concerned with protein synthesis. Ribosomes act as an assembly line where aminoacids are joined together into peptide chains and proteins. The process is directed by messenger RNA (mRNA), which carries the code for such synthesis from the nuclear DNA. mRNA attaches to ribosomes where the transcribed code is translated into appropriate protein synthesis. *Antimicrobials can bind to ribosomes and may interfere with the synthesis of peptide chains in bacteria or the transcription mechanisms.*

Mechanisms of action of various antimicrobials are summarised in Box 43.2.

Box 43.2 Mechanism of Action of Antimicrobial Drugs

- **Interference with cell wall synthesis:** Penicillins, cephalosporins, carbapenem, monobactam, bacitracin, vancomycin, ticloplanin and cycloserine
- **Damage to the cytoplasmic membrane:** Polymyxins, colistin, polyene antibiotics and detergents
- **Inhibition of protein synthesis and impairment of function of the ribosomes:** Aminoglcosides, tetracyclines, chloramphenicol, macrolides, linezolid, sodium fusidate, quinpristin-dalfopristin and lincomycin
- **Interference with transcription/translation of genetic information:** Quinolones, metronidazole, azoles and rifampicin
- **Antimetabolite action:** Sulphonamides, sulphones, PAS and trimethoprim
- **Inhibition of viral enzymes:** Protease inhibitors, acyclovir, zidovudine and nevirapine

The therapeutic efficacy of an antimicrobial agent depends not only on the sensitivity of the organism, but also on its concentration and duration at the site of infection. Thus, the antimicrobial effect could be '**concentration dependent**' or '**time dependent**'. In case of former, efficacy of the drug depends mainly upon the peak concentration achieved at the site of infection in relation to its minimum inhibitory concentration (MIC). With drugs like aminoglycosides or fluoroquinolones, the inhibitory effect of a single dose is prolonged and the postantibiotic effect (PAE) persists till next dose is administered. On the other hand, with beta lactam and macrolide antibiotics, whose actions are time dependent, the PAE is modest and hence for optimising its activity, it is necessary to maintain the drug concentration above MIC for a period between two doses.

Classification of Antimicrobial Agents

The organisms susceptible to the inhibitory or lethal effect of an antimicrobial agent constitute its 'spectrum'. Antimicrobials can be classified according to their mechanism of action (Box 43.2). Clinically, they are classified according to their spectra:

I. **Antimicrobials mainly effective against Gram-positive bacteria:**
   - **For systemic infections**, e.g. penicillins, macrolides (erythromycin), lincomycin, vancomycin, novobiocin and fucidin
   - **For topical use**, e.g. bacitracin

II. **Antimicrobials mainly effective against Gram-negative bacteria:**
   - **For systemic infections**, e.g. streptomycin, and other aminoglycosides
   - **For local use in the intestines**, e.g. neomycin

III. **Antimicrobials effective against both Gram-positive and Gram-negative bacteria:**
   - **For systemic infections**, e.g. ampicillin, amoxicillin, carbencillin, cephalosporins, rifamycins, imipenem
   - **For topical use**, e.g. neomycin, tyrothricin and framycetin

IV. **Antimicrobials effective against both Gram-positive and Gram-negative bacteria, rickettsiae and chlamydia (Broad spectrum)**, e.g. tetracyclines and chloramphenicol

V. **Antimicrobials effective against acid fast bacilli**, e.g. aminoglycosides (streptomycin), rifampicin, INH, fluoroquinolones

VI. **Antimicrobials effective against fungi**, e.g. nystatin, amphotericin B, griseofulvin
VII. **Antimicrobials effective against protozoa**, e.g. metronidazole, paromomycin, tetracyclines
VIII. **Antimicrobials effective against viruses**, e.g. acyclovir, ribavarin, zidovudine
IX. **Antimalignancy antibiotics**, e.g. actinomycin D, mitomycin and azaserine (Chapter 59)

SULPHONAMIDES

SULPHONAMIDES are the antimicrobial compounds containing a sulfonamido (SO_2NH_2) group (Fig. 43.2). This group is also present in other non-antibacterial compounds like the antidiabetic sulphnonyl ureas, diuretics like thiazides and their congeners, furosemide and acetazolamide.

Classification

I. **Those administered for the treatment of systemic infections**
- **Short acting:** Sulphadiazine, sulphadimidine (sulphamethazine), sulphacetamide, sulphafurazone (sulphisoxazole) and sulphamethizole
- **Intermediate acting:** Sulphamethoxazole
- **Long acting:** Sulphadoxine, sulphamethoxy pyridazine, sulphadimethoxine

  Their use as single agents in therapy is discouraged because they can cause bacterial resistance. However, they are used in combination with other drugs such as trimethoprim (see section, Cotrimoxazole).

II. **Those administered orally for the treatment of ulcerative colitis:** Sulphasalazine
III. **Those used topically:** Mafenide, Silver sulphadiazine, sulphacetamide

Mechanism of action: Sulphonamides, because of their structural similarity to PABA, compete with and substitute for it in the bacterial metabolism (Woods–Fields theory) (Fig. 43.2).

Folic acid derived from PABA is important in bacterial metabolism. Sulphonamides compete with PABA for the enzyme folic acid synthase which is involved in the conversion of PABA to folic acid (Fig. 43.3). Inhibition of this enzyme causes folic acid deficiency resulting in injury to the bacterial cell that can be easily phagocytosed.

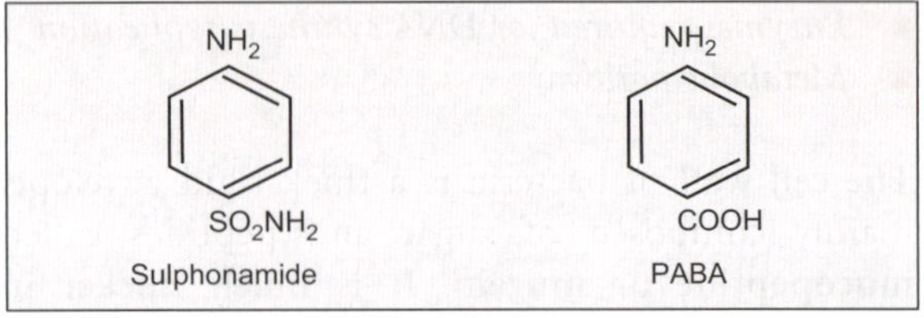

FIG. 43.2 Chemical structures of sulphonamide and PABA

Sulphonamides are ineffective in the presence of pus and tissue breakdown products which contain large amounts of PABA. Their bacteriostatic action can be countered by PABA; microorganisms resistant to sulphonamides often show enhanced PABA synthesis.

Sulphonamide resistance: A variety of microorganisms, such as Staphylococci, Streptococci, Pneumococci, Meningococci, Gonococci and *Escherichia coli* can acquire resistance to sulphonamides. Resistance in all enterobacteria is now common, and in *Shigella sonnei*, it is almost invariable. Resistance can be chromosomally mediated or transferred by 'R' factors (Chapter 49). Some of the resistant strains synthesise a folic acid synthase with a lowered affinity for sulphonamides, whereas some others overproduce PABA.

Pharmacological actions: They are effective against a variety of Gram-positive, Gram-negative organisms and chlamydia:

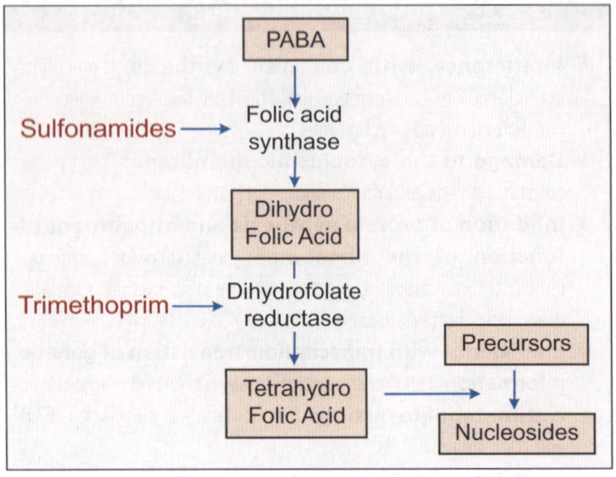

FIG. 43.3 Mode of action of sulphonamides – trimethoprim combination.

1. *Streptococci, Staphylococci (some strains), Gonococci, Pneumococci and Meningococci.*
2. *Clostridia, Bacillus anthracis.*
3. *Haemophilus influenzae, H. ducreyi, Vibrio cholerae, E. coli, Pastuerella pestis, Shigella, Donovania granulomatosis.*
4. *Nocardia and Actinomyces.*
5. *Chlamydia organisms causing lympho-granuloma venereum, psittacosis and trachoma.*
6. *In combination with drugs that inhibit folic acid synthesis, sulphonamides are effective against protozoal infections, e.g. malaria and in toxoplasmosis.*

They are mainly **bacteriostatic,** but occasionally, in very high concentrations, particularly in the urinary tract, they may be bactericidal.

Absorption, fate and excretion: Sulphonamides intended for systemic use are well absorbed; 70%–90% of the dose reaches the blood stream. The absorption of topical sulphonamides is variable, but sufficient to cause sensitisation and toxicity.

In the blood, these drugs are bound to albumin. Protein binding of sulphonamides is important for several reasons:

- **The bound sulphonamide** cannot pass into tissue fluids or cross the BBB which accounts for its less bacteriostatic activity.
- **Protein binding helps to prolong their action**
- **Protein binding results in low plasma levels of free sulphonamide as a result of which they are not so effective in the treatment of acute infections.**

The free form of sulphonamides is uniformly distributed throughout all the tissue fluids. These drugs readily cross the placental barrier and are also secreted in milk.

Sulphacetamide and sulphadiazine readily penetrate into the aqueous humour.

They are metabolised in the liver by acetylation. Individuals can be differentiated into two distinct groups:

- **Rapid acetylaters** acetylate 62%–90% of sulphadimidine
- **Slow acetylaters** acetylate only 40%–53% of sulphadimidine
  The acetylated form:
  a. Is devoid of antibacterial activity.
  b. Possesses the toxic potentialities of the parent drug.
  c. In addition, certain acetylated products are poorly soluble in acidic urine and may cause crystalluria and renal complications.

The urinary solubility of acetylated derivatives of sulphadiazine is increased in alkaline urine; the free and the acetylated sulphonamides are mainly eliminated in urine, mostly by glomerular filtration; the urinary concentration is higher than their plasma levels. Short-acting sulphonamides are concentrated by the kidney, and hence even their low plasma levels are adequate to produce therapeutic benefits in urinary tract infections (UTI). The excretion of the intermediate and the long-acting sulphonamides is slow.

Preparations and dosage:

i. **Short acting (5–6 h):**
   Sulphisoxazole (Sulphafurazole): Dose: Initial 1–2 g, then 0.5–1 g 12 hourly.
ii. **Intermediate acting (10–12 h):**
   Sulphamethoxazole: Used only as a component of cotrimoxozole.
iii. **Long acting (7–9 days):**
   a. Sulphadoxine (250, 500, 750 mg tablets) Plasma t½ 150–200 h. Used in combination to treat malaria.
   b. Sulphasalazine (Salazopyrine): It is available as 500 mg and 1g tablets. See text.
iv. **Topical:**
   a. Mafenide propionate: It is also available as 1% mafenide acetate cream.
   b. Silver sulphadiazine: Used as 1% cream.
   c. Sulphacetamide: Used as 6% eye ointment and 10%, 20%, 30% eye drops.

Adverse reactions: *Unfortunately, there is a tendency to exaggerate the ill effects of sulphonamides which were used extensively in the past and are still valuable.* However, the potential of these drugs to cause adverse effects should be remembered and their indiscriminate use avoided.

- **Allergy:** This can occur at any time during therapy. The commonest allergic symptoms are drug fever, skin rash and eosinophilia. Rarely, severe exfoliative dermatitis may develop. Serum sickness, characterised by fever, joint pains, urticaria, bronchospasm and leucopenia sometimes develops within the first two weeks of therapy. The **uncommon allergic manifestations** include cutaneous photosensitisation, a fatal necrotising arteritis resembling polyarteritis nodosa, acute toxic hepatitis and rarely fatal hepatic necrosis, toxic nephrosis, and acute haemolytic anaemia. A severe exudative type of erythema multiforme, associated with widespread lesions of the skin and mucous membranes, termed **Stevens Johnson syndrome,** has been reported. The syndrome is usually self-limiting but can occasionally be fatal.
  Cross-sensitivity among various sulphonamides and between sulphonamides and other drugs containing the sulfonamido (SO_2NH_2) group is known. Local application of sulphonamides to skin can sensitise the patient.
- **GI symptoms:** They commonly produce nausea and vomiting, but these are rarely troublesome. *Unlike the broad spectrum antibiotics, sulphonamides do not usually produce troublesome disturbances in the gut flora.*
- **Renal toxicity:** In the presence of acid urine, the acetylated form of the drug may be precipitated, mainly in the collecting tubules and the calyces and may precipitate renal colic. Crystalluria, albuminuria and haematuria can rarely occur. These can be minimised by
  a. Adequate fluid intake to maintain urine output of 1200 mL per day.
  b. Making the urine alkaline to increase the solubility of the conjugation products.
  c. Use of sulphonamides with acetylated metabolites soluble in acid urine, e.g. sulphisoxazole.
- **Haemopoietic toxicity:** This includes thrombocytopenia, granulocytopenia and rarely aplastic anaemia. Sulphonamides tend to oxidise haemoglobin to methaemoglobin. In patients with G6PD deficiency, they may cause haemolysis.
- **Bilirubin metabolism:** Sulphonamides compete with serum bilirubin for albumin binding sites. Administered during late pregnancy, they may displace bilirubin from albumin binding sites in the fetus. The free bilirubin, by crossing the BBB, which is permeable to bilirubin only in fetuses and infants, causes kernicterus. *They should not be given to neonates, and to pregnant women.*
- **Nervous system toxicity:** These include CNS disturbances like confusion, depression, ataxia, tinnitus, fatigue and acute psychotic episodes.
- **Miscellaneous:** Rarely they can cause goitre and hypothyroidism.

Drug interactions: See Table 43.1.

Indications: Sulphonamides are relatively cheap, broad spectrum chemotherapeutic agents. *Their use as single agents in therapeutics has diminished because of the development of resistance by a variety of organisms and availablity of safer bactericidal agents.* They are now used in combination with trimethoprim or pyrimethamine.

- **Burns:** Mafenide propionate and silver sulphadi-

Table 43.1 Interactions of Sulphonamides

Interfering Drug	Result
Sulphonylureas	ID displaced from plasma protein binding, with possible hypoglycaemia
Coumarin anicoagulants, methotrexate, phenytoin, thiopental	ID activity enhance
Phenylbutazone, salicylate, probenecid	S displaced from plasma binding, with enhancement of S activity
Methenemine	Certain S are precipitated in urine
PABA-containing local anaesthetics, e.g. procaine	Direct inhibition of S activity

ID, interfering drug; S, sulphonamide.

azine are used **topically** as prophylactic antimicrobials in burns to prevent colonisation by Gram-positive and Gram negative bacteria. Silver sulphadiazine, which is less toxic with wide antibacterial spectrum, is preferred.

- **Bacterial conjunctivitis:** Sodium salt of **sulphacetamide** has almost neutral pH and better tissue penetration and hence preferred. It is also used as an adjunctive drug in trachoma.
- **Urinary tract infections:** See Chapter 50.
- **Inflammatory bowel disease (IBD):** See Chapter 39.
- **Toxoplasmosis and malaria:** Sulphonamides in combination with pyrimethamine are used in the treatment of resistant malaria and toxoplasmosis (Chapters 54 and 56).
- **Acute bacillary dysentery:** Used as cotrimoxazole. See Chapter 47.
- **Chancroid:** See Chapter 51.
- ***Pneumocystis jiroveci* pneumonia:** See under the section Co-trimoxazole.
- **Nocardiosis:** Sulphadiazine in combination with ampicillin or ciprofloxacin is used for several months. Co-trimaxozole is also preferred.
- **Rheumatoid arthritis:** Sulphasalazine therapy has been found useful (Chapter 73).

Although sulphonamides are mainly bacteriostatic, they do not antagonise the bactericidal effects of penicillin and can be combined with it for treating susceptible infections with beneficial effects.

COTRIMOXAZOLE

TRIMETHOPRIM and COTRIMOXAZOLE: Trimethoprim, a pyrimidine derivative, is effective against many common pathogenic bacteria. Given alone, it is either bacteriostatic or bactericidal. In *in vitro* studies, it is

1. Effective against *Staph, aureus, Streptococci, C. diphtheria, E. coli, Salmonella, Shigella, H. influenzae, K. pneumoniae, Proteus* and *V. cholerae.*
2. *Somewhat less effective against N. gonorrhoeae, N. meningitidis, Cl. welchii* and *B. pertussis.*

Its action may be inhibited in necrotic wounds containing pus and other cellular debris, which contains thymine and thymidine.

Mechanism of action: Bacteria and protozoa synthesise folic acid from PABA, which is necessary for their growth. *Trimethoprim inhibits dihydrofolate reductase, which converts dihydrofolate (DHF) to tetrahydrofolate (THF), thus interfering with nucleic acid synthesis* (Fig. 43.3). The bacterial enzyme is far more susceptible to trimethopim than the enzyme in human cells. Any depressant effect of this drug on human folate metabolism can be countered by administering exogenous folate.

Since sulphonamides act by inhibiting the incorporation of PABA into dihydrofolate by organisms, *a combination of trimethoprim and sulphonamide acts sequentially in the same metabolic pathway in the synthesis of nucleotides* (Fig. 43.3). Hence, trimethoprim which is 20–100 times more potent than the sulphonamide is combined with sulphamethoxazole. *This combination, known as* **Cotrimoxazole**, *is synergistic and is bactericidal.* Bacterial resistance to this combination develops less frequently than when either drug is used alone.

Absorption, fate and excretion: Cotrimoxazole contains trimethoprim 80 mg with sulphamethoxazole 400 mg (1:5). Given orally it has been shown to give the optimum synergistic ratio in the plasma against common pathogens.

Trimethoprim is rapidly and almost completely absorbed from the intestines. Sulphamethoxazole has absorption and excretion characteristics very close to those of trimethoprim. The half-lives of trimethoprim and sulphamethoxazole are 16 and 10 h, respectively.

Trimethoprim is distributed more widely than sulphamethoxazole which essentially remains in the ECF. This explains the higher optimum (20:1) sulphonamide: trimethoprim ratio in the plasma than that (5:1) in the tablets. *Because of their differences in the distributions, different ratios may be observed in different tissues.* Adequate concentration is reached in CSF, bile, prostatic fluid and vaginal secretions.

Trimethoprim is a weak base and hence, its excretion increases markedly with acidification of urine, due to its ionisation. About 70% of the oral dose of trimethoprim is excreted in the urine within 24 h; about 80% of this is in an unchanged form.

Adverse reactions: These are due to the following:

1. **Sulphonamide component,** described earlier
2. **Trimethoprim:** The combination can cause nausea, vomiting, abdominal pain and diarrhoea. Allergic reactions are more common with the combination than with individual agents. Glossitis and stomatitis are relatively common. Trimethoprim may precipitate megaloblastic anaemia in persons with pre-existing folic acid deficiency. Serious toxicity (raised liver enzymes, hyperkalaemia and hyponatraemia) appears to be more common in patients with AIDS. Dosages must be reduced in presence of kidney damage.

   Development of bacterial resistance is its major drawback. *Its use in pregnant women should be avoided because of the teratogenicity of large doses of trimethoprim in animals.*

Preparations and dosage:

i. Cotrimoxazole contains trimethoprim 80 mg + sulphamethoxazole 400 mg; dose two tablets (three tablets in severe infection) twice daily for 10–14 days for the management of most infections. A double-strength formulation (trimethoprim 160 mg + sulphamethoxazole 800 mg) is also available. Paediatric tablets contain trimethoprim 20 mg + sulphamethoxazole 100 mg. Suspension of 40 mg trimethoprim + 200 mg sulphamethoxazole per 5 mL is also available. The drug can also be used intramuscularly or intravenously in the dose of 960 mg (equivalent to two tablets) every 12 h.
ii. Trimethoprim 100 mg, 200 mg tablets; 1–1½ tablets every 12 h. It is also available as 10mg/ml oral suspension.

Indications for cotrimoxazole:

- **Urinary tract infection** due to *E. coli* and *Proteus* group of organisms (Chapter 50).
- **Prostatitis:** It is the therapy of choice. Trimethoprim alone has also been used in treating UTI and prostatitis.
- **Respiratory tract infections such as bronchitis, sinusitis, whooping cough and otitis media.**
- **GI infections such as shigellosis.**
- **Typhoid fever** (Chapter 47).
- **STD such as gonorrhoea, chancroid, granuloma inguinale** (Chapter 51).
- **Serious infections such as meningitis and osteomyelitis** due to susceptible Gram-negative organisms.
- ***Pneumocystis jiroveci* pneumonia:** It is used in high doses (15–20 mg/kg/day of trimethoprim plus 75–100 mg/kg/day of sulphamethoxazole) and if required IV to treat *Pneumocystis jiroveci* infection in immunocompromised patients where it is the drug of choice. Low dose therapy has been used for prophylaxis of *P. jiroveci* in severely neutropenic patients.
- **Miscellaneous:** Plague, brucellosis and nocardiosis (Chapter 45).

Advantages of cotrimoxazole:

- It is a **broad spectrum** antibacterial drug.
- It is relatively **safe and well-tolerated.**
- It is highly **cost-effective** in many common infections in practice.

However, bacteria can develop resistance to this combination.

Indications for trimethoprim: The indications for trimethoprim given alone are similar to those of cotrimoxazole. Concentrations achieved in renal and prostatic tissues are higher and it causes less ADR than cotrimoxazole. However, due to development of bacterial resistance it is not used except in a few cases of UTI and prostatitis. It is given in the dose of 100–200 mg b.i.d.

NITROFURANS

Though usually bacteriostatic, the nitrofurans can be bactericidal in high concentrations.

Mechanism of action: They undergo enzymatic reduction, resulting in a highly reactive intermediate that damages the bacterial DNA. They also possess radiomimetic and mutagenic properties.

Pharmacological actions: Nitrofurans acts against a variety of Gram-positive and Gram-negative organisms including *Staphylococci, Streptococci, E. coli, Salmonella* and *Shigella*. Some compounds, particularly furazolidone, inhibit the growth of *Trichomonas vaginalis*, a protozoal organism, whereas nifuroxime is effective against *Candida albicans* and other fungi.

Bacterial resistance can develop and cross-resistance among the various compounds is also known.

Adverse reactions: These include abdominal discomfort, nausea, vomiting and rashes of various types. Rarely, haemolytic anaemia may develop in individuals with G6PD deficiency. Immunological reactions such as pulmonary infiltration and fibrosis, chronic active hepatitis, and SLE-like reaction have been rarely reported. The drug may precipitate antabuse-like reactions in alcoholics. Polyneuritis is an important adverse effect which particularly occurs in the presence of impaired renal function. These compounds are avoided during pregnancy and infancy.

Preparations: Nitrofurans are yellow, crystalline compounds, and need to be protected from light.

NITROFURANTOIN: It is rapidly and completely absorbed from the GI tract. *Food increases its bioavailability.* It does not achieve a bacteriostatic concentration in the plasma but approximately 40% of the drug is excreted unchanged by the kidney, **achieving a bactericidal concentration in the urine**. The drug is effective against many common urinary pathogens, including *E. coli* and *Aerobacter*, and is **used exclusively as a urinary antiseptic** (Chapter 50). Its activity decreases at alkaline pH. *Therefore, the urine should not be alkalinised during nitrofurantoin therapy. It does not appear in the urine in severe renal failure and in azotemic patients, and hence should be avoided.*

It is administered orally with food in the dose of 50–100 mg 6 hourly. The comparable dose in children is 50 mg up to 1 year, 75–100 mg from 1 to 5 years and 150–200 mg from 6 to 12 years in three or four divided doses. The drug should not be given for more than 2 weeks. The dose for long suppression of susceptible urinary tract pathogens is 100 mg once a day. *The drug colours the urine brown.*

FURAZOLIDONE: This compound has been employed effectively in the treatment of GI infections such as bacterial enteritis, bacillary dysentery and giardiasis. It is used along with nifuroxime, in the treatment of bacterial, trichomonal and monilial vaginitis. It is bactericidal. The dose is 100 mg q.i.d. orally for 5–7 days.

NIFUROXIME: The compound is effective against the fungus *Candida albicans*, a common vaginal pathogen, and is employed locally usually along with furazolidone.

NITROFURAZONE is available as 0.2% solution and ointment for topical application for the treatment of superficial wounds and skin infections. It is used systemically in trypanosomiasis (Chapter 56).

QUINOLONES

Quinolones, particularly the **fluoroquinolones** with their broad antimicrobial activity, are considered as a distinct therapeutic advance.

Mechanism of action: Quinolones inhibit enzymes:

1. DNA gyrase (topoisomerase II) and
2. DNA topoisomerase IV leading to arrest of DNA replication.

The activity of quinolones against:

a. Gram-negative bacteria is primarily due to their direct action on DNA gyrase,
b. Gram-positive bacteria is primarily due to their action on topoisomerase IV.

NALIDIXIC ACID: This 4-quinolone derivative is effective against certain Gram-negative bacteria, especially *E. coli*, shigella and many strains of Proteus. *It is relatively ineffective against Gram-positive organisms.* Bacteria can develop resistance fairly rapidly.

Adverse reactions include allergic reactions, nausea, vomiting and diarrhoea. The CNS manifestations include headache, malaise, drowsiness, myalgia and convulsions with overdosage. It may cause haemolytic anaemia and increase in intracranial pressure (pseudotumour cerebri) in young children. **Because of its toxicity and availability of fluoroquinolones, use of nalidixic acid has now diminished.**

FLUOROQUINOLONES: They are, chemically related to nalidixic acid and have fluorine in their chemical structure; (Fig. 43.4) hence termed as Fluoroquinolones. Fluorine increases their activity manifold and broadens the spectrum. They are:

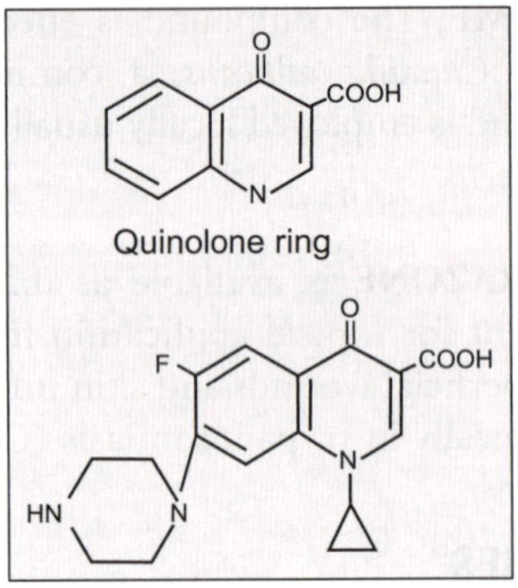

FIG. 43.4 **Fluoroquinolone.**

Mechanism of action – fluoroquinolones.

- **Highly effective orally**
- **Rapidly bactericidal with broad antibacterial spectrum**
- **Effective against bacteria resistant to beta-lactam and aminoglycoside antibiotics**
- **Relatively safe**

Antibacterial activity: They are highly active against many Gram-negative and some Gram-positive organisms, in a concentration-dependent manner.

- They possess excellent activity against the Enterobacteriaceae (*E. coli, Klebsiela and Proteus mirabalis*) including many organisms resistant to penicillins, cephalosporins and aminoglycosides.
- They are highly effective against Shigella species, Salmonellae (including those resistant to chloramphenicol), *H. ducrei. H. influenzae, B. catarrhalis* and Neisseria species including penicillinase producing gonococci.
- *P. aeruginosa* is inhibited in the urinary tract but not in other tissues/sites due to inadequate concentrations at the sites.
- Intracellular pathogens such as legionella, brucella, chlamydia and mycoplasma pneumoniae are inhibited to variable degrees.
- They are also effective against *M. tuberculosis* and *M. avium complex.* **They are not effective against anaerobes.**
- *Most of them are much less active than penicillin against Gram-positive organisms.* However, staphylococci including MRSAs are well inhibited. They have high activity against streptococci including *Strept. pneumoniae.*
- Bacteria, can develop resistance to fluoroquinolones, generally by genetic mutation and cross-resistance amongst various groups is common.
- The activity of fluoroquinolones diminishes in acidic urine.

Absorption, fate and excretion: The oral bioavailability of fluoroquinolones is excellent (Table 43.2); and the plasma levels after oral administration are similar to those after IV administration. *Hence, their IV administration is rarely indicated.* The simultaneous administration of compounds of aluminium, magnesium (antacids), zinc, iron and calcium reduce their bioavailability. *Food delays their absorption.* They are widely distributed in various tissues and are concentrated in urine, kidney, prostatic tissue and achieve therapeutic levels in lungs and bones. There is substantial excretion and reabsorption in the colon.

Metabolism of the fluoroquinolones varies considerably (Table 43.2). Thus:

1. Levofloxacin, ofloxacin and lomefloxacin are entirely eliminated by the kidneys, and a dose adjustment is a must with reduced renal function.
2. Pefloxacin, gemifloxacin, moxifloxacin and sparfloxacin are mostly eliminated by the liver.
3. Ciprofloxacin and norfloxacin are eliminated by both, liver and kidneys.

Quinolones such as ciprofloxacin are potent liver **enzyme inhibitors** and can reduce the metabolism of warfarin, theophylline and sulphonyluereas.

Due to differences in the pharmacokinetic properties, **norfloxacin** is effective in infections of the urinary and GI tracts; **its serum levels are relatively low and therefore, it is not recommended for systemic infections.**

Preparations and dosage: See Table 43.2.

Nadifloxacin is available as 1% cream for topical application to the skin. **Gatifloxacin** is available as 0.5% ophthalmic solution.

Adverse reactions: In general, these drugs are well-tolerated.

Table 43.2 Fluoroquinolone Generations: Pharmacokinetic Features, Doses and Indications

Name	Oral Bioavailability %	t½ (h)	Metabolism/ Clearance	Dose	Indications
Second generation: Class I					
Norfloxacin	30–40	3–4	R/H	400 mg b.i.d.	UTI, prostatitis
Lomefloxacin[a]	About 90	6–8	R	400 mg o.d., 400 mg IV	
Second generation: Class II					
Ciprofloxacin[a]	60–70	3.3–4.9	R/H	250 mg o.d., 250–750 mg b.i.d., 200–400 mg by IV infusion (over 30–60 min) b.i.d.	UTI, typhoid, gonorrhoea, gastroenteritis, skin, soft tissue, bone and joint infections, especially with Gram-negative organisms
Ofloxacin[a]	About 95	5–7	R	200–400 mg o.d.	
Pefloxacin[a]	About 90	8–13	H	400 mg b.i.d.; 400 mg by IV infusion (over 1 h) b.i.d.	
Third generation: Class III					
Sparfloxacin[b]	>90	21	H	200–400 mg in one or two divided doses per day	Like Class II. Preferred in community acquired pneumonia
Levofloxacin[a,b]	> 90	6 -8	R	250 mg/ 500 mg o.d. for 7–14 days	
Moxifloxacin[a,b]	90	12	R/H	400 mg o.d.	
Gemifloxacin[b]	70	7	H	320 mg o.d.	

Notes: Nalidixic acid and cinoxacin are first generation quinolones.
R, renal; H, hepatic.
[a]Also available for IV infusion.
[b]These are termed *respiratory fluoroquinolones* because of their excellent antipneumococcal activity.

- **GI toxicity:** Anorexia, nausea, vomiting, abdominal discomfort and diarrhoea are common. Trovafloxacin can cause severe hepatotoxicity.
- **CNS toxicity:** They cause mild headache, dizziness, nervousness and insomnia. Neuropsychiatric disturbances like confusion, delirium, memory impairment agitation, hallucinations and rarely seizures.
- **Tendon and cartilage damage:** Rupture of shoulder, hand and Achilles tendons have been reported with these drugs especially in the elderly, those on glucocorticoids and those with renal insufficiency. Treatment is discontinued if the patient experiences pain, inflammation and rupture of a tendon. Because of the cartilage damage in weight bearing joints of young animals, their use is restricted in pregnant and nursing mothers and in young children.
- **Cardiac toxicity:** Lomefloxacin, sparfloxacin and moxifloxacin can prolong QTc interval in patients on class III or class IA antiarrhythmic drugs (Chapter 28).
- **Hypoglycemia:** Fluoroquinolones can cause hypoglycemia, which may be fatal. Most of the incidences are seen with levofloxacin, followed by ciprofloxacin moxifloxacin and ofloxacin.
- **Miscellaneous:** Allergic reactions such as skin

Box 43.3 Conditions in which Fluoroquinolones Are Preferred IM 3.12

- ***Complicated urinary tract infections*** (Chapter 50), especially those caused by *P. aeruginosa* or other drug-resistant Gram-negative pathogens
- ***Bacterial gastroenteritis*** in patients ill enough to merit empiric therapy, especially salmonella gastroenteritis
- ***Typhoid fever*** and the faecal carrier state of *S. typhi* (for which they are the drugs of choice)
- ***Invasive otitis media*** by *P. aeruginosa*
- ***Gram-negative osteomyelitis and soft tissue infection***
- ***Respiratory infections*** including acute pneumonias, acute exacerbations in chronic bronchitis, mycoplasma infections
- ***Multidrug resistant tuberculosis***
- ***Atypical mycobacterial (M. avium complex) infection.***
- ***Leprosy***
- ***Anthrax*** prophylaxis and treatment
- ***Meningococcal carriers*** for eradication.
- ***Neutropenics*** for infection prophylaxis
- ***Empiric treatment of septicemia in emergency***
- ***Prophylaxis for close contacts of cases of meningococcal meningitis or septicaemia*** (Single dose ciprofloxacin 500 mg p.o.)

rash, arthralgia and photosensitivity have been reported. Rarely, leucopenia and renal damage with acute renal failure can occur.

Indications: Because of their pharmacokinetic properties (superior bioavailability, tissue distribution and penetration) broad spectrum, and bactericidal activity against most aerobic Gram-negative and many aerobic Gram-positive bacteria, fluoroquinolones are useful in treating a wide variety of infections, in many anatomical sites. Box 43.3 lists the conditions for which the fluoroquinolones are preferred.

Because of their complete GI absorption, they are routinely prescribed orally. However, they can be administered by IV infusion (Table 43.2) in serious conditions.

The later generation fluoroquinolones like high-dose **levofloxacin** and **moxifloxacin** are used to treat multidrug resistance tuberculosis (Chapter 52) and **ofloxacin** for treatment of leprosy (Chapter 53). The third generation of fluoroquinolones are recommended for atypical pneumonia (chlamydia, mycoplasma and legionella).

Though effective, fluoroquinolones should not be used for the routine treatment of uncomplicated UTI, mild-to-moderate GI infections, skin infections and other sundry infections, where an equally effective and cheaper drug such as cotrimoxazole is available. Their extensive misuse has already resulted into the development of drug resistance, thus rendering them ineffective in the treatment of serious conditions.

ANTIMICROBIAL AGENTS

Antimicrobials mainly effective against Gram-positive bacteria

For systemic infections

- Penicillins
- Macrolides (erythromycin)
- Lincomycin
- Vancomycin
- Novobiocin
- Fucidin

For topical use

- Bacitracin

Antimicrobials mainly effective against Gram-negative bacteria

For systemic infections

- Streptomycin
- Gentamicin
- Amikacin

For local use in the intestines

- Neomycin

Antimicrobials effective against both Gram-positive and Gram-negative bacteria

For systemic infections

- Ampicillin
- Amoxicillin
- Carbencillin
- Cephalosporins
- Rifamycins
- Imipenem

For topical use

- Neomycin
- Tyrothricin
- Framycetin

Antimicrobials effective against both Gram-positive and Gram-negative bacteria, rickettsiae and chlamydia (Broad spectrum)

- Tetracyclines
- Chloramphenicol

Antimicrobials effective against acid fast bacilli

- Aminoglycosides (Streptomycin, Amikacin, Capreomycin, Kanamycin)
- Rifampicin
- INH
- Fluoroquinolones (Levofloxacin, Moxifloxacin)

Antimicrobials effective against fungi

- Nystatin
- Amphotericin B
- Griseofulvin

Antimicrobials effective against protozoa

- Metronidazole
- Paromomycin
- Tetracyclines

Antimicrobials effective against viruses

- Acyclovir
- Ribavarin
- Zidovudine

Antimalignancy antibiotics

- Actinomycin D
- Mitomycin
- Azaserine

Bactericidal and bacteriostatic drugs

Bactericidal

- Penicillin
- Aminoglycosides
- Rifampicin
- Cephalosporins
- Metronidazole
- Cotrimoxazole
- Fluoroquinolones

Bacteriostatic

- Sulphonamides
- Nitrofurans
- Erythromycin
- Tetracyclines
- Chloramphenicol
- Lincomycin
- Trimethoprim

SULPHONAMIDES

Those employed for the treatment of systemic infections

Short acting
- Sulphadiazine
- Sulphadimidine
- Sulphacetamide
- Sulphafurazone
- Sulphamethizole

Intermediate acting
- Sulphamethoxazole

Long acting
- Sulphadoxine
- Sulphamethoxy pyridazine
- Sulphadimethoxine

Those employed orally for the treatment of ulcerative colitis

- Sulphasalazine

Those used topically

- Mafenide
- Silver sulfadiazine
- Sulphacetamide

FLUOROQUINOLONES

Second generation: Class I
- Norfloxacin
- Lomefloxacin

Second generation: Class II
- Ciprofloxacin
- Ofloxacin
- Pefloxacin

Third generation: Class III
- Sparfloxacin
- Levofloxacin
- Moxifloxacin
- Gemifloxacin

CHAPTER 44

Penicillins and Other Antibiotics Effective Mainly against Gram-Positive Organisms

Learning Objectives

This chapter will enable reader:

1. To enlist different classes of beta-lactam antibiotics.
2. To explain the mechanism of action of penicillin and different mechanisms by which bacteria acquire resistance to penicillin.
3. To state the antibacterial spectrum, salient pharmacokinetic features, ADR and indications for penicillin G and its repository preparations.
4. To classify semisynthetic penicillins according to their spectrum of antimicrobial activity and compare and contrast them with respect to degradation by gastric acid, susceptibility to beta-lactamase, ADR and indications.
5. To enlist beta-lactamase inhibitors and explain the rationale of combining them with semisynthetic penicillins.
6. To explain the mechanism of action, salient pharmacokinetic features, ADR and indications of macrolides, lincosamide antibiotics, cyclic lipopeptides, streptogramins and oxazolidinones.

KEY TERMS

beta-lactam antibiotics, p. 651
benzylpenicillin, p. 652
allergy and anaphylaxis, p. 653
ampicillin, p. 658
amoxicillin, p. 659
extended spectrum penicillins, p. 659
beta-lactamase inhibitors, p. 660
macrolides, p. 661
clindamycin, p. 663
vancomycin, p. 664
quinupristin/dalfopristin, p. 666
linezolid, p. 666
pleuromutilins, p. 666
bacterial endocarditis, pharmacotherapy, p. 667

PENICILLIN, the most important of the antibiotics, was first extracted from the mould *Penicillium notatum*. Subsequently, a mutant of a related mould, *P. chrysogenum*, was found to give the highest yield of penicillin and is employed for its commercial production.

Penicillins belong to a group of antibiotics called **beta-lactam** antibiotics; the other members include **cephalosporins, cephamycins, monobactams** and **carbapenems.** Its basic structure consists of a thiazolidine ring fused with a **beta-lactam ring** which is essential for antibacterial activity. The two rings constitute the fundamental nucleus of all the penicillins, namely, 6-aminopenicillanic acid (6-APA) (Fig. 44.1). Both the 6-APA nucleus and the side chain are essential for the antibacterial activity. In addition, the side chain determines the stability of the penicillin against degradation by gastric acid and by the enzyme **beta-lactamase (penicillinase)** produced by certain microorganisms such as *Staphylococcusaureus, Pseudomonas, Enterobacter* and some strains of *H. influenzae* and *N. gonorrhoea.*

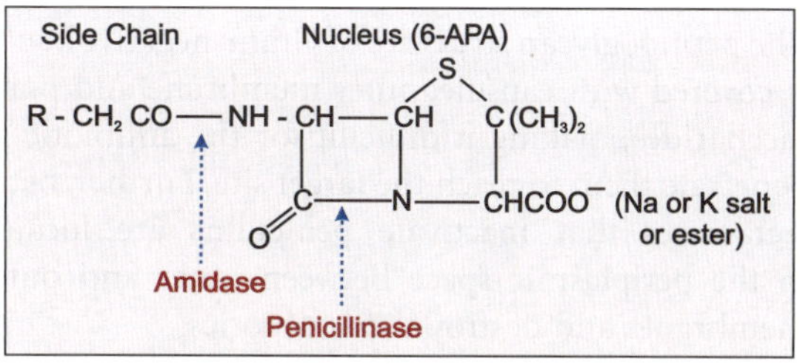

FIG. 44.1 Basic structure of penicillins

Mechanism of action: The action of penicillins requires the presence of a cell wall that contains peptidoglycans. (a) **Peptidoglycan** is a major structural component of the bacterial cell wall that is cross-linked into a net like structure that surrounds the bacterial cell. It provides strength and rigidity to it and protects the cell from osmotic rupture. (b) **Transpeptidase**, involved in crosslinking and other enzymes located on the cell membrane are called Penicillin Binding Proteins **(PBP)**. These enzymes act as binding sites for beta-lactams. (c) Inactivation of transpeptidase inhibits the peptidoglycan biosynthesis. This weakens the bacterial cell wall and makes the organisms vulnerable to rupture. (d) As cell wall synthesis occurs during the growth phase, the antibiotic is most effective against actively multiplying organisms.

Mechanism of action – lactams.

In addition, penicillins block the effects of cell membrane associated holin-like proteins which are responsible for maintaining the membrane potential.

Penicillins are bactericidal. The effect continues for a period of 3–8 h after withdrawing penicillin G and a bacteriological cure is assured if adequate plasma penicillin levels are maintained for 6 h per day. The best effect occurs at a concentration 5–20 times greater than MIC.

Bacterial resistance: Bacterial resistance to penicillin can be:

- **Natural** or
- **Acquired**

The peptidoglycan structure of Gram-negative bacilli is covered with capsule, outer membrane and polysaccharides, making it difficult for the antibiotic to penetrate them to reach the target site. Further, beta-lactamases that inactivate penicillins are located in the periplasmic space between inner and outer membranes and destroy the antibiotics.

Fortunately, bacteria do not acquire resistance to penicillin easily and sensitivity of many of the susceptible pathogens has so far remained unchanged. The resistance to penicillin develops stepwise. Staphylococci *resistant to penicillin are common*. *Streptococcus viridans* also develops resistance but to a lesser extent. Partially resistant strains of gonococci, meningococci and pneumococci are also encountered.

The important mechanism of bacterial resistance to the beta-lactams is bacterial production of beta-lactamases, that hydrolyse the beta-lactam ring and render the drug inactive. Microorganisms such as staphylococci, *E. coli, M. tuberculosis, B. anthracis* and *A. aerogenes* produce beta-lactamases (penicillinases). Presence of beta-lactamase elaborating bacteria in a mixed infection may cause rapid destruction of penicillin with a consequent reduction in its therapeutic efficacy. *Thus, penicillin may not be effective in the treatment of Strep. pyogenes pharyngitis if beta-lactamase elaborating staphylococci are also present in the throat.* Some staphylococci that do not produce beta-lactamase may also develop resistance to penicillin *in vitro* due to mutation which alter the PBPs.

BENZYLPENICILLIN: Benzylpenicillin is available in the form of its water soluble sodium and potassium salts. One milligram of sodium salt is equivalent to 1667 units of penicillin.

Antibacterial activity: It is one of the most potent antimicrobial agents and inhibits the bacterial growth of susceptible organisms *in vitro* in a concentration as low as 1 in 50 million.

- **It is effective mainly against Gram-positive cocci and bacilli and some Gram-negative cocci.** Thus, majority of streptococci with the exception of D strains (enterococci) are highly susceptible. Staphylococci, gonococci, pneumococci and meningococci have acquired resistance on a large scale. *Bacillus anthracis, Corynebacterium diphtheriae* and most anaerobic microorganisms, including the *Clostridium* species, are highly sensitive;
- Among the **spirochaetes, *Treponema pallidum*** is extremely sensitive to penicillin while leptospira infection responds moderately. Although penicillin is effective in actinomycosis, it is not useful against fungi.

Absorption, fate and excretion: Given orally, benzylpenicillin is largely inactivated by the gastric acid and by the intestinal bacterial flora. It is rapidly absorbed after SC or IM administration. Peak plasma level is reached within 15 to 30 minutes and the drug disappears from the plasma within 3 to 6 hours. Plasma protein binding is 60%.

Penicillin is widely distributed in the body with very high concentrations detected in the kidneys, but its concentrations in ocular, pericardial, pleural and peritoneal fluids is low. However, in the presence of inflammation, its concentration in these fluids is higher. *The drug does not readily cross the BBB, but therapeutically adequate CSF concentration is achieved in the presence of meningeal inflammation.* It crosses the placental barrier.

Nearly 30% of a single parenteral dose is metabolised. *The major portion is eliminated by the kidneys* by tubular secretion and only 10 to 15% by glomerular filtration. *The t½ is about 30 minutes. It is important to note that doubling the dose does not double the duration of effect, and that for continuous effect, large and frequent doses are essential.*

Its rapid urinary elimination necessitates 4-6 hourly parenteral administration. Repository preparations are relatively insoluble and release benzylpenicillin slowly when injected. They thus produce relatively low but prolonged plasma concentration. These agents, however, are not useful for treating severe infections where an immediate, high plasma concentration of benzylpenicillin is desirable. Neonates and infants in whom renal function is not adequately developed and individuals with renal insufficiency show prolonged and higher plasma levels and require 12 hourly administration.

Preparations and dosage:

i. Benzylpenicillin (Penicillin G) (sodium and potassium salts) injection 4,00,000; 5,00,000 and 10,00,000 units per millilitre.

The repository preparations:

i. **Procaine benzylpenicillin** powder to be suspended in distilled water, prior to injection. Dose: 6,00,000 to 12,00,000 units IM daily. After a single dose, the peak plasma level is reached within 1 to 3 hours. The drug remains in blood for 8 to 12 hours, and in some patients for 24 hours.
ii. **Fortified benzylpenicillin** is a mixture of 3,00,000 units of procaine benzylpenicillin and 1,00,000 units of benzylpenicillin per millilitre. It achieves a quick and high serum penicillin concentration on IM injection which persists for 12 to 24 hours.
iii. **Benzathine penicillin,** a salt of benzylpenicillin, has a very poor water solubility and is administered IM in the dose of 6,00,000 to 24,00,000 units. With the dose of 6,00,000 units, blood levels persist for 10 days and the drug is detected in the plasma for 2 weeks. A dose of 1.2 million units produces detectable blood levels for 3 weeks.

Benzathine penicillin should be used only in conditions where the infecting microorganism is exquisitely sensitive to low concentrations of penicillin *viz.*

a. for treatment and prophylaxis of pharyngitis due to group A beta-hemolytic streptococci;
b. for treatment of pyoderma due to group A beta-hemolytic streptococci; and
c. for treatment of syphilis not involving the CNS.

Probenecid, a uricosuric agent, competes with penicillin for tubular transport and delays its excretion (Chapter 73). Administered orally in the dose of 2 g per day, in divided doses, along with penicillin, it raises its plasma level twofold to fourfold which is maintained for approximately twice as long as without probenecid. Hence it is sometimes used for this purpose. It is not recommended in children below two years.

Adverse reactions: Penicillin is a remarkably safe drug. The only important reaction to be feared in practice is anaphylaxis.

- **Allergy and anaphylaxis:** The risk of allergic reactions is 5 to 10% with benzathine penicillin, 2 to 5% with procaine penicillin and $<$ 3% following benzylpenicillin. As a generalisation, the incidence of these reactions is considerably greater when benzylpenicillin is used either topically or in an aerosol form, and is least when it is taken orally. However, fatalities have occurred following ingestion.

Some individuals are so sensitive that the mere handling of penicillin tablet or even a skin test dose may precipitate immediate severe reaction. Further, severe reactions have been recorded following first dose of penicillin, in persons who had never received the drug before. This is probably because many of us are exposed and slightly sensitised to various common air-borne moulds that readily grow on and elaborate penicillin and penicillin-like substances in foodstuffs such as bread, fruit, and oil, with or without decay.

Penicilloic acid, *a metabolite of penicillin, either alone or linked to a plasma protein is probably responsible for allergic reactions. A person known to be allergic to one penicillin will also be allergic to other penicillins.* Partial cross allergy is seen between penicillin and cephalosporins. Carbapenams and the monobactam, however, carry much less risk.

The important allergic reactions are:

- **Skin rashes** of various types associated with pruritus are the most common reactions.
- **A serum sickness like syndrome,** characterised by rash, fever, eosinophilia lymphadenopathy, angioneurotic edema, bronchospasm and arthralgia.
- **Renal disturbances** like hematuria and albuminuria.
- **Hemopoietic disturbances** like hemolytic anemia and neutropenia, which occur very rarely.
- **Anaphylaxis** is the most serious reaction but occurs in fewer than 0.01% of patients. The symptoms of anaphylaxis usually begin within a few minutes after penicillin administration. It is characterised by an acute cardiovascular collapse, bronchospasm, and angioedema, particularly edema of the larynx (see Chapters 2 and 23). *Antihistaminics do not decrease the incidence of penicillin anaphylaxis;* however, they are valuable in controlling minor allergic reactions.

Tests for detection of penicillin allergy: A reliable method of detecting penicillin allergyis not available. History of allergy or even a positive skin test is not in itself a complete evidence of allergy, nor does a negative history or negative skin test indicate the safety of penicillin administration.

Skin tests: One method of skin testing is to scratch the skin through a drop of solution containing 10,000 units of benzylpenicillin per ml. If a central wheal due to local edema (not diffuse erythema) occurs after 15 minutes, it is considered a positive reaction. *A positive skin reaction is a relatively reliable indicator of potentially serious penicillin allergy.* Rarely even the small amount of penicillin used for the test may itself rarely produce severe reaction.

Another skin test involves the administration of 0.05 ml of **penicilloyl-polylysine intradermally** and subsequent observation of the inflammatory response. This test is often combined with benzylpenicillin scratch test. Combination of these two tests will predict virtually all reactions to all the types of penicillin.

Even in patients in whom the skin test is negative, most physicians administer a test dose of 1000–2000 units of penicillin andproceed to higher doses if no reaction occurs.

Except for above-mentioned allergic reactions, benzylpenicillin, even in large doses, is almost devoid of toxic manifestations provided kidney function is normal. The other rare and minor ADR are as follows:

- **Jarisch-Herxheimer reaction** is a rare reaction reported in patients with syphilis treated with penicillin (Chapter 51).
- **Superinfection:** Long term use of penicillin may suppress the sensitive coccal members of the bacterial flora, and encourage superinfection in the form of bacteremia, urinary infection or pneumonia owing to overgrowth of such resistant microorganisms as *Klebsiella, Aerobacter, Pseudomonas* and *Candida.*
  Stomatitis, glossitis and a black hairy tongue are known to develop after local use of penicillin troches and lozenges.
- **Minor reactions:** Prolonged administration of IV benzylpenicillin may lead to thrombophlebitis; accidental IV administration of procaine benzylpenicillin can cause anxiety, mental disturbances, paraesthesiae and seizures, due to procaine.
- **Acute non-allergic reactions:** Intramuscular aqueous procaine penicillin sometimes produces acute non-allergic reaction, which could be serious. It is characterised by transient palpitation, hypertension, twitchings, auditory and visual disturbances, headache, and dizziness. In addition, psychiatric symptoms like fear of imminent death and acute depersonalisation may occur.
- **Neurotoxicity:** When given by intrathecal route, the drug may cause arachnoiditis, *convulsions and encephalopathy*. Large doses may also cause neurotoxicity.

Indications

The various penicillin regimens can be summarised for practical purposes as shown in Box 44.1.

Box 44.1 Penicillin Regimens

- ***Regimen 1 (oral):*** Penicillin V 250–500 mg or benzylpenicillin 400,000–800,000 units orally every six hours.
- ***Regimen 2 (IM small dose, repository penicillin):*** Fortified benzyl penicillin (procaine benzylpenicillin 600,000 units + benzylpenicillin 200,000 units) IM once a day.
- ***Regimen 3 (IM large dose benzyl penicillin):*** Benzylpenicillin 1–2 million units IM every 4–6 hours (4–12 million units per day).
- ***Regimen 4 (IV large dose benzyl- penicillin):*** Benzylpenicillin 4 million units IV every 4 hours (24 million units per day).

Regimen 1 or 2 is used in mild infection such as streptococcal pharyngitis. Regimen 3 or 4 are needed in severe infections such as severe pneumonia, empyema, meningitis and bacterial endocarditis. The choice of the regimen in each individual infection is indicated in Table 44.1.

- **Pneumococcal infections:** *Benzylpenicillin continues to be the drug of choice for sensitive strains of S. pneumoniae.*
- **Streptococcal infections:** *Infections due to S. pyogenes* that respond satisfactorily to penicillin, are listed in Table 44.1. Penicillin G is also used in the treatment and prophylaxis of Streptococcal subacute bacterial endocarditis (Refer section on Pharmacotherapy of subacute bacterial endocarditis). Acute rheumatic fever is an autoimmune response to infection with Gp A Streptococci (GAS), i.e. *S. pyogenes*. Role of penicillin in its pharmacotherapy is described in the present section below under Penicillin prophylaxis.
- **Staphylococcal infections:** A major problem is the development of penicillin resistant staphylococci which limits its utility in staphyloccocal infections. Box 44.2 lists the drugs currently recommended in community-acquired staphylococcal infections. For serious systemic staphylococcal infections, see Tables 44.1 and 49.2.
- **Meningococcal meningitis:** See Chapter 46.

Table 44.1 Choice of Penicillin Regimen in the Common Infections — IM 3.12, IM 3.13

Organisms	Regimens 1 and 2	Regimens 3 and 4
S. pneumoniae	Pneumonia (mild-moderate), until afebrile for 4 days	Empyema, pericarditis, osteomyelitis, arthritis* (2–4 weeks), meningitis (7–10 days)
S. pyogenes, S. viridans, Group A beta-hemolytic streptococci	Pharyngitis**, erysipelas, pyoderma (7–10 days), otitis media (2 weeks)	Mastoiditis (2 weeks) osteomyelitis, arthritis* (2–4 weeks), meningitis (7–10 days), SBE (4–6 weks)
Type D streptococci (enterococci)	—	Meningitis (14–21 days with gentamicin)
S. aureus	—	—
N. gonorrhoeae	Gonorrhoea (uncomplicated: single injection; complicated: 14 days)	—
Treponema pallidum	Syphilis (single dose or weekly for 3 weeks)	—
Actinomyces israeli	Actinomycosis (2 weeks with sulfadiazine 4 g)	—
Nocardia brasilliensis	Nocardiasis	—
Corynebactrium diphtheriae	Diphtheria (10–12 days)	—
Clostridium tetani	Tetanus (10–12 days)	—
Clostridium species		Gas gangrene (1–2 weeks)
Fusospirochetal infection	Gingivostomatitis (trench fever) and pharyngitis (Vincent's angina)	Lung abscess
Pasturella multocida	—	2–4 weeks
Listeria monocytogenes	—	Listeriasis (2 weeks)
Streptobacillus moniliformis muris and Spirillium minus	—	Rat-bite fever (7–10 days)

SBE = Subacute bacterial endocarditis. * Intracavitary local injection
** = Single injection of 1.2 megaunits, benzathine penicillin

Box 44.2 Drugs for Community-Acquired Staphylococcal Infections

- Antistaphylococcal penicillins
- Cephalosporins
- Co-trimoxazole
- Minocycline
- Gentamicin; and
- Fluoroquinolones

Penicillin is the drug of choice in meningitis caused by meningococci sensitive to penicillin (Table 46.2). But, penicillin and its derivatives do not effectively eradicate this organism from the nasopharynx with short courses, and hence they are not recommended for prophylaxis in close contacts of patients with meningococcal infections.

- **Sexually transmitted diseases (STD):** Penicillin is the drug of choice in the treatment of syphilis (Chapter 51).
- **Actinomycosis:** Penicillin is the agent of choice in this condition (Table 44.1).
- **Anthrax:** Benzylpenicillin is useful for sensitive strains. In case of severe infection, IV doses are given with clindamycin ± rifampicin. Ciprofloxacin 500 mg bid or doxycycline, 100 mg bid for 60 days is currently preferred.
- **Diphtheria, tetanus and gas gangrene:** (Table 44.1) Diphtheria and tetanus in addition to penicillin, require the administration of the specific antiserum (Chapter 71). Administration of penicillin helps to eliminate the bacilli from the lesions and terminate the carrier state.
- **Miscellaneous infections:** These are shown in Table 44.1.
- **Penicillin prophylaxis:** IM 1.27

Rheumatic fever: The diagnosis of acute rheumatic fever is entirely clinical without any laboratory support and no treatment has been shown to reduce prognosis of rheumatic disease. Antibiotics neither modify its course of rheumatic fever nor influence the subsequent development of carditis. Yet, it is customary to give antibiotics in rheumatic fever. Box 44.3 illustrates **treatment and prevention** of acute rheumatic fever and its associated manifestations. The role of antibiotics mentioned under the treatment is essentially prophylactic as given below:

Box 44.3 Pharmacotherapy of Acute Rheumatic Fever IM 4.22, IM 1.27

Eradication of GAS Infection

Benzathine penicillin 1.2 million units IM single dose

Or

Phenoxymethly penicillin 500 mg t.i.d orally for 10 days

Or

Amoxicillin 35–40 mg/kg/day orally for 10 days

Or

Cephalexin 15–20 mg/kg twice a day orally for 10 days

Or

Azithromycin 500 mg orally once daily for 5 days

Or

Erythromycin 40 mg/kg/day orally in divided doses for 10 days

Symptomatic and Supportive Care

- *Arthralgia and arthritis* (during acute episode)
  - Aspirin 80–100 mg/kg/day in 3–4 divided doses for 1–4 weeks depending on response

    Or

    Naproxen 20 mg/kg/day in two divided doses
  - Steroid therapy (it induces rapid fall in ESR but causes rebound increase on stopping)
- *Carditis with mitral regurgitation* (during acute episode)
  - ACEI (Chapter 30)
  - Diuretics (furosemide 0.5–2 mg/kg/day)
    - Venodilators (sodium nitroprusside), if pulmonary edema
- *Chorea* (weeks and months after GAS infection)
  - Mild isolated: no treatment
  - if treatment in needed,
  - Antiepileptics: Carbamazepine (7–20 mg/kg/day)/sodium valproate (15 mg/kg/day) is the most preferable therapy

    Or
  - Dopamine antagonists: Haloperidol (0.25–0.5 mg/kg/day)/chlorpromazine (EPR is the limiting factor)

    Or
  - Prednisolone 2 mg/kg/day/for 4 weeks (steroidal ADR are the limiting factors)

Prevention of Progression to Rheumatic Heart Disease

- Anti-inflammatory drugs like steroids/aspirin (no conclusive data to support)

Prevention of Recurrent GAS Infection

- Secondary prophylaxis with antibiotics (see Text), improve living conditions

(i) To eradicate rheumatogenic group A streptococci (GAS) **in the tonsils and the pharynx**, in order to prevent the spread of the organism to close contacts. **Benzathine penicillin is preferred as it is**

cost-effective. A single injection is needed with no issues of compliance as seen with oral antibiotics. It is also used for secondary prophylaxis. In patients known to have minor hypersensitivity, cephalosporins are used. Those having history of allergy/anaphylaxis wih penicillins, macrolides are the choice.

(ii) To prevent recurrence of rheumatic fever (**secondary prophylaxis**). **Benzathine penicillin** IM 1.2 million units every 3 weeks provides the best protection. Oral penicillin V may also be used in the dose of 125 mg 12 hourly in cooperative patients. In patients allergic to penicillin, **erythromycin** 250 mg twice daily may be used. The prophylactic therapy is continued for 10 years in children without evidence of carditis. In those who develop carditis, it is continued till the age of 40 years. *In patients with valvular disease, it should preferably be life long.*

II. **Streptococcal infections:** Oral penicillin or a single injection of benzathine penicillin offers satisfactory protection from pharyngeal infections due to *S. pyogenes* during outbreaks of streptococcal disease in close populations, e.g. institutionalised children.

III. **Bacterial endocarditis:** Refer section on pharmacotherapy of subacute bacterial endocarditis.

IV. **Syphilis:** Chapter 51.

V. **Recurrent lymphangitis:** Benzathine benzylpenicillin, 600,000 units, administered IM once a month is effective in preventing recurrent lymphangitis and consequent lymphedema in patients who have congenital abnormalities of the lymphatic system and in filariasis. Other drug used is doxycycline.

SEMISYNTHETIC PENICILLINS

The major drawbacks of benzylpenicillin are:

- **Inactivation by the gastric acid.**
- **Short duration of action.**
- **Poor penetration into the CSF.**
- **Narrow spectrum of activity.**
- **Development of resistant organisms, especially staphylococci;** and
- **Possibility of anaphylaxis.**

Attempts, therefore, have been made to synthesise penicillins free from such drawbacks (Box 44.4) by altering composition of side chain attached to 6-APA nucleus.

Box 44.4 Classification of Penicillins

I. **Penicillin G and its esters**
Penicillin G (Benzyl penicillin)
Procaine penicillin G
Benzathine penicillin G

II. **Acid-resistant penicillins:**
Phenoxymethlypenicillin (penicillin V)*

III. **Penicillinase-resistant penicillins****
a. ***Acid labile:*** Methicillin, Nafcillin
Cloxacillin, Dicloxacillin
b. ***Acid resistant:*** Flucloxacillin

IV. **Penicillins effective against Gram-positive and some Gram-negative organisms:**
Ampicillin, Amoxicillin
Talampicillin, Pivampicillin

V. **Extended spectrum penicillins:**
(1) ***Antipseudomonal penicillins***
a. Carboxypenicillins
Carbenicillin, Ticarcillin
b. Ureidopenicillins
Piperacillin, Mezlocillin, Azlocillin
(2) ***Amidinopenicillins***
Mecillinam, Pivmecillinam

VI. **Penicillins with beta-lactamase inhibitors:**
Amoxicillin-clavulanic acid
Ticarcillin-clavulanic acid

Groups other than III are not resistant to penicillinase (beta-lactamase) and not effective against *S. aureus*.
*Not available
**Antistaphylococcal penicillins, not effective against MRSA.

All synthetic penicillins, however, are capable of producing allergic reactions similar to those caused by penicillin G.

I. **Acid resistant penicillins:** These penicillins are relatively resistant to inactivation by gastric acid and hence, can be given orally.

II. **Beta-lactamase (Penicillinase) resistant penicillins:** These resist the action of beta-lactamase and are effective in the treatment of infections due to beta-lactamase producing organisms. These are:

METHICILLIN: *As several strains of staphylococci have developed resistance to methicillin, it is now rarely used except for laboratory testing for MRSA. The term methicillin resistant Staphylococcus aureus (MRSA) is used to refer to beta-lactam antibiotic resistant (i.e., penicillinase producing) staphylococci.*

Most of MRSA strains are resistant to cloxacillin, flucloxacillin and all beta-lactam antibiotics (penicillins, cephalosporins and imipenem) and often to other classes of antimicrobial agents.

CLOXACILLIN: This drug has a weaker antibacterial activity than benzylpenicillin but is 5 to 10 times more active than methicillin against resistant staphylococci. It is also acid resistant. Food interferes with its absorption.

After a single oral dose, plasma levels persist for 4 to 6 hours. Nearly 30% of a single dose is excreted in the urine. Significant amounts are excreted in the bile.

The initial oral dose of cloxacillin varies from 0.5 to 1 g 6 hourly, and the maintenance dose is 250 mg given at the same intervals. In children, the dose varies from 50 to 100 mg per kg daily (according to severity of infection) divided into 4–6 portions. *The drug should be administered 1 hour before or 2 hours after a meal to ensure adequate absorption.* It can also be given IM and by slow IV bolus, 250–500 mg 4–6 hourly.

FLUCLOXACILLIN is similar to dicloxacillin but is relatively less protein bound, and hence may be preferred to dicloxacillin. It sometimes causes cholestatic jaundice.

NAFCILLIN: Its GI absorption is slow, irregular and incomplete. Intramuscular injection yields quicker and higher plasma levels. Approximately 87% of the drug is protein bound. *It is predominantly excreted by the liver in bile and may be preferred in patients with renal damage.* The oral doses are similar to those of cloxacillin.

Initial treatment of a severe staphylococcal infection should always be with one of the beta-lactamase resistant penicillins or a cephalosporin. **Staphylococci resistant to the above penicillinase-resistant penicillins have been reported.**

III. Penicillins effective against Gram-positive and Gram-negative organisms:

AMPICILLIN: Ampicillin is water soluble and acid resistant. Its antibacterial activity is generally similar to that of benzylpenicillin; *in addition, it is highly effective against various Gram-negative bacteria.* The drug is effective against *H. influenzae, Strep. viridans, Proteus mirabilis, Neisseria gonorrhoea, Salmonella typhi*, many strains of *E. coli* and several strains of *Shigella.* It is moderately effective against Klebsiella, certain strains of *Aerobacter and Enterococci.* The Gram-positive cocci are less sensitive to ampicillin than to benzylpenicillin.

Ampicillin is inactivated by beta-lactamase and, therefore, is ineffective against staphylococci resistant to benzylpenicillin. Bacteria can develop resistance to ampicillin, and many strains of salmonella, shigella, *E. coli* and proteus resistant to this drug have been isolated. Hence, it is combined with sulbactam, a beta-lactamase inhibitor (see under section beta-lactamase inhibitors).

Absorption, fate and excretion: It is readily but incompletely absorbed on oral administration. *Food interferes with its absorption*. The portion not absorbed is inactivated by beta-lactamase of the colonic bacterial flora and hence, the drug rarely produces superinfection.

Peak plasma levels are reached within 2 hours and 1 hour respectively after a single oral or IM dose. The drug persists in the plasma for 6–8 hours. Only 20% is bound to plasma proteins. *About 1/3rd of the dose is excreted unchanged in urine and high concentrations are present in the bile*. In premature and very young infants, excretion of ampicillin is delayed. It crosses the placental barrier and achieves therapeutic concentrations in the amniotic fluid.

Adverse reactions: These are similar to those of penicillin G; however, *skin rashes usually maculopapular are more common.* The onset is delayed. Diarrhoea is common with oral ampicillin and its derivatives. It is sometimes associated with *Clostridium difficile* infection.

Preparations and dosage: The ampicillin capsule contains ampicillin hydrate equivalent to 250/500 mg of the base. It is also available 25, 50 and 100 mg/ml oral solution and 250, 500 mg powder for solution as injection. The usual adult dose by all routes is 250 to 500 mg 6 hourly; doses as large as 1 g 6 hourly may be required for more refractory Gram-negative infections. In

children < 13 years, the daily oral dose is 50 to 200 mg per kg. Parenterally 25 to 50 mg per kg may be given per day in divided doses. Higher doses are used in the treatment of meningitis and bacterial endocarditis.
Stability of sodium ampicillin in solution decreases markedly and storing of solutions even at refrigeration temperature results in deterioration of activity; the presence of dextrose and lactate accelerates the loss of potency.

Indications:

- **Urinary tract infections** caused by *E. coli, P. Mirabilis,* non-hemolytic *streptococci* and *enterococci.* (Chapter 50).
- **Respiratory tract infections:** It is preferred particularly in mixed infections with *H. influenzae and P. pneumoniae.*
- **Meningitis and subacute bacterial endocarditis:** See Chapter 46 and Table 44.2.
- **Biliary tract and intestinal infections:** Ampicillin can be used against intestinal infections due to *E. coli, enterococci, salmonella* and *shigella.* Although it is effective in typhoid fever, it is not a preferred drug (see Chapter 47).
- **Miscellaneous:** Ampicillin is preferred to tetracyclines in pregnant women and in infants to avoid tetracycline deposition in bones and teeth. It can be used in the treatment of whooping cough. The other drugs useful in whooping cough are azithromycin (the drug of choice), erythromycin and cotrimoxazole.

TALAMPICILLIN: This carboxylic ester of ampicillin is a prodrug. It is hydrolysed by tissue esterases in the intestinal wall to release ampicillin into the circulation. It has no intrinsic antibacterial activity and hence, is unlikely to have direct effect on the gut bacterial flora.
Pivampicillin has properties similar to those of talampicillin.

AMOXICILLIN: This structural analogue of ampicillin (amino-p-hydroxy-benzylpenicillin) has properties and uses similar to those of ampicillin. However, it has **certain advantages:**

- It is almost completely absorbed and the blood levels on oral administration are twice as high as those of ampicillin.
- **Its absorption is not influenced by food.**
- It is less protein bound and the urinary excretion is higher than that of ampicillin.
- The incidence of diarrhoea is less.

It is more expensive. It is available as 250 mg capsules. The usual oral dose in adults is 250–500 mg 8 hourly. In severe or recurrent purulent, respiratory infections doses as large as 3 g 12 hourly are recommended. It can also be given IM or IV but offers no advantage over parenteral ampicillin. Amoxicillin is available in combination with clavulanic acid, a beta-lactamase inhibitor (see under section beta-lactamase inhibitors).

IV. Extended Spectrum Penicillins, also known as antipseudomonal penicillins:

(1) The **carboxypenicillins** and the **ureido-penicillins** (Box 44.4), are considered extended spectrum penicillins, because **they inhibit a wide variety of aerobic Gram-negative bacilli, including *P. aeruginosa.*** They have the following properties:

- They are acid labile and susceptible to beta-lactamase.
- **They are highly active against anaerobes.**
- They are most useful in infections caused by *P. aeruginosa* and other Gram-negative rods.
- They are much less active than penicillin G against Gram-positive organisms and are not reliable for treating staphylococcal infections.
- The CNS penetration of the carboxy- and the ureido-penicillins is about 10% of their serum levels, and hence they are not recommended for the treatment of meningeal infections.
- They act synergistically with aminoglycoside antibiotics, particularly against *P. aeruginosa* and the Enterobacteriaceae.
- They may inactivate the aminoglycoside antibiotics *in vitro* when mixed together in the same bottle.

  P. aeruginosa may develop resistance to these drugs, which may be prevented by concurrent administration of an aminoglycoside.

CARBENICILLIN: It has a similar spectrum as but weaker antibacterial activity than ampicillin.

Its important advantage over ampicillin is that it is effective against all strains of *Proteus* and *P. aeruginosa.*
It is now replaced by more active analogue, ticarcillin.

TICARCILLIN: This thienyl analogue of carbenicillin is:

- twice as active against *P. aeruginosa.*
- effective against some anaerobes, including many forms of *Bacteroides fragilis*
- much less active than ampicillin against streptococci, pneumococci and penicillin sensitive staphylococci.

It diffuses well into the CSF, pleural fluid and sputum and is excreted by the kidneys. It can be used in the treatment of severe UTI. It is usually combined with clavulanic acid to increase effective blood levels. Because of its high sodium content, it may cause sodium overload in patients with cardiac or renal damage.

PIPERACILLIN: This ureidopenicillin has a **broad spectrum** activity against Gram-negative bacilli, particularly *P. aeruginosa* (against which it is three times as active as ticarcillin). It is regarded as one of the most broadly active of the currently available penicillins with regard to other bacterial species, especially *Proteus, Klebsiella, Bacteroides fragilis, H. influenzae and Gonococci.*
Piperacillin is given parenterally. It is mainly eliminated in the urine (70%–90%) and adjustmentof its dose is needed in the presence of renal damage. Piperacillin crosses the BBB and may be useful in neonatal meningitis. Adverse effects are similar to those of other penicillins. However, it is less likely to cause sodium overload.
Although it is useful in a variety of infections, its use should be reserved for serious infections, especially those due to P. aeruginosa.
Azlocillin and **mezlocillin** have similar indications as piperacillin.

(2) **Amidinopenicillins:**

MECILLINAM: Mecillinam has no therapeutic activity against Gram-positive organisms but is effective against Gram-negative organisma such as *E. coli,* (including those resistant to ampicillin), *Klebsiella* species, *Shigellae* and *Salmonellae. Proteus* is less susceptible; *it has no action on Pseudomonas.* It is poorly absorbed orally and is given intramuscularly. Its ester **pivmecillinam** is better absorbed orally and is hydrolysed to mecillinam. These compounds have been used in UTI and in typhoid fever, but are not superior to the other commonly used drugs.

BETA-LACTAMASE INHIBITORS

CLAVULANIC ACID: This penicillin analogue produced by *Streptomyces clavuligerus* has the following properties:

- **It is a potent and irreversible inhibitor of many beta-lactamases and protects beta-lactam antibiotics from inactivation, when combined with them.**
- **It is well absorbed on oral administration but has only a weak antibacterial activity.**
- **Combined with amoxicillin, it widens the antibacterial spectrum of the latter to include beta-lactamase producing strains of *S. aureus, H. influenzae, N. gonorrhoea, E. coli, Proteus, Klebsiella, M. catarrhalis and Bacteroides species.***

It is used in combination with amoxicillin or ticarcillin.

SULBACTAM is another beta-lactamase inhibitor penicillin analogue similar in action to clavulanic acid, and it is combined with ampicillin and cefoperazone. **Tazobactam** is a penicillanic acid sulfone, beta-lactamase inhibitor. It is combined with piperacillin or ceftolozane, a third generation cephalosprin.

For some newer beta-lactamase inhibitors devoid of beta-lactam structure, which are combined with cephalosprins and carbapenem, see Chapter 46.

However, these combinations are expensive and are not cost-effective for routine infections. They should be reserved for infections due to beta-lactamase producing organisms.

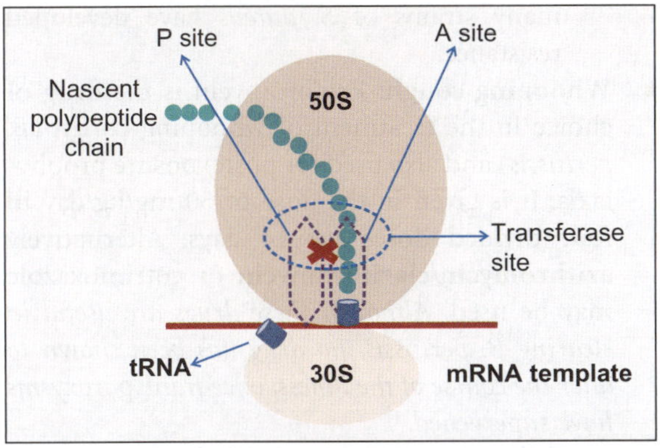

FIG. 44.2 Mechanism of action of macrolides. Macrolides bind reversibly to the 50S ribosomal subunit and inhibit the translocation of the nascent polypeptide chain from the A (acceptor) site to the P (peptidyl) site (denoted by X) and thus inhibit protein synthesis.

The beta-lactamases produced by P. aeruginosa and by Enterobacter species are resistant to clavulanic acid and sulbactam. Further, MRSA are not susceptible to antimicrobials containing clavulanic acid or sulbactam.

MACROLIDES

Erythromycin and **spiramycin** constitute the macrolide group of antibiotics, so named because of the presence of a large lactone ring in their chemical structure. They have similar antibacterial spectra, erythromycin being the most effective of all.

Mechanism of action: Macrolides act by inhibiting the protein synthesis by binding to the 50S ribosomal subunits (Fig. 44.2). Depending upon its concentration, the antibiotic can be bacteriostatic or bactericidal. Bacteria can develop resistance to macrolides by mutation. Active efflux of macrolides and their enzymatic inactivation are other two mechanisms of resistance.

Mechanism of action – macrolides.

ERYTHROMYCIN is derived from the fungus *Streptomyces erythreus*. Its **antibacterial spectrum resembles that of penicillin**. It is mainly effective against the Gram-positive cocci including the Streptococci, Staphylococci and Pneumococci. Neisseria, some strains of *H. influenzae, C. diphtheriae, Campylobacter jejuni, Listeria, P. multocida, Mycoplasma pneumoniae, Rickettsiae* and *Treponema* are also inhibited by low concentration. The drug is effective against penicillin resistant staphylococci. However, staphylococci and hemolytic streptococci can develop resistance to it.

Absorption, fate and excretion: Erythromycin is mainly absorbed from the small intestine. The drug is partially destroyed by the gastric juice and, therefore, is administered in the form of enteric coated tablets. The ester form, erythromycin estolate, is more resistant to inactivation by the gastric acid and is absorbed better than the base.

Peak plasma levels are reached within 2 to 4 hours after a single oral dose and the levels decline within 6 to 8 hours; hence, it is given 6 hourly.

Erythromycin readily diffuses into the body fluids but the penetration into the CSF is poor. It is concentrated in the liver, and the levels of the active form in bile are significantly high. Most of the drug (95%) is metabolised in the liver. It can pass into the foetal circulation.

Adverse reactions: Serious adverse effects are uncommon. Allergic reactions include fever, eosinophilia, urticaria, dermatitis and lymph-adenopathy. *Nausea, vomiting, epigastric pain and diarrhoea are common.* **Hepatic dysfunction, particularly cholestatic hepatitis and jaundice**, has been described **following of erythromycin estolate.** It usually clears up

Box 44.5 Drug Interactions with Erythromycin

- ***Reduction in plasma clearance with increased plasma levels and increased toxicity of:*** Ketoconazole, theophylline, carbamazepine, cyclosporine, digoxin, warfarin, disopyramide, methylprednisolone.
- ***Interference with the action of chloramphenicol and clindamycin*** as these drugs compete for the same bacterial binding sites.
- ***Physical/chemical incompatibility (in solution) between parenteral forms of Erythromycin*** and vitamin B complex, ascorbic acid, tetracycline, colistin, chloramphenicol, heparin, metaraminol and phenytoin.

within a few days after discontinuation of therapy. Hepatic dysfunction is a relative contraindication for erythromycin therapy.

Drug interactions: *Erythromycin is a potent inhibitor of hepatic microsomal CYP3A4*, thereby interfering with the metabolic degradation of number of drugs such as ketoconazole and cimetidine (Box 44.5). Some of them have been documented for other macrolide antibiotics as well.

Preparations and dosage:

i. Enteric coated tablets contain 250 mg of erythromycin base. Dose: 250–500 mg administered 6 hourly. *Food should not be given immediately after its administration*. The dose in children is 5 mg per kg 6 hourly in children below 1 year, 10 mg per kg 6 hourly in children upto 8 years and 15 mg per kg in children between 8 and 12 years.
ii. Erythromycin estolate tablets contain the equivalent of 125 and 250 mg of erythromycin base. It is administered in similar dosage. It is tasteless and resistant to gastric acid. Food does not interfere with its absorption.
iii. Erythromycin stearate filmtabs and capsules, contain 250 mg of the base. Dose in children: 30–50 mg/kg per day in divided doses.
iv. Erythromycin ethylsuccinate for IM injection 2 ml containing 100 mg of the base. It is also available as 25, 50 and 100 mg/ ml oral suspension.
v. Erythromycin lactobionate available as 1 gm powder for solution as IV infusion.

Indications:

- **As a substitute for penicillin:** Erythromycin is valuable in patients allergic to penicillins and in those in whom organisms have developed resistance to penicillin.
  (i) For **subacute bacterial endocarditis** due to *S. viridans,* in a penicillin allergic individual.
  (ii) **Diptheria carrier state:** Erythromycin in the dose of 250 and 500 mg every 6 hours for 10–12 days eradicates the carrier state in children and adults, respectively.
  (iii) **Prophylaxis against streptococcal infection and rheumatic fever.**
  (iv) **Skin and soft tissue infections:** Though erythromycin is an alternative to penicillin, many strains of *S. aureus* have developed resistance.
- **Whooping cough:** Erythromycin is the drug of choice in the treatment of whooping cough (*B. pertussis*) and also used for postexposure prophylaxis. It is given in the dose of 50 mg/kg/day in four divided doses for 14 days. Alternatively **azithromycin/clarithromycin** or cotrimoxazole may be used. *Although these drugs are useful in clearing B. pertussis, no drug has been shown to alter the course of the illness, once frank paroxysms have supervened.*
- **Mycoplasma and chlamydial infection:** *It is the drug of choice in the treatment of mycoplasma pneumoniae.* It is preferred in chlamydial pneumonia in infancy and in urogenital infections, particularly during pregnancy.
- **Diarrhoea due to *Campylobacter jejuni*.** It is the drug of choice (Chapter 39).
- **STD:** See Chapter 51.
- **Acne:** See Chapter 69.

Spiramycin is used to treat toxoplasmosis (Chapter 56).

Roxithromycin, azithromycin, clarithromycin and **fidaxomicin** are **azalides**, with a similar spectrum of activity as erythromycin. However,

- **They are resistant to acid hydrolysis.**
- **They are absorbed better and give higher tissue levels;** and
- **They have longer duration of action and can be given once daily.**
- **Azithromycin and clarithromycin** are also active against *H. influenzae, M. catarrhalis, T. gondii* and *M. avium complex.*

ROXITHROMYCIN: This substituted erythromycin has antibacterial spectrum and Indications similar to those of erythromycin.

AZITHROMYCIN: This is an azalide antibiotic. It:

- Has similar activity and toxicity as erythromycin.
- Acts against certain Gram-negative bacilli including *H. influenzae* and *C. trachomatis.* It also shows activity against *M. avium* complex.
- Penetrates the tissues better, concentrates in polymorphs.

- Has a longer half life (68–72 h) and is given OD and
- Is largely not metabolised and excreted in bile and faeces.
- Should not be administered with food. It is given 1 h before food or 2 h after food.
- Should be used cautionsly in patients with CVS risk factors, as it can cause QT prolongation and cardiac arrhythmia.

Indications: Its uses are similar to erythromycin.

- **Respiratory infections:** For pharyngitis, acute bacterial sinusitis, pneumonia, chronic bronchitis, a loading dose of 500 mg, followed by 250 mg 12 hourly for 2–5 days, is usually recommended.
- **Nongonococcal urethritis (NGU) and genital chlamydial infections:** It is given in a single 1 g dose (see Chapter 51).
- **Chlamydial infections:** For trachoma and lymphogranuloma venereum, three oral doses of 1 g, given at weekly intervals, are highly effective.
- **Rickettsial disease:** Azithromycin 500 mg in a single dose for five days is an alternative to doxycycline. **It is the drug of choice in pregnant woman.**
- **Avian complex in AIDS:** It is a first line drug for prophylaxis and treatment.
- **Other infections:** Otitis media, atypical pneumonia due to mycoplasma, whooping cough, toxoplasmosis, and Legionnaire's disease.

CLARITHROMYCIN:

- It has good activity against *H. influenzae, N. gonorrhoea, L. pneumophiliae* and chlamydia. It is better than azithromycin against MAC (Chapter 52) and *H. pylori.*
- The drug is absorbed rapidly and almost completely from the gut but undergoes first pass metabolism, has a short half-life (3–7hours) and has better tissue penetrability than erythromycin.
- *Food does not interfere with its absorption.*
- It is metabolised to 14-hydroxy-clarithromycin, which is active, and is excreted by renal and extrarenal mechanisms.
- Clarithromycin is administered orally in the dose of 500 mg bid.

Indications:

- The uses of clarithromycin are similar to azithromycin.

Clarithromycin, though very expensive, is the macrolide of choice for the treatment of H. pylori while azithromycin is preferred for the treatment of Chlamydia trachomatis infections.

FIDAXOMICIN is the narrow spectrum macrolide which is minimally absorbed on oral administration. It inhibits the bacterial RNA polymerase and is bactericidal.

Its oral toxicity is similar to vancomycin. Vomiting is the primary ADR. Given orally in the dose of 200 mg bid for 10 days, *it selectively eradicates Clostridium difficile without affecting the other bacterial species in the intestine.*

KETOLIDE ANTIBIOTICS

TELITHROMYCIN: This first **ketolide** antibiotic is related to erythromycin with similar antibacterial spectrum. However, it is also effective against macrolide resistant pneumococci. Adverse reactions include **diarrhoea,** blurred vision, diplopia and QTc prolongation. It can cause exacerbation of myasthenia gravis. Hepatotoxicity limits its use. The drug is a potent inhibitor of CYP3A4.

LINCOSAMIDE ANTIBIOTICS

LINCOMYCIN: Lincomycin, elaborated by *Streptomyces lincolenesis,* acts by binding to ribosome and interfering with protein synthesis. It is bacteriostatic with spectrum similar to that of erythromycin, e.g. staphylococci. Enterococci, meningococci, hemophilus and gonococci and many clostridia are resistant. Development of resistance by staphylococci has been reported. Cross resistance with macrolide antibiotics may occur. Lincomycin has been replaced by its derivative clindamycin.

CLINDAMYCIN: This is 7-chloro-7-deoxylincomycin, a semisynthetic derivative of lincomycin. It is bacteriostatic at low concentrations and bactericidal at slightly higher ones. It has antibacterial spectrum similar to that of lincomycin. However, it is:

- Much better absorbed orally and undergoes entero-hepatic circulation.
- Absorbed adequately in presence of food.
- Highly protein bound.
- Mostly metabolised in the liver (t½ 3h).
- Distributed throughout the body and is concentrated in the liver, spleen, kidneys, lung and bone. It also crosses the placental barrier.
- Accumulated in neutrophils and alveolar macrophages.
- Administered orally and intravenously.

Like lincomycin, it also achieves high levels in bone and bile.

Adverse reactions: The major adverse reaction is diarrhoea due to pseudomembraneous colitis in 20% of patients. It is due to superinfection with *C. difficile* and *C. sordellii* which secrete exotoxins with a necrotizing effect on the colonic mucosa. The organisms are sensitive to vancomycin. *However, metronidazole 250 mg tid for 10–14 days is equally effective.* Other ADR include nausea, vomiting and abdominal pain. Hypersensitivity reactions, elevation of liver enzymes and jaundice can occur. Local thrombophlebitis can occur with intravenous injections.

Preparation and dosage:

Clinamycin palmitate or hydrochloride: The dose of this oral formulation varies between 150 and 450 mg four times daily. In children and infants, it is given in the dose of 10–20 mg/kg daily in 3 to 4 divided doses.

Clindamycin phosphate: It is administered intramuscularly or by IV infusion, in a dose of 600–1200 mg per day 6, 8 or 12 hourly. For life-threatening infections in adults, doses upto 4.8 g by IV infusion have been used. It is also available as topical formulation.

Indications: It is used to treat:

- **Infection caused by Gram-positive organisms, which are resistant to penicillin or cephalosporins.**
- Anaerobic infections, e.g. peritonitis due to mixed infection, wherein it is given in a combination with an aminoglycoside. It is also used for anaerobic lung and pleural space infection.
- Staphylococcal bone and joint infections, lung abscess, actinomycosis, anthrax and diptheria.
- Malaria, toxoplasmosis (Chapter 54, 56) and *P. jiroveci* pneumonia, in combination with other drugs.
- Acne, wherein it is applied locally (Chapter 69).
- Bacterial vaginosis, wherein it can be used vaginally or orally.

GLYCOPEPTIDE ANTIBIOTICS

VANCOMYCIN: Vancomycin is obtained from the fungus *Streptomyces orientalis*. It is highly effective against Gram-positive cocci, MRSA and *Enterococcus fecalis*. The drug is bactericidal. Bacteria (enterococci and staphylococci) can develop resistance to vancomycin.

Mechanism of action: It acts on the cell wall by interfering with transglycosylase reaction, the last step in the cell wall synthesis.

Absorption, fate and excretion: Vancomycin is not absorbed orally and IM administration is very painful. It is given intravenously. It crosses BBB, if the meninges are inflammed. Approximately 80% of the drug is eliminated in urine within 24 hours.

Adverse reactions: These include local thrombophlebitis, generalised cutaneous reactions (**Red Man Syndrome**) due to massive histamine release and renal/auditory damage. The drug is mainly eliminated by the kidney.

Indications:

- **It is mainly used to treat multi-resistant staphylococcal and *E. fecalis* infections.**
- It may also be used in penicillin and cephalosporin resistant infections, e.g. skin and soft tissue infections, bone/ joint infections, pneumonia and meningitis caused by penicillin-resistant *S. pneumoniae* and nosocomial meningitis by *S. aureus*. For endocarditis, refer to Table 44.2. It is given IV in the dose of 500 mg over 60 minutes every 6 hours or 1 g every 12 hours.
- Oral dose of 125 mg 6 hourly adequately controls acute staphylococcal enterocolitis, and pseudo-

membranous colitis caused by the toxins of *C. difficille. However, metronidazole is equally effective and cheaper.*

TEICOPLANIN: It is produced by *Actinoplanes teicomyetius* and is structurally related to vancomycin and has similar properties. Unlike vancomycin, it can be given safely by IM injection. It is highly (90%) protein bound with t½ of 50 hours. It is used in preference to vancomycin in the dose of 6–30 mg/kg/day to treat **MDR infections caused by staphylococci, streptococci and enterococci.**

Telavancin, dalbavancin and **oritavancin** are semisynthetic lipoglycopeptides.

TELAVANCIN, derived from vancomycin, acts similar to vancomycin. In addition, it can cause direct disruption of the bacterial membrane and shows rapid antibacterial effect. Given IV once daily, it acts against Gram-positive bacteria including VRSA. It can cause QT prolongation and is teratogenic.

DALBAVANCIN is derived from teicoplanin and shares the same mechanism of action. It has activity against Gram-positive bacteria including MRSA and VRSA. The drug has a **long t½ (or approx 14 days) and therefore is administered once weekly IV infusion.** The common ADR include nausea, diarrhoea and headache. Redman syndrome can also occur.

Oritavancin also has a long t½, which allows weekly dosing and is highly (>90%) protein bound. It has a large volume of distribution (~1 L/kg). Careful monitoring is required if the patient is on warfarin.

Bacteria can develop resistance to all the glycopeptides.

MISCELLANEOUS ANTIBIOTICS

DAPTOMYCIN: This bactericidal antibiotic produced by *Streptomyces roseosprous* belongs to a new class called **cyclic lipopeptides**.

Mechanism of action: It binds to the bacterial plasma membrane. causing membrane depolarisation and release of intracellular ions. This causes cell damage.

Its spectrum is similar to that of vancomycin and includes *Gram-positive bacteria including MRSA, VRSA, penicillin resistant S. pneumoniae and vancomycin resistant E. faecalis.*

Absorption, fate and excretion: Its oral absorption is poor hence it is administered IV It has plasma **t½ of nine hours. It is inactivated by pulmonary surfactant. Hence it does not achieve adequate concentration in the lungs.** It is largely excreted by the kidney.

Adverse reactions: include GI disturbances, rash, headache and dose related muscle pain/weakness. Hence CPK monitoring is advisable.

The drug appears to be similar to vancomycin in efficacy against vancomycin sensitive organisms, but **is also useful to treat MRSA and VRSA skin and soft tissue infections**. It is usually administered in the dose of 4–6 mg/kg IV od.

SODIUM FUSIDATE: Fucidin, the sodium salt of fucidic acid, is obtained from the parasitic fungus *Fusidium coccineum.* It has a steroidal structure. The drug is effective mainly against Gram-positive organisms and is used *against beta-lactamase producing staphylococci.* It is bacteriostatic. *However, staphylococci rapidly develop resistance to this antibiotic by mutation.* The antibiotic exerts a synergistic effect when combined with flucloxacillin and erythromycin.

Adverse reactions: These include skin reactions, nausea, vomiting, epigastric pain, diarrhoea and hepatic dysfunction.

Indications: In resistant staphylococcal infections, sodium fusidate may be administered orally or IV infusion as diethanolamine fusidate. It is employed locally as 2% sodium fusidate in a neutral ointment base to treat staphylococcal skin lesions.

BACITRACIN: Bacitracin is a polypeptide antibiotic obtained from *Bacillus subtilis.* It resembles penicillin in antibacterial activity. *It is effective against Gram-positive organisms like Streptococci, Staphylococci, Pneumococci and Enterococci. Corynebacterium, Gonococci, Meningococci, C. tetani, C. difficile, Treponema and H. influenzae are highly sensitive.* Microorganisms do not readily develop resistance to bacitracin.

Bacitracin is not much absorbed orally. Parenterally, it is nephrotoxic. Acute tubular necrosis and anuria may occur. It is **used only topically as an antiseptic in combination**.

MUPIROCIN: This antibiotic is obtained from the cultures of *Pseudomonas fluorescens*. It is bactericidal. It is most active against Gram-positive bacteria but also has activity against Gram-negative aerobic organisms. *It is used as 2% ointment to treat localised superficial skin infections caused by Staphylococci and Streptococci, and for eradication of nasal colonisation by S. aureus.*

STREPTOGRAMINS

QUINUPRISTIN (Q)/DALFOPRISTIN (D) is a combination of streptogramin B with streptogramin A in the ratio of 30:70. They are semisynthetic **derivatives of pristinamycin** which had been in use in France for over 30 years. They act on different sites of 50S ribosomal subunit synergistically to disrupt protein synthesis. The combination is bactericidal. It is active against *E. faecium, S, aureus, S. epidermidis, S. pneumoniae, N. meningitidis, Moraxella catarrhalis, Legionella, Mycoplasma pneumoniae* and *C. perfringens*. The combination is administered by IV infusion in 5% dextrose (not in saline). Both have elimination half life of about one hour. They are metabolised in the liver. Bacteria can develop resistance to these drugs.

Adverse reactions: Locally, the combination causes inflammation, pain and thrombophlebitis. Other ADR reported are arthralgia and myalgia. Both the drugs are potent inhibitors of CYP3A4 and hence may increase the blood levels of co-administered drugs.

Indications: The combination is used *to treat the Vancomycin resistant Enterococcus faecium (VREF) and complicated skin infections caused by multidrug resistant (MDR) S. aureus and S. pyogenes, nosocomial pneumonia with S. pneumoniae and MRSA.* Because of high incidence of ADR, drug interactions and very high cost, their routine use is to be avoided.

OXAZOLIDINONES

LINEZOLID: This antibacterial drug belongs to a new chemical class called oxazolidinones.

Mechanism of action: It acts by preventing initiation of protein synthesis. **Because of its unique binding site (on 50S subunit), there is no cross-resistance with other drug classes.** Bacteria can develop resistance to this drug by mutation.

It is bacteriostatic against Staphylococci and Enterococci and bactericidal against Streptococci and Pneumococci. **Its main advantage is that it is active against *E. faecium*, MRSA and VRSA. It also acts against penicillin-resistant Pneumococci and *M. tuberculosis*.**

Absorption, fate and exeretion: Given orally, the drug is rapidly and completely absorbed. It undergoes nonenzymatic oxidation in the liver and excreted in urine, 30–35% being in an active form. It has a half life of about 5 hours. It can also be given intravenously. The drug gets decomposed by light. No dose adjustment is recommended in chronic renal failure.

Adverse reactions: These include diarrhoea, nausea, vomiting, headache, rash, thrombocytopenia, leucopenia and rarely bone marrow suppression and neuropathy. The drug is an MAO inhibitor.

Indications: It should be reserved for the treatment of well documented serious VREF and VRSA infections, MDR respiratory infection and chronic osteomyelitis. *It is now advocated in the treatment of MDR TB* (Chapter 52). It is given in the dose of 400–600 mg 12 hourly. It is expensive.

Tedizolid, a new oxazolidinone, is an active moiety of a prodrug tedizolid phosphate. The action, and antibacterial spectrum, indications and ADR are similar to linezolid.

PLEUROMUTILINS

Retapamulin and **Lefamulin:** These are new bacterial protein synthesis inhibitors, which act on the 50S ribosomal subunit. They inhibit peptide bond formation. They have bactericidal effect on Gram-positive organisms, Staphylococci, including MRSA, and Streptococci, with the exception of Enterococci. They show some activity against Gram-negative organisms like *H. influenzae* and *M. catarrhalis*. They are also

Table 44.2 Antibiotic Regimens for the Treatment of Bacterial Endocarditis IM 3.12, IM 3.13

Organism	Antibiotic regimen
Streptococcus. viridans (Alpha-hemolytic)	Penicillin G 10–20 million units/day IV in six equal doses, *plus* gentamicin 1 mg/kg IV or IM 8 hourly. (Avoid gentamicin in patients over 65 years and in presence of renal failure or eighth nerve damage.) Penicillin alone may be used for 4 weeks or in combination for two weeks In patients allergic to penicillin: Ceftriaxone 2 g IV or IM once daily or Vancomycin 30 mg/kg (not to exceed 1 g) IV 12 hourly. Duration: 4 weeks.
Streptococcus pyogenes (Beta-hemolytic, Group A)	Pencillin G 2 million units IV 6 hourly. OR Cefazolin 2 g IV 8 hourly Duration: 2–4 weeks.
Streptococcus fecalis ***(Enterococcus fecalis)*** (Beta-hemolytic, Group D)	Penicillin G 4 million units/Ampicillin 2 g IV 4 hourly *plus* gentamicin 1 mg/kg IV 8 hourly for 4–6 weeks, OR Vancomycin 30 mg/kg (not to exceed 1g) IV 12 hourl *plus* gentamicin as above. Duration: 4–6 weeks.
Staphylococcus aureus	Nafcillin 2 g IV 4 hourly, for 4–6 weeks. In complicated cases, Nafcillin as above *plus* gentamicin 1 mg/kg IV 8 hourly for the first 3–5 days. In patients allergic to penicillin, Cefazolin 2 g IV 4 hourly OR vancomycin as above for 4–6 weeks.
HACEK organisms	Fluoroquinolone OR Cephalosporin IV

effective against *Chlamydophila, Mycoplasma,* and *Legionella.*

Retapamulin is used topically (1% cream twice daily) for the treatment of impetigo. It may get absorbed from thin skin as in children or broken skin.

Lefamulin is used orally and intravenously for the treatment of community-acquired bacterial pneumonia. It has low bioavailability. It is highly protein bound (~95%), and has t½ of 12 h. It gets excreted largely unchanged in faeces. The oral dose is 600 mg twice daily and IV dose is 150 mg. Lefamulin is well tolerated and common ADR include nausea and diarrhea. QT prolongation has been reported.

Most of the newer antimicrobial drugs are reserved for infections not responding to the existing and commonly used antimicrobials, and that too after identification of organisms and determination of their sensitivity to these antimicrobials. They are very expensive.

PHARMACOTHERAPY OF SUBACUTE BACTERIAL ENDOCARDITIS (SBE)

The alpha-hemolytic streptococci (*S. viridans*) account for the majority of cases of SBE.

Therapeutic response in bacterial endocarditis depends upon the proper selection of antibiotics, the stage at which treatment is begun and its thoroughness. If the diagnosis and consequently the treatment are delayed, irreversible cardiac damage occurs. In principle, high doses of bactericidal drugs are given initially IM/IV to achieve high peak concentration. In all cases therapy is continued for a minimum period of 4–6 weeks and monthly blood cultures are done for at least 3 months to detect a recurrence.

Regimens for the treatment of the common forms of bacterial endocarditis are given in Table 44.2. The choice of the antibiotic(s) and duration of therapy depend upon the type of organism and the nature of underlying lesion (whether rheumatic valve disease or prosthetic valve).

Prophylaxis of SBE: Prophylactic penicillin is indicated in individuals with rheumatic or congenital heart disease, who have to undergo surgical procedures like tooth extraction, dental scaling, and procedures involving the lower genitourinary tract. Recommended drug for this is **oral amoxicillin** 2 g in adults and 50 mg/kg in children given 1 hour before the procedure.

The alternatives are:

a. **Azithromycin** or **clarithromycin** 500 mg in adults and 15 mg/kg in children; or
b. **Clindamycin** 600 mg in adults and 20 mg/kg in children; or
c. **Cephalexin** 2 g in adults or 50 mg/kg in children, given similarly. In each case, ½ the dose is repeated once, 6 hours after the procedure.

When **parenteral administration** is indicated, give IM or IV (½ hour before the procedure) either:

a. **Ampicillin** 2 g in adults and 50 mg/kg in children; or
b. **Clindamycin** 600 mg in adults and 20 mg/kg in children; or
c. **Cefazolin** 1 g in adults and 25 mg/kg in children.

In MDR cases and those allergic to penicillin, a combination of vancomycin and gentamicin is used. *These regimens are used even in patients on rheumatic fever prophylaxis with penicillin.*

PENICILLINS

Penicillin G and its esters
- Penicillin G (Benzyl penicillin)
- Procaine penicillin G
- Benzathine penicillin G

Acid-resistant penicillins
- Phenoxymethlypenicillin (penicillin V)

Penicillinase-resistant penicillins**
- *Acid labile*: Methicillin, Nafcillin, Cloxacillin, Dicloxacillin
- *Acid resistant*: Flucloxacillin

Penicillins effective against Gram-positive and some Gram-negative organisms
- Ampicillin
- Amoxicillin
- Talampicillin
- Pivampicillin

Extended spectrum penicillins

Antipseudomonal penicillins
- *Carboxypenicillins*: Carbenicillin, Ticarcillin
- *Ureidopenicillins*: Piperacillin, Mezlocillin, Azlocillin

Amidinopenicillins
- Mecillinam
- Pivmecillinam

Penicillins with beta-lactamase inhibitors
- Ampicillin-sulbactam
- Amoxicillin-clavulanic acid
- Ticarcillin-clavulanic acid

CHAPTER 45

Aminoglycosides and Other Antibiotics Effective Mainly Against Gram-Negative Organisms

Learning Objectives

This chapter will enable the reader:

1. To mention the common features of aminoglycosides group of antibiotics.
2. To classify aminoglycosides.
3. To explain the mechanism of action of aminoglycosides and different mechanisms by which bacteria acquire resistance to them.
4. To describe the salient pharmacokinetic features, ADR and indications for aminoglycosides.
5. To explain the mechanism of action, antibacterial spectrum, ADR and indications for nonaminoglycoside agents, e.g. polypeptides, spectinomycin, fosfomycin.
6. To state advantages and limitations of monobactams.

KEY TERMS

Aminoglycosides form an important group of antibiotics (Box 45.1), useful mainly against aerobic Gram-negative bacteria. They are protein-synthesis inhibitors, interfering with ribosomal function. *Compounds derived from Streptomyces are called* **'mycins'** *(e.g. streptomycin) whereas those derived from Micromonospora are called* **'micins'** *(e.g. gentamicin).*

The aminoglycosides have certain common features:

- *Chemically, they are polycations having amino sugars linked to a hexose (aminocyclitol) ring by glycoside bonds.*
- *They are bactericidal* and their activity is maximum in an alkaline medium.
- *They have similar spectrum of activity.* They are highly effective in infections caused by *Gram-negative microorganisms,* **and are not effective in infections due to anaerobes.**
- *They are highly polar (water soluble) and* **are not absorbed orally**. *Their distribution is essentially extracellular,* and penetration into the CSF (except in the neonate) and into the eye is poor on systemic administration.
- *They are excreted unchanged relatively rapidly by the kidneys by glomerular filtration* and dosage adjustment is a must in patients with renal impairment and in old people.
- *Bacteria develop resistance to them fairly rapidly* and may even exhibit cross resistance among different aminoglycosides.
- *They exhibit synergism when combined with a beta-lactam antibiotic such as a penicillin or a cephalosporin.*
- *They cause* **nephrotoxicity** and **ototoxicity** (eighth cranial nerve damage). They also have **curarimimetic** properties.
- *They should be avoided in pregnancy because of their ADRs.*

Classification of Aminoglycosides: Refer Box 45.1

Mechanism of action: Aminoglycosides diffuse through the outer cytoplasmic membrane and are transported to ribosomes. Ribosomes manufacture enzymes as per the directions from messenger RNA (mRNA) (Fig. 45.1). Aminoglycosides **bind mainly to 30S ribosomes** and interfere with initiation of

Box 45.1 Classification of Aminoglycosides Based on Clinical Use

For topical use in the eye and on the skin: Neomycin, framycetin, gentamicin
For GI infections and gut sterilisation: Neomycin, paromomycin
For systemic use: Streptomycin, gentamicin, kanamycin, amikacin, tobramycin, netilmicin

protein synthesis, block the translation of mRNA and prematurely terminate the synthesis. Incorrect amino acids get incorporated in the protein chain, leading to production of abnormal proteins. These proteins, on insertion into the cell membrane, cause its disruption (Fig. 45.1). They exhibit **concentration-dependent killing**. Their bactericidal activity persists even after fall in the serum concentration below the minimum inhibitory concentration (MIC); the duration of this postantibiotic effect is also concentration dependent.

Hence, the present trend is to administer these antibiotics in a single daily high dose which probably reduces the incidence of ototoxicity and renal toxicity.

Aminoglycoside resistance: The microorganisms readily develop resistance to aminoglycosides. Some important examples are *Streptococcus pneumoniae, Mycobacterium tuberculosis, Proteus, Escherichia coli, Aerobacter, Haemophilus influenzae, Brucella, Staphylococcus aureus and Streptococcus faecalis.*

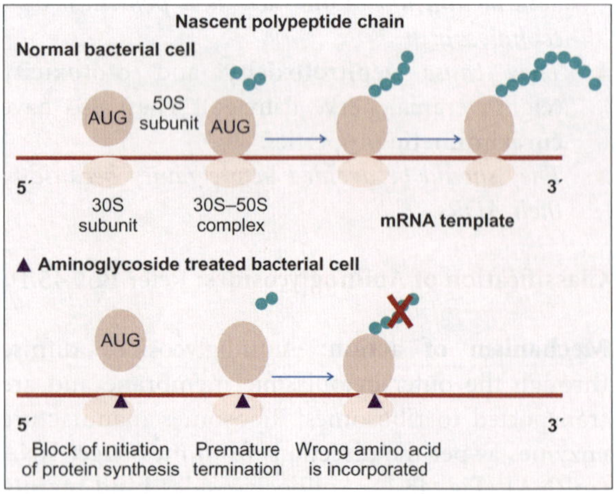

FIG. 45.1. Mechanism of action of aminoglycosides.

Resistance to aminoglycosides arises from several different mechanisms.

- **Low-level resistance** is due to decreased cell permeability to the antibiotic, thus, preventing the drug reaching the drug-sensitive ribosomes.
- **High-level resistance** results from a single-step mutation which affects the ribosomal proteins. This affects the affinity for aminoglycoside binding. It is not a common mechanism.
- **'R' factor-mediated resistance** (see Chapter 49) is **clinically significant**. The genetic material transferred during conjugation confers on the recipient cell the capacity to synthesise specific enzymes which destroy the aminoglycoside.

Adverse reactions:
Local irritation: Pain at the site of injection is common. Sterile abscess can occur.

Allergy: The manifestations include various skin rashes, eosinophilia, drug fever and lymphadenopathy. Serious manifestations like angioedema, pericarditis, exfoliative dermatitis and blood dyscrasias are rare.

Ototoxicity: The incidence of this ADR is dependent on the drug, dose and duration of therapy. The likelihood of ototoxicity is greater in infants, elderly patients and those with impaired renal function. High concentrations of aminoglycosides are found in the endolymph and the perilymph of the inner ear and may result in cochlear or vestibular dysfunction or both. It may be reversible or irreversible. The risk factors for ototoxicity are presented in the Box 45.2.

Aminoglycosides cause degeneration of sensory hair cells and neurons in the cochlea, which results in deafness. This is usually preceded by tinnitus. High-frequency hearing loss occurs first, and therefore may not be recognized by the patients. Hence, serial audiometry needs to be done to identify the deficit. The vestibular dysfunction presents itself with a moderately severe headache followed by nausea, vomiting, giddiness, ataxia and nystagmus develop. These persist for 8–15 days. The acute stage is usually followed by chronic labyrinthitis and ataxia. With stoppage of the drug, recovery usually occurs within 12–18 months.

Use of streptomycin or gentamicin is associated with vestibular dysfunction whereas amikacin, kanamycin or neomycin cause mainly auditory dysfunction. Tobramycin can affect both. The risk of ototoxicity is highest with streptomycin and least with netilmicin.

Nephrotoxicity: Aminoglycosides accumulate in the proximal tubular cells and damage them. They also reduce the sensitivity of the collecting ducts to vasopressin and interfere with renal concentrating ability.

Mild albuminuria, cylindruria or acute tubular necrosis may occur in patients receiving aminoglycosides though azotaemia is rare. Dosage adjustment must be made in patients with renal insufficiency. On withdrawal of aminoglycosides, reversal of toxic effects are seen because proximal tubules have capacity to regenerate. Risk factors for nephrotoxicity are presented in the Box 45.3.

Streptomycin is the least nephrotoxic aminoglycoside. Neomycin exhibits the highest nephrotoxic potential. Dose adjustment is needed for aminoglycosides if creatinine clearance of a patient is <80-100 mL/min.

Neuromuscular blockade: All aminoglycosides have a potential curarimimetic action, producing neuromuscular block and respiratory arrest on intrapleural or intraperitoneal instillation. They probably act by both, inhibition of ACh release at the neuromuscular junction through competition with calcium ions and decreasing the sensitivity of postsynaptic NM receptors to ACh. The blockade can be antagonised by calcium salts and by neostigmine.

Box 45.2 Risk Factors for Ototoxicity

- High serum levels of aminoglycoside
- Intravenous injections given over multiple days or as multiple courses
- Advanced age
- Renal dysfunction
- Pre-existing auditory impairment
- Concurrent use of loop diuretics e.g. ethacrynic acid and furosemide
- Possibility of potential genetic predisposition

The risk is maximum with neomycin and the least with tobramycin. Neuromuscular blockade is manifested in the postoperative setting. The risk is more if aminoglycosides are administered as intrapleural or intraperitoneal injections but can occur after IV and IM injections. Patients having myasthenia gravis are more susceptible.

STREPTOMYCIN: This antibiotic, obtained from *Streptomyces griseus*, is an organic base.

Antibacterial activity: The organisms usually sensitive to streptomycin are: *M. tuberculosis, Shigella species, E. coli, Proteus, Pseudomonas aeruginosa, Aerobacter aerogenes, H. influenzae, Haemophilus ducreyii, Yersinia pestis, Francisella tularensis, Brucella, Actinobacillus mallei, Listeria and Nocardia.*

The moderately sensitive organisms include *Staphylococci, Streptococcus pyogens, S. faecalis, Streptococcus viridans, S. pneumoniae, Vibrio comma* and the *Salmonella* organisms.

Streptomycin is bacteriostatic in low and bactericidal in high concentrations. Its bactericidal action increases progressively with rise in concentration.

Absorption, fate and excretion: Given intramuscularly, peak plasma level is reached within 30–60 min and the activity persists for 6–8 h. The drug is well absorbed when instilled intrapleurally. About 30%–35% of the drug is bound to plasma proteins. It diffuses into the synovial, pericardial and peritoneal fluids but repeated systemic administration is necessary to produce a high concentration in the pleural fluid. It is concentrated mainly in kidneys, liver and skeletal muscles. It does not readily cross the BBB; however, in the presence of meningeal inflammation, higher CSF concentrations are usually

Box 45.3 Risk Factors for Nephrotoxicity

- Total amount and duration of aminoglycoside
- Advanced age
- Concurrent medication with nephrotoxic potential e.g. amphotericin B, vancomycin, ACEIs, cisplatin, cyclosporine
- Volume depletion and K^+ loss with furosemide
- Comorbid conditions such as liver disease, diabetes mellitus, septic shock

achieved. It crosses the placental barrier and the cord blood concentration is similar to that of the maternal blood.

Streptomycin is excreted unchanged by glomerular filtration. Approximately 50%–60% of the drug is eliminated in urine in an active form within 24 h.

Adverse reactions: Streptomycin exhibits all the ADRs described above. Given below is the description of its ototoxic effect.

- **Eighth cranial nerve damage:** This is the most serious adverse effect of streptomycin. Streptomycin is more prone to impair the vestibular function; however, the symptoms of vestibular damage are usually reversible. Streptomycin causes deafness, preceded by tinnitus. A few cases of congenital loss of hearing have been reported following its administration during pregnancy. Other rare toxic effects include optic neuritis and peripheral neuritis.
- **Superinfection:** Superinfection with *S. aureus* and *Candida* has been reported.

Preparations and dosage: Streptomycin sulphate injection (0.75g/ 1g): Dose: 0.5–1 g of the base daily by deep intramuscular injection.

Indications:

- **Tularemia:** This infection is highly sensitive to streptomycin and most cases respond to IM dose of 1–2 g (15-25 mg/kg) daily for 10-14 days.
- **Plague:** Streptomycin is highly specific and the drug of choice in the treatment of plague. It is administered in the dose of 30 mg/kg/day IM in two divided doses for 10-14 days. Streptomycin may be used in pregnant women, old people and children with pneumonic plague. For optimum results, **doxycycline** is combined with streptomycin, in the dose of 100 mg twice a day (or 200 mg once a day), preferably intravenously (or orally).
  Alternatives to streptomycin are gentamicin or fluoroquinolones. In meningitic plague, chloramphenicol-streptomycin is the preferred regimen.
  Contacts of a case of pneumonic plague should be treated with either tetracycline (250 mg q.i.d. orally) or cotrimoxazole (250-mg q.i.d. orally) for 5–10 days.
- **Brucellosis:** Brucellosis is transmitted to humans from the cattle and camel through contaminated dairy products, especially fresh cheeses. **Streptomycin** 0.75–1 g IM daily for 3 weeks **plus doxycycline** 100 mg b.i.d. for 6 weeks is recommended as the treatment of choice. In case of complicated brucellosis or in noncompliant patients, rifampicin 600 mg once daily for 6 weeks is added. **Doxycycline** plus **rifampicin** 3–6 weeks can be used as prophylaxis. Cotrimoxazole in high doses can also be used if doxycycline is contraindicated.
- **Enterococcal infections:** Streptomycin is sometimes used in serious infections with susceptible enterococci. It exhibits synergistic effect with penicillin G. For resistant strains, gentamicin is used.
- **Tuberculosis:** Streptomycin though used earlier as a first line drug is now used in the MDR – TB chemotherapy. It is used only if amikacin is not available or there is a confirmed resistance to it (Chapter 52).

KANAMYCIN: This aminoglycoside is derived from *Streptomyces kanamyceticus*. Its antibacterial spectrum, pharmacokinetics and toxicity are similar to those of streptomycin. However, it is much more toxic and hence no longer recommended.

GENTAMICIN: This aminoglycoside antibiotic is produced by *Micromonospora purpura.*

Antibacterial activity: Gentamicin is highly effective against *Pseudomonas, E. coli, Proteus, A. aerogenes, Klebsiella pneumoniae, salmonellae* and Group A *beta haemolytic streptococci. Staphylococci* are also highly sensitive including those resistant to penicillin. *M. tuberculosis and Mycoplasma pneumoniae* are also highly sensitive. Bacterial resistance develops slowly. **It acts synergistically with beta-lactams and metronidazole**.

Absorption, fate and excretion: Given intramuscularly, the peak plasma levels are reached within 60–90 min and therapeutically effective concentration persists for 6–8 h. Approximately, 25%–30% of the drug is bound to plasma proteins. It is excreted largely unchanged by glomerular filtration. *Its urinary concentration ranges from 50 to 100 times that in the plasma.*

Adverse reactions: It is much less toxic than kanamycin and streptomycin. Allergic skin reactions and possibly photosensitivity reactions have occurred following topical gentamicin. Parenteral therapy, particularly in the presence of renal impairment, may produce vestibular damage and ototoxicity. Dizziness is the main presenting symptom. A transient rise in blood urea nitrogen has also been reported in some patients.

Preparations and dosage: It is available as sulphate. Administration of entire dose (5.5 mg/kg over 30–60 min) once daily is effective and is less toxic. **High concentration achieved by the single dose accounts for higher efficacy and is also cost effective.** If creatinine clearance is low then dosing interval should be extended. The IM or slow IV dose of the drug is 2–5 mg/kg/day in divided doses, for patients with normal renal function. The dose should be reduced in the presence of renal damage.

A 0.3% cream, ointment or eye drops is used for topical application.

Indications:

- **Topical use:** Gentamicin has been employed in a variety of skin infections, in cases of burns infected with pseudomonas, bed sores, the nasal carriers of staphylococci and ocular infections.
- **Urinary tract infections:** It is an alternative for complicated urinary tract infections including pyelonephritis (Chapter 50).
- **Systemic infections:** It is used as a single agent or in combination therapy for variety of infections caused by Gram-negative organisms. It is often a part of initial empiric therapy in hospital acquired infections before the causative agent is identified:
- **Adjunct to provide synergistic bacterial killing with:**
    - Penicillin G or ampicillin in the treatment of **bacterial endocarditis** caused by *S. viridans* and *S. faecalis*, respectively. Ampicillin and gentamicin combination is also used for Listeria meningitis.
    - Carbenicillin or a cephalosporin in treating **serious multidrug-resistant Gram-negative bacillary infections** especially those caused by *P. aeruginosa, enterobacter, Klebsiella* and *Serratia* and by other species. The infections so treated include urinary tract infections, peritonitis, meningitis, osteomyelitis, septic burns, otitis, pneumonia and septicemia.
    - Carbenicillin or piperacillin to treat pseudomonas infection.

Tetracyclines and chloramphenicol should not be used together with gentamicin as they reduce its therapeutic efficacy.

NETILMICIN (Netromycin): This semisynthetic aminoglycoside has activity similar to gentamicin but is effective against some Gram-negative bacilli resistant to gentamicin and tobramycin. It is less active than gentamicin against pseudomonas. It is not metabolised by most aminoglycoside-inactivating enzymes.

TOBRAMYCIN: This drug, belonging to the **family of nebramycins,** is derived from the actinomycetes *Streptomyces tenebrarius.* Its antibacterial spectrum, pharmacodynamic properties and toxicity are similar to those of gentamicin. Clinically, it is:

- Four times as active as gentamicin against *Pseudomonas* and hence preferred with antipseudomonal beta-lactam antibiotics
- Relatively less toxic
- Active against a number of bacterial strains with acquired resistance to gentamicin
- Less active against proteus and enterococci and ineffective against mycobacteria

It is administered intramuscularly or intravenously in the dose of 3–5 mg/kg/day in 3–4 equal doses. Higher doses of tobramycin (10 mg/kg) are used to treat infection causing acute exacerbations in patients with cystic fibrosis. Inhalational formulation is also available for this purpose. Ophthalmic ointment and solution are also available.

AMIKACIN is a semisynthetic derivative of kanamycin A with pharmacokinetic properties similar to those of kanamycin. **It has the broadest spectrum antibacterial activity** among the aminoglycosides. Its uses and adverse effects are similar to those of gentamicin. **It is not much affected by most of the enzymes that degrade gentamicin and tobramycin.** *Hence, it is active against gentamicin-resistant organisms such as P. aeruginosa, Klebsiella, E. coli and Proteus.*

It is much more expensive than gentamicin and is usually reserved for hospital-acquired Gram-negative infections which are resistant to gentamicin and tobramycin, in MDR TB and atypical mycobacterial infections. It is given intramuscularly or by slow IV drip in the dose of 15 mg/kg/day in two divided doses.

Among gentamicin, amikacin and tobramycin, gentamicin is the most active against all gentamicin sensitive bacilli except P. aeruginosa which is more sensitive to tobramycin.

Plazomicin a new aminoglycoside has been approved for treatment of adults with complicated UTI. It is administered IV and is active against MDR enterobacteriaceae, including strains resistant to other aminoglycosides.

NEOMYCIN: This antibiotic obtained from *Streptomyces fradiae*, is a polybasic, water soluble substance relatively stable to heat and changes in pH. It is used as a sulphate complex.

Antibacterial activity: Neomycin is effective against a wide variety of Gram-positive and Gram-negative organisms including *Enterococci, Streptococci, Staphylococci, Bacillus anthracis, Corynebacterium diptheriae, H. influenzae, H. pertussis, Proteus, Pasteurella, Vibrio comma, Salmonella* and *Shigella.* Resistance to the antibiotic is known and the resistant organisms show cross resistance to kanamycin and streptomycin.

Neomycin is poorly absorbed orally. It is used mainly for sterilization of bowels prior to surgery. It is administered orally in the dose of 1 g 4–6 hourly. It is also used locally for skin, eye and ear infections.

Adverse reactions: Its toxicity on parenteral administration is qualitatively similar to **but more severe** than that of streptomycin. Hence, *it is not used systemically.*

Indications: IM 5.16

- **For topical application to the skin and eye,** it is usually combined with other antibiotics like bacitracin or polymyxin to prevent the emergence of resistant strains and to widen the spectrum;
- **For preparation of bowel** prior to colonic surgery and for suppression of intestinal flora in hepatic failure It is also used for "selective digestive decontamination" to reduce the risk of ventilator-associated pneumonia.
- **For irrigation of the urinary bladder.** Neomycin along with polymyxin B are used in patients with indwelling catheter to prevent bacteriuria and bacteremia.

FRAMYCETIN: This antibiotic, produced by *Streptomyces decaris*, is used as the water soluble sulphate salt. Its antimicrobial spectrum, uses and toxicity are similar to neomycin. Framycetin sulphate, as a 0.5% ointment, cream or solution is used for staphylococcal skin infections, in the treatment of nasal carriers of staphylococci and for ear and eye infection.

PAROMOMYCIN: This antibiotic, obtained from a strain of *Streptomyces rimosus*, has a similar spectrum of activity and toxicity as neomycin. It also shows considerable activity against *Entamoeba histolytica, G.lamblia, Cryptosporidium and Leishmania.* The drug is not absorbed orally. Adverse effects of oral therapy include headache, emesis, diarrhoea and skin rashes; superinfection with Candida may occur after prolonged oral therapy.

Indications:

- **Intestinal amoebiasis:** (Chapter 55)
- **Giardiasis:** (Chapter 56)
- **Leishmaniasis:** Given intramuscularly for 21 days, it has been claimed to be effective in treating visceral leishmaniasis. It can be used topically for cutaneous leishmaniasis (Chapter 56).
- **Cryptosporidiosis:** It is used to treat chronic watery diarrhoea in immunocompromised

patients with AIDS caused by intestinal protozoa, *Cryptosporidium parvum*.

ARBEKACIN: See Chapter 46.

NONAMINOGLYCOSIDE AGENTS

COLISTIN (Polymyxin E): This polypeptide antibiotic is obtained from the bacterium *Aerobacillus colistinus*.

Mechanism of action: It binds with the anionic phospholipids from the outer cell membrane of gram-negative bacteria because of its cationic detergent property. The resultant permeability changes cause leakage of cell contents and cell death.

Antibacterial activity: Colistin is bactericidal to many Gram-negative organisms, e.g. *H. pertussis, Pseudomonas, E. coli, A. aerogenes, K. pneumoniae, H. influenzae* and *Shigella*. Resistance to the antibiotic appears slowly. There is a complete crosssusceptibility as well as cross resistance between colistin and polymyxin B.

Absorption, fate and excretion: Colistin is not significantly absorbed orally. It is given parenterally for systemic infections. It is largely excreted unchanged by the kidneys.

Adverse reactions: These occur in a large proportion of patients and include local pain, circumoral and lingual paraesthesiae, nausea, skin rash, pruritus, vertigo, ataxia, nystagmus (**neurotoxicity**) and acute tubular necrosis (**nephrotoxicity**). Other serious toxic effects include partial deafness, neutropenia, hepatotoxicity and transient disturbances of vision and speech. It can cause neuromuscular blockade, which can lead to respiratory failure or apnoea.

Preparations and dosages: Two forms of colistin are available commercially for therapeutic use:

(i) Colistin sulfate: It is a cationic stable formulation for oral or topical use.
(ii) Colistimethate sodium: It is an anionic prodrug given as intravenously/intrathecally/intraventricularly. It gets hydrolyzed to sulfomethylated derivatives and colistin.

The two formulations are not interchangeable and have different pharmacokinetic profile.

Indications:

- **MDR Gram-negative bacilli infections:** Colistimethate is one of the last reserve drugs for variety of multidrug-resistant infections including ventilator associated pneumonia and MDR meningitis caused by pseudomonas, klebsiella, acinetobacter and Eneterobacteriaciae. The IV dose is 4 to 8 mg/kg of colistimethate sodium per day in divided doses. It can also used as a nebuliser (80–160 mg twice daily) to treat resistant psuedomonas pulmonary infections in patients with COPD or cystic fibrosis.
- **Bowel decontamination:** Colistin sulfate is used orally for this purpose.

POLYMYXIN B: Polymyxin is the generic name for a group of closely related polypeptide antibiotics elaborated by various strains of *Bacillus polymyxa*. Of these polymyxin B is used, which has antibacterial spectrum, absorption, metabolism and toxicity similar to those of colistin.

In addition, it binds to the lipopolysaccharide (endotoxins) present in Gram-negative organisms and inactivates it. Polymyxin B does not get absorbed from intact or denuded skin or mucous membranes and hence no systemic ADR are observed on topical use. It is prescribed as spray, cream or powder for local application, for skin, ear and eye infections, especially caused by *P. aeruginosa*.

CYCLOSERINE: This antibiotic, obtained from *Streptomyces orchidaceus* is mainly used for MDR TB (Chapter 52) and in UTI due to resistant *E. coli* (Chapter 50).

SPECTINOMYCIN: This antibiotic derived from *Streptomyces spectabillis* has moderate *in vitro* activity against many Gram-positive and Gram-negative bacteria. *It is bactericidal for both penicillin sensitive and penicillin resistant strains of gonococci.* **Hence, it is mainly used to treat uncomplicated gonorrhoea, as an alternative to penicillin.** It is usually administered in the dose of 2–4 g deep IM as a single dose.

Adverse effects reported include nausea, insomnia and allergic reactions.

FOSFOMYCIN: This antibiotic has **bactericidal** action against many urinary pathogens: *E. coli, Enterococcus faecalis, Klebsiella, P. aeruginosa*, enterobacter, enterococci including vancomycin resistant *Enterococcus faecium* (VREF) and staphylococci. *Its combination with beta-lactam antibiotics, aminoglycosides or fluoroquinolones is synergistic against Gram-positive and Gram-negative organisms.*

Mechanism of action: As a phosphonic acid derivative, fosfomycin inhibits bacterial cell wall synthesis (bactericidal) by inactivating the enzyme, pyruvyl transferase, which is critical in the synthesis of cell walls by bacteria.

Absorption, fate and excretion: It is well absorbed orally and high concentrations are achieved in the urine. Antacids or calcium salts may decrease its absorption. Protein binding is minimal. Half-life is 4–8 h. **It is excreted unchanged in the urine; high urinary levels (100 mcg/mL) persist for more than 48 h.**

Adverse reactions: These are headache, rash, diarrhoea, nausea, vomiting, abdominal discomfort, anorexia, dizziness, drowsiness, fatigue, pruritus. No dosage adjustment is required in hepatic impairment.

Indications: It is currently used in the therapy of uncomplicated UTI in women. It is administered as single dose of 3 g in 100 mL of water. Multiple doses, 3 g every 3 days for 3–7 doses, are used in complicated UTI.

For **extended spectrum penicillins** effective against Gram-negative organisms, see Chapter 44.

MONOBACTAMS

AZTREONAM: This synthetic antibiotic belongs to the class of **beta-lactam** antibiotics, referred to as monobactams. The monobactams are produced by bacteria in the soil. The word monobactam is derived from *mono* (a single ring), *bact* (produced by bacteria) and *am* (a beta lactam). Aztreonam is produced by *Chromobacterium violaceum.*

Like other beta-lactam antibiotics, **it acts on the bacterial cell wall and is bactericidal. It has activity only against aerobic Gram-negative species;** *E. coli, Klebsiella, H. influenzae* and *Proteus* are highly sensitive. Higher concentrations are effective against *Pseudomonas*. *It has negligible activity against anaerobes.*

Its advantages are:

- *Lack of cross allergenicity with penicillins and cephalosporins, except for ceftazidime with which it shares an identical side chain.*
- Resistance to hydrolysis by most of the beta-lactamases.
- Lack of ototoxicity and nephrotoxicity.

Absorption, fate and excretion: It is not absorbed orally and is largely excreted unchanged in urine.

Adverse reactions: Toxicity reported so far is mild and includes skin rashes, GI upset, neutropenia and rarely hepatotoxicity.

Indications:

- **As an alternative to aminoglycosides** in severe infections caused by susceptible **Gram-negative organisms,** e.g. complicated UTI (Chapter 50). It is administered intramuscularly or by IV infusion in the dose of 1–2 g every 8–12 h. Higher doses are used in systemic *P. aeruginosa* infection and in lung infection in patients with cystic fibrosis. Inhalational formulation is also available to treat lung infections.
- **In neonatal Gram-negative infections,** in conjunction with ampicillin
- **In patients who are allergic to penicillin and cephalosporins.**

AMINOGLYCOSIDES BASED ON CLINICAL USE

For topical use in the eye and on the skin	For GI infections and gut sterilisation	For systemic use
Neomycin Framycetin Gentamicin	Neomycin Paromomycin	Streptomycin Gentamicin Kanamycin Amikacin Tobramycin Netilmicin

CHAPTER 46

Antibiotics Effective Against Both Gram-Positive and Gram-Negative Organisms

Learning Objectives

This chapter will enable reader:

1. To enlist antibacterial drugs effective against both Gram-positive and Gram-negative bacterial infections.
2. To explain the mechanism of action of cephalosporins and different mechanisms by which bacteria acquire resistance to them.
3. To compare various generations of cephalosporins (giving examples of drugs in each generation) with respect to antibacterial spectrum, salient pharmacokinetic features, ADR and indications.
4. To explain the mechanism of action, antibacterial spectrum, ADR and indications for carbapenems.
5. To explain the mechanism of action and indications for rifamycins.
6. To outline the drug therapy of bacterial meningitis.

KEY TERMS

Antibiotics which are effective in both Gram-positive and Gram-negative infections are:

- Semisynthetic penicillins, e.g. ampicillin, and carbenicillin (Chapter 44)
- Rifamycins (see section, Rifamycins)
- Cephalosporins
- Carbapenam
- Arbekacin
- Tetracyclines (Chapter 47)
- Chloramphenicol (Chapter 47)

The last two are also effective against certain protozoa and rickettsiae and hence are called 'broad spectrum antibiotics'.

CEPHALOSPORINS

Cephalosporins were isolated from fungus *Cephalosporium acremonium.*

Cephalosporins have 7-amino cephalosporanic acid nucleus (Fig. 46.1), which bears close resemblance to the 6-APA nucleus of penicillins. Structurally, they contain beta-lactam and dihydrothiazine rings. They are water soluble and stable to changes in pH and temperature. The various cephalosporins, however, differ in their antibacterial spectrum and their resistance to beta-lactamases.

Cephamycins are similar to cephalosporins but they are derived from an actinomycete. Examples are cefoxitin and cefotetan.

Antibacterial activity: Cephalosporins possess a wide range of activity against Gram-positive and Gram-negative bacteria.

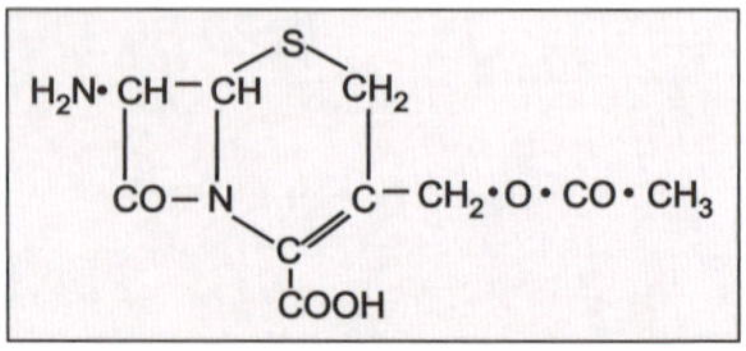

FIG. 46.1 7-amino cephalosporanic acid

The **first-generation cephalosporins** are active against **Gram-positive organisms** like staphylococci (except MRSA), pneumococci and *Group A* and *beta haemolytic streptococci*. They have modest activity against Gram-negative organisms like *Escherichia coli, Proteus mirabilis* and *Klebsiella pneumoniae*.

The **second-generation cephalosporins** have better activity against Gram-negative organisms including *H. influenzae, Moraxella catarrhalis*, indole-positive Proteus spp., and Klebsiella.

However, they are less active than the first-generation cephalosporins against Gram-positive bacteria Cefotetan, cefoxitin and cefmetazole are also effective against *Bacteroides fragilis*.

The **third-generation cephalosporins** have much better activity than earlier generations **against** *Pseudomonas aeruginosa, enterobacteriaceae* and *bacteroides* but are less effective against Gram-positive organisms. However, ceftriaxone and cefotaxime have excellent activity against *Neisseria gonorrhoea*, streptococci and staphylococci, but not against MRSA. Amongst third-generation agents, **ceftazidime and ceftolozane are antipseudomonal having activity against MDR and ESBL** (extended spectrum beta-lactamase)-**producing enterobacteriaceae**.

The **fourth-generation cephalosporins** have similar spectrum-like anti-pseudomoanl agents, whereas their Gram-positive activity is similar to cefotaxime. Cefiderocol is a siderophore cephalosporin. Siderophores are iron chelators. Thus, it binds to free extracellular iron and enters the periplasmic space of bacteria via iron transport channels. Once inside, it dissociates to exert its antibacterial effect. The resultant high concentrations and its stability against beta-lactamases contribute to its efficacy against carbapenem-resistant *enterobacteriaceae*.

The **fifth-generation agents** are the **extended spectrum, anti-MRSA cephalosporins**. Although they are effective against other organisms, their use is restricted to MRSA infections (Table 46.1).

Mechanism of action: Cephalosporins act by inhibiting bacterial cell wall synthesis in a manner similar to penicillins, and are bactericidal.

Resistance to cephalosporins develops slowly and is mediated either by bacterial beta-lactamases or by lack of bacterial permeability to the drug or altered targets, the PBPs. Cross resistance for other beta-lactam agents also occurs. Compared to the first-generation cephalosporins, the second generation *viz.* cefoxitin and cefuroxime, and the third-generation cephalosporins are more resistant to hydrolysis by the beta-lactamases produced by Gram-negative bacteria. *Cefepime, ceftolozane, and cefiderocol are even more resistant than are the third-generation drugs. But they are susceptible to degradation by carbapenemases.*

Absorption, fate and excretion: Cephalosporins are administered either orally or intravenously; IM administration is painful. Their distribution is similar to that of penicillin. There are significant differences among the various cephalosporins regarding their pharmacokinetics.

Amongst cephalosporins, cefotaxime has an active metabolite but the activity is lesser than the parent compound. Cephalosporins are eliminated mainly by renal tubular secretion and *high concentrations are achieved in the urinary tract*. Renal tubular blocking with probenecid increases the plasma levels significantly. The renal excretion is markedly reduced in renal insufficiency. Therefore, their dose should be appropriately reduced in case of renal impairment. Concentration in the bile is similar to that in the plasma. *Unlike other cephalosporins, cefpiramide and cefoperazone are excreted predominantly in the bile.* Ceftriaxone has both renal and nonrenal elimination.

Adverse reactions: In general, cephalosporins are well tolerated.

- **Local reactions:** IM injections are painful and IV injections can cause thrombophlebitis.
- **Allergy:** Maculopapular skin rash, urticaria, anaphylaxis, bronchospasm, fever, serum sickness, eosinophilia, neutropenia, transient splenomegaly and increased SGOT levels.
- **Drug fever:** Cephalosporins are among the common causes of drug fever.
- **Superinfection:** Superinfection with resistant organisms can occur during therapy, generally with broad spectrum third-generation agents.

Table 46.1 Cephalosporins – Bacterial Sensitivity, Pharmacokinetics and Doses

Drug	*S. aureus*	*H. influenzae*	*Enterobacter*	*P. aeruginosa*	*B. fragilis*	Protein Binding (%)	Plasma Half-life (h)	Disposal	Urinary Excretion (%)	Dose
						I Generation				
Oral										
Cefalexin	++	0/+	++	0	0	14	0.9	R	91	0.25–0.50 g q 6–8 h
Cefadroxil	++	0/+	++	0	0	18–20	1.6	R	88	0.5–1.0 g q 12 h
Cefradine	+	++	++	0	0	8–12	1	H/R	90	250–500 mg 6 h
Parenteral										
Cefazolin	+++	+++	++	0	++	80	1.8	R	90	0.25–1.5 g IM/IV q 6–8 h
						II Generation				
Oral										
Cefaclor	++	++	++	0	0	40	0.6	R	60	0.25–0.5 g q 8 h
Cefuroxime axetil	++	+++	+++	0	+	40	1.3	R	50	0.25–0.5 g q 12 h
Cefprozil	++	++	++	0	0	30–45	1–1.4	R	60	500 mg OD
Loracarbef	++	++	++	0	0	25	1	R	80–90	200–400 mg 12 h
Parenteral										
Cefamandole	++	+++	+++	0	+	70	0.8	R	75	0.5–2.0 g IM/IV q 4–8 h
Cefoxitin	++	++	+++	0	+++	75	0.7	R	90	1–2 g IV q 6–8 h
Cefuroxime	++	+++	+++	0	0	35	1.4	R	80	0.75–1.5 g IM/IV q 8 h
Cefotetan	++	++	+++	0	+++	88	3–4.6	H/R	50–80	1–2 g 12 h
Cefmetazole	++	++	+++	0	+++	65–85	1.1–1.5	H/R	85	0.5–1 g IM/IV 12 h
						III Generation				
Oral										
Cefixime	+	+++	+	+	+	67	3.5	H/R	18	100–400 mg/day in 1–2 div. doses
Ceftibuten	0	++	0	0	0	65	2.4	H/R	56	400 mg o.d.
Cefdinir	+	+++	+	+	+	89	1.4–1.5	H/R	13–23	600 mg o.d.
Cefpodoxime proxetil	+	+	++	+++	+++	25	2.2	H/R	30	200–400 mg q 12 h

Table 46.1 Cephalosporins – Bacterial Sensitivity, Pharmacokinetics and Doses—cont'd

Drug	*S. aureus*	*H. influenzae*	*Enterobacter*	*P. aeruginosa*	*B. fragilis*	Protein Binding (%)	Plasma Half-life (h)	Disposal	Urinary Excretion (%)	Dose
Cefditoren pivoxil	++	+	0	0	0	88	1.6	R	12-20	200–400 mg 12 h
Parenteral										
Cefotaxime[a]	+	+++	+++	++	+	40	1.0	H/R	90	1–2 g IM/IV q 8 h
Ceftriaxone[a]	+	+++	+++	++	+	95	8.5	H/R	60	1–2 g IM/IV q 12–24 h
Cefaperazone	+	+++	++	+++	+	90	1.7	H/R	25	1–2 g IM/IV q 8–12 h
Ceftazidime[a]	0	+++	+++	++++	0	21	1.6	R	85	1–2 g IM/IV q 8–12 h
Ceftizoxime[a]	+	+++	+++	++	++	30	1.8	R	80	1–2 g IM/IV q 8–12 h
Ceftolozane (with tazobactam)	0	+++	+++	+++++	+	20	2.5	R	95	1.5 g IV infusion 8 h
IV Generation										
Cefepime[a]	+	+++	+++	+++	0	16-19	2.0	R	80	0.5–1g IM/IV q 8–12 h
Cefpirome	+	+++	+++	++++	0	10	2	R	80	1-2g IM/IV q 12 h
Cefiderocol	0	+++	+++	++++	0	57.8	2.26	R	90.6	2g q IV infusion 8h
V Generation										
Ceftaroline fosamil	++	++	0	0	+	<20	2.6	R	50	600 mg IV 12 h (for community-acquired pneumonia) 600 mg IV every 8 h (for MRSA infections)
Ceftobiprole	++	+++	+++	++++	–	15–20	3	R	80–90	500 mg IV 8 h

q 6–8 h = every 6–8 h. R = renal. H = hepatic.

[a]Good CNS penetration. *Penetration of others is not enough to treat meningitis.*

- **Diarrhoea:** is more common with cefoperazone, which undergoes biliary excretion.
- **Nephrotoxicity:** Large doses can cause nephrotoxicity. It is probably dose related and is potentially reversible on drug withdrawal; it is enhanced by loop diuretics such as furosemide.
- **CNS toxicity:** Signs of cerebral irritation, nystagmus and hallucinations may occur following intrathecal administration. Cefepime, can cause encephalopathy and nonconvulsive status epilepticus in patients with renal damage, preexisting brain injury or in case of overdosing.
- **Haematological toxicity:** Impairment of normal haemostasis may result from hypo-prothrombinaemia and abnormalities in platelet aggregation. Parenteral vitamin K therapy will correct the abnormality and is recommended prophylactically when moxalactam, cefazolin, cefaperazone, cefotetan and cefamandole (with methyltetrazole moiety) are used for prolonged periods. Thrombocytopenia, neutropenia and haemolytic anaemia may rarely occur.
- **Neonatal jaundice:** Ceftriaxone can displace bilirubin from serum albumin in neonates causing jaundice. Hence cefotaxime is preferred. Ceftriaxone has higher biliary concentration and has affinity for calcium and may cause biliary pseudolithiasis.
- **Disulfuram-like reaction:** Cefoperazone, cefamandole and cefotetan cause disulfiram-like effect when ingested with alcohol.

  In patients with a history of allergy to penicillin, the risk of crossreaction to cephalosporin is very low. However, they should be avoided in patients with skin-test reactivity to antigen of penicillin metabolite.

Preparations and dosage: Table 46.1 shows various available cephalosporins.

Indications:: They should not be used routinely for infections that respond to older, cheaper and equally effective antibiotics because bacteria can develop resistance to them and they are expensive. For the general practitioner, it is enough to remember a few guiding principles about using cephalosporins, (Box 46.1.).

- **First-generation cephalosporins: Cefalexin** and **cefadroxil** are useful in treating community-acquired, respiratory and urinary tract infections, and skin and soft tissue infections caused by *S. pyogenes* and methicillin-susceptible *S. aureus.* **Cefazolin** (1 to 2 g IV or IM) is considered the agent of choice for antimicrobial prophylaxis in most surgical procedures because of its activity against most of the skin pathogens that cause infection of surgical wounds. It can be used against systemic infections including endocarditis caused by *S. pyogenes* or methicillin susceptible S. aureus (Chapter 44, Table 44.2). However, *they are not considered the agents of choice for empiric treatment of any serious systemic infections because of the limited spectrum and poor efficacy against beta-lactamase producing organisms.*
- **Second-generation cephalosporins** are useful in the treatment of Gram-negative infections, especially those caused by beta-lactamase producing organisms, including *H. influenzae.* They are used for respiratory tract infections and otitis media. Cefoxitin, cefotetan and loracarbef are used to treat anaerobic infection caused by *B. fragilis* such as peritonitis and pelvic inflammatory disease. They are used prophylactically for patients undergoing abdominal or pelvic surgery.
- **Third-generation cephalosporins: They are drug of choice to treat serious Gram negative infections and have almost replaced the second-generation cephalosporins for this purpose. Often they are combined with gentamicin or amikacin.**

Box 46.1 Guiding Principles for the Use of Cephalosporins

- Cephalosporins are expensive and should not be used where an equally effective, alternative antibiotic is available
- None of them is effective against infections by enterococci *(Strep. fecalis), L. monocytogenes, the atypical respiratory pathogens (Legionella pneumophila, Mycoplasma pneumoniae, Chlamydophila pneumoniae) and Campylobacter jejuni.*)
- None of them is the agent of choice against anaerobic infections e.g. *C. difficile.*
- Except for cefotaxime, ceftriaxone, ceftazidime, ceftizoxime and cefepime, the CNS penetration of cephalosporins is poor. However, these five are the drugs of choice in Gram-negative bacillary meningitis (see Tables 46.1 and 46.2)

Ceftriaxone has sufficiently long half-life to permit once a day administration in gonorrhoea and in Lyme disease. Moreover, this drug as well as cefotaxime are used to treat meningitis and community-acquired pneumonia. Ceftriaxone is an effective alternative to rifampicin for prophylaxis of close contacts of patients with meningococcal meningitis.

The third generation agents are not indicated for routine surgical prophylaxis.

Antipseudomonal cephalosporins (e.g. ceftazidime, ceftolozane) are mainly indicated for the empirical treatment of nosocomial infections, which are aminoglycoside resistant or MDR Gram-negative bacillary systemic infections such as pneumonia, urinary tract infections, and intra-abdominal infections. However, they have variable activity against ESBL producing Enterobacteriaceae.

Ceftazidime is also available in combination with **avibactam**, a beta-lactamase inhibitor. Avibactam restores the activity of ceftazidime against many *Enterobacteriaceae* and therefore the combination can be used against multidrug-resistant Gram-negative infections.

Ceftolozane- tazobactum is used for complicated intra-abdominal infections or complicated UTI including pyelonephritis.

- **Fourth-generation cephalosporins: Cefepime** has properties like those of the third-generation antipseudomonal cephalosporins, but *it is more resistant to some beta-lactamases.* Its main use is in serious Gram-negative infections, including infections of the CNS into which it has excellent penetration.

  Cefpirome also has similar properties and uses as cefepime.

  Cefiderocol is usually reserved for treatment of complicated urinary tract infections, hospital acquired and ventilator-associated bacterial pneumonia caused by extensively drug-resistant (especially carbapenem resistant) Gram-negative pathogens against which few or no options are available.

- **Fifth-generation cephalosporins:** They serve as anti-MRSA cephalosporins. Both, **Ceftaroline fosamil** and **Ceftobiprole medocaril** are prodrugs, which are rapidly converted to active moieties (ceftaroline and ceftobiprole) on IV administration. They are useful for MRSA induced skin and soft-tissue infections and for pneumococcal pneumonia.

  Ceftobiprole is also effective against penicillin-resistant *Streptococcus pneumoniae, Enterococcus faecalis Pseudomonas aeruginosa* and enterococci. It is used to treat community- as well as hospital-acquired pneumonia (excluding ventilator associated pneumonia).

  It is advisable to identify the organisms before using the fourth and fifth generation cephalosporins. They are expensive and should be kept reserved for use in infections resistant to other antibiotics.

CARBAPENEMS

This group of **beta-lactam antibiotics** are obtained by modification of a parent antibiotic thienamycin, derived from *Streptomyces cattleya.* Thienamycin itself is chemically unstable.

Mechanism of action: *Like penicillin, carbapenems act by inhibiting cell wall synthesis*. They are bactericidal with a **wider antibacterial spectrum** than cephalosporins due to their non-susceptibility to beta-lactamases. They are highly active against Gram-negative aerobes including *P. aeruginosa, Enterobacteriaceae*, Gram-positive aerobes and many anaerobes (e.g. *B. fragilis*). They are active against enterococci *except Enterococcus fecium and non–beta-lactamase producing penicillin-resistant strains*. They show activity against staphylococci including penicillinase-producing strains **but not MRSA.** They are also effective against *Listeria*, Nocardia and some species of rapidly growing mycobacteria. *However, they are not active against chlamydia and mycoplasma species.* There is an emerging resistance due to carbapenemase-producing *Enterobacteriaceae*, Pseudomonas and Acinetobacter.

IMIPENEM: It is not absorbed orally and is administered parenterally. It does not penetrate intracellularly. It is hydrolysed by a dehydropeptidase found in the brush border of proximal renal tubule and therefore the concentration of the active drug in the kidney is less than that in the plasma. *It is always combined with* **cilastatin**, *an inhibitor of the renal* *dehydropeptidase, which prevents inactivation of imipenem and prolongs its t1/2.* Cilastatin has no antimicrobial activity.

Adverse reactions: Imipenem has most of the adverse effects of other beta-lactam antibiotics. They include nausea, vomiting, allergic reactions and transient elevation of liver enzymes in the blood. It can cause **pseudomembranous colitis**. In high doses, it can cause convulsions, especially in patients of renal insufficiency and those with CNS lesions. Leucopenia and granulocytopenia have been reported. Cross allergy with penicillin can occur.

Indications: It is used either empirically or as a definitive therapy in:

- Seriously ill and/or hospitalised patients with UTI, lower respiratory infections, abdominal and pelvic infections, musculoskeletal and joint infections due to Gram-positive and Gram-negative aerobes and anaerobes (including all subspecies of *B. fragilis*), which are likely to be resistant or who have received other beta-lactam antibiotics.
- Multidrug resistant Gram-negative infections including those due to pseudomonas

It should be avoided in meningitis because of its epileptogenic properties.

It is administered in the dose of 500–1000 mg (in terms of imipenem) by deep IM injection 6–8 hourly; it can also be administered by IV infusion in the dose of 1–2 g daily, in 3–4 divided doses.

Recently, **imipenem – cilastatin combination is coformulated with relebactam**, a novel beta-lactamase inhibitor, which widens its spectrum against carbapenemase producing organisms including *Enterobacteriaceae*. However, its effects against imipenem resistant Pseudomonas are variable. It is used against Gram-negative pathogens resistant to all other antibiotics. .

Meropenem It is a dimethyl-carbamoyl derivative of thienamycin.

- It is not susceptible to renal dipeptidase and does not require coadministration with cilastatin.
- Its antibacterial spectrum is similar to that of imipenem, but less effective against Gram-positive organisms and more effective against Gram-negative organisms including imipenem-resistant *P. aeruginosa*.
- Its ADR are similar to imipenem. It is less likely to induce seizures and hence if carbapenem is required in the treatment of meningitis, then it can be used.
- Meropenem is used intravenously 1-2 g every 8 h in the treatment of hospital acquired respiratory infections, skin and skin structure infections, intra-abdominal infections, and bacterial meningitis when organisms resistant to penicillin or cephalosprins are suspected.
- It can be coformulated with vaborbactam, a beta-lactamase inhibitor (**in a ratio1:1**) which restores its activity against many carbapenem-resistant *Enterobacteriaceae*. Merpenem- vaborbactam is reserved for treatment of infections caused by multidrug-resistant *Escherichia coli, Klebsiella pneumoniae,* or *Enterobacteriaceae.*

Doripenem has properties and uses similar to those of meropenem.

Ertapenem has a long t½ and hence is used once daily IV It is not active against enterococci, Pseudomonas and Acinetobacter species. However, because of its activity against enterobacteriaceae and anaerobes, it is used in intra-abdominal, pelvic and urinary tract infections.

Feropenem: This is the only **orally effective** carabapenem which is administered in a dose of 150 mg t.i.d.

A carbapenem is the reasonable first choice for empiric monotherapy of serious, complicated, intra-abdominal infections. Other alternatives are: piperacillin – tazobactam; a fluoroquinolone + metronidazole; or tigecycline.

RIFAMYCINS

These are a group of macrocyclic antibiotics derived from a strain of *Streptomyces mediterranei*. **Rifampicin** (Rifampin) is a semisynthetic derivative of rifamycin B, whereas **rifabutin** is a derivative of rifamycin S. Both these drugs bind to DNA-dependent RNA polymerase and inhibit RNA polymerase, thereby suppressing RNA synthesis. They have action against certain Gram-positive and Gram-negative bacteria and mycobacteria. They are mainly used in the treatment of tuberculosis, leprosy, atypical mycobacterial infections and infections with *S. aureus* (Chapters 52 and 53). Rifampicin is used prophylactically for meningococcal infections and *H. influenzae* meningitis.

Rifapentine is a cyclopentyl derivative of rifampicin with a longer half-life ($t½$ = 20h) than rifampicin ($t½$ = 3 h). This permits dosing of rifapentine once or twice weekly. Rifapentine is approved for use in treating active as well as latent tuberculosis (Chapter 52). Rifapentine is an intermediate between rifabutin and rifampicin in activity as an inducer of the CYP450 enzymes.

Rifabutin is a substrate of CYP3A, and therefore if given with CYP3A inhibitors, such as protease inhibitors, a dose reduction is needed.

Rifaximin is an oral, nonabsorbable rifampin derivative, used to treat infective diarrhoeas (Chapter 39).

ARBEKACIN: This semisynthetic **aminoglycoside has broad spectum antibacterial activity.** It is effective against Gram-negative bacteria such as *Escherichia coli*, *Pseudomonas aeruginosa*, *Klebsiella pneumoniae* and *Acinetobacter baumannii*, and also Gram-positive bacteria including MRSA. It causes membrane damage and **binds to both, the 50S and the 30S ribosomal subunits**, resulting in codon misreading and inhibition of translation. It is stable against the aminoglycoside-inactivating enzymes. It is nephrotoxic and ototoxic. It is available as 200mg/4ml to be given as 150–200 mg/day IV infusion in normal saline for 30 min–2 h. Arbekacin is reserved for patients with pneumonia or sepsis caused by MRSA and MDR Gram-negative bacterial infections due to *A. baumannii* and *P. aeruginosa* in combination with beta-lactams like aztreonam.

DRUG THERAPY OF BACTERIAL MENINGITIS

IM 17.13

Acute bacterial meningitis is a medical emergency.

- **In adults** the commonest organisms are *Strep. pneumoniae* and *N. meningitidis,* with Gram-negative bacilli, staphylococci and streptococci following suit.
- **In neonates**, the vast majority of infections are due to Gram-negative bacilli like *E. coli* and streptococci, commonly nonhaemolytic. Listeria infections are also common.
- **In children** (<15 years) the majority of cases are due to *Strep. pneumoniae, N. meningitidis* and *H. influenzae.*

  Staphylococci and Gram-negative meningitis (especially due to *P. aeruginosa*) should be thought of in the setting of head injury, neurosurgical procedures, diabetes mellitus, cirrhosis of the liver and renal failure. To be effective, the appropriate antibiotic treatment must be started immediately, before the full identification of the causative pathogen is available. The treatment should be preferably carried out in an ICU, under expert supervision.

The recommended empirical therapy of severe meningitis is a combination of third or fourth-generation cephalosporin (ceftriaxone/cefotaxime/cefepime) + vancomycin ± ampicillin (all given intravenously). These antibiotics penetrate the CSF adequately and should be administered parenterally in high doses. In patients with otitis, sinusitis and mastoditis, Gram-negative anaerobes should be suspected and metronidazole is added to the above-mentioned empirical regimen.

In the neonate, the preferred empirical regimen is cefotaxime + ampicillin with or without gentamicin. In children the initial treatment should be with a third-generation cephalosporin with vancomycin or with ampicillin + chloramphenicol.

If nosocomial infection is suspected or neutropenia is present, then a triple regime consisting of ceftazidime/cefepime/meropenem + vancomycin + ampicillin is preferred.

After detecting the causative organisms, specific therapy can be started as mentioned in Table 46.2.

Table 46.2 Drug Therapy of Specific Forms of Bacterial Meningitis (Adult Doses)

Organism	Preferred Regimen	Other Regimens
Meningococci[a]		
Penicillin sensitive	a. Penicillin G 4 million units IV q 4 h for 7 days.[b] After the patient becomes afebrile, ampicillin (2 g q 4 h) b. Amoxicillin/ampicillin 2 g q 4 h	Cefotaxime 2 g IV q 6 h/ceftriaxone 2 g IV q 12 h with or without ampicillin In patients allergic to penicillin, chloramphenicol 4–6 g IV q 6 h for 7 days
Penicillin resistant	Cefotaxime/ceftriaxone	Cefepime 2 g q 8 h/meropenem 1 g IV q 8 h/chloramphenicol
Cephalosporin resistant	Vancomycin 1 g q 12 h + third generation cephalosporins	
Pneumococci		
Penicillin sensitive and resistant	Same as meningococcal meningitis	
Cephalosporin resistant	Vancomycin + third-generation cephalosporins for 10–14 days	If highly resistant, Vancomycin + third-generation cephalosporins + rifampicin 600 mg/day. Moxifloxacin in nonresponders
H. influenzae		
Beta-lactamase negative	Ampicillin-sulbactam 4 g q 8 h for 7 days	Cefotaxime/ceftriaxone/cefepime/chloramphenicol/aztreonam 50 mg/kg IM q 8 h for 10–14 days
Beta-lactamase positive	Cefotaxime/ceftriaxone	Cefepime/chloramphenicol/aztreonam
Beta-lactamase negative and ampicillin resistant	Meropenem 1 g IV q 8 h	Fluoroquinolone
Enterococci	Penicillin G as above + gentamicin 1 mg/kg IV q 8 h for 14–21 days	Vancomycin + gentamicin. If resistant, quinpristin/dalfopristin 7.5 mg/kg IV over 1 h, q 8 h or tigecycline 100 mg IV infusion followed by 50 mg IV infusion q 12 h
Staphylococcus aureus		
Methicillin sensitive	Nafcillin or oxacillin 2 g IV q 4 h for 14 days	Vancomycin/linezolid 600 mg IV q 12 h/daptomycin 6 mg/kg IV infusion q 24 h
Methicillin resistant	Vancomycin ± rifampicin	Cotrimoxazole/linezolid/daptomycin
Gram-negative bacilli other than P. aeruginosa	Cefotaxime/ceftriaxone for 21 days	Cotrimoxazole 10–20 mg/kg IV q 12 h/(ampicillin-sulbactam)/meropenem/aztreonam
P. aeruginosa	Ceftazidime 2 g IV q 8 h/cefepime for 21 days	Aztreonam/meropenem
Bacterioides fragilis and Fusobacterium spp.	Metronidazole 0. 5 g q 6 h for 7 days	
Listeria monocytogenes	Amoxicillin/ampicillin for 3 weeks In critically ill, add gentamicin	In patients allergic to penicillin, cotrimoxazole 6 hourly

Note: **Penicillin should not be injected intrathecally.**

[a]Close contacts and family members should receive prophylaxis with rifampicin 600 mg orally b.i.d. for 2 days; alternatively, ceftriaxone 250 mg single IM dose or ofloxacin 400 mg single oral dose may be used. These drugs, in short courses, achieve long-term (3–4 weeks) eradication of meningococci from the pharynx. The index case should also be treated with rifampicin before discharge.

[b]2 g IV q 4 h = 2 g intravenously every 4 h.

Dexamethasone, 10 mg IV is used as adjunctive therapy 20 min before, or at least concurrently with the first dose of antibiotics and then repeated every 6 h for 4–5 days, to decrease cytokine-induced inflammation and neurological morbidity. However, it may not be helpful for patients presenting late with advanced disease, malnourishment, HIV coinfection and those pretreated with antibiotic.

CEPHALOSPORINS

I Generation

Oral
- Cefalexin
- Cefadroxil
- Cefradine

Parenteral
- Cefazolin

II Generation

Oral
- Cefaclor
- Cefuroxime axetil
- Cefprozil
- Loracarbef

Parenteral
- Cefamandole
- Cefoxitin
- Cefuroxime
- Cefotetan
- Cefmetazole

III Generation

Oral
- Cefixime
- Ceftibuten
- Cefdinir
- Cefpodoxime proxetil
- Cefditoren pivoxil

Parenteral
- Cefotaxime
- Ceftriaxone
- Cefaperazone
- Ceftazidime
- Ceftizoxime
- Ceftolozane (with tazobactam)

IV Generation
- Cefepime
- Cefpirome
- Cefiderocol

V Generation
- Ceftaroline fosamil
- Ceftobiprole

CHAPTER 47

Tetracyclines and Chloramphenicol

Learning Objectives

This chapter will enable the reader:

1. To explain the mechanism of action of tetracyclines and different mechanisms by which bacteria acquire resistance to them.
2. To state the antibacterial spectrum, salient pharmacokinetic features, ADR, drug interactions and indications for tetracyclines used in clinical practice.
3. To mention the salient pharmacokinetic features, ADR and indications for semisynthetic tetracyclines.
4. To describe the mechanism of action, advantages and limitations of chloramphenicol.
5. To outline the treatment of typhoid fever.
6. To outline the management of chronic bronchitis.

KEY TERMS

broad spectrum antibiotic, p. 689
superinfection, p. 690
doxycycline, p. 692
cholera, p. 692
chloramphenicol, p. 694
bone marrow toxicity, p. 695
typhoid fever, p. 696
chronic bronchitis, p. 697

Systematic screening of a multitude of soil microorganisms for potential antibiotic activity resulted in the discovery of tetracyclines. The first member chlortetracycline was isolated from *Streptomyces aureofaciens*, followed by oxytetracycline derived from *Streptomyces rimosus* and tetracycline was prepared synthetically.

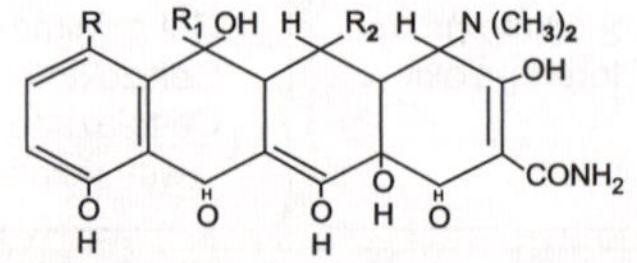

	R=	R_1=	R_2=
TETRACYCLINE	H	CH_3	H
CHLORTETRACYCLINE	Cl	CH_3	H
OXYTETRACYCLINE	H	CH_3	OH
DEMETHYLCHLORTETRA-CYCLINE	Cl	H	H

FIG. 47.1 Basic structure of tetracyclines.

TETRACYCLINES

The tetracyclines are naphthacene derivatives, made up by fusion of four partially unsaturated cyclohexane radicals and hence the name tetracyclines (Fig. 47.1). Tetracyclines are more stable at acid pH. They are:

- Orally active
- Broad spectrum
- Bacteriodstatic
- Protein synthesis inhibitors

Classification of Tetracyclines

I. **Group I (half life : 6-9 hours):** Chlortetracycline, oxytetracycline, tetracycline
II. **Group II (half life: 16-18 hours):** Demeclocycline, methacycline
III. **Group III (half life: 18-24 hours):** Doxycycline, minocycline
IV. **Group IV:** Newer tetracyclines, e.g. tigecycline, eravacycline, omadacycline

Antibacterial spectrum: Various tetracyclines have similar antibacterial spectrum. **They are bacteriostatic.**

The Gram-positive and Gram-negative organisms inhibited by tetracyclines include methicillin-sensitive and -resistant *S. aureus*, some strains of alpha haemolytic streptococci, *H. influenzae, H. ducreyi, Brucella,*

Vibrio cholerae, Donovania granulomatis, B. anthracis, C. jejuni, H. pylori, F. tularensis, Y. pestis, Fusobacterium, Pasteurella multocida, Listeria monocytogenes and some atypical mycobacteria. They have poor activity against Proteus and Pseudomonas. In addition to a number of Gram-positive and Gram-negative organisms, they are highly effective against certain actinomyces, rickettsiae and chlamydia organisms.

Other organisms which respond satisfactorily are *Mycoplasma pneumoniae*, Legionella and spirochetes such as *Leptospira icterohaemorrhagiae*, *Borrelia recurrentis, Borrelia burgdorferi* (*Lyme disease*) *and T. pallidum*. Amongst the protozoa, it has action against *E. histolytica* and plasmodia. Hence they are termed as **broad spectrum antibiotics**.

Mechanism of action: The susceptible bacteria accumulate the antibiotic by an active transport system. Tetracyclines bind to 30S ribosomes and interfere with protein synthesis by preventing addition of amino acids to the growing peptide chain (Fig. 47.2). Tetracyclines also chelate calcium and magnesium ions, which may contribute to its action.

Tetracycline resistance: Resistance may occur through several mechanisms and can be passed from one organism to another by transfer of plasmids. In resistant organisms, accumulation of the drug is absent due to either decreased influx or increased efflux by active transport protein pump. Tigecycline is a poor substrate for this pump. Bacteria form proteins/enzymes that interfere with binding to ribosomes or displace tetracycline from its site of action or inactivate the drug. Partial cross resistance occurs between tetracyclines and chloramphenicol.

Absorption, fate and excretion: The absorption of oral tetracyclines is variable but adequate (Table 47.1). The tetracyclines form insoluble complexes by chelation with calcium, magnesium and aluminium, and hence substances like milk that contain calcium, antacids and sucralfate reduce their absorption. Ingestion of food and iron also interferes with their absorption. Hence tetracyclines should be taken ½ h before or 2 h after food.

The tetracyclines are mainly absorbed from the duodenum and the upper small intestine. Absorption is better on empty stomach. With larger doses, proportionately more of the drug escapes absorption and may cause gastrointestinal disturbances.

After oral administration of a single therapeutic dose

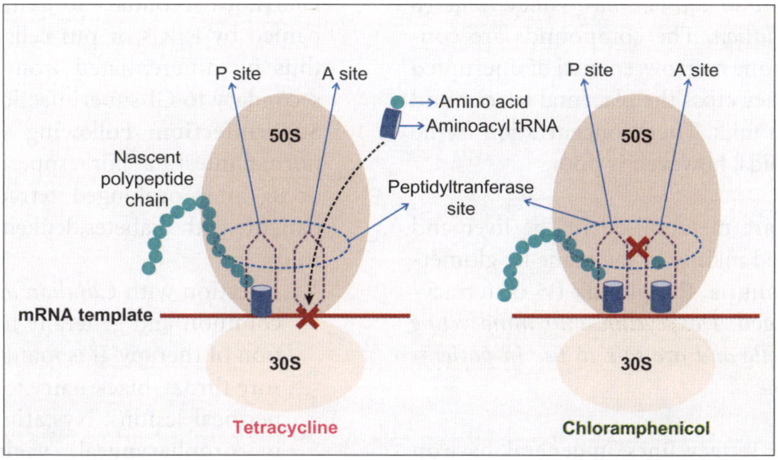

FIG. 47.2 Mechanism of action of tetracyclines and chloramphenicol. Messenger RNA (mRNA) attaches to the 30S subunit of bacterial ribosomal RNA. The P (peptidyl) site of 50S ribosomal RNA subunit contains the nascent polypeptide chain; normally the aminoacyl tRNA carrying the next amino acid to be added to the chain moves into the A (acceptor) site. Tetracyclines inhibit bacterial protein synthesis by binding to the 30S subunit and blocking binding of the amino acid containing end of the aminoacyl tRNA to the A site. Chloramphenicol binds to 50S ribosomal subunit at the peptidyltransferase site and inhibits the peptide bond formation between the growing peptide chain and new amino acid (transpeptidation reaction). The red cross indicates site of action of the drugs.

Table 47.1 Properties of Commonly Used Tetracyclines

	Tetracycline	Oxytetracycline	Doxycycline	Minocycline	Tigecycline
Stability	Less	Less	More	More	More
Absorption	77%	58%	> 90%	> 90 %	poor, hence given IV
Plasma protein binding	65%	35%	90%	76%	> 80%
Urinary recovery	60%	70%	< 40%	6%	33%
CSF level	+	+	++	+++	+
Half-life (h)	8	9	16–22	14–22	36–42
Effect on bone	+++	+++	++	+	–
Relative *in vitro* activity[a]	100	80	110	200[b]	250[b]
Usual oral dose	250–500 mg 6–8 hourly		200 mg loading 100 mg daily	100 mg b.i.d.	100 mg IV loading and then 50 mg 12 h

–, Nil; +, low/less; ++, moderate; +++, high.
[a]Against *S. aureus*.
[b]Active against organisms resistant to other tetracyclines.

of tetracycline and oxytetracycline, peak plasma level is reached within 3–4 h. They are usually administered at 6 hourly intervals in order to maintain their therapeutic plasma concentration. Oxytetracycline and tetracycline, given intramuscularly, produce peak plasma levels within 1 h, and adequate levels are maintained for 12 h.

The tetracyclines are widely distributed in the body similar to that of penicillin. Concentrations in the bile are 5–20 times those in the plasma as they undergo enterohepatic circulation. The compounds are concentrated in liver, bone marrow, enamel of unerupted teeth and lungs. They cross the placental barrier and are also secreted in milk. Their concentration in the CSF and ocular fluids, however, is poor.

The tetracyclines are metabolised in the liver and metabolites excreted mainly in the urine by glomerular filtration. In anuria, the plasma t½ of tetracyclines gets prolonged. *Doxycycline and minocycline are eliminated in bile and are safe to use in patients with renal impairment.*

Adverse reactions: Tetracyclines, in general, have an acceptable toxicity. The adverse effects are as follows:

- **Allergy:** Skin rashes may develop mainly on topical application of these agents. Severe allergic reactions, however, are rare.
  Photosensitivity is manifested by marked erythema and even vesicular exanthema. A brown-black discolouration and loosening of nails may also occur. It is common with demeclocycline and doxycycline.
- **GI tract:** Nausea, vomiting, epigastric distress and loose stools are relatively common. Nausea and vomiting may be prevented by taking these drugs after meals. Mild diarrhoea appears to be dose-dependent and is more common following daily doses over 2 g.
  Diarrhoea secondary to irritation is not accompanied by RBCs or pus cells in faeces, and can thus be differentiated from serious diarrhoea secondary to GI superinfection.
- **Superinfection:** Following suppression of the normal intestinal flora, superinfection is liable to occur after prolonged tetracycline therapy, in patients with diabetes, leukemia or those on steroids.
  i. Infection with *Candida albicans* is especially common and generally limited to the duration of therapy. It is manifested as diarrhoea, sore throat, black hairy tongue, vaginitis and perineal lesions. Nystatin is effective locally in oropharyngeal, vaginal and perineal lesions.
  ii. Superinfection with resistant *S. aureus* occurs more frequently in hospitalised patients and causes **staphylococcal enteritis**. Immediate stoppage of tetracyclines, institution of antistaphylococcal therapy and correction of

dehydration and electrolyte imbalance are recommended.

iii. **Pseudomembranous colitis** characterised by profuse diarrhoea and fever may occur due to superinfection with *Clostridium difficile.* The stools contain shreds of mucous membrane and blood (also see Chapter 44).

- **Teeth and bones:** Tetracyclines chelate calcium, forming a tetracycline-orthophosphate complex and are deposited in bones and teeth, especially in children. **They should be avoided in infants and in children below 8 years.**

  Administration of these antibiotics to pregnant women may lead to yellow staining of the teeth of the infants, defective formation of enamel and hypoplasia of the teeth. Pigmentation of permanent teeth and increased risk of caries may occur in children. **Even a short course given after the 14th week of pregnancy can be damaging.**

  Tetracyclines may reduce the foetal linear bone growth. They are also deposited in nails.
- **Antianabolic effect:** Since tetracyclines inhibit protein synthesis, their prolonged use produces an antianabolic effect and weight loss.
- **Liver:** Fatal hepatic dysfunction with pancreatitis may occur with large doses of tetracyclines over short periods, particularly by IV route. Such patients develop jaundice, azotemia and coma. **Tetracyclines should be avoided in pregnancy in the interest of both mother and fetus.**
- **Kidney:** In patients with significant renal impairment, tetracyclines may cause an aggravation of azotemia due to its **antianabolic effect**.

  A reversible **'Fanconi-like' syndrome**, may develop after ingestion of outdated tetracycline capsules. It is attributed to a degradation product, epianhydrotetracycline.
- **Benign intracranial hypertension:** Some patients may develop pseudomotor cerebri (false brain tumour) manifesting as increased intracranial pressure.
- **Miscellaneous:** IV tetracyclines may cause local thrombosis. They may interfere with blood coagulation. This effect is probably secondary to chelation of calcium.

  Thrombocytopenia, steatorrhoea and deficiency of vitamin K may occur after prolonged tetracycline therapy.

Box 47.1 Drug Interactions of Tetracyclines

- ***Decreased bioavailability of tetracyclines:*** Divalent or trivalent cations (Ca^{++}, Mg^{++}, Fe^{++}, Zn^{++}, Al^{+++}); milk and milk products; antacids, vitamin or mineral products and cathartics containing divalent or trivalent cations; bismuth subsalicylate
- ***Decreased half-life of tetracyclines:*** Carbamazepine; phenytoin; barbiturates; chronic ethanol ingestion
- ***Interference with the bactericidal action of penicillin***
- ***Potentiation of the anticoagulant action of coumarin drugs,*** e.g. warfarin

Drug interactions: See Box 47.1.

Preparations and dosage:

i. *For fetal oral administration*: Oxytetracycline hydrochloride, tetracycline hydrochloride capsules or tablets 250 mg. The dose varies between 1 and 2 g per day in 3–4 divided doses.

ii. *For parenteral administration*: Oxytetracycline and tetracycline are available for IM and IV administration. The usual IM dose is 100 mg at 8 hourly intervals. The total daily IV dose of oxytetracycline and tetracycline for most acute infections in adults is 1–2 g in two equal doses at 12 hourly intervals. *The tetracyclines are never administered intrathecally.*

iii. Ophthalmic ointments and eye drops containing tetracyclines (0.5%–1%).

iv. Topical skin preparations are available but they should be used with precaution due to their propensity to cause phototoxicity.

SEMISYNTHETIC TETRACYCLINES

DEMECLOCYCLINE (Demethylchlortetracycline): As the drug is slowly excreted by kidneys the therapeutic blood levels are maintained for at least 24 h after cessation of treatment. Concentration in the CSF is poor.

It is available as 150 mg and 300 mg capsules and as a syrup. The usual adult dose is 600 mg daily in two or three divided doses.

Demeclocycline is useful in the **treatment of chronic hyponatremia due to Syndrome of Inappropriate Antidiuretic Hormone secretion (SIADH).** The drug produces unresponsiveness to ADH. Its action is dose-dependent and reversible. However, now vasopressin antagonists are preferred.

Methacycline has activity similar to demethyl-chlortetracycline. It gives higher and more sustained blood levels. **Lymecycline** is a tetracycline made soluble by combining it with the amino acid lysine. It is claimed to be almost completely absorbed on oral administration.

DOXYCYCLINE: It is well absorbed from the gut and is more slowly excreted than other tetracyclines (Table 47.1). **With a single dose of 500 mg serum level of 1 mcg/mL has been reported to be present up to 4 days.** It is metabolised in the liver and excreted in faeces as an inactive conjugate. *Its plasma half-life is not significantly affected by renal insufficiency and the drug does not aggravate azotemia.*

Doxycycline has similar toxicity as the conventional tetracyclines. However, **it has many advantages**. These are as follows:

- **Better GI absorption** and hence smaller doses
- **Longer half-life** (t½ 16 h), permitting less frequent dosing schedule
- **Higher lipid solubility**, leading to higher tissue concentrations
- **Elimination independent of renal function**; hence, it can be used in patients with impaired renal function
- **Less propensity to cause diarrhoea.**
- **Can be administered intravenously.**

Preparations and dosage:

The drug is available in 100 mg capsules. The recommended dose in adults is 200 mg (single dose) on day one and then 100 mg once a day. In severe infections, a dose of 100 mg every 12 h is recommended. For children, a dose of 3–4 mg/kg daily is given initially in two divided doses. In severe infections, a larger dose may be given. Subsequently, a maintenance dose of 1–2 mg per kg is administered either as a single dose or divided into two doses. Doxycycline can also be given intravenously by infusion.

MINOCYCLINE: This tetracycline is absorbed completely from the GI tract and exhibits greater antibacterial activity than older tetracyclines. *It is retained in fat; hence, it is long acting with t½ of 16 h.* It is metabolised in the liver and excreted in bile and faeces. The drug has better tissue penetration. Minocycline achieves satisfactory levels in the CNS. **It is effective against tetracycline-resistant** *S. aureus, S. pyogenes,* **Enterococci, Meningococci and** *E. coli* and exhibits a significant activity against Acinetobacter, nocardia, asteroides and **nontuberculous mycobacteria**.

It is used in prophylaxis of meningococcal meningitis. It causes reversible vestibular toxicity such as vertigo, dizziness, ataxia, nausea and vomiting. The dose is 100 mg b.i.d.

Indications for tetracyclines: Although tetracyclines are effective against a wide range of organisms, they are not to be preferred routinely against the organisms that are highly sensitive to other equally safe and bactericidal agents like penicillin, cotrimoxazole and fluoroquinolones. **Doxycycline is commonly used and is a first line drug for:**

- **Rickettsial infections:** They are very effective in rickettsial infections like murine, epidemic and scrub typhus, Q fever and Rocky mountain spotted fever. Relapses are rare. Doxycycline is used as 200 mg/day in two divided doses for seven days. The alternative is azithromycin (Chapter 44). In complicated cases doxycycline is used as intravenous infusion initially followed by oral treatment for 7-15 days.
- **Primary atypical pneumonia:** This condition, caused by *Mycoplasma pneumoniae*, responds satisfactorily to doxycycline.
- **Cholera:** Cholera is caused by strains of Gram-negative *Vibrio cholerae* and is characterised by severe diarrhoea, leading to rapid dehydration, and shock. *Hence, rapid rehydration is the mainstay of treatment*, for which WHO ORS formulation is preferred (Chapter 39). Patients in shock will need initially IV fluids and correction of acidosis with IV Ringer lactate and oral potassium supplements.

  The organisms respond to a single oral dose of **doxycycline** 300 mg or **ciprofloxacin** 1 g as a single dose. For children, oral doxycycline 2–4 mg/kg as

Box 47.2 Drugs Used in Chlamydial Infections IM 3.12, IM 3.13

- Doxycycline/tetracycline
- Erythromycin, azithromycin
- Ofloxacin
- Sulphonamides

a single dose is used; other alternatives are azithromycin 20 mg/kg (max 1 g) or ciprofloxacin 20 mg/kg (max 1 g) as single oral dose. In patients with multidrug-resistant cholera, **azithromycin** 1 g as a single dose is reported to be highly effective.

- **Chlamydia infections:** *Chlamydia trachomatis* causes trachoma, nongonococcal urethritis (NGU), cervicitis, epididymitis, inclusion conjunctivitis, lymphogranuloma venereum and infant pneumonia (Chapter 51). Box 47.2 lists the drugs used in chlamydial infections.
  Use of tetracyclines in **lymphogranuloma venereum** and NGU is discussed in Chapter 51.
  In **trachoma, doxycycline** 100 mg b.i.d. for 7 days is used. Though **azithromycin** 1 g single oral dose is preferred by some, 7 day course is more effective. In endemic areas it may be used as ointment, applied twice daily on every alternate day for 6 months. In children, **azithromycin** given as single dose is preferred.
- **Lyme's disease:** Doxycycline is the drug of choice for this and other infections due to Borrelia.

The other indications include:

- **Sexually transmitted diseases:** They are now less preferred due to resistance (Chapter 51).
  Patients with primary, secondary, or latent syphilis, who are allergic to penicillin, can be treated with doxycycline for 2 weeks (Chapter 51). But tetracyclines should not be used for neurosyphilis.
- ***H. pylori infection:*** See Chapter 41.
- **Bacillary infections:** Although tetracyclines are effective in tularemia, streptomycin is usually preferred. They can also be used in **infections due to** *H. influenzae* but either ampicillin or chloramphenicol is preferred.
- **Brucellosis:** In combination with rifampicin or streptomycin, doxycycline is used for acute and chronic infections caused by Brucella (Chapter 45).
- **Plague:** See Chapter 45.
- **Acne vulgaris:** Doxycycline in low dose, 25 mg orally twice a day is used. Chapter 69.
- **Prophylaxis of drug-resistant malaria:** See Chapter 54.
- **Leptospirosis:** Mild cases respond to doxycycline 100 mg b.i.d. or ampicillin 500–750 mg q.i.d. Severe cases need IV penicillin G 1.5 million units q.i.d. or IV ampicillin 1 g q.i.d. or ceftriaxone 1 g o.d. Doxycycline 200 mg/week appears to be adequate for prophylaxis.
- **Atypical mycobacterial infections:** Tetracyclines can be used for these infections including swimming pool granuloma caused by *Mycobacterium marinum*.
- **Miscellaneous:** Other infections which respond to tetracyclines include anthrax, actinomycosis and yaws, but penicillin is preferred. Doxycycline is used in the treatment of tropical sprue, blind loop syndrome, bronchitis and community acquired pneumonia, skin and soft-tissue infections caused by MRSA and various periodontal infections. It is also indicated for prevention or treatment of anthrax.

TIGECYCLINE is a glycylcycline, a derivative of minocycline with a broad spectrum.

Mechanism of action: It is similar to that of other tetracyclines. But it has less affinity for efflux pump and more affinity towards ribosome target site. Hence it is highly effective against MRSA, VRSA and vancomycin-resistant enterococci (VRE), penicillin-resistant staphylococci, *Streptococcus pneumoniae* and many Gram-negative bacilli resistant to older tetracyclines. It is also effective against Gram-positive and -negative anaerobes, and rapidly growing mycobacteria.

Absorption, fate and excretion: Given intravenously, it has a $t½$ of 42 h. About 80% is excreted unchanged via the biliary route into the faeces and 20% in urine. Dose adjustment is needed in hepatic failure.

Adverse reactions: It is generally well tolerated but may cause nausea and vomiting. *C. difficile*–associated diarrhoea and pancreatitis have been reported. It should not be used in children and pregnant women.

Indications:

- Life-threatening skin and soft tissue infection

- Complicated intra-abdominal infections
- Community acquired pneumonia
- Other MDR infections

Eravacycline, a fluorocycline and **omadacycline**, a aminomethylcycline are the newer tetracycline congeners with broad-spectrum activity and are effective against tetracycline-resistant organisms. Their spectrum is similar to that of tigecycline.

Eravacycline is available as parenteral formulation to be administered intravenously in a dose of 1 mg/kg every 12 h. It undergoes hepatic metabolism to some extent and hence frequency adjustment (every 24 h) is needed in hepatic diseases.

Oral absorption of omadacycline is poor (33%) and food further interferes with it. Hence it should be administered 2h before or 4 h after food intake as a 450 mg loading dose for 2 days followed by 300 mg/day. It can be given IV as 200 mg on first day followed by 100mg/day. It is eliminated unchanged through bile and kidney.

CHLORAMPHENICOL

Chloramphenicol is a broad spectrum antibiotic derived originally from *Streptomyces venezuelae.* The commercial preparation, however, is entirely synthetic. It is a derivative of dichloroacetic acid, containing a nitrobenzene moiety (Fig. 47.3). Compared to tetracyclines, it is better diffusible in tissues, causes less GI disturbances and can be used for similar indications; but because of its bone marrow toxicity, its use is now restricted to life threatening conditions wherein safer antibiotics cannot be used because of resistance or allergy.

Antibacterial activity: The antibacterial spectrum of chloramphenicol is **similar to that of tetracyclines.** It is **bacteriostatic** but can be *bactericidal against common meningeal pathogens – H. influenzae, N. meningitidis and S. pneumoniae. S. typhi, H. influenzae,* and *B. pertussis* are more susceptible to chloramphenicol than tetracycline. The bacteroides, some staphylococci resistant to penicillin, a few strains of streptococci, including multidrug-resistant *E. faecium, and V. cholerae* are also inhibited. Pseudomonas are, however, resistant. It is effective against rickettsiae, chlamydiae of the psittacosis-lymphogranuloma group and *Mycoplasma pneumoniae.*

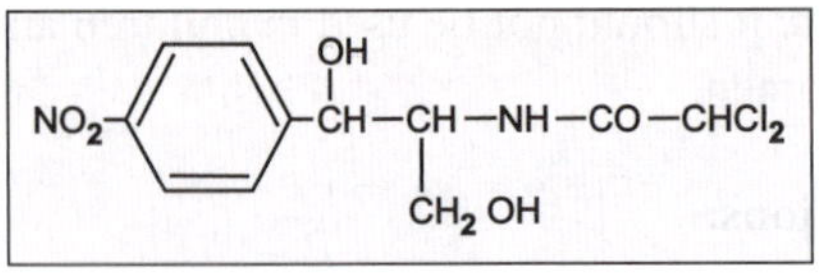

FIG. 47.3 Chloramphenicol.

Mechanism of action: Chloramphenicol readily penetrates into the bacterial cell by facilitated diffusion and **acts by interfering with the synthesis of bacterial proteins by binding to 50S ribosomes and preventing transpeptidation** (Fig. 47.2). It can inhibit mitochondrial protein synthesis of erythropoietic cells of the host.

Resistance develops slowly. However, resistant strains of *E. coli,* Salmonella, Shigella and other Gram-negative bacteria have been reported. Resistance is usually due to plasmid–encoded acetyltransferase that inactivates the drug. It can also occur due to ribosomal mutation or decreased permeability into the cell.

Absorption, fate and excretion: Unlike tetracyclines, **chloramphenicol is completely absorbed from the gut and is better diffusible into the various tissues including brain.** The CNS concentrations are equal to those in serum. *Blood levels of chloramphenicol after oral administration are superior to those after IM administration. Being poorly water soluble, its absorption depends to a great extent on particle size.*

Given orally, peak plasma levels are reached within 2 h; it has a plasma t½ of 1½–3½ h. About 60% of plasma chloramphenicol is bound to protein.

Chloramphenicol palmitate, the paediatric oral preparation, is a prodrug. It is slowly hydrolysed by pancreatic lipases to release free chloramphenicol for absorption. Chloramphenicol sodium succinate, the parenteral preparation, is also a prodrug which undergoes hydrolysis by esterases to liberate chloramphenicol. In neonates, poor renal function can increase the levels of the chloramphenicol but poor esterase activity prolongs time to reach peak levels.

Chloramphenicol is largely inactivated by hepatic conjugation to glucuronide and excreted by the kidney. *Hence, chloramphenicol can be relatively safely administered in patients with renal impairment but not in those with hepatic insufficiency.*

Adverse reactions:

- **Allergy:** This is relatively uncommon. However, skin rashes, drug fever, angioneurotic oedema, exfoliative dermatitis, atrophic glossitis and, Jarisch–Herxheimer reaction have been reported.
- **Bone marrow toxicity:** Aplastic anaemia, reported in all age groups, is an idiosyncratic reaction; its incidence is between 1:10,000 and 1:100,000.
  Many patients may develop less pronounced haemopoietic changes (leucopenia, anaemia or thrombocytopenia) which are dose dependent and reversible. This is due to inhibition of mitochondrial protein synthesis in erythroid precursors. Pancytopenia occurs more commonly after prolonged therapy and with large doses. Conversion of the nitro group to a toxic intermediate by intestinal bacteria is one of the contributory factors.
  It must be noted that *the risk of this complication should not prevent the use of chloramphenicol in life-threatening situations.*
- **Grey baby syndrome:** This complication with high mortality is observed in neonates and infants. The initial manifestations are seen 2-9 days after starting the therapy and include refusal to suck vomiting, lethargy, anorexia, abdominal distension and shallow irregular respiration. Later, the condition worsens, leading to hypothermia, flaccidity, ashen grey cyanosis and shock. The factors incriminated are:
  - Deficient conjugation of chloramphenicol in the liver due to a low level of hepatic glucoronyl transferase enzyme activity.
  - Immaturity of the renal tubules leading to impairment of excretion of the free form.
- **Liver toxicity:** Liver damage with chloramphenicol is rare.
- **CNS toxicity:** It may cause headache, peripheral neuritis, mental confusion, depression and delirium. Optic neuritis, probably secondary to drug induced pyridoxine deficiency, may occur rarely. The drug may also affect the cochlear function if used locally, for ear infections.
- **Miscellaneous:** A 'typhoid shock' syndrome may develop in patients having typhoid fever, on administration of a large loading dose. It is attributed to excessive release of endotoxin from the microorganisms.

Drug interactions: It inhibits hepatic microsomal enzymes that metabolise drugs and prolong their t½, whereas microsomal enzyme inducers reduce the concentration of chloramphenicol to subtherapeutic levels.

Preparations and dosage:

i. Chloramphenicol 250 mg capsules. Dose: adults, 1–3 g daily in divided doses. For children, 25–50 mg/kg daily in divided doses.
ii. Chloramphenicol palmitate oral suspension: 125 mg of chloramphenicol base in each 5 mL. The preparation is tasteless and, therefore, is preferred in children.
iii. Chloramphenicol monostearoylglycolate used in the form of a dry syrup.
iv. Chloramphenicol sodium succinate has a high aqueous solubility and is administered SC, IM or IV slow infusion. The doses are similar to those given orally. *Absorption from SC and IM sites is unreliable.*
v. Chloramphenicol 1% ophthalmic ointment, as applicaps and as eye drops 0.5%.

Indications:

- **Rickettsial infections**: Though tetracyclines are preferred, chloramphenicol can be substituted for tetracyclines. in patients allergic to tetracyclines, in pregnant women, and in children less than 8 years of age, chloramphenicol is an alternative therapy. It is used in the dose of 50 mg/kg per day divided into 6-h intervals till the patient is afebrile for 24-48 h.
- **Meningitis:** It is an alternative drug for meningitis caused by H. influenzae, N. meningitidis, and S. pneumoniae (Chapter 46).
- **Plague:** It is used in combination with streptomycin in meningitic plague (Chapter 45).
- **Typhoid fever:** Refer section on Pharmacotherapy of typhoid fever..
- **Ophthalmic infections:** Because of its satisfactory penetration into the intraocular fluid on local and

systemic administration, chloramphenicol is employed in the treatment of ocular infections.

- **Miscellaneous:** It is also used in chronic otorrhea, particularly due to Gram-negative organisms. Though effective in brucellosis, rifampicin is preferred.

PHARMACOTHERAPY OF TYPHOID FEVER

Typhoid fever is caused by *S. typhi*. The organisms attack the intestinal mucosa (mainly terminal ileum) and invade the regional lymph nodes and other tissues. Ideally, the antibiotic should be selected based on antibiotic sensitivity test. However, such facility is not available in a large part of the world where the disease pattern is endemic. **Drugs effective in treating typhoid fever are listed in Box 47.3.**

Ciprofloxacin with its bactericidal action, shorter duration of therapy (5–7 days) and acceptable toxicity is preferred. With the dose of 500 mg b.i.d.,the cure rate is almost 98% with relapse rate and faecal carrier state of 3% if organisms are susceptible. Short course of **ofloxacin** is equally useful. The clinical improvement is seen within 48–72 h. Temperature returns to normal within 3–5 days. Clinical cure is achieved before the GI ulcerations have healed and haemorrhage and perforation can occur during therapy even in an afebrile patient. However, because of extensive empirical use of fluoroquinolones, drug resistance is a major problem. If the isolates show reduced susceptibility to ciprofloxacin, then high-dose ciprofloxacin (750 mg PO bid or 400 mg IV q 8h for 10–14 days) can be used.

Cotrimoxazole in the dose of 2 tablets b.i.d., continued for 5–7 days after defervescence, is also effective, but to a lesser magnitude.

Amoxicillin (1 g t.i.d. for 12–14 days) has also been used to treat typhoid fever. The therapeutic response, however, is slower in onset and often inadequate.

Chloramphenicol, though effective against sensitive strains, **is no more considered a drug of first choice** because of longer duration of therapy (14–21 days), toxicity and possible drug resistance.

In endemic areas with high prevalence of MDR *S. typhi*, the treatment of choice is combination of cephalosporin and azithromycin. The preferred cephalosporins in this combination therapy are ceftriaxone (2 g/day IV for 10–14 days) or cefotaxime or oral cefixime. **Azithromycin** in a dose of 1 g/day for 5 days is administered orally as a part of this combination therapy. *However, these drugs are less effective in achieving clinical cure and relapse rate is 3–5%.*

Patients with severe typhoid fever (diarrhoea, persistent vomiting, delirium, obtundation, stupor, coma or shock) may need parenteral therapy for 7–10 days and total therapy for 14 days.

A short course of **glucocorticoid** may be added to antibiotic therapy in severe typhoid fever and in those with shock-like syndrome. *Their routine use in all cases is, however, not recommended.*

Supportive therapy includes maintenance of adequate nutrition and antipyretics. Soft diet should be given to the patient along with plenty of fluids to avoid dehydration. Either ibuprofen or paracetamol 6 hourly may be given till 36 h after defervescence.

In addition to S. typhi, campylobacter and yersinia infections can progress to 'enteric fever' by penetrating the intestinal cells and causing systemic infection. **Thus, typhoid is an enteric fever but all enteric fevers are not typhoid.**

Box 47.3 Drugs Effective in Typhoid Fever IM 3.12,IM 3.13

Against sensitive organisms:
- Ciprofloxacin
- Chloramphenicol
- Ampicillin/amoxicillin
- Cotrimoxazole

Against multidrug-resistant organisms:
- Ceftriaxone (IV)
- Azithromycin (oral)

Empirical treatment:
- Ceftriaxone
- Azithromycin

Treatment of carriers: Carriers are defined as patients who continue to excrete the organisms in the stool for more than 3 months after recovery. Chloramphenicol does not prevent or eliminate the carrier state. The treatment of choice is **ciprofloxacin** 750 mg twice daily for 28 days. The other drugs effective are ampicillin or amoxycillin (2 g q.i.d. for 4 weeks) and cotrimoxazole (2 tablets b.i.d. for 4 weeks), which are secreted in bile.

Paratyphoid fever, though usually a milder disease, is treated similarly.

PHARMACOTHERAPY OF CHRONIC BRONCHITIS

Chronic bronchitis is a clinical condition involving small bronchioles. It presents as chronic cough with sputum. Its aetiology is not known. Chronic bronchitis with airflow obstruction leads to COPD, characterised by irreversible air flow resistance. In many elderly patients, *it is progressive and incurable, terminating eventually in right heart failure.*

Patients with chronic bronchitis should receive a prophylactic dose of **pneumococcal vaccine** (Chapter 71).

Pharmacotherapy of chronic bronchitis is directed primarily towards the inflammation and infection which are controllable. *The pathological changes associated with emphysema, however, are irreversible.*

The treatment can be divided into the following:

1. **Treatment of acute exacerbations:**
   Antimicrobial therapy: *Acute exacerbations of chronic bronchitis* should be treated promptly with an antibiotic to minimise further bronchopulmonary damage. *The antibiotic regimens recommended* **in the absence of pneumonia** are (i) tetracycline 250 mg q.i.d.; (ii) doxycycline 150 mg once daily; (iii) ampicillin/amoxicillin 250 mg q.i.d. and (iv) cotrimoxazole, 2 tablets b.i.d. All these regimens are given from 7-10 days. They are equally effective and any one may be selected. Some patients may need erythromycin, azithromycin, a respiratory fluoroquinolone (Chapter 43) or a cephalosporin, depending upon the causative organism.
   Patients with pneumonia need amoxicillin (with or without clavulinic acid), a fluroquinolone, a second or third generation cephalosporin, azithromycin/clarithromycin or cotrimoxazole depending on the nature of the infecting organism. **Beta-lactam antibiotics are preferred over macrolides due to high prevalence of macrolide resistance in *S. pneumoniae* in India.**

   Symptomatic therapy: Bronchodilators counter the bronchospasm. For liquefaction of thick and sticky secretions, mucolytic agents may be useful (Chapter 26). Steam, inhalation and expectorants facilitate the expulsion of secretions.
   In severe respiratory distress with resting hypoxemia and signs of pulmonary hypertension or right heart failure, oxygen has to be given continuously (Chapter 75). Such oxygen therapy has been shown to decrease mortality.

2. **Management of chronic state:** It is important to avoid all irritants to the respiratory tract, especially smoke, dust, chemicals and environmental pollutants. Breathing exercises, postural drainage and bronchodilators are beneficial. For details of management of COPD, see Chapter 27.

TETRACYCLINES

Group I
- Chlortetracycline
- Oxytetracycline
- Tetracycline

Group II
- Demeclocycline
- Methacycline

Group III
- Doxycycline
- Minocycline

Group IV
- Tigecycline
- Eravacycline
- Omadacycline

CHAPTER 48

Antifungal Agents

Learning Objectives

This chapter will enable the reader:

1. To enlist fungi causing superficial and invasive infections.
2. To classify antifungal drugs based on their target sites.
3. To classify azole derivatives.
4. To describe the mechanism of action, antifungal spectrum, salient pharmacokinetic features, formulations, ADR and indications for (a) griseofulvin, (b) amphotericin B, (c) antifungal azoles, (d) terbinafine and (e) echinocandins.
5. To compare and contrast ketoconazole, fluconazole, posaconazole and voriconazole.
6. To state the drug of choice for various types of fungal infections giving rationale for the same.

KEY TERMS

nystatin, p. 700
candidiasis, localised p. 700
griseofulvin, p. 700
dermatophytes, p. 700
amphotericin B, p. 701
clotrimazole, p. 703
fluconazole, p. 704
terbinafine, p. 706
echinocandins, p. 706
choice of antifungal agents, p. 706

Fungal infections are common (Box 48.1), both as primary diseases and secondary to oral antibiotics therapy. Individuals suffering from malignancy, diabetes mellitus, those on corticosteroids and immunocompromised subjects are more prone to fungal infections.

Fungi occur as either rounded budding forms (*yeast-like*) or hyphi (*moulds*).

DR 7.3

Classification of Antifungal Agents

I. **Those employed topically:** These include many synthetic drugs such as azoles, tolnaftate, undecyclenic acid, terbinafine and ciclopirox (Chapter 69). Only nystatin, an antibiotic, is discussed here.

II. **Those used systemically:**
Antibiotics: Griseofulvin and amphotericin B
Antimetabolites: Flucytosine
Azole derivatives: Clotrimazole, ketoconazole, itraconazole and fluconazole
Allylamine: Terbinafine
Echinocandins: Caspofungin

Box 48.1 Types of Fungi Infecting the Humans (with fungal diseases)

I. ***Responsible for superficial fungal infections (skin and mucus membrane)***

Surface: *Malassezia furfur (Tinea versicolor or Pityriasis versicolor)*

Cutaneous: *Dermatophyte species (dermatophytosis or ringworm infection)*

II. ***Responsible for invasive fungal infection***

a. Opportunistic:

- ***Yeasts:*** *Candida sp. (candidiasis) and Cryptococcus sp. (cryptococcosis)*
- **Mycelial or Filamentous Fungi:**
  (a) *Zygomycetes* – Mucor sp., Rhizopus sp., Conididiobolus, Basidiobolus (zygomycosis),
  (b) *Pseudallescheria boydii* (mycetoma and maduromycosis)
  (c) *Aspergillus spp.* (aspergillosis)
- ***Protozoan-like fungi:*** *Pneumocystis jiroveci* (pneumonia)

b. True pathogenic:

1. Common: *Histoplasma capsulatum* (histoplasmosis), *Blastomyces dermatitidis* (blastomycosis), *Coccidioides immitis* (coccidioidomycosis)

- *Rare: Paracoccidiodies brasiliensis* (paracoccidioidomycosis), *Cladophialophora carrionii*, (chromomycosis chromoblastomycosis), *Sporothrix schenckii* (sporotrichosis), *Trichosporon* sp. (trichosporonosis)

Mechanism of action – antifungal drugs.

I. Agents employed topically:

NYSTATIN: This antibiotic, obtained from *Streptomyces noursei*, contains many double bonds in its chemical structure and hence, is called a polyene antibiotic. It rapidly loses its activity in the presence of water or plasma.

Antifungal activity: Nystatin shows inhibitory activity against several fungi *in vitro; Candida, Histoplasma, Blastomycoses, Trichophyton* and *Microsporum audouini* are sensitive.

Mechanism of action: Nystatin binds to ergosterol present in the cell membrane of the yeast and creates pores/channels, thus increasing the membrane permeability. Depending upon concentration, it can act either as a fungistatic or a fungicidal.

It is not absorbed from the gut, the skin or the mucous membranes. On parenteral administration, it produces a variety of toxic effects including serious nephrotoxicity; its activity is reduced in the presence of plasma. Hence, it is not used for systemic infections.

Adverse reactions: Adverse effects are usually mild. It has a bitter taste. Oral administration may cause nausea, vomiting and diarrhoea.

Preparations and dosage:

i. Nystatin tablet 500,000 U. Dose: 5,00,000–10,00,000 U 8 hourly in adults. In children and infants it can be given as 1,00,000 U suspension 4 times daily.
ii. Nystatin suspension 1,00,000 U/mL for oral topical application.
iii. Nystatin pessary or vaginal tablet 1,00,000–2,00,000 U/day.
iv. Nystatin ointment 1,00,000 U/g.

Indications:

- **Localised candidiasis** of vagina, mouth, skin and the gut. Imidazoles or triazoles are more effective agents than nystatin for vaginal candidiasis

II. Agents employed systemically:

GRISEOFULVIN: Griseofulvin, isolated from *Penicillium griseofulvium* is the first oral compound to cure effectively infections due to the superficial dermatophytes (ringworm).

Antifungal activity: It is fungistatic against various species of dermatophytes *viz Trichophyton, Microsporum* and *Epidermophyton. It is not useful for superficial candidiasis, Tinea versicolor* and invasive fungi (Chapter 69).

Mechanism of action: Dermatophytes specifically attack the keratinous tissue. Griseofulvin binds to the keratinocyte precursor cells and gets incorporated into keratin of the skin, hair and nails. It damages the microtubular protein of dermatophytes in keratin tissue, and prevents fungal mitosis, mainly in the growing fungal cells, thereby inhibiting fungal cell division. *The already established fungus is not affected. Hence, the treatment takes a long time to ensure cure.* It also has a weak anti-inflammatory action.

Absorption, fate and excretion: Small particles (microsize and ultramicrosize) are better absorbed than large particles; divided oral doses achieve higher level than a single dose; and a diet rich in fat enhances its absorption. It is metabolised in the liver; t1/2 is 1 day and 50% get excreted in the urine as metabolites.

Adverse reactions: These are as follows:

- Mild reactions such as headache, epigastric distress, nausea, vomiting and diarrhoea.
- Allergic and photosensitivity reactions. Cross allerginicity with penicillin, as griseofulvin is derived from a penicillium.
- Nervous system disturbances such as peripheral neuritis, vertigo, psychomotor incoordination, lethargy and blurred vision.
- Leukopenia, neutropenia, punctate basophilia, and monocytosis can occur, which disappear despite continued treatment. However, it is advisable to do weekly hemogram.
- Superinfection with *C. albicans.*
- Rarely, severe angioedema, hepatotoxicity, proteinuria, gynaecomastia and pigmentation of the genitalia are reported.

Drug interactions: Concurrent administration of griseofulvin and phenobarbitone may retard the absorption of the former from the GI tract. **It is a hepatic microsomal enzyme inducer** and hence it depresses the blood levels of drugs like warfarin and oral contraceptives. It can cause antabuse like reaction with alcohol.

Preparations and dosage: Griseofulvin is available as 125, 250, 375 and 500 mg tablets. The adult dose is 500 mg daily in two or four divided doses. In certain infections like *Tinea capitis*, a larger dose of 1 g daily may be necessary. Children are given 10 mg/kg daily, administered as a single dose or in divided doses.

Indications: Griseofulvin has made clinical control of some chronic resistant ringworm infections possible. Nevertheless, its narrow spectrum and high cost demand that it should not be used unless the cheaper and well-established topical therapy fails (see Chapter 69) or the lesion is known to be resistant to such therapy. The indications are as follows:

- **Tinea capitis** – ringworm of the scalp, where clinical cure usually occurs within 4–6 weeks of therapy.
- **Tinea barbae** – fungus infection of the beard caused by *Trichophyton faviforme, Trichophyton mentagrophytes* and *Microsporum canis.*
- **Tinea cruris** and **tinea corporis** – ringworm of the groin and the body.
- **Tinea pedis** and **tinea manus** – ringworm of the feet and hands. Griseofulvin is more effective in chronic fungal infections at these sites than in the acutely inflamed forms.

In all above conditions, the treatment is continued for some weeks after both clinical and microscopic evidence of infection has disappeared. Usually, this takes 4–8 weeks.

- **Onychomycosis:** It is more useful for fungal infection of fingernails than toenails which may respond minimally. Treatment is given for 6-9months for infection of finger nails and 10–12 months for toenails. Itraconazole or terbinafine is much more effective for onychomycosis. *Since chronic fungal infections tend to cause hyperkeratosis, concomitant topical keratolytic therapy with salicylic acid is beneficial.*

AMPHOTERICIN B: This polyene antibiotic, obtained from *Streptomyces nodosus*, is amphoteric and hence the name. Its **mechanism of action is similar to that of nystatin**. In addition, it also causes oxidative damage to fungi cells.

Antifungal activity: Amphotericin B has a broad spectrum antifungal activity. It inhibits the growth of *Histoplasma capsulatum, Cryptococcus neoformans, Sporothrix schenkii, Coccidioides immitis, Paracoccidiodies brasiliensis* and *Blastomycosis dermatitidis* in low concentrations. Candida responds to a slightly higher concentration. Depending upon the concentration, it can be fungistatic or fungicidal. Candida may develop resistance to this antibiotic *in vivo.*

Absorption, fate and excretion: Amphotericin B is poorly absorbed from the gut. The IM administration is painful. The drug, therefore, is given by IV infusion. Only 5% of the therapeutic dose is found in urine within 24 h. *It is concentrated in liver, spleen, kidney and lungs and remains in the body for several weeks.* Its CSF, vitreous humour and amniotic fluid concentration is poor. Its metabolic fate is unknown.

Adverse reactions: These include:

- Infusion-related local reaction like phlebitis, nausea, anorexia, vomiting, profound generalised malaise and weight loss.
- Chills, fever, tachypnea, respiratory stridor, modest hypotension as a result of proinflammatory reaction by the immune cells. This reaction resolves on its own within 30-45 min. Pretreatment with paracetamol, ibuprofen or hydrocortisone decreases this reaction. Patients with preexisting cardiac or pulmonary disease may develop hypoxia or hypotension.
- Headache, skin rash, diplopia, vertigo, convulsions, myalgia and peripheral neuritis. Arachnoiditis may occur following intrathecal administration
- Nephrotoxicity. *It is recommended that one litre of normal saline should be infused on the day of amphotericin therapy, to reduce the risk of nephrotoxicity.* Irreversible renal damage may occur if the cumulative dose exceeds 3 to 4 g.

  Renal tubular acidosis and renal wasting of K^+ and Mg^{++} may be seen. K^+ supplementation is needed in patients on prolonged therapy.

- Hypochromic, normocytic anaemia due to decreased production of erythropoietin
- Rarely, haemorrhagic gastroenteritis, thrombocytopenia, hepatic failure, hypotension and ventricular failure may occur.

Preparations and dosage:

i. Amphotericin B lotion 3% and topical gel 0.1 %/ 5 g.

ii. Amphotericin B deoxycholate (IV): A concentration of 0.1 mg/mL in 5% dextrose is given by slow IV infusion. Dose is 0.6 mg/kg.
   Following are the **lipid formulations** of amphotericin B. Infusion reactions and risk of acute kidney injury are lesser with these but they are very expensive.

iii. Amphotericin B colloidal dispersion: It contains equimolar amounts of amphotericin B and cholesteryl sulfate. It is reconstituted in aqueous solution and forms colloidal solution. Larger doses (4-6 mg/kg) are required to achieve plasma levels comparable to amphotericin B deoxycholate. Febrile reaction is more with this formulation but it is claimed to be less nephrotoxic.

iv. Amphotericin B lipid complex: It is a complex of amphotericin B with two phospholipids.
   The dose is 5 mg/kg in 5% dextrose in water, infused intravenously once daily over 2 h. The levels of amphotericin B are much lower than those with amphotericin B deoxycholate.

v. Liposomal amphotericin B (AmBisome; 50 mg lyophilized powder to be reconstituted with sterile water for IV infusion; 5 mg/kg). The drug is released slowly from these formulations and hence causes less toxicity.It is possible to use higher doses to achieve optimal blood levels of amphotericin B.

Indications:

- **Topically,** the antibiotic is useful in the treatment of candida lesions and as eyedrops to treat fungal corneal ulcers and keratitis.
- **For systemic therapy,** the patient should be hospitalised. Though toxic, it could be lifesaving. *Its toxicity could be reduced by using (a) smaller doses in combination with other systemic antifungal agents or (b) lipid formulations (liposomes).*

Amphotericin IV is the treatment of choice in the primary, cutaneous and disseminated forms of blastomycosis, histoplasmosis, cryptococcosis, candidiasis, sporotrichosis, aspergillosis, chromoblastomycosis and occasionally in phycomycosis and maduramycosis. It may be administered with flucytosine in the treatment of cryptococcal meningitis. It can be given intrathecally in meningitis that does not respond to IV therapy. It is used to treat mucormycosis in diabetics.

Lower doses are required for candida esophagitis than for deeply invasive mycoses

It is also used in treatment of leishmaniasis (Chapter 56).

FLUCYTOSINE: This prodrug is a synthetic fluorinated pyrimidine. It is taken up by fungal cells and converted to 5-fluorouracil. **The antifungal activity is due to 5-fluorouracil, an antimetabolite, which produces active metabolites that inhibit DNA and RNA synthesis.** Human cells do not convert the drug to active metabolites. Given orally, it is well absorbed and reaches adequate concentrations in the blood and CSF. It is mostly excreted unchanged by glomerular filtration, and hence requires dose reduction in patients with renal impairment. Its t½ is 3-6 h.

Adverse reactions include rash, nausea, vomiting, diarrhoea and severe enterocolitis, reversible elevation in liver transaminases and bone marrow suppression causing neutropenia and thrombocytopenia. **It is less toxic than amphotericin B.**

Indications: The drug is useful in cryptococcal meningitis and systemic candidiasis, including UTI. Used alone, it can lead to rapid emergence of drug resistance. Hence, it is usually combined with amphotericin B or fluconazole. It is administered daily, in the oral dose of 50–150 mg/kg in four divided doses. It can also be given by IV infusion.

AZOLE DERIVATIVES

Azoles possess a five member azole ring that is attached by a carbon-nitrogen bond to other aromatic rings as their unit (Fig. 48.1). Therapeutically, they are classified as follows:

I. **Antibacterial** and **antiprotozoal agents,** e.g. metronidazole and tinidazole (Chapter 55)

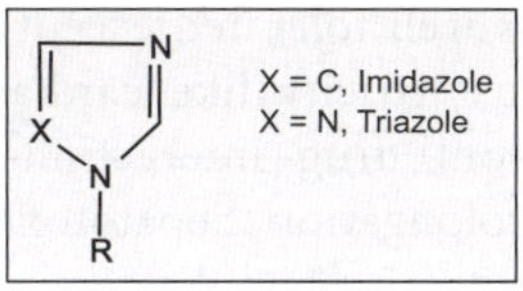

FIG. 48.1 **Azole nucleus.**

II. Anthelmintic agents, e.g. mebendazole, albendazole (Chapter 58)

III. Antifungal azole agents

Antifungal azoles are further classified into:

- **Imidazoles** indicating two nitrogen atoms in the azole ring, e.g. clotrimazole, miconazole, ketoconazole, econazole, butoconazole, oxiconazole, sertaconazole, sulconazole, tioconazole, and luliconazole.
  They are generally used topically to treat superficial mycoses, and cutaneous and vaginal candidiasis.
- **Triazoles** with three nitrogens in the azole ring, e.g. terconazole, itraconazole, fluconazole, voriconazole, posaconazole, and isavuconazole. They have greater volume of distribution, slower rate of metabolism, greater selectivity and better CNS penetrability than imidazoles. They are also considered to be less toxic as they have less effect on human sterol synthesis and cause less endocrinal disturbances.

Mechanism of action: Azoles act by inhibiting synthesis of ergosterol, an important constituent of the fungal cell membrane. Among the series of enzymatic steps leading to ergosterol synthesis, azoles inhibit 14-α-sterol demethylase. This enzyme belongs to CYP 450 family.

There is an accumulation of 14-α-methylsterols, which disrupt the close packing of acylchains of phospholipids and and disturb the function of membrane bound enzymes. Some azoles affect the membrane permeability but at higher concentrations, which can be achieved if used topically. They have a broad spectrum antifungal and antibacterial activity and are effective against dermatophytes, Microsporum, Candida, Cryptococcus, Blastomyces, Coccidioides, Paracoccidioides, Madurella and Nocardia. The activity is less against *Candida glabrata*. Mucormycosis exhibits resistance against most of the azoles.

- *All azoles are potentially embryotoxic and teratogenic and should be avoided during pregnancy and lactation.*
- *The azoles used systemically are potent inhibitors of hepatic microsomal enzymes and can increase the blood levels and toxicity of several drugs. Inducers of CYP such as carbamazepine and rifampicin can reduce the concentrations of the azoles.*
- *Combination of azoles with certain drugs is contraindicated (Box 48.2)*

CLOTRIMAZOLE: *This drug is not used for systemic infections because of its toxicity.* Its topical use for cutaneous and vaginal candidiasis has been described in Chapter 69.

Uses of many other imidazoles are similar (Chapter 69).

MICONAZOLE: This imidazole has a broad spectrum antifungal and Gram-positive antibacterial activity. However the latter activity is not sufficient for clinical use. High concentrations are trichomonicidal.

For systemic fungal infections, it is given has been used intravenously and sometimes intrathecally. But the IV miconazole induces allergic reaction and may also cause liver damage and pruritus, nausea, blood dyscrasias, hyponatraemia, hyperlipidaemia and arrhythmias. Hence now it is mainly used topically for skin or mucosal fungal infection (Chapter 69).

Box 48.2 Contraindicated combination of azoles with some drugs

- Simvastatin
- Salmeterol
- Nisoldipine
- Rifapentine
- Ritonavir
- Tolvaptan and conivaptan
- Silodosin
- Sirolimus and everolimus
- Dronedarone
- Nilotinib

KETOCONAZOLE: This imidazole was the first azole available for oral use to treat systemic fungal infections. It is effective against several fungi. It is water soluble and well absorbed from the gut. However, because of its poor efficacy and toxicity, it has been largely replaced by itraconazole and fluconazole though it is relatively much cheaper.

In large doses, ketoconazole inhibits several biosynthetic steps in the synthesis of adrenal and gonadal steroids. **It can thus reduce the plasma levels of cortisol and testosterone.**

Adverse reactions: The drug can cause headache, gastric irritation, allergic reactions, gynaecomastia (due to impairment of testosterone synthesis) and acute hepatic necrosis. It is a CYP3A4 inhibitor and inhibits the metabolism of many drugs such as warfarin, phenytoin and oral contraceptives. Cyclosporin and astemizole compete with ketaconazole and increase its plasma levels. H_2 receptor antagonists and antacids interfere with its absorption.

Indications:

- **As a topical antifungal agent** (Chapter 69)
- **Familial testotoxicosis** (gonadotropin independent activation of Leydig cells)
- **Cushing syndrome**
- **Prostatic cancer**

ITRACONAZOLE: This broad spectrum antifungal triazole, related to ketoconazole, exerts both topical and systemic activity. However, **it lacks effects on adrenal and gonadal steroid synthesis.** Its spectrum is similar to ketaconazole but it is also effective against Aspergillus.

It is given orally or intravenously. *However, its bioavailability is variable. A super-bioavailable (SUBA)-itraconazole is available to overcome this problem.* It is metabolised mostly in the liver to its metabolite, which is also active (t½ 30–40 h). Loading dose is needed when treating deep mycoses. It is both a substrate for and a potent inhibitor of CYP3A4. It does not appear in the urine or the CSF and it does not inhibit the production of steroids.

Itraconazole is well tolerated except for GI disturbances. Serious toxicity like cardiac arrhythmias may result from drug interactions. Other ADR include QT prolongation, hepatotoxicity, skin rash, hypertriglyceridemia, hypokalaemia and with IV use, HF in patients with impaired ventricular function.

Indications

- **Oropharyngeal and oesophageal candidiasis:** 100 mg of the solution once or twice a day for 2 to 4 weeks for and
- **Subungual onychomycosis:** 200 mg capsuless once daily for 12 weeks.
- **Indolent, nonmeningeal invasive aspergillosis and mild to moderate true pathogenic fungal infections:** It is the drug of choice. However, loading dose of 200 mg three times daily for the first 3 days, followed by 200-mg twice daily is required for longer periods (6–12 months) to treat these deep fungal infections. Long-term therapy with itraconazole is helpful in allergic bronchopulmonary aspergillosis to decrease the dose of glucocorticoids and to reduce attacks of acute bronchospasm.

FLUCONAZOLE: This triazole derivative undergoes complete absorption and is effective both, orally and by IV infusion. It has plasma t½ of 25–30 h and is given once daily. Its bioavailability is not affected by food or gastric pH. *It penetrates readily into the CSF.* Unlike itraconazole, almost 90% of the drug is eliminated in the urine unchanged. It inhibits CYP3A4, CYP2C9 and CYP2C19. However, **drug interactions are uncommon unless patient is on high dose** (>400 **mg daily**) or has elevated fluconazole levels due to azotaemia.

Because of fewer hepatic enzyme interactions and GI disturbances, it is preferred to itraconazole in the treatment of:

- **Severe/widespread dermatophytosis:** 150 mg once or twice a week needs to be given for 4–8 weeks.
- **Local and systemic candidiasis:** For Oropharyngeal candidiasis 100 to 200 mg daily for 7 to 14 days is effective whereas vaginal candidiasis needs

a single dose of 150 mg. Treatment of candidemia requires a loading dose of 800 mg followed by 400 mg daily. However, the drug of choice is an echinocandin.

- **Cryptococcal infections including meningitis:** In patients with cryptococcal meningitis following initial therapy with amphotericin B for 2 weeks, 400 mg fluconazole is used daily for 8 weeks. In patients with AIDS the dose is then reduced to 200 mg daily and continued indefinitely to prevent relapse. Instead of amphotericin B, fluconazole can be used in combination with flucytosine in the initial period.
- **Coccidioidomycosis:** Its activity is comparable to itraconazole. It is the drug of choice for coccidioidal meningitis because of its good CSF penetrability and lesser ADR compared to amphotericin B.
- **Blastomycosis:** Fluconazole is an alternative; the drug of choice is itraconazole.

It is less effective against Candida glabrata and Candida krusei. It is not active against aspergillosis, mucormycosis and other true pathogenic fungi.

Fluconazole can be given as IV infusion in saline and in dextrose solution. Dose varies with the infecting organism from 50–400 mg once daily. A loading dose of twice the daily maintenance dose is needed on the first day of therapy.

The drug may cause headache, nausea, GI disturbances, abnormalities of liver enzymes and with prolonged therapy at high doses (400 mg daily), alopecia, muscle weakness and skin rash. Rare incidences of hepatic failure and Stevens-Johnson syndrome have been reported. Fluconazole should be avoided in pregnancy. It causes inhibition of CYP3A4 and CYP2C9, especially when used at doses higher than 400 mg daily or in patients with azotemia.

POSACONAZOLE, an oral triazole, is related chemically to itraconazole. It has similar spectrum as itraconazole but greater activity against yeasts and filamentous fungi, including some of the fungi that cause mucormycosis. Its bioavailability is increased by food. It has a long t½ (25–31 h), a large volume of distribution and high protein binding. It undergoes glucuronidation Majority of the administered drug is excreted in faeces.

It is well tolerated. Common ADR include nausea, vomiting, diarrhoea, abdominal pain, and headache. It can prolong the QTc interval. Like itraconazole, it inhibits CYP3A4. Hence it should not be coadministered with drugs that are CYP3A4 substrates and also prolong the QTc interval e.g. methadone, quinidine, risperidone, tacrolimus.

It is particularly useful in the prevention and treatment of invasive fungal infections, including oropharyngeal candidiasis refractory to fluconazole. It is the drug of choice for invasive aspergillosis. It is used to treat mucormycosis in patients not tolerating amphotericin B. It is preferred to amphotericin-B for the treatment of zygomycete infection.

It is administered orally in the dose of 200 mg three times a day. The IV dose is 300 mg twice on day 1 and 300 mg daily thereafter.

VORICONAZOLE: It has structural similarity to fluconazole but has an expanded spectrum and poor aqueous solubility. High-fat meal reduces its bioavailability so oral administration should be either 1 h before or 1 h after meals. It undergoes extensive tissue distribution and crosses CSF barrier. It is metabolised by CYP2C19, CYP2C9 and CYP3A4; the metabolites are excreted in urine (t½ is 6 h). It exhibits nonlinear metabolism. Genetic polymorphisms in CYP2C19 causes variations in plasma levels. 20% of Asians are homozygous poor metabolizers. TDM is advisable for voriconazole. The drug and its major metabolite inhibit the above CYP enzymes and interact with many drugs which get metabolised by these CYPs.

Voriconazole is generally well tolerated but can cause hepatotoxicity, skin rashes (including photosensitivity) and prolongation of QTc interval. With IV infusion, transient visual or auditory hallucinations and anaphylactoid reactions may occur. Oral voriconazole is preferred to IV infusion if creatinine clearance is less than 50 mL/min. Omeprazole (40 mg/day or more) and voriconazole increase each other's concentrations in plasma and hence omeprazole dose needs to be reduced by half when initiating voriconazole therapy.

It is active against fluconazole resistant candida (including *C. glabrata* and *C. krusei*) and is preferred in invasive aspergillosis as posaconazole. It is also used in esophageal candidiasis and initial treatment of candidemia. Therapy is usually started with IV infusion of 6 mg/kg every 12 h for two doses, followed by 3 - 4 mg/kg every 12 h. As the patient improves, 200 mg orally every 12 h is recommended.

ISAVUCONAZOLE: This triazole is a broad spectrum antifungal agent, effective against most yeast species, including *Candida, Cryptococcus* and *Aspergillus* and most of the fungi causing mucormycosis.

It is available as oral or IV isavuconazonium sulfate, which is a prodrug. On oral administration it is rapidly hydrolyzed to the active form, *isavuconazole.* It *undergoes* metabolism by CYP3A4 and CYP3A5. It has a long plasma half-life (~130 h). Common ADR include GI disturbances including constipation, headache, fever, hypokalemia, and cough. It is an inhibitor of CYP3A4. It causes a dose-related shortening of QTc.

It is used for the treatment of invasive aspergillosis and invasive mucormycosis.

TERBINAFINE: This synthetic allylamine is keratophilic like griseofulvin but is **fungicidal**. It inhibits the enzyme squalene epoxidase thus, blocking ergosterol biosynthesis. The accumulated squalene is cytotoxic. It is effective orally and topically. It is extensively metabolised in the liver. **Topically, it is used to treat dermatophyte infections of the skin, especially tinea capitis.** Oral treatment with 250 mg daily has been reported to cure onychomycosis in about 6-12 weeks as against 18 months required by griseofulvin. It is available as nail lacquer for onychomycosis. It is generally well tolerated but should not be used in patients with renal or hepatic failure. Adverse effects include GI distress, headache and rash.

ECHINOCANDINS

These are cyclic lipopeptides with a nucleus.

CASPOFUNGIN: This agent belongs to a group of new antifungals called **echinocandins.**

Mechanism of action: They act on the fungal cell wall to block the synthesis of β1 (1–3) glucans. They are fungicidal against *Candida and fungistatic for Aspergillus.*

Caspofungin, micafungin and **anidulafungin** are the three semisynthetic echinocandins. They are:

- Not absorbed orally and are used only intravenously
- Extensively protein bound (>97%)
- Not able to penetrate into CSF
- Not eliminated by kidney
- Administered once daily
- Well tolerated. Phlebitis can occur at the infusion site and rapid infusion results in histamine-like effects. It may cause hypercalcaemia.
- Contraindicated in pregnancy as they are embryotoxic
- Very expensive

Table 48.1 Choice of Antifungal Agents

Type of Infection	Drug(s) Preferred
Tinea pedis/cruris	Topical azoles
Tinea corporis	Oral azole/terbinafine
Onychomycosis	Terbinafine/topical efinaconazole/ oral azole; griseofulvin
Cutaneous candidiasis	Topical azoles/nystatin
Vulovaginal candidiasis	Topical azoles/nystatin; fluconazole (oral single dose); if required 7 days course
Oral candidiasis	Topical nystatin or amphotericin B; systemic fluconazole (in immunocompromised patients)
Oesophageal candidiasis	Systemic fluconazole; echinocandin; newer triazoles if indicated
Microsporidiosis	Albendazole (Chapter 58); fumagillin
Pneumocystis jirovecii pneumonia	Cotrimoxazole (Chapter 43); Pentamidine (Chapter 56)

Notes: For invasive fungal infection, see text.

Caspofungin is metabolised by CYP3A4 and requires dose reduction in moderate hepatic impairment. Micafungin to some extent is metabolized in the liver by arylsulfatase and COMT. No dose reduction is required in hepatic impairment. Both are inhibitors of CYP3A4 and exhibit drug interaction. Anidulafungin undergoes chemical degradation. It does not exhibit any drug interaction.

Indications:

- **Invasive Candidiasis:** They are the drug of choice for the initial treatment of candidemia. They are also used for the treatment of intra-abdominal abscess, peritonitis and esophageal candidiasis.
- **Invasive aspergillosis:** They are used in amphotericin B or voriconazole resistant or intolerant patients.

FUMAGILLIN: It is an acyclic polyene macrolide, which is used orally to treat intestinal microsporidiosis in immunocompromised patients. It is available as topical formulation to treat keratoconjunctivitis. Its ADR include GI disturbances and reversible thrombocytopenia and neutropenia.

Table 48.1 outlines the choice of antifungal agents in superficial fungal infection.

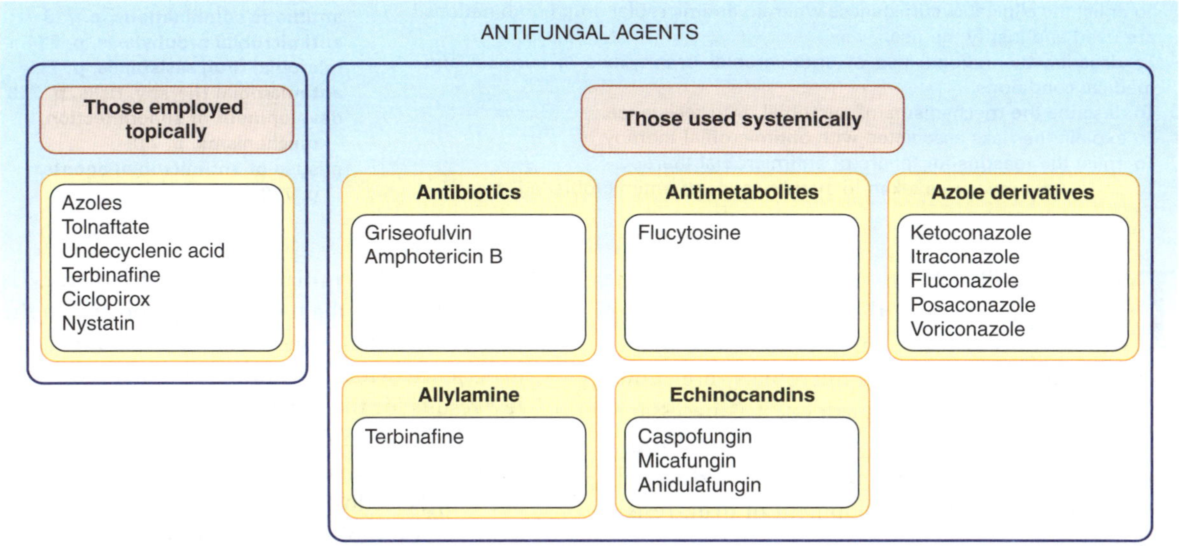

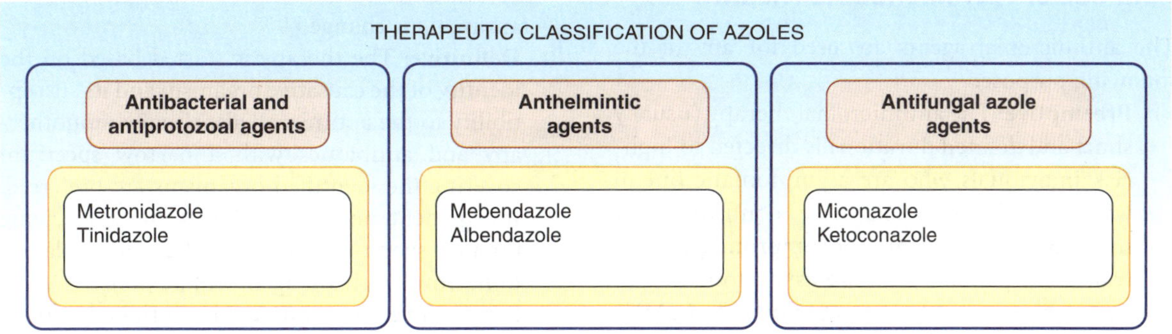

CHAPTER 49

PH 1.42

General Principles of Chemotherapy of Infections

Learning Objectives

This chapter will enable the reader:

1. To discuss the host-/pathogen-/drug-related factors involved in selection of an antimicrobial agent.
2. To mention the antimicrobial drug of choice for various bacterial infections.
3. To enlist the clinical circumstances wherein antimicrobial drug combinations are used and justify the use.
4. To describe the rational use of antimicrobial prophylaxis in surgical and medical conditions.
5. To describe the mechanisms of microbial drug resistance.
6. To explain the risks associated with antimicrobial therapy.
7. To enlist the reasons for failure of antimicrobial therapy.
8. To enumerate measures taken to avoid misuse of antimicrobial agents.

KEY TERMS

host-related factors, p. 709
pathogen-related factors, p. 709
drug-related factors, p. 709
antibiotic combinations, p. 713
antimicrobial prophylaxis, p. 714
microbial drug resistance, p. 715
antimicrobial therapy, risks, p. 718
development of superinfection, mechanisms, p. 718
misuse of antimicrobial agents, p. 718

Infections still remain a major problem in medical practice, and their rational treatment with drugs is of prime importance. Since many therapeutically effective antimicrobials are now available and more are being added, it is necessary to lay down certain guiding principles for tailoring a rational therapeutic regimen for an individual patient and to avoid the development of drug-resistant organisms.

PURPOSE OF ANTIMICROBIAL THERAPY

The antimicrobial agents are used for any of the following purpose:

i. **Preemptive:** The antimicrobial therapy (usually short and defined duration) is directed to high-risk individuals who are asymptomatic but in whom laboratory tests have confirmed the infection e.g., in immunocompromised liver transplant patients who are asymptomatic but show presence of cytomegalovirus (CMV) viremia, antiviral drugs are used till the tests are negative for CMV.

ii. **Empirical:** The initial antimicrobial therapy is directed against the most likely pathogens in the first 24–48 hours based on clinical judgment and experience while awaiting the microbiological test results for the organisms and their antibiotic sensitivity. Antibiotic selection depends on various factors and has been discussed under the Section, 'Selection of antimicrobial agent.' Many a times the antibiotic used in the empiric therapy is continued till the patient is cured. If definitive microbiological results show different organisms or resistance to the selected antibiotic, then the antibiotic is changed.

iii. **Definitive:** The therapy is started based on the identity of the causative organism and its susceptibility to the antimicrobials. Usually monotherapy and antibiotics with a narrow spectrum covering the identified organisms are preferred. If a patient on empirical therapy is receiving broader spectrum antibiotic then de-escalation to narrow spectrum agent can be done.

iv. **Suppressive:** The treatment is continued at lower doses in patients for suppression of the infection which is not completely eradicated by the initial definitive therapy especially in immunocompromised individuals. Doses used in suppressive therapy are lower than that used for definitive therapy and sometimes route of administration or even the antibiotic is different. This therapy is used in patients suffering from recurrent urinary tract infection.

v. **Prophylaxis:** The antimicrobial therapy is given to individuals who are not infected or do not have any evidence of development of disease due to infected organisms (See under the section Antimicrobial prophylaxis). This is termed as primary prophylaxis.
Sometimes a patient cured following an antibiotic therapy, is prescribed an antibiotic to prevent new infection, if he is at high risk of contracting it. This is termed as secondary prophylaxis.

SELECTION OF ANTIMICROBIAL AGENT

PH 1.43

The choice of an antimicrobial agent is decided by the following.

1. **Host-related factors:**
   - **Age of the patient:** Lower doses are needed in infants and elderly because of deficient hepatic and renal function, e.g. chloramphenicol may cause serious toxic effects in infants in whom liver enzymes/renal function are not fully developed. A significant reduction of hepatic and renal function is observed in people over 80 years (see Chapter 3).
   - **Pregnancy and neonatal period:** Most antimicrobial agents cross the placenta and can reach therapeutic concentrations in fetal tissues. Hence, they should be avoided during pregnancy. Penicillins, cephalosporins, erythromycin (except estolate which is hepatotoxic), lincomycin, clindamycin, azithromycin, INH, ethambutol and probably sulphonamides (for short term) can be safely used in pregnancy (Chapter 78).
   - **Immunocompetency status of the patient.** Bactericidal agents are always preferred in immunocompromised patients.
   - **Severity of the infection and general condition of the patient:** A mild case of bacillary dysentery in an otherwise healthy individuals usually responds satisfactorily to ORT, whereas in severe cases, a fluoroquinolone is necessary in addition. More aggressive treatment is needed in the presence of diabetes mellitus, immunosuppression and in those on corticosteroids.
   - **History of allergic reaction or intolerance** to the antimicrobial agent: Elicitation of a proper history avoids adverse reactions in patients.
   - **Hepatic and renal status:** In compromised hepatic and renal functions, dose reduction of antimicrobial agents or use of safer alternatives is preferred.
2. **Pathogen-related factors:**
   - **The probable causative organism and the expected clinical course of the infection:** One must decide whether the given illness is likely to be due to a microorganism susceptible to one of the available antimicrobials. *Antibiotics are not nonspecific antipyretics and their use in all cases of fever is to be deprecated.* Many cases of fever such as due to common cold are due to viruses that are not susceptible to antibiotics. Routine use of antibiotics in all such cases may cause drug toxicity and promote drug resistance (Chapter 46).
   - **Identification of the causative microorganism and its sensitivity to antimicrobial drugs:** Though ideal, this may not always be possible owing to lack of facilities. In certain cases, e.g. tuberculosis and viral infections, polymerase chain reaction (PCR) studies using tissue material, e.g. pleural fluid, CSF are valuable for identifying specific microbes.
   - **Possibility of drug resistance**, e.g. if the infection is due to drug-resistant TB, malaria or Staphylococci, alternative therapy with another antibiotic will have to be used.
   - **Nature and site of infection:** In case of obstructive lesions, necrotic and pyogenic infections (such as abscesses, empyema) surgical drainage in addition to antimicrobial therapy may be needed.
3. **Drug-related factors:**
   - **Nature of the drug** (Table 49.1). **Bactericidal drugs are always preferred to bacteriostatic agents. Carriers should be treated only with**

Table 49.1 Commonly Used Bactericidal and Bacteriostatic Drugs

Bactericidal	Bacteriostatic
Penicillin	Sulphonamides
Aminoglycosides	Nitrofurans
Rifampicin	Erythromycin
Cephalosporins	Tetracyclines
Metronidazole	Chloramphenicol
Cotrimoxazole	Lincomycin
Fluoroquinolones	Trimethoprim

bactericidal drugs since bacteriostatic agents are not so effective.

- **Concentration-dependent** or **time-dependent killing:** The antimicrobials which eradicate pathogenic bacteria by achieving high concentration at the binding site/s of organisms are termed as **concentration-dependent antibiotics.** To achieve the best kill, their concentration should be ≥10 times above the MIC (minimum inhibitory concentration) of the target organism (e.g. aminoglycosides, flouroquinolones). Those classes of antibiotics whose killing response is dependent on the extent of time they remain bound to target sites at concentration above MIC of the organism are termed **time-dependent antibiotics.** Therefore, optimal responses to these antimicrobial agents are dependent on the time the serum concentrations remain above the MIC during the dosing interval. **Higher concentration of such drugs does not result in greater killing of organism,** e.g. penicillins, cephalosporins, carbapenems, monobactams, clindamycin, macrolides, linezolid.
- **Risk of drug toxicity**, particularly in the presence of cardiac, liver or kidney damage. The risk involved in using a more toxic drug in preference to less effective but less toxic agent is justified only if the infection is severe.
- **Pharmacokinetic properties of the drug**, e.g. tissue penetration; metabolism; duration of action and its elimination. Biofilm producing bacteria (e.g. Staphylococci) and fungi (e.g. Candida) hamper penetration of antibiotics. Exopolysaccharide matrix of biofilms binds to antibiotics and prevents their access to the organisms.
- **The cost of therapy:** This is particularly important where many equally effective drugs are available for a given infection. Newer drugs are always costly and not necessarily superior than established ones.
- **Drug compliance by the patient** (Chapter 4).

Although Antibiotic sensitivity tests give important information, they are neither necessary nor practicable in daily practice. Sometimes, they can even be misleading and hence, **the physician should use his clinical judgement in selecting the antibiotic and not depend blindly on the results of such tests.** It must be realised that the organisms isolated by the bacteriologist may not be the prime cause of the disease under treatment. This is particularly so in case of organisms cultured from sputum and faeces. Similarly, **the sensitivity data obtained from *in vitro* studies do not necessarily hold true *in vivo*.** Bacterial sensitivity tests, however, are useful in selecting a proper regimen in chronic diseases like MDR TB or UTI, resistant Staphylococcal infections, endocarditis and chronic osteomyelitis.

ANTIBIOTIC USE IN THE PRESENCE OF ORGAN DYSFUNCTION

Many drugs are metabolised by the liver to inactive products and although these metabolites accumulate in the presence of renal failure, they are not so harmful (Box 49.1). In contrast, other antimicrobial drugs (Box 49.2) are removed almost entirely by the kidney and accumulate in the blood in the active form in patients with impaired renal function. Many of these agents, e.g. aminoglycosides are

Box 49.1 Antimicrobials Cleared by Nonrenal Mechanisms

- Erythromycin, azithromycin
- Chloramphenicol
- Doxycycline, tigecycline
- Rifampicin
- Cefoperazone, ceftriaxone
- Linezolid
- Metronidazole

Box 49.2 Antimicrobials Eliminated by Renal Excretion

- Penicillins
- Aminoglycosides
- Most cephalosporins
- Fluoroquinolones
- Colistin
- Polymyxins
- Vancomycin, daptomycin
- Amphotericin B
- Amantadine

highly effective against Gram-negative organisms but are also nephrotoxic and neurotoxic. Such drugs need reduction in doses in the presence of renal damage, as guided by the plasma creatinine level. **In such patients therapeutic drug monitoring (TDM) may be useful.**

In patients with impaired renal function, the renal clearance of drugs like penicillins, aminoglycosides, most of the cephalosporins and tetracycline is reduced by the same proportion as the reduction from 100 mL/min in the measured or calculated creatinine clearance (Chapter 1).

In the case of penicillin G, no adjustment is required if the daily dose is 1.2 MU or less; it is required in case massive doses are being used. Following generalisations can be made while using antimicrobials in patients with renal impairment:

- Antibiotics like ampicillin, cloxacillin, carbenicillin and other penicillins can be used safely but **need substantial reduction in dosage**, in patients with chronic kidney disease (CKD).
- The tetracyclines increase protein catabolism. Further, accumulation of protein metabolites in the uraemic patient would make the condition worse. This may result in liver failure. It is advisable, therefore, to avoid tetracyclines (except doxycycline) in CKD.
- Fluoroquinolones can accumulate in the presence of renal damage and need dose adjustment.
- The renal/hepatic elimination mechanisms in neonates and in premature infants are not well developed. Hence, antimicrobials, essentially eliminated by them tend to accumulate, leading to toxicity. Their doses for newborns and premature infants should, therefore, be reduced and spacing between doses increased compared to those advocated for adults (see also Chapter 78).
- The elderly have diminished renal function, and antimicrobials which are disposed of largely by the kidneys should be administered in reduced doses.
- It takes longer to reach a steady state if the t½ is prolonged due to renal damage, e.g. amoxicillin and gentamicin.

Antimicrobials of choice in various infections are given in Table 49.2.

The selected drug should be given in adequate doses for a sufficient period depending upon the type of case. **In majority of the uncomplicated acute infections and even in certain chronic conditions, orally effective, relatively nontoxic and inexpensive drugs should be preferred.** Parenteral therapy is inconvenient, more expensive, and needs medical supervision. It should be reserved for:

- *Emergency and serious cases with bacteraemia/shock*
- *Patients who cannot take oral therapy or in whom the drugs are not likely to be absorbed orally*
- *Those in whom the organisms have developed resistance to orally used drugs*

Drugs used commonly to treat infections with common Gram-negative anaerobes are listed in Box 49.3.

Community-associated MRSA is often a cause of skin and soft tissue infections. These organisms are resistant to fluoroquinolones. Oral agents preferred in these conditions are clindamycin, doxycycline/

Box 49.3 Drugs Used to Treat Infections with Common Gram-Negative Anaerobes

- Metronidazole
- Fluoroquinolones
- Ticarcillin-clavulanic acid
- Piperacillin-tazobactam
- Imipenem
- Monobactams
- Ampicillin-sulbactam

Table 49.2 Antimicrobial Drugs of Choice — IM 3.12, IM 3.13

Organism	Antimicrobial Agents: First Choice	Antimicrobial Agents: Other Effective Drugs
Actinomyces israeli (bovis)	Penicillin G, amoxicillin	Tetracycline, erythromycin, clindamycin
Anaerobes (other than clostridia)	Metronidazole, penicillin G, cefoxitin, carbapenems, ampicillin – sulbactam, piperacillin – tazobactam	Chloramphenicol, clindamycin
Bacillus anthracis	Ciprofloxacin, doxycycline	Clindamycin ± rifampicin, penicillin G
Bordetella pertussis	Azithromycin	Cotrimoxazole, Erythromycin, Clarithromycin
Brucella	Doxycycline + streptomycin/ gentamicin	Doxycycline + rifampicin, cotrimoxazole + rifampicin, ciprofloxacin + rifampicin
Candida albicans	Fluconazole, voriconazole	Echinocandins, nystatin
Chlamydia trachomatis	Azithromycin	Ofloxacin, doxycycline, erythromycin
Clostridium difficile	Metronidazole, vancomycin	Nitazoxanide, bacitracin, fusidic acid, rifaximin
Clostridium tetani	Penicillin G, metronidazole	Clindamycin
Corynebacterium diphtheriae	Procaine penicillin, erythromycin	Rifampicin, clindamycin
Donovan bodies of granuloma inguinale	Azithromycin, doxycycline	Erythromycin, cotrimoxazole, chloramphenicol, norfloxacin
Enterococcus (Streptococcus faecalis)	Penicillin G/vancomycin + gentamicin	(Ampicillin – sulbactum) + imipenem, (ampicillin – sulbactum) + ceftriaxone linezolid, daptomycin
Escherichia coli	Fluoroquinolones	Amoxicillin – clavulanic acid, amikacin, cephalosporin, tigecycline, polymyxin B
Fusospirochetes	Penicillin G	Erythromycin, clindamycin, metronidazole
Gardnerella vaginalis	Metronidazole	Clindamycin
Haemophilus ducreyi	Azithromycin	Fluoroquinolone, erythromycin, ceftriaxone
Haemophilus influenzae	Third-generation cephalosporin	Fluoroquinolones, chloramphenicol, amoxicillin – clavulanic acid, azithromycin
Klebsiella pneumoniae in seriously ill patients	Imipenem, amikacin	Third-generation cephalosporin, cotrimoxazole
Legionella pneumoniae	Azithromycin/clarithromycin, fluoroquinolones	Doxycycline, cotrimoxazole
Mycoplasma pneumoniae	Azithromycin/clarithromycin, fluoroquinolones	Third-generation cephalosporin, doxycycline
Micrococcus catarrhalis	Cotrimoxazole	Amoxicillin, erythromycin, tetracycline, cephalosporin
Neisseria gonorrhoeae	Ceftriaxone, cefixime, doxycycline/ azithromycin	Cephalosporin (cefotaxime, ceftizoxime, cefotetan) + probenecid, spectinomycin
Neisseria meningitidis (intracellularis)	Penicillin G, third-generation cephalosporin	Carbapenem, chloramphenicol

Continued

Table 49.2 Antimicrobial Drugs of Choice—cont'd

Organism	Antimicrobial Agents	
	First Choice	**Other Effective Drugs**
Yersenia pestis	Streptomycin, doxycycline	Cotrimoxazole, chloramphenicol gentamicin, ciprofloxacin
Francisella tularensis	Gentamicin, chloramphenicol	Ciprofloxacin, doxycyline, levofloxacin
Pneumocystis jiroveci	Cotrimoxazole	Trimethoprim + dapsone, atovaquone, clindamycin + primaquine, pentamidine, trimetrexate + leucovorin
Proteus mirabilis and Proteus vulgaris	Amikacin, cotrimoxazole, imipenem	First-generation cephalosporin
Pseudomonas aeruginosa	Ceftazidime, cefepime, amikacin + (carbenicillin, carbapenem/ piperacillin)	Fluoroquinolones
Rickettsiae	Doxycycline	Chloramphenicol, erythromycin
Salmonella typhi	Fluoroquinolones, chloramphenicol	Cefoperazone, ceftriaxone, cotrimoxazole, amoxicillin, azithromycin
Shigella	Ciprofloxacin	Azithromycin, ceftriaxone, pivmecillinam
Spirillum minus	Penicillin G	Streptomycin, a tetracycline
Staphylococcus aureus	**Sensitive to pencillin:** Penicillin G **Sensitive to methicillin:** Methicillin **MRSA:** Vancomycin **VRSA:** Linezolid, tigecycline	**Sensitive to methicillin:** Nafcillin, oxacillin **MRSA:** Daptomycin, quinupristin + dalfopristin, arbekacin
Streptococcus pneumoniae	Penicillin G, amoxicillin	Third-generation cephalosporins, fluoroquinolones, azithromycin, doxycycline
Streptococcus pyogenes	Penicillin G or V	Cephalosporin, erythromycin, azithromycin, clindamycin
Streptococcus viridans	Penicillin G alone or with (gentamicin or streptomycin)	Cephalosporin, vancomycin
Toxoplasma gondii	Sulphadiazine – pyrimethamine, clindamycin	Atovaquone – pyrimethamine spiramycin, cotrimoxazole
Treponemapallidum	Penicillin G	Doxycycline, ceftriaxone, azithromycin
Vibrio cholerae	Doxycycline, tetracycline	Cotrimoxazole, chloramphenicol, fluoroquinolone, azithromycin

minocycline, linezolid and cotrimoxazole, which are to be given for 5–10 days. Rifampicin is used only in combination with other agents. In patients with severe systemic illness, parenteral agents like vancomycin, daptomycin, ceftaronil fosamil, telavancin and tigecycline are used.

ANTIMICROBIAL COMBINATIONS

As a rule, antimicrobials should not be combined unless therapeutic effect to one of the drugs in the combination is known to be unsatisfactory or proven to be so in a given patient. When indicated, the best known combination should be selected. Fixed dose combinations should not be used routinely, as they do not allow adequate doses of the major drugs and it is difficult to make dose adjustment of individual drugs. *Furthermore, one should be critical of the combinations recommended on the basis of laboratory data alone.*

Antibiotics may, however, be combined under certain circumstances for the following reasons:

- **To achieve an additive or synergistic effect against a single organism:** A combination of gentamicin with carbenicillin acts synergistically against pseudomonas infection. Brucellosis responds better to streptomycin + doxycycline combination than to streptomycin alone. It should be noted, however, that for a given antibiotic combination the dose of the individual antibiotic needed to accomplish synergism varies according to the type of organism.
- **To accelerate killing of microbes:** Artemisinin-based combination therapy (ACT) for falciparum malaria (Chapter 54).
- **In mixed infections with bacteria sensitive to different drugs:** Penicillin or metronidazole is combined with an aminoglycoside in peritonitis to control certain aerobes as well as anaerobes.
- **To delay the development of or to overcome the drug resistance** as in HIV, tuberculosis and malaria (see Chapters 51, 52 and 54).
- **To decrease the adverse reactions** to an individual drug, another agent may be added so that the doses of each drug can be reduced and possible dose-dependent toxicity avoided, e.g. flucytosine + amphotericin B for cryptococcal meningitis.
- **When etiological diagnosis is not known, the infection is severe and the body defence is poor** (as in malnourished patients, chronic alcoholics, patients with chronic renal failure, immunosuppressed patients and in neutropenic patients), empirical combined antimicrobial therapy may be given based on clinical assessment in order to cover a range of organisms. However, in such cases, the appropriate regimen should be instituted as soon as the organisms are identified.

It is not possible to predict which combination will have a synergistic effect and which will be antagonistic. The laboratory data are not always applicable to the disease processes in humans.

- **Combination of bacteriostatic drug with a bactericidal agent can cause:**
  1. **Drug antagonism:** If the bacteria are highly sensitive to the bactericidal drug
  2. **Additive effect:** If the bacteria are relatively resistant to the bactericidal drug

The bactericidal drugs more effectively attack the multiplying bacteria and hence, if a bacteriostatic drug is used along with a bactericidal agent, inhibition of bacterial multiplication may reduce the efficacy of the bactericidal agent. Combination of penicillin with chlortetracycline has been shown to produce antagonistic effect in pneumococcal meningitis. Significant antagonism occurs if patients are exposed to a broad spectrum bacteriostatic antibiotic before the institution of penicillin therapy. However, there are exceptions to such antagonism, e.g. combination of rifampicin (bactericidal) and fusidic acid (bacteriostatic) is recommended for methicillin-resistant staphylococcal skin infections.

- **Combining bacteriostatic drugs** usually leads to an additive effect; the effect may sometimes be synergistic as with the combination of sulphamethoxazole and trimethoprim.
- **Combination of bactericidal drugs among themselves may cause synergistic effect particularly with the drugs with different mechanisms of action.** Thus, gentamicin added to penicillin has a synergistic effect in the treatment of enterococcal endocarditis. Further, a combination of either ampicillin or carbenicillin with an aminoglycoside has been shown to act synergistically against susceptible *Escherichia coli*, *Klebsiella*, *Proteus*, *Providencia* and *Pseudomonas*. This is because penicillins promote the entry of the aminoglycoside through the microbial cell wall. A combination of ampicillin and clavulanic acid acts synergistically since the latter drug inhibits beta-lactamase production by the organisms and thus protects ampicillin.

Risks of Antimicrobial Combination Therapy

- *Emergence of organisms resistant to the multiple drugs used*
- *Increased risk of adverse reactions*
- *Increased risk of superinfection by resistant organisms*
- *Sense of false security* which may lead to incomplete evaluation and inadequate therapy
- *Increase in the cost of therapy*

ANTIMICROBIAL PROPHYLAXIS

It must be remembered that a drug which can cure a disease does not necessarily prevent it. Antimicrobials are not likely to be useful in chemoprophylaxis, if they are given as a blanket cover to prevent colonisation by various organisms in the internal and external environments of a patient. **They are, however, useful when used as single specific agents to prevent or destroy the infection due to specific organisms.** Further, short-term prophylaxis is more likely to be successful than prolonged prophylaxis because resistant organisms are likely to emerge during prolonged prophylaxis. Circumstances where such chemoprophylaxis may be useful are:

- **Prophylaxis following exposure to infective organisms:** For preventing meningococcal infection in healthy children during an epidemic; for prevention of diseases like syphilis, gonorrhoea, malaria and filariasis; for preventing recurrent UTI and HIV.
- **Prophylaxis in immunocompromised states:** Patients with neutropenia as in AIDS or those who have undergone organ transplant and are on immunosuppressants benefit from chemoprophylaxis. Microbial complications like bronchopneumonia, e.g. in severe cases of measles and tetanus, are prevented by instituting antimicrobial prophylaxis.
- **Prophylaxis for endocarditis:** Minor surgical procedures like tonsillectomy or tooth extraction in patients with cardiac lesions/prosthesis require prophylaxis 1 h before the procedure or within 2 h of the procedure. It is also given for preventing repeated attacks of streptococcal infection particularly in patients with history of rheumatic fever.
- **Pre-surgical prophylaxis:** For preventing invasion of blood stream by pathogens during certain surgical manipulations, e.g. catheterisation in patients with UTI, colonic surgery. **Routine prophylaxis in all ordinary operative procedures is unnecessary.** Such prophylaxis is, however, useful in surgery of the GI tract, biliary tract, uterus, and vagina; in joint replacement; and in open heart surgery. *Prophylaxis should be started not more than 1 h before surgery and should not be continued for more than 24 h after surgery in majority of cases. Care should be taken that throughout the surgery the concentration of chosen antimicrobial remains above its MIC, and therefore based on the t½, the dosing frequency of the antimicrobial drug is decided.*
- **Prophylaxis for trauma patients:** In patients with compound musculo-skeletal injury, penetrating wounds and skull injuries with rhinorrhoea and otorrhoea. For those puncture wounds that are at high risk for infection, e.g. contaminated wounds, deep wounds, wounds to the forefoot and wounds in individuals with diabetes mellitus or peripheral vascular disease.
- **Prophylaxis following bites:** Animal and human bites, as they are at high risk for infection by the oral flora.
- **Prophylaxis during hepatic failure:** Neomycin is administered orally to inhibit ammonia-producing intestinal pathogens which prevents the development or worsening of coma in hepatic failure.
- **Prophylaxis in comatose or paralytic states:** In poisoning cases prophylactic antimicrobials may be administered to prevent aspiration bronchopneumonia. *However, their routine use in all unconscious patients is of no benefit and may cause adverse effects.*

The indiscriminate prophylactic use of antibacterial agents may cause adverse and allergic reactions, produce resistant organisms, disrupt microbiome and cause superinfection due to other non-susceptible pathogens. This adds to the financial burden. As pointed out in an editorial in the Lancet "*the unwarranted use of antibiotics and particularly broad-spectrum antibiotics in a mistaken prophylactic attempt is a sin, and it would be wise to 'avoid not only the sin but also the occasions of sin' by better understanding of the epidemiology of Gram negative bacteria and the application of aseptic and other methods designed to prevent these bacteria colonising or infecting patients*'".

MICROBIAL DRUG RESISTANCE MI 1.6

Bacterial drug resistance is a major problem in chemotherapy. The host defence, environmental factors and the properties of the drug used influence the development of bacterial resistance to a drug.

Bacterial resistance can be **natural** or **acquired**.

In organisms which are **naturally resistant,**

1. The target sites for antibiotic may be altered or exist with low affinity.
2. The drug may fail to reach the target due to permeability barrier or absence of transport mechanisms or presence of efflux pumps.
3. Some naturally resistant organisms may elaborate

a substance which destroys the antibiotic, e.g. *E. coli* produce beta-lactamase which destroys penicillin.

Following the use of an antimicrobial agent which destroys the sensitive strain, these naturally resistant variants multiply and become dominant.

Acquired microbial resistance occurs following exposure to the drug or acquisition of genes that code for resistance.

Mechanisms for Acquiring drug Resistance

- **Genetic mutation**, i.e. by alteration in the structure of their own DNA. Such random mutations occur when microorganisms are under threat of antibiotic and need mechanisms to survive. As a result of mutations, changes may occur either in the transport protein, target protein or expression of inactivating enzymes so that the given antibiotic fails to act. The number of resistant mutants thus remain and increase as the trait is passed to the daughter cells.

In **genetic mutation**, the resistance is usually of a low level, to a single drug, and involves commonly non-enzymatic mechanisms such as decreased permeability to the antibiotic, e.g. methicillin resistance of *Staphylococcus aureus*. However, *M. tuberculosis* demonstrate high degree of resistance to isoniazid due to katG, Ser315 mutations. **Resistance due to genetic mutation is not transferable to other bacteria.** In some cases, the mutant bacteria even possess the capacity to multiply in the presence of higher concentrations of the drug concerned, e.g. streptomycin-resistant mutants.

- **Genetic exchange**, i.e. *by acquisition of extrachromosomal DNA from other bacteria*

Genetic exchange is the most important cause of serious clinical drug resistance because it can produce epidemic resistance to multiple drugs due to horizontal transfer. In genetic exchange, the resistance genes are transferred from one bacterial species to another by means of discrete, movable, extrachromosomal DNA elements called **plasmids.** The plasmids that encode for resistance to antimicrobial drugs are called **R-plasmids or R-factors.** *A plasmid* can reproduce itself and in the case of plasmid transfer, the replicating plasmid donates one copy to the new recipient cell. Transfer of R-plasmids between bacteria can occur by:

- **Conjugation**, i.e. direct physical mating between bacteria.
- **Transduction**, i.e. through the agency of bacteriophages.
- **Transformation,** where resistance genes from chromosomes may be transferred directly through a sex pilus without the mediation of a vector (plasmid or phage)., e.g. in Streptococci, Pneumococci, and some species of Haemophilus, Clostridia and Bacteroids.
- **Transposition**, which occurs independent of R-plasmids. **Resistance determinants (transposons) have the ability to 'hop' from one plasmid to another plasmid, or to a chromosome, or to a bacteriophage.** After entry into the host cell, the plasmid and the phage may be lost, leaving the transposons permanently in the plasmids or the chromosomes of the host cell. *Since transposons may carry multiple resistances, the recipient bacteria can acquire resistance to multiple drugs.*

Plasmid (R-factor) and/or transposon-mediated resistance results in the following:

- **Decreased bacterial cell wall permeability** to the antibiotic, e.g. resistance to penicillin and chloramphenicol
- **Active extrusion of the antibiotic from the bacterial cell**, e.g. resistance to tetracycline
- **Extracellular inactivation of the antibiotic**, e.g. enzymatic degradation or modification of penicillin, cephalosporins, aminoglycosides and chloramphenicol by resistant strains
- **Intracellular inactivation of the antibiotic**; this inactivated part then binds to the bacterial ribosomes and prevents them from taking up the active drug, e.g. resistance to aminoglycosides
- **Change in the bacterial ribosomes which are no longer susceptible to the action of the antibiotic**, e.g. resistance to macrolides
- **Synthesis of a drug-resistant enzyme** in place of the drug-sensitive enzyme in the biosynthetic pathway of the bacterial cell, e.g. resistance to sulphonamides and trimethoprim

R-factor–mediated resistance is often lost spontaneously. In contrast, the resistance due to genetic mutation is liable to be permanent.

R factors are found in intestinal bacteria, especially in *E. coli, Enterobacter aerogenes, Klebsiella pneumoniae, Salmonella, Shigella, Proteus* and *Pseudomonas.* R factors can be transferred from one bacterial species to another, e.g., from resistant *E. coli* to *Salmonella* or *Shigella.* In the case of some bacteria the R-factor may carry up to 8–10 different R-determinants, each responsible for resistance to a different drug.

Clinically, resistant Gram-negative bacteria carrying R factors present a serious problem because their resistance to multiple drugs can spread in epidemic proportions. Widespread outbreaks of bacillary dysentery caused by multiple drug resistant (MDR) Shigellae have been reported from Japan, Bangladesh and South America. In Mexico, MDR *Salmonella typhi* produced the worst epidemic of typhoid fever; and MDR-resistant *S. typhi* strains have been isolated from India. Transferable drug resistance is frequent in Gram-negative bacilli causing urinary infections.

Organisms that become resistant to one drug may exhibit cross resistance to other related compounds, e.g. cross resistance is seen between kanamycin and neomycin.

The organisms which are naturally resistant or those which develop resistance after exposure to the drug *in vivo* usually remain resistant and do not again become susceptible.

Antibiotic Stewardship Program PH 1.43

It is known that resistance genes and plasmids were present in bacteria even before the advent of antibiotics. These genes can then be transferred to the human pathogens. The excessive and indiscriminate use of antimicrobials in humans in the hospitals and in the community and in animals has encouraged the development of resistance. Many hospital strains of staphylococci, certain strains of *E. coli* and pseudomonas have become resistant to multiple antimicrobial agents. On the other hand, antimicrobial drug development has slowed down. Hence it is essential to conserve the existing antimicrobials we have in practice today. Thus, antibiotic stewardship programs are implemented to promote the optimal use of antimicrobials, improve patient outcomes, reduce antimicrobial resistance and decrease the spread of infections caused by MDR organisms. There are 2 major approaches to antimicrobial stewardship:

- **Front-end or pre-prescription approach:** It imposes restriction on the use of certain antimicrobials by making prior authorization for use mandatory.
- **Back-end or post-prescription approach:** It uses prospective review and feedback. The antimicro-

Box 49.4 Measures taken in Antibiotic Stewardship Programme

Educational:

- **Continuous education:** Clinicians are educated about **appropriate and rational use of antimicrobials** for specific infections. Emphasis is given on:
  - Using antibiotics only when necessary
  - Selecting the appropriate antibiotic and using it for an adequate period of time
  - Using a drug combination when it is known to delay the development of drug resistance (e.g. treatment of TB). However, remember that incidence of bacterial resistance parallels the number of antibiotics used in a given patient

Managerial:

- **Establishment of Hospital Infection Committee (HIC) and Drugs and Therapeutic Committee (DTC)** for:
  - **Prescription audit** to check antimicrobial usage and give feedback
  - **Pharmacodynamic dose optimization** based on time or concentration based killing optimal dose of an antibiotic
  - **Regular monitoring of drug resistance pattern** in hospitals and the community, and **antibiotic cycling** on a regular basis. It involves scheduled removal and substitution of specific antimicrobials or antimicrobial classes in a given patient care unit.
  - **Clinical guidelines/treatment algorithms designing:** specific to hospital based on local trends in antimicrobial resistance and national recommendations to make guideline-based antibiotic choices
  - **Computer-assisted decision support program institution:** to provide guidance to clinicians

Regulatory:

- **Formulary restriction:** to allow prescription of only selected antibiotics
- **Prescribing and dispensing control:** Authorization of faculty to prescribe or approve prescription or appointing dispensing physicians to counter-check prescription

bial steward reviews current antibiotic orders and provides recommendations to clinicians whether to continue, adjust, change, escalate /de-escalate or discontinue the therapy based on the available antimicrobial sensitivity results and clinical features of the patients.

Most of the times, combination of both the approaches is used. Most of the programs include measures depicted in Box 49.4. These programs have shown to reduce antibiotic misuse/ overuse/ abuse, treatment failure, adverse effects, hospital stay and cost of treatment.

RISKS OF ANTIMICROBIAL THERAPY

Antimicrobials are potentially harmful. The harmful effects are:

- **Development of allergic and anaphylactic reactions**
- **Selective organ/tissue toxicity,** e.g. diarrhoea, ototoxicity, thrombophlebitis
- **Life-threatening toxicity,** such as aplastic anaemia, hepatic failure or nephrotoxicity, wherein the toxicity is more serious than the infection being treated
- **Development of superinfection**
- **Development of MDR organisms**
- **Deficiency of certain vitamins**, e.g. vitamins K and folic acid because of the destruction of nonpathogenic bacteria in the intestine, which synthesise these vitamins
- **Fetal damage** by transplacental passage of certain antimicrobials
- **A false sense of security in the patient as well as the physician,** leading to the neglect of the need to establish the exact diagnosis. Similarly, strict asepsis may be neglected by a surgeon who relies too much on antimicrobials

Superinfections are defined as new infections that occur during chemotherapy of primary infection. They are manifested by new clinical symptomatology usually related to intestinal, renal and respiratory tracts or to blood stream. The organisms most commonly encountered are *Staphylococci, Candida albicans, E. coli, Proteus* and *Pseudomonas*. Some of the superinfections can be dangerous and may cause fatal results, e.g. resistant Staphylococcal enterocolitis and systemic fungal infections. The mechanisms are given in Box 49.5. **Superinfections are usually related to the dose and duration of antimicrobial therapy.** Infants, patients with pulmonary diseases, diabetics and immunocompromised patients are more prone to get superinfections.

Box 49.5 Mechanisms of Development of Superinfection

- Eradication of susceptible organisms in a patient with a mixed infection leaving the resistant strains to multiply
- Destruction of normal nonpathogenic bacterial flora, thus creating a bacterial vacuum leading to overgrowth of resistant organisms
- Colonisation of the lesion with resistant exogenous organisms from the environment

Failure to respond to antimicrobial therapy: When a patient does not respond to antibiotic therapy, the case should be reviewed with a view to answer the questions listed in Box 49.6.

MISUSE OF ANTIMICROBIAL AGENTS

The present total consumption of antimicrobials in relation to the known incidence of infections is very much in excess, indicating that antimicrobials are often misused. This obviously would create many problems as discussed above.

The various conflicting advertised claims of superiority of a newer antibiotic over the older one used for a similar purpose should be critically evaluated before accepting the change in established

Box 49.6 Failure of Antimicrobial Therapy — Why?

- Was an antibiotic really necessary?
- Is the right antibiotic being used?
- Is the bacterial strain isolated really responsible for the illness? Or, is a previously unsuspected infection present?
- Is the antibiotic being given in adequate doses and by proper route?
- Is the antibiotic reaching the site of infection?
- Is drainage necessary?
- Does the patient have resistant organisms or a superinfection?
- Is the fever due to the underlying disease, a drug reaction or an iatrogenic complication such as phlebitis?
- Is diabetes mellitus or AIDS present?

prescribing practice. Thus, cotrimoxazole may work out to be as effective and safe as and cheaper than a cephalosporin or a fluoroquinolone in the treatment of uncomplicated UTI or bacillary dysentery.

From the various antimicrobials now available, one needs to know only the important representative of each class. It is suggested that the family physician familiarises himself/herself thoroughly with the use of the following drugs for day-to-day practice: cotrimoxazole, ampicillin/amoxicillin, cephalexin, azithromycin, doxycycline, gentamicin/amikacin, ciprofloxacin and metronidazole.

Once started, the drug must not be changed without valid reasons. Too large or too low a dosage should be avoided as it may either produce toxicity or cause bacterial resistance. If any adverse effect is observed during the therapy, the drug should preferably be withdrawn instead of using another compound to suppress toxicity.

Antibiotics should not be used routinely in patients with fever without understanding its nature, simply to give 'quick benefits' of chemotherapy.

CHAPTER 50

Chemotherapy of Urinary Tract Infections

Learning Objectives

This chapter will enable the reader:

1. To be aware of the aetiopathogenesis, clinical features and diagnostic investigations for acute and chronic urinary tract infection (UTI).
2. To state the therapeutic goals for the treatment of various types of UTI.
3. To explain the general principles of use of antimicrobial agents in the treatment of UTI.
4. To classify drugs used in the treatment of UTI.
5. To explain the pharmacological basis for use of cotrimoxazole/ampicillin/carbenicillin/aminoglycosides/fluoroquinolones/cephalosporins/other beta lactam antibiotics/urinary antiseptics in the treatment of UTI.
6. To discuss the management of lower UTI.
7. To explain the antimicrobial regimens used for treatment of upper UTI.
8. To enumerate the indications and drug regimens used for prophylaxis of UTI.

KEY TERMS

significant bacteriuria, p. 721
cotrimoxazole, p. 721
fluoroquinolones, p. 721
piperacillin, p. 722
aminoglycosides, p. 722
cephalosporins, p. 722
nitrofurantoin, p. 722
choice of therapy in UTI, p. 724
acute uncomplicated cystitis, p. 724
recurrent infection, p. 725
chronic persistent infection, p. 725
acute pyelonephritis, p. 726

Urinary tract infection (UTI) is a common disorder at all ages and in both sexes. A healthy and normal urinary tract is generally resistant to infection. However, for anatomical reasons, the female lower urinary tract is more susceptible to infection.

UTI may present itself in acute or chronic form:

Acute infection: Infection localised to the urethra and bladder (**cysto-urethritis, lower UTI**) causes increased frequency and urgency of micturition, dysuria and pain in the perineum. Fever, chills and leucocytosis are generally absent. Such infections are generally self-limiting. If the **kidneys are involved** (**pyelonephritis, upper UTI**), the patient may have loin pain, fever, chills and leucocytosis. Urine is usually loaded with pus cells. Urine culture shows 'significant bacteriuria' (see subheading, Pathogenesis and bacteriology).

Inadequately treated acute UTI may lead to chronic pyelonephritis. Many patients with chronic infection, however, do not give a history of acute UTI.

Chronic infection: Patients with chronic infection may have few urinary symptoms unless renal failure has supervened. It must be remembered that *chronic pyelonephritis is an important cause of hypertension and chronic renal failure.* The urine may show a few pus cells. Significant bacteriuria is demonstrable in most patients with active infection and is essential for diagnosis.

In infants and children, UTI often masquerades as fever of unknown origin, failure to thrive, unexplained vomiting or as vague abdominal pain. Hence, the diagnosis can be easily missed. Elderly patients with UTI may present with altered mental status without usual signs and symptoms of UTI.

Pathogenesis and Bacteriology

The bacteria commonly found in UTI originate in the rectum. Bladder infection in females is often preceded by the establishment of the infecting organisms in the vaginal introitus. From there, the organisms ascend to the urethra and the bladder.

Ninety-five per cent of the cases of uncomplicated UTI in women are due to Gram-negative bacilli. E. coli is the commonest offender (80%), and next to it are Proteus mirabilis, Klebsiella, Aerobacter and Pseudomonas aeruginosa. In men, Gram-negative bacilli are responsible for about 75% of UTI, and *E. coli* causes less than half of the infections. Bacilli particularly involved include *Proteus* sp. and, to a smaller extent, *Providencia* sp. Gram-positive organisms account for about a fifth of infections. Hospital infections are generally by organisms other than *E. coli*. Mixed infections are likely to be present in chronic cases, in diabetics, in those with obstructive uropathies and in those with indwelling bladder catheters. Such infections are more difficult to treat.

For chlamydia, see below.

Significance of bacteria in the urine: The normal urinary tract, except for the distal urethra, is sterile. A few bacteria may, however, be sometimes found even in properly collected urine of apparently healthy individuals. Colony counts equal to and above 10^5/mL are designated as **significant bacteriuria** and are diagnostic of infection. Those on corticosteroid therapy may have **asymptomatic bacteriuria.** On the other hand, women with frequency of urination, dysuria and pyuria due to urethritis (*acute urethral syndrome*) may have fewer than 10^5 bacteria per mL or even a sterile urine on *routine* cultures (**symptomatic abacteriuria**). Many of them have gonococcal or chlamydial urethritis.

Classification of drugs used in UTI PH 1.48

I. **Bacteriostatic agents** such as doxycycline and nitrofurantoin
II. **Bactericidal agents** such as cotrimoxazole, ampicillin, extended spectrum penicillins, aminoglycosides, fluoroquinolones, cephalosporins and azithromycin

Urinary antiseptics are the drugs which act as antibacterial agents only in the urinary tract, e.g. nitrofurantoin, methenaminemandelate and nalidixic acid.

COTRIMOXAZOLE: This combination of sulphamethoxazole and trimethoprim (Chapter 43) is a potent and cost-effective bactericidal agent against *E. coliand Proteuss* pecies *but not Pseudomonas.* In acute uncomplicated UTI, it is used in the dose of 2 tablets (1 tablet contains sulphamethoxazole 800 mg + trimethoprim 160 mg) b.i.d. for 7–10 days. In smaller doses (as low as one tablet twice a week), it has been claimed to be effective in eliminating chronic bacteriuria. *Cotrimoxazole should be avoided during pregnancy.* Renal insufficiency leads to retention of trimethoprim, altering its ratio with sulphamethoxazole in urine, hence cotrimoxazole is likely to be less effective in renal insufficiency. As trimethoprim concentrates in the prostate much better than most other drugs, cotrimoxazole is useful for eradicating the prostatic focus of infection, often responsible for recurrent UTI.

Trimethoprim alone 100 mg b.i.d. is also used.

AMPICILLIN and **AMOXICILLIN:** These are effective both orally and parenterally. They are bactericidal to *E. coli*, *Aerobacter*, certain strains of *Proteus* and *Enterococci*. *Pseudomonas* is resistant. Both produce good tissue levels and are excreted unchanged in the urine in high concentrations.

When ampicillin is used in a dose of 0.5–1 g 6 h (or amoxicillin as 0.5–1 g 8 h) for 7–10 days, it eradicates majority of UTI due to *E. coli*. Both are useful for treatment of UTI in pregnant women. *However, many infections with E. coli, especially those acquired in the hospital are reported to be resistant to ampicillin/amoxicillin.* Ampicillin-sulbactum or amoxicillin–clavulanic acid may be used if resistance is suspected. They have low rate of pathogen eradication and higher rates of relapse.

FLUOROQUINOLONES: These are considered **ideal agents for nosocomial pyelonephritis and complicated UTI. They are useful even if renal function is very low**. The high tissue and urine concentrations even in acid urine far exceed the bactericidal concentrations against most pathogens including *Pseudomonas*(Chapter 43). *They should not be used routinely in uncomplicated UTI for fear of emergence of drug resistance.* Misuse of fluoroquinolones has already resulted in resistance. Risk of Achilles tendon rupture and irreversible neuropathy are the additional concerns regarding its use.

CEPHALOSPORINS: These drugs are valuable in infections with *E. coli* and *Proteus*, resistant to other antibiotics. *They are the drugs of choice in klebsiella infections. The third generation cephalosporins are particularly effective against multi-resistant enterobacteria and Pseudomonas resistant to other antibiotics.* Cephalosporins are particularly indicated in septicemic UTI (Chapter 46). They are ineffective against *Enterococci*.

FOSFOMYCIN: It is administered as single dose of 3 g. See section, Treatment of lower UTI. In addition, see Chapter 45.

PIPERACILLIN: It has a broad spectrum of activity against Gram-negative organisms, **especially *P aeruginosa*.** It is given intravenously in divided, daily, adult doses of 4–8 g for moderate infections in persons with normal renal function; the dose is raised to 12–16 g/day in life threatening infections. It can be combined with gentamicin with synergistic effects. **It is particularly useful in patients with renal impairment where aminoglycosides are to be avoided.** *Its use should be limited to severe UTI with life threatening septicemia* (Chapter 44). Piperacillin-tazobactum combination is used in drug resistant cases.

AMINOGLYCOSIDE ANTIBIOTICS: Gentamicin (160 mg IM/IV) and **amikacin** (5 mg/kg in two divided doses as IM/slow IV bolus/infusion) are commonly used in UTI. They are effective against *E. coli*, *Proteus* and *Pseudomonas*. They can cause ototoxicity and renal toxicity. *The nephrotoxicity can be considerably reduced by giving the entire daily dose as a single dose.* Their use is reserved for complicated UTI (Chapter 45).

CARBAPENEMS: These compounds are reserved for complicated UTI due to *Pseudomonas* and *Enterococci*. They can be combined with aminoglycosides (Chapter 46).

MONOBACTUM: Aztreonam (0.5–1 g t.i.d or b.i.d), active against Gram-negative organisms including *Pseudomonas* is given for nosocomial infection where aminoglycosides are to be avoided.

AZITHROMYCIN: It is commonly used for chlamydial urethritis (Chapter 51).

DOXYCYCLINE: See Chapter 47.

URINARY ANTISEPTICS

NITROFURANTOIN: It is effective against commonly occurring urinary pathogens such as *E. coli* and *Aerobacter*. However, it is mainly bacteriostatic. Most strains of *Pseudomonas* and some strains of *Proteus are* resistant (Chapter 43). *It is useful in the treatment of acute cystitis caused by susceptible strains of E.coli.* Though it achieves a high urinary concentration, it has *poor tissue levels* (due to extensive protein binding), and is therefore **unsuitable for the treatment of renal parenchymal infections.**

Absorption, fate and excretion: It is rapidly and completely absorbed from the GI tract. *Food increases its bioavailability*. It does not achieve a bacteriostatic concentration in the plasma but approximately 40% of the drug is excreted unchanged by the kidney, **achieving a bactericidal concentration in the urine(luminal effect)**. Its activity decreases at alkaline pH. *Therefore, the urine should not be alkalinised during nitrofurantoin therapy. It does not appear in the urine in severe renal failure and in azotemic patients, and hence should be avoided.*

Preparation and dosages: available as capsules (50 mg and 100 mg), it is administered orally with food in the dose of 50–100 mg 6 hourly for 7 days. The comparable dose in children is 50 mg up to 1 year, 75–100 mg from 1 to 5 years and 150–200 mg from 6 to 12 years in three or four divided doses. The drug should not be given for more than 2 weeks. The dose for long suppression of susceptible urinary tract pathogens is 100 mg once a day in patients with genitourinary abnormalities to prevent frequent/ recurrent UTI (**chronic suppressive therapy'**).

Adverse reactions: The most frequent adverse events are nausea, vomiting, headache, and flatulence. It can cause diarrhoea, dyspepsia, abdominal pain, dizziness, drowsiness, amblyopia and allergic manifestations e.g., acute pulmonary hypersensitivity reaction ,and urticaria. Occasionally nitrofurantoin can cause alopecia, fever, chills, malaise and rarely cholestatic jaundice, hepatitis and pulmonary toxicity.

The drug colours the urine brown. It is generally safe in pregnancy.

Nitrofurantoin exhibits therapeutic antagonism with nalidixic acid.

METHENAMINE MANDELATE (Mandelamine): This drug is a salt of mandelic acid and methenamine, and combines the antibacterial properties of both the drugs. It is rapidly absorbed from the GI tract and is excreted in urine. **At an acid pH of less than 5.5, methenamine liberates formaldehyde which acts against many Gram-negative pathogens and *C. albicans*.** Mandelic acid helps to lower the urine pH. *Bacteria do not develop resistance to it.*

It is sometimes used in chronic suppressive therapy.

The drug is available as 500 mg and 1 g tablets. It is used in a dose of 500 mg four times a day.

Adverse reactions: Except gastric discomfort, they are rare. Large doses can cause acute inflammation of the urinary tract.

NALIDIXIC ACID: This drug, available in 0.5 g tablets, is sometimes used for chemoprophylaxis in the dose of 0.5–1 g/day (Chapter 43). If used for treatment, the dose is 1 g q.i.d for 7 days.

Investigations in a Case of UTI

In every patient with recurrent UTI, it is essential to look for a predisposing cause, especially diabetes mellitus, congenital anomalies and obstructive lesions in the urinary tract.

- **Urine obtained by midstream technique or by suprapubic bladder puncture is examined** for:
  a. Microscopic urine analysis (2–5 WBCs or $\geq$ 15 bacteria/hpf indicate UTI) and
  b. Urine culture to identify bacteria and to test sensitivity of isolated microorganism **to various antibacterial drugs.**

Pretreatment urine culture is not required in the first attack in young women as such attacks are usually due to *E. coli. Urine culture should be done only if the UTI is recurrent!*

In pregnant women, incidence of bacteriuria is high and may cause growth retardation in fetus. Asymptomatic bacteriuria can also progress to pyelonephritis. Hence regular screening is required.

UTI is uncommon in men under the age of 50 years. Urine culture should always be done for these patients. In such patients:

- **Diabetes mellitus must be ruled out.**
- **Detailed urological investigation** is mandatory for all men and in children with single attack and in women who get more than two recurrences in 1 year to detect parenchymal disease.
- **Infective focus in the prostate should be ruled out** in men with UTI.

Even a single UTI infection is a potentially serious condition and failure to treat it may lead to development of serious chronic pyelonephritis, hypertension and renal failure.

DRUG THERAPY OF UTI

Goals for the Treatment of UTI are as follows:

1. To eradicate the infecting organisms
2. To provide symptomatic relief by altering the pH of urine and/or giving phenazopyridine
3. To prevent and treat recurrence
4. To identify and treat predisposing factors

General Principles of Therapy: PH 1.1

- **In acute cases,** *an appropriate drug may be started as soon as the urine has been collected for bacteriological examination.* When the results of drug sensitivity of the pathogen grown are available, another drug may be substituted for the first one, if necessary. Although the symptoms are relieved quickly, the pyuria takes a longer time to clear.
- **In chronic cases,** mixed infection is more likely and concomitant renal failure may modify drug therapy. In such cases, *there is no desperate hurry to start drug treatment before the case is investigated.*
- The significant infection is in the tissues and not in the luminal urine alone. *Hence, the drug must achieve adequate concentration in the tissues as well as in the urine.* Further, the effects of the antimi-

crobial agent on the vaginal flora are also important in the lasting eradication of bacteriuria. The concentration of trimethoprim and fluoroquinolones in the vaginal secretions is high enough to eradicate the *E. coli.*

- *Bactericidal drugs are to be preferred for treatment. The drug must be used in adequate doses and for adequate periods.* The last dose should be given immediately *before retiring, having emptied the bladder completely.* This is important because the diminished urinary flow and frequency at night encourage bacterial growth.
- **All pregnant women should be screened for bacteriuria in the first trimester** and should be treated, if found, to reduce their increased risk of acute pyelonephritis, premature delivery and low birth-weight newborn. In such cases, a 7- to –14-day course is recommended. Follow-up is necessary in order to detect a recurrence.
- The growth of *E. coli* is optimum at pH 5.0–6.0 and is inhibited at pH below 5.5 and above 7.5. **Alkalinisation of the urine (pH > 7.5) must also be maintained at a level that would permit optimum antibacterial activity of the drug used.** Alkalinisation also helps to reduce irritation of the urinary tract. It is achieved by the administration of 2 g (½ teaspoon) of sodium bicarbonate, sodium citrate or potassium citrate, 4–6 times a day. *Alkalinisation of urine enhances the antibacterial activity of penicillins, erythromycin and aminoglycosides.*
- It must be emphasised that infections due to *Proteus* and sometimes other coliforms, *S. albus* and some diphtheroids, give rise to alkaline urine. This is because these organisms produce urease, an enzyme which splits urea to form ammonia.
- *The fluid intake should be liberal as frequent emptying of the bladder* (every 2–3 h) helps to reduce the bacterial counts in the urine and the growth of *E. coli.*
- There is no satisfactory antibacterial drug to which all the strains of *E. coli*, the commonest causative organism, are invariably sensitive. *Hence, the initial choice of the drug depends upon the relative cost and the known adverse effects of the drugs.*

Choice of Therapy: Choice of antibacterial therapy of UTI is determined by:

- *The site of the infection*
- *Whether a predisposing cause such as diabetes mellitus or an abnormality of the urinary tract is absent (uncomplicated UTI) or present (complicated UTI)*
- *Whether the infection is caused by drug-sensitive or drug-resistant organisms*

Factors influencing the choice of therapy are shown in Box 50.1. Lower UTI is often an uncomplicated infection, whereas upper UTI is commonly a complicated infection in this sense.

Box 50.1 Factors Influencing Choice of Therapy

- ***The patient:*** Site of infection in urinary tract, symptomatic or not, age, sex, pregnancy, first attack or a recurrence, underlying abnormality of the urinary tract, renal function and associated diseases such as diabetes mellitus
- ***The organisms (expected or isolated):*** Their identity, single or multiple species and their drug sensitivity
- ***The drug:*** The route of administration, cost and adverse effects

TREATMENT OF LOWER UTI

- **Acute uncomplicated cystitis-urethritis:** *The first attack in a young, healthy woman is treated by 3-day antibiotic therapy which reduces the rectal carriage of Gram-negative bacteria and is not associated with increased recurrence rate in UTI.*

Cotrimoxazole is perhaps the best initial choice for empirical therapy in a non-pregnant woman. It is cost-effective and relatively safe. When low resistance to *E. coli* is known, **nitrofurantoin** 100 mg b.i.d. for 5–7 days is equally effective. More expensive alternative is fosfomycin 3 g as a single dose. The regimens used are shown in Box 50.2. *Fluoroquinolones are not recommended as first-line empirical treatment of uncomplicated cystitis.*

Three-day therapy provides complete symptomatic relief but may not achieve 100% bacteriological cure. Hence, therapy for 7–14 days which achieves both clinical and bacteriological cure is preferred in the following:

- *Failure of the 3-day regimen*

Box 50.2 Suggested Oral Antimicrobial Regimens for Acute Uncomplicated Cystitis

- Cotrimoxazole 2 tablets b.i.d.[a]
- Trimethoprim 100 mg b.i.d.[a]
- Nitrofurantoin 100 mg b.i.d. (50 mg b.i.d. if weight is <50 kg)[b]
- Ampicillin 250–500 mg q.i.d.[a]

[a]for 3days or 7-14 days
[b]for 7 days

- *Symptomatic men*
- *Recurrences in both men and women*
- *Elderly (age more than 65 years)*
- *Symptoms persisting more than 7 days*
- *Pregnant women*
- *Children*
- *Patients with underlying renal disease, urinary tract obstruction/abnormalities and diabetes mellitus*

Although a single-dose cotrimoxazole, ampicillin/amoxicillin or fosfomycin has been used to treat first attack of UTI, such therapy gives low cure rate and leads to frequent recurrences. It fails to eradicate Gram-negative bacteria from the rectum, the major reservoir for recruitment of ascending uropathogens, and hence, should not be recommended.

In pregnant woman with cystitis, amoxicillin (±clavulanic acid), cephalexin, Cefotaxime, ceftibuten and nitrofurantoin are treatment options. Single-dose therapy with fosfomycin tromethamine (3 g) has been advocated for uncomplicated, first attack of infection in a pregnant woman. Follow-up urine culture is done 1–2 weeks after treatment and then monthly until delivery.

Cotrimoxazole and fluoroquinolones should be avoided during pregnancy (Chapter 78).

- **Recurrent infection**, manifested by repeated bacteriuria usually within 2 weeks of apparently successful treatment, is caused by the same organism which caused the first infection. *Recurrence should be documented by a culture at least once before starting therapy.* Such women should receive treatment for at least 4–6 weeks with either cotrimoxazole or a fluoroquinolone. Other expensive alternatives are: amoxicillin + clavulanic acid; a third generation cephalosporin such as cefixime or cefpodoximeproxetil. *It is important to eliminate the vaginal colonisation by E. coli.* Also, hidden source of infection or a urological abnormality should be looked for.

In patients with **suspected prostatic focus** of infection, urine culture and antibiotic sensitivity is to be done. Drugs like trimethoprim, fluoroquinolones, doxycycline and aminoglycosides are recommended for 2 – 4 weeks. Despite prolonged therapy (6–12 weeks), the failure rate in chronic bacterial prostatitis is usually 30%–40%. *It should be remembered that nonbacterial prostatitis is far commoner than proven bacterial prostatitis.*

Where bacteriuria cannot be eradicated, chronic suppressive therapy with 1 tablet of cotrimoxazole or 50–100 mg of nitrofurantoin once daily can suppress symptomatic infection. *Trimethoprim alone should be avoided for suppression for fear of development of drug resistance.*

- **Chronic persistent infection** should be treated with one of the 7- to 14-day regimens given above. *Long-term continued administration of antibacterial agents only leads to the emergence of drug resistant organisms.* Attempt should be made to discontinue the catheter prior to starting therapy.
- **Asymptomatic bacteriuria** is often transient and resolves without treatment. Treatment is appropriate:
  a. In patients with congenital or acquired abnormality of the genitourinary tract and those undergoing urologic surgery.
  b. In infection with virulent microorganisms.
  c. In immunocompromised host e.g. neutropenic / renal transplant recipients. Neutropenic patients with asymptomatic bacteriuria are treated for 6 weeks.

Children and pregnant women with asymptomatic bacteriuria must be treated adequately to prevent chronic renal infection.

- **Postcoital cystitis:** should be initially treated by a full course of a suitable antibacterial drug as in acute uncomplicated UTI. Following this, she should be advised to apply 0.5%cetrimide cream to the periurethral area before coitus and to empty her bladder immediately after the sexual act. A *single dose* of ampicillin 250 mg, nitrofurantoin 100 mg or a cotrimoxazole tablet may be prescribed after each coitus.
- **Acute urethral syndrome** in women is often due to **chlamydial infection**. Its treatment is discussed in Chapter 51.

TREATMENT OF UPPER UTI

This is usually due to the same pathogens that cause lower UTI but is a more serious condition.

- **Acute pyelonephritis** is commonly associated with a predisposing factor such as obstructive uropathy or diabetes mellitus (complicated UTI). The patient may be septicaemic and severely ill. *Urine and blood cultures are mandatory before starting the therapy; the results are helpful in modifying the initial therapy which is started without waiting for the culture report.*

The drugs used in **mild cases (uncomplicated)** are: ciprofloxacin 500 mg b.i.d.; cotrimoxazole 2 tablets b.i.d.; amoxicillin-clavulanate 500 mg b.i.d. or ampicillin 1–2 g orally or intravenously (especially in infection due to enterobacter) or a cephalosporin (Chapter 46). The duration of treatment is 10–21 days or longer.

Follow up urine culture is recommended after 2 weeks of therapy. In pregnant women, a parenteral cephalosporin and/or an extended spectrum penicillin are indicated.

In severely ill patients and in those with recurrent, complicated UTI, empirical IV treatment should be started with:

1. A fluoroquinolone.
2. A carbapenem.
3. Piperacillin –tazobactam.
4. Cefotaxime/ceftriaxone 1 g IV followed by oral therapy with a fluoroquinolone.

The definitive treatment and its duration is guided by urine culture and is usually longer than 21 days.

- **Chronic pyelonephritis:** This serious condition can lead to chronic renal failure and secondary hypertension. An underlying cause such as obstruction must be carefully searched for. The antibacterial treatment is prolonged and the choice of the drug is governed by the identity of the organisms and their drug sensitivity, and by the extent of renal impairment (see below).

It is difficult to treat. It is important to detect drug failure early so that an ineffective drug is discontinued. In such cases, it may be better to use antimicrobials only during acute episodes. Suppressive therapy is rarely effective.

In patients with **renal impairment**, the dose of aminoglycosides and cephalosporins must be scaled down. *Nitrofurantoin does not achieve adequate urinary concentration in patients with renal failure and may cause toxicity.* Tetracyclines, except doxycycline, are avoided in chronic renal failure.

Follow-up: Successful treatment of an acute attack with an antibacterial agent leads to disappearance of bacteriuria within 24 h; but pyuria and symptoms take longer to disappear. Patients should be followed up for at least 6 months after treatment and urine cultures should be repeated at 1–2 month intervals. Cases with recurrent acute infection or with chronic infection need prolonged suppressive drug therapy (6–12 months) after the initial treatment. In such cases, follow-up cultures should be done for about 2 years.

Unarrested or repeated kidney infection not only leads to chronic pyelonephritis but also prevents the kidney growth in children.

ANTIMICROBIAL PROPHYLAXIS

This is indicated:

- *Following instrumentation of the urinary tract.*
- *In patients with uncorrectable congenital anomalies of the urinary tract.*
- *In patients with 3 or more symptomatic UTI attacks/ year.*
- *In chronic prostatitis and pregnant women with asymptomatic bacteriuria.*

Before starting antimicrobial prophylaxis, the preceding attack of UTI, if any should be treated. **Low dose cotrimoxazole (40/200 mg), nitrofurantoin (50-100 mg), trimethoprim (100 mg) and norfloxacin (200 mg)at bedtime or three times / week are the most commonly employed** agents for this purpose. It must be remembered, however, that doses which are employed for long-term prophylactic therapy may not produce adequate tissue levels. Although the urine may remain sterile, infection may continue to progress without being detected. Short-term catheterisation may be covered by giving the patient nitrofurantoin.

Catheter associated UTI: Urine culture sensitivity needs to be done to decide antibacterial therapy. Catheter may be removed or replaced. Asymptomatic patients with candiduria may recover without treatment once catheter is removed or replaced. In case of symptomatic candiduria fluconazole 200-400 mg /day for 14 days is recommended.

PHENAZOPYRIDINE: This azo dye is used in the dose of 200 mg three times a day to relieve pain, burning, urgency and frequency associated with lower UTI. *It does not act as a urinary antiseptic but can give symptomatic relief.* The drug colours the urine red or orange and can stain clothing. Therapy with this drug is generally limited to 1 week.

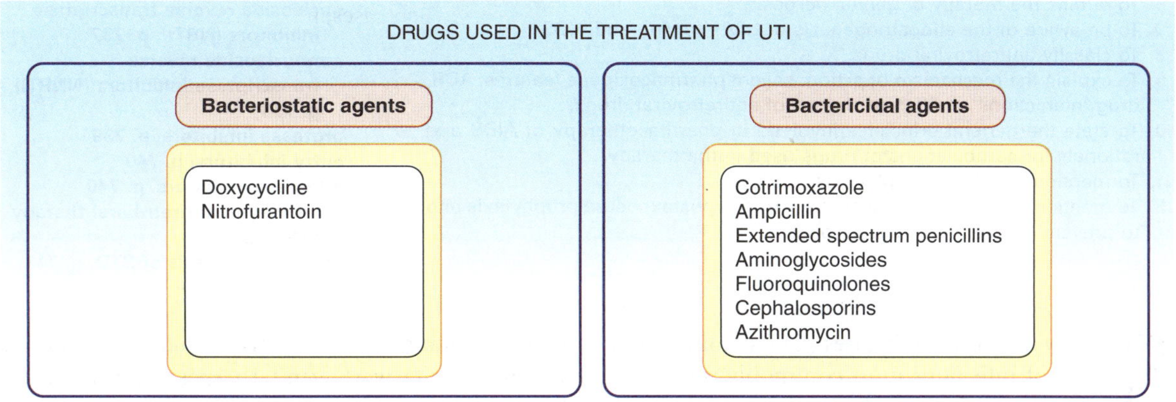

CHAPTER 51

Chemotherapy of Sexually Transmitted Diseases

Learning Objectives

This chapter will enable the reader:

1. To enlist the clinical syndromes that can present as sexually transmitted diseases (STD).
2. To outline the principles and drug regimens used in the treatment of different types of syphilis.
3. To explain the antimicrobial regimens for acute uncomplicated/complicated gonorrhoea.
4. To outline the treatment for nongonococcal urethritis.
5. To mention the drug/s of choice for lymphogranuloma venereum, chancroid, granuloma inguinale, vaginitis and genital warts.
6. To outline the therapy of genital herpes.
7. To be aware of the etiopathogenesis of HIV infection and AIDS.
8. To classify antiretroviral drugs.
9. To explain the mechanism of action, salient pharmacokinetic features, ADR, drug interactions of different classes of antiretroviral drugs.
10. To state the general principles involved in pharmacotherapy of AIDS and rationale for combinations of drugs used in the therapy.
11. To mention the chemoprophylaxis of STD.
12. To mention drug regimens used for pre- and postexposure prophylaxis and to prevent vertical transmission of HIV.

KEY TERMS

syphilis, drug therapy, p. 729
Jarish–Herxheimer reaction, p. 732
acute pelvic inflammatory disease (PID), p. 732
acute gonorrhoea, uncomplicated/complicated, p. 733
nongonococcal urethritis, p. 733
bacterial vaginitis, p. 734
viral STD, p. 735
nucleoside reverse transcriptase inhibitors (NRTI), p. 737
nonnucleoside reverse transcriptase inhibitors (NNRTI), p. 738
protease inhibitors, p. 739
entry inhibitors, p. 740
integrase inhibitors, p. 740
combination antiretroviral therapy (ART), p. 741
chemoprophylaxis of STD, p. 743

Sexually transmitted diseases (STDs) comprise a group of infections most commonly transmitted by sexual contact; accidental infection through fomites and infection of laboratory workers are rare modes of transmission. In the case of syphilis and AIDS, transplacental transmission to the foetus can occur.

Survey by WHO has indicated a worldwide rise in the prevalence of STDs. Hence, chemotherapy will continue to play an important role in their treatment. The concurrent presence of AIDS (HIV infection) complicates the management of STD by suppressing the immune system.

The **important STDs** are syphilis, gonorrhoea, nongonococcal urethritis (NGU), chancroid, lymphogranuloma venereum, granuloma inguinale, vaginitis, genital warts, genital herpes, AIDS (acquired immunodeficiency disease) and hepatitis B.

Aetiological diagnosis of STD is problematic due to constraints on time, resources, costs and access to treatment.

Since more than one type of STDs may commonly be present in a person at the same time, ideally all patients with suspected STD should be screened for HIV, syphilis, gonorrhoea and chlamydia. However, this is beyond the means of most third world countries. In addition, the sensitivity and specificity of available diagnostic tests can vary significantly. To overcome this, a syndrome-based approach to the management of these infections was developed by

WHO and promoted in many developing countries. Accordingly, the signs and symptoms are classified into a few 'Clinical syndromes' such as:

- **Anogenital ulcer**
- **Urethral discharge, dysuria and increased frequency** (urethritis)
- **Vaginal discharge** (vaginitis)
- **Lower abdominal pain/dyspareunia** (pelvic inflammatory disease, PID)
- **Warty lesion** (genital warts)

Each of these syndromes is then treated with multiple drugs that will deal with the majority organisms responsible for producing that syndrome. The National AIDS Control Organization (NACO) provides colour-coded treatment kits under the National AIDS Control Programme (NACP) for syndromic management of sexually transmitted infections (STIs) based on the 'National Guidelines on Prevention, Management and Control of Reproductive Tract Infections including STIs'. Though syndromic management has been shown to decrease the disease burden in developing countries because of prompt treatment of infection without the necessity of undergoing laboratory investigations, there are certain limitations e.g. asymptomatic patients do not receive treatment; it does not distinguish between cervicitis and vaginitis and may lead to overtreatment in some individuals.

Hence clinical features, responsible organisms and the definitive evidence-based therapy of various STDs is described first followed by the information on the treatment kits and drugs therein. The important points to remember about treatment of STDs are outlined in Box 51.1.

Box 51.1 Points to Remember about the Management of STDs

- STDs often occur concurrently
- Compliance with treatment and follow up are often dismal
- It may be better to treat even when an STD is suspected, preferably with single dose therapy (see Table 51.2)
- Serious complications including infertility may occur from lack of adequate treatment
- Perform serological test for syphilis on patients with other STDs
- Perform pregnancy test on all females with STD
- Counsel patients about STD prevention and importance of HIV testing
- Advise all patients of bacterial STI and trichomoniasis that the sexual partner must be treated to prevent reinfection without waiting for laboratory test results

PH 1.48, DR 10.3

DRUG THERAPY OF SYPHILIS

Syphilis is caused by the spirochete *Treponema pallidum.* **Penicillin is the drug of choice for all stages of syphilis.** With adequate treatment of early cases, almost 90% of cases can be cured. Penicillin resistant *T. pallidum* is so far unknown.

Clinically, syphilis manifests as:

1. **Primary syphilis,** characterised by genital or extragenital, painless, nontender, indurated ulcer (chancre), occurs within 3 weeks after the infection. This can be diagnosed easily by dark-field microscopy or direct fluorescent antibody test of the exudates.
2. **Secondary syphilis,** characterised by skin and mucosal lesions occurring within 6 weeks to 6 months after the infection. This is diagnosed by serological tests (see below). Both these stages can resolve even without treatment.
3. **Latent syphilis is asymptomatic** but with positive serological evidence. **Early latency** is diagnosed if the infection has been acquired within the preceding 1–2 years (WHO classification). After that, it is considered as **late latency**.
4. **Tertiary syphilis,** which manifests 4–5 years after the infection, and includes neurosyphilis (GPI, Tabes dorsalis), cardiovascular syphilis and gummatous syphilis. It is not contagious but needs more prolonged treatment with higher doses of penicillin and still complete cure may not be possible. *Syphilis is considered a great imitator, and almost every organ in the body can be affected.*

Principles of therapy:

- **Before starting treatment, the diagnosis must be established with certainty.** Dark-field microscopy of material from surface lesions is a must in the case of primary chancre and secondary syphilis. When surface lesions are absent, one has to rely on serological tests.
- **Treated cases should be followed up for adequate period.**
- **It is necessary to trace and treat contacts.**

Table 51.1 Drug Therapy in Sexually Transmitted Diseases

Clinical condition with Organisms	Regimen of choice	Alternatives
	Syphilis	
Primary, secondary syphilis (early syphilis) and early latent syphilis (< 1 year)	Procaine penicillin 600,000 U IM daily × 10–15 days If allergic to penicillin, Doxycycline 100 mg po bid × 14 days	Benzathine penicillin 2.4 MU IM (1.2 MU in each buttock) in a single dose/ Ceftriaxone 1–2g daily IM or IV × 10–14 days
Latent syphilis (> 1 year)	Procaine penicillin 600,000 units IM daily × 15 days. If allergic to penicillin, Doxycycline 100 mg po bid × 28 days	Benzathine penicillin 2.4 MU IM (1.2 MU in each buttock) once weekly for 3 weeks
Neurosyphilis, ocular or oto syphilis	Penicillin G 18–24 MU daily in 6 divided IV bolus or as infusion, × 10–14 days.	Procaine penicillin 2.4 MU IM once a day, together with probenecid 500 mg po qid, × 10 days.
	Gonorrhoea	
Uncomplicated urogenital, rectal, pharyngeal	Ceftriaxone 500 mg IM once	Cefixime 800 mg po once If severely allergic, Gentamicin 240 mg IM once + Azithromycin 2g po
Epididymitis, proctitis (often associated with Chlamydial infection)	Ceftriaxone 500 mg IM once + Doxycycline 100 mg po bid x 10 days	
Complicated with PID [a]		
Intravenous therapy[b]	Ceftriaxone 1g IV every 24h + Doxycycline 100 mg po or IV bid + Metronidazole 500 mg po or IV every 12 h OR Cefotetan 2 g IV every 12h or cefoxitin 2 g IV every 6h + Doxycycline 100 mg po bid or IV	Ampicillin/sulbactam 3 g IV every 6h + Doxycycline 100 mg po bid or IV + Metronidazole 500 mg orally twice a day OR Clindamycin 900 mg IV every 8h + Gentamicin loading dose 2 mg/kg IV or IM once, then 1.5 mg/kg IV every 8h. Single daily dosing (3-5 mg/kg) can be substituted
Intramuscular or Oral	Ceftriaxone 500 mg IM once + Doxycycline 100 mg po bid + Metronidazole 500 mg bid[c] OR Cefoxitin 2 g IM once + Probenecid 1 g po once + Doxycycline 100 mg po bid + Metronidazole 500 mg po bid	Levofloxacin 500 mg po once/day + Metronidazole 500 mg po bid x 14 days[d] Levofloxacin can be replaced by Moxifloxacin 400 mg po once/day[d] OR Azithromycin 500 mg IV once/day x 1-2 doses,then 250 mg po once/day (total 7 days) + Metronidazole 500 mg po bid[d]
NGU	Doxycycline 100 mg po bid x 7 days	Azithromycin 1 g po once
	Chlamydial infection	
Oropharyngeal, urogenital, rectal	Doxycycline 100 mg po bid x 7 days	Levofloxacin 500 mg po once/day x 7 days / Azithromycin 1 g po once
Lymphogranuloma venereum	Doxycycline 100 mg po bid x 21days	Azithromycin 1 g po once/day x 21 days / Erythromycin base 500 mg po qid x 21 days

Table 51.1 Drug Therapy in Sexually Transmitted Diseases

	Chancroid	
	Single dose Azithromycin 1 g po / Ceftriaxone 500 mg i.m.	Cotrimoxazole 2 tablets bid for 7 days / Erythromycin 500 mg qid for 7–10 days / Ciprofloxacin 500 mg bid for 3 days
	Granuloma inguinale	
	Azithromycin 1 g once a week x 4 weeks	Doxycycline 100 mg bid / Cotrimoxazole 2 tablets bid / Erythromycin base 500 mg po 4 times a day / Ciprofloxacin 750 mg po twice a day / Ampicillin 500 mg 6 hourly for 3–4 weeks
	Trichomoniasis	
	Metronidazole 500 mg po bid x 7 days (women) and 2 g po once (men)	Tinidazole 2 g po once (women and men)
	Viral infections	
Anogenital warts	Podophyllotoxin 0.5% solution / gel applied twice daily for 3 consecutive days each week for 10–15 weeks	Imiquimod 5% cream, applied three times a week on alternate days for 16 weeks / Sinecatechins 15% tid up to 16 weeks
Genital herpes	Acyclovir 400 mg po tid x 7-10 days / Famciclovir 250 mg po tid x 7-10 days / Valacyclovir 1 g po bid x 7-10 days	

po= per oral IM= intramuscular; IV= intravenous
[a]Duration of therapy should be 14 days.
[b]Intravenous therapy can be stopped 24-48 h after clinical improvement and oral doxycycline 500 mg bid and oral metronidazole 500mg bid should be started.
[c]Other parenteral third-generation cephalosporin (e.g., ceftizoxime or cefotaxime) + Doxycycline 100 mg orally twice a day plus Metronidazole 500 mg orally twice a day can be used.
[d]If the patient is allergic to cephalosporin and if gonococcal infection is unlikely and patient can be followed.

Drug therapy of syphilis:

I. **Primary and secondary syphilis (early syphilis) and early latent syphilis of less than 1 year's duration:** See Table 51.1.
The drug of choice is **procaine penicillin** which is administered for 10-15 days to maintain the concentration as it follows *time-dependent killing*. **Benzathine penicillin** is an alternative and is less likely to be painful. Patients allergic to penicillin are treated with **doxycycline.**
All treated patients must be examined clinically and a quantitative serological test carried out at regular intervals for at least 4 years from the beginning of the disease. The CSF must be examined at the end of the first year to rule out neurological involvement. If there is a relapse or a rise in the titre of the serological test, the penicillin course must be repeated.

II. **Syphilis (except neurosyphilis) of more than 1 year's duration**: See Table 51.1. It is treated with either **procaine penicillin** or **benzathine penicillin**. The latter needs to be given as 3 doses, a week apart between the doses.

III. **Neurosyphilis:** All clinical types of neurosyphilis are associated with CSF changes, and CSF cell count provides good monitoring for judging the effects of therapy. The drug of choice is **penicillin G.** Alternatively, it may be treated with **procaine penicillin.**

Patients are followed clinically, serologically and with CSF examination at frequent intervals. *Persistently positive serology alone is not an indication for more treatment.* If, however, the test becomes positive in a higher titre or if CSF abnormalities persist, treatment should be repeated.

Syphilis in HIV positive patients usually progresses rapidly and has higher risk of neurological complications and treatment failure.

Pregnancy and syphilis: Congenital syphilis is a completely preventable disease. Hence, syphilis detected during pregnancy should be treated with any of the regimes of penicillin described above for primary syphilis. Patients allergic to penicillin should be treated with erythromycin or ceftriaxone. Alternatively, after skin testing and desensitization, penicillin G is given.

Congenital syphilis detected in infants and children can be treated by injecting benzyl penicillin for 10 days. Interstitial keratitis, a complication of congenital syphilis, needs additional treatment with local or systemic glucocorticoids.

Adverse reactions to penicillin are described in Chapter 44. Jarisch–Herxheimer reaction, which is observed in syphilitic patients, is described below:

- **Jarisch–Herxheimer reaction:** *This consists of an initial exacerbation of lesions at any stage of syphilis following the first dose of a quick acting spirocheticidal drug like penicillin. Any reaction that occurs after subsequent injections of penicillin is unlikely to be due to Herxheimer phenomenon.* It is due to a rapid destruction of a large number of spirochetes with release of the endotoxin. It occurs in many cases of **early syphilis**, and leads to an aggravation of the mucocutaneous lesions and a mild systemic illness consisting of malaise, tachycardia and fever. Lymph nodes are enlarged and tender. **It lasts for 2–6 h and is harmless.** The patient should, however, be forewarned about it as, otherwise, he might feel that wrong treatment was administered. **The treatment with penicillin must be continued despite the reaction.**

A sharp febrile reaction occurring within 24 h of the use of penicillin in gonorrhoea suggests the possibility of concurrent syphilis as Jarisch–Herxheimer reaction is known to occur even in the incubation period of syphilis.

In cardiovascular and neurosyphilis, however, a Herxheimer reaction may precipitate severe angina or CHF; and psychosis, convulsions, coma or optic atrophy respectively. Fatalities have occurred due to laryngeal oedema or coronary occlusion.

Herxheimer reaction is an all or none phenomenon and cannot be prevented. Even a small first spirocheticidal dose is likely to precipitate it. An attempt can be made to prevent it in cardiovascular and late neurosyphilis by starting prednisolone in the single, daily dose of 30 mg in the morning, 2 days before starting penicillin. From the 7th day, the prednisolone dose can be tapered and the drug omitted with the end of penicillin therapy.

PH 1.48, DR 10.8

DRUG THERAPY OF GONORRHOEA

Gonorrhoea is caused by gonococci. *Though previously, most strains were sensitive to penicillin, resistance, over the years resistance has been developed against penicillin, tetracycline and fluoroquinolones.* Recently decreased susceptibility against azithromycin, cefixime and ceftriaxone is also reported, which are currently the agents of choice. Chlamydial and gonococcal infection may coexist.

Gonococcal infection is more difficult to diagnose and treat in females than in males. **Acute PID** (pelvic inflammatory disease) **may be caused by other organisms** (*Chlamydia trachomatis, Mycoplasma hominins, Hemophilus* species, vaginal flora including anaerobes, Gram-negative organisms such as *Escherichia coli* and Group B streptococci) in addition to the gonococci; and hence, *the treatment will need multiple drugs covering potential pathogens.*

Before starting chemotherapy, the diagnosis must be established by smear and culture of material obtained from the urethra and by prostatic massage in the males and the urethra, vagina, cervix or Bartholin glands in the females.

Acute uncomplicated urogenital, rectal or pharyngeal gonorrhoea: Eradication of acute, uncomplicated gonococcal infection caused by penicillin sensitive organisms is relatively easy and **procaine penicillin is a drug of choice.** *Benzathine penicillin which gives low but prolonged plasma penicillin levels should not be used to treat gonorrhoea.*

The initial therapy with penicillin may mask the early manifestation of concomitant syphilitic infection. Therefore, *penicillin should be used in full doses as recommended for syphilis, in all cases.*

However, now presence of multidrug resistant (MDR) gonococci necessitates use of 500 mg IM **ceftriaxone** or 800 mg oral **cefixime** in a single dose. The response to treatment is usually prompt and dramatic.

Previously this regime included azithromycin because NGU is known to be commonly associated with gonorrhoea. But now resistance of gonococci to azithromycin is increasing and therefore coadministration of azithromycin is not recommended. If chlamydial infection cannot be excluded then ceftriaxone therapy should be followed by a 7-day course of doxycycline 100 mg twice a day.

If the patient is severely allergic to cephalosprins then a single dose of IM gentamicin along with azithromycin is effective for urogenital or rectal gonorrhoea.

The sex partner should be treated with ceftriaxone or cefixime. The patient should be advised abstinence from alcohol for about 2 weeks. Though no testing is required for treated patients with urogenital or rectal gonorrhoea, it is needed to confirm cure in pharyngeal gonorrhoea. Sexual abstinence is required till the cure is achieved. As chances of reinfection are high, rescreening after 3 months for gonorrhoea is essential in all treated patients.

Complicated gonorrhoea: When there is bacteremia and/or the spread of gonococci to joints and tissues then it is called as complicated infection. The regimens shown in Table 51.1 have been recommended in gonorrhoea complicated by acute PID.

Treated patients are followed up clinically, bacteriologically and serologically at frequent intervals for at least six months before they are declared as 'cured'.

DRUG THERAPY OF NONGONOCOCCAL URETHRITIS (NGU)

No pathogen is detected in 40-50% patients with NGU. The infection may be due to the following:

- **Infection with *Trichomonas vaginalis*** (Chapter 56) or ***Mycoplasma genitalium.***
- **A generalised urinary tract infection** (Chapter 50).
- **Nonspecific urethritis: This common STD is caused by** *C. trachomatis* **in about 50% of the cases.** The final diagnosis is by exclusion of gonococcal and trichomonal infections in cases of urethritis. See the section on Drug therapy of Chlamydial infection for drug therapy (Table 51.1)

The presumptive treatment of choice for NGU, including chlamydial infection is **doxycycline** 100 mg twice a day for 7 days. **Azithromycin,** in the single oral dose of 1 g, which is also highly effective and safe during pregnancy. Repeated infections may be due to *M. genitalium*. In these patients, doxycycline course should be followed by moxifloxacin for 7 days.

DRUG THERAPY OF CHLAMYDIAL INFECTION

Chlamydial infections are usually asymptomatic and present as oropharyngeal, urogenital and rectal infections. The treatment of choice is oral **doxycycline** for 7 days (Chapter 48). The effective alternative is **levofloxacin** (Table 51.1). Azithromycin though used as a single dose is less effective than these antibiotics against rectal chlamydial infections and both, rectal and urogenital infections coexist. However, **azithromycin remains a choice in pregnant woman.** The less effective alternative is amoxicillin.

Neonates of women having cervical chlamydial infection are at the risk of conjunctivitis and pneumonia, which are treated with systemic erythromycin for 14 days. Alternative is azithromycin for 3 days (Table 51. 1). Milder cases can be treated with topical erythromycin. DR 10.8

Lymphogranuloma venereum is a more invasive disease caused by chlamydia and causes proctocolitis or genital ulcer with lymphadenopathy. **Doxycycline 100 mg b.i.d. for 21 days is effective** in curing the acute inguinal disease. **Alternatives are azithromycin or erythromycin**. In the chronic hypertrophic type, surgery may be needed in addition to doxycycline for 6–8 weeks. Alternatively, erythromycin may be used. The prognosis in chronic cases is poor.

The sexual partner of the patient with chlamydial infection should be treated at the same time with a 7 day course of doxycycline, to prevent reinfection. During therapy, the patient should abstain from sexual intercourse and alcohol which may aggravate urethritis.

PH 1.48, DR 10.8

DRUG THERAPY OF CHANCROID

Chancroid or soft sore is **caused by *H. ducreyi*.** Clinically, it causes multiple, painful, pulsed out penile ulcers with fluctuating inguinal lymphadenopathy (bubo).

The treatment of choice is single dose of **azithromycin** or **ceftriaxone**. Alternative regimens are, cotrimoxazole; or erythromycin; or ciprofloxacin (Table 51.1) Ampicillin and tetracycline should not be used as resistance is likely to be present. In HIV positive patients or uncircumcised patients, longer antibiotic courses are required.

DRUG THERAPY OF GRANULOMA INGUINALE

Granuloma inguinale (Donovanosis) is caused by *Calymmatobacterium granulomatis*. The drug of choice is **azithromycin** 1 g once a week for 4 weeks. Alternatively either of the following antimicrobials, doxycycline, cotrimoxazole, erythromycin, ciprofloxacin or ampicillin are also effective (Table 51.1). They are continued if reepithelialization is incomplete. If the ulcers do not respond to above therapy within the first few days, gentamicin is added. Relapse may occur after 6-18 months later. In such cases, treatment is reinitiated.

VAGINITIS – DRUG THERAPY

This is a common condition predominantly caused by three types of organisms

- ***C. albicans*** (fungus)
- ***T. vaginalis*** (protozoon)
- ***Gardenella vaginale*** (bacteria) and a**naerobic organisms**

Candidial vaginitis responds to intravaginal therapy with **triazole compounds** (Chapter 48), once each night for 3–7 days. **A single oral dose (150 mg) of fluconazole** is as effective as several days of clotrimazole and miconazole locally. Asymptomatic carriers need no treatment.

Metronidazole is the drug of choice for trichomoniasis (Chapter 56). **Single dose of metronidazole or tinidazole is recommended for the male partner** (Table 51.1). *According to the current guidelines there is no need for abstinence form alcohol as disulfiram like reaction does not occur with metronidazole in clinical practice.* Reinfections are common and retesting after 3 months should be done. Trichomoniasis has adverse outcomes in pregnancy and hence should be treated with metronidazole, which appears to be safe in pregnancy. However, safety of tinidazole is not established. **Bacterial vaginitis** also responds to **metronidazole** 500 mg b.i.d. for 7 days. Alternatively, **clindamycin** 2% cream at bedtime for 7 days may be used. Similar regimens should be used to treat male partners, since 90% of them are urethral carriers of *G. vaginale*.

Table 51.2 lists the single dose regimens for the various STDs.

Table 51.2 Single Dose Regimens for Treatment of STDs

Syphilis (early)	Benzathine penicillin 2.4 MU in two IM injections, one on each buttock once
Gonorrhoea	Ceftriaxone 500 mg IM (or cefixime 400 mg orally)
Chlamydial NGU	Azithromycin 1 g po
Chancroid	Azithromycin 1 g po/ceftriaxone 500 mg IM
Trichomoniasis	Tinidazole 2 g po
Candidial vaginitis	Fluconazole 150 mg po

Po= per oral IM= intramuscular

DRUG THERAPY OF VIRAL STD

Anogenital Warts

This condition is due to local human papilloma virus (HPV) infection and is sexually transmitted in 60% of cases (condylomata acuminata). The warts grow rapidly in the presence of moisture and are inhibited by dryness. The virus may cause cervical dysplasia or cancer. No treatment eradicates HPV or modifies the risk. Recurrence is common after treatment.

The warts are treated either by electric cautery under local anaesthesia or by applying **podophyllum resin** (20% suspension in liquid paraffin or alcohol) or **trichloracetic acid** weekly. **The surrounding skin must be protected by application of soft paraffin. Cryotherapy with liquid nitrogen is also effective.**

Self-treatment is possible with podophyllotoxin (Podofilox) (Table 51.1) or **imiquimod**. Imiquimod can eradicate about 50% of these anogenital warts. It acts by inducing the local production of interferon α along with proinflammatory cytokines IL- 1, -6 and -α8, and TNF-α. Both the drugs should be avoided during pregnancy.

Imiquimod (1% cream) applied three times a day for 5 days a week also resolves the lesions of a disease, molluscum contagiosum.

Sinecatechines is a watery extract of green tea leaves (*Camellia sinensis*); 15% ointment is used locally for external genital and perianal warts. The drug may cause erythema, pruritus, rash and erosions.

All self-application drugs should be avoided in pregnancy.

Genital Herpes

Herpes simplex 1 (HSV 1) and *Herpes simplex* 2 (HSV 2) are known to infect the anogenital areas. Of these, HSV 2 causes most of the recurrent infections associated with itching, parasthesia, and maculovesicular eruptions. HSV is one of the important causes of genital ulcers. The drugs used are **acyclovir** 400 mg orally t.i.d., or **famciclovir** 250 mg t.i.d. or **valaciclovir** 1 g b.i.d., for 7–10 days. Similar treatment for 5 days is given for recurrences (Chapter 57). Higher doses with longer duration of treatment are needed in patients with HIV. Oral acyclovir is safe in pregnancy.

Table 51.3 presents the treatment regimens enclosed in the colour coded kits for syndromic management of sexually transmitted infections (STI).

DRUG THERAPY OF HIV

Human immunodeficiency virus (HIV) infection and AIDS is caused by a retrovirus, HIV-1 and -2 which is most commonly transmitted by sexual intercourse. The other modes of transmission are by contaminated syringes and needles, by blood transfusions and by blood products. It is also transmitted from an infected mother to the foetus during pregnancy, during childbirth or breast feeding. *The virus is not spread by casual contact such as handshake with a sufferer, nor by aerial transmission, nor by fomites.*

HIV REPLICATION CYCLE

1. On entering the body, viral outer glycoprotein (gp120) of HIV binds to CD4 receptors on the surface of T lymphocytes, monocytes, macrophages and brain dendritic cells (Fig. 51.1). This is followed by binding to other chemokine receptors on the cell surface, i.e. CCR5 and CXCR4.

Table 51.3 Syndromic Management of STI: Possible Pathogens and Drug Regimens

Kit No. and Colour	Syndrome (Consistent group of symptoms and signs)	Common Organisms for syndrome	Drugs and Regimen
Kit 1: Grey	Urethral discharge, Cervical discharge, Ano-rectal discharge, Painful scrotal swelling	*Chlamydia trachomatis (D-K), Neisseria gonorrhoeae*	Tablet Azithromycin 1 g once and Tablet Cefixime 400 mg once
Kit 2: Green	Vaginal discharge	*Trichomonas vaginalis, Candida albicans, anaerobic bacteria, Chlamydia trachomatis (D-K), Neisseria gonorrhoeae, Mycoplasma genitalium*	Tablet Secnidazole 2 g once and Tablet Fluconazole 150 mg once
Kit 3: White	Genital ulcer, non-herpetic	*Treponema pallidum, Haemophilus ducreyi, Klebsiella granulomatis, Chlamydia trachomatis*	Inj. Benzathine penicillin 2.4 MU once and Tab. Azithromycin 1 g once
Kit 4: Blue	Genital ulcer, non-herpetic and the patient allergic to penicillin	-do-	Tab. Doxycycline 100 mg bid x 15 days and Tab. Azithromycin 1 g once
Kit 5: Red	Genital Ulcer Disease- Herpetic	*Herpes simplex virus*	Tab. Acyclovir 400 mg tds x 7 days
Kit 6: Yellow	Lower abdominal pain (PID)	*Neisseria gonorrhoeae, Chlamydia trachomatis (D-K)* and other bacteria like Mycoplasma, Gardnerella, anaerobic bacteria etc.	Tab. Cefixime 400 mg once and Tab.Metronidazole 400 mg bid x 14 days and Cap. Doxycycline 100 mg bid x 14 days
Kit 7: Black	Inguinal bubo	*Haemophilus ducreyi, Chlamydia trachomatis*	Cap. Doxycycline 100 mg bid x 21 days and Tablet Azithromycin 1 g once

2. After attachment to CD4 and chemokine receptors, the virus fuses with the cell through viral glycoprotein, gp41 and the viral contents like single-stranded RNA, an RNA-dependent DNA polymerase (also known as **reverse transcriptase**), and other enzymes are internalised.
3. From the single-stranded viral RNA, reverse transcriptase synthesises a complementary strand of DNA and later a double-stranded DNA. *Many mutations can occur in the conversion of RNA to DNA, which are responsible for HIV's ability to develop drug resistance.*
4. The double stranded DNA migrates to the host cell nucleus and is integrated by an HIV enzyme called **integrase** into the host cell chromosome. This process is termed as strand transfer.
5. On activation of the cell by antigens or cytokines, HIV replication starts using host DNA polymerase. This enzyme transcribes viral DNA into messenger RNA, and mRNA is then translated into viral proteins.
6. These proteins assemble beneath the host cell membrane. The viral nucleocapsid is formed surrounding these proteins, and the virus buds from the cell.
7. After budding, the virus maturation takes place. HIV protease enzyme cleaves large polypeptides into smaller functional proteins. Newly formed virus can infect other cells only after maturation.

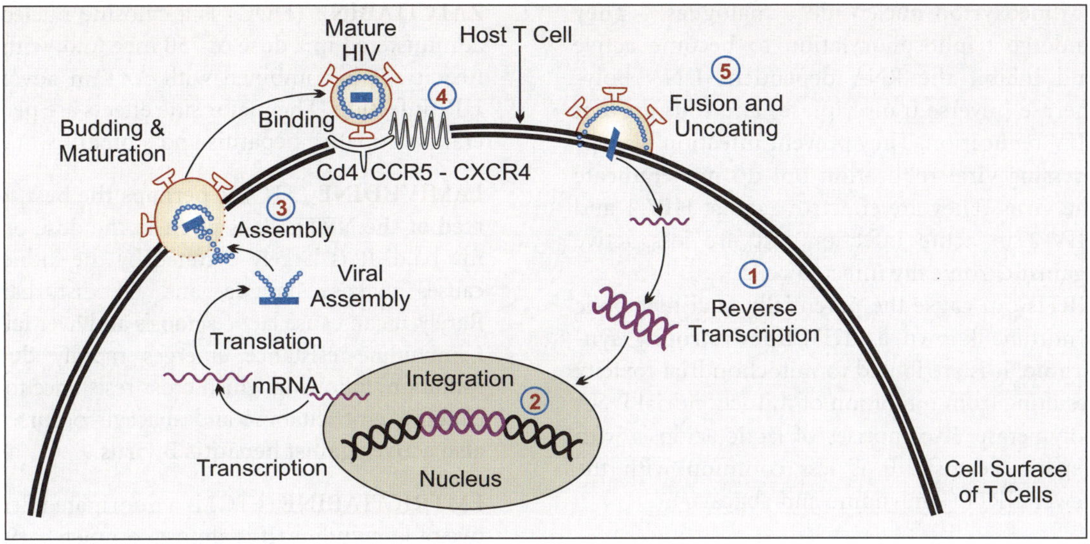

FIG. 51.1 Life cycle of HIV and site of action of antiretroviral drugs. CCR5, CXCR4 = chemokine receptors; target sites: (1) for NRTI, NNRTI and NTRI, (2) for integrase inhibitors, (3) for protease inhibitors, (4) for chemokine receptor antagonist, (5) for fusion inhibitors.

The antiretroviral drugs act on various steps of the viral replication (See under Classification of Antiretroviral Drugs; Fig. 51.1).

During the process of viral replication, the CD4 cells suffer from functional impairment. Impaired CMI makes the patient susceptible to opportunistic infections.

Antibodies to HIV develop in 2–8 weeks after infection. The viruses are also killed by cytotoxic T-lymphocytes or undergo apoptosis. However, within some cells, they may stay dormant for several years. *Most of the subjects remain asymptomatic carriers for prolonged periods and can transmit the disease;* a few develop a short febrile illness.

The next stage is of high rate of viral replication in lymph nodes and the development of a persistent generalised lymphadenopathy with or without infections such as oral candidiasis and herpes zoster.

In **the final stage (AIDS),** the body cannot replenish T lymphocytes and the CD4 counts drop to <200 cells/mm3. The patient suffers from several opportunistic infections (tuberculosis, candidiasis, *Pneumocystis jiroveci* pneumonia, cryptococcal meningitis and CNS toxoplasmosis), repeated chronic GI infections and malignancies. Severe neurological disorders such as dementia, encephalitis and meningitis can also occur. Death is inevitable.

Classification of Anti-Retroviral Drugs

I **Nucleoside reverse transcriptase inhibitors (NRTI):** Azidothymidine*, didanosine, zalcitabine, stavudine, lamivudine*, emtricitabine, abacavir*

II **Non-nucleoside reverse transcriptase inhibitors (NNRTI):** Nevirapine*, efavirenz,* delaviridine, etravirine, rilpivirine

III **Nucleotide reverse transcriptase inhibitor (NTRI):** Tenofovir disoproxil* /alafenamide

IV **Protease inhibitors (PI):** Ritonavir*, amprenavir, lopinavir*, atazanavir*, darunavir*

V **Entry inhibitors:** Enfuvirtide, maraviroc, fostemsavir, ibalizumab (IBA)

VI **Integrase strand transfer inhibitor (INSTI):** Raltegravir*, dolutegravir*, elvitegravir

The drugs which have been marked as * are included in the National guidelines for HIV care and treatment.

Salient Pharmacological Features of Antiretroviral Drugs PH 1.48

I. **Nucleoside reverse transcriptase inhibitors (NRTI):** All these drugs are 2′,

3′-dideoxyribo-nucleoside analogues. They undergo triphosphorylation to become active and inhibit the RNA dependent DNA polymerase (reverse transcriptase) and thus prevent HIV replication. They prevent infection by suppressing viral replication but do not eradicate the virus. They are effective against HIV-1 and HIV-2 in acute infection but are less active against chronically infected cells.

NRTIs can cause the potentially fatal metabolic syndrome known as **HIV lipodystrophy syndrome.** It is attributed to mitochondrial toxicity resulting from inhibition of mitochondrial DNA polymerase. It comprises of lactic acidosis with hepatic steatosis. It is less common with the newer NRTI (lamivudine and abacavir).

AZIDOTHYMIDINE (AZT, Zidovudine): Given orally, 3′-azido-3′-deoxy thymidine gets incorporated into DNA of the HIV and terminates chain synthesis of viral DNA. The viral DNA polymerase is more susceptible than of mammalian cells.

AZT is well absorbed orally; it can also be given intravenously. It is mostly metabolised in the liver. (t½ 1 h). It penetrates into CSF and amniotic fluid.

It causes GI upset, headache, myalgia and insomnia. Serious ADR include severe anaemia, granulocytopenia and thrombocytopenia. Rarely agitation, seizures, hepatotoxicity and myopathy have been reported.

The drug has been used in the dose of 300 mg orally, b.i.d. Considering the safety of AZT, no change is required in pregnancy.

DIDANOSINE (ddI): This nucleoside analogue of deoxyadenosine, with similar actions as AZT, has longer duration of action. It is nontoxic to the haemopoietic cells but can cause pancreatitis and peripheral neuropathy. The other ADR are headache, diarrhoea, nausea/vomiting, asthenia, insomnia, CNS depression, aches and pains, loss of taste, arthritis, alopecia, dizziness, retinal depigmentation and optic neuritis.

***STAVUDINE** (d4T) has properties similar to those of didanosine, and should not be combined with it, as toxicity of the combination is more.* Stavudine also exhibits pharmacodynamic antagonism with AZT.

ZALCITABINE (DDC) is a cytosine nucleoside administered in a dose of 750 mcg t.i.d; with less toxicity. It is combined with AZT in advanced HIV infection. The major side effects are peripheral neuropathy, hepatitis and stomatitis.

LAMIVUDINE (3TC) is **perhaps the best tolerated of the NRTIs.** It is given in the dose of 150 mg b.i.d. It is largely excreted by the kidney. It causes malaise, fatigue, and GI disturbances. Rarely, it can cause lactic acidosis and liver failure. Lamivudine-resistance emerges rapidly due to mutation, following which cross resistance to zalcitabine, emtricitabine and abacavir occurs. **It is also active against hepatitis B virus.**

EMTRICITABINE (FTC) is a fluorinated derivative of lamivudine. It is almost completely (93%) absorbed and has intracellular t½ of 39 h. Hence, it is given once daily. It is hepatotoxic.

ABACAVIR (ABC) is a well-tolerated NRTI with high therapeutic efficacy. Dose is 300 mg b.i.d/ 600 mg o.d. The ADR include hypersensitivity reactions, sometimes fatal; this is genetically associated with HLA-B*5701 typing.

II. **Non-nucleoside reverse transcriptase inhibitors (NNRTI):** These drugs, like NRTIs, inhibit reverse transcriptase but by a different mechanism, which does not require their metabolic conversion. Hence, **they are usually combined with an NRTI.** They are more selective for HIV-1 reverse transcriptase and therefore are **effective only against HIV-1.** They do not inhibit human DNA polymerase. HIV isolates resistant to NRTIs remain sensitive to these drugs. They are metabolised in the liver. They cause skin rash, hepatotoxicity and multiple drug interactions.

DELAVIRDINE (DLV)**:** This NNRTI has high bioavailability and plasma protein binding capacity. ADR include headache, fatigue and diarrhoea. It is also an inhibitor of CYP3A4 and CYP2C9 and can cause potential drug interactions. The drug is teratogenic in rats and should be avoided in pregnancy.

EFAVIRENZ (EFV): This NNRTI administered as 600 mg o.d., **crosses the BBB, which most other anti-HIV drugs fail to do.** The development of resistance to this drug is claimed to be slower than to the older drugs. It is given once a day (t½ 52 h). The adverse reactions comprise dizziness, insomnia, hallucinations, abnormal dreams and rarely pancreatitis. The drug is teratogenic in animals but the available data suggests that exposure to EFV does not result in increased birth defects. It is a mixed inducer and inhibitor of CYP3A4.

NEVIRAPINE (NVP) is more effective and penetrates the CNS well. It is started in a dose of 200 mg o.d. for 2 weeks and if no rash then it is increased to 200 mg b.i.d.

Etravirine (ETV) and **rilpivirine** (RPV) are other NNRTI usually used in combination with NRTI to treat resistant HIV infection. Long acting formulation (IM depot injection) of rilpivirine is available. **Doravirine** (DOR) exhibits efficacy against HIV strains that are resistant to efavirenz and other earlier NNRTI. It has minimal CNS ADR and has better safety profile than other drugs in this class.

III. **Nucleotide, reverse transcriptase inhibitor (NTRI):** Like NRTI, **tenofovir inhibits a variety of DNA polymerisation reactions and hence is prone to cause more toxicity**. It appears to be effective against HIV strains resistant to other drugs. It is also effective in hepatitis B. **Tenofovir disoproxil** (TDF) is a prodrug, which gets hydrolysed in plasma to tenofovir while **tenofovir alafenamide** (TAF) is taken up by the cells, wherein it gets converted into tenofovir. Though both the salts are well tolerated except for flatulence, nephrotoxicity can occur in patients with pre-existing renal damage. TDF can cause lactic acidosis, pancreatitis, hepatitis, rhabdomyolysis, osteomalacia and asthenia.
Both the salts are given as 300 mg once daily.

IV. **Protease inhibitors (PI):** These drugs are listed in Table 51.4 and they:
a. Inhibit aspartyl protease which cleave viral proteins and effectively arrest replication
b. Block the infectivity of the nascent virions
c. Prevent subsequent waves of infection

They have no effect on cells already harbouring integrated proviral DNA. They are effective against HIV-1 and HIV-2. Orally, they are well tolerated and metabolised by hepatic CYP3A4 (except Nelfinavir). **Most of them inhibit CYP3A4; the most potent being ritonavir.** Ritonavir allows reduction in the doses of other PI like lopinavir, and atazanavir, when used concurrently. This **boosted PI regimen is currently preferred.**

Table 51.4 Currently Available Protease Inhibitors

Drug	Dose	Remarks
Amprenavir (APV)	1200 mg b.i.d.	NOT to be given with RTV *Now rarely used*
Indinavir (IDV)	800 mg t.i.d.	B.i.d. therapy, if with RTV *Now rarely used*
Nelfinavir (NFV)	750 mg t.i.d.	*Now rarely used*
Saquinavir (SQV)	1000 mg t.i.d.	*Now rarely used*
Ritonavir (RTV)*	600 mg b.i.d.	Not used alone because of GI ADR
Lopinavir (LPV))*	400 mg b.i.d.	Always with RTV
Atazanavir (ATV))*	400 mg o.d.	300 mg o.d., if with RTV
Darunavir (DRV)*	600 mg b.i.d.	For HIV resistant to other PI Structural similarity to sulphonamide
Fosamprenavir (FPV)	1400 mg b.i.d.	700 mg b.i.d., if with RTV Prodrug of amprenavir with better solubility and has replaced the latter *Now rarely used*
Tipranavir (TPV)	500 mg b.i.d.	*Now rarely used*

Note: RTV, ritonavir (100–200 mg)
* Available in the National programme

Adverse reactions: Commonly, they cause nausea, vomiting, diarrhoea and parasthesiae. GI symptoms are less with the newer drugs like atazanavir and darunavir. Hepatotoxicity, insulin resistance, hyperglycaemia, dyslipidaemia, lipodystrophy (buffalo hump) and pancreatitis can occur. Indinavir may cause nephrolithiasis. Darunavir and fosamprenavir contain sulpha moiety, which is responsible for skin rashes. **Drug interactions are common with all the PIs.**

They are mainly used as second line drugs.

V. **Entry inhibitors:**

The entry inhibitors are reserved for patients resistant to other drugs. Four drugs are available in this class, each with different mechanism of action.

ENFUVIRTIDE (ENF) is a synthetic HIV-derived peptide which **selectively inhibits membrane fusion of HIV (fusion inhibitor) with cells and prevents their entry into cells**. It is not active against HIV-2. It is administered in a dose of 90 mg subcutaneously twice daily. Apart from local reactions, it may cause lymphadenopathy, peripheral neuropathy, pneumonia and suppression of IL-12.

Maraviroc (MUC): This drug is a chemokine receptor-5 (CCR-5) antagonist and prevents entry of CCR-5 tropic virus in the host cell. However it has no activity against CXCR-4 tropic viruses or dual tropic viruses. It can cause dose dependent orthostatic hypotension. As it is metabolized by CYP3A4 , drug interactions with CYP inducers and inhibitors can occur. It is administered as 300 mg orally twice daily.

FOSTEMSAVIR: This prodrug gets rapidly hydrolysed to release temsavir, which binds to the viral envelope protein gp120. This prevents the attachment to CD4 cells and virus cannot enter the cell. It is used only in MDR- HIV-1 infection, wherein other ARV are already tried. It elevates hepatic transaminases and prolongs QT interval. Temsavir is a CYP3A4 and p-glycoprotein substrate and is prone for drug interactions.

IBALIZUMAB: This is a humanized monoclonal antibody . It binds to extracellular domain of CD4 cells. It does not prevent attachment of viral gp120 to CD4 cell but prevents subsequent conformational change that is necessary for fusion and entry. It is also termed as '**post-attachment maturation inhibitor**'. It does not interfere with host immune response as it binds to CD4 at a site different from MHC class II binding site.

It is also used for MDR- HIV-1 infection. Resistance can develop to it rapidly. It is given as IV infusion every 2 weeks. It is well tolerated.

VI. **Integrase strand transfer inhibitors (INSTI):** They bind to the active site of HIV-1 and -2 integrase, an enzyme needed for viral DNA insertion into the host genome. This prevents integrase from binding to HIV DNA, and blocks the strand transfer step, which is essential for HIV replication.The viral load declines rapidly with these drugs over 3–4 months. Their antiretroviral activity and safety profile is better. Hence they are used to treat new cases of HIV who are not on any treatment.

RALTEGRAVIR (RAL)**:** It is used orally (400 mg b.i.d) in combination to treat patients with MDR HIV-1 strains. It causes insomnia and has certain toxic effects of concern such as rhabdomyolysis, myopathy, myalgia, diarrhoea, fever, rash, Stevens-Johnson's syndrome, hepatitis and liver failure.

DOLUTEGRAVIR (DTG): This drug causes rapid suppression of virus by reducing the viral burden to <50 copies/ml within 4 weeks and thus decreases the chances of transmission. It is effective against HIV-2. It has high genetic barrier. It is more potent (50 mg once daily) and **currently preferred drug for treatment of HIV-positive adults, adolescents and children** (aged more than 6 years with bodyweight more than 20 kg) under the National programme because of ease of administration. It has better tolerability than raltegravir and NNRTI-based regimens. Its ADR include insomnia, headache, dizziness, tiredness, allergic reactions and weight gain. It has minimal drug interactions.

If HIV and TB coexists then rifampicin-based regimens can be used with DTG-based ART regimen but an additional dose of DTG 50 mg should be used 12 hours later daily for entire duration of antiTB therapy. This is necessary to maintain DTG levels because rifampicin reduces the bioavailability of DTG.

However it is costly and not easily available in many countries.

Elvitegravir (EVG), another INSTI, is administered with a pharmacokinetic enhancer cobicistat, which is an inhibitor of CYP3A4, CYP2D6 and P-glycoprotein. As elvitegravir is metabolised by CYP3A4, coadministration with cobicistat increases its concentration favouring once daily administration. The combination is contraindicated with drugs which are metabolised by CYP3A4 (e.g. statins). **Cabotegravir (CAB)** and **bictegravir (BIC)** are yet other INSTI, which are highly effective, safe and given once daily. But they are expensive.

Long acting formulation of cabotegravir is available in combination with LA rilpivirine as a nanocrystalline suspension for IM injection given as monthly depot preparation.

PH 1.55, IM 6.17, DR 11.3

PHARMACOTHERAPY OF HIV

The treatment of HIV is challenging because:

- *It is difficult to eradicate HIV since the virus becomes an integral part of the T cells it infects;* drugs only suppress the viral replication
- *HIV infects the brain cells and many antiretroviral drugs do not cross the BBB.*
- *The available drugs are toxic.*
- *The virus can develop drug resistance.*

None of the currently used drugs can eradicate HIV infection; but when used in combination of at least three antiretroviral drugs from different classes, they decrease the viral replication, reduce viremia to undetectable levels, improve immunologic status by an increase in the CD4 count, reduce frequency of OIs, delay onset of AIDS, improves the quality of life and prolong survival. Thus, their use has turned this disease as 'chronic manageable illness'. The aim is to maintain viral load at undetectable level or <1000 copies/mL throughout the treatment course.

The patients should be treated for opportunistic infections, if any, before starting ART except for mycobacterium avium complex infection and progressive multifocal leukoencephalopathy. Those who have CD4 count < 350 cells/mm^3 or in clinical stage 3 and 4 are given cotrimaxozole prophylaxis along with ART. *All patients should be screened for TB and those who do not have TB are started with TB prophylaxis in addition to ART.*

Antiretroviral therapy (ART) is recommended for all HIV-infected individuals, regardless of CD4 T lymphocyte cell count, and should be started as early as possible, preferably within seven days from the day of HIV diagnosis.

As the chances of development of resistance to antiretroviral drug is very high, combination therapy is always preferred. The National guideline recommends that ARV should be from two different classes *viz.* **two NRTI**, preferably non-thymidine (Tenofovir plus Lamivudine) **plus a third drug, INSTI**, preferably DTG (Table 51.5).

They are prescribed as a fixed-dose combination which is to be taken as a single tablet once daily, preferably at bedtime. This improves long-term compliance and helps to reduce the viral load and emergence of resistant strains.

The above regimen is modified in case of underweight people, patients with serum creatinine levels (creatinine clearance > 30ml/min) or with TB. Treatment failure, adverse reactions, drug interactions, poor patient compliance are the other reasons for alteration in regimen. **Alternatives to DTG are efavirenz or ritonavir boosted lopinavir.**

In children below 10 years and weight < 30 kg, abacavir is used instead of tenofovir disoproxil fumarate because of safety concerns like proximal renal tubulopathy and reduced bone mineralization in children. DTG can be given to children ≥ 6 years and above 20 kg. LPV/r is prescribed in children < 6 years and weighing < 20 kg till the availability of paediatric formulations of DTG under the National programme.

Adequate counselling of patients prior to prescription and during therapy is essential. So also adequate follow -ups with careful clinical and laboratory monitoring, especially in patients with diabetes and hypertension.

Table 51.5 Drug Therapy Regimens for HIV infection PH 1.55, IM 6.17, DR 11.3

Therapy	Regimen
First line therapy for ART-naïve: All PLHIV with age >10 years and weight >30kg and Pregnant and breast feeding women	Tenofovir (TDF 300 mg) + Lamivudine (3TC 300 mg) + Dolutegravir (DTG 50 mg) (TLD) as FDC in a single pill once a day
Second line therapy for treatment failure	A. If DTG in first line, switch to ATV/r. Use LPV/r for pregnant women or HIV-2. If ATV/r or LPV/r in first line, switch to DTG. B. If AZT is used in first line, switch to TDF. If TDF/ABC is used in first line, switch to AZT. C. Continue Lamivudine
Third line for second line treatment failure	New drugs with minimal risk of cross-resistance to previously used regimens such as INSTIs and second-generation NNRTIs and PIs

The response to drug therapy is judged by measuring CD4 count every 6 months and viral load after 6 months, 12 months and then yearly.

Sometimes, **immune reconstitution inflammatory syndrome (IRIS)** precipitates within the first 4-8 weeks of initiation of ART, especially in patients with advanced disease having subclinical mycobacterial, fungal and viral infections. The rapid increase in CD4 count results in a sudden increase in the inflammatory response which is manifested as non-specific symptoms such as fever or a paradoxical worsening of pre-existing signs and symptoms of infective or non-infective conditions or development of disease due to occult infections. IRIS may last for few weeks to a year and needs therapy with steroidal or nonsteroidal anti-inflammatory agents. ART may be temporarily stopped if there is potential life threatening IRIS.

The response to therapy is considered as adequate if the plasma viral load decreases to <1000 copies/mL and CD4 count increases by at least 50 cells/mm^3 at 6 months of ART initiation.

Higher plasma viral load (≥1,000 copies/ml at or after 6 months of ART) is a first and most sensitive indication of treatment failure and can be detected 6 months in advance to immunological decline (CD4 count) or appearance of clinical symptoms and signs. For HIV-2, because viral load measurement is not possible, CD4 count and clinical signs- symptoms are monitored. If response is found to be inadequate then adherence to the therapy should be reviwed first. Drug-drug interactions should be ruled out. Any opportunistic infection or malignancy should be treated. Repeat viral load testing is done 3 months after ensuring >95% treatment adherence and if still high then the treatment is switched to second line drugs (Table 51.5).

As the HIV mutates during replications, some patients on second-line ART may develop resistance to their regimen. For these patients, third line therapy is initiated includes new drugs with minimal risk of cross-resistance to previously used regimens.

The objective of second or third line therapy is to prolong the patient survival as much as possible with complete suppression of viral replication. Hence regular monitoring with viral load assessment every 6 months should be done for all these patients.

Remember that recommendations for drug therapy of HIV are constantly revised.

STD – PROPHYLAXIS

Avoidance of promiscuous sexual contact is the best-method of preventing STD. Failing this, physical methods such as the use of a **condom** and **thorough washing of the genitals** and the surrounding areas with soap and water after an intercourse is recommended.

Chemoprophylaxis of STD: **Pre-exposure vaccination is the effective method for the prevention of transmission of hepatitis A, hepatitis B, human papillomavirus (HPV), and *N. meningitides*** (See Chapter 71).

Post-exposure prophylaxis of syphilis is indicated in exposed contacts who might be incubating infection but are not symptomatic or infectious. If the last sexual contact with the patient was within the past 90 days presumptive treatment (even in the absence of clinical or serologic findings) is given. Doxycycline, 200 mg, given within 24 h (but no later than 2 h) after a sexual encounter resulted in a 73% reduction in the risk of syphilis. However, no treatment is required if the sexual contact history is beyond 90 days and if the person is asymptomatic and nonreactive serologically.

For post- exposure prophylaxis of gonorrhoea and Chlamydia, as they commonly exist as dual infection, heterosexual partners should be treated with **ceftriaxone** 500 mg IM (or Cefixime 400 mg orally) plus a single dose of **azithromycin** 1 g orally. **Doxycycline** (two 100 mg tab) taken once within 72 hours of a condomless sexual exposure has also shown to reduce the incidence of chlamydia and syphilis. However, *N. gonorrhoeae* are resistant to it.

Metronidazole or tinidazole 2 g is recommended as a single dose for postexposure prophylaxis of bacterial vaginitis and trichomoniasis.

PH 1.55, IM 6.18

Chemoprophylaxis of HIV: Since no single strategy provides complete protection against HIV infection, a combination of methods is needed to help reduce HIV transmission.

The general principles of prevention of STD also apply to AIDS. In addition, sterilisation of needles and syringes (preferably the use of disposable material), good blood banking practices and avoidance of pregnancy by women known or suspected to harbour the virus are important measures to check its spread. HIV is killed by sterilisation with pressurised steam (in an autoclave or pressure cooker) at 121°C for at least 20 min and with boiling water (100°C) for at least 20 min.

Indications for antiretroviral drugs:

- *Early treatment of the infected partner in a sero-discordant couple.*
- *Preventing parent-to-child transmission* **(PPTCT).**
- *Pre-exposure prophylaxis* **(PrEP).**
- *Postexposure prophylaxis* **(PEP).**

In serodiscordant couples, one partner has HIV and other does not. WHO recommends immediate ART, irrespective of CD4 count, for the HIV-infected partner. ART in these patients includes 2 NRTI drugs along with efavirenz. PrEP is offered to HIV-negative partners of serodiscordant couples and includes tenofovir and emtricitabine.

PMTCT: The transmission of HIV from a HIV-positive mother to child during pregnancy, labour, delivery or breastfeeding is called as mother to child transmission. **'Fixed Drug Combination (FDC)' triple-drug ART regimen (Table 51.5) should be initiated in all pregnant and breastfeeding women regardless of CD4 cell count** or clinical stage, both for reducing maternal viral load and to prevent vertical HIV transmission. It should be continued lifelong.

Viral load testing of all HIV-positive pregnant women is done during 32 to 36 weeks of pregnancy (regardless of duration of ART). Accordingly the infants born to HIV-positive mothers are categorised as low and high –risk infants. All infants born to HIV-positive mothers should receive a short course of antiretroviral treatment as soon as possible after birth (Table 51.6).

HIV test of the infant should be done at 6 weeks and 18 months after birth.

PrEP is recommended to those healthy individuals who are at substantial risk of getting HIV due to sexual habits or injection drug use. Dual antiretroviral regimen of tenofovir(TDF; 300 mg) and emtricitabine (200 mg) or tenofovir(TDF; 300 mg) and

Table 51.6 Prophylaxis of Infants Born to HIV positive Mothers

Low-risk infants (born to mothers with viral load of <1000 copies/mL done any time during 32-36 weeks of pregnancy)	**Single drug ARV prophylaxis** Syrup Nevirapine (2 mg/kg) once daily from birth till six weeks
High risk infants (born to mothers with viral load > 1000 copies/mL done any time during 32-36 weeks or if mother has not received ART or not undergone viral load testing)	**Dual drug ARV prophylaxis** Syrup Nevirapine (2 mg/kg) and syrup AZT (twice daily 5–15 mg/dose twice daily depending on weight). – If exclusively breastfed (EBF), then duration is from birth till12 weeks – If exclusively on replacement feed (ERF), then the duration is from birth till six weeks

lamivudine (300 mg) as a single tablet once daily is used.

PEP is recommended in uncommon situations right after a potential HIV exposure, e.g. in health care workers following needle stick injury or individual getting exposed through unprotected sex or sexual assault. **PEP is not intended for long-term use.** The first dose should be given as soon as possible after exposure, ideally within 72 h and the risk is evaluated. If the risk is not significant, then it is discontinued. Continuation of PEP is decided based upon type of exposure and HIV status of the individual. The preferred three drug PEP regimen as per National guidelines is tenofovir DF 300 mg + lamivudine 300 mg + dolutegravir (50 mg) administered as a single FDC once daily for 28 days. Dolutegravir may be substituted with ritonavir-boosted lopinavir (100 mg/400 mg twice daily) or efavirenz (600 mg). Children > 6 years or > 20 kg are given AZT + Lamivudine (doses as per weight band) + Dolutegravir (50 mg). If Hb is, 9gm% then AZT is substituted by abacavir. For children below 6 years or having weight below 20 kg, AZT and lamivudine with ritonavir-boosted lopinavir is preferred.

ANTIRETROVIRAL DRUGS

Nucleoside reverse transcriptase inhibitors (NRTI)

Azidothymidine
Didanosine
Zalcitabine
Stavudine
Lamivudine
Emtricitabine
Abacavir

Non-nucleoside reverse transcriptase inhibitors (NNRTI)

Nevirapine
Efavirenz
Delaviridine
Etravirine
Rilpivirine

Nucleotide reverse transcriptase inhibitor (NTRI)

Tenofovir disoproxil
Tenofovir alafenamide

Protease inhibitors (PI)

Saquinavir
Ritonavir
Indinavir
Amprenavir
Nelfinavir
Lopinavir
Atazanavir
Fosamprenavir
Tipranavir
Darunavir

Entry inhibitors

Enfuvirtide
Maraviroc
Fostemsavir
Ibalizumab

Integrase strand transfer inhibitor (INSTI)

Raltegravir
Dolutegravir
Elvitegravir
Cabotegravir
Bictegravir

CHAPTER 52

Chemotherapy of Tuberculosis

Learning Objectives

This chapter will enable the reader:

1. To enumerate the challenges faced while treating tuberculosis (TB).
2. To classify anti-TB drugs.
3. To discuss the mechanism of action, salient pharmacokinetic features, ADR, drug interactions of different classes of anti-TB drugs.
4. To state the rationale for combination therapy for TB.
5. To write the drug regimens as per National Tuberculosis Elimination Programme (NTEP).
6. To state the response indicators for chemotherapy.
7. To outline the management of multidrug-resistant TB.
8. To discuss the treatment of extrapulmonary TB.
9. To enumerate the indications and contraindications for the use of glucocorticoids in treatment of TB.
10. To state the chemoprophylaxis of TB.
11. To outline the treatment of nontuberculous mycobacterial infections.
12. To discuss the anti-TB treatment strategy in special patient populations, i.e. HIV patients, pregnant ladies.

KEY TERMS

Tuberculosis (TB) is an infectious disease, caused by several species of mycobacteria. The important human pathogens of this class are *Mycobacterium tuberculosis* and *Mycobacterium bovis*. TB is a systemic disease, the commonest form in a man being pulmonary TB. Unlike other bacterial infections, TB is a difficult disease to treat. The reasons are:

- **Tubercle bacilli grow slowly, dividing only once in 1–2 days, even in the most favourable circumstances** such as in an open cavitatory pulmonary lesion. In less favourable circumstances, such as a closed, caseous lesion, the bacteria become metabolically dormant, stop multiplying and may 'persist' (**persisters**) for many years. They exhibit multidrug tolerance and survive treatment by all known antimicrobials. In an open cavity, there may be many bacilli resistant to one drug even before drug therapy is commenced.
- **The caseation and fibrosis tend to block the blood vessels supplying the necrotic area,** making penetration by drugs difficult. The caseated material itself is not impenetrable to many anti-TB drugs.
- **Tubercle bacilli remain viable and multiply even when ingested by macrophages.** The chemotherapeutic agents [except isonicotinic acid hydrazide (INH), rifampicin, and pyrazinamide] penetrate poorly into the macrophages.

- **CMI develops 2–8 weeks after the infection** in most infected patients. This gives some protection from its spread. Deficient CMI as in AIDS accelerates the spread.
- **The organisms tend to develop resistance to the chemotherapeutic agents** by spontaneous chromosomal mutation. **Multidrug-resistant (MDR) TB is now a major problem.**

Classification of Anti-Tuberculosis Drugs CT 1.14

I. **First-line drugs:**
   - **Bactericidal:** Isonicotinic acid hydrazide (H), rifampicin (R) and pyrazinamide (Z)
   - **Bacteriostatic:** Ethambutol (E)

II. **Second-line drugs:**

Oral

- **Bactericidal:** Fluoroquinolones (FQ-levofloxacin: Lfx and moxifloxacin: Mfx); bedaquiline (Bdq); delamanid (Dlm)
- **Bacteriostatic:** Ethionamide (Et), cycloserine (C), terizidone (Trd), clofazimine (Cfz), linezolid (Lzd), thiacetazone (T), paraminosalicylic acid (PAS)

Injectables

Bactericidal: Aminoglycosides [e.g. amikacin (Am) and streptomycin (S)]; carbapenems [imipenem plus cilastatin (Ipm–Cln), meropenem (Mpm)]

The second line drugs are used for multidrug resistant (MDR) and extensively drug resistant (XDR) TB.

FIRST-LINE DRUGS PH 1.44

Salient properties of first line anti-tuberculosis drugs are summarised in Table 52.1.

ISONICOTINIC ACID HYDRAZIDE (INH): This is the cheapest and one of the most effective antituberculous drugs (Fig 52.1). It is bactericidal and 'decimates' the population of tubercle bacilli within a few days of starting the treatment. It:

- **Acts on the bacilli multiplying in the walls of the cavities, as well as those inside the macrophages.**
- **Is more effective than other drugs in preventing drug resistance.**

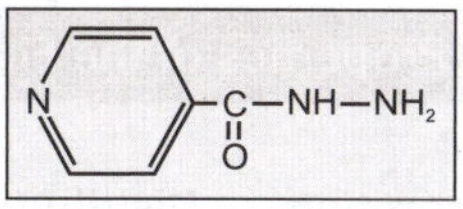

FIG. 52.1 **Isonicotinic acid hydrazide.**

- **Is well tolerated, cheap and safe even in pregnancy.**
- **Does not eliminate the persisters.**

Mechanism of action: INH is a prodrug. It is activated by the mycobacterial catalase-peroxidase to an active compound, which **inhibits the synthesis of mycolic acid, a unique constituent of the mycobacterial cell wall.** In addition, the drug inhibits the same catalase-peroxidase and makes the organisms susceptible to oxidative mechanisms. Although INH is an excellent bactericidal drug, *it has poor sterilising activity as it fails to kill all viable organism.*

INH resistance: Used alone, the mycobacteria rapidly develop resistance to INH by mutation *in vitro*. It does not correlate with the drug response in patients, where the drug can still remain effective. INH, therefore, should not be discontinued because of apparent failure to achieve the therapeutic objectives. However, mutations in katG gene, which encodes catalase- peroxidase, confer high-level INH resistance because then conversion of INH to biologically active form is not possible.

Absorption, fate and excretion: INH is rapidly and completely absorbed on oral administration. Peak plasma levels are reached within an hour and effective blood levels may persist for as long as 24 h. *The absorption of the drug from the GI tract is so complete that oral and parenteral doses produce comparable plasma and tissue levels.* Antacids interfere with its GI absorption. It is distributed throughout the body and penetrates well into the saliva, milk, pleural fluid and CSF. Its concentration in CSF is about 20% of the plasma levels but increases (50%) in the presence of tubercular meningitis. It can cross the placental barrier freely. Its concentration in breast milk is similar to that in the plasma.

INH penetrates and acts intracellularly and diffuses into macrophages and the necrotic centres, and even after its disappearance from tissues like brain and muscles, tissues like liver, skin, lungs and caseous material still retain an appreciable amount of the drug.

Table 52.1 Properties of the First-Line Anti-tuberculosis Drugs

Drug	Oral Absorption	Distribution	Disposal	Action	Action on Persisters	CSF Level	Serious Toxicity
H	90%	Wide (IC)	Hepatic	Cidal	None	Good	Neuro, hepato
R	90%	Wide (IC)	Hepatic	Cidal	Yes	Good	Hepato, immuno
Z	Good (70%)	Wide (IC)	Hepatic	Cidal (IC)	None	Excellent	Hepato
E	Good (77%)	All tissues except CSF	Renal	Static	None	Fair	Ocular

Notes: IC, intracellular; EC, extracellular; neuro, neurotoxicity; hepato, hepatotoxicity; nephro, nephrotoxicity; immuno, immunological toxicity; cidal, bactericidal; static, bacteriostatic. For full forms of drug names, see text.

It is mainly metabolised in the liver by acetylation. Approximately, 75%–95% of orally administered INH is excreted in the urine within the first 24 h, mainly as acetyl isoniazid and isonicotinic acid. Acetyl isoniazid can get converted to acetyl hydrazine and then to toxic metabolites by CYP2E1. Small quantities are excreted after conjugation with glycine and as isonicotinoyl hydrazone. Individuals may differ in their ability to metabolise INH and can be:

- **Rapid acetylators**
- **Slow acetylators**

Acetylation status is a genetically determined character. Rapid acetylation is of no therapeutic importance when doses are administered daily. *Incidence of neuropathy is more in slow acetylators.*

INH is safe in chronic renal failure and 300 mg/day can be administered when plasma creatinine is less than 12 mg%. Dose adjustment (⅓ to ½) is necessary in the presence of liver damage.

Adverse reactions: In general, **INH is a remarkably safe drug.** The clinically important ADR involve mainly the peripheral and the central nervous systems. They are:

- **Allergy:** These include fever, malaise, skin eruptions, sometimes, lymphadenopathy and jaundice and rarely blood dyscrasias and diffuse vasculitis.
- **Peripheral neuropathy:** Being a structural analogue of pyridoxine, **it promotes excretion of pyridoxine.** Thus, it causes peripheral neuritis leading to anaesthesia, paraesthesiae, burning and pain in extremities, sometimes accompanied by anaemia. Neuropathy is dose related. It is rare with the 200–300 mg/day regimen. *In the dose of 10–15 mg per day, pyridoxine prevents such neuropathy.* Rarely optic neuritis leading to atrophy may develop; hence, it should be discontinued if visual disturbances develop.
- **Central nervous system:** INH stimulates the CNS. Psychotic behavior and seizures may be seen in patients with a history of psychosis and epilepsy respectively. The psychic disturbances consist of euphoria, transient loss of memory, loss of self-control and personality changes. Large doses may cause ataxia, muscle twitching and toxic encephalopathy.
- **Liver damage:** The incidence of hepatitis is highest in individuals older than 50 years. The liver shows multilobular necrosis. Toxic metabolites of acetylhydrazine may have some role to play. Patients receiving INH should be monitored for possible hepatotoxicity and the drug should be stopped if the SGPT increases to more than three times the upper limit of normal. Slow acetylators are more prone to hepatotoxicity. Similarly, CYP2E1 inducers (e.g.rifampicin) may potentiate this toxicity.
- **Miscellaneous:** These include dryness of mouth and GI discomfort. **INH inhibits CYP2C19 and CYP3A.** It may thereby raise the plasma levels of **phenytoin, carbamazepine and ethosuximide.** INH also interacts with disulfiram. Toxic doses (40 mg/kg or higher) may cause severe metabolic acidosis, hyperglycaemia, seizures and coma.

Preparations:

i. Isoniazid tablet 50, 100 and 300 mg
ii. Isoniazid syrup, 50–100 mg per 5 mL
iii. Isoniazid injection, 25 mg/mL

RIFAMPICIN (R): It is a semisynthetic derivative of rifamycin B, isolated from *Streptomyces mediteranei*. It is:

- **Effective orally against TB and leprosy.**
- **Bactericidal and acts against both intra and extracellular organisms.**
- **Faster than INH in sterilising effect.**
- **Effective against tubercle bacilli resistant to other standard drugs and against some of the atypical mycobacteria.**
- **The only drug which acts on the persisters.**

Other bacteria: It is also active against *Staphylococcus aureus* and *albus, Clostridium welchii Streptococcus viridans* and *beta haemolyticus, Pneumococci, Bacillus anthracis, Corynebacterium diphtheriae, Haemophilus influenzae, Neisseria gonorrhoeae* and meningococci. It is only moderately active against *Streptococcus faecalis*. It is active in vitro against many **Gram-negative bacilli** like *Escherichia coli*, Proteus, Salmonella, Shigella, *Pseudomonas aeruginosa* and Brucella. However, organisms rapidly develop resistance to rifampicin.

Mechanism of action: Rifampicin inhibits bacterial DNA-dependent RNA polymerase and thus blocks RNA synthesis. Human RNA polymerase is not inhibited. *Compared to INH, rifampicin is less bactericidal but has potent sterilising activity.*

Absorption, fate and excretion: Rifampicin is well absorbed from the gut. After a dose of 600 mg orally, given at least ½ h before breakfast, the peak level is achieved within 2–3 h and **therapeutic concentration persists for more than 12 h.**

Food interferes with its absorption. Almost 85% of the drug gets bound to serum proteins. It is widely distributed throughout the body and is present in effective concentrations in many tissues and body fluids including the CSF. It crosses the placenta. The drug is largely metabolised in the liver to an **active metabolite desacetyl rifampicin** which undergoes enterohepatic circulation. High concentrations of the drug occur in the bile and the saliva. It is largely (60%) excreted in faeces as desacetylated form. Only small amount is excreted in the urine unchanged. *Hence, dosage adjustment is not necessary in the presence of renal damage.*

Adverse reactions: These occur in less than 5% of patients with the usual doses. They include skin rashes, diarrhoea, ataxia, hepatitis, jaundice, proteinuria, leucopenia and thrombocytopenia. *It is advisable to check hepatic function before starting the drug. Patients on rifampicin therapy should be told that there will be orange red discoloration of their urine, faeces, saliva, sputum, tears, sweat and even contact lenses, which is harmless.*

Acute hepatic and renal failure, allergic reactions including shock and a flu-like syndrome have been reported in patients taking **large doses of rifampicin** (>900 mg) **intermittently**. Some of these may have immune mechanisms. *However, intermittent therapy with smaller doses (450–600 mg) appears to be safe.*

Rifampicin is a potent hepatic microsomal enzyme inducer (CYPs 3A4, 2E1, 1A2, 2C9 and 2C19),and thus increases metabolism of several drugs, e.g. hydrocortisone, oral contraceptives, phenytoin, sulphonylureas, warfarin, digoxin, dapsone, verapamil, zolpidem, simvastatin, methadone, theophylline, non-nucleotide reverse transcriptase inhibitors and most protease inhibitors. *This action is of less clinical importance when the drug is administered once a month as in leprosy.*

Preparations:

i. Rifampicin caps 150, 300, 450 and 600 mg
ii. Rifampicin syrup (100 mg/5 ml) for children
iii. Rifampicin infusion vials containing 600 mg powder

Indications:

- **Tuberculosis:** Because of the likelihood of the emergence of resistant bacteria and availability of other potent antibiotics for the Gram-positive and negative organisms, rifampicin is mainly reserved for the treatment of TB (see section, Management of pulmonary tuberculosis).
- **Leprosy** (Chapter 53).
- **Serious staphylococcal septicaemia** resistant to the conventional drugs

- **Prophylaxis of meningococcal infection and infection with *H. influenzae (type B) because of high concentration of rifampicin in the saliva.***
- **Brucellosis** (Chapter 45)
- **Legionnaire disease**

Other Rifamycin Derivatives

RIFAPENTINE: This semisynthetic rifamycin has a spectrum similar to that of rifampicin but it is longer acting. Given orally, it is readily absorbed and is metabolised in the liver to the active metabolite 25-desacetyl rifapentine. The *t*½ of both rifapentine and its active metabolite is 13 h. It is highly protein bound and is mostly (70%) cleared by the liver. It is also an enzyme inducer. Its toxicity is similar to that of rifampicin. It is administered in the dose of 600 mg once or twice weekly.

RIFABUTIN: See section on Nontuberculous mycobacterial infections.

RIFAXIMIN: It is used for Traveller's diarrhoea. See Chapter 39, Section on Drug therapy of diarrhoea.

PYRAZINAMIDE (Z): This drug, related chemically to thiosemicarbazones and nicotinamide, is effective orally against *M. tuberculosis* of human type resistant to streptomycin and INH.

- **It is bactericidal and reaches all the sites within the lung harbouring tuberculous bacilli.**
- **It is effective only against tubercle bacilli within macrophages** (Intracellular effect) **as well as persisters in the caseous material.**
- **It has good meningeal penetration.**
- **In combination with streptomycin, INH and rifampicin, pyrazinamide exerts a potent sterilising effect on the tuberculous lesions during the first 2 months of therapy.**

Mechanism of action: It is a prodrug and is converted by pyrazinamidase to the bioactive compound pyrazinoic acid (POA) in the mycobacterial cell. POA binds with the active site on mycobacterial PanD, which encodes L-aspartate decarboxylase and competitively inhibits it. L-aspartate decarboxylase converts l- aspartate to beta- alanine. This step is crucial in the biosynthesis of pantothenate (vitamin B 5) and then of CoA, which is a cofactor for number of metabolic pathways (Fig 52.2). PanD gets degraded by a caseinolytic protease complex attached to it. POA binding promotes this degradation and serves as a selective bacterial '**target degrader**.' In addition, there is a possibility that mycobacteria metabolise POA and the resultant products are toxic.

Pyrazinamidase is encoded by the gene PncA, mutations of which are responsible for pyrazinamide

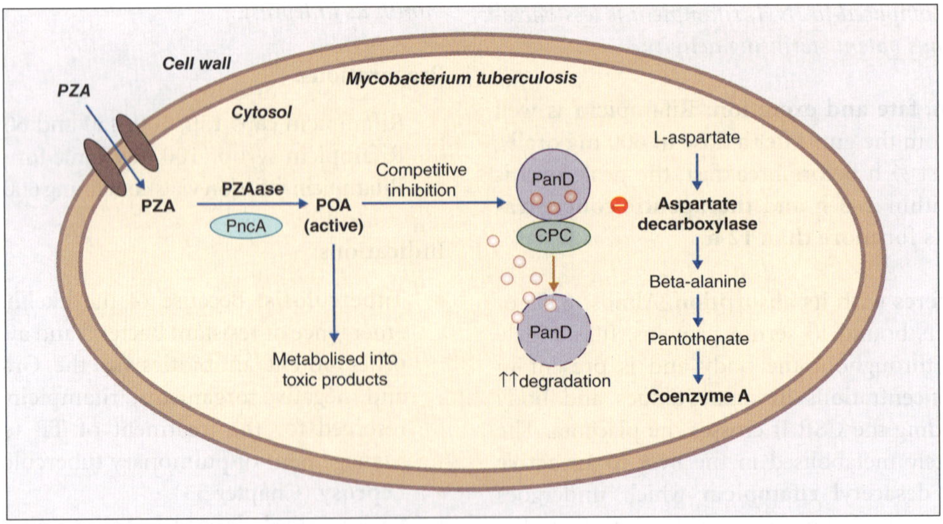

FIG. 52.2 Mechanism of action of pyrzinamide PZA= Pyrizinamide; PZAse=pyrazinamidase; POA =Pyrazinoic acid; CPC= caseinolytic protease complex; – sign = inhibits At the place -sign, use red symbol with – sign in it.

resistance. However, other mechanisms also contribute to resistance.

Absorption, fate and excretion: Pyrazinamide is rapidly absorbed from the GI tract. The peak plasma levels are reached within 1–3 h, and the drug can be detected in the plasma up to 15 h. It is widely distributed in the body and *achieves a concentration in the CSF almost equal to the plasma levels.* The drug is deaminated in the liver and metabolites and free drug excreted in urine.

Adverse reactions: These include anorexia, nausea, vomiting, malaise, fever, arthralgia, dysuria and mild skin rashes. Rarely, it can cause photosensitivity resulting in bright red-brown discolouration of the exposed parts of the body.

Serious hepatotoxicity is major disadvantage. Toxic hepatitis may occur at any time and is not dose related. The drug, therefore, is contraindicated in the presence of hepatic insufficiency.

Hyperuricemia due to increased tubular reabsorption of urates and gouty arthritis may occur.

Preparations and dosage: It is available as 500, 750, 1000, 1200 and 1500 mg tablets. Dose 25 mg/kg/day (not exceeding 1.5 g/day) in one or two divided doses. For children: 15–30 mg/kg daily.

ETHAMBUTOL (E): Ethambutol is the dextrorotatory isomer of 2,2′ (ethylenediamine)-di-L-butanol (Fig. 52.3). The levorotatory form is inactive.

- **It is effective orally against mycobacteria resistant to INH, streptomycin and ethionamide as well as against many atypical mycobacteria.**
- **It is bacteriostatic.**
- **Primary resistance to this drug has not been reported.**
- **When used in combination, the bacterial resistance to other drugs is greatly delayed.**

Mechanism of action: It acts mainly against rapidly multiplying organisms in the walls of the cavities. **It disrupts the synthesis of bacterial cell wall** by inhibiting the enzyme arabinosyl transferase. This

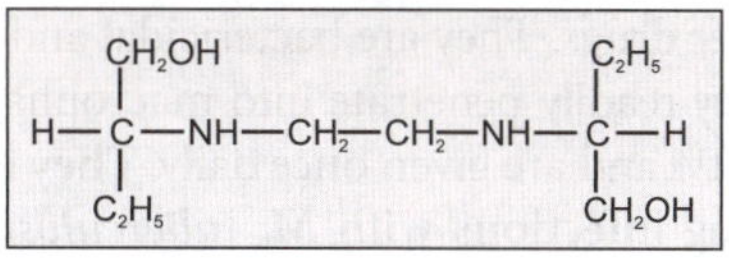

FIG. 52.3 Ethambutol.

enzyme is essential to transfer arabinose to form arabinogalactan in cell wall.

Absorption, fate and excretion: Nearly 70% of the drug is absorbed after oral administration. Erythrocytes serve as the depot, from which it is released into the circulation. **It, however, does not persist in other tissues and body fluids**; the CSF level is only 50% of the plasma level.

Approximately 50% of the oral dose is eliminated unchanged in urine within 24 h; 15% of the drug is excreted in the form of two metabolites. It accumulates in the presence of renal damage.

Adverse reactions: *The main adverse effect is retrobulbar optic neuritis on prolonged therapy.* The early symptoms are blurring and haziness, followed by progressive decrease in visual acuity, contraction of the visual fields, and poor colour discrimination. The symptoms usually disappear when the drug is discontinued. **It is rare in patients receiving 15 mg/kg/day.** Peripheral neuritis has also been reported. It is avoided in children below 8 years because of the difficulty in identifying early reduction in visual acuity. Tests for visual acuity should be done before, during and after the treatment.

Other ADR include nausea, anorexia, confusion, headache and allergic reactions.

Preparations: Ethambutol as 100, 200, 400, 800 and 1000 mg tab. For doses, see Table 52.3.

SECOND-LINE DRUGS PH 1.45

Majority of these antitubercular drugs are less effective and more toxic than the first drugs.

FLUOROQUINOLONES (FQ): See Chapter 43. **Levofloxacin (Lfx), moxifloxacin (Mfx)** and **ofloxacin** are active against *M. tuberculosis*, even those resistant to the other drugs. They are bactericidal and are given orally. They readily penetrate into macrophages. They have long t½ and are given once daily. **They are useful for treating infections with *M. tuberculosis* and M. avium complex (MAC)** (see Section, Nontuberculous mycobacterial infections) which are resistant to first-line drugs.

BEDAQUILINE (Bdq): This diarylquinoline **acts by inhibiting mycobacterial ATP synthase, an enzyme essential for energy production in tuberculous bacilli.** It is bactericidal against sensitive and MDR tuberculous bacilli. **It also acts on dormant bacilli so has sterilising effect.** It has been shown to improve the sputum conversion time significantly in patients with multidrug resistant (MDR)TB.

It is metabolised by CYP3A4. It has long *t*½ of 5.5 months. It accumulates in tissues.

ADR include nausea, anorexia, hepatic damage and arthralgia. QT prolongation can occur resulting in fatal arrhythmias. Therefore, ECG monitoring is recommended daily in the first 2 weeks, every 2 weeks for the next 3 months and then monthly.

It is indicated in adult patients with MDR TB, who are resistant to all FQ and/or second-line anti-TB drugs or treatment failures of MDR TB. It is given orally in the dose of 400 mg o.d. for initial 2 weeks (in the hospital setting) followed by 200 mg thrice weekly for 22 weeks along with at least four second-line drugs based on drug sensitivity testing. After 6 months, it is discontinued. There is no adequate evidence on safety and efficacy for using bedaquiline beyond 6 months and for children < 6 years.

Recent data indicates that pregnant or lactating women, and stable- arrhythmia patients can also be prescribed bedaquiline albeit after approval of specialist considering the risk-benefit ratio.

Delamanid (Dlm): This bicyclic nitro-imidazole derivative is a mycolic acid and protein synthesis inhibitor. It generates reactive nitrogen species (NO-) and kills intracellular tuberculous bacilli. It has a t½ of 36 hours. Given as an add-on therapy in a dose of 100 mg twice daily for 6 months, it has shown to increase sputum conversion rate among patients with MDR pulmonary TB. QT prolongation, however, is of concern.

Like bedaquiline, it is indicated in MDR-TB patients. It should not be used beyond 6 months and in children below the age of 6 years. It is administered in the dose of 50 mg twice daily (for 6-11 years) and 100 mg twice daily (for 12 years and above).

Delamanid is not recommended in pregnancy.

ETHIONAMIDE (Eto): Ethionamide is structurally related to INH with the same mechanism of action. It is effective against tubercle bacilli resistant to other drugs and in infections due to atypical mycobacteria. Resistance can develop. Such organisms show cross resistance to thiosemicarbazones.

Absorption, fate and excretion: It is absorbed fairly rapidly from the gut but is a GI irritant. Its distribution is similar to that of INH. It is metabolised in the liver to several metabolites. Only 1% is excreted in the active form in urine.

Adverse reactions: Its toxicity makes drug withdrawal mandatory in about 30% of cases. Allergic manifestations include skin rashes and alopecia; occasionally, serious manifestations like purpura and anaphylactoid shock may develop. GI disturbances are common. The neurological disturbances are similar to those observed following INH. The drug also causes toxic hepatitis.

The miscellaneous adverse effects include endocrinological disturbances like gynecomastia, menorrhagia and impotence. Pellagra-like symptoms including stomatitis and diarrhoea have been reported.

Ethionamide is contraindicated in pregnancy up to 32 weeks of gestation.

Preparations and dosage: Ethionamide 250 mg tablets. The optimum dose of the drug is 1 g daily. It is administered initially in the dose of 250 mg twice daily and increased gradually by 250 mg every fortnight.

CYCLOSERINE (Cs): It is used in the treatment of tuberculous as well as for Gram-negative infections. It is tuberculostatic. **Cycloserine acts by inhibiting**

the peptidoglycan synthesis and disrupts the bacterial cell wall. It is effective against tubercle bacilli resistant to INH or streptomycin and against atypical mycobacteria, although it is less active.

Absorption, fate and excretion: Cycloserine is rapidly absorbed from the gut. Repeated administration leads to accumulation of the drug in the plasma. It is distributed throughout the body and achieves similar concentration in the CSF as in the plasma. Approximately 50% of the orally administered drug appears in the urine unchanged within 12 h, and 65% is excreted by the kidney within 72 h. **Renal impairment leads to high plasma concentrations.**

Adverse reactions: The use of cycloserine is limited by its **psycho-neuro-toxicity.** The neurological effects include peripheral neuropathy, ataxia, slurred speech and seizures. The risk of seizures may increase in alcoholics. The psychic effects include nervousness, insomnia, anxiety, psychotic reactions, and suicidal ideations. Pyridoxine 150 mg/day may help to reduce neurotoxicity. It should be avoided in patients with a history of epilepsy, psychosis, depression and those with renal impairment.

Preparations and dosage: Cycloserine tartrate 250 mg. The recommended dose of the drug is 0.5–1 g daily, administered in two divided doses.

TERIZIDONE (Trd): This derivative of cycloserine is effective against *M. tuberculosis* and *M. avium*. It has higher concentration in blood and urine and hence useful in urogenital TB. Its ADR are lesser than cycloserine and is better tolerated by patients with psychiatric comorbidity or chronic alcoholics. It is recommended for MDR and XDR TB.

Clofazimine (Cfz): This antileprosy drug (Chapter 53), given in combination is used in MDR-TB.

Linezolid (Lzd) (Chapter 44) is used in combination with other drugs for MDR/XDR infection (300–600 mg o.d.). Though bacteriostatic, it achieves adequate intracellular concentration. Toxicity is dose-related and includes anaemia, neuropathies, hyperlactataemia and myelosuppression.

THIACETAZONE (T): This thiosemicarbazone derivative, is used as a companion drug to INH. It is bacteriostatic. Given orally, it rapidly diffuses into the various body tissues and crosses the placenta. It is partly metabolised, and about 40% is excreted in urine within 48 h. It is also secreted in milk.

Adverse reactions: Anorexia, nausea and vomiting are common. Fever, skin rashes and Stevens–Johnson syndrome appear occasionally. The serious toxic manifestations include progressive anaemia, granulocytopenia and agranulocytosis; it also causes kidney and liver damage. *It should never be used in HIV patients as it can cause severe and fatal skin reactions.*

Its dose is 150 mg (2 mg/kg) once daily given with INH. Thiacetazone and INH tablet contains 50 mg of thiacetazone and 100 mg of isoniazid. It is difficult to get quality assured formulation of thiacetazone.

PARA-AMINOSALICYLIC ACID (PAS): It is a bacteriostatic agent used for TB since 1940. **It is a folate acid synthesis inhibitor** but other mechanisms may be responsible for its effects. Its potency is much less than other drugs but may be useful in combination in the treatment of MDR TB. The usual adult dose is approximately 2–3 g four times a day (150 mg/kg/day), which is too bulky. The common ADR include nausea, vomiting, diarrhoea and occasionally hepatitis.

MACROLIDES: Newer macrolides, **azithromycin** and **clarithromycin** (Chapter 46) have action against acid-fast bacilli. They are used to treat atypical mycobacterial infections (see section, Nontuberculous mycobacterial infections) and patients with relapse.

INJECTABLE ANTI TB DRUGS

AMINOGLYCOSIDES: These drugs are discussed in detail in Chapter 45.

- **They are not absorbed orally and must be administered intramuscularly. The injection is painful.**
- **They are bactericidal** to the tubercle bacilli rapidly multiplying at neutral pH in the walls of the tuberculous cavities.
- **They do not penetrate into the macrophages nor into caseous material.** They are less effica-

cious than INH and rifampicin.

- **Their concentration in the CSF is poor.**
- **They are much more toxic than INH and rifampicin.**

Amikacin and **streptomycin** are the only two aminoglycosides currently considered to be used in anti-TB regimens for multidrug resistant tuberculosis (See the section, Management of MDR/RR TB).

Amikacin (Am), though active against mycobacteria resistant to streptomycin, INH and cycloserine, is not recommended for drug-sensitive TB due to its ADR.

NEWER DRUGS

Pretomanid: It is a nitroimidazo-oxazole, which is structurally similar to delamanid and has similar mechanism of action. In addition, it leads to ATP depletion. It is active against both, replicating and non -replicating organisms. It is well tolerated Most common adverse reactions (≥10%) are myelosuppression, peripheral and optic neuropathy; commonly manifested are anaemia and GI disturbances such as dyspepsia, decreased appetite, nausea, vomiting, diarrhea and abdominal pain and increased liver enzymes. Other ADR include pleuritic pain, lower respiratory tract infection, back pain, hypoglycemia, lactic acidosis and loss of weight.

It needs further evaluation and is **reserved the TB regimens for MDR or XDR TB** if appropriate criteria are met and after informed consent (**conditional access**). The effective dose is 100–200 mg daily.

MANAGEMENT OF PULMONARY TUBERCULOSIS PH 1.55, PE 34.3, CT 1.15

In India, under **National Tuberculosis Elimination Programme (NTEP)** universal access to TB diagnostics and treatment is provided to all patients with pulmonary and extrapulmonary TB, including those having drug-resistant and HIV-associated TB. The programme is made domiciliary by appointing health workers or trained volunteers for direct observation of treatment (DOT). The programme involves use of advanced and effective interventions and technologies for diagnosis, treatment and care of TB cases. This programme is responsible for carrying out the Government of India's five-year National Strategic Plan for TB elimination (2017–25) which was, launched to eliminate TB in India by 2025. In 2020, another 'NSP India 2025' has been introduced to make this aim feasible.

The presence of active pulmonary TB can be suspected from clinical features and routine laboratory investigations like the ESR; nevertheless, it should be confirmed by a chest X-ray, repeated sputum examinations culture and polymerase chain reaction (PCR) for mycobacterial antigen. *It is important to remember that an active disease can exist even in the absence of significant symptomatology.* PH 1.1

Chemotherapy is the mainstay of the treatment of TB and nonpharmacological measures like high protein diet and bed rest are adjuvant to chemotherapy. Majority of the patients can now be treated successfully as out-patients and up to 95% of drug-responsive new cases can be cured by first line drugs. However, patients in the communicable stage of the disease should be strictly isolated from infants for a few weeks.

The aims of chemotherapy are:

- **To kill the dividing bacilli in the lung lesions** so as to render the sputum negative and the patient noninfectious
- **To kill the 'persisters' so as to avoid relapse and to ensure total cure**
- **To prevent the emergence of drug resistance**

Selection of Chemotherapeutic Regimen

INH, rifampicin, ethambutol and pyrazinamide are the four antituberculous drugs preferred for initial therapy in patients with sensitive mycobacterial infection. They are always administered in **combination** as single dose, half an hour before breakfast. in order to:

- **Delay the development of acquired resistance and prolong the effective therapy.**
- **Eliminate persisters.**
- **Shorten the course of therapy.**
- **Reduce ADR.**

Table 52.2 Regimen of NTEP for sensitive strains of mycobacteria PH 1.55

Patient Type	Regimen[a] (Duration in Months) Intensive	Maintenance
Newly diagnosed, treatment naive or received anti-TB treatment < 1 month or previously treated	HRZE (2)	HRE (4)

[a]All drugs are administered daily according to the weight range, e.g. within the weight range of 46-70 kg the dosage used are H-300 mg, R-600 mg, Z-1500 mg, E-1200 mg.

On the large populations of bacilli actively multiplying at neutral pH in the walls of pulmonary cavities, INH and rifampicin are bactericidal and ethambutol is bacteriostatic; The most active drug against the small bacterial population that multiplies inside macrophages in an acid medium is pyrazinamide, followed by INH and rifampicin. **Rifampicin and pyrazinamide are active against intermittently multiplying persisters in solid caseous lesions;** therefore, they are particularly effective in preventing a relapse.

TB is one of the diseases where the use of fixed dose drug combinations is justified. Its advantages are as follows:

- **Reduction in the number of pills to be swallowed**
- **Improvement in drug compliance**
- **Convenience in the mass-treatment of populations**

The regimen used is as follows (Table 52.2):

A 6-month course consisting of daily H + R + Z + E for **2 months**, followed by H + R + E daily for **4 months** is the regimen for patients with drug sensitive organisms (DS-TB; *usually newly diagnosed cases and also previously treated patients when there is no resistance to H and R*). The dosages of these drugs are given in Table 52.3.

During the initial intensive phase, most of the growing tubercle bacilli are killed and the patient becomes noninfectious. The **continuation or sterilising phase (4 months) is necessary to eliminate the persisters and reduce the failure.** The duration of treatment must never be shorter than 6 months.

In patients with risk factors like big cavity, extensive disease, immunosuppression, as well as those with bone or joint TB, tubercular meningitis, miliary TB and those with HIV infection, it is advisable to extend the continuation phase by 3–6 months.

Tuberculosis in children: Treatment regimens, except for dosage, are generally the same for children and adults.

Table 52.3 Dosage of Commonly Used Drugs

Drug	Adults (Daily Dosage) body wt. <50 kg	body wt. >50 kg	Children (Daily Dosage)
Rifampicin (R)	450 mg	600 mg	10 mg/kg; Max. 600 mg
Isoniazid (H)	300 mg	300 mg	5–10 mg/kg; Max. 300 mg
Pyrazinamide (Z)	1000 mg	1500 mg	15–30 mg/kg
Ethambutol (E)	25 mg/kg (see text)	–	Not recommended
Streptomycin (S)	0.75 g	1.0 g	20–30 mg/kg; Max. 0.75 g

Notes: 1. All drugs are given in a single dose. 2. Use pyridoxine 10 mg daily as supplement when high doses of INH are used, as in miliary tuberculosis and meningitis. 3. Before starting streptomycin, check kidney function, particularly in patients over 60 years of age; reduce the dose accordingly, if necessary.

Tuberculosis during pregnancy: This should be treated with standard regimen mentioned above. The patient should be followed up monthly. Pyridoxine needs to be supplemented. USG is advised at 18–22 weeks of pregnancy to diagnose congenital anomalies if any. After delivery, the treatment to the mother continues. Breast feeding should not be stopped. Chemoprophylaxis is given to the neonate after ruling out active TB.

- **Monitoring of drugs response:**
  The response to chemotherapy depends on the duration of the lesion rather than the extent of the lesion. Lesions of recent origin, even though extensive, may be completely reversible. The response can be gauged by:
  i. **Clinical improvement:** (usually within 2–3 weeks) as shown by improvement in appetite, weight gain and a feeling of well-being.
  ii. **Bacteriological improvement: Adequate chemotherapy makes sputum-positive patients 'noninfectious' within 3–6 weeks.** Smear negativity is checked at the end of induction phase and further at end of continuation phase in patients with DS-TB. Negative sputum cultures on two occasions, one of which is at the end of 3 months of therapy, is considered as cure.
  iii. **Radiological improvement:** With adequate chemotherapy, cavity closure/its disappearance has been reported in 75%–90% of patients within 3–6 months.
  iv. **Periodic determination of ESR.**
  v. ***In vitro* susceptibility tests** to *determine* the bacterial sensitivity to the drugs should be carried out before and during the therapy. This is often impractical. PH 1.7
- **Monitoring of ADR:** The patients should be monitored for possible serious toxicity of drugs. The common ADR caused by anti-TB drugs are enlisted in Table 52.4. If hepatitis develops, all the antiTB drugs should be stopped till symptoms resolve and liver enzymes return to baseline levels. Treatment is restarted with one drug at a time starting with R, H and lastly Z. In decompensated liver disease, R should be avoided. However, *S, E and FQ can be used in subjects with fulminating liver disease. The usual dose of H, R, Z can be given in renal failure* as they are eliminated in bile or metabolised to nontoxic products. S and E must be used with caution in these patients. Induction of autoimmune thrombocytopenia by R, impaired vision by E or H and gouty arthritis by Z mandate their withdrawal.
- **Adjuvant therapy:** Well balanced nutritious

Table 52.4 Common Adverse Effects of Anti-TB Drugs

Antituberculosis Drug	Common Adverse Effects
Isoniazid (H)	Peripheral neuropathy, skin rash, hepatitis, sedation, lethargy
Rifampicin (R)	Abdominal pain, nausea, vomiting, hepatitis, generalised cutaneous reactions, thrombocytopenic purpura
Pyrazinamide (Z)	Arthralgia, hepatitis, abdominal pain
Ethambutol (E)	Retrobulbar neuritis
Streptomycin (S)/Kanamycin (K)/ Capreomycin (Cm)	Ototoxicity, nephrotoxicity, vertigo, electrolyte imbalance
Fluoroquinolones (FQ)	Diarrhoea, abdominal pain, dizziness, convulsions, phototoxicity, tendinitis, rash, QT prolongation, arthralgia
Ethionamide (Eto)	Epigastric pain, anorexia, nausea, vomiting, metallic taste, salivation, peripheral neuropathy, hallucination, depression, hepatitis, hypothyroidism, gynaecomastia, menstrual disturbances, impotence, acne
Cycloserine (Cs)	Dizziness, slurred speech, convulsions, headache, tremor, insomnia, confusion, depression, suicidal tendency
PAS	Anorexia, nausea, vomiting, abdominal pain, skin rash, hepatitis, hypokalemia, hypothyroidism

diet is recommended. The patients should avoid smoking and respiratory irritants. Secondary respiratory infection must be promptly treated with appropriate antibiotics; so also associated diseases like DM.

Dry, hacking, spasmodic cough can be controlled by antitussives. However, over-suppression of the cough reflex favours atelectasis.

Pulmonary haemorrhage leading to haemoptysis needs prompt evacuation of the bronchopulmonary secretions to prevent aspiration and bronchial spread of the disease.

Rifampicin may interact with contraceptives, which decreases their efficacy against pregnancy. In these patients, oral contraceptive having a higher dose of estrogen (50 µg) or other forms of contraception viz. barrier methods (condoms/diaphragms), IUCDs (CuT) or depot-medroxyprogesterone (depo-provera) are recommended.

- **Failure to obtain reversal of infectiousness after 3 months of therapy:** Failure of drug therapy is likely to be due to several causes (Box 52.1) of which **noncompliance is the most important.**

In patients who have failed to respond to or shown relapse after first course of chemotherapy, drug resistance to R or H may be suspected. This could be due to:

- **Inadequate/irregular drug therapy or poor quality drugs.**
- **Patients coming from an area with high prevalence of drug resistance.**
- **Known exposure to a patient with drug-resistant disease.**

The major difficulty is how to persuade patients to take drugs regularly for adequate periods of time. Majority of treatment failures are due to either failure to take prescribed therapy or infection with resistant bacilli.

Box 52.1 Causes of Failure of Drug Treatment of Tuberculosis

- Failure of the patient to take the drugs (noncompliance)
- Incorrect prescribing of drugs
- Primary drug resistance
- Secondary drug resistance
- Persisters which are dormant and therefore have not been affected by the drugs
- Poor general health due to malnutrition, diabetes or chronic alcoholism
- Associated disease such as diabetes mellitus or AIDS

Programmatic Management of Drug Resistant TB (PMDT) of India PH 1.55, PE 34.3, CT 1.15

Drug resistant TB (DR-TB) includes all tuberculous diseases caused by *M. tuberculosis* complex resistant to any anti-TB medicine. The increasing burden of DR-TB has led development of special services for its prevention, diagnosis and management, which are termed as PMDT. These are updated from time to time.

- Biological samples of all the patients with presumptive TB, all notified patients with TB and non-responders to earlier anti-TB treatment are subjected to 1. rapid molecular drug resistance testing (DRT; genotypic tests) to detect genetic mutations associated with drug resistance and 2. growth based phenotypic drug susceptibility testing (DST; phenotypic tests), wherein bacilli are grown and subsequently tested for drug susceptibility. Both identify resistance to the anti-TB drugs sequentially from rifampicin, INH and fluoroquinolones, if any.
- On confirmation of diagnosis of drug resistant TB, pre-treatment evaluation is done to identify potential risk factors and then the patient is switched to anti-TB regimen under PMDT based on the resistance pattern (Table 52.5).

INH resistance

A TB patient, whose biological specimen shows resistance to isoniazid and susceptibility to rifampicin may be resistant to either INH alone (H mono resistance) or to additional first-line anti-TB drugs (H poly resistance).

For H mono-/poly-resistance, FQs are to be used. It

Table 52.5 Treatment Regimens for Drug Resistant (DR) TB (PMDT 2021) PH 1.45

Resistance Type	Drugs	Duration (months)
H mono/poly[a] DR TB (No R resistance)	Lfx, R, E, Z	6[b]
MDR/RR TB		
Shorter oral Bedaquiline-containing regimen	**Induction phase:** Bdq, Lfx, Cfz, Z, E, Hh, Eto	4-6 months
	Continuation phase: Lfx, Cfz, Z, E,	5 months
All oral longer MDR TB regimen	Bdq, Lfx, Lzd, Cfz, Cs	18- 20 Bdq: 6
Shorter injectable MDR TB regimen (when oral BDq regimen cannot be given)	**Induction phase:** Mfx^h, Am/Km, Eto, Cfz, Z, H^h, E	4-6
	Continuation phase: Mfx^h, Cfz, Z, E	5

[a]Resistance to more than one first-line anti-TB drug, other than both, INH and Rifampicin.
[b]The duration is increased to 9 months if there is resistance to Lfx or Z or any of the replacement drugs, and in patients with extensive disease, uncontrolled comorbidity,extra-pulmonary TB and if smear at the end of 4th month is found positive; In CNS, skeletal and milliary TB, duration may be extended to a year.
RR= Rifampicin resistant with or without resistance to other anti-TB drugs excluding INH; Mfx^h= high dose moxifloxacin; H^h= high dose INH.
The above mentioned regimens are modified if there is additional resistance, treatment failure, drug intolerance, if the treatment is interrupted for > 1 month or any exclusion criteria to the regimen emerges.

consists of levofloxacin, ethambutol, rifampicin and pyrazinamide (Table 52.5) for 6 months. Positive sputum smear at the end of month 5 or later is 'treatment failure' and mandates diagnostic reevaluation.

Rifampicin is a key component in H-resistant TB regimens. As it decreases drug levels of bedaquiline, the latter is not used in H-resistant TB.

Rifampicin resistance (RR): Tuberculous organisms resistant to rifampicin may be susceptible or resistant to INH. The latter are termed as **multidrug resistant (MDR)**. It is now widespread globally, often remaining undiagnosed. *Treatment of MDR tuberculosis is complex, needs elaborate evaluation and is best left to experts.* Management of both, RR and MDR TB remains the same.

PH 1.55, PE 34.3, CT 1.15

MDR/RR TUBERCULOSIS MANAGEMENT

For MDR/RR-TB, two oral regimens are advocated which are completely oral (Table 52.5):

1. Bdq-containing shorter oral regimen, and
2. All oral longer regimen

- **Bdq-containing shorter oral MDR/RR TB regimen:** is recommended to all DR TB patients fulfilling the criteria mentioned in Box 52.2. All the 7 drugs of intensive phase are given for 4 months. At the end of 4 months if sputum microscopy is negative then, INH and ethionamide are stopped and then for next 2 months 5

Box 52.2 Inclusion Criteria for Shorter Oral Regimen of MDR/RR TB

- R resistance plus H resistance detected with Kat G or Inh A mutation (not both) and no evidence of resistance to fluoroquinolones
- No history of prior exposure to drugs in shorter oral regimen (Bdq, Lfx, Eto or Cfz) for 1 month or more (unless susceptibility to these medicines is confirmed)
- No risk of toxicity from a drug in the shorter regimen (e.g. drug–drug interactions)
- No bilateral lung cavities, extensive parenchymal damage (indicative of extensive TB). In children under 15 yrs, no evidence of cavities or bilateral disease
- No severe extrapulmonary TB such as miliary/meningeal/CNS TB. In children no extrapulmonary TB except lymphadenopathy
- Children more than 5 years of age and weighing at least 15 kg
- Pregnancy more than 32 weeks
- Lactating mothers ready to use formula feeds

drugs are continued, after which bedaquiline is stopped. (i.e. at the end of 6th mth).The remaining 4 drugs are continued for next 5 months (Table 52.5).

- **All oral longer MDR TB regimen** is initiated for those who cannot be selected for a shorter MDR TB regimen due to:- intolerance to any drug in the shorter MDR-TB regimen or risk of toxicity from a drug in the shorter regimen. Those who cannot fulfil the criteria for Bdq containing shorter oral therapy (Box 52.2) are also the candidates for longer oral therapy.
  Table 52.6 provides guidance for the drug combinations used to treat MDR TB. The treatment is given for 18–20 months with 5 drugs (3 drugs from Group A and both the drugs from Group B). Linezolid dose is reduced to 300 mg after 6 to 8 months. The patient receives only 4 drugs after 6 months. There is no separate intensive or continuous phase.
  If resistance to these drugs is detected in addition, then the MDR TB regimen is appropriately modified using the guidelines of PMDT 2021. The drugs are replaced by the specialist based on their efficacy, absence of demonstrable resistance, evidence of prior use, ADR profile and background level of resistance. Combined use of bedaquiline and delamanid is recommended for those M/XDR-TB patients in whom an appropriate regimen cannot be designed using all 5 drugs from Group A and B.

- **Shorter injectable containing MDR/RR-TB regimen**
  This was the earlier regimen. Currently, a state-wise transitioning is going on in a phased manner from this regimen to the shorter oral Bdq-containing MDR/RR-TB regimen in patients >5 years of age weighing 15kg or more. Till all the states get covered with Bdq-containing shorter oral regimen, the shorter injectable containing MDR TB regimen continues. It involves 4-6 months of intensive phase with 7 drugs containing injectables followed by 5 months of continuous phase with 4 drugs (Table 52.5). In case the intensive phase is prolonged, the injectable is administered only three times a week.

All the drugs are administered as single daily dose with 100 mg pyridoxine.

Table 52.6 Anti-Tuberculous Drugs Recommended for MDR-TB Regimens PH 1.45

Class	Anti-Tuberculous Drugs	Recommendations for Regimen
A	levofloxacin (Lfx) or moxifloxacin (Mfx) Bedaquiline (Bdq) Linezolid (Lzd)	Include all the 3 unless contraindicated
B	Clofazimine (Cfz) Cycloserine (Cs) or terizidone (Tzd)	Add one or both as second choice
C[a]	Ethambutol (E) Delamanid (Dlm) Pyrazinamide (Z) Imipenem–cilastatin (Ipm–Cln)[b] or meropenem (Mpm)[b] Amikacin (Am) or Streptomycin (S) Ethionamide (Eto) or Prothionamide (Pto) Para-aminosalicylic acid (PAS)	Used when medicines from Groups A and B cannot be used Can be added to complete the regimen based on individual factors

[a]In decreasing order of preference based on benefit to harm ratio. Imp-Cln is to be used as the last resort.
[b]Imipenem–cilastatin and meropenem requires clavulanic acid with every dose. As the latter is available only in FDC with amoxicillin–clavulanic acid, the FDC is used. But remember this FDC itself is not an anti-tuberculous drug and should not be used alone.

Standardized monthly treatment boxes are provided to the patient according to weight band.

- The treatment strategy remains the same for extra-pulmonary MDR-TB, provided the patients do not have any of the exclusion criteria.
- If there is an interruption in treatment for more than 2 months, then it is considered as lost-to-follow-up.
- The patient monitoring is done using a digital e-Nikshay system. Sputum smear is examined at each month and later at 6 monthly intervals.

Pre-extensively and extensively drug resistant tuberculosis (Pre-XRD and XRD-TB) Management

Pre-XDR TB is defined as TB caused by *Mycobacterium tuberculosis* strains that are multi-drug resistant/rifampicin- resistant (MDR/RR) and are also resistant to any fluoroquinolone.

XDR-TB is defined as TB that fulfills the definition of pre-XDR TB and in addition, the organisms are resistant to at least one Group A drug (presently to either bedaquiline or linezolid or to both).

Current pre-XRD and XDR-TB regimen is all oral longer regimen described above but for 20 months duration.

Bone marrow suppression and anaemia can occur due to linezolid. Cycloserine can cause depression and suicidal tendency. Clofazimine can cause skin discolouration. Frequent monitoring of haemogram, serum creatinine, liver function tests and chest X-ray is needed in these patients.

- **DR-TB in Children** The principles of management remains the same as adults. Both shorter or longer oral MDR/RR-TB regimens can be used for children above 5 yrs with weight at least 15 kg but the dosages are given according to weight bands. *Child-friendly formulations should be used whenever possible.* Children below 5 years are given short course injectable till further evidence on use of bedaquiline is available.
- **DR-TB in Pregnancy** For a pregnant woman with DR-TB medical termination of pregnancy (MTP) is advisable provided the pregnancy is < 20 weeks. However, if there is unwillingness for MTP or if pregnancy is > 20 weeks then a **modified all oral longer regimen** is administered after counselling with monthly follow up. This regimen consists of levofloxacin, linezolid, clofazimine, cycloserine and pyrazinamide for 18-20 months and is modified suitably if any other drug resistance/intolerance is detected. Post-delivery care remains the same as drug sensitive TB.

BPaL regimen

This regimen is under evaluation. It consists of 3 drugs viz. bedaquiline (B) + pretomanid (Pa) + linezolid (L) and is given for 6 months. All 3 drugs contribute to bactericidal and curative activity.

It is indicated in :

- Pre-XDR TB patients, with no or < 2 weeks exposure to bedaquiline and linezolid
- Patients with MDR/XDR TB who are non-responsive or intolerant to longer oral anti- TB regimen

This regimen is not indicated in drug sensitive, latent or extrapulmonary TB.

OTHER FORMS OF TUBERCULOSIS OR 3.1

Drug regimens proven effective in pulmonary TB are effective in extrapulmonary TB as well. **Severe forms of TB like meningitis, skeletal TB, pericarditis, and acute miliary TB require continuation phase extended by 3–6 months.** Based on the clinical decision, a longer treatment with three or four drugs for 12 months may be needed. IM 17.13

Tuberculous meningitis: H + S + R + Z is the preferred initial combination in this disease. INH is used in the dose of 10–15 mg/kg/day. Intensive chemotherapy is administered till CSF returns to normal, followed by maintenance therapy. Total duration of chemotherapy may be of 2 years. Pyridoxine is prescribed to prevent INH neurotoxicity.

Steroids should be used in all severely ill patients, in those with a suggestion of cerebrospinal block. The initial adult dose of prednisolone is 80 mg per day (1 mg/kg in children) in four equally divided doses. The dose should then be gradually reduced till a maintenance level of 25–30 mg daily is reached within 2–3 weeks. For withdrawal of glucocorticoids see Chapter 64.

The same regime including steroids is also applicable to miliary TB, tuberculous pericarditis and tuberculous pneumonia.

Tuberculous lymphadenitis: This condition which is often due to atypical mycobacteria usually responds unsatisfactorily to chemotherapy (see section, Nontuberculous mycobacterial infections). If no progress is apparent within 6–8 weeks, the glands may be removed surgically.

Miscellaneous tuberculous infections: TB of the genitourinary tract, bones, joints, skin, larynx and intestine responds well to routine chemotherapy. For ocular TB, topical and systemic glucocorticoid therapy may be required in addition to systemic chemotherapy.

For extrapulmonary DR-TB longer oral M/XDR-TB regimen can be given. In case of MDR/RR TB meningitis this regimen must be modified as per the replacement table because some dugs do not cross the BBB e.g., Ethambutol. Data regarding the CNS penetration of Cfz, Bdq or Dlm is insufficient. On the other hand, Lfx, Mfx, Lzd and Eto, Cs, and Imp-Cls have good penetration across the BBB. Meropenem is preferred in TB meningitis and in children as imipenem is more likely to cause seizures.

Treatment of TB is essentially medical. Moreover, it must be emphasised that surgical removal of the lesion does not mean that the disease is completely eradicated. Therefore, the patient must be treated with adequate chemotherapy before, during and after such procedures.

GLUCOCORTICOIDS IN TUBERCULOSIS

Glucocorticoids impair host defence mechanism and promote dissemination of infection. However, their anti-inflammatory action may be helpful. Their **short-term use reduces excessive inflammatory reaction** which is likely to threaten life or lead to extensive fibrosis on healing. *They must never be used without cover of effective antitubercular chemotherapy.* The indications are as follows:

- **To relieve toxic symptoms and hypoxemia in fulminating, rapidly progressive infection in pulmonary TB, tuberculous pneumonia or miliary TB.**
- **To prevent bronchial stenosis in endobronchial TB.**
- **To reduce toxemia, hasten the absorption of the exudate and prevent the formation of adhesions, arachnoiditis and hydrocephalus in tuberculous meningitis.**
- **To hasten the reabsorption of fluid in TB of the serous membranes like the pleura and the pericardium.** Use of glucocorticoids in abdominal TB, may be dangerous as it may lead to intestinal perforation.
- **As an adrenal cortical hormone replacement,** e.g. in Addison disease, when it occurs with TB elsewhere in the body.
- **To counter the hypersensitivity reactions to antituberculous drugs.**
- **To arrest the dire consequences in rapidly enlarging mediastinal tuberculous lymph nodes.**
- **To prevent the serious consequences of fibrosis in ocular and genito-urinary TB.**

In addition, see Chapter 64.

PE 34.4

CHEMOPROPHYLAXIS OF TUBERCULOSIS

Chemoprophylaxis of TB means the use of antituberculous drugs for its prevention (TB preventive therapy- TPT). INH is the ideal drug for this purpose as it is cheap, effective orally and has acceptable toxic effects. However, recently newer shorter TPT regimens are emerging. Active TB needs to be ruled out before starting TPT. Two regimens are recommended under NETP:

1. INH monotherapy: The recommended dose is 5 mg/kg daily for children $\geqslant$ 10 years and for adults and 10 mg/kg daily for children less than $<$ 10 years. The maximum dose of INH is 300mg/kg. It is given for 6 months (6H). It can be used safely in pregnant women. No interactions are observed in HIV patients on ART. ADR of H monotherapy can be peripheral neuropathy. However, it occurs infrequently and is reversible on INH withdrawal or giving 100-200 mg / day pyridoxine. Pyridoxine supplementation is required for those with malnutrition, chronic alcoholics, patients with HIV, renal failure or diabetes, or pregnant or breastfeeding women. These prophylactic doses are 10mg/day in children and 25 mg/day in adults. The dose is 50mg/day in an adult HIV patient. The other ADR include hepatitis, GI disturbances and rash.

2. INH and rifapentine: These are given weekly for 12 weeks (3 HP). For adolescents > 14 years and adults, the doses of INH and rifapentine are 900mg each. For children from 2–14 years, the dosage varies according to weight bands. INH and rifapentine are also available as FDC. Though the pill burden and treatment duration is less with this regimen, experience with it is less. Its safety in pregnancy is not known. It is contraindicated in HIV patients on PI, NVP/NNRTI and TAF. Other drugs like TDF, EFV (600 mg), DTG, RAL can be used without dose adjustment. ADR include flu-like syndrome, hypersensitivity reactions, GI upset, orange discolouration of body fluids and rash but chances of hepatitis is less.

The efficacy of both the regimens is similar but rifapentine based therapy has advantages of better adherence due to the shorter duration and at least 20% greater treatment completion rate.

TPT is indicated for children and adult household contacts of pulmonary TB as well as patients with HIV and silicosis, those receiving immunosuppressive therapy, anti-TNF treatment, dialysis and transplants. It is also indicated in HIV patients who have completed antiTB therapy as recurrence of TB is high among them (post-treatment TPT). Choice of regimen for TPT depends on availability and tolerance to drugs. However, in children below 2 years and in children living with HIV, only INH monotherapy is used.

CHEMOPROPHYLAXIS TO CONTACTS OF DR-TB PATIENTS

Contacts of patients with INH-resistant TB can be treated with daily 10mg/kg rifampicin for 4 months. MDR- TB contacts should receive 6 months of levofloxacin in the dose of 750 mg/day if the weight is < 45 kg and 1g/day if ≥ 45 kg.

For RR-TB contacts, INH and levofloxacin are administered for 6 months.

Current National guidelines recommend that the contacts should be monitored for active TB during TPT.

PH 1.54, PE 34.4

BCG VACCINE: BCG is prepared from *Bacille Calmette Guerin,* a strain of bovine tubercle bacillus with greatly attenuated virulence, developed in France by Calmette and Guerin. The aim of the vaccination is to increase the patient's resistance by producing artificial primary tuberculous infection with an organism which causes only a local lesion and some swelling of the adjacent lymph nodes. *It is probably the safest among vaccines in use today.*

Before vaccination, a tuberculin skin test (TST) is carried out where 0.0001 mg or 5 test units of purified protein derivative (PPD) obtained from the mycobacterium is injected intradermally on the ventral surface of the forearm. If the test is negative, it is repeated after 6 weeks. If the TST still remains negative, 0.1 mL of the vaccine is injected intradermally in the deltoid region. This leads to the formation of a papule followed by an ulcer within 4–6 weeks. The regional glands are slightly enlarged. Healing occurs gradually thereafter, but the papule may be detectable up to a period of 12 months. After vaccination, the TST becomes positive within 6–12 weeks indicating the development of immunity.

A rare complication of BCG vaccination is a glandular cold abscess. This should be treated with antimicrobials. *Just an enlargement of lymph nodes needs no treatment.* Individuals with hypogammaglobulinaemia or eczema should not be vaccinated.

BCG vaccination is useful in:

- **TST negative school children**
- **Contacts of cases with active TB**
- **Persons living in TB endemic areas**

Ideally, it is given within first 6 months of life. *Pretesting with PPD is not needed if BCG is given immediately after birth.* During mass vaccination programme also pretesting is not necessary as BCG is not hazardous to tuberculin positive children.

BCG has contributed to the control of TB. But, the

efficacy of different BCG vaccines varies in different populations. Its efficacy is about 70% against serious form of disease in children (meningitis and miliary TB) but variable against pulmonary TB in adults. *It must not be given to anyone with symptomatic HIV infection.* BCG gives relative degree of resistance to clinical TB. The protection, is 'not complete, nor permanent, nor predictable, nor measureable'. Further, the presence of infection with mycobacteria other than tubercle bacilli can interfere with the protection given by BCG.

BCG and host defence: It enhances the host defence mechanisms. It stimulates the RES and acts as immunostimulant against bacterial and viral infections. Its administration can prevent the growth and cause regression of transplanted tumours in animals. Local intralesional injection of BCG or PPD produces beneficial effects in superficial bladder cancer, malignant melanoma and reticulum cell sarcoma.

The mechanism of its **anticancer action** is not well understood. As an immunostimulant, it activates the natural killer cells and the production of haemopoietic stem cells. Macrophages activated by BCG become more active killer cells and more effectively clear antigens and immune complexes.

NONTUBERCULOUS MYCOBACTERIAL (NTM) INFECTIONS

These infections caused by organisms such as *Mycobacterium kansasii, M. abscessus, M. xenopi, M. avium, M. marinum and M. scrofulaceum* are grouped under **atypical mycobacterial infections.** Of these, *M. scrofulaceum* causes cervical lymphadenitis especially in children; and *M. marinum* causes skin disease. Clinical signs and symptoms of *M. kansasii* infection resembles TB. **MAC infection is caused by** *M. avium, M. intracellulare* and *M. chimaera*, among others. Though they can affect lungs of immunocompetent persons, the infection is disseminated in patients with HIV.

The atypical mycobacteria are, in general, of low virulence but the disease caused is usually resistant to antituberculous drugs. Whenever possible, surgical removal of the infected tissue is recommended, followed by chemotherapy. Most of the pulmonary cavitary NTM including. **MAC** respond to the 3 drug combination therapy with first-line drugs, *viz.* **clarithromycin** (500 mg)/**azithromycin** (250 mg), **ethambutol** (15 mg/kg) and **rifamycins** [rifampicin (600 mg)/rifabutin (300 mg)] given daily. Amikacin (15 mg/kg) thrice weekly is administered for severe or macrolide resistant MAC. An intermittent (3 times per week) can be used for nodular/bronchiectatic MAC infection. However the doses are higher (1000 mg clarithromycin or 500 mg azithromycin + 25 mg/kg ethambutol and 600 mg rifampicin). *M. kansasii* can be treated with INH instead of a macrolide but in that case daily triple therapy is recommended. Daily therapy as described above is recommended for patients who have severe pulmonary disease or a history of treatment failure. The duration of therapy is for 12 months after sputum conversion to negative.

Long-term outcome of NTM infection is poor despite the treatment.

Fluoroquinolones such as ciprofloxacin, ofloxacin and moxifloxacin are considered as second-line drugs against MAC. Ciprofloxacin is used in the dose of 750 mg b.i.d. and levofloxacin in the dose of 500 mg/once a day.

RIFABUTIN: is a semisynthetic antibiotic derived from rifamycin S. Its action is similar to that of rifampicin. **It is more active than rifampicin against MAC and even against MAC strains resistant to rifampicin.** It is readily absorbed and tissue levels are 5–10 times higher than plasma concentration. CSF concentration is 30%–70% that of the plasma. Its plasma $t½$ is 45 h, compared to 3–5 h of rifampicin. It is mainly eliminated in bile and no dose adjustment is needed in the presence of kidney damage.

Adverse reactions: These include GI disturbances, neutropenia, myalgia and impairment of taste. Other adverse effects are similar to those of rifampicin. It too induces hepatic microsomal enzymes.

Indications: It is given in a dose of 300–600 mg/day along with other drugs in pulmonary MAC infection for up to 6 months. Smaller doses are used for treating pulmonary TB and as a single agent for prophylaxis against MAC. It is used in place of rifampicin to treat

HIV patients taking protease inhibitors as it does not affect the serum level of these drugs.

CLARITHROMYCIN: This macrolide (Chapter 44) is used in combination with ethambutol and rifampin. It is more potent than azithromycin but the latter has better intracellular penetration, lesser dose frequency and drug-drug interactions. Hence azithromycin is preferred.

TUBERCULOSIS AND HIV INFECTION

HIV infection causes a specific and progressive destruction of the helper T lymphocytes (CD4 cells) and impairs the function of the B lymphocytes and macrophages (Chapter 51). This makes an HIV infected person:

- **More liable to have recurrence even after successful treatment**
- **To get a fresh infection**
- **To progress rapidly from latent infection to active clinical TB**

Further, the severity of TB increases as the destruction of the immune system by HIV progresses. TB also increases HIV replication and aggravates it. Both *M. tuberculosis* and the MAC can infect these patients, much before the other opportunistic infections do. About 25% of patients with HIV may have undiagnosed active but subclinical TB. *Hence, screening for TB is recommended for all patients with HIV infections.*

Treatment of active TB is with the **first-line four drug regimen** (INH, rifabutin, E and Z) for 9–12 months, pyrazinamide being dropped after the first 2 months. *Rifampicin, being hepatic enzyme inducer, renders protease inhibitors and NNRTI (except efavirenz) ineffective.* Efavirenz regime is compatible with the rifampicin containing therapy.

WHO recommends that HIV infected persons with positive tuberculin skin test but without active TB and living in high burden population are to be treated with any one of the following regimes:

1. Daily INH 300 mg for 6 months.
2. INH + rifampicin combination daily (INH: 300 mg + R: 600 mg) or supervised twice weekly (INH: 900 mg + R: 600 mg) for 3 months.

The antiretroviral therapy (Tenofovir + Lamivudine + Efavirenz) is started within the first 8 weeks after the initiation of anti-TB treatment. But patients with CD4 positive cell count <50/mm³ should receive such therapy within 2 weeks. Patients who are already receiving antiretroviral therapy should continue the same when treatment of TB is instituted. Occasionally, these patients may show temporary exacerbation of TB due to **immune restitution inflammatory syndrome (IRIS),** which can be treated with glucocorticoids.

In H mono/poly Dr-TB patients with HIV coinfection, ART should be started within 8 weeks of TB treatment initiation (regardless of CD4 count). In HIV patients with MDR/RR-TB, both the shorter or longer oral MDR-TB regimen can be used along with ART. Anti TB therapy is started first and within first 2 weeks, ART is initiated irrespective of CD4 count. Close monitoring is required due to additive toxicities or drug drug interactions e.g., ritonavir may increase bedaquiline related ADR.

In general, the treatment of MAC associated with HIV is complex and should be left to the special clinics.

Prophylaxis against MAC with 300 mg rifabutin daily is started if CD4 count is <50mm³. It is continued for life time unless active MAC develops, which needs multiple drug therapy. Other alternatives are 1200 mg azithromycin weekly, 600 mg azithromycin/ 500 mg clarithromycin twice-weekly.

ANTI-TUBERCULOSIS DRUGS

First-line drugs

- **Bactericidal**
  - Isonicotinic acid hydrazide (H)
  - Rifampicin (R)
  - Pyrazinamide (Z)
- **Bacteriostatic**
  - Ethambutol (E)

Second-Line Drugs

Oral

- **Bactericidal**
  - Fluoroquinolones
    - Levofloxacin (Lfx)
    - Moxifloxacin (Mfx)
  - Bedaquiline (Bdq)
  - Delamanid (Dlm)
- **Bacteriostatic**
  - Ethionamide (Et)
  - Cycloserine (C)
  - Terizidone (Trd)
  - Clofazimine (Cfz)
  - Linezolid (Lzd)
  - Thiacetazone (T)
  - Paraminosalicylic acid (PAS)

Injectables

- **Bactericidal**
  - Aminoglycosides
    - Amikacin (Am)
    - Streptomycin (S)
  - Carbapenems
    - Imipenem plus Cilastatin (Ipm-Cln)
    - Meropenem (Mpm)

CHAPTER 53

Chemotherapy of Leprosy

Learning Objectives

This chapter will enable the reader:

1. To be aware of different clinical types of leprosy.
2. To enlist the aims of leprosy treatment.
3. To enumerate the drugs used in the treatment of leprosy.
4. To discuss the mechanism of action, salient pharmacological features, adverse drug reactions and indications for antileprosy agents.
5. To describe the pharmacotherapy of multibacillary and paucibacillary leprosy.
6. To enlist the drugs giving rationale for their use in treatment of lepra reactions.

KEY TERMS

dapsone, p. 767
multibacillary leprosy, p. 767
paucibacillary leprosy, p. 767
rifampicin, p. 768
clofazimine, p. 768
Leprosy management, p. 768
U-MDT, p. 770
ROM therapy, p. 770
Drug resistant leprosy, p. 771
lepra reactions, p. 771
Leprosy prophylaxis, p. 772
thalidomide, p. 772

Leprosy is caused by *Mycobacterium leprae* which produces characteristic lesions in the skin and the peripheral nerves. *M. leprae* are obligate intracellular acid fast bacilli and their ability to survive within the macrophages and Schwann cells is a key feature of their pathogenicity. The disease is common in Southeast Asia, Africa and other tropical and subtropical countries.

Human leprosy bacilli from the nasal washings and skin biopsies, cultivated in the foot pads of mice, have been successfully transmitted to some species of armadillo. The infected armadillo tissues contain a large number of leprosy bacilli, which provide a good experimental model of human leprosy.

Types of leprosy: Clinically, there are four main types of leprosy:

- **Lepromatous (LL)**
- **Tuberculoid (TL)**
- **Indeterminate (IL)**
- **Dimorphic (borderline, BL)**

They are determined by the degree of cell mediated immunity (CMI) in the host against the lepra bacilli.

In **LL**, the **CMI is low** (**negative lepromin test**), the lesions abound in lepra bacilli and the disease progresses rapidly. *The nerves are affected late in the disease.* The disease affects mainly the face, nose, ears, eyes and lymph glands. The typical lesion of LL is a macule, a hypopigmented, circular, erythematous patch not associated with itching or hypoalgesia. Macules are usually small, smooth and symmetrically distributed. Eventually, the skin becomes furrowed and nodulated, giving a peculiar 'leonine facies'. Eyelashes fall off. Later, ulceration occurs with marked tissue destruction involving eyes, nose and larynx. **Histologically, the lesion of LL is essentially a granuloma consisting of many macrophages, called lepra cells, containing numerous bacilli.**

In **TL**, the **CMI is intact** (**strongly positive lepromin test**), **the organisms are few, nerves are predominantly affected first**, and the progress of the disease is slow. The typical TL lesion is a large, flat, atrophic, hairless, hypopigmented skin area, with red, raised margin showing marked impairment of sensation. The peripheral nerves are thickened. The prognosis is better than in LL and gross mutilation occurs only secondary to nerve destruction and anaesthesia. **Histologically,** the lesion consists of focal masses of epitheloid cells and giant cells with lymphocytic infiltration. Since this picture resembles to that seen in tuberculosis, it is called **TL leprosy**.

IL or the confusing form is an early stage where the lesions are vague hypopigmented macules and do not give a clue about the type of disease.

BL is an unstable condition, where immunity is low and which becomes LL if left untreated.

LL and BL forms have plenty of bacilli in the lesions and are called **multibacillary leprosy,** whereas TL and IL with fewer bacilli are called **paucibacillary leprosy**.

The diagnosis of leprosy is essentially clinical, supported by bacteriological evidence from smears from the lesions, nodules, earlobes, or from scrapings of the nasal mucosa. **All smear positives are multibacillary type.**

All patients with active leprosy should be treated with chemotherapy. **It is, however, unjustifiable and even dangerous to treat this disease on mere suspicion.** This not only exposes the patient to prolonged therapy with potentially toxic drugs but can also cause severe psychological trauma. In case of doubtful diagnosis, it is better to wait for definite diagnosis because little harm occurs by waiting.

PH 1.46, DR 9.5

Classification of Anti-Leprosy Drugs

I. **Sulfone:** Dapsone (DDS)
II. **Phenazine derivative** Clofazimine.
III. **Antitubercular Drugs:** Rifampicin
IV. **Fluoroquinolones:** Ofloxacin, Pefloxacin
V. **Other Antimicrobials:** Minocycline, Clarithromycin

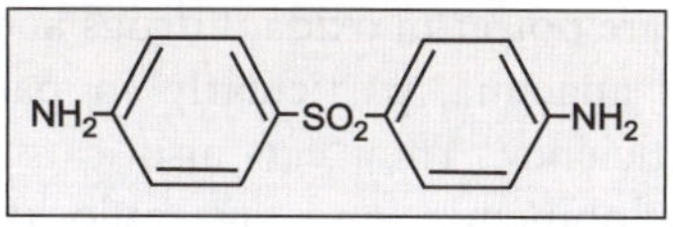

FIG. 53.1 **Diamino-diphenylsulphone (DDS).**

SULPHONES: Sulphones are derivatives of 4-4'-diamino-diphenyl sulphone (DDS, **Dapsone**) (Fig. 53.1). Sulphones are chemically related to sulphonamides, and are highly effective in the treatment of leprosy **in small doses.** Among the various sulphones, **dapsone** still remains the drug of choice.

Mechanism of action: Sulphones are essentially bacteriostatic and act by inhibiting the *de novo* synthesis of folic acid by *M. leprae*. The action of DDS is antagonised by para-amino-benzoic acid similar to sulphonamides.

Sulphones are bacteriostatic against other bacteria susceptible to sulphonamides and against the tubercle bacilli. They are, however, not used in other infections because of their toxicity which occurs at the doses used.

Absorption, fate and excretion: DDS is slowly but completely absorbed from the GI tract. The peak plasma level is reached within 1–3 h and the drug remains detectable in the plasma for 8–12 days (t½ 27 h). Sulphones are cumulative drugs. They are distributed throughout the body fluids and tissues and can be detected in the tissues up to 3 weeks after stoppage of therapy. They are metabolised in the liver and excreted in urine as glucuronic acid conjugates. Large quantities are also excreted in bile; this portion however, is reabsorbed. Excretion also occurs in human milk.

Dapsone resistance: Both primary and secondary resistance of *M. leprae* to dapsone is well documented, and is associated with **gene mutation**. However, primary resistance to dapsone is rare.

Adverse reactions: These are similar to those due to sulphonamides (Chapter 43). They commonly cause anorexia, nausea and vomiting. They can give rise to allergic reactions like dermatitis and drug fever. Fatal exfoliative dermatitis (Stevens–Johnson syndrome) associated with drug fever, hepatitis and psychosis can rarely occur.

Sulphones are powerful oxidant drugs and can cause haemolytic anaemia, particularly in patients with G6-PD deficiency. They can also cause anaemia, methaemoglobinemia and agranulocytosis. Mild anaemia is not a contraindication to dapsone therapy. Dapsone may be used (along with haematinics) to treat a patient with haemoglobin more than 8gm%.

Other toxic effects include haematuria, liver damage and goitrogenesis.

Although the list of toxicity is formidable, sulphones, in the dosage recommended in leprosy, are remarkably well tolerated by most of the patients.

Contraindications to DDS:

- Patient allergic to sulpha drugs: Clofazamine may be an alternative to dapsone.
- Patients with Hb< 8gm%: Treatment of anaemia should be started and dapsone is withheld till Hb rises above 8gm%.

Preparations and dosage:

i. Dapsone (DDS): 50–100 mg tablets. It is given in the dose of 100 mg daily.
ii. Dapsone injection is a 20% w/v suspension in arachis oil. Dose: 0.2 mL IM weekly, gradually increased to a maximum of 0.8 mL weekly.

Other indications of sulphones:

- **Dermatitis herpetiformis** is a chronic disease characterised by intensely itching papules, urticaria-like lesions, vesicles and bullae on the extensor surfaces of the body. Dapsone, in the dose of 50 mg orally, daily, increased by 25 mg (daily dose) once in 10–15 days to 25 mg three to four times daily, rapidly controls the skin lesions.
- *Pneumocystitis jiroveci* infection Dapsone used as second line drug for prophylaxis (50 mg twice daily) and treatment for mild/moderate disease in the dose of 100 mg daily with trimethoprim (15 mg daily) and atovaquone (750 mg BID)
- MDR falciparum malaria: Dapsone is used in combination with pyrimethamine(Chapter 54).

RIFAMPICIN: This antituberculous antibiotic has been discussed in Chapter 52. It is bactericidal, highly effective and safe. *Few toxic effects have been reported so far in the case of monthly administration. Supervised administration of 600 mg of rifampicin single dose once a month is equally effective as daily administration.* It is a drug of choice. Bacterial resistance to rifampicin can occur.

CLOFAZIMINE: This red-purple phenazine dye is well absorbed after oral administration. It is principally retained in tissues of the reticuloendothelial system and concentrated by macrophages of the skin. It acts by **inhibition of mycobacterial DNA synthesis**. It is probably bactericidal and has action against dapsone resistant organisms. It also **possesses anti-inflammatory properties.** Bacterial resistance to clofazimine is rare. Its t½ is 70 days and is excreted in the urine slowly for several weeks. In the dose of 100 mg three times a day, it is useful in lepra reactions because of its simultaneous bactericidal and anti-inflammatory actions. It is also claimed that the drug enhances the ability of human macrophages to kill listeria.

Adverse reactions: Clofazimine imparts a reddish black hue to the skin, which persists for several months. It is also deposited in the intestine where it may cause segmental thickening leading to crampy pain and diarrhoea. Otherwise, it is remarkably safe.

It is also used in MDR-TB (Chapter 52).

Other drugs: Ofloxacin/pefloxacin(400 mg/day), **minocycline**(100 mg/day), **clarithromycin, ethionamide, prothionamide, have demonstrated *in vitro* bactericidal activity against *M. leprae.*** They are described in the respective Chapters 43, 47 and 52. These drugs are particularly useful in patients allergic to DDS and those with resistant infection. Ethionamide was considered earlier, if patients cannot accept or tolerate clofazimine. However, WHO does not recommend its use due to serious hepatotoxicity.

MANAGEMENT OF LEPROSY PH 1.55, DR 9.6

Leprosy, which was once considered to be an incurable disease, **can now be cured completely**. The disease is transmitted by prolonged and intimate contact with untreated, open LL patients whose cutaneous lesions and mucosal discharges teem with leprosy bacilli. As in the case of tuberculosis, the main difficulty in the treatment of leprosy is in persuading the patient to continue the drug therapy regularly for a prolonged period. In majority of the patients, the medical treatment of leprosy can be wholly undertaken by practitioners or by trained medical auxiliaries.

Aims of therapy:

- **To achieve clinical cure**
- **To achieve bacteriological cure**
- **To treat physical deformities resulting from nerve and tissue damage**

The psychosocial aspect of the patient and his environment also need attention. Leprosy treatment is offered under out-patient services. Isolation is indicated only in patients with LL who are untreated or in whom treatment has lapsed.

Rifampicin, dapsone and **clofazimine** *are the first line drugs in leprosy*. The multiplication time of *M. tuberculosis is* 18 h whereas that of *M. lepraeis* 12 days. **Therefore, rifampicin has to be given daily in tuberculosis whereas in leprosy even once a month regime is effective.** *A single dose of 600 mg rifampicin kills >95% of lepra bacilli within 4 days and hence there is no public health problem after 4 days of therapy.*

Although approximately 99.9% of leprosy bacilli are killed in about 3–4 months by dapsone or clofazimine given daily and within 3–7 days by rifampicin given in a single dose of 600 mg, some bacilli may still persist for a long time. This is probably because, the bacilli, though drug sensitive, are not metabolically active. **These persisters can cause relapse over 3–30 years.** So far, no drug given alone can eliminate all "persisting" *M. leprae*. Hence, as in TB, **combination of drugs** is recommended in order to:

- **Render the patient non infectious and limit the spread.**
- **Eliminate persisting organisms.**
- **Prevent drug resistance to monotherapy.**
- **Decrease the required duration of therapy.**
- **Reduce the progression and prevent complications.**

Table 53.1 National Leprosy Eradication Programme (NLEP) PH 1.55

Leprosy Type	Drugs	Duration
Tuberculoid (paucibacillary)	Dapsone 100 mg/day, + Rifampicin 600 mg monthly	6 months
Lepromatous (multibacillary)	Dapsone 100 mg/day + clofazimine 50 mg/day and rifampicin 600 mg + clofazimine 300 mg monthly	12 months

Drug regimens used in leprosy: *All patients should* receive **multidrug therapy (MDT)** (Table 53.1). *Tuberculosis must be excluded before starting monthly rifampicin. If TB co exists, rifampicin is administered in the dose required for the treatment of TB.*

A patient with low body weight (less than 35 kg) having **multibacillary leprosy** is given 450 mg of rifampicin as single monthly dose (supervised) and dapsone in the dose of 50 mg daily. Similar doses are used for adolescents. It is recommended that MDT be given for 1 year and be continued, when possible, up to smear negativity in LL cases. In case clofazimine is not acceptable, ofloxacin (400 mg daily), minocycline (100 mg daily), and clarithromycin (500mg) are established second-line drugs.

Studies indicate that 100 mg of **minocycline** with 500 mg of **clarithromycin** given daily produces beneficial effects. However, minocycline may cause hyperpigmentation of skin lesions, so it may not be an appropriate substitute for clofazimine if pigmentation is to be avoided.

In case of **paucibacillary** leprosy (TL and IL), NLEP recommends rifampicin 600 mg once a month (supervised) and dapsone 100 mg daily (self-administered) for six months. In all cases, the maximum dosage of dapsone should be used from the start and need not be reduced during lepra reaction.

Table 53.2 Suggested Doses for Leprosy in Children PH 1.55

Drug	Age: 10–14 Years	Age: < 10 Years
Multibacillary leprosy		
Dapsone	50 mg/day	2 mg/kg day
Rifampicin	450 mg/month	10 mg/kg/month
Clofazimine	150 mg/month and 50 mg on alternate days	6mg/kg/ month and 1 mg/kg/day (to be given weekly capsule as the lowest strength of available capsule is 50 mg)
Paucibacillary leprosy		
Dapsone	50 mg/day	2 mg/kg day
Rifampicin	450 mg/month	10 mg/kg/month

The drug regimens in children remain the same as those in adults, however, the doses differ and are given in Table 53.2.

Recently WHO has advocated clofazimine even for paucibacillary leprosy as in multibacillary leprosy but only for 6 months (Uniform MDT; U-MDT). The studies have shown that U-MDT can be a better option in countries wherein leprosy is endemic. Hence from 1st April 2025 onwards it will be included in the NLEP.

WHO recommends one time dose for treating a single skin lesion of paucibacillary leprosy, using **rifampicin 600 mg + ofloxacin 400 mg + minocycline 100 mg,** all taken together (ROM therapy). Smaller doses are used in children. There are studies done in multibacillary leprosy wherein ROM therapy was given for 6 or 12 months, which demonstrated similar cure rate, relapse rate and lower rate of adverse effects when compared with MDT. However, large clinical studies have not been conducted to substantiate these benefits of multiple ROM therapy.

Since leprosy is exacerbated during pregnancy it is important to continue the treatment with dapsone, rifampicin and clofazimine. MDT is safe in pregnancy.

All patients should be periodically tested for sensory and motor nerve involvement in all four limbs. *Usually, the patients developing reactions during drug therapy (Table 53.3) and those with impending eye or nerve damage need hospitalisation.* **Prednisolone** (20–40 mg/day) should be added to the specific chemotherapy promptly on suspicion of sensory or motor involvement. It should be tapered over a period of 8–12 months. Local treatment may be necessary for neuropathic ulcerations of the extremities.

Following drug therapy, early lesions disappear completely. Late cutaneous lesions in LL show atrophy, tissue paper like wrinkling and scarring. In TL, nerves already damaged may remain permanently thickened. *Prognosis with early drug therapy is excellent and recovery is almost complete without any residual damage.* The disease is considered inactive when during a 12-month period:

- **The disease is clinically inactive.**
- **No acid fast bacilli are demonstrated by the slit-and-scrape samplings from the skin sites.**
- **Skin biopsies are negative for acid-fast bacilli.**

Clinical activity in TL is denoted by:

1. Increase in the size of previous lesions or the appearance of new ones
2. Persistence of erythema or infiltration in the lesions
3. Progressive sensory impairment and motor loss
4. Continuation or worsening of local tenderness of peripheral nerves

In LL, clinical activity is indicated by:

1. Continued presence of hypopigmented macules or nodules
2. Tenderness on peripheral nerves

In case of paucibacillary leprosy if patients miss > 3 months of therapy and in multibacillary > 6 months of therapy, they are considered as defaulters. They need re-examination to re start the regimen. Such patients can be rapidly rendered noninfectious by using rifampicin.

Following adequate MDT, the **TL or IL leprosy rarely**

Table 53.3 Common Adverse Effects of Anti -Leprosy Drugs PH 1.46, DR 9.5

Adverse drug reactions	Implicated drug	Action taken
Anaemia	Dapsone	Give antihelminthic therapy Treat anaemia Stop dapsone if Hb<8gm%
Reddish discoloration of secretions and/or skin	Rifampicin, clofazimine	Reassure the patient that the skin discolouration will fade after completion of therapy
Allergic skin rash	Rifampicin	Stop rifampicin
Icthyosis	Clofazimine	Reassure the patient Apply oil to the dry skin
Exfoliative dermatitis	Dapsone	Stop dapsone. Refer to hospital immediately Not to restart dapsone
Dryness of conjunctiva	Clofazimine	Administer moistening drops
Hepatitis	Dapsone, rifampicin	Stop dapsone and rifampicin Wait for resolution to re start the therapy

recurs and usually no treatment is necessary after the clinical cure. In case of **LL leprosy**, patients should be followed up at regular intervals for detecting a possible recurrence. This may be due to drug resistance, inadequate therapy, persisters or re infection. Patients with relapse are treated with regimen for multibacillary leprosy irrespective of their previous / current leprosy type. *Impairment of nerve function can occur even during or after MDT, and needs to be monitored for 2–3 years.*

Minocycline and a fluoroquinolone can be substituted in **dapsone-resistant cases. In case of rifampicin resistance,** at least two of the following drugs are used: clarithromycin, minocycline or a fluoroquinolone (ofloxacin, levofloxacin or moxifloxacin). In addition, daily clofazimine should be given for initial 6 months. This is followed by clofazimine plus one of the second-line drugs daily for an additional 18 months.

However, **if there is resistance to rifampicin and ofloxacin,** then fluoroquinolone should not be used. Hence clarithromycin, minocycline and clofazimine may be used for 6 months, followed by clarithromycin or minocycline plus clofazimine for an additional 18 months.

Lepra Reactions DR 9.4

The acute exacerbation that occurs during the course of leprosy is called lepra reaction. They are usually precipitated by anxiety, malaria, helminth infestation, acute infections and during treatment with sulphones. Treatment of precipitating factors helps in early resolution of lepra reactions.

They are of **two types: type I** and **type II.**

Type I reaction (reversal reaction):

1. It occurs in patients with good CMI towards *M. leprae.*
2. Existing lesions show increased erythema, swelling and tender peripheral nerves. Loss of nerve function may occur.
3. The constitutional symptoms are not marked.
4. Often it leads to a decrease in the number of bacilli in the lesions.

This type of reaction usually occurs in TL leprosy. The mechanism of type I reactions is thought to be delayed type of hypersensitivity. **The treatment is mainly directed at controlling acute inflammation, reversing the eye and nerve damage.**

Type II reaction:

1. *This is more severe than the first one.*
2. It occurs usually in about 20% of LL leprosy and is characterised by **erythema nodosum leprosum** (ENL). The basic lesion is a

vasculitis following deposition of (antigen + antibody) immune complexes. Suddenly, many crops of bright erythematous nodules and raised patches appear and the existing lesions become worse.

3. It may be associated with fever, iritis, neuritis, arthritis orchitis and lymphadenitis.
4. **It is difficult to treat and lesions may actually spread.**

Management of lepra reactions

The patient is advised rest and analgesics to immobilise the joints near the affected nerve.

The drugs used are as follows:

- **Clofazimine and prednisolone:** They are administered in **both types of reactions.** They act as anti-inflammatory agents. **Prednisolone** in the dose of 40 mg/day (preferably in the morning after breakfast as single dose) × 2 weeks, 30 mg/day × 2 weeks, 20 mg/day × 2 weeks, 15 mg/day × 2 weeks, 10 mg/day × 2 weeks and then 5 mg/day. The treatment is continued for 3–12 months, depending on the severity of the reaction and may be prolonged if there is neuritis. The early use of prednisolone helps to prevent permanent nerve damage.
- **Clofazimine** is given in the dose of 100 mg t.i.d. (maximum for 1 month), following which it is tapered to 100 mg / day for several days; however it is less potent then prednisolone and takes 4-6 weeks to develop its full effect. It is useful for reducing / withdrawing prednisolone in steroid dependent patients. The total duration of therapy should not exceed > 12 months.

DDS is continued in full doses throughout both types of lepra reactions.

- **Thalidomide,** a selective **TNF alpha inhibitor** (Chapter 72), in the dose of 400 mg daily, is very **useful and even better than steroids for managing acute severe and chronic ENL.** It causes dryness of mouth, constipation and diarrhoea. *The drug is highly teratogenic and is absolutely contraindicated in pregnancy.* In chronic ENL, thalidomide may have to be given for many years. *Severe type II reactions need prolonged treatment with both, prednisolone and thalidomide.*

LEPROSY PROPHYLAXIS

Antitubercular **BCG vaccine** (Chapter 52) has been shown to endow some protection against leprosy. Single dose rifampicin is recommended for chemoprophylaxis to contacts of leprosy patients. The dose is 600 mg for adults (above 35 kg), 450 mg for those having body weight 20 to 35 kg, and 10–15 mg/kg for those with <20 kg.

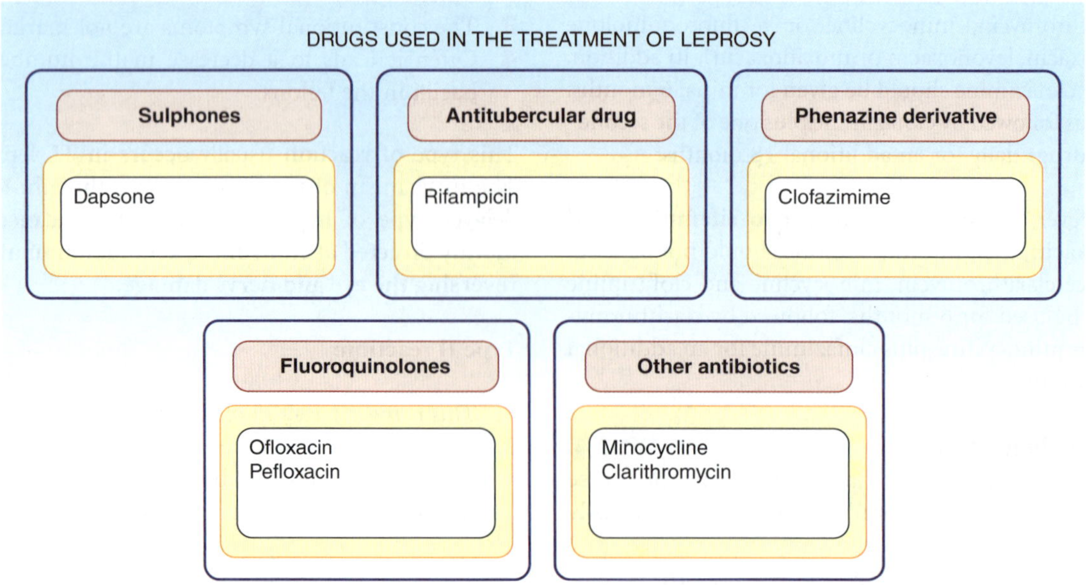

CHAPTER 54

Chemotherapy of Malaria

Learning Objectives

This chapter will enable the reader:

1. To be aware of the life cycle of the causative organism – plasmodia.
2. To classify antimalarial drugs based on their clinical use in malarial prophylaxis and treatment
3. To discuss the mechanism of action, antiprotozoal spectrum, pharmacological effects, salient pharmacokinetic features, ADR, and indications of rapidly acting erythrocytic schizonticides
4. To enumerate slow-acting erthrocytic schizonticides and state their mechanism of action, pharmacological effects, ADR and indications.
5. To state the drug regimens used for prophylaxis of malaria.
6. To outline the treatment of chloroquine sensitive and chloroquine resistant malaria.
7. To give examples of artemisinin combination therapies available for treatment of malaria.
8. To outline the treatment of malaria in special populations, i.e. children, pregnant ladies and G6PD deficient patients.
9. To enumerate measures to eradicate malaria.
10. To enlist various mosquito repellents.

KEY TERMS

plasmodium life cycle, p. 773
chloroquine, p. 775
primaquine, p. 778
artemisinin, p. 779
acute attack of malaria treatment, p. 784
severe malaria treatment, p. 785
artemisinin-based combination therapy (ACT), p. 786
drug resistant malaria, p. 786
malaria prophylaxis, p. 788
malaria elimination, p. 789

Malaria is caused by parasitic protozoa of the genus *Plasmodium* and is characterised by fever with rigor, anaemia and splenomegaly. The World Malaria Report, 2019 estimated global prevalence of 228 million cases of malaria from 89 countries. India represented 3% of the global malaria burden and is the highest malaria burden country of the Southeast Asia region, **Nearly 50% of the cases the world over are caused by *Plasmodium falciparum.***

Life cycle of Plasmodium: There are four major types of plasmodia which infect man:

- *P. vivax*
- *P. falciparum*
- *P. ovale*
- *P. malariae*

P. vivax causes **benign tertian malaria** which, though mild, has a tendency to relapse. *P. falciparum* infection results in **malignant tertian malaria**, a fulminating infection, which, if not treated, may result in death; but the disease, once cured, has no tendency to relapse. In both infections, the infected individual develops pyrexia with rigors every 3rd day, and hence the term 'tertian'. *P. ovale* and *P. malariae* infections are usually mild; the individual develops pyrexia every 4th day, and hence, it is described as '**benign quartan**'. Recently, *P. knowlesi* has been shown to infect human beings.

An individual is infected by malarial parasites through the bite of a **female Anopheles mosquito**. The disease can also be transmitted by transfusion of infected blood and from mother to the fetus across the placenta. The salivary glands of the infected mosquito contain a large number of *sporozoites,* which are introduced into of the host during mosquito bite. After entry, into the blood stream of the host, the sporozoites develop further through various stages (Fig. 54.1).

1. **Pre-erythrocytic stage**

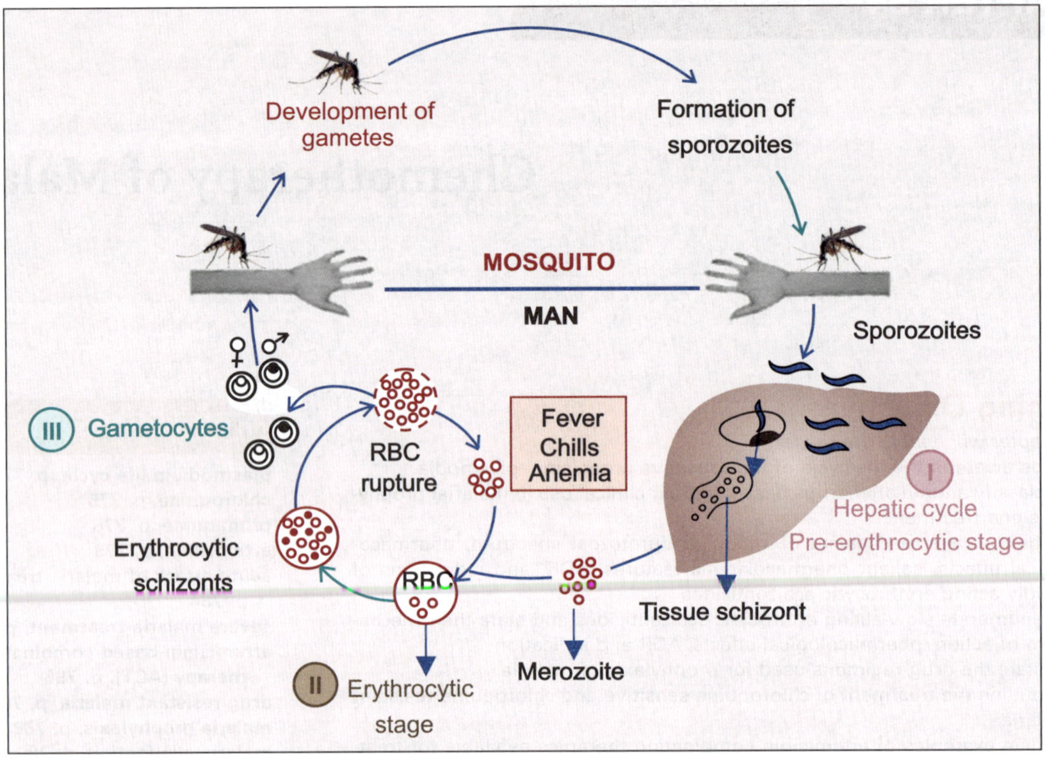

FIG. 54.1 **Life cycle of malarial parasite (*P. falciparum*).**

2. **Erythrocytic stage**
3. **Development of sexual forms**

In the **pre-erythrocytic stage,** sporozoites disappear rapidly from the circulation and invade the hepatic cells **(Hepatic cycle – Site I).** *The host does not develop any symptoms during this phase.* At the completion of this phase, the infected reticuloendothelial cell, termed **tissue schizont** (*primary exoerythrocyte form*), releases thousands of **merozoites** into the blood stream.

In the **erythrocytic stage (Site II),** merozoites invade the erythrocytes and undergo further development and multiplication, giving rise to **erythrocytic schizonts** *(asexual erythrocyte forms).* The infected RBCs eventually rupture, and release thousands of merozoites into the blood. This periodic release of merozoites is associated with paroxysms of fever with rigor. The released merozoites invade fresh RBCs and the cycle of erythrocytic schizogony repeats.

Some of the merozoites develop into **male (macro) and female (micro) gametocytes (sexual forms-Site III).** During a mosquito bite, the gametocytes are sucked in from the blood and they mature into gametes in the mosquito gut. The female gamete is fertilised by the male gamete to form a **zygote.** The zygote invades mosquito gut wall to form an **oocyst. The mature oocyst contains thousands of sporozoites.** After about 1–4 weeks, depending upon the species of plasmodium, the oocyst ruptures releasing **free sporozoites** which reach the salivary glands of the mosquito, ready to be injected in the host.

The above cycle in case of *P. falciparum*, terminates at this point. **However, *P. vivax* and *P. ovale* have persistent hepatic cycle due to** presence of **hypnozoites,** also known as latent tissue phase or **exoerythrocytic phase.** The delayed formation of tissue schizonts from such latent hypnozoites explains the relapses of *P. vivax* and *P. ovale* malaria.

Clinical Classification of Antimalarial Drugs

I. **True causal prophylactics:** These are the drugs that would destroy the sporozoites before their invasion of the host reticuloendothelial cells. *However, no such drug is currently available.*
II. **Causal prophylactics (primary tissue schizonticides):** These drugs *prevent the maturation of or destroy the sporozoites within the infected hepatic cells (Site I) and* **thus prevent erythrocytic invasion. Primaquine, pyrimethamine**

and proguanil act as causal prophylactics against *P. falciparum* but their efficacy against *P. vivax* is doubtful.

III. **Suppressives (schizonticides):** These drugs **inhibit erythrocytic schizogony (Site II)** *and prevent the rupture of the infected erythrocytes.* This leads to freedom from rigors and pyrexia (**clinical cure**). However, **they do not eradicate the infection.**

Suppressives can cure P. falciparum infection as the parasite does not undergo secondary exoerythrocytic schizogony but they do not affect the persistent tissue phase of P. vivax (hypnozoites) and hence relapses can occur with the stoppage of suppressive therapy. The suppressive agents include:
- **Rapidly acting** schizonticides: **quinine, 4-aminoquinolines, mefloquine, artemisinin, atovaquone** and **halofantrine**
- **Slowly acting** schizonticides: **proguanil, pyrimethamine, sulphadoxine and tetracycline**

IV. **Radical curatives:** These drugs **eradicate both, erythrocytic and secondary exoerythrocytic schizogony** so that relapse does not occur. For radical cure of vivax infection, **primaquine** and **proguanil** are effective (see section, Management of malaria). *Radical cure of falciparum malaria can be achieved with suppressives alone.*

V. **Gametocytocidal drugs: Primaquine** is highly effective against gametocytes of all species, including *P. falciparum.* The suppressives such as **chloroquine, quinine** and **artesunate** *are effective against gametocytes of all species except P. falciparum.*

Proguanil and **pyrimethamine** *do not destroy gametocytes* but prevent their development in the mosquito. They are also known as **sporonticidal drugs.**

Chemical Classification

I. **Quinoline derivatives:**
   a. **4-Aminoquinolines:** Chloroquine, amodiaquine and pyronaridine
   b. **8-Aminoquinolines:** Primaquine, tafenoquine and bulaquine
   c. **Quinoline methanol:** Mefloquine

II. **Artemisinin compounds:** Artesunate, arteether and artemether

III. **Cinchona alkaloids:** Quinine and quinidine

IV. **Phenanthrene methanol:** Halofantrine and lumefantrine

V. **Antifolates:**
   a. **Biguanides:** Proguanil
   b. **Diaminopyrimidines:** Pyrimethamine
   c. **Sulphonamides:** Sulphadoxine

VI. **Antimicrobials:** Doxycycline, clindamycin and atovaquone

Table 54.1 summarises the actions of the commonly used antimalarials.

4-AMINOQUINOLINES PH 1.47, IM 4.22

The 4-aminoquinolines constitute the mainstay of suppressive therapy of malaria. The therapeutically useful compounds of this class are **chloroquine, hydroxychloroquine** and **amodiaquine.**

CHLOROQUINE: This is the most frequently used drug (Fig. 54.2).

Pharmacological actions:

Antimalarial activity: As a **suppressive,** chloroquine is superior to quinine.

1. It kills the erythrocytic forms of *P. vivax* and *P. falciparum.*
2. It is also effective against the gametocytes of *P. vivax, P. ovale* and *P. malariae.*

However, *it has no effect on the sporozoites, the pre-erythrocytic stage and the persistent tissue forms.*

Mechanism of action: Malarial parasites digest haemoglobin in their lysosomes to utilise amino acids. The released haem is highly toxic but is converted by the parasitic polymerase to nontoxic hemozoin.

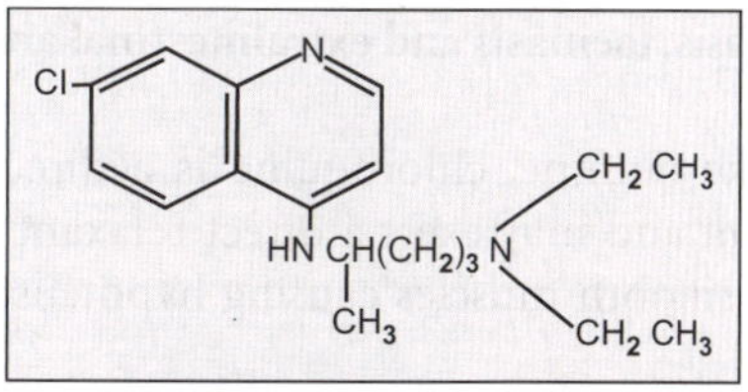

FIG. 54.2 **Chloroquine.**

Table 54.1 Actions of Commonly Used Drugs on the Life Cycle of the Malarial Parasites

Drug	Hepatic Phase	Erythrocytic Phase: Asexual Parasites	Erythrocytic Phase: Sexual Forms (Gametocytes)	Latent Tissue Phase (Responsible for Relapse)	Development of Gametocytes in the Mosquito (Sporonticidal Action)
Chloroquine amodiaquine	No action	Fast action	As quinine	No action	No action
Primaquine	Active and can be used for prophylaxis	Weakly active	Direct and fast action on all species but particularly *P. falciparum*	Highly active	Highly active
Artesunate	No action	Fastest acting	Active against *P. vivax*	No action	No action
Quinine	No action	Fast action	Active against *P. vivax* and *P. malariae*. No direct action on *P. falciparum*	No action	No action
Proguanil	Active particularly on *P. falciparum*	Active but relatively *slow*	No direct action	No action	Highly active
Pyrimethamine	As proguanil	As proguanil	No evidence of direct action	Some action on *P. vivax*	Little evidence
Sulphones and sulphonamides	Possible action	Action slow	As pyrimethamine	Little evidence	–
Mefloquine	No action	Marked but slow	As quinine	No action	No action
Atovaquone	No	More active than chloroquine	No	No	No

Chloroquine, being a basic drug, concentrates in the acidic lysosomes and binds to released haem, thus preventing its polymerisation. This results in oxidative damage to parasites, causing their death.

Resistance to chloroquine by *P. falciparum* develops due to an efflux mechanism by which the parasite pumps the drug out of the cell. Such organisms exhibit cross-resistance to other 4-aminoquinolines.

Other antiparasitic actions: The drug is also **effective in giardiasis, taeniasis and extraintestinal amoebiasis.**

CVS: Like quinine, chloroquine is a direct cardiac depressant and may exert a direct relaxant effect on vascular smooth muscles causing hypotension.

Miscellaneous actions: It has some **anti-inflammatory**, antihistaminic and local anaesthetic activities.

Absorption, fate and excretion: Chloroquine is rapidly and almost completely absorbed from the gut. Effective plasma concentration is attained within 2–3 h of oral dose and within 15 min of IM administration. About 55% of the drug in plasma is protein bound. It is highly concentrated in the liver, spleen, kidney, lung and leucocytes. The brain and the spinal cord levels, however, are only 10–30 times the plasma levels. **Because of its high volume of distribution, a loading dose is necessary to initiate therapy.** Due to its affinity for the tissue proteins, the drug persists in the body for a long time after discontinuation. It is metabolised in the liver to the active metabolite 4-hydroxychloroquine. Acidification of urine hastens its renal excretion.

Adverse reactions: *Chloroquine* **used as an antimalarial is a relatively safe drug.** Commonly, it causes nausea and vomiting, headache, urticaria and pruritus. The drug, however, may produce serious toxicity when used in large doses for prolonged periods as in RA. The important toxic manifestations are:

- **Intolerance:** Skin rashes with or without pruritus, angioneurotic oedema, photosensitivity, pigmentation and even exfoliative dermatitis have been reported. Long term treatment may lead to bleaching of hair. Rarely, thrombocytopenia, and pancytopenia may occur.
- **Eye:** Ocular complications can occur with the high dosage, prolonged chloroquine therapy of RA, and lupus erythematosus. Temporary loss of accommodation with blurring of vision or diplopia may develop. Retinopathy with abnormal blue-black pigmentation of the retina, depigmentation of the macula and macular degeneration, lenticular opacities and posterior subcapsular cataracts have been reported. The field of vision is constricted. *These changes are not reversible and need immediate discontinuation of the drug.* Because of its prolonged sojourn in the body, the ocular changes may appear even a few years after discontinuation. **Hence, patients on long term chloroquine therapy should undergo periodic ophthalmoscopic examination.**
- **Central nervous system:** Confusion, convulsions, myopathy and peripheral neuropathy may occur and are reversible once the drug is withdrawn. Overdosage may rarely cause neuropsychiatric disturbances including suicidal ideation. Ototoxicity has also been reported.
- **Cardiovascular system:** Abnormalities of ST segment and T waves are reported. *Hypotension, arrhythmias and cardiac arrest have been observed when high doses are administered rapidly intravenously.*

Preparations and dosage:

i. Chloroquine phosphate tablet 250 mg (150 mg of the base). For dose, see Box 54.1. Chloroquine phosphate oral suspension 16 mg/ml or 50 mg/ml is also available.
ii. Chloroquine sulphate tablet contains 150 mg of chloroquine base. Dosage: same as above.
iii. Chloroquine injection contains chloroquine phosphate or sulphate equivalent to 40 mg of the base per mL. Dose: 200–300 mg of the base IM divided between two injection sites, or intravenously, slowly, diluted with 100 mL of glucose saline. The total parenteral dose within 24 h should not exceed 900 mg.

Indications

- **Malaria:** It is still the first line of treatment for *P. vivax* malaria and uncomplicated falciparum malaria due to sensitive strains (see section, Management of malaria). *Chloroquine and amodiaquine are considered safe antimalarials during pregnancy.*
- **Hepatic amoebiasis:** Chapter 55.
- **Giardiasis:** Although chloroquine phosphate is effective, metronidazole is preferred (Chapter 56).
- **Clonorchis sinensis (Chinese liver fluke) infestation:** Chloroquine phosphate, 250 mg daily, is given for 6 weeks.
- **Rheumatoid arthritis (RA):** Chapter 73.
- **Discoid lupus and disseminated lupus erythematosus:** Chloroquine is useful only in the milder forms of this disease and as a supplementary therapy to glucocorticoids in severely ill patients.

HYDROXYCHLOROQUINE: This drug is has similar properties and uses as chloroquine.

AMODIAQUINE: This drug is as effective as chloroquine, in a single oral dose. Its pharmacological actions are similar to those of chloroquine. It is rapidly absorbed and is concentrated in the liver and the spleen. It is largely metabolised in the liver. The adverse effects include GI disturbances, headache, photosensitivity reactions and rarely, agranulocytosis.

Amodiaquine tablet contains 250 mg of the salt. Dose: as a suppressive in an acute attack of malaria: 600 mg followed by 200 mg (base) on Day 1; 400 mg once a day on Day 2 and 3 (i.e 25 – 35mg/kg over 3 days.).

P. falciparum strains resistant to chloroquine may still be sensitive to amodiaquine. *However, it is not recommended for prophylactic (chronic suppressive) therapy because of possible hepatitis and agranulocytosis.*

Amopyroquine has similar properties as amodiaquine but can also be given parenterally.

Pyronaridine, structurally related to amodiaquine, developed in China, is given orally as well as parenterally. It has schizonticidal activity against *P. falciparum* and *P. vivax* and is effective against chloroquine-resistant parasites when administered with artemisinin.

8-AMINOQUINOLINES

PRIMAQUINE: This drug (Fig. 54.3) is effective against:

- **The pre-erythrocytic (hepatic) and sexual forms (gametocytes) of all species of human malarial parasites**
- **The persistent tissue forms of *P. vivax***

Mechanism of action: Its precise mechanism of action is not known. It probably acts by generating toxic, reactive species and/or by interfering with electron transport in the parasite.

Primaquine destroys only a proportion of gametocytes in the blood, whereas the rest are rendered incapable of undergoing further maturation in the mosquito. The drug has a weak schizonticidal activity against *P. vivax* but exerts no effect on the schizonts of *P. falciparum. It is, therefore, not effective as a suppressive.* **It is usually combined with a 4-aminoquinoline, to achieve radical cure in P. vivax infection.**

Absorption, fate and excretion: Given orally, it is rapidly and completely absorbed and is concentrated in the liver. Large amounts are also present in the lung, brain, heart and the skeletal muscle. It is rapidly metabolised in the liver, and the products excreted in the urine; only 1% of the drug is excreted unchanged.

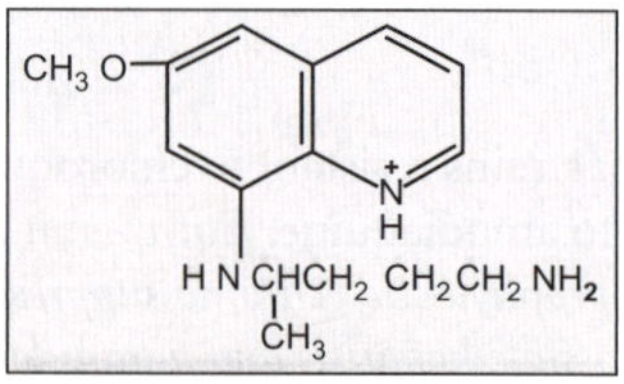

FIG. 54.3 Primaquine.

Adverse reactions: At the recommended dosage, toxicity is uncommon. The ADR are as follows:

- **Gastrointestinal:** Epigastric distress and abdominal cramps can be minimised by taking the drug with or after food and by antacids.
- **Haemopoietic:** *Moderate doses* cause mild anaemia and leucopoenia. *Large doses* may cause methaemoglobinemia, cyanosis and agranulocytosis. It can cause haemolysis in G6PD-deficient patients.
- **In patients with G6PD deficiency,** it can cause intravascular haemolysis (Chapter 36).

Although it has not been established that primaquine is teratogenic in humans, its use should be postponed till after delivery.

Preparations and dosage: Primaquine tablet contains 2.5/7.5/15/45 mg of primaquine base. The dose for radical cure of vivax malaria is 15 mg of the base for 14 days. In earlier days the gametocytocidal dose for falciparum malaria was 45 mg (0.75mg base /kg). However WHO has recommended reduction of this dose to 0.25 mg base /kg as this dose gives maximum gametocytocidal effect and is considered safe even in G6PD deficient individuals and does not require testing for the same.

Bulaquine, an analogue of primaquine, is claimed to be as effective as primaquine.

Tafenoquine is a new, long-acting, potent, primaquine-like drug which achieves radical cure in 3 days.

QUINOLINE METHANOL

MEFLOQUINE is a quinoline methanol derivative. It probably acts like chloroquine. It:

- **Acts on the erythrocytic stage.**
- **Is highly effective in a single dose against *P. falciparum* including chloroquine resistant and MDR strains.**
- **Can be given 12 h after the last dose of quinine. However, because of long half-life of mefloquine, quinine should not be administered after it as both are cardiotoxic.**
- **Has no action on the persistent tissue forms.**

Given orally, mefloquine is rapidly and completely absorbed, is highly protein bound and is extensively distributed in the tissues. *It has a very long plasma t½ of about 20 days.* It is eliminated slowly in faeces. The parasites can develop resistance to it.

Adverse reactions:

- **GI tract:** Mefloquine commonly causes dizziness, nausea, vomiting, diarrhoea or abdominal pain; these generally resolve without specific treatment.
- **Neuropsychiatric disturbances:** The most common of these are affective disorders, anxiety disorders, hallucinations and sleep disturbances. A single dose may cause light headedness and loss of concentration. Transient depressive feeling occurs more commonly with mefloquine than with chloroquine. Rarely, psychosis, toxic encephalopathy and convulsions have been reported.
- **CVS:** Like chloroquine and halofantrine, mefloquine causes **bradycardia** and **sinus arrhythmia**. Patients who have recently received mefloquine should not receive halofantrine, which hastens QT prolongation.
- **Teratogenicity: Mefloquine is teratogenic** *and should be avoided in the first trimester of pregnancy.* However, it may be used in the second and third trimesters. *The nonpregnant women of childbearing age should be advised to avoid pregnancy for 3 months after the treatment.* Women treated with mefloquine may continue breast-feeding.
- **Miscellaneous:** Allergic skin reactions, hepatitis and blood dyscrasias can occur.

Preparations and dosage: Mefloquine is available as 250 mg tablets. A single dose of 750 mg (15 mg/kg) orally is sufficient in most areas to treat uncomplicated malaria. However, in certain areas, the same dose may have to be repeated in 6 h to ensure a cure. In the single dose of 1.5 g, mefloquine is uniformly effective in curing multidrug resistant (MDR) malaria in almost 100% of patients. *However, such a dose invariably causes severe nausea and vomiting.*

Due to fear of the development of drug resistance, it is not recommended as a single drug for prophylaxis in endemic areas.

ARTEMISININ COMPOUNDS

ARTEMISININ: This is an active principle obtained from the Chinese plant *Artemisia annuta* (Qinghaosu, sweet worm wood). It is a sesquiterpene lactone endoperoxide. Derivatives of artemisinin include **artesunate** (water soluble), **arteether** and **artemether** (both lipid soluble).

Mechanism of action: Artemisinin and related compounds covalently bind to parasitic proteins. **Intraparasitic haem iron catalyses cleavage of endoperoxide bridge in artemisinin. The resultant free radicals damage parasitic proteins.**

Artemisinin compounds act as **schizonticides** against all malarial parasites, including those resistant to chloroquine and quinine. They rapidly reduce parasitaemia. They have no effect on the hepatic stage.

Absorption, fate and excretion: Orally, they are well absorbed and are metabolised to the active form, dihydroartemisinin. **They cross BBB. The t½ of artesunate is short – about 23 min, whereas that of artemether is about 45 min.**

Adverse reactions: No serious adverse reactions have been reported. ADR include nausea, vomiting, abdominal pain, anorexia and leucopoenia. Higher doses may produce bradycardia, prolongation of PR and QT intervals and transient increase in SGOT/SGPT. They should be preferably avoided during the first trimester of pregnancy, during lactation and in children $\leq$5 kg.

Preparations and dosage:

i. Artesunate 50 mg tablets.
   Artesunate injection for IV/IM use contains 60 mg. It is administered in a dose of 120 mg on day 1, followed by 60 mg 12 h later and 60 mg once daily for the next 4 days.
ii. Arteether is a synthetic ethyl derivative of artemisinin. Dose is 150 mg IM once daily for 3 days. Children are given 3 mg/kg for 3 days.
iii. Artemether injection containing 80 mg/mL in arachis oil.
iv. They are also available as rectal suppositories containing 100 mg of artesunate.

Indications: Artemisinin and its derivatives are safe and effective alternative to quinine in the treatment of **falciparum malaria**. However, their use should be restricted to the treatment of MDR malaria. They are also useful in cerebral malaria.

It is recommended that oral artemisinin derivatives should not be administered as monotherapy. They are rapidly acting schizonticides with short half life. They are always administered along with another antimalarial drug which is preferably a long acting erythrocytic schizonticide. This ensures the clearance of the remaining parasites after rapid reduction by artemisinin. Such artemisinin combination therapy (ACT) enhances the efficacy of the regime, prevents or slows down the rate of emergence and spread of resistance and reduces the overall malaria transmission.

For use of artemether in schistosomiasis, see Chapter 58.

CINCHONA ALKALOIDS

QUININE is an alkaloid isolated from the bark of the cinchona tree, originally a native of Peru, South America. Quinine, the oldest of all the therapeutic agents used to treat malaria is still useful **in the treatment of cerebral malaria and chloroquine-resistant *P. falciparum* infection.**

Pharmacological actions:

Antimalarial action: Quinine is **schizonticidal** and is useful only as a suppressive. **It is also gametocytocidal against all species except *P. falciparum*.** It has no effect on the sporozoites, the pre-erythrocytic stage and the persistent tissue forms.

Mechanism of action: It is similar to that of chloroquine (see section, 4-Aminoquinolines), but as the drug is not extensively concentrated in the parasites, other mechanisms may also be involved.

Quinine has been termed a 'general protoplasmic poison'. It depresses various enzymatic processes, reduces ciliary activity and inhibits phagocytosis and the growth of fibroblasts.

Local irritant action: Quinine causes pain, oedema and reactive fibrosis. Sterile injection abscesses and venous thrombosis may occur.

GI tract: Quinine has an intensely bitter taste and can cause nausea, vomiting and epigastric pain.

Cardiovascular actions: Like quinidine (Chapter 28), another cinchona alkaloid, quinine is also a **direct depressant of the myocardium**. It reduces excitability, conductivity and lengthens the refractory period. Intravenous quinine can produce profound **hypotension** due to cardiac depression and dilatation of the arterioles.

Miscellaneous actions: It has a **mild analgesic and antipyretic activity**. It stimulates the uterine smooth muscle. However, in the doses used in malaria, it has hardly any adverse effect on the pregnant uterus. It has a **curarimimetic action** on the skeletal muscles.

Absorption, fate and excretion: It is almost completely and rapidly absorbed from the small intestine, and the peak plasma levels are reached within 1–3 h. It readily crosses BBB and the placental barrier.

Quinine is mainly metabolised in the liver. Its plasma t½ is about 10 h, Approximately 5% of the total dose appears unchanged in urine.

Adverse reactions: The major reason for the decline in popularity of quinine is its toxicity. The salient toxic manifestations are as follows:

- **Cinchonism:** This syndrome, occurs when quinine is administered for a long time. Mild symptoms consist of ringing in the ears, nausea, headache and visual impairment. With large doses, tinnitus, deafness, vertigo, blurred vision, disturbances of colour vision and photophobia appear. **Toxic amblyopia** occasionally leading to total blindness has been rarely reported.
  Severe intoxication causes vomiting, diarrhoea, confusion, delirium, hypotension and respiratory arrest. Even if the patient recovers, visual and auditory impairment may not be entirely corrected. The treatment is essentially symptomatic.
- **Idiosyncrasy:** The commonest manifestation is intense flushing, pruritus and urticaria. Quinine

may precipitate angioneurotic oedema or asthmatic attacks in sensitive individuals. Rarely, it causes thrombocytopenic purpura, haemolytic anaemia and agranulocytosis.

- **Cardiovascular toxicity:** Quinine is a myocardial depressant and can cause cardiac arrest *when given intravenously.*
- **Black water fever:** It is characterised by **acute intravascular haemolysis, haemoglobinuria, fever and acute renal failure**. It is encountered with chronic *P. falciparum* malaria. Focal hepatic necrosis may develop in severe cases. Blackwater fever may occur during the natural course of malaria and is often triggered by quinine treatment. The reaction probably has an immunological basis and is caused by a state of hypersensitivity attributable to the presence of incompletely suppressed falciparum infection. The patient should also be evaluated for his G6PD status.
- **Hypoglycaemia:** Quinine can cause hypoglycaemia **by releasing insulin** from the pancreatic beta cells.
- **Miscellaneous:** Quinine IV may cause convulsions.

Preparations and dosage:

i. Quinine sulphate tablet 100mg, 200 mg, 300 mg, 600 mg. Dose: 300–600 mg. Quinine sulfate oral suspension- 150 mg/5ml is also available.
ii. Quinine hydrochloride injection: 300 mg/ml. Dose: 300–600 mg.
iii. Quinine sulphate injection 300 mg/mL. It can be administered by IV infusion or by deep IM route. Dose: 300–600 mg.

Indications:

- **Malaria:** It is an important drug for treating severe falciparum infection (see section, Management of malaria). Quinine (650 mg of salt), 1 tablet thrice daily for 7 days in combination with either doxycycline or clindamycin.
- **Myotonia congenita:** Quinine has been used in the treatment of this hereditary myopathy, characterised by tonic spasm of skeletal muscles.
- **Cramps:** The drug has been used in the dose of 200–300 mg at bedtime to prevent nocturnal muscle cramps.

PHENANTHRENE METHANOL

HALOFANTRINE: It is:

- **An erythrocytic schizonticide and is as effective as chloroquine against chloroquine sensitive strains of *P. falciparum***
- **Also effective against strains resistant to chloroquine, pyrimethamine and quinine**

It acts like other quinolines.

Given orally, it is slowly and variably absorbed with peak concentration at 4–6 h. The drug should not be taken along with fatty foods. Its plasma t½ is about 1–2 days, although its active *N*-desbutyl metabolite has a longer t½ of 3–5 days. It is given in three doses of 500 mg 6 h apart, repeated after 1 week, if necessary. It is available for parenteral use.

Adverse reactions: These include nausea, vomiting, abdominal pain, diarrhoea and rise in liver enzymes. **It causes prolongation of QT interval and even fatal ventricular arrhythmias;** *it should not be used in patients receiving quinine, chloroquine or quinidine, antidepressants and antipsychotics. It is not suitable for prophylaxis.*

Lumefantrine is structurally similar to halofantrine. **Used in combination with artemether**, it is well tolerated. The combination is used for uncomplicated falciparum malaria, and when resistance to monotherapies is observed. It can also be combined with mefloquine.

BIGUANIDES

PROGUANIL (Chloroguanide): It is a prodrug and is converted into a cyclic ring triazine metabolite, **cycloguanil**. This compound binds to an enzyme dihydrofolate reductase, which converts folic acid to folinic acid. Deficiency of folinic acid prevents the completion of schizogony. **As the sulphonamides prevent the conversion of PABA into folic acid, they synergise with its antimalarial effect.** It:

- **Is an effective schizonticide against both *P. vivax* and *P. falciparum***; but its action is slower than that of 4-aminoquinolines.

- **Is effective against the primary pre-erythrocytic forms of *P. falciparum***, and for causal prophylaxis of falciparum malaria.
- **Prevents the development of gametes encysted in the gut wall of the mosquito.** It is, thus, valuable in **sporonticidal prophylaxis.**

Plasmodia can develop an *acquired resistance* to this agent due to mutation.

Absorption, fate and excretion: It is rapidly and adequately absorbed, mostly from the small intestine. Approximately 75% is bound to proteins. Its elimination is slow, mainly in the urine, with plasma t½ of 12–21 h.

Adverse reactions: In therapeutic doses, proguanil is free from significant toxic effects. GI disturbances, stomatitis, and mouth ulcers may develop occasionally. A reduction in the leucocyte count and megaloblastic anaemia may occur rarely.

Preparations and dosage: Proguanil hydrochloride tablets 100 mg.

Indications: Given alone, it is not so useful for controlling an acute attack. It can be used for causal prophylaxis, (100–200 mg daily) in an area with sensitive strains of plasmodium.

Malarone, a **combination of proguanil 100 mg with atovaquone 250 mg is used for treating MDR falciparum malaria** (for doses, see Box 54.2). *The drug appears to be safe during pregnancy but data is inadequate.* It can be combined with folinic acid 5 mg daily, to prevent megaloblastic anaemia.

DIAMINOPYRIMIDINES

PYRIMETHAMINE (Fig. 54.4): Like proguanil, **it selectively binds to dihydrofolate reductase**. It is more potent than proguanil. Its antimalarial activity is enhanced by combination with sulphonamides. Unlike other antimalarials, it is tasteless and, therefore, suitable for children.

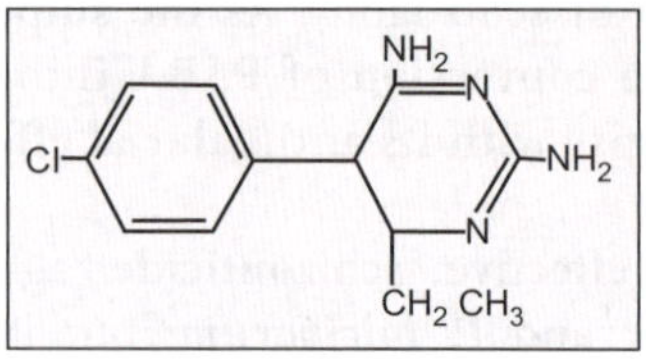

FIG. 54.4 Pyrimethamine.

Development of resistance to the drug *in vivo* has been reported and some degree of cross-resistance between pyrimethamine and proguanil can also occur. Chloroquine-resistant strains of *P. falciparum* are frequently resistant to proguanil and pyrimethamine.

Absorption, fate and excretion: Pyrimethamine is completely but relatively slowly absorbed from the small intestine. It is extensively metabolised and excreted slowly. Following a single dose of 25 mg, it persists in the plasma and gets excreted in the urine for more than 14 days.

Adverse reactions: The drug is relatively safe. It can cause GI disturbances, ataxia and megaloblastic anaemia, which responds to oral folic acid. *The drug appears to be safe in antimalarial doses during pregnancy.*

Preparations and dosage: Pyrimethamine tablet 25 mg.

Indications:

- **Malaria:** It is generally **used in combination with 500 mg sulphadoxine or with sulphadimethopyrazine**; dose: 2–3 tab once weekly. Combination of pyrimethamine 12.5 mg with dapsone 100 mg was used earlier **for prophylaxis** of *P. falciparum*.
- **Toxoplasmosis:** Chapter 56.
- **Polycythemia vera:** Chapter 59

SULPHONAMIDES: Sulphonamides and sulphones have antimalarial activity similar to pyrimethamine, but their mechanism of action is different (Chapter 43). *They potentiate the action of pyrimethamine or proguanil (DHF-reductase inhibitors).* A long-acting sulphonamide such as **sulphadoxine** (t½ 200 h) with **pyrimethamine** is usually preferred. *These combinations have been used to treat P. falciparum infection resistant to chloroquine.*

Sulphonamide-containing combinations are no longer recommended for prophylaxis because of Stevens–Johnson syndrome.

ANTIMICROBIALS

DOXYCYCLINE: This drug exerts a slow but potent action against the **blood schizonts and the primary exo-erythrocytic forms** of *P. falciparum*, including those resistant to chloroquine and proguanil. It is **used in combination in resistant cases** as resistance to tetracyclines is rare (see Box 54.2).

CLINDAMYCIN has also been found useful in combination with other drugs (see Box 54.2).

ATOVAQUONE: This is a highly lipophilic, hydroxynaphthoquinone compound which has potent activity against *P. jiroveci*, *Plasmodia* and *T. gondii.* It acts by selectively interfering with mitochondrial electron transport in susceptible parasites. **Proguanil potentiates its antimalarial activity.** Used alone, the parasites develop resistance to it rapidly, by mutation.

Its oral absorption is slow and incomplete but is increased threefold by fatty foods. Its plasma t½ is 2–3 days and it is excreted, mostly unchanged, in faeces.

Adverse reactions: These include fever, vomiting, anorexia, headache, diarrhoea, dose-related maculopapular rash, anaemia and neutropenia.

Indications:

- **Atovaquone + proguanil** are useful as a **prophylactic against *P. falciparum* and in treating *MDR malaria.*** The combination is active against the circulating parasites but not the hepatic stage of plasmodium..
  The combination contains atovaquone 250 mg +proguanil 100 mg for adult use and atovaquone 62.5 mg +proguanil 25 mg for paediatric use. For **prophylaxis**, the dose is one tablet daily taken with food. For **treatment of MDR malaria**, it is 4 tablets as a single dose for 3 consecutive days.
- In the dose of 750 mg t.i.d. for 21 days, it is helpful in treating **mild to moderate *P. jiroveci* pneumonia in AIDS patients.**
- It is also used in **toxoplasmosis** (Chapter 56).

Table 54.2 Half-life of the Commonly Used Antimalarial Drugs

Drug	Half-life
Chloroquine and amodiaquine	3 weeks
Mefloquine	15–33 days
Primaquine	8.5 h
Artesunate	23 min
Quinine	10–12 h
Pyrimethamine	80–100 h
Proguanil	12–21 h
Sulphadoxine	100–200 days
Atovaquone	2–3 days
Doxycycline	18–22 h

Table 54.2 shows the plasma t½ of the commonly used antimalarial drugs.

MANAGEMENT OF MALARIA

Objectives for the pharmacotherapy of Malaria are presented in Table 54.3

Principles of therapy

1. Diagnosis and treatment should be prompt to prevent progression to severe malaria and deaths.
2. No single drug is effective against all stages of parasites that co exist. Therefore for complete

Table 54.3 Pharmacotherapy of Malaria: Objectives, Target Sites and Agents Used

Objective	Target site	Agents used
1. Alleviate all symptoms and ensure clinical and parasitological cure	Blood schizonts	Blood schizonticides
2. Prevent relapse of *P. vivax* (radical cure)	Liver hypnozoites	Hepatic schizonticide(Primaquine)
3. Prevent transmission of malaria	Gametocytes	Primaquine for *P. falciparum*, Chloroquine for all other species

cure, one has to use combination therapy with at least two effective antimalarials having different mechanisms of action.

2. Rational selection of the antimalarial drug is based on the type of infection, severity of infection, status of the host and associated co-morbidities.

Under the National Vector borne disease control program (NVBDCP), strategies have been formulated for elimination of malaria from India by 2030 (National Framework for Malaria Elimination). Currently 5 year national strategic plan for malaria elimination (2017-2022) is followed. **This malaria elimination plan is based on 3 aspects:**

- Universal access to malaria diagnosis and treatment
- Strengthening the surveillance
- Acceleration towards malaria elimination

PH 1.55, IM 4.23

Treatment of an Acute Attack

The diagnosis of malaria is confirmed by microscopy of blood films. If the species is uncertain, it should be considered to be *P. falciparum*. The prognosis worsens with *P. falciparum* infection, higher parasitic counts and more mature parasites. In serious cases, smear examination should be repeated every 12 h for monitoring the efficacy of therapy.

The **drug regimens used in an acute clinical attack of malaria with** *P. vivax*, *P. ovale* and *P. malariae*, in adults, are shown in **Box 54.1**. Since latent exoerythrocytic forms persist in the liver in infections with *P. vivax* and *P. ovale*, **delayed true relapses occur in the majority of patients.** In such cases, radical cure can be obtained by **primaquine** in the dose of 7.5–15 mg daily for 14 days, started either from day 1 or after treating the acute attack. In this dosage, the drug is generally well tolerated and haemolysis, if it occurs, is mild and self-limiting. In some cases, higher doses of primaquine (30 mg daily for 14 days) may be needed; such regimen, however, needs supervision for ADR.

When haemoglobin continues to fall in the absence of bleeding, and asexual forms of the malarial parasite persist along with symptoms, after 48 h of treatment, chloroquine resistance can be suspected and patient should be treated accordingly (Box 54.1). *The persistence of gametocytes for several weeks after treatment does not represent failure of treatment.*

The **drug regimens used in an acute clinical attack of malaria with** *P. falciparum* in adults, are shown in Box 54.2. *P. falciparum* has acquired resistance to chloroquine in India and in many other countries and hence ACT based regimens are used. In *P. falciparum* malaria primaquine is used in a single dose to destroy falciparum gametocytes.

There is a possibility of mixed infection. For this, ACT containing lumefantrine is advocated in North- East states and Artesunate + SP combination in other states for 3 days along with primaquine 15 mg (0.25mg/kg) for 14 days.

Postural hypotension is common in uncomplicated malaria and is exacerbated by chloroquine. Febrile

Box 54.1 Treatment of Acute Malaria due to *P. vivax, P. ovale, P. malariae*

- ***Uncomplicated chloroquine sensitive:***
  In patients who can take orally medication:
  Chloroquine (base) 600 mg (4 tablets of 150 mg base each) taken immediately, followed by 600 mg on day 2 and and 300 mg on day 3 (10mg/kg on day 1and 2 followed by 5mg/kg on day 3)
- ***In patients who cannot take orally medication:***
  Chloroquine IM 2.5 mg/kg every 4 h or 3.5 mg/kg every 6 h (total dose not to exceed 25 mg/kg base)
  OR
  Chloroquine IV 10 mg/kg base over 4 h, followed by 5 mg/kg base (given in a 2 h infusion) every 12 h (total dose not to exceed 25/mg/kg base)
  In addition, all patients should receive:
  - Primaquine 0.25mg /kg daily for 14 days starting from day 1
- ***Uncomplicated chloroquine resistant:***
  ACT regimens containing lumefantrine, mefloquine or piperaquine (refer Box 54.2).

Notes: 1. Primaquine is contraindicated in infants, pregnant women and individuals with G6PD deficiency.
2. ACT containing SP should be avoided in *P. vivax* as parasites have developed resistance to SP.

Box 54.2 Treatment of acute attack of Chloroquine Resistant *P. falciparum* Malaria

- **Uncomplicated malaria:**
  In all states and union territories of India except North- East
  - Artesunate SP regimen: Sodium artesunate(4 mg/kg) 100 mg orally 12 hourly for 3 days plus sulphadoxine 25mg/kg (750 mg)+ pyrimethamine 1.25 mg/kg (37.5 mg) 2 tabs as single dose on day one

  In North- East states
  - Artmether (20 mg) + lumefantrine (120 mg) 4 tabs twice daily for 3 days

  In addition, all patients must receive:
  - Primaquine(0.75 mg/kg) 45 mg (6 tablets with 7.5 mg base each), given as a single dose on second day of treatment, to prevent spread.

  In case of treatment failure to ACT, then administer
  - Quinine 600 mg thrice a day + doxycycline 100 mg once daily / clindamycin 10 mg/kg twice daily for 7 days

patients, should therefore lie in the horizontal position.

Most of these antimalarial drugs are very bitter and hence, they may be given along with milk or fruit juice. Care must be taken to ensure that the patient swallows the tablets and does not vomit later. *If vomiting occurs within 1 h of drug ingestion, the full dose of the drug is administered.* If vomiting occurs after 1 h, it is not necessary to repeat the drug.

PH 1.55, IM 4.23

Treatment of severe malaria

Severe falciparum malaria is characterised by presence of one / more of the following features, occurring in the absence of another alternative cause and presence of *P. falciparum* parasitemia:

Impaired consciousness, generalised weakness, multiple convulsions, acidosis, hypoglycaemia, severe anaemia, hyperparasitemia (>10%), pulmonary edema, renal impairment and shock

Severe vivax malaria may also present with similar features but cerebral malaria, renal failure and/or shock are less common and there is no defined parasite density threshold. The treatment remains the same as for falciparum malaria, however patients must receive radical cure with primaquine.

Patient with severe malaria should be hospitalised for evaluation, treatment and monitoring. *In case of severe P. falciparum infection, particularly in a non-immune individual, treatment must be immediate.*

Patients with severe malaria are treated with injectable artemisinin followed by oral ACT (Box 54.3). If parenteral artemisinin is not available, alternatively parenteral quinine in high dilution can be started followed by oral quinine +doxycycline or clindamycin. If there are no facilities for IV infusion, quinine can be given in the dose of 0.25–0.5 g in 20 mL glucose saline IV, over not less than 10 min by the clock. *More rapid injection may cause a fall in BP, cardiac arrhythmias and cardiac arrest.* Alternatively, quinine can be given intramuscularly provided the solution is sterile and nearly neutral in reaction.

For falciparum malaria, a single dose of primaquine is given on day 2 while for vivax malaria, primaquine is given for 14 days to achieve radical cure (Box 54.3).

Cerebral malaria, a medical emergency, occurs as a complication of *P. falciparum* infection and has a high mortality. It needs to be treated in the ICU. Cerebral malaria sometimes causes coma and shock. Blood pressure should be maintained by IV fluids and dopamine. Management of coma is similar to that of coma due to other causes.

Glucocorticoids, urea and mannitol which were used in the past to treat the cerebral oedema of falciparum malaria, are of doubtful value and in fact may have deleterious effects in these cases; they are better avoided.

Hypoglycaemia, sometimes fatal, has been reported in patients with cerebral malaria; this complication may not respond well to glucose by IV bolus and to glucagon. *A somatostatin analogue*

Box 54.3 Treatment of Complicated (Severe) Falciparum and Vivax Malaria

- **Artesunate IV/IM 2.4mg/kg at 0,12, 24 and 48 h**
  OR
- **Artemether IM 3.2mg/kg (total dose administered as 1.6 mg/kg /day for 2 days).**
  When condition improves to take oral therapy;
- **Oral ACT (Box 54.4)**

If parenteral artemisinin is not available then administer:
- **Quinine hydrochloride IV infusion 20mg/kg** in 500 mL of 5%dextrose-saline over 4 h; followed by 10 mg/kg infused over 2 h, every 8 h, until the patient is able to swallow and parasite density is <1%.

When condition improves to take oral therapy:
- **Quinine (600 mg) or 10mg/kg 8h till total duration of 7 days**
  plus
- **Doxycycline 100 mg twice a day for 7 days**
  OR
  Clindamycin 10 mg/kg twice a day for 7 days

In addition,
For falciparum malaria:
- **Primaquine 0.75mg/kg on day 2**

For vivax malaria:
- **Primaquine 0.25mg/kg /day for 14 days**

Notes: Clindamycin is preferred in pregnant women and children where doxycycline is contraindicated
Total quinine therapy is for 7 days inclusive of the parenteral therapy

octreotide which inhibits the stimulatory effect of quinine on the beta cells of the pancreas may be useful.

Children and pregnant women often present with severe malaria.

Treatment of malaria in children is essentially similar to that in adults, however care should be taken to ensure that the pediatric dose never exceeds the adult dose. **Quinine** is better tolerated by children but its parenteral use is associated with high toxicity. **Chloroquine** injection may cause convulsions in infants and small children, and should be avoided. *Febrile babies should not be carried vertically, especially after any of the above drugs is given parenterally*. In children aged 6 months to 6 years, rectal artemisinin suppositories can be used immediately at home before transferring the child to the hospital.

Primaquine should be avoided in the neonates for fear of haemolysis. For details, see Table 54.4.

In pregnant women with malaria, chances of abortion is common in early pregnancy. In addition, there is also an increased incidence of still birth, intrauterine growth retardation and low birth weight.

Acute malaria during pregnancy can be treated with chloroquine or quinine in the usual doses. In first trimester quinine 10mg/kg three times daily should be given along with clindamycin 10 mg/kg 12h for 7 days. However, quinine can produce hypoglycaemia and hence should not be administered on an empty stomach.

Use of ACT is safe in second and third trimester. In severe malaria benefits of artemisinin derivatives outweigh the possible side effects. ACT containing lumefantrine is recommended in North-East states while in other states any ACT is recommended except ACT containing SP.

Mefloquine is contraindicated in first trimester, SP in first and last trimesters while halofantrine, primaquine and doxycycline are contraindicated throughout the pregnancy. To prevent the relapse of *P. vivax* malaria, 500 mg of chloroquine is administered weekly as suppressive chemoprophylaxis.

Malaria in G6PD-deficient persons should be treated with the usual doses of either chloroquine or quinine. In patients with milder G6PD deficiency, primaquine can be given as 0.75 mg/kg **once a week** for 8 weeks for radical cure in vivax malaria.

PH 1.55, IM 4.23

DRUG RESISTANT MALARIA

It is always treated with drug combinations (Box 54.4).

In **Artemisinin-based combination therapy (ACT)**, an artemisinin derivative is given in

Table 54.4 Dosage Schedule for Oral Treatment of Moderate and Severe Malaria in Children

Drug	Dose (mg)					Regimen
	Up to 1 Year	1–3 Years	4–6 Years	7–11 Years	12–14 Years	
Quinine	100–200	200–300	300–500	500–1000	1000–2000	Daily dose to be divided into 3 parts and continued for 7 days
Chloroquine (base) in mg	75	150	300	300	400–600	i. Loading dose
	75	150	150	150	225–300	ii. Second-one follow 6 h after first
	37	75	150	150	150–300	iii. One dose daily on days 2 and 3
Amodiaquine	50	100	150	200–300	400–600	i. Dose for first day
	50	50	300	50–200	250–400	ii. Daily dose for days 2 and 3
500 mg sulphadoxine + pyrimethamine 25 mg per tablet	½ tab	½ tab	1 tab	1 tab	2 tab	Single dose

Source: Modified from *The Clinical Management of Acute Malaria,* WHO Reg. Pub., South East Asia Series No. 9, New Delhi.

Box 54.4 Currently Used Antimalarial Drug Combinations for Resistant Falciparum Malaria

- Artemisinin-based Combination Therapy)
  - Artesunate + SP (refer Box 54.2)
  - Artemether + Lumefantrine (refer Box 54.2)
  - Artesunate 100 mg + Mefloquine 220 mg
  - Artesunate 200 mg + Amodiaquine 600 mg for 3 days
  - Dihydroartemisinin 120 mg + Piperaquine 960 mg for 3 days
  - Sodium artesunate 100 mg orally 12 hourly for 3 days plus mefloquine 750 mg on day 2 and then 500 mg on day 3
- Quinine + Doxycycline/Clindamycin (refer Box 54.3)
- Atovaquone (250 mg) + Proguanil (100 mg) x 4 times a day x 3 days

Notes: SP is always given as a single dose. All other drugs are given for 3 days, except quinine + doxycycline/clindamycin combination, which is given for 7 days.

combination with a long-acting antimalarial (amodiaquine, lumefantrine, mefloquine or sulphadoxine-pyrimethamine) for 3 days or with rapidly eliminated agents (doxycycline, clindamycin) for 7 days. ACT available in India is listed in Box 54.4, of which artesunate + sulphadoxine-pyrimethamine (SP) and artemether + lumefantrine are used in the National Malaria Programme of India.

Recrudescence: This indicates a repeat attack of malaria due to the survival of malaria parasites in red blood cells (comprising of the same genotype that caused the initial illness). This may be due to inadequate /ineffective therapy. This must be differentiated from reinfection, wherein the repeat attack of malaria is not caused by same genotype. It should be treated with artemisinin.

Relapse is defined as the occurrence of repeated attack of malaria due to persistent hepatic schizonts (after complete treatment of the blood infection) Hence relapses are seen in *P. vivax* and *P. ovale* infections but not with *P. falciparum*.

Chronic malaria is commonly associated with iron-deficiency anaemia, which responds to oral

Table 54.5 Drug Regimens for Malarial Prophylaxis IM 4.26

Drug, Dose and Frequency	When to Start before Entering Endemic Area	How Long to Continue after Leaving the Area	Remarks
Chloroquine sensitive *P. falciparum*[a] and *P. vivax/P. ovale*			
Chloroquine (base) 300 mg once weekly	1 week	4 weeks	Choice for infants/children/pregnant women and lactating mothers
Proguanil 200 mg o.d.	2 days	4 weeks	
Chloroquine-resistant *P falciparum* and MDR strains[a]			
1. Atovaquone 250 mg + proguanil 100 mg; one tablet per day[c]	1–2 days	7 days	Not in children <5 kg/ pregnant and lactating women
2. Doxycycline 100 mg one tablet / day	1–2 days	4 weeks	Not in children <8 years/ pregnant and lactating women
3. Mefloquine 250 mg mg once a week	1 week	4 weeks	In mefloquine sensitive areas
Terminal prophylaxis to prevent relapse of *P. vivax/P. ovale* (after leaving the endemic area)			
Primaquine 30 mg once daily		14 days along with postexposure prophylactics (or after its completion)	Not in pregnancy; In infants, children and lactating mothers, after ruling out G6PD deficiency

[a]If the traveller cannot tolerate any of these regimens, Primaquine 30 mg 1–2 days before, throughout the stay and 7 days after leaving.

iron therapy. Severe anaemia may need blood transfusion.

PROPHYLAXIS IM 4.26

Malaria can be prevented by offering protection against mosquito bite. For this the traveller should be urged to avoid contact with the night biting anopheles in the endemic area by covering exposed parts, Putting net over the bed, closing window doors, fitting window-screens, using insecticides and mosquito repellents (Chapter 60).

Chemoprophylaxis is advocated to:

- Non-immune travellers to an endemic area
- Non-immune residents shifting to an endemic area for fixed period
- High risk individuals (pregnant ladies, elderly and patients with end organ failure) residing in endemic areas.

When residents of a nonendemic area wish to travel to an endemic area, antimalarial drug(s) are recommended to prevent or suppress symptoms caused by malarial parasites. The choice depends on the likely strain of malarial parasites in the region and its known sensitivity pattern (Table 54.5). The therapy should be started before the start of the travel, continued during travel in the endemic area and even after departure from the area. Presumptive anti-relapse terminal prophylaxis to eliminate hepatic forms of *P. vivax/P. ovale* is indicated for persons who have had prolonged exposure in malaria-endemic areas.

All infants and children travelling to endemic areas need antimalarial prophylaxis. *Chloroquine is the drug of choice.* For areas with resistant strains, mefloquine is an option. To use doxycycline, the age of the child should be above 8 years and for atovaquone/proguanil, weight should be at least 5 kg.

Ideally, **pregnant women** should be advised to avoid travel to an endemic area. If it is not possible, chemoprophylaxis is given, which reduces the incidence of severe maternal anaemia and other adverse outcomes like abortion, still birth, prematurity, and low birth weight. *Chloroquine remains the drug of choice for sensitive organisms, whereas mefloquine is currently the only medication recommended for chloroquine resistant organisms.* Doxycycline is contraindicated and atovaquone/proguanil is not used but the limited data available suggest that it is not harmful to the fetus.

Very small amounts of chloroquine and mefloquine are excreted in the breast milk and hence can be given for prophylaxis in lactating women. Atovaquone/proguanil is not recommended. Limited data are available for doxycycline. Before giving primaquine both the mother and infant should be tested for G6PD deficiency.

Such chemoprophylaxis is not 100% effective; hence, malaria should be one of the differential diagnosis in a patient with fever who had recently visited an endemic area even if he had taken chemoprophylaxis.

CHEMOPROPHYLAXIS IN INDIA

This is advocated for selected groups in high *P. falciparum* endemic areas e.g. military troops/paramedical staff. These regimens include:

1. Short term chemoprophylaxis (upto 6 weeks): For this doxycycline 100 mg once daily to be started 2 days before travel and continued for 4 weeks after leaving that area.
2. Long term chemoprophylaxis (> 6 weeks): For this mefloquine 250 mg for adults to be started 2 weeks before and continued for 4 weeks after leaving that area.

Malaria elimination

To achieve malaria elimination vigorous attack on the parasites in patients with the suppressive, causal prophylactic and radical curative drugs is necessary. In additioneradication of mosquitoes, the vector for plasmodium species, is also essential which can be achieved using insecticides or larvicides. Mosquito repellents, can be used to protect individuals from mosquito bite (Chapter 60).

ANTIMALARIAL DRUGS

Clinical

True causal prophylactics
- No drug available

Causal prophylactics
- Primaquine
- Pyrimethamine
- Proguanil

Suppressives (schizonticides)

Rapidly acting
- Quinine
- 4-Aminoquinolines
- Mefloquine
- Artemisinin
- Atovaquone
- Halofantrine

Slowly acting
- Proguanil
- Pyrimethamine
- Sulphadoxine
- Tetracycline

Radical curatives

Against P. vivax infection
- Primaquine
- Proguanil

Gametocytocidal drugs

Against all species except P. faciparum
- Primaquine
- Chloroquine
- Quinine
- Artesunate

Chemical

Quinoline derivatives

4-Aminoquinolines
- Chloroquine
- Amodiaquine
- Pyronaridine

8-Aminoquinolines
- Primaquine
- Tafenoquine
- Bulaquine

Quinoline methanol
- Mefloquine

Artemisinin compounds
- Artesunate
- Arteether
- Artemether

Cinchona alkaloids
- Quinine
- Quinidine

Phenanthrene methanol
- Halofantrine
- Lumefantrine

Antifolates

Biguanides
- Proguanil

Diaminopyrimidines
- Pyrimethamine

Sulphonamides
- Sulphadoxine

Antimicrobials
- Doxycycline
- Clindamycin
- Atovaquone

CHAPTER 55

Chemotherapy of Amoebiasis

Learning Objectives

This chapter will enable the reader:

1. To be aware of the pathogenesis and clinical manifestation of amoebiasis.
2. To be aware of the life-cycle of *Entamoebahistolytica*.
3. To classify antiamoebic drugs.
4. To explain the mechanism of action, antimicrobial spectrum, pharmacological effects, salient pharmacokinetic features, ADR, drug interactions and indications for metronidazole.
5. To compare and contrast metronidazole, tinidazole, secnidazole and ornidazole.
6. To state the limitations of emetine as an antiamoebic drug.
7. To explain the role of quinoline derivatives, diloxanide furoate, paramomycin and tetracyclines in the treatment of amoebiasis.
8. To outline the management of: an acute attack of amoebiasis, cyst passers and extraintestinal amoebiasis.

KEY TERMS

luminal amoebicides, p. 791
tissue amoebicides, p. 792
metronidazole, p. 792
chloroquine, p. 794
acute intestinal amoebiasis, treatment, p. 795
cyst passers, treatment, p. 796
hepatic amoebiasis, p. 796

Amoebiasis is an infectious disease caused by the protozoon, *Entamoeba histolytica*. The disease, though labelled as 'tropical', is not uncommon in temperate zones. It primarily affects the colon, but other organs like liver, lung and brain may get secondarily involved. *E. histolytica* usually lives as a harmless commensal in the lumen of human bowel, a state termed as **asymptomatic amoebiasis**. The parasite subsists on debris and bacteria and not on the tissues of its host. When it becomes a pathogen, the trophozoites become larger and haematophagous, having many erythrocytes in the endoplasm, and cause **invasive amoebiasis**. Invasion is mediated by the destruction of epithelial cells and killing of neutrophils and lymphocytes.

Intestinal amoebiasis is characterised by gastrointestinal and constitutional symptoms and has a tendency to chronicity. Acute amoebic dysentery is associated with bloody, mucoid stools, abdominal pain and tenesmus. These are due to ulceration of the colon. Involvement of the caecum and appendix may cause appendicitis. A granulomatous lesion of the caecum gives rise to a lump in that region **(amoeboma).** Many infected persons (>80%), who pass the cysts in faeces, however, remain asymptomatic 'carriers'.

Life cycle of *E. histolytica*: *E. histolytica* exists in two forms:

- **The trophozoites,** present in the intestinal lumen and in infected tissues
- **The cysts,** which develop from the trophozoites within intestinal lumen

The trophozoites with amoeboid movements are the active form. However, they die rapidly after elimination in the stool. The **cysts represent a dormant stage** and are resistant to freezing and partial drying and transmit infection from person to person.

In the intestine of the host, the cyst wall is weakened by the intestinal enzymes and the trophozoites released invade the wall of the colon and enteroportal circulation. The organism may then find its way to the liver and other tissues, giving rise to **extraintestinal amoebiasis.**

Antiamoebic Drugs: Clinical Classification

I. **Drugs used only in intestinal amoebiasis (luminal amoebicides):** Halogenated hydroxyquinolines, diloxanide furoate, paramomycin and kurchi

II. **Drugs used in both intestinal and extraintestinal amoebiasis (tissue/mixed amoebicides):** Emetine, dehydroemetine, metronidazole, tinidazole, secnidazole

III. **Drugs used only in extraintestinal amoebiasis:** Chloroquine

Chemical Classification

I. **Imidazole derivatives:** Metronidazole, tinidazole, secnidazole

II. **Quinoline derivatives:**
- **Halogenated hydroxyquinolines:** Diiodohydroxyquinoline, iodochlorohydroxyquinoline
- **4-Aminoquinolines:** Chloroquine

III. **Emetine group:** Emetine, dehydroemetine and its resinate

IV. **Antibiotics:** Tetracyclines, paromomycin

V. **Miscellaneous:** Diloxanide furoate, nitazoxanide and kurchi

PH 1.47

IMIDAZOLE DERIVATIVES

METRONIDAZOLE: Metronidazole, a nitroimidazole derivative (Fig. 55.1), **is the drug of choice in most forms of amoebiasis** except in asymptomatic cyst passers. It is:

- **A potent amoebicide**
- **Effective in both intestinal and extraintestinal amoebiasis**
- **Relatively less toxic and cost-effective**
- **Also highly effective against:**
  1. ***Anaerobic protozoa*** (*Trichomonas vaginalis, Giardia lamblia* and *Balantidium coli)*
  2. ***Nonsporing, anaerobic, Gram-positive and Gram-negative bacilli*** such as bacterioides, including the *Bacteroides fragiles* group, *Clostridium difficile* and *Helicobacter pylori*

Metronidazole also has a radiosensitising effect on hypoxic tumour cells.

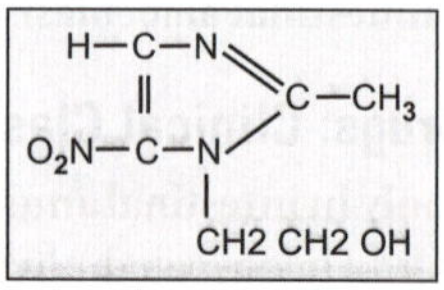

FIG. 55.1 Metronidazole.

Mechanism of action: *E. histolytica* derive energy from anaerobic oxidation of pyruvate. This reaction is caused by an enzyme, **pyruvate ferredoxin oxidoreductase (PFOR)**. Ferredoxins are the electron transport components of susceptible amoebae. Metronidazole diffuses across cell membranes of amoebae. PFOR system in the mitochondria transfers single electron to metronidazole, which results in liberation of highly toxic nitroradicals, which damage the microbial DNA and other biomolecules. Metronidazole acts specifically against anaerobic organisms including amoebae.

Resistance to metronidazole has been reported in *T. vaginalis* and *G. lamblia* infections but not in *E. histolytica* infection.

Absorption, fate and excretion: Metronidazole is rapidly and almost completely (80%) absorbed from the small bowel. **It is, therefore, relatively ineffective in the asymptomatic cyst-passers and in chronic intestinal amoebiasis.** Food does not affect its bioavailability. Protein binding is 20% and the drug diffuses into all tissues except placenta. It also achieves concentrations lethal to the sensitive organisms in CSF, bile, bone and abscesses. It is metabolised mainly in the liver. Its t½ is 8 h. The metabolites are excreted by the kidneys, imparting a red colour to urine. Renal insufficiency does not significantly alter its kinetics, but hepatic insufficiency prolongs its plasma t½. The drug is secreted in the milk.

Adverse reactions: These are mild and seldom necessitate discontinuation of therapy. They include the following:

- **Common:** Marked nausea, anorexia, abdominal pain and metallic taste in the mouth
- **Less common:** Vomiting, diarrhoea, headache, stomatitis, cystitis, dizziness, vertigo, ataxia, urticaria, pruritus and flushing
- **Rare:** Muscular weakness, seizures and incoordination. **Mild blood dyscrasia** in the form of neutropenia. It is reversible
- **Antabuse-like reactions** on alcohol consumption (Chapter 6), during and for up to 3 days of metronidazole therapy

Classification of Drugs used in Leishmaniasis:

I. **Pentavalent antimony compounds:** Sodium stibogluconate, meglumine antimonate
II. **Diamidine derivatives:** Dihydroxystibamidine isethionate, pentamidine isethionate
III. **Miscellaneous:** Amphotericin B, paromomycin (aminosidine), miltefosine

Their dosage regimens are summarised in Table 56.1.

Salient Pharmacological Features of Antileishmanial Drugs PH 1.47

I. PENTAVALENT ANTIMONY COMPOUNDS

The pentavalent antimony compounds, discovered in 1912, exhibit little activity against the leptomonad forms of Leishmania *in vitro*. Their efficacy *in vivo* suggests their reduction into **trivalent antimony compounds** in the body.

SODIUM STIBOGLUCONATE: This is the most preferred drug for the treatment of leishmaniasis. It act as a prodrug, which is reduced to the more toxic Sb^{3+} species that kill the amastigotes. *It also acts by suppressing both glycolysis and fatty acid metabolism and by diminishing the next generation of ATP and GTP in the amastigotes.* Given intravenously/intramuscularly, it is excreted in two phases: a short phase with t½ of 2 h and long phase with t½ of more than 24 h (33–76 h). The latter reflects slow release of trivalent antimony from the tissues, which contributes to prolonged effects of the drug. Leishmania can develop resistance to antimonials.

Adverse reactions: The common adverse effects include a metallic taste in mouth, nausea, vomiting, diarrhoea, giddiness and local thrombosis. Myalgia, arthralgia, hepatitis, pancreatitis and rarely arrhythmia may occur. ECG may show flattening or inversion of *T* waves, and prolongation of QT interval. A few cases of anaphylactoid shock and renal failure have been reported.

Table 56.1 Drugs for Leishmaniasis

Drug	Dose (Adults and Children)
Sodium stibogluconate	20 mg of Sb/kg/day, IV slowly over 5 min or IM for 28–30 days
Meglumine antimonate	Same as above
Amphotericin B	0.5–1.0 mg/kg IV, every second day for 15 infusions
Liposomal amphotericin B	3 mg/kg/day on days 1–5, 14 and 21 (total 21 mg/kg)
Pentamidine	2–4 mg/kg daily or every second day IV or IM up to 15 doses
Miltefosine	2.5 mg/kg/day for 4 weeks

II. DIAMIDINE DERIVATIVES

These drugs are **more potent but more toxic** than the antimony compounds. **They are not so effective in Indian Kala-azar.** The mechanism of action is not known. They interfere with amino acid transport, disrupt the mitochondria and **inhibit the transformation of amastigotes to promastigotes.** They are also useful for prophylaxis against *Trypanosoma gambiense* and in the treatment of early Gambian trypanosomiasis before CNS involvement.

PENTAMIDINE: Two pentamidine salts are available, isethionate (Pentamidine) and mesylate (Lomidine). They are administered intramuscularly.

Pentamidine is concentrated in the liver; very little gets into the brain tissue. It can be detected in the urine for 6–8 weeks.

Adverse reactions: Following the IM injection, it may cause local irritation, breathlessness, nausea, vomiting, facial flushing, pruritus, arthralgia, myalgia, tachycardia, arrhythmia and hypotension. The systemic toxicity includes hepatotoxicity, leukopenia, thrombocytopenia and nephrotoxicity. About 5% of patients may develop insulin dependent diabetes mellitus. It appears to have a direct action on the pancreatic beta cells, resulting in initial insulin release followed by impaired insulin secretion.

Indications:

- **Visceral and mucocutaneous leishmaniases** resistant to antimonials
- ***Pneumocystis jiroveci* pneumonia:** It is less

Possible tumorigenic and mutagenic effects occur in experimental animals but are not reported in humans.

Preparations and dosage:

i. Tablets 200, 400 and 500 mg for oral use
ii. Paediatric suspension 200 mg/5 mL
iii. Vaginal tablets containing 500 mg and vaginal gel: 7.5 mg/1 g
iv. Rectal suppositories 0.5 and 1 g
v. Solution for IV use as 5 mg/ml

For doses, see text.

Indications:

- **Intestinal and hepatic amoebiasis:** It is the drug of choice (See section, Management of amoebiasis).
- **Anaerobic infections:** Metronidazole is effective in chemoprophylaxis and treatment of infections due to **nonsporing, Gram-negative anaerobes** (**bacteroides**) and has been used in combination with other antimicrobials in gynaecological and colorectal surgery. Initially, it is given rectally as suppositories in the dose of 1 g 8 hourly until oral feeding begins. It is then administered orally in the dose 800 mg initially, followed by 400 mg 8 hourly for 7–10 days. It can also be administered by IV infusion in the dose of 15 mg/kg followed by 7.5 mg/kg 6–8 hourly. Each dose is infused over a period of 1 h. In severe abdominal and pelvic sepsis, gentamicin with either metronidazole or clindamycin is synergistic. It can also be used for surgical prophylaxis in the dose of 400 mg, 24 h and 8 h before surgery.
  For its use in **pseudomembranous colitis,** see Chapter 47.
- **Ulcerative gingivitis** (Vincent's stomatitis): The causative organisms are a spirochaete, *Treponema vincenti* and Gram-negative bacilli, *Leptotrichia buccalis*. The preferred treatment is with penicillin G. Metronidazole orally in the dose of 200 mg thrice daily for 3–7 days is also useful. Tetracycline and clindamycin are other drugs used.
- ***H. pylori infection:*** Chapter 41
- **Trichomoniasis and giardiasis:** Chapter 56
- **Dracunculosis:** Chapter 58

TINIDAZOLE: It is an analogue of metronidazole with long t½ (13 h) and is probably better tolerated than metronidazole. In acute amoebic dysentery, it is given in the dose of 600–800 mg orally t.i.d. for 5 days or in the dose of 2 g (50 mg/kg in children) once daily for 3 days. In anaerobic infections, it is used orally in the dose of 2 g initially, followed by 1 g daily (single dose) for 5–6 days. For surgical prophylaxis, it is administered in the dose of 2 g once 12 h before surgery.

SECNIDAZOLE: This analogue of metronidazole also has a longer t½ (17–29 h) and similar uses. In acute amoebic dysentery, it is administered orally in a single dose of 2 g. In children a single dose of 30 mg/kg is used. In hepatic amoebiasis, the dose is 1.5 g per day for 5 days. In giardiasis, the single oral doses are: 2 g in adults; 500 mg in children weighing 10–15 kg; 750 mg in children weighing 16–26 kg and 1 g in those weighing over 26 kg. Secnidazole oral tablet/ granules as 2-gram single dose is effective in bacterial vaginitis too.

ORNIDAZOLE: is an imidazole with similar properties as secnidazole. Its t½ is 13 h. It is available as 500 mg tablets. The dose is 500 mg b.i.d. for 5–10 days. A single daily dose of 1.5 g for 3 days is also effective.

QUINOLINE DERIVATIVES

Amongst these, **diiodohydroxyquinoline, iodochlorohydroxyquinoline** and **broxyquinoline** are halogenated hydroxyquinolines, whereas **chloroquine** is a 4-aminoquinoline derivative. *They act by direct contact with the trophozoites of E. histolytica.* All the halogenated oxyquinolines also have some **antibacterial and antifungal properties**. The mechanism of action of halogenated oxyquinolines is unknown.

DIIODOHYDROXYQUINOLINE: This halogenated quinoline (Fig. 55.2) is an **effective luminal amoebicide,** against both motile and cystic forms of the protozoan, more so against the former. Clearance of cysts is partially due to elimination of trophozoites. **It is not effective in extraintestinal amoebiasis.**

Absorption, fate and excretion: Diiodohydroxyquinoline is insignificantly absorbed from the intestinal tract and 90% of it is excreted in faeces.

Adverse reactions: These are mild and uncommon. The drug may occasionally cause headache, nausea, vomiting and diarrhoea. Chills, fever, skin eruptions and iodine dermatitis have been reported. It is contraindicated in patients with iodine intolerance.

Preparations and dosage: Diiodohydroxyquinoline tablet 300 mg. Dose: 600 mg thrice daily for 15 days. It may be repeated after 2–3 weeks.

IODOCHLOROHYDROXYQUINOLINE: This drug resembles diiodohydroxyquinoline in antiamoebic action. It is not much absorbed from the GI tract. It is probably **more useful in cyst carriers**. It also has antibacterial, antifungal and antitrichomonal actions.

Adverse reactions: These are usually mild and include diarrhoea or constipation, abdominal pain, anal pruritus and mild iodism. A neurological syndrome consisting of myelitis, peripheral neuritis and sometimes optic nerve involvement (subacute myelo-optic neuropathy – SMON) has been reported in patients receiving this drug over prolonged periods. These cases were mostly reported from Japan in 1960. *They are very rarely reported from other areas.* Usually, oral daily doses of up to 750 mg for 8–10 days are considered relatively safe in adults. **Larger doses (>2 g per day) and frequent/prolonged (>20 days) use should be avoided.**

Preparations and dosage:

i. Iodochlorohydroxyquinoline tablets 250 mg. Dose: 750 mg daily in 3 divided doses for 10 days. The course may be repeated once after a week.
ii. Iodochlorohydroxyquinoline 3% cream for topical dermal use

Indications: Besides its use as luminal amoebicide, it is also used topically in fungal infections of the skin (Chapter 68). *The major disadvantage of topical application is yellow staining of clothes and linen.*

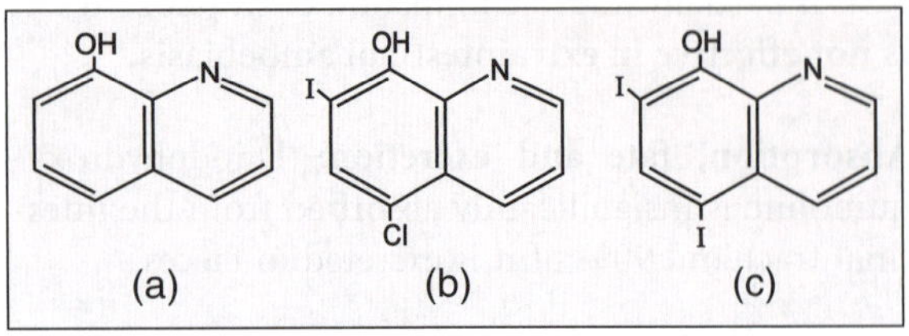

FIG. 55.2 **(a) Hydroxyquinoline nucleus, (b) iodochlorohydroxyquinoline, (c) diiodohydroxyquinoline.**

CHLOROQUINE: The pharmacology of chloroquine is discussed in Chapter 54. Given orally, it is completely absorbed from upper intestine and **concentrated in the liver.** It has a minimal effect in intestinal amoebiasis because of poor concentration in colonic lumen and wall. Its use in **hepatic amoebiasis** has declined following the availability of metronidazole.

EMETINE GROUP

EMETINE: Emetine is an alkaloid obtained from roots of ipecac (*Cephalis ipecacuanha*).

Antiamoebic action: It inhibits protein synthesis in trophozoites, which arrests their multiplication and leads to their phagocytosis. **It has, however, little effect on the cystic forms.**

Absorption, fate and excretion: Emetine has a bitter taste and is absorbed from the gut but because of its irritant nature, it is administered by deep IM injection. The drug gets concentrated in the liver. It is slowly eliminated in urine and repeated injections cause cumulation.

Adverse reactions: The major drawback of emetine is its toxicity, mainly cardiovascular toxicity due to which it is not preferred in clinical practice. The adverse reactions include

- local painful reactions at the site of injection
- Vomiting and diarrhoea (due to gastric irritation and stimulation of the CTZ)
- Muscle weakness (due to neuromuscular blockade)
- Cardiotoxicity: Emetine may cause tachycardia, precordial pain, hypotension, myocarditis and pericarditis. The ECG offers an early index of cardiotoxicity.

Emetine should be avoided in patients with cardiac or renal damage, in pregnant women, in geriatric and pediatric patients.

Indications:

It was used earlier as a tissue amoebicide (see section, Management of amoebiasis), for lung and liver fluke infestations (Chapter 58) and as an emetic (in form of Ipecacuanha syrup; See Chapter 39). It is now rarely used because of its toxicity.

DEHYDROEMETINE: This semisynthetic drug, claimed to be less toxic than emetine, is preferred to emetine. Dehydroemetine injection contains 60 mg/ml. Dose: 1 mg/kg IM daily for 5–7 days. Dehydroemetine resinate is a slow release preparation given orally in the dose of 50 mg daily for 10 days.

ANTIAMOEBIC ANTIBIOTICS

TETRACYCLINE: The intestinal bacteria are essential for the production of intestinal amoebic lesions. They probably act by creating an environment congenial to the growth of amoebae, by manufacturing certain metabolites and vitamins on which the protozoa thrive, and by producing secondary infection. Tetracycline, though exhibiting an antiamoebic action *in vitro* in large doses, **probably acts *in vivo* by altering the intestinal bacterial flora and creating a medium unfavourable for the growth of amoebae.** It may be administered in the dose of 0.25 g 6 hourly for 10–15 days, in combination with metronidazole to treat amoebic liver abscess particularly when bacterial coinfection is suspected.

PAROMOMYCIN: This aminoglycoside antibiotic (Chapter 45) given orally, is not absorbed. In the dose of 500 mg t.i.d. for 10 days, it is effective as **luminal amoebicide** (cure rate 80%). It has also been used parenterally in the treatment of leishmaniasis (Chapter 56).

MISCELLANEOUS AGENTS

DILOXANIDE FUROATE: This potent direct amoebicidal drug (Fig. 55.3) is **highly effective in chronic intestinal amoebiasis,** in cyst passers and partially useful in mild acute cases. It is of no value in extraintestinal amoebiasis.

Given orally it is hydrolysed to diloxanide which is partly absorbed. Nonabsorbable portion acts as a luminal amoebicide. *The drug is well tolerated, safe and almost nontoxic.* The adverse effects reported are mild and include mainly GI disturbances, particularly flatulence.

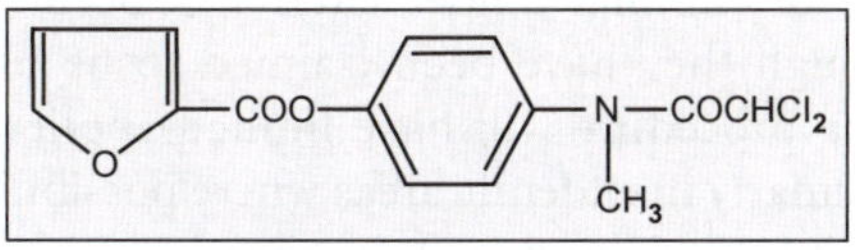

FIG. 55.3 Diloxanide furoate.

Diloxanide furoate is available as 500 mg tablets. Dose: 500 mg 3 times daily for 5–10 days. A second course may be given immediately following the first course.

Nitazoxanide can also be used for amoebiasis (Chapter 56).

KURCHI: Kurchi consists of the dried stem bark of *Holarrhena antidysenterica.* Kurchi has mild antiamoebic activity and is useful only in mild intestinal amoebiasis. It may produce nausea and vomiting but is otherwise well tolerated. Powdered roots of this plant are used as a household remedy in India for ages for 'abdominal pain and diarrhoea'.

MANAGEMENT OF AMOEBIASIS IM 16.13

Amoebiasis, in general, is a difficult disease to treat because of its tendency to chronicity and the inability of various drugs to eradicate the cystic forms of the parasite completely.

Table 55.1 summarises the suggested treatment of amoebiasis.

Acute Intestinal Amoebiasis

Metronidazole in the dose of 400–600 mg (15 mg/kg in children) t.i.d. for 5–7 days is the treatment of choice. Almost 90% of patients with moderate amoebic dysentery respond clinically to oral metronidazole. The symptoms are relieved within 24 h. Severe cases may need IV infusion of metronidazole. **Additional advantage of this drug is its effectiveness in hepatic amoebiasis which can never be entirely excluded in patients with amoebic dysentery.**

Parasites persist in the intestine in almost 30%–40% of the patients who receive only metronidazole. Therefore, **metronidazole therapy should always be followed by a course of a luminal amoebicide to ensure a cure.** For this purpose, **diloxanide furoate** 500 mg t.i.d. for 10 days or diiodohydroxyquinoline 600 mg b.i.d. or 500 mg t.i.d. for 15 days is used.

In patients presenting with fulminating amoebic colitis with toxic symptoms, it is advisable to use oral tetracycline in addition, to eliminate the intestinal bacteria. *Emetine, though controls symptoms rapidly, is no more recommended due to its cardiotoxicity.*

Table 55.1 Summary of Suggested Treatment of Amoebiasis

Cyst passers	Diloxanide furoate 500 mg t.i.d. for 10 days OR Diiodohydroxyquinoline 650 mg t.i.d. for 15–20 days OR Iodochlorhydroxyquinoline 250 mg t.i.d. for 10 days
Invasive	Metronidazole 400–800 mg t.i.d. for 5 days OR Tinidazole 2 g daily for 2–3 days OR Secnidazole 2-g single dose followed by a luminal amoebicide for 10–20 days
Severe cases and hepatic abscess	Metronidazole IV OR Dehydroemetine IM for 5 days (see text)

Adjuvant therapy includes the use of antispasmodics for relief of colicky pain and correction of dehydration in severe cases.

Asymptomatic Cyst Passers and Chronic Intestinal Amoebiasis

The drug regimens recommended in such cases are:

1. **Diloxanide furoate** 500 mg t.i.d. for 10 days.
2. A combination of diiodohydroxyquinoline 1.8 g daily and tetracycline 1 g daily, in divided doses for 10 days.
   Chronic amoebic colitis is sometimes difficult to treat and usually more than one drug, given in rotation, is needed to achieve success. Some of the symptoms of colitis may not regress rapidly, even after the colon is cleared of pathogens. Symptomatic therapy such as a high fibre diet and antispasmodics may be needed in such cases.

Hepatic Amoebiasis

Metronidazole is the drug of choice. Emetine hydrochloride and chloroquine diphosphate are other alternatives.

Metronidazole (800 mg three times a day for 10 days) rapidly controls hepatic amoebiasis in majority of cases. An alternative regime is 2.4 g (30 mg/kg) in a single daily dose for 2 successive days. In this dose nausea is likely to be severe and should be prevented by administration of metoclopramide. Metronidazole may also be administered intravenously in the dose of 15 mg/kg (0.75–1 g for an adult) as a loading dose, followed by 7.5 mg/kg every 6 h for 7–10 days. Each dose is infused slowly over 1 h. Neutralised solutions should not be refrigerated, lest precipitation occurs.

Aspiration is usually necessary in addition to chemotherapy whenever an abscess is present. Simultaneous use of tetracycline is beneficial.

Chloroquine diphosphate is much less potent than metronidazole. It is given in the dose of 500 mg thrice daily for 2 days followed by 250 mg twice daily for 2–3 weeks; however, the relapse rate is high.

In patients in whom the diagnosis between amoebic and pyogenic liver abscess is not certain, metronidazole alone should be avoided because a pyogenic liver abscess may temporarily respond to metronidazole.

Other forms of extraintestinal amoebiasis: These respond well to metronidazole.

Criteria for cure of amoebiasis: Failure to detect *E. histolytica* in stool specimens obtained at regular intervals for next 2 years is taken as the criterion for cure of amoebic infection. Clinical cure does not signify cure of the disease and relapses can occur.

Prevention

The cysts responsible for propagation of the disease are resistant to the agents routinely used to purify water, e.g. chlorine. It is, therefore, necessary to avoid faecal contamination of water. Fly control and detection and treatment of carriers are equally important. *The surest way to eliminate cysts from water is to boil it. There is no effective prophylactic therapy.* Prophylactic use of small doses of luminal amoebicides has been tried. Although they have been claimed to be useful, such a procedure will have limited application, particularly in endemic areas where possibility of frequent reinfection is always present.

ANTIAMOEBIC DRUGS

Clinical

Drugs used only in intestinal amoebiasis (luminal amoebicides)

- Halogenated hydroxyquinolines
- Diloxanide furoate
- Tetracycline
- Paramomycin
- Kurchi

Drugs used in both intestinal and extraintestinal amoebiasis (tissue/mixed amoebicides)

- Emetine
- Dehydroemetine
- Metronidazole
- Tinidazole
- Secnidazole

Drugs used only in extraintestinal amoebiasis

- Chloroquine

Chemical

Imidazole derivatives

- Metronidazole
- Tinidazole
- Secnidazole

Quinoline derivatives

Halogenated hydroxyquinolines

- Diiodohydroxyquinoline
- Iodochlorohydroxyquinoline

4-Aminoquinolines

- Chloroquine

Emetine group

- Emetine
- Dehydroemetine

Antibiotics

- Tetracyclines
- Paromomycin

Miscellaneous

- Diloxanide furoate
- Nitazoxanide
- Kurchi

CHAPTER 56

Chemotherapy of Other Protozoal Infections

Learning Objectives

This chapter will enable the reader:

1. To be aware of clinical syndromes of leishmaniasis and the life cycle of *Leishmania donovani.*
2. To classify drugs used in leishmaniasis.
3. To mention the mechanism of action, pharmacological effects, ADR and indications for antileishmanial drugs, e.g. antimonials, pentamidine, amphotericin B and miltefosine.
4. To enlist the drugs used in the treatment of trypanosomiasis.
5. To discuss the drug regimens used in the treatment of toxoplasmosis.
6. To outline the management of trichomoniasis.
7. To enlist drugs used in the treatment of giardiasis.

KEY TERMS

sodium stibogluconate, p. 799
amphotericin B, p. 800
toxoplasmosis, treatment, p. 802
leucorrhoea, treatment, p. 803
trichomoniasis, treatment, p. 803
metronidazole, p. 804
nitazoxanide, p. 804
giardiasis, treatment, p. 804

Leishmaniasis is a vector-borne infection caused by **intracellular protozoa** of the genus *Leishmania.* From 30 mammalian-infecting species of leishmania, 21 are responsible for human disease.

Leishmaniasis presents as several clinical syndromes. The most common are:

1. Visceral leishmaniasis (VL)
2. Cutaneous leishmaniasis (CL; Oriental sore)
3. Mucocutaneous (MCL) leishmaniasis resulting from pathological changes in reticulo-endothelial organs, dermis and muco-oropharynx, respectively

VISCERAL LEISHMANIASIS OR KALA-AZAR

This form of the disease, produced by *Leishmania donovani* and *Leishmania infuntum* (India, Nepal, Bangladesh and Sudan) and *Leishmania chagasi* (Latin America) is transmitted by Phlebotomus sandflies. In most leishmania infections, dogs and rodents act as reservoir. Only patients with post-kala-azar dermal leishmaniasis (PKDL) and those with CL act as human reservoir for *L. donovani* and *Leishmania tropica*, respectively.

VL can be asymptomatic, subclinical and self-resolving or it can run an aggressive fatal course. Clinically, it is characterised by weight loss, hepatosplenomegaly, irregular fever, anaemia, leukopenia and hypergamma-globulinaemia and suppressed cellular immunity.

Life cycle: During its life cycle, the protozoan exists in two forms:

1. **Leishmania forms (amastigotes), found within the reticuloendothelial cells** of the liver, spleen and lymph nodes, and within the macrophages of the infected person
2. Motile flagellated **leptomonad forms (promastigotes)** which develop from the leishmania forms within the digestive tract of the sandfly. The development of the leptomonad forms takes about 10 days. They are injected by the sandfly into man during its bite, whereupon they attack the reticuloendothelial cells, are phagocytosed by macrophages and get transformed into the leishmania forms.

effective than cotrimoxazole. It is also used for prophylaxis. The other drugs used for the same purpose are daily cotrimoxazole and weekly combination of sulphadoxine and pyrimethamine (Chapter 54).

- **Trypanosomiasis:** See section, Trypanosomiasis

DIHYDROXYSTILBAMIDINE ISETHIONATE: This is given intravenously in the dose of 250 mg daily for 10 days. The course may be repeated after an interval of 2 weeks and a total dose of 7.5 g, should be given over a period of 4–5 weeks. Its toxicity is similar to that of pentamidine.

III. MISCELLANEOUS

AMPHOTERICIN B: This antifungal antibiotic, (Chapter 48) is useful in patients not responding to antimony compounds. However, it is expensive, toxic and not easily available. The doses vary in different regions probably because differences in leishmania species and their susceptibility. **It is effective against antimony-resistant organisms.**
Amphotericin damages an ergosterol-like membrane steroid of leishmania. It is considered the drug of choice for Indian Kala-azar. Amphotericin B is also used in the treatment of cutaneous or mucosal leishmaniasis and is effective in immunocompromised patients. The disease can relapse but responds to repeat therapy. Freedom from relapse for 6 month indicates cure.

Preparations:

i. Conventional amphotericin B (C-AMB; complex with bile salt deoxycholate)
ii. Amphotericin B colloidal dispersion (ABCD)
iii. Amphotericin B lipid complex (ABLC) available as 5mg/ml for infusion
iv. Liposomal preparations (L-AMB): available as 50mg powder for solution as IV *They are less toxic as they are targeted specifically towards macrophages, and may be preferred.*

MILTEFOSINE: This phosphocholine derivative is the **first oral drug**, which is effective against Indian visceral and cutaneous leishmaniasis.

Mechanism of action: It acts by interfering with cell signalling pathways. This possibly results in altered lipid metabolism, inhibition of mitochondrial function, modulation of macrophage response and induction of apoptosis. It is administered as 50 mg b.i.d. for 4 weeks. For those with weight more than 50 kg, 50 mg t.i.d. is recommended. Response rate to miltefosine is variable (60%–90%).

Absorption, fate and excretion: After oral absorption, it is widely distributed. It is metabolised by the liver and **has a long t½ of 1–4 weeks.** The drug cannot be given intravenously because it has hemolytic activity.

Adverse reactions: They include vomiting, diarrhoea and transient hepatic and renal damage. **It is teratogenic** *and should be avoided in pregnancy. While on miltefosine therapy, women should be advised not to conceive and use adequate contraception during therapy for 5 months after the therapy is discontinued.* **Rapid development of drug resistance is a major disadvantage.** In such resistant cases a combination of miltefosine with paromomycin is preferred.

PAROMOMYCIN (Aminosidine): This broad spectrum aminoglycoside antibiotic (Chapter 45) has been claimed to be useful in the treatment of visceral leishmaniasis. It is given in the dose of 15–20 mg/kg/day, in three divided doses intramuscularly, for 21 days. The short treatment duration and lower cost, favour the usage of this drug. It can be used in combination with sodium stibogluconate. It is also considered as an alternative for visceral leishmaniasis resistant to classical drugs. It can be used orally as second line drug to treat amoebiasis, cryptosporidiosis, and giardiasis. Topical formulations have been used to treat trichomoniasis and cutaneous leishmaniasis.

ORIENTAL SORE

This condition is caused commonly by *L. tropica (L. major)*. It is characterised by nodular skin lesion that later ulcerates. Mild lesions may be left to heal by themselves. More severe cases require local as well as systemic antimonial therapy. Ketoconazole in the dose of 200–400 mg/day for 4–6 weeks may be useful.

Sores on the face and hands often get secondarily infected and tend to become chronic. This would need additional antibiotic therapy.

MUCOCUTANEOUS LEISHMANIASIS

It is caused by *Leishmania brasiliensis and Leishmania mexicana.* It is characterised by skin granulomas and ulcerative lesions of the nose, mouth and pharynx. The treatment is similar to that of visceral leishmaniasis. However, **the disease is relatively resistant to antimonials.** Amphotericin B is perhaps the best alternative.

Currently used drugs for leishmaniasis are generally toxic, need to be given for long time and do not eliminate persistent forms of the parasite from the host. There is a variation in therapeutic response to different leishmanial species and drug resistance to Leishmania has been reported.

TRYPANOSOMIASIS

This disease, caused by parasites of the genus *Trypanosoma*, is characterised by chronic irregular fever, skin eruptions, lymphadenitis and physical and mental lethargy. It can be divided into the following:

1. **African trypanosomiasis** (**Sleeping sickness**) is caused by *T. gambiense* and *Trypanosoma rhodesiense* transmitted by tse-tse and open woodland flies, respectively
2. **South American trypanosomiasis** caused by *Trypanosoma cruzi* transmitted by blood sucking Reduviid bugs

African trypanosomiasis: Therapeutic response is better if the treatment of sleeping sickness is undertaken in its earlier stage when the parasite has not invaded the CNS.

SURAMIN SODIUM: This drug, a complex organic urea compound, is particularly useful in treating the more acute rhodesian form of African trypanosomiasis and early infections with *T. gambiense.* It is a useful prophylactic agent but has been replaced by pentamidine for this purpose.

Mechanism of action: It is selectively taken up by the parasite and causes inhibition of trypanosomal enzymes, receptors and lysosomal functions. Parasites treated with the drug lose their infectivity but still survive *in vitro* for over 24 h after exposure. In addition to trypanocidal activity, the drug is effective against the adult forms of *Onchocerca volvulus.*

Absorption, fate and excretion: Suramin is administered intravenously; IM administration is painful. It gets extensively bound to plasma proteins and **persists in the plasma for as long as 3 months after a single dose.** *It does not cross the BBB and is, therefore, not useful in the encephalitic stage.* The drug is excreted in urine.

Adverse reactions: These include nausea, vomiting, dermatitis, chills, fever, pruritus, paraesthesias, photophobia, polyuria and sometimes loss of consciousness. Blood dyscrasias may develop occasionally. The drug is nephrotoxic and may give rise to cylindruria, albuminuria and haematuria.

Preparations and dosage: The initial dose is 0.5 g followed by 1 g in subsequent IV injections at intervals of 5–7 days for 5–6 injections. For use of suramin in onchocerciasis (Chapter 58).

PENTAMIDINE ISETHIONATE: This drug may be used as a substitute for suramin. Dose is 3–4 mg per kg body weight IV on every alternate day for 10 doses. It has been shown to protect against the Gambian but not the Rhodesian disease. Hypotension and hypoglycaemia are common adverse effects. *The drug doses not cross the BBB*.

The organic arsenical compounds used in African trypanosomiasis are **Mel B** and **Mel W.** These compounds are toxic and are mainly used **to treat meningo-encephalitic stage of the disease.** They are:

MELARSOPROL (Mel B): This trivalent organic arsenical, dissolved in propylene glycol, is administered intravenously, slowly, in increasing doses of 0.36–3.6 mg/kg (up to a maximum of 200 mg). The injection is given on alternate days for 3 days. *The course may be repeated after an interval of 3 weeks in cases with involvement of the CNS.* Nearly 95% of the patients can be cured without serious complication, whereas 1%–5% die during treatment. The toxic manifestations include vomiting, abdominal colic, proteinuria, neuritis, blood dyscrasias, myocardial damage and arsenical encephalopathy. Although melarsoprol is also effective against late-stage West African trypanosomiasis caused by *T. brucei* or *T. gambiense*, NECT and fexinidazole have become the first-line treatments of this disease.

MELARSONYL POTASSIUM (Mel W): This water soluble derivative of Mel B is given as a 5% solution, by IM injection. The first dose is 2 mg/kg; 4 mg/kg/day for 3 days. The preparation is probably less toxic but also less effective than the parent compound in advanced *T. rhodesiense* infection, but may be equally effective in *T. gambiense* infection. The drug is also useful in onchocerciasis.

NITROFURAZONE: The drug has been employed for trypanosomiasis in patients who have relapsed after other forms of treatment. **It is given orally** in doses of 500 mg t.i.d. for 7–10 days. For children, a dose of 30 mg/kg is recommended. The adverse manifestations include GI disturbances, peripheral neuritis, seizures and haemolysis in G6PD deficient patients.

EFLORNITHINE HYDROCHLORIDE (difluoromethylornithine, DFMO) has been shown to give **high cure rates** in late stages of gambian trypanosomiasis. **It causes irreversible inhibition of synthesis of polyamines required for cell division and differentiation.** The drug can cause headache, alopecia, diarrhoea, anaemia, leucopoenia and thrombocytopenia. Hallucinations, convulsions and hearing loss may occur. It is teratogenic. It is administered by IV infusion in the dose of 400 mg/kg/day in four divided doses for 14 days. It is an alternative for patients who relapse after melarsoprol.

Eflornithine in combination with nifurtimox (Nifurtimox-eflornithine combination therapy – NECT) is currently the drug of choice for the treatment of severe late-stage (CNS involvement) West African (Gambian) trypanosomiasis in adults and children. The combination has better cure rate then individual agents. **Eflorinthine cream** has been found useful in reducing the rate of growth of facial hair in women; however it needs to be used for prolonged period (Chapter 67).

South-American Trypanosomiasis (Chagas' disease): There is no effective and safe agent available for the treatment of this condition. Two drugs **nifurtimox** and **benznidazole,** effective orally, appear to kill circulating trypanosomes. They are not useful in chronic disease.

Nifurtimox is given orally in a dose of 8–10 mg/kg/day in 4 divided doses, for 90–120 days. The drug may cause GI disturbances, weight loss, insomnia, arthralgia, neuropathy, leucopoenia and seizures.

FEXNIDAZOLE

It is a nitroimidazole similar to nifurtimox. It is the first oral treatment for both early and late (CNS) stages of West African trypanosomiasis in adults and children aged > 6 years or older and weighing >20 kg.

This prodrug is bioactivated by nitroreductases in trypanosomatids that use NADH as a reductive cofactor to perform electron oxidation reactions. These reactive molecules interact with multiple targets in the cell and cause DNA modification and breakage.

The dose of fexinidazole in adult patients is 1800 mg (3 tablets of 600 mg each) once a day for 4 days, followed by 1200 mg (2 tablets of 600 mg each) fpor 6 days.

The common adverse effects include headache, tremor, dizziness and gastrointestinal effects such as vomiting and decreased appetite.

Benznidazole is administered in a dose of 5–10 mg/kg/day in two divided doses for 60 days. Generally it is well tolerated. It can cause GI disturbances, polyneuropathy and bone marrow suppression.

TOXOPLASMOSIS

Toxoplasmosis is a common disease of birds and mammals, caused by infection with the obligate **intracellular protozoan** *Toxoplasma gondii.* The organisms are arc shaped (toxon = arc; gondii = the name of a North American rodent).

Infection in animals occurs by ingestion of cysts that contain sporulated oocytes (**bradyzoites**) by an intermediate host such as the rat or the sheep. The bradyzoites released in the gut enter the epithelium of the small intestine and transform into rapidly dividing **tachyzoites,** which can infect all mammalian cells except the RBCs. The parasites' sexual phase (feline phase) takes place in the definitive host like the cat which ingests the infected rats. The infected cats may excrete millions of sporozoites containing oocytes which may remain viable for many years in the soil. Human infection occurs following ingestion of either soil contaminated with sporulated oocytes or undercooked meat containing tachyzoites.

Toxoplasmosis is largely asymptomatic and self-limiting, but a small percentage of patients get lymphadenopathy, fever and malaise. **Retino-choroiditis forms an important manifestation (25%–35%) in children but is rare in adults.** Encephalitis, myocarditis and pneumonitis can occur. *Repeated abortions can occur in infected women.*

There is no drug which will kill the trophozoites or eradicate the cysts. Spontaneous cure is known. Asymptomatic infection in immunocompetent subjects need no treatment as the disease is self-limiting.

For symptomatic patients, either of the combination treatment regimens for 6 weeks is needed:

1. **Pyrimethamine** (100 mg loading dose orally followed by 25–50 mg/day) **plus sulphadiazine** (2–4 g/day divided 4 times daily)
2. **Pyrimethamine** (100-mg loading dose orally followed by 25–50 mg/day) **plus clindamycin** (300 mg orally 4 times daily)
3. **Pyrimethamine** (100-mg loading dose orally followed by 25–50 mg/day) **plus azithromycin** 500 mg once daily
4. **Pyrimethamine** (100-mg loading dose orally followed by 25–50 mg/day) **plus atovaquone** 750 mg twice daily

Patients may receive in addition, **trimethoprim** (10 mg/kg/day) **sulphamethoxazole** (50 mg/kg/day) for 4 weeks.

Azithromycin and **atovaquone** are the drugs of choice in patients who are allergic to sulphadiazine and clindamycin.

Folinic acid (leucovorin) (10–25 mg/day) may be administered to all patients to prevent haematologic toxicity of pyrimethamine.

If the patients exhibit clinical deterioration or elevated intracranial pressure despite 48 h of therapy, steroids are indicated.

Patients with AIDS need higher doses of pyrimethamine (initial dose 200 mg followed by 50-75 mg/day) and sulphadiazine (4-8 g/day) for 6 weeks, followed by lifelong suppressive therapy (pyrimethamine 50 mg/day orally plus sulphadiazine 1-1.5 g/day) with folinic acid (10 mg/day).

The regimen recommended in affected pregnant woman is **spiramycin** (Chapter 44) 1 g t.i.d. orally continued throughout the pregnancy. However, if amniotic fluid test is also positive for *T. gondii*, pyrimethamine (50 mg/day) with sulphadiazine is given for 3 weeks along with folinic acid, followed by spiramycin 1 g t.i.d. for 3 weeks. Both the regimes are repeated alternatively till delivery. Another option is to give only pyrimethamine (25 mg/day) and sulphadiazine till delivery.

Congenitally infected neonates are treated aggressively with oral pyrimethamine (1.0–2.0 mg/kg/day) for 2 days followed by sulphadiazine (100 mg/kg/day) along with folic acid for 1 year. In patients allergic to sulphonamides, sulphadiazine may be substituted by spiramycin or clindamycin.

TRICHOMONIASIS

PH 1.48

Vaginal discharge is a common complaint in general practice. It must be emphasised that **many discharges are non-infective**, and hence, it is wrong and may even be harmful to use systemic or local antimicrobial drugs unless proper diagnosis is made.

In women of the child-bearing age excessive vaginal discharge (**leucorrhoea**) may simply be due to pelvic congestion or increased secretion of the cervical glands as in *cervical erosion or during oral contraceptive medication.* In such cases, bacteriological examination is negative and no drugs are indicated. *What is needed is reassurance and advice on simple hygiene and cauterisation of the cervical erosion.*

Vaginal discharge due to infection should be treated according to the causative organism. *Trichomonas vaginalis* is by far the commonest one, followed by *Candida albicans.* Typically,

- **Trichomoniasis** presents as an **intense vaginitis** with a purulent, greenish yellow profuse, frothy, **offensive discharge.** Other symptoms include pruritus, burning, oedema, dyspareunia and urinary frequency.
- **Candidial vaginitis** is **less intense** with thin and curd like or **'cheesy' discharge** and adherent plaques on the vaginal wall

T. vaginalis is the infectious protozoon most commonly associated with vulvovaginitis during reproductive years. *Infection in males is often asymptomatic.*

Drugs for local treatment: They are useful when extravaginal sources of reinfection are not present. They include:

- **Halogenated hydroxyquinolines** like iodochlorohydroxyquinoline, diiodohydroxyquinoline
- Agents like **furazolidone, surfactants like sodium lauryl sulphate, dioctyl sodium sulphosuccinate, triclobisonium and povidone iodine**

These drugs are discussed elsewhere (See Chapters 54 and 60). They are often combined with deodorisers like thymol, menthol, or eucalyptol. Other local agents like vinegar, boric acid and lactic acid are used to lower the vaginal pH to its usual acidity (3.5–4.5). This facilitates the growth of the normal vaginal flora and results in suppression of the trichomonal infection.

Drug for systemic therapy: Oral metronidazole is **the drug of choice for trichomoniasis** (Chapter 55).

It is given in the dose of 400 mg twice daily for 7 days. A second course may be instituted after 4–6 weeks. *A single dose of 2 g has also been reported to give equally good results. Since trichomoniasis is a urogenital infection, using local pessaries without systemic therapy is unsatisfactory.*

Trichomoniasis is sexually transmissible and it is advisable to administer a course of metronidazole to the sexual consorts of the infected persons. It is advisable to avoid sexual intercourse until cure has been confirmed.

Infections due to *C. albicans* and gonococcal and puerperal infections need appropriate antibiotic therapy (Chapter 51).

Nonspecific vaginitis: Metronidazole, given in the dose of 400 mg twice daily for 7 days, is also useful in the treatment of mixed vaginitis due to an aerobe (*Gardnerella vaginalis*) and anaerobes. The infection causes a malodorous, off-white, vaginal discharge of high pH, giving a positive amine test. There is no inflammation of the vaginal wall.

Tinidazole and **secnidazole:** These imidazoles are effective in a single oral dose of 2 g in the treatment of vaginal trichomoniasis and giardiasis (Chapter 55).

GIARDIASIS

Giardia lamblia is a flagellate protozoan parasite of the small intestine. Like *Entamoeba histolytica*, it has no animal host and is transmitted from man to man by faecal contamination of food and water. It can cause diarrhoea, anorexia, nausea, vomiting, abdominal pain and weight loss. Both the cysts and trophozoites may be found in the stools. *Giardiasis is quite common and often exists in association with E. histolytica infection.*

Metronidazole is the drug of choice in giardiasis. It is given in the dose of 200 mg t.i.d. for 5 days in adults and 15 mg/kg/day in 3 divided doses for 5 days in children.

Nitazoxanide, a nitrothiazolebenzamide compound, is active against *Cryptosporidium parvum and* G. *Lamblia.*

It is a prodrug, which on oral absorption, gets converted to an active metabolite, tizoxanide. The latter acts like metronidazole and inhibits pyruvate-ferredoxin oxidoreductase (PFOR), an enzyme essential to anaerobic energy metabolism. Its precise mechanism for antianthelmintic activity is still unclear.

Food increases the absorption of nitazoxanide. It is extensively bound to plasma protein (99%) It is generally well tolerated. ADR include mild GI disturbances.

The adult dose is 500 mg (and for children 100–200 mg) b.i.d. for 3 days.

Other drugs used are **tinidazole**, 2 g single dose, **furazolidone** (100 mg q.i.d. for 7 days) and **paromomycin**.

DRUGS USED IN THE TREATMENT OF LEISHMANIASIS

Pentavalent antimony compounds	Diamidine derivatives	Miscellaneous
Sodium stibogluconate Meglumine antimonate	Dihydroxystibamidine isethionate Pentamidine isethionate	Amphotericin B Paromomycin (aminosidine) Miltefosine

CHAPTER 57

Chemotherapy of Viral Infections

Learning Objectives

This chapter will enable the reader:

1. To enumerate clinically important RNA and DNA viruses and state challenges in treating viral infections.
2. To classify antiviral drugs based on their mechanism of action.
3. To explain the mechanism of action, pharmacological effects, ADR and indications for drugs used in the treatment of herpes and CMV infections.
4. To enlist drugs used in the treatment of viral hepatitis giving their mechanism of action.
5. To enumerate anti-influenza drugs and mention their mechanism of action, pharmacological effects and ADR.
6. To explain mechanism of action of interferons and state their ADR.
7. To enlist various interferon formulations and their uses.

KEY TERMS

A virus is made up of a nucleic acid and nucleoproteins, which constitute the core of viral particle. This core is enclosed in a protein coat called **capsid**, which consists of repeating, identical subunits termed as **capsomeres**. Some viruses are, however, more complex and have additional outer lipid containing coats. *In general, the viruses with lipid coats (e.g. HIV, herpes, hepatitis and influenza) are sensitive to lipid solvents and nonionic detergents which dissolve the coating.* Viruses with only nucleocapsid are resistant.

Viruses are of two types (Box 57.1):

I. **Deoxyribonucleic acid (DNA) viruses**
II. **Ribonucleic acid (RNA) viruses**

Box 57.1 DNA and RNA Viruses

DNA viruses: Herpes simplex virus (HSV), varicella zoster virus (VZV), smallpox virus, hepatitis B virus (HBV), cytomegalovirus (CMV) and adenovirus

RNA viruses: Rabies virus, measles virus, mumps virus, rubella virus, dengue virus, yellow fever virus, poliomyelitis virus, human immunodeficiency virus (HIV), influenza virus and rotavirus

Most viruses survive outside the host cell only for a short time. After penetration into the target cell, viral replication occurs in the following steps:

1. Uncoating of viral nucleic acid strands
2. Synthesis of early regulatory proteins
3. Replication of viral DNA/RNA
4. Synthesis of late structural proteins
5. Coating and maturation of viral particle
6. Release from the target cell

Antiviral drugs can act at any of these steps.

The major difficulties encountered in the chemotherapy of viral infections are as follows:

- Viruses, unlike bacteria are intimately parasitic on host cells. They are obligatory intracellular agents. Hence, a drug that is expected to destroy the virus is likely to damage the normal host cells as well.
- Certain viruses multiply in the cytoplasm, whereas others do so in the nucleus of the infected cell. A drug which acts on a virus in the cytoplasm may

not necessarily act on a virus that multiplies in the nucleus and *vice versa*.

- Precise diagnosis of many viral infections is difficult. Further, *in vitro* efficacy of a new drug may not predict its therapeutic efficacy.
- In many viral infections, the greater part of the viral multiplication takes place before the clinical diagnosis can be made. The antiviral compounds are usually most effective during the stage of replication of the virus, which is difficult to detect clinically.
- Antiviral drugs **inhibit viral replication.** However, viruses start replicating after stopping the drug. This is a common problem in immunocompromised patients. Moreover, antiviral drugs may not eliminate latent viruses.
- Viruses have high mutation rates and hence develop drug resistance rapidly

Viruses cause cell injury by:

- **Direct lysis resulting from viral replication**
- **Lysis induced by antiviral antibody and the complement system**
- **Cell-mediated immune mechanisms**
- **Transforming host cells which proliferate and produce tumours**, e.g. papilloma virus causing cervical cancer

Since the multiplication of a virus is heavily dependent on host cell mechanisms, an effective antiviral agent must act intracellularly and selectively.

Classification of Antiviral Drugs

I. **Inhibitors of nucleic acid synthesis,** e.g. idoxuridine, acyclovir, ribavirin, trifluridine and azidothymidine (AZT)
II. **Inhibitors of attachment/penetration,** e.g. amantadine, rimantadine
III. **Inhibitors of viral enzymes**
   i) **Reverse transcriptase inhibitors,** e.g. lamivudine
   ii) **Neuraminidase inhibitors,** e.g. oseltamivir
   iii) **Protease inhibitors,** e.g. lopinavir
IV. **Immunological agents,** e.g. interferon, gamma globulin and monoclonal antibodies

ANTI-HERPES AND ANTI-CMV DRUGS

PH 1.48

IDOXURIDINE (5-Iodo-2′-Deoxyuridine): This compound, related to thymidine, acts by competing with it in the synthesis of DNA, and prevents the utilisation of thymidine. The drug interferes with the synthesis of host cellular DNA and, hence is too toxic for systemic use. It has been **employed locally** as 0.5% drops or ointment in the treatment of herpetic keratitis.

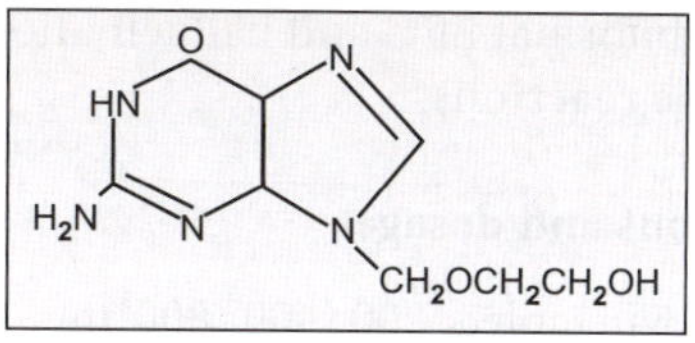

FIG. 57.1 Acyclovir.

TRIFLURIDINE: This nucleoside analogue has been used as 0.5% ophthalmic ointment to treat ocular herpes. It is less specific.

ACYCLOVIR: This guanosine analogue (Fig. 57.1) is a **potent antiviral drug of low toxicity.**

Mechanism of action: The drug is phosphorylated by viral-specific thymidine kinase to monophosphate derivative. Further phosphorylation by host cell kinases leads to the formation of **acyclovir triphosphate, which specifically inhibits virus induced DNA polymerase and thus inhibits viral DNA synthesis.**

The antiviral spectrum includes Herpes simplex virus (HSV) 1 and 2, Varicella zoster virus (VZV) and Epstein–Barr virus (EBV). HSV and VZV can develop resistance to acyclovir.

Absorption, fate and excretion: Given orally, it has a bioavailability of 15%–30%; the CSF level of the drug is 50% that of plasma. Hence, for viral encephalitis it is given intravenously. Its t½ is 3 h. **It is mostly excreted unchanged in the urine**; 15% is metabolised in the liver.

Adverse reactions: Locally, it may cause stinging and reversible superficial keratopathy. Orally, the drug is generally well tolerated. Given intravenously, it may cause headache, thrombophlebitis and elevation of blood urea and creatinine (**crystalline nephropathy**). CNS toxicity includes lethargy, tremors, abnormal EEG and hallucinations (**neuropsychiatric reaction**).

Preparations and dosage

i. Acyclovir tablets 200, 400, 800 mg. Dispersible tablets also available. Dose 200–400 mg 4–5 times a day.
ii. IV infusion as lyophilized powder 250/500 mg or as solution 25/50 mg/ml. Dose 5–10 mg/kg over 1 h at 8 h interval.
iii. Acyclovir eye ointment 3%
iv. Acyclovir cream 5% for skin application

Both, HSV and VZV produce their effects by destroying the epithelial cells by replicating in them. Once the damage is done:

- The healing time in an **immunocompetent** individual is unrelated to the virus. **Hence, to be effective, treatment must be started within 24 h of the onset of the rash.** Most of the herpes simplex lesions are mild and heal without any problems. They do not need the drug.
- In an **immunocompromised** person, however, failure to curtail viral replication may lead to prolongation of the local lesions and dissemination of infection. In such patients, treatment with acyclovir should be begun at any stage of the infection. Acyclovir reduces visceral complications but has no effect on healing of skin lesions or pain.

Indications:

- **Herpes simplex virus infection:**
  a. **Primary and recurrent genital infections:** It is highly effective in an oral dose of 200 mg 5 times a day for 7 days. Duration of therapy increased if new lesions appear during treatment or if healing incomplete.
  b. **Gingivostomatitis and pharyngitis:** also responds to above-mentioned regime
  c. **Keratoconjunctivitis:** It is used topically
  d. **Meningitis and encephalitis: Acyclovir IV is the treatment of choice**
- **Varicella zoster virus infection:** VZV causes varicella (**chicken pox**) **as primary infection. Reactivation of the virus**, which remains latent in dorsal root ganglia, **results in herpes zoster.**
  a. **Varicella:** Acyclovir is not routinely used if VZV infection is uncomplicated in children. In adults, 800 mg orally 5 times a day for 5 days decreases time to crusting, its eruption and duration of fever. Treatment should be started within 24 h of rash. Severe varicella pneumonia and encephalitis need IV therapy.
  b. **Localised herpes zoster:** Oral treatment with acyclovir in *immunocompetent individuals* should probably be reserved for those who have very early lesions and for those in whom the attack threatens to be widespread or in a critical area such as the face.

If acyclovir is given within 72 h of rash, in the dose of 800 mg 5 times a day for 7–10 days, it decreases pain and healing time but does not reduce the intensity of postherpetic neuralgia. It also decreases ocular complications of keratitis or uveitis. Given by IV infusion, it may be lifesaving in patients with encephalitis.

Both varicella and herpes zoster in the immunocompromised patient should always be treated with IV acyclovir.

- **Prophylaxis with acyclovir:** Prophylactic treatment with acyclovir is given to immunocompromised patients.

Penciclovir has similar mechanism of action but its triphosphate has less affinity for viral DNA polymerase than acyclovir. It achieves higher concentration in cells and has intracellular half-life of 7–20 h. **Valacyclovir** and **famciclovir** are prodrugs for acyclovir and penciclovir, respectively.

DOCOSANOL: It is a saturated 22-carbon aliphatic alcohol and an over-the-counter (OTC) product, available as 10% cream to be applied 5 times a day until healing. It is used **for recurrent orolabial herpes simplex**. It blocks the fusion between cellular and viral envelope membranes and thus inhibits viral replication.

The use of glucocorticoids in herpes zoster is best left to the specialists.

GANCICLOVIR: It is an acyclic nucleoside analogue of guanine with action similar to that of acyclovir but has higher intracellular concentration, which remains for 24 h. It is given orally or by IV infusion. It is excreted unchanged in urine.

ADR include GI disturbances, myelosuppression and aspermatogenesis. CNS symptoms include headache, behavioural changes and convulsions. It may also cause liver and renal dysfunction. It is carcinogenic, teratogenic and mutagenic in animals. Because of its toxicity, its use is limited to immunocompromised host with serious cytomegalovirus (CMV) infection of the retina and colon.

Valganciclovir is a prodrug for ganciclovir.

CIDOFOVIR: This acyclic cytosine nucleotide has similar mechanism as ganciclovir, but *does not require viral enzymes for phosphorylation; hence, it is active against resistant CMV and HSV*. Its active metabolite contributes to longer duration of action (intracellular t½ 17–65 h). Its CSF penetration is poor. The drug is eliminated by active renal tubular secretion.

The drug causes dose dependent renal tubular nephropathy. The other ADR include uveitis, iritis, ocular hypotony and neutropenia.

It is used intravenously for CMV retinitis.

It can also be used to treat Molluscum contagiosum in immunocompromised patients.

Letermovir is a novel inhibitor of the CMV viral enzyme DNA terminase, which is responsible for the cleavage of newly synthesized CMV DNA into individual viral genomes. It is indicated for prophylaxis of CMV infection and disease in adult CMV-seropositive recipients undergoing hematopoietic stem cell transplantation.

FOSCARNET SODIUM: This drug, an inorganic pyrophosphate compound, is given by IV infusion to treat **CMV retinitis** in patients with AIDS. It has potent activity against HIV as well. It inhibits DNA polymerase. *It does not require activation by viral thymidine kinase and is effective against acyclovir- and ganciclovir-resistant strains.* The drug can cause GI toxicity, nephrotoxicity, anaemia and CNS disturbances. Hypocalcaemia, hypokalaemia and hypomagnesemia have also been reported.

FOMIVIRSEN, an oligonucleotide agent, is used intravenously for the treatment of difficult cases of CMV retinitis.

SORIVUDINE is a pyrimidine nucleoside analogue which can be used in both immunocompromised and immunocompetent patients with herpes zoster infection.

ANTIHEPATITIS B DRUGS

Hepatitis B virus (**HBV**) infection is a global public health problem. Treatment of acute infection is mainly with supportive therapy and not with antiviral drugs. The therapy of chronic HBV infection depends on factors like clinical presentation, risk factors, immunological response, the HBV viral load and genotype. The main goal of therapy is to improve survival and quality of life by preventing disease progression, and consequent development of hepatocellular carcinoma. When the therapy is indicated, there are broadly two treatment options:

1. Nucleoside/nucleotide analogues (NA)
2. Pegylated interferon (IFN) alpha

1. Nucleoside/nucleotide analogues (NA): Mechanism of action of NA is represented in the Fig. 57.2.

LAMIVUDINE, an anti-HIV drug, has also been used for treating chronic HBV infection (Chapter 51).

ADEFOVIR is available as a prodrug, adefovir dipivoxil. It is phosphorylated by cellular kinases to active form. It is effective against HBV, HIV and herpes virus. It has prolonged intracellular t½ and is administered once daily. It is excreted by kidneys and requires dose adjustment in renal failure. It is nephrotoxic. Other ADR include headache, diarrhoea, asthenia, lactic acidosis and occasionally hepatic steatosis. It is not a preferred drug because of associated ADR and emergence of viral resistance.

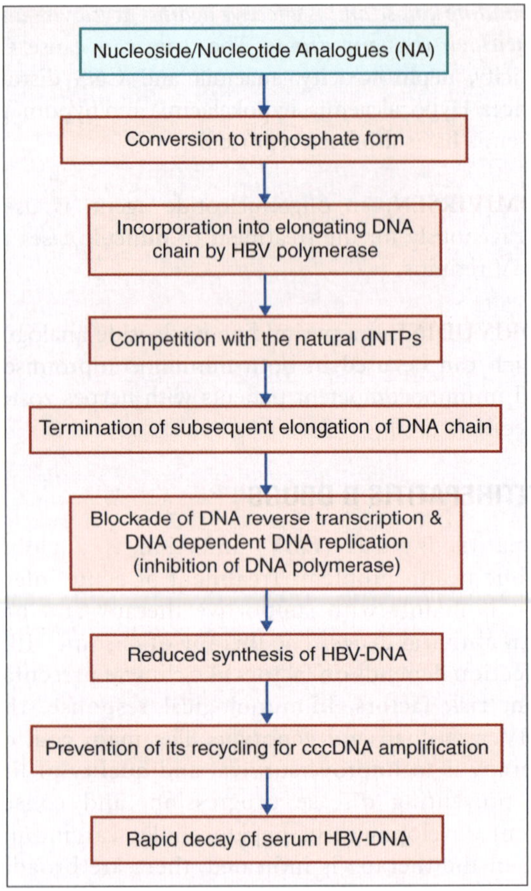

FIG. 57.2 Mechanism of Action of Nucleoside/Nucleotide Analogues (NA). HBV= Hepatitis B virus; dNTPs = Deoxyribonucleotide triphosphates; cccDNA=covalently closed circular DNA

ENTECAVIR is an orally administered guanosine nucleoside that competitively inhibits HBV DNA polymerase. This reduces the synthesis of HBV-DNA and its recycling for covalently closed circular DNA (cccDNA) formation. This results in HBsAg loss. Bioavailability is 100% but decreases with food. It is eliminated by kidneys. The ADR include headache, fatigue, nausea, and dizziness. It can cause drug interactions with drugs that compete for tubular secretion.

TELBIVUDINE, a thymidine nucleoside analogue, with similar action as entecavir, has bioavailability unaffected by food. It is widely distributed and has no documented drug interactions. Adverse effects are mild like fatigue, headache and GI intolerance. Lactic acidosis, hepatic steatosis and peripheral neuropathy may occur.

TENOFOVIR, an antiretroviral NRTI (Chapter 51) can be used for chronic HBV infection. It shows better activity than adefovir. It is useful against lamivudine and entecavir resistant organisms.

Tenofovir is available as: 1. Tenofovir disoproxil fumarate (TDF), 2. Tenofovir alafenamide fumerate(TAF), which is prodrug and claimed to have safer kidney and bone profile, and 3. Tenofovir exalidex, a lipid conjugate.

Entecavir and tenofovir (TDF or TAF) are the preferred NA regardless of the severity of liver disease. NA therapy may be required for at least 4–5 years of treatment, and in some life long therapy.

NA therapy suppresses viral replication and serum HBV-DNA remains undetectable. It also promotes seroconversion from HBeAg to antiHBe, which slows down the disease progression and reduces the risk of complications. Thus, high long-term efficacy, sustained virologic response, favourable safety profile and low potential for the development of resistance are the advantages of NA therapy. However, the cost of this prolonged therapy is high. The decline of serum HBsAg and of liver cccDNA is slow and usually incomplete. Low-level HBV replication persists and naïve hepatocytes get affected.

2. Pegylated IFN alpha (See section on Interferons): It clears infected hepatocytes and enhances cell mediated immune response. It is used to induce long-term immunological control. However, responses can be highly variable and safety profile is unfavourable.

A combined therapy (NA + IFN) may be used.

However, with both the therapies, though HBV DNA becomes undetectable, loss of HBsAg remains incomplete. Moreover, HBV genetic reservoir (cccDNA) remains within the nuclei of infected hepatocytes. It transcribes HBV pregenomic RNA (pgRNA) and other viral mRNAs. Chromosome integrated viral genome produces large amounts of viral subunit antigens (HBe, HBs), which are secreted in the blood stream. This exhausts HBV-specific T and B cell immunity. Currently there is no drug that will eliminate HBV cccDNA from the host and lead to complete functional cure.

ANTIHEPATITIS C DRUGS PH 1.48

Chronic hepatitis C virus (HCV) infection (with virus genotypes 1–6) is a leading cause of liver cirrhosis and hepatocellular carcinoma. Use of directly acting antivirals (DAA) orally for 8–12 weeks has improved the virological response >95% for most genotypes and offered a good tolerability.

Three nonstructural proteins in the genome of HCV (NS3/4A, NS5A, and NS5B) play a role in HCV replication, and serve as targets for drugs.

Classification of Directly Acting Antivirals Drugs for HCV

I. **NS3/4A Protease Inhibitors**
   Simeprevir, asunaprevir, paritaprevir, grazoprevir

II. **NS5A inhibitors**: Daclatasvir, ledipasvir, ombitasvir, elbasvir, velpatasvir

III. **NS5B RNA-dependent RNA polymerase inhibitors**
   a. *Nucleoside/nucleotide analogues (NPIs):* Sofosbuvir
   b. *Non-nucleoside analogues (NNPIs):* Dasabuvir

I. NS3/4A PROTEASE INHIBITORS

NS3/4A protease impairs induction of IFN and thereby prevents viral elimination by host cells. NS3/4A protease inhibitors block the NS3 catalytic site or the NS3/4A interaction. Inhibition of the NS3/4A protease enhances host immunological response.

SIMEPREVIR: This second-generation NS3/4A protease inhibitor is effective against HCV genotypes 1a and 1b. Simeprevir absorption is increased with food. It is metabolised primarily by CYP3A and excreted in faeces. It is a weak inhibitor of intestinal CYP3A4 and p-glycoprotein, Simeprevir is not recommended with ritonavir, efavirenz, nevirapine and cyclosporine. No dose adjustment is required in renal and mild hepatic impairment, but is contraindicated in moderate and severe hepatic impairment. The adverse effects reported when it is combined with RBV/IFN are nausea, myalgia, rash, photosensitivity, pruritus and dyspnoea.

Other drugs, **asunaprevir, paritaprevir, grazoprevir** are similar to simeprevir. All are administered orally with food. Asunaprevir is a moderate inhibitor of CYP2D6 and weak inducer of CYP3A4 while grazoprevir is a weak inhibitor of CYP3A. Paritaprevir is neither enzyme inducer nor inhibitor.

II. NS5A INHIBITORS

These drugs inhibit both viral RNA replication and virion assembly by binding to the NS5A (a replication regulator), causing structural distortions that interfere with its functions. They are potent and effective across all genotypes, but resistance can develop. The adverse effect profile is variable.

DACLATASVIR: It is well absorbed orally. Fatty meal decreases its bioavailability. It is highly bound to plasma protein (99%) and gets metabolised primarily by CYP3A4 and eliminated in the faeces. Its t½ is about 13 hours.

Generally, daclatasvir is well tolerated. The most common ADR include headache, fatigue, nausea and diarrhoea. Severe bradycardia has been reported when it was co-administered with amiodarone and sofosbuvir. It is an inhibitor of P-glycoprotein and organic anion transporting polypeptide. It is contraindicated with CYP 3A4 inducers like phenytoin, carbamazepine and rifampicin, whereas a dose reduction is recommended when it is used with CYP3A4 inhibitors. No dosage adjustment is required for patients with renal or hepatic impairment.

The other NS5A inhibitors, **Ledipasvir** and **Velpatasvir** are available only as a fixed-dose combination with sofosbuvir.

III. NS5B INHIBITORS

NS5B (RNA dependent RNA polymerase) has a catalytic site to which nucleoside/nucleotide polymerase inhibitors (NPI) bind causing chain termination. Non-nucleoside polymerase inhibitors (NNPI) bind to other sites causing allosteric alterations. The structure of this polymerase enzyme is common across all the HCV genotypes. Thus, the drugs that inhibit NS5B are effective against all the six genotypes of HCV.

SOFOSBUVIR: This pyrimidine nucleotide analog is phosphorylated within the cell and gets incorporated into the growing viral RNA strand and terminates HCV RNA strand synthesis prematurely.

Sofosbuvir is effective in combination with pegIFN and RBV. It is an excellent alterative if IFN therapy is contraindicated or stopped because of adverse effects.

Sofosbuvir can be administrated with/without food. Following a single 400 mg oral dose, 80% of the drug gets eliminated in the urine. No dosage adjustments are recommended for hepatic or mild-to-moderate renal impairment.

The most common ADRs are fatigue, headache, nausea, insomnia, pruritus, irritability, anaemia, asthenia, and diarrhoea.

Fixed Drug Dose Combinations for HCV Infection

Many fixed dose combinations of directly acting antiviral agents are available, which offer synergistic effects e.g., velpatasvir and ledipasvir (NS5A inhibitors) with sofosbuvir (NS5B RNA polymerase inhibitor), **Glecaprevir** (NS3 protease inhibitor) with **Pibrentasvir** (NS5A inhibitor), **Grazoprevir** (NS3 protease inhibitor) with elbasvir (NS5A inhibitor). Tripple drug combination of **Voxilaprevir** (NS3 protease inhibitor), velpatasvir and sofosbuvir is also available. But none of them offers permanent cure.

> In the treatment of chronic HCV infection, especially with decompensated liver cirrhosis, addition of ribavirin to the directly acting antivirals (DAAs) helps in enhancing sustained virological response rate.

ANTI-INFLUENZA DRUGS

PH 1.48

RIBAVIRIN (RBV): This purine nucleoside analogue has a broad spectrum antiviral activity against DNA and RNA viruses. It is administered orally or by inhalation. Aerosol therapy is generally well tolerated and its systemic toxicity is less because of poor systemic absorption. It has been shown to be of some use against influenza A and B infections, respiratory syncytial virus (RSV) infection, Lassa fever and hepatitis C.

Adverse reactions: It causes dose dependent anaemia, bone marrow suppression, cardiac and neurological toxicity. Ribavirin has been shown to be teratogenic, mutagenic, embryotoxic and gonadotoxic in small animals, and is contraindicated in pregnancy. *A woman must avoid conception for 6 months after cessation of ribavirin.* Further, passive exposure to aerosolised ribavirin should be avoided by pregnant women.

Antiviral monoclonal antibody palivizumab is used for prevention of RSV (Chapter 72).

AMANTADINE (1-Admantanamine hydrochloride): This drug acts by inhibiting uncoating of viral RNA of influenza A virus within infected cells, thus inhibiting early step in viral replication. **Clinically, it is useful in the prophylaxis and treatment of influenza A, but not of influenza B.** Its therapeutic usefulness, however, appears to be limited. To be effective, it must be administered within the first 24–48 h after the onset of symptoms.

The drug is administered orally in the dose of 100 mg once or twice daily for 5–7 days.

Adverse reactions: It causes anticholinergic effects (see Chapter 15). It can also cause confusion, high headedness, slurred speech, insomnia, hallucinations, urinary retention and skin rash.

It is also used in parkinsonism (Chapter 15).

RIMANTADINE: It has actions similar to those of amantadine but is 4–10 times more active. It has a long t½ of 24–36 h. No dosage adjustment is necessary in patients with renal impairment except in those with end stage renal failure.

Both the drugs show high drug resistance and are teratogenic in animals.

OSELTAMIVIR is a prodrug of oseltamivir carboxylate, the **first orally active, specific inhibitor of influenza neuraminidase.** This enzyme cleaves sialic acid residues on new virons to set them free from infected cells. Oseltamivir, by inhibiting the enzyme, prevents release of progeny virions and their spread to other cells.

It is effective against **both types of influenza viruses (including the avian H5N1, swine origin H1N1 and H9N2 strains)**. Given orally in a dose of 75 mg b.i.d. within 36 h of onset of symptoms, it can decrease the severity of influenza and reduces respiratory complications. The duration of therapy is for 5 days. For chemoprophylaxis, it can be administered 75 mg once a day for 7 days to contacts of patients within 48 h of the onset of symptoms.

Adverse reactions: The ADR include GI disturbances e.g. nausea, vomiting, diarrhoea and abdominal pain. It should be taken with food. Rarely, it may cause hepatitis, allergic rash, toxic epidermal necrolysis, seizures, and confusion. In high risk pregnant patient it may be preferred to zanamivir.

Is decreased in patients with renal damage to 30 mg b.i.d. or OD.

ZANAMIVIR: This drug is a potent inhibitor of the viral neuraminidase. Used within 48 h, it is useful against both types of influenza viruses and oseltamivir resistant infection. *It is given as dry powder inhalation (10 mg b.i.d. for 5 days)*. It can be used prophylactically once daily by inhalation. The drug can cause nausea, vomiting and bronchospasm. Both oseltamivir and zanamivir appear to be safe for use in pregnancy.

Both zanamivir and oseltamivir remain effective against viruses resistant to amantadine and are the drugs of choice. **There is no need to provide prophylaxis with antiviral drugs to healthy individuals exposed to influenza.**

Peramivir, another potent viral neuraminidase inhibitor is available for IV administration. Its efficacy and safety is comparable to oseltamivir.

Baloxavir, is an oral selective inhibitor of influenza capsid dependent endonuclease. It blocks influenza proliferation by inhibiting the initiation of mRNA synthesis. It is active against both, type A and type B influenza. It is indicated for the treatment of acute uncomplicated influenza in patients, who have been symptomatic for up to 2 days and for those at high risk of developing influenza-related complications. It is also approved for post-exposure prophylaxis of influenza.

DRUGS AGAINST CORONAVIRUS PH 1.48

Coronavirus, is a family of single-stranded, **RNA viruses** that cause wide range of illnesses ranging from common cold to severe acute respiratory syndrome (SARS). The highly pathogenic viruses amongst them responsible for respiratory virus epidemics include SARS- Coronavirus (SARS-CoV), Middle East Respiratory Syndrome Coronavirus (MERS-CoV) and the novel corona virus detected in 2019, SARS-CoV-2. These viruses can be transmitted through direct and indirect contact of the mucous membranes of the nose, mouth, or eyes.

There is currently no clinically proven specific antiviral agent available for these viral infections. Management of infected patients focuses on supportive therapy with use of antipyretics and analgesics, adequate nutrition and hydration, antitussives if required, oxygen therapy based on clinical monitoring, and control of co-morbid conditions. Antibiotics should be used only if there is a clinical suspicion of secondary bacterial infections. Systemic corticosteroids are not indicated in mild disease. In patients with moderate to severe disease, dexamethasone 6 mg/day or methylprednisolone (32 mg in 4 divided doses) is administered usually for 5 to 10 days or until discharge, whichever is earlier. There remains a risk of secondary infection such as invasive mucormycosis if steroids are used at higher dose or for longer time. The patients with moderate to severe disease are at a high risk of developing thromboembolic complications and need prophylactic UFH or LMWH (e.g. enoxaparin 0.5mg/kg per day SC). Most importantly, care should be taken to prevent transmission to others. The risk of transmission can be reduced by isolation of the patient, use of masks, proper and frequent washing of hands with soap, sanitization of surfaces in contact with the patient, and social distancing. These measures are often more important than the drug therapy.

SARS-CoV-2 was responsible for the global pandemic of 2020 and cause the disease designated as COVID-19, which is characterised by fever, sore throat, cough, myalgia, diarrhoea and dyspnea. Loss of smell (anosmia) or loss of taste (ageusia) may precede respiratory symptoms.

Though a number of drugs were advocated and tested during COVID pandemic, currently only the following agents are recommended:

RITONAVIR-BOOSTED NIRMATRELVIR

Nirmatrelvir is an oral viral protease inhibitor, which plays an essential role in viral replication by cleaving the viral polyproteins. Nirmatrelvir is combined with ritonavir, a strong cytochrome CYP3A4 inhibitor that serves as a pharmacokinetic booster by inhibiting metabolism of the co-administered CYP3A4 substrate(Chapter 51). It thus increases nirmatrelvir concentrations to the target therapeutic range. The recommended dose is nirmatrelvir 300 mg with ritonavir 100 mg orally twice daily for 5 days in non-hospitalized adults and children (aged ≥12 years and weighing ≥40 kg) with mild to moderate COVID-19 and are at high risk of disease progression. Treatment should be initiated as soon as possible and within 5 days of symptom onset. The ADR include change in taste sensation, diarrhea, hypertension, myalgia, allergic reactions and hepatotoxicity. It has a high potential for serious drug interactions due to presence of ritonavir, which can inhibit metabolism of concomitant medication administered to the patient.

REMDESIVIR

It is an adenosine analogue that can target the RNA dependent RNA polymerase and block viral RNA synthesis. It has shown antiviral activity against SARS-CoV-2 *in vitro*. It has antiviral potential against various RNA viruses including SARS and MERS-CoV *in vitro* and animal studies. It is administered intravenously. The reported ADR include nausea, vomiting, and transaminase elevations.

In non-hospitalized patients with mild to moderate COVID-19, who are at high risk of progressing to severe disease, remdesivir should be started within 7 days of symptom onset and administered for 3 days. The dose of remdesvir is 200 mg IV on Day 1, followed by 100 mg IV once daily on Days 2 and 3. Each infusion is administered over 30–120 minutes and patients are observed for ≥1 hour after completion of the infusion. Hospitalized patients should receive remdesivir for 5 days or until hospital discharge, whichever is earlier. In all these patients RFT and LFT should be monitored.

MOLNUPIRAVIR

Molnupiravir serves as an alternative therapy when neither of the above two therapies are available, feasible to use, or clinically appropriate. It is a prodrug of beta-D-N4-hydroxycytidine (NHC), a ribonucleoside that has shown antiviral activity against SARS-CoV-2 *in vitro* and in clinical trials. It is used for the treatment of adults with mild to moderate COVID-19, who are within 5 days of symptom onset. *It is administered orally* in the dose of 800 mg twice daily for 5 days. The reported ADR include diarrhea, nausea and dizziness. There are concerns regarding use of this drug as it can cause mutagenicity and genotoxicity.

The ICMR has issued guidelines for management of COVID-19, which are being revised time to time (https://www.icmr.gov.in/pdf/covid/techdoc/COVID_Clinical_ Management _19032023.pdf dated 05.01.2023).

These guidelines recommend remdesivir in those having moderate to severe disease, who are on supplemental oxygen. In patients who are having severe, rapidly progressing COVID-19, i.e. needing oxygen supplementation or invasive mechanical ventilation, having high CRP and/or IL-6 and not responding adequately to steroids, **tocilizumab** 4 to 6 mg/kg (400 mg in 60 kg adult) in 100 ml NS over 1 hour is recommended. It is preferably given within 24-48 hours of onset of severe disease/ ICU admission along with steroids. Before its administration active TB, fungal or systemic bacterial infection should be ruled out and these patients need long term follow up later on for reactivation of TB or flaring of herpes.

INTERFERONS

Interferons (IFNs) are **species specific cellular glycoproteins, produced naturally by virus-infected cells,** and have antiviral protective action. They can interfere with a wide variety of DNA and RNA viruses. They are considered as potent, broad spectrum, antiviral compounds with a high therapeutic ratio. The IFNs vary from species to species but each species produces at least three types of IFNs:

- **Alpha** and **Beta** from nearly all cell types induced by viruses, double stranded RNA and cytokines like Il-1, Il-2 and TNF.
- **Gamma** from immunologically stimulated T lymphocytes and NK cells.

Each of these can now be produced by recombinant DNA technology. Alpha and beta IFNs have 166 amino-acids and molecular weight, ranging from 16,000 to 26,000. Gamma interferon has 146 amino-acids with molecular weight 20,000–25,000; it has less antiviral and more immunoregulatory properties.

Certain agents like the live attenuated measles virus, microbial extracts and anionic polysaccharides can stimulate the production of endogenous interferon.

Mechanism of action: IFNs act by binding to specific, cell-surface receptors and inducing the production of new cellular RNA and proteins, which in turn inhibit protein synthesis of viruses. They inhibit several steps of viral reproduction. IFNs also act as an immune modulator, thus increasing cytotoxic T lymphocyte activity, enhancing NK cell activity and activating macrophages. **IFNs have no effect on extracellular virus.**

Table 57.1 Therapeutic Uses of the Commonly Used Antiviral (Non-HIV) Drugs

Drug	Route	Indications
Idoxuridine	T	HSV keratitis
Trifluridine	T	HSV keratitis, dermatitis
Acyclovir	T, O	Herpes genitalis; mucocutaneous HSV; local herpes zoster
	IV	Herpes simplex encephalitis; severe herpes genitalis; herpes zoster in the immunocompromised
Ganciclovir	IV	CMV infections
Foscarnet	IV	CMV retinitis; acyclovir resistant HSV infection
Amantadine	O	Influenza A
Rimantadine	O	Influenza A
Zanamivir	Inhalation	Influenza A and B
Oseltamivir	O	Influenza A and B
Adefovir	O	HBV infection
Lamivudine	O	HBV infection
Entecavir	O	HBV infection
Tenofovir	O	HBV infection
Simeprevir	O	Hepatitis C infection
Daclatasvir	O	Hepatitis C infection
Sofosbuvir	O	Hepatitis C infection
Ribavirin	Aerosol	Respiratory syncytial virus infection
Pegylated interferon alpha 2a/2b	SC,	Chronic hepatitis B, C and D; condyloma acuminata

Notes: T, topical; O, oral; IV intravenous; SC subcutaneous; CMV, cytomegalovirus; HIV, human immunodeficiency virus; HSV, herpes simplex virus.

They do not penetrate CSF readily.

Adverse reactions: These include hypersensitivity reactions, fever, flu-like syndrome, lethargy, myalgia, arthralgia and ocular symptoms. Dose-related myelosuppression, nephrotoxicity and hepatotoxicity have also been reported. Larger doses cause alopecia, neurotoxicity, personality changes, depression, reversible hearing loss, retinopathy, thyroid dysfunction, azotaemia and impaired fertility. Antibodies to IFNs can decrease their therapeutic effect.

Preparations and dosage:

- **IFN-alpha 2a and 2b** are available as only pegylated IFN-alpha 2a and 2b. They have prolonged absorption and reduced clearance resulting into increased t½. The higher and more sustained plasma levels allow once weekly dosages. They are administered subcutaneously as a single dose once a week.
- **IFN-beta 1a:** It is a glycosylated recombinant product from mammalian cells available for IM or SC administration.
- **Peginterferon–beta 1a:** It is available as SC injection.
- **IFN-beta 1b:** It is a nonglycosylated recombinant product from mammalian cells available for SC injection.
- **IFN-gamma 1b:** It is administered subcutaneously.
- **IFN-alpha n3:** is available for intralesional administration of twice weekly for a maximum of 8 weeks.

Indications:

- **Chronic hepatitis B:** Recombinant IFN-alpha 2b to prevent progressive liver damage
- **Chronic hepatitis C and D:** All forms of IFNs (see Table 57.1)
- **Condyloma acuminata:** Intralesional IFN-alpha n3
- **Hairy cell leukaemia:** IFN-alpha 2a and 2b
- **Chronic myelogenous leukaemia to induce remission:** IFN-alpha 2a
- **Kaposi sarcoma (in patients with HIV):** IFN-alpha 2a and 2b
- **Multiple sclerosis:** IFN-beta 1a and 1b are currently recommended for relapsing/remitting MS (Chapter 15).
- **Chronic granulomatous disease and malignant osteopetrosis:** IFN gamma 1b
- **All severe viral infections:** IFNs are given empirically.

Partially purified IFNs have shown. Antitumour effects in osteogenic sarcoma, multiple myeloma, lymphoma and breast cancer nodules.

GAMMA GLOBULIN: It prevents viral adsorption to and their penetration into the target cell (see Chapter 72).

Important uses of antiviral drugs are summarised in Table 57.1.

Antiviral drugs used to treat AIDS (HIV infection) are discussed in Chapter 51.

MANAGEMENT OF DENGUE, CHIKUNGUNYA AND ZIKA VIRUS INFECTION

Dengue, chikungunya, and Zika infections pose threat to public health world-wide. They are arthropod-borne viral diseases caused by arboviruses. There may be overlapping symptoms in these 3 diseases.

Dengue may present as a life-threatening infection. Symptoms suggestive of progression to severe disease in dengue include persistent vomiting, progressive abdominal pain, irritability, drowsiness, mucosal bleeding, clinical or radiological evidence of fluid accumulation, hepatomegaly, and progressive increase in haematocrit. Detection of these symptoms and warning signs are crucial in diagnosis and prognosis of Dengue.

Chikungunya manifests as fever associated with arthralgia, rash and headache. This may lead to a subacute phase lasting for 3 months. Infection may be life threatening in neonates, elderly, pregnant women and those with comorbidity due to failure organ system/s. It can lead to chronic, debilitating arthritis/arthralgia in up to 40% of infected individuals affecting their quality of life and may last for 6 years.

Many a times no symptoms are developed following infection with Zika virus. Fever, rash, headache, arthralgia/myalgia and conjunctivitis may be experienced. They are usually mild.

There is no vaccine or specific antiviral treatment for these infections and the emphasis is on control of fever and muscle aches with antipyretics (preferably with paracetamol 500 mg every 6 hours), adequate oral fluid intake, and sufficient rest. Physiotherapy may be advocated for Chikungunya. **NSAIDs may be given for Chikungunya or Zika virus infection after ruling out Dengue.**

Those with severe dengue, having warning signs, with comorbidity such as diabetes, children, elderly and pregnant women should be hospitalised and monitored for disease worsening and complications.

Intravenous fluid therapy with crystalloids is initiated in dengue patients with at least one warning feature, especially if the patient presents with shock. Transfusion of blood components (platelet concentrate, fresh frozen plasma) is not recommended to dengue patients with thrombocytopenia irrespective of platelet counts. They are used if the patient presents with bleeding or with a condition that poses a high risk of bleeding such as pregnancy. **It is necessary to avoid NSAIDs such as ibuprofen and aspirin, steroids and anticoagulants in dengue patients.**

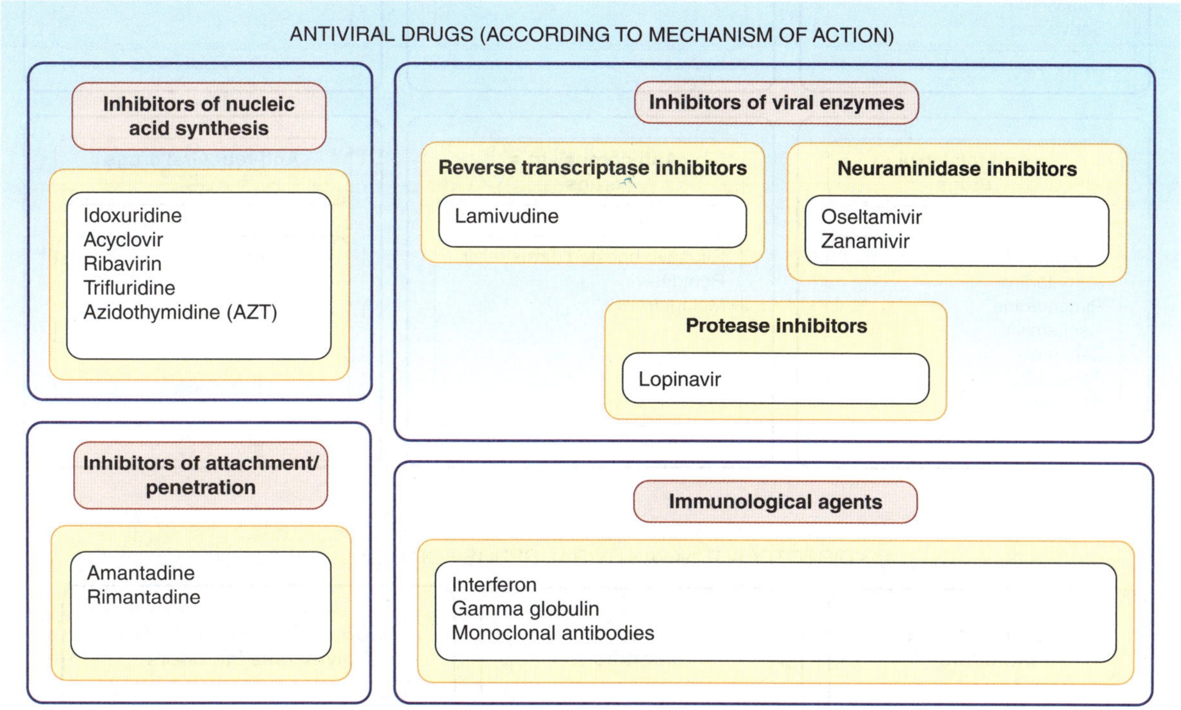

ANTIVIRAL DRUGS (CLINICAL CLASSIFICATION)

Anti-herpes and anti-CMV drugs

- Idoxuridine
- Trifluridine
- Acyclovir
- Penciclovir
- Valacyclovir
- Famciclovir
- Docosanol
- Ganciclovir
- Cidofovir
- Letermovir
- Foscarnet sodium
- Fomivirsen
- Sorivudine

Anti-hepatitis B drugs

- Lamivudine
- Adefovir
- Entecavir
- Telbivudine
- Tenofovir
- Pegylated IFN alpha

Anti-hepatitis C drugs

See the flow chart below

Anti-influenza drugs

- Ribavirin
- Amantadine
- Rimantadine
- Oseltamivir
- Zanamivir
- Peramivir
- Baloxavir

Anti-corona virus drugs

- Ritonavir boosted nirmatrelvir
- Remdesivir
- Molnupiravir

Anti-retroviral drugs

See Chapter 51

DIRECTLY ACTING ANTIVIRAL DRUGS FOR HCV

NS3/4A Protease inhibitors

- Simeprevir
- Asunaprevir
- Paritaprevir
- Grazoprevir

NS5A inhibitors

- Daclatasvir
- Ledipasvir
- Ombitasvir
- Elbasvir
- Velpatasvir

NS5B RNA-dependent RNA Polymerase inhibitors

Nucleoside/nucleotide analogues (NPIs)

- Sofosbuvir

Non-nucleoside analogues (NNPIs)

- Dasabuvir

CHAPTER 58

Chemotherapy of Helminthiases

Learning Objectives

This chapter will enable the reader:

1. To classify the drugs used in the treatment of helminthiasis as per their mechanism of action.
2. To explain the pharmacological effects, anthelmintic spectrum, adverse effects, indications and drug interactions of mebendazole.
3. To enlist the drug regimens for the treatment of (a) roundworm, (b) hookworm, (c) pinworm, (d) strongyloides and (e) guinea worm infestation.
4. To discuss the mechanism of action, pharmacological effects, ADR, indications, and contraindications of diethylcarbamazine.
5. To explain the pharmacological basis for use of ivermectin, albendazole and doxycycline in filariasis.
6. To outline pharmacotherapy of tapeworm infestation giving rationale for the agents used.
7. To discuss the mechanism of action, pharmacological effects, ADR, indications for praziquantel.

KEY TERMS

Worm infestation (helminthiasis) is one of the major global public health problems, more so in tropical countries. Besides the environmental conditions peculiar to tropics, poverty, illiteracy, lack of adequate sanitary facilities and pure water supply render total eradication of helminthiasis very difficult. The commonest parasites observed are roundworms, hookworms, threadworms, tapeworms, filarial worms and schistosomes.

Worms can cause various GI and general symptoms. In addition, some of them cause blood loss, nutritional deficiencies, urticaria and other allergic manifestations, intestinal obstruction and hepatosplenomegaly. Roundworms have been implicated in the pathogenesis of bronchial spasm in endemic areas. Peripheral blood eosinophilia occurs in all nematode infestations (except enterobiasis). A vigilant stool examination may often spare the unnecessary removal of teeth and tonsils, usually blamed for 'septic foci', in cases with 'resistant urticaria' which may be the only presenting complaint in helminthiasis.

The helminths are multicellular organisms possessing three germ layers and exhibiting a bilateral symmetry. They are classified into two major phyla (1) **phylum Nemathelminthes** (roundworms: **nematodes**) and (2) **phylum Platyhelminthes** (flat worms: **cestodes and trematodes** (Table 58.1)).

Anthelmintics are drugs used in the treatment of helminthiasis. In endemic areas, the main aim of anthelmintic treatment should be to reduce the load of infection below the level of clinical significance. Complete parasitological cure is often not possible due to surrounding environmental factors.

An anthelmintic drug which kills the worm is called **vermicidal,** while that which facilitates the easy expulsion of the worm without killing it is known as a **vermifuge**.

The anthelmintic drugs used commonly for therapy are listed in Table 58.1.

Table 58.1 Common Forms of Helminthiasis and the Drugs Used in their Treatment PH 1.47

Helminth	Common Name	Drug of Choice	Alternative Drugs
Nematodes (Intestinal)			
Ascaris lumbricoides	Roundworm	Albendazole, mebendazole	Pyrantel, piperazine
Ancylostoma duodenale	Hookworm	Albendazole, mebendazole	Pyrantel, thiabendazole
Enterobius vermicularis	Pinworm	Albendazole, mebendazole	Pyrantel, piperazine
Trichuris trichura	Whipworm	Mebendazole	Albendazole, thiabendazole
Strongyloides stercoralis	Threadworm	Ivermectin	Thiabendazole, albendazole
Trichinella spiralis	Pork roundworm	Albendazole	Thiabendazole, mebendazole
Nematodes (Somatic)			
Wuchereria bancrofti	Lymphatic filarial worm	Diethylcarbamazine	Ivermectin
Onchocerca volvulus	Oculodermal filarial worm	Ivermectin	Diethylcarbamazine
Onchocerca Loa loa	Oculodermal filarial worm	Ivermectin	Diethylcarbamazine
Dracunculus medinensis	Guineaworm	Metronidazole	Mebendazole
Cestodes			
Taenia saginata	Beef tapeworm	Praziquantel	Niclosamide
Taenia solium	Pork tapeworm	Praziquantel	Niclosamide
Cysticercus cellulosae[a]	Larva of *T. solium*	Albendazole	Praziquantel
Diphyllobothrium latum	Fish tapeworm	Praziquantel	Niclosamide
Hymenolepis nana	Dwarf tapeworm	Praziquantel	Niclosamide
Echinococcus granulosus	Hydatid larva	Albendazole	Mebendazole
Trematodes			
Schistosoma haematobium	Blood flukes	Praziquantel	Metrifonate
S. mansoni	Blood flukes	Praziquantel	Oxamniquine
S. japonicum	Blood flukes	Praziquantel	
Flukes			
Fasciola hepatica and Fasciola gigantica	Liver fluke	Praziquantel	Triclabendazole Niclosamide
Clonorchis sinensis	Chinese liver fluke	Praziquantel	Niclosamide
F. busci	Giant intestinal fluke	Praziquantel	Niclosamide
Paragonimus westermani	Lung fluke	Praziquantel	Triclabendazole Niclosamide

[a]Glucocorticoids are administered concurrently to reduce oedema.

Mechanisms of action of common anthelmintics are summarised in Table 58.2.

PH 1.47

DRUG THERAPY OF ROUNDWORMS

Benzimidazoles: These are broadspectrum anthelmintics. They include mebendazole, albendazole and thiabendazole.

MEBENDAZOLE: This drug (Fig. 58.1) given orally, is poorly (<10%) absorbed. It inhibits microtubule polymerisation in cytoskeleton by binding to beta-tubulin. The drug is slow acting and it may take 2–3 days for parasitic clearance from the gut. It also adversely affects the ova of the trichuris and the hookworm. It is effective *in vivo* against the larvae of *Trichinella spiralis* and exerts a lethal effect on the

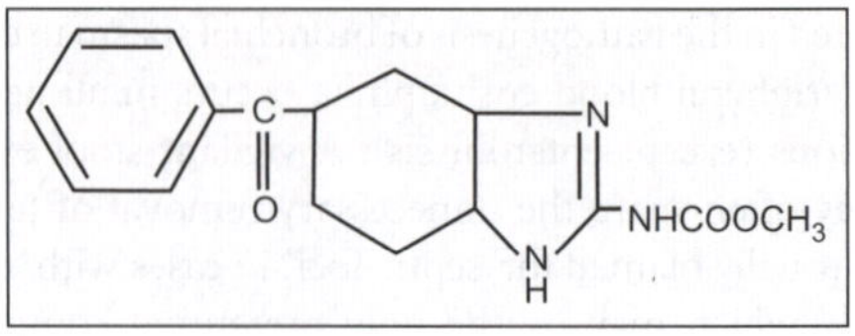

FIG. 58.1 Mebendazole.

Table 58.2 Mechanisms of Action of Common Anthelmintics

Site	Drug(s)	Mechanism
Neuromuscular Transmission		
a. Ganglionic nicotinic ACh receptors at neuromuscular junction[a]	Levamisole, pyrantel pamoate	Stimulation produces persistent depolarisation resulting in muscular contracture/paralysis
b. GABA receptors at neuromuscular junction	Piperazine	GABA agonist causing hyperpolarisation and flaccid paralysis
c. Glutamate-gated, chloride channel at neuromuscular junction in invertebrates	Ivermectin	Causes tonic paralysis of microfilariae which are then immobilised and phagocytosed by RE cells
Acetyl cholinesterase	Metrifonate	Inhibition, causing muscular contracture
Cell membrane	Praziquantel	Increases Ca^{++} influx leading to muscular contracture
Microtubules in cytoskeleton	Mebendazole, albendazole, thiabendazole, triclabendazole	Bind to beta-tubulin and inhibit polymerisation of microtubules
Mitochondria	Niclosamide	Inhibition of anaerobic phosphorylation of ADP leading to death

[a]The agonists cause contractions of the worm. Experimentally, it can be reversed by the ganglionic blocker, mecamylamine.

germinal membrane of the larvae of *Echinococcus granulosus* (Hydatid Worm).

It is highly effective in ascariasis, enterobiasis, trichuriasis and in hookworm infestation.

Adverse reactions: These are usually mild and consist of abdominal pain, nausea and diarrhoea. Large oral doses may cause vertigo, dizziness, headache and arthralgia. Benzimidazoles are embryotoxic and teratogenic in animals, and should be avoided in pregnancy.

Preparation and dosage: It is available as 100-mg tablets and liquid suspension.

Indications:

- **Enterobiasis:** A single dose of 100 mg repeated after 1 week. It is a drug of choice.
- **Hookworm and round worm infestation:** 100 mg b.i.d. for 3 days
- **Trichuriasis:** It is a drug of choice. See under the section, Drug therapy of trichuriasis.
- **Taenia infestation:** 300 mg t.i.d. for 3 days
- **Hydatid cysts of the liver:** 400–600 mg t.i.d. for 21–30 days for regression of hydatid cysts. Such treatment, though rarely, may cause bone marrow aplasia. *Hence, albendazole is preferred.*

ALBENDAZOLE: This has actions similar to those of mebendazole. It also has **larvicidal actions** in hydatid disease, ascariasis and ankylostomiasis and **ovicidal properties** in ascariasis, ankylostomiasis and trichuriasis. It is a drug of choice.

Given orally, it is rapidly absorbed and has better bioavailability than mebendazole. *After absorption, it undergoes first pass metabolism in the liver to its active metabolite, albendazole sulphoxide.* It is well distributed in tissues, bile, CSF and hydatid cyst. It has plasma t½ 8–12 h. **Its major advantage is that it is effective against many common intestinal worms in a single dose and is cost effective.**

The drug is well tolerated and adverse reactions are mild, mainly GI disturbances. Long term administration as in hydatid disease may cause alopecia, liver damage and bone marrow depression. It should be avoided in pregnancy.

Indications:

- **Ascariasis, ankylostomiasis and trichuriasis:**

Usually 400 mg single dose. Hookworm and trichuriasis may need a repeat dose.

- **Enterobiasis:** 400 mg single dose, repeated after 4 weeks
- **Hydatid disease:** 400 mg b.i.d. for 1 month, repeated if necessary.
- **Strongyloidiasis:** 400 mg twice daily for 3 days, repeated after 3 weeks if necessary
- **Trichinellosis:** 400 mg b.i.d. for 8–14 days
- **Cysticercosis: It is considered the drug of choice** because of short course, better penetration into CSF, less toxicity, and cost. It is given as 15mg/kg/day for 8 days. Treatment may be continued up to 30 days, if necessary. A glucocorticoid is started prior to albendazole to reduce the intensity of the inflammatory reaction to the dead parasites.
- **Other infections:** Albendazole, 400 mg/day, has been used for therapy of certain microsporidial intestinal infections in patients with AIDS. Infection with *Capillaria philippinensis* can be treated with a 10-day treatment regimen of albendazole (400 mg/day).

PYRANTEL PAMOATE: This pyrimidine-derivative is highly effective against round worms and pin worms and a little less effective against hookworms. It has a *depolarising, neuromuscular blocking action on nicotinic receptors of worms and causes spastic paralysis*. It is not much absorbed from the gut.

In ascariasis and enterobiasis, it is usually given in a single dose (10 mg/kg up to a maximum of 1 g); for hookworm infestation, the same dose is repeated on three successive days. The dose can be repeated after 2 weeks, if needed. **It can be used in pregnancy.**

Adverse reactions: These are usually mild and include GI disturbances, abdominal pain, headache, drowsiness and skin rashes.

Oxantel pamoate, an analogue of pyrantel, is also claimed to be useful in trichuriasis. It is given in a single dose.

PIPERAZINE: This drug (Fig. 58.2) was extensively used in the therapy of ascariasis and enterobiasis.

Mechanism of action: It acts as a *GABA agonist and causes hyperpolarisation of ascaris muscle resulting in*

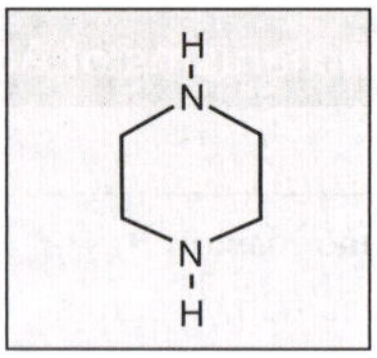

FIG. 58.2 Piperazine.

flaccid paralysis of the worms which are then easily expelled by peristaltic movements.

Absorption, fate and excretion: Piperazine is absorbed from the gut, to the extent of about 30%. The drug is partly metabolised in the body and partly excreted unchanged in the urine.

Adverse reactions: Piperazine has a wide margin of safety. Adverse effects are uncommon. They include nausea, vomiting, diarrhoea and urticaria. Neurotoxic effects, observed rarely; include vertigo, muscular incoordination, hypotonia, ataxia of cerebellar type (*worm—wobble*), and, blurring of vision. **The drug appears to be safe during pregnancy.**

Preparations and dosage: A variety of piperazine salts are available for therapy. They are equally effective.

i. Piperazine hydrate. Dose: Adults, 4 g as a single dose. Children, 120 mg/kg, up to a total dose of 4 g.
ii. Piperazine citrate as 300-mg tablets (equivalent to about 250 mg of piperazine hydrate), as an elixir and as a mixture for infants (750 mg per 5 mL)

For ascariasis in adults, a single dose of 5 g is administered.

For use of piperazine in enterobiasis, see section, Drug therapy of pinworms.

LEVAMISOLE: Levamisole is l-tetramisole (Fig. 58.3) and accounts for most of the antehelmintic activity of

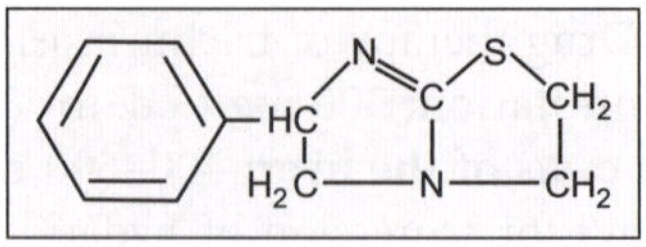

FIG. 58.3 Levamisole.

the racemic mixture, tetramisole. Like pyrantel, it causes sustained contracture of somatic muscles of the worm by an *irreversible, noncompetitive, depolarisation type of neuromuscular block.* It is rapidly and considerably absorbed and about 60% is excreted in the urine, mostly as metabolites, within 24 h.

Levamisole also has **immunostimulant** properties (Chapter 72).

Levamisole is available as a single-dose tablet containing 150 mg for adults and 50 mg for children. In **ascariasis,** it is given as a single dose of 2.5–5.0 mg/kg. It is also effective against **hookworms** though to a smaller extent. In **trichostrongyloidiasis**, a single dose is effective in over 95% of the cases. *These drugs are not active against larvae.*

Adverse reactions reported are usually mild and include nausea, vomiting, abdominal pain, diarrhoea, giddiness and drowsiness.

DRUG THERAPY OF HOOKWORMS PH 1.47

Ancylostoma duodenale infestation is very common in tropical countries and represents an important cause of iron deficiency anaemia due to intestinal blood loss. Acute clinical manifestations can be due to larval migration through various tissues and skin.

The infestation co-exists with ascariasis. It is preferable to treat ascariasis first, as drugs used solely against ancylostomiasis may irritate the roundworms causing their migration or aggregation into ball-like masses, which may precipitate acute appendicular or intestinal obstruction. Hence, drugs effective against both roundworms and hookworms are to be preferred.

It should be noted that a single course of therapy does not eradicate all the hookworms in 100% cases, and it is necessary to repeat the same drug or give another drug after an appropriate interval. **Albendazole** (400 mg single dose), **mebendazole** and **pyrantel pamoate** are the preferred drugs in ancylostomiasis (see above).

Adjuvant treatment: Regular, oral administration of **iron** daily can prevent the anaemia and maintain the haemoglobin levels without immediate treatment of worms. Provision of footwear to avoid larval penetration should be encouraged in endemic areas.

DRUGS THERAPY OF PINWORMS PH 1.47

E. vermicularis is a common parasite found in the caecum and the vermiform appendix. The infestation is more common in children. The majority of cases are asymptomatic. The gravid female worm deposits eggs on the perianal and perineal skin leading to intense itching. Gravid female worms sometimes migrate into the female genital tract, causing pelvic pain, vulvovaginitis, pruritus and even granuloma.

Antihistaminic cream may be applied around the anus to relieve itching. In recurrent cases, besides the drug therapy, additional measures are desirable, e.g. at night, the patient should wear gloves and pants under the pyjamas. Patients should be advised to boil the clothes. It may be useful to treat the whole family simultaneously.

Mebendazole 100 mg, or **albendazole** 400 mg single dose, repeated after 2 weeks, and **pyrantel pamoate** are the drugs of choice. Single doses of mebendazole produce 90%–100% cure rates.

DRUG THERAPY OF STRONGYLOIDIASIS PH 1.47

The adult female of *S. stercoralis* lives in the mucosal epithelium of the duodenum and the jejunum. Ova passed by the adult worm develop into larvae in the intestine. These larve develop into infective form either after their passage in the stool, in the soil and invade the human host by penetrating the skin or in the intestine itself; the latter penetrate the intestinal wall to reach the circulation (*internal autoinfection*). Internal autoinfection leads to persistence of the infection for up to 20 years.

The intestinal parasites cause epigastric pain and diarrhoea; heavy infections may produce malabsorption. In immunosuppressed or malnourished patients internal autoinfection may assume massive proportions with ectopic migration of larvae, resulting in *hyperinfection syndrome*. Hyperinfection syndrome is a serious complication with acute onset of fever, abdominal pain and distension, often accompanied by shock and pneumonitis.

IVERMECTIN in the dose of 100–200 mcg/kg daily for 2 days is considered the therapy of choice

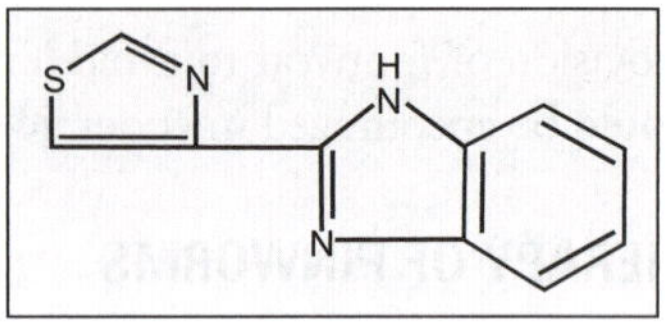

FIG. 58.4 Thiabendazole.

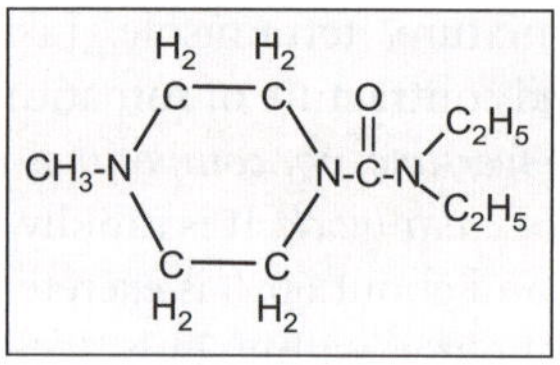

FIG. 58.5 Diethylcarbamazine.

(see section, Drug therapy of filiariasis).

Albendazole is another alternative (see section, Drug therapy of roundworms).

THIABENDAZOLE: This drug (Fig. 58.4), has a broad spectrum of activity and is effective against roundworms, hookworms, pinworms and strongyloid worms. It acts in the same way as other benzimidazoles.

Adverse reactions: These occur in 15%–30% of patients and include skin reactions, anorexia, nausea, vomiting, epigastric distress, dizziness and fever. Other adverse effects are hypotension, hypoglycaemia, disturbances of colour vision, liver damage and crystalluria.

Because of its toxicity, it is now rarely used.

DRUG THERAPY OF TRICHURIASIS (WHIPWORM) PH 1.47

Trichuriasis caused by *Trichuris trichura* (whipworm) is frequently co-exists with roundworms and hookworms. Children are unusually susceptible and develop anaemia.

Rarely, the worms may cause peritonitis.

Mebendazole is highly effective. It is given orally as 100 mg twice daily for 3 days or as a single 500 mg dose. A second course may be given after 3 weeks with a cure rate of almost 90%.

Albendazole is less effective; it is given in a single daily dose of 800 mg for 4 days.

DRUG THERAPY OF FILARIASIS PH 1.55

Filarial infections are caused by parasitic tissue-dwelling filarial nematodes, which are transmitted by biting insects (Table 58.3).

Different varieties of this worm infect over 250 million people in the world, causing hydrocoele, elephantiasis and blindness in severe cases. In case of lymphatic filariasis, the adult worm resides within lymphatics and can remain active for 5–8 years without causing any symptoms. About 4% of global cases of lymphatic filariasis are in India. In case of onchocerciasis, the adult worm resides in the subcutaneous or deeper tissues, forms a nodule and releases microfilariae that migrate to the skin and eye. Over 95% of global onchocerciasis burden exists in Africa and is a major cause of blindness.

The drugs used are **diethylcarbamazine, ivermectin, albendazole** and **doxycycline**.

DIETHYLCARBAMAZINE (DEC): This piperazine derivative (Fig. 58.5), is inactive *in vitro*. It leads to a rapid disappearance of microfilariae of *Wuchereria bancrofti, Brugia malayi* and *Loa loa* from the human peripheral blood after oral administration. It has some action in ascariasis.

Mechanism of action: The drug probably acts by sensitising the microfilariae so that they become susceptible to phagocytosis and are trapped by the

Table 58.3 Types of Filariasis

Type	Species	Vector
Lymphatic	*W. bancrofti, B. malayi*	Mosquitoes
Subcutaneous and ocular	*O. volvulus*	Blackfly (simulium)
Dermal	*L. loa*	Biting flies (chrysops)
Asymptomatic/ pruritus, arthralgia, neurologic or ocular	*M. perstans*	Infected midge/ black fly

fixed reticuloendothelial cells in the liver sinusoids. DEC also enhances cell mediated immunity (CMI) of the human host and thus resistance to the infestation. *The microfilariae of W. bancrofti in a hydrocoele, however, are not affected.* The drug also kills the adult worms of *B. malayi* and *L. loa* and possibly those of *W. bancrofti.* However, this action is slow and longer/repeated courses are needed. **It has no action against the adult worm of *O. volvulus.***

Absorption, fate and excretion: Diethylcarbamazine is rapidly absorbed from the GI tract. It is uniformly distributed in the body with the exception of fat. It is metabolised in the liver and eliminated in urine within 30 h.

Adverse reactions: The drug is usually well tolerated. The common ADR include anorexia, nausea, vomiting, headache and drowsiness. Allergic reactions, due to release of foreign proteins in the tissues by the death of larvae or adult worms, include fever, tachycardia, bronchospasm, lymphadenopathy, muscular pains, arthralgias and urticaria. In onchocersiasis the severe allergic reactions may involve the eyes (**Mazzoti reaction**). This may start within a few hours of first oral dose and persist for 3–7 days. It is recommended, therefore, to start the therapy with a small dose (50 mg, single dose) and then increase it gradually. Ocular reactions can be controlled by instillation of 5% hydrocortisone drops. Administration of antihistaminics or glucocorticoids can minimise systemic allergic effects. Large doses may cause muscle tremors and convulsions.

Preparations: Diethylcarbamazine citrate as 50 mg or 100 mg tab and 10 mg/mL or 120mg/ 5ml as syrup.

Indications:

- **Filariasis:** DEC is a drug of choice for active lymphatic filariasis (*W. bancrofti* and *L. loa* infestation). The recommended dose is 6 mg/kg body weight in single or divided doses daily for 10–12 days. The course may be repeated after 1 month. Although a single dose of 6 mg/kg may be useful, daily doses for 10–12 days are considered more effective. Combination of DEC with ivermectin or albendazole is synergistic. Daily DEC + albendazole for 7–10 days has significant macrofilancidal action.

  DEC has microfilaricidal effect in onchocerciasis, however, ivermectin is preferred as DEC may cause various ADRs, including worsening of the ocular condition.
- **Mass treatment of filariasis:** See later
- **Tropical eosinophilia:** Classical tropical eosinophilia with typical mottling in the lung, fever, anorexia, weight loss and attacks of dyspnoea resembling bronchial asthma is an *inflammatory response to microfilaria. It is associated with leucocytosis and marked eosinophilia (more than 3000/mm^3).*

  DEC in doses of 6 mg/kg body weight daily orally for 7–10 days is highly effective. Resistant cases may need double the dose.

  Pulmonary eosinophilia resulting from parasitic infestation, on the other hand, occurs as mild illness with fever and cough that lasts for a few days (*Loeffler syndrome*). This is due to transient allergic pneumonitis in response to parasitic antigens during the invasive stage of larval migration of roundworm and hookworm. This responds to appropriate anthelmintic treatment.

- **Larva migrans** (creeping eruption): In this condition, a dose of 3 mg/kg is given daily for 10–15 days. **Albendazole** 400 mg daily for 3 days or **ivermectin**, 200 mcg/kg as a single dose, is considered the treatment of choice.

IVERMECTIN: Ivermectin was originally obtained from *Streptomyces avermitilis* found in the soil sample of a Japanese golf course by Satoshi Omura and William Campbell (2015 Nobel prize winners). This macrocyclic lactone has been found to be highly effective against a broad range of parasites and arthropods, and is extensively used in veterinary medicine. *Ivermectin is the drug of choice in onchocerciasis.*

Mechanism of action: It activates glutamate gated chloride channel and causes hyperpolarisation. This leads to tonic paralysis of microfilariae, which are then phagocytosed by reticuloendothelial system. Its efficacy to eliminate the microfilarie from the skin and ocular tissues is as good as that of DEC but perhaps more sustained. *In addition, it has the* *advantage of being effective in a single dose.* However, the drug has no lethal effect against adult worms.

Absorption, fate, excretion: It is well absorbed and is highly protein-bound in the plasma. More than 97% is metabolised in the liver and is mostly eliminated in the faeces. Its elimination t½ is 12–56 h.

Adverse reactions: Compared with DEC, it is better tolerated. It may cause itching, skin oedema, arthralgia, headache and fever. The ADRs are mostly due to the death of microfilariae (Mazzoti reaction), which causes ocular inflammation that may rarely, lead to blindness. Ivermectin has GABA agonistic activity, and hence, it should be avoided in meningitis and along with CNS depressants.

Indications:

- **Onchocerciasis:** A single dose of 150 mcg/kg is highly effective. However as the adult worm is not killed, it is advisable to repeat the same dose once in 6–12 months for 10–14 years. If symptoms recur, then the same dose is given every 3 months instead of once a year, for the rest of the period. It appears that a single dose of ivermectin once every 6–12 months is useful in preventing this disease. When onchocerciasis and loiasis coexist, a single annual dose of 400 mcg/kg can be used.
  As a curative treatment of severe onchocerciasis, suramin (Chapter 56) is sometimes used. It kills the worm but is highly toxic. Doxycycline 200 mg daily for 6 weeks is claimed to be macrofilaricidal.
- **Lymphatic filariasis:** Ivermectin in a single dose of 100–200 mcg/kg is highly effective against the microfilariae of *W. bancrofti*. Single annual doses of 400 mcg/kg are effective and safe for prophylaxis.
- **Intestinal nematode infection:** Ivermectin as a single dose of 100 mcg/kg is used for strongyloidiasis. A higher dose of 150–200 mcg/kg is used when ascariasis, trichuriasis and enterobiasis coexist.
- **Scabies and head-lice infestation:** Given as a single oral dose (150–200 mcg/kg) it has been found to be highly effective.

This drug has shown broad spectrum antiviral activity *in vitro* and has been used with doxycycline in the treatment of SARS-CoV-2. Additional studies are needed to confirm its anri-COVID-19 potential.

Moxidectin, a macrocyclic lactone related to ivermectin, is used for the treatment of onchocerciasis due to *O. volvulus* in patients aged > 12 years. It has greater activity than ivermectin. It has a very long t½ of 23 days. It is a poor substrate for p-glycoproteins and is also less prone to cause drug interactions with CYP3A4 substrates.

It is also useful in the treatment of trichuriasis when given with albendazole and has excellent activity in strongyloidiasis. A single dose of 8 mg (four tablets, each containing 2 mg of moxidectin) is recommended. Moxidectin is also used to treat scabies and head lice (Chapter 69).

ALBENDAZOLE 400 mg given in combination with DEC or ivermectin reduces the peripheral microfilarial load for longer time than monotherapy. There is no added effect on adult worm.

DOXYCYCLINE: Filariae act as a host to endo-symbiotic *Wolbachia* bacteria. The growth, reproduction and survival of adult worm depend on *Wolbachia*. Wolbachia lipoprotein has been blamed for promoting chronic disease by provoking inflammatory reaction. The release of *Wolbachia* from dying microfilariae induces the systemic inflammatory response.

Doxycycline 200 mg/day for 6 weeks is reported to cause a long-term sterilising effect in bancroftian filariasis; eventually causing death of the adult worm. Similar macrofilaricidal effect has been reported in onchocerciasis, with doxycycline 100 mg/day for 6 months. However, it is not the drug of choice for treating filariasis, nor it is useful for mass treatment. It may be used to treat individual cases. It is contraindicated in children and pregnant women (see Chapter 47).

Mass Treatment of Filariasis PH 1.55

In endemic areas, mass treatment is given with the objective of reducing microfilariae to subinfective levels. DEC incorporated in table salt (0.2%–0.4% of the base by weight) has been found to reduce the prevalence. Either (DEC 6 mg/kg + albendazole 400 mg) or (ivermectin 200 mcg/kg + albendazole 400 mg) in single doses every 6–12 months has shown to be more effective than either drug used alone in controlling the transmission of filariasis, including lymphatic filariasis. The combination of DEC 6 mg/kg and ivermectin 400 mcg/kg, given as a single dose, once a year, is also reported to be effective. Recent Egyptian studies indicate that yearly rounds of DEC + albendazole for 5 consecutive years can possibly eliminate filariasis from an endemic area.

Mansonelliasis infection: *Mansonella perstans* is usually asymptomatic and considered as minor filariasis. It is common in Africa.

Effective treatment is, however, lacking. DEC is often ineffective. Long-term doxycycline (200 mg daily for 6 weeks) has been claimed to be effective.

DRUG THERAPY OF GUINEA WORM

Dracunculus medinensis infestation is transmitted by drinking of water containing infected cyclops (water flea). The adult female usually remains in subcutaneous tissue and may come out through a small ulcer, usually on the foot.

The treatment mainly consists of mechanical removal of the worm. **Metronidazole** is helpful in this process. **Mebendazole** in the dose of 200 mg t.i.d. orally for 7–10 days is also claimed to be effective in helping easy expulsion. The important treatment of dracontiasis is preventive. This is very simple as the intermediate host, cyclops, can easily be filtered out from the drinking water by using a piece of cloth.

DRUG THERAPY OF TAPEWORMS

This infestation is transmitted by ingestion of infected beef or pork and can be prevented by avoiding the ingestion of suspected meat or by its thorough cooking.

PRAZIQUANTEL: It is the drug of choice in taeniasis. In a single dose of 10 mg/kg it is highly effective against intestinal taeniasis, *Taenia saginatum, Taenia solium* and *Diphyllobothrium latum* – infections, as well as in cysticercosis of the brain. A single dose of 25 mg/kg is used to treat H. nana infection. For details, see section, Drug therapy of schistosomiasis.

MEBENDAZOLE/ALBENDAZOLE: These drugs are used to treat hydatid disease of the liver.

NICLOSAMIDE (Chlorsalicylamid): This drug (Fig. 58.6) is effective in *T. saginata, T. solium, D. latum* and *H. nana* infestations. Given orally, it is not absorbed. It inhibits anaerobic phosphorylation of ADP by the parasitic mitochondria.

Niclosamide is a vermicidal drug. The segments of the worm which are voided after its administration are partially digested by the action of the intestinal proteolytic enzymes; this makes identification of the scolex impossible. The criterion for cure with this drug, therefore, is absence of eggs and proglottids in the stools for 3–4 months after therapy. This is the period required for *T. saginata* to mature and shed mature proglottids from the scolex.

In *T. solium* infestation, identification of scolex is important as cysticercosis, (i.e. harbouring of the larval forms, cysticerci in the tissues) may develop, if the infestation is not completely eradicated. This makes it mandatory to use a purge within 1–2 h after niclosamide is given, in order to prevent digestion of the segments. As niclosamide does not affect the ova, regurgitation of viable ova can result in autoinfection with larvae and thus cysticercosis. *Niclosamide is not effective against cysticercosis. Hence, in the treatment of infection with T. solium, praziquantel is preferred.*

The major advantage of niclosamide is its lack of serious toxicity. It causes mild GI disturbances.

The patient is advised to take a light meal on the previous day and fast overnight, following which 2 tablets of the drug (1 g) are given in the morning on an empty stomach. The tablets should be chewed and not swallowed. Another 1 g is given after 1 h. A

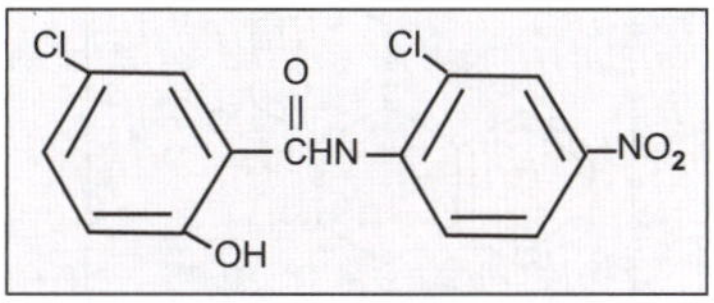

FIG. 58.6 Niclosamide.

saline purge may be given 1–2 h after the second dose but is not essential except in *T. solium* infestation. The dosage in children is 1 g for those between 2 and 8 years and 0.5 g under 2 years. Infestation with *H. nana* requires treatment for 5–7 days.

DRUG THERAPY OF SCHISTOSOMIASIS

Schistosomiasis (bilharziasis) is caused by blood flukes (Schistosomes) that reside as parasites in the venous channels. The three common species are *Schistosoma haematobium*, *S. mansoni* and *S. japonicum*. The parasites are localised in organs other than the gut. Free living cercariae, emerging from the water snail (intermediate host), penetrate the human skin and mature into the adult worms. The infection causes:

- **Cercarial dermatitis (Swimmer's itch)** due to repeated exposure to larvae
- **Acute schistosomiasis or Katayama fever,** a serum sickness-like illness, more common with *S. japonicum*
- **Chronic illness associated with the formation of egg granuloma** as in various tissues such as urinary bladder and intestines, leading to obstructive and inflammatory lesions. *S. mansoni* causes intestinal and hepatic schistosomiasis, whereas *S. haematobium* causes urinary disease.

PRAZIQUANTEL: This drug (Fig. 58.7) is highly effective against:

1. **Trematodes** including **Schistosomes (blood flukes),** and **tissue flukes** (liver, lung and intestinal)
2. **Cestodes**

Mechanism of action: The drug *increases the permeability of cell membrane to calcium ions,* leading to strong muscular contractions and tegumental damage causing the schistosomes to detach from the wall of the vein. **It has negligible effect on ova.**

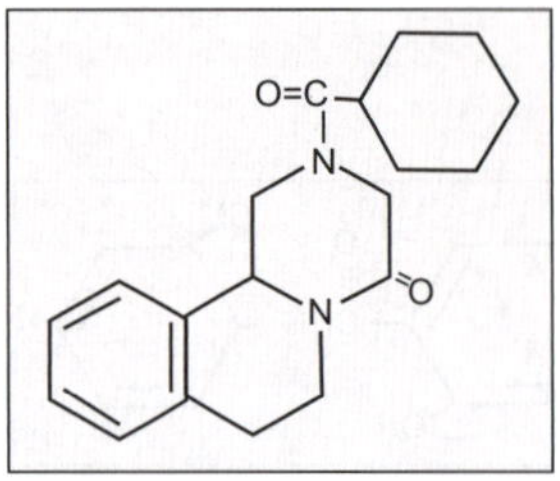

FIG. 58.7 **Praziquantel.**

Absorption, fate and excretion: Given orally, praziquantel is rapidly absorbed, but a significant proportion of the drug is metabolised during the first pass. Its absorption is increased by a high carbohydrate meal. **It acts within 1 h of ingestion.** Its plasma t½ is 1–1.5 h. Approximately 70%–80% of a dose is excreted in urine within 24 h.

Adverse reactions: These are dose dependent and are usually mild such as headache, anorexia, drowsiness, dizziness, lassitude, colic and allergic reactions. *It is considered safe in children and pregnant women.*

Indications:

- **Schistosomiasis:** It is the drug of choice and is given orally in the dose of 40 mg/kg for *S. haematobium* infection and 60 mg/kg for *S. mansoni* and *S. japonicum* infections. The total dose may also be divided into two doses given 4 h apart. It is very bitter and the tablet should be swallowed. A cure rate of 80%–90% has been claimed in *S. haematobium* infection and more than 60% in infection with the other species, at one year follow-up. Even in those in whom the disease is not cured, the egg count drops by more than 90%. The dose may be repeated after 6–8 weeks. Because of its short t½, it is not used for prophylaxis.

Praziquantel cannot kill the schistosomules (migrating larvae) that are 3–21 days old. **Artemether** (Chapter 54) does kill them during the first 21 days in the body, and may be given in the dose of 6 mg/kg every 2 weeks. *A combination of artemether and praziquantel is synergistic in killing the adult worm.*

Katayama fever is treated with a glucocorticoid along with praziquantel.

- **In taeniasis**, a single dose of 10 mg/kg produces high cure rates. *Praziquantel does not* *kill the ova and hence a post-treatment purge is advised in T. solium infection.* A single dose of 20 mg/kg is highly effective in *H. nana* infection. Although it is effective in the treatment of cerebral cysticercosis in the dose of 50 mg/kg/day in three divided doses for 14–30 days, albendazole is usually preferred (see Albendazole).

- **In fluke infestations:** See section, Drug therapy of flukes
- **Hydatid disease:** It may be used as an adjunct to albendazole

OXAMNIQUINE: This, tetrahydroquinoline derivative, is well absorbed when given orally. *It is effective only against S. mansoni (African) infestation.* ADR include dizziness, somnolence, abdominal pain, headache and diarrhoea. It is better tolerated after meals. Rarely, it causes hallucinations and seizures. The urine may be coloured red. It should be avoided during pregnancy. The dose varies according to the geographical region. The cure rate is 60%–90%.

METRIFONATE: This prodrug owes its effects to its metabolite dichlorovas, which is an organophosphorous cholinesterase inhibitor (Chapter 19). It is effective only in *S. haematobium* infestation with a cure rate of 40%–80%. The ADR are mild and transient, usually GI disturbances. However, it is not commercially available.

DRUG THERAPY OF TISSUE FLUKES

PRAZIQUANTEL: **This is a drug of choice against lung and intestinal flukes.** The recommended dose is 75 mg/kg, divided into three doses given on the same day. The dose may be repeated (see above).

Thiabendazole, as a single dose of 10 mg/kg for liver and lung flukes infestation, is also useful.

Bithionol 30 mg/kg daily for 5 days is also effective but more toxic. Also see Chapter 60.

TRICLABENDAZOLE

This is a narrow spectrum benzimidazole derivative. It is used in the treatment of fascioliasis, which is caused by flatworms, *Fasciola hepatica* or *Fasciola gigantica*, the liver flukes.

Mechanism of action: The precise mechanism of action is unknown but current evidence indicates that triclabendazole primarily binds to beta-tubulin and prevents the polymerization of microtubules. This prevents the movement of secretory granules to the tegmental surface, which causes disruption of tegmental integrity. It inhibits adenylate cyclase activity which affects various essential cellular processes such as energy metabolism or neuromuscular co-ordination. The sulphoxide metabolite appears to have a delayed but more potent effect on parasite motility than triclabendazole itself.

Absorption, fate and excretion: Given orally, triclabendazole is rapidly absorbed and reaches peak in 2-3 h. It undergoes pre-systemic biotransformation in plasma to sulfoxide metabolite. Food enhances the AUC of sulfoxide metabolite increasing its t½ to 11h. Hence triclabendazole should be administered with food. The parent drug along with sulfoxide metabolite undergo biliary elimination in the faeces.

Adverse reactions: The drug is generally well tolerated. Urticaria, pruritus and rash have been reported after its use. The uncommon adverse effects include headache, dizziness and vertigo. Biliary colic like symptoms may appear 3-7 days after the treatment and may be related to the expulsion of dead or dying flukes into biliary ducts. The abdominal pain may be associated with raised hepatic enzymes and alkaline phosphatase suggestive of obstructive jaundice. The colic is treated with antispasmodics.

Indications:

- **Fascioliasis:** Triclabendazole is administered in a single dose of 10 mg/kg and repeated after a day in patients with high infection intensity.
- **Lung fluke infestation:** It is an alternative drug to praziquantel.

ANTHELMINTIC DRUGS

Against nematodes (Intestinal)

- Albendazole
- Mebendazole
- Pyrantel pamoate
- Piperazine
- Ivermectin (against *Strongyloides stercoralis*)
- Thiabendazole

Against nematodes (Somatic)

- Diethylcarbamazine
- Ivermectin
- Metronidazole (against *Dracunculus medinensis*)
- Mebendazole (against *Dracunculus medinensis*)

Against cestodes

- Praziquantel
- Niclosamide
- Albendazole (against Cysticerci and *Echinococcus granulosus*)

Against trematodes

- Praziquantel
- Metrifonate
- Oxamniquine

Against tissue Flukes

- Praziquantel
- Niclosamide
- Triclabendazole (against *Paragonimus westermani*)

CLASSIFICATION OF ANTHELMINTHICS BASED ON MOA

At neuromuscular transmission

- **Ganglionic nicotinic ACh receptors agonists**
  - Levamisole
  - Pyrantel pamoate
- **GABA receptors agonists**
  - Piperazine
- **Glutamate-gated, chloride channel**
  - Ivermectin

Acetyl cholinesterase inhibitors

- Metrifonate

At microtubules

- **Polymerisation inhibitors**
  - Mebendazole
  - Albendazole
  - Thiabendazole

At cell membrane

- **Increase in calcium ion influx**
  - Praziquantel

At mitochondria

- **Inhibition of anaerobic phosphorylation**
  - Niclosamide

CHAPTER 59

Chemotherapy of Malignancy

Learning Objectives

This chapter will enable the reader:

1. To state the differences between cancer chemotherapy and antimicrobial chemotherapy.
2. To describe various stages of the cell cycle and specify anticancer drugs effective in each stage of cell cycle.
3. To compare and contrast cytotoxic chemotherapy and targeted chemotherapy.
4. To classify anticancer drugs based on their mechanism of action giving examples of drugs from each class.
5. To state common toxicity of cytotoxic drugs.
6. To explain the salient pharmacokinetic features, ADR and indications for alkylating agents, antimetabolites, radioactive isotopes, cytotoxic antibiotics, antimitotic natural products, hormones and their antagonists.
7. To explain the role of tyrosine kinase inhibitors and monoclonal antibodies in the management of cancer.
8. To discuss the principles of management of cancer with chemotherapeutic agents.
9. To state the palliative symptom control measures in terminally ill cancer patients.

KEY TERMS

cytotoxic drugs, p. 833
targeted cancer therapy, p. 833
cyclophosphamide, p. 834
mesna, p. 835
cisplatin, p. 836
methotrexate, p. 836
6-mercaptopurine, p. 837
5-fluorouracil, p. 838
gemcitabine, p. 838
radioiodine, p. 839
doxorubicin, p. 840
hormones and antihormonal drugs, p. 841
monoclonal antibodies, p. 844
tyrosine kinase inhibitors, p. 845
metronomic chemotherapy, p. 846
chemotherapy principles, p. 847
palliative symptoms control, p. 848

Recent advances in both medical and surgical therapies for cancer have markedly improved the mortality and morbidity in cancer. Almost over 60% of patients diagnosed early with cancer can now be cured. The aetiology of cancer is complex. Various multiple factors are implicated in carcinogenesis; only in about 10% cases, it is genetically inherited.

Chemotherapy of malignancy differs in some respects from that of infection:

- In infections, the invading microbe is biologically 'foreign' to the host and its metabolic reactions are so different from those of the host tissue cells that a chemotherapeutic agent can attack it selectively without affecting the host tissue cells. No such clear-cut differences in metabolic reactions have been demonstrated between malignant and normal cells.
- In infections, the body helps the antimicrobial drug with its own defence system in the form of antibodies, phagocytosis, etc. Although antibodies have been demonstrated against certain cancer cells, such host defence is usually lacking or ineffective.

Cancer of the epithelial tissues is called **carcinoma** and that of the nonepithelial (mesenchymal) tissues is known as **sarcoma**.

The characteristics which distinguish the cancer cells from normal cells are as follows:

- **Uncontrolled (autonomous) proliferation**
- **Dedifferentiation and loss of function**
- **Tissue invasiveness/metastasis**

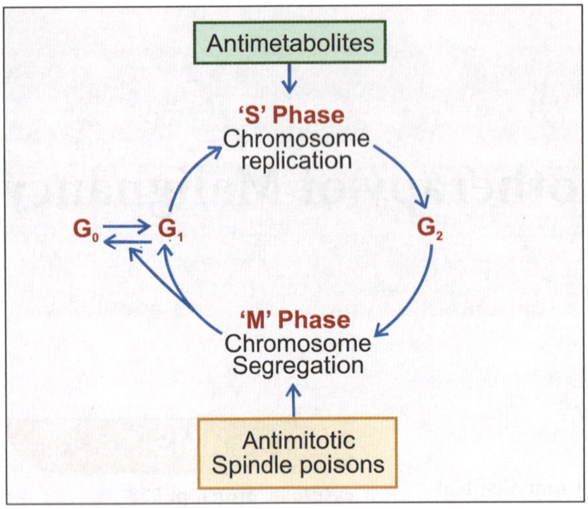

FIG. 59.1 **Cell cycle and sites of action of drugs.**

The normal cell proliferates through a definite **cell cycle**, which causes programmed DNA replication. The mechanism of cell division is divided into five phases (Fig. 59.1). Thus, the cell successively goes through:

1. **G_0 (gap 0 or resting) nonproliferative phase,** which may last for few hours to years
2. **G_1 (gap 1, i.e. presynthetic) phase,** during which the cell synthesizes proteins needed for DNA synthesis; the cells grow larger and it lasts for 18-30 h
3. **S (synthetic) phase**, during which chromosomes start to divide and copy. This lasts for 18-20 h.
4. **G_2 (gap 2, i.e. postsynthetic) phase**, during which the accuracy of DNA replication is determined, and errors are corrected. Synthesis of cellular component needed for mitosis also starts. This stage lasts for 2-10 h.
5. **M (mitotic) phase**, during which the replicated chromosomes are separated into two nuclei along with cytoplasmic division for the two daughter G_1 cells. This lasts for 30-60 min.These cells may re-enter the cycle or pass into the resting G_0 phase. Drugs can block any of these phases and inhibit the cell growth.

Topoisomerases I and II play an important role during DNA replication. The cell-cycle transition between G_1 and S and that between G_2 and M are so well regulated that the cell divides properly with a minimum of errors. Check points in G_1 and G_2 determine whether the cell will enter S and M, respectively. **These check points are regulated by protein kinases (cyclin-dependent kinases, cDK) and kinase-associated proteins called cyclins.**

In the cancer cell, deregulation of the cell cycle control occurs by:

- **Abnormal growth factor function**
- **Abnormal cyclins and/or cDK function**
- **Abnormal DNA synthesis**
- **Abnormal decreases in negative regulatory factors due to mutation in the tumour suppressor gene p53**

Apoptosis acts as the first line of defence against mutations and renewal of cells with abnormal DNA that could become malignant.

The treatment approaches to cancer can be following:

1. **Kill or remove the cancer cells:** This can be achieved by:
   a. **Cytotoxic chemotherapy:** These drugs act on all rapidly dividing normal and cancerous cells and kill them. Their action is thus not specific for cancer cells. They are mostly effective during S phase of cell cycle and many of these drugs cause DNA damage, which results in initiation of apoptosis and cell kill. Hence the term 'cytotoxic'.
   b. **Radiotherapy.**
   c. **Targeted cytotoxic agents,** e.g. antibodies linked to toxins. See below.
   d. **Surgery**
2. **Targeted cancer therapy:** It uses drugs that block the growth and spread of cancer by interfering with specific molecules (**'molecular targets'**) that are involved in the growth, and spread of cancer. Thus, the targets are identified first (specific genes, proteins, or the tissue environment) and the drugs are designed to interact with the targets. These are often **cytostatic (block tumour cell proliferation)**. Two types of drugs are used in targeted therapies:
   a. **Small molecules** which can enter the cells to act on the target located within the cells
   b. **Monoclonal antibodies**, which are relatively large and act on the targets on the cell surface.
3. **Metronomic therapy:** This regimen involves the frequent uninterrupted oral administration of cytotoxic chemotherapeutic agents at very low

doses especially for cancers with high risk of recurrence or with metastasis.

Cytotoxic Chemotherapy

Cytotoxic chemotherapy can be 1. phase specific or 2. phase nonspecific:

I. **Phase specific**
- **S phase:** Antimetabolites, camptothecins
- **G_1 phase:** Asparginase, steroids
- **M phase:** Taxanes and vinca alkaloids
- **G_2 phase:** Bleomycin, epipodophyllotoxins (etoposide)

These injure DNA at a specific phase of cell cycle but do not act on the resting phase.

II. **Phase nonspecific,** e.g. alkylating agents, antitumour antibiotics, platinum analogues, and doxorubicin. These injure DNA at any phase of the cell cycle including the resting phase (G_0) to block the check points before the cell division.

Classification of Cytotoxic Drugs

I. **Alkylating agents:**
- **Nitrogen mustards,** e.g. mechlorethamine, cyclophosphamide, melphalan and chlorambucil
- **Ethylenimines,** e.g. triethylenethiophosphoramide (Thio-TEPA)
- **Alkyl sulphonates,** e.g. busulfan
- **Methylhydrazine derivative,** e.g. procarbazine
- **Triazenes,** e.g. dacarbazine (DTIC) and temozolomide
- **Nitrosoureas,** e.g. carmustine (BCNU) and bendamustine
- **Platinum coordination complexes,** e.g. cisplatin, carboplatin and oxaliplatin

II. **Antimetabolites:**
- **Folic acid antagonists,** e.g. methotrexate
- **Purine antagonists,** e.g. 6-mercaptopurine and azathioprine
- **Pyrimidine antagonists,** e.g. fluorouracil, fluorodeoxyuridine and cytosine arabinoside
- **Deoxycytidine analogues,** e.g. cytarabine and gemcitabine

III. **Radioactive isotopes,** e.g. radioiodine, radiogold and radiophosphorus

IV. **Cytotoxic antibiotics,** e.g. actinomycin-D, mitomycin-C, rubidomycin, doxorubicin, bleomycin and mithramycin

V. **Antimitotic natural products** (Spindle poisons), e.g. vinca alkaloids (vinblastine, vincristine, vindesin), eribulin, taxanes (paclitaxel, docetaxel), podophyllotoxin derivatives (etoposide, teniposide) and camptothecin analogues (irinotecan, topotecan)

VI. **Miscellaneous,** e.g. hydroxyurea, mitotane, L-asparaginase, tretinoin and arsenic trioxide

Cytotoxic agents can be targeted towards tumour cells by tagging them to carriers, namely radioactive substance, chemical or monoclonal antibodies. After binding to the target site, the cytotoxic agent linked to the carrieris released, taken up by the cancer cell to cause its death.

All the above-mentioned cytotoxic drugs have common toxicity related to their action on various rapidly dividing cells such as:

- **Bone marrow and immuno-lympho-reticular system suppression**
- **Damage to GI mucosa** (enteritis and ulceration), nausea and vomiting
- **Loss of hair** (alopecia)
- **Specific organ damage,** e.g. gonads and lungs
- **Impaired wound healing**
- **Growth inhibition** in children
- **Teratogenicity**

Targeted Cancer Therapies

These include:

- **Hormone therapies** to slow or stop the growth of tumours which require certain hormones to grow (hormone sensitive), e.g. breast cancer and prostate cancer
- **Signal transduction inhibitors** to block the components of oncogene signaling pathway, e.g. inhibitors of tyrosine kinase, cyclins, cDKs and Ras
- **Immunotherapies** to trigger the immune system to destroy cancer cells, e.g. monoclonal antibodies that directly cause destruction of cells or cytokine-based therapies that modulate immune cells
- **Angiogenesis inhibitors** that inhibit vascular endothelial growth factor (VEGF) or other molecules and block the growth of new blood vessels in and around tumours, thereby preventing their oxygen and nutrient supply
- **Apoptosis inducers** to cause cancer cells to undergo a process of controlled cell death

- **Gene expression modulators** to restore function of tumour suppressor gene, e.g. gene therapy

PH 1.49

Classification of Targeted Cancer Therapies

I. **Hormones and antihormones:**
   - **Glucocorticoids**, e.g. prednisolone
   - **Estrogens and progestins**
   - **Antiestrogens**, e.g. tamoxifen and flutamide
   - **Aromatase inhibitors**, e.g. letrozole
   - **GnRH agonists**, e.g. leuprolide and goserelin
   - **GnRH antagonist**, e.g. abarelix
   - **Somatostatin analogues**, e.g. octreotide

II. **Signal transduction inhibitors,** e.g. tyrosine kinase inhibitors (Imatinib)

III. **Immunotherapies:**
   - **Monoclonal antibodies**, e.g. trastuzumab and rituximab
   - **Biological response modifiers**, e.g. interferons (Chapter 56), interleukins, BCG, levamisole (Chapter 75)

IV. **Angiogenesis inhibitors,** e.g. bevacizumab

V. **Apoptosis inducers,** e.g. proteasome inhibitors (bortezomib, carfilzomib)

Chemotherapy of cancer is a specialised field, to be handled only by an oncologist. Its detailed discussion is beyond the scope of this book. Hence, some important drugs used are described below.

ALKYLATING AGENTS

PH 1.49

Nitrogen mustards, first used in chemical warfare, have anticancer properties.

Mechanism of action: Nitrogen mustards are called alkylating agents because these compounds can transfer an alkyl radical to a suitable receptor site. Alkylating agents, in neutral or alkaline solution, form highly reactive quaternary ammonium derivatives, ethyleniminium cations (Fig. 59.2). These cations react with

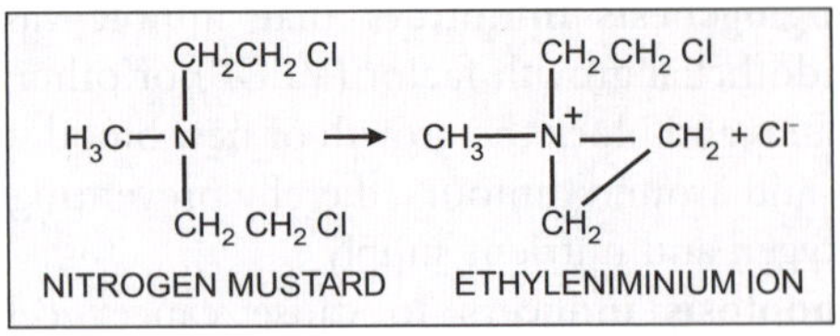

FIG. 59.2 Mechanism of action of nitrogen mustard.

(alkylate) groupings like amino, sulphhydryl, hydroxy or phosphate in the physiologically important molecules in the cells and render them unavailable for the normal metabolic reactions.

Alkylating agents are **cell cycle phase nonspecific** drugs. They inhibit DNA synthesis and also bring about a cross-linkage of DNA strands and thus interfere with cell replication.

Pharmacological actions common to various alkylating agents are as follows:

- **Cytotoxic action:** The haemopoietic system is highly susceptible to this action. Thus, they cause leucopenia, anaemia, thrombocytopenia and, in toxic doses, aplasia of the bone marrow. Chlorambucil is more effective against the cells of lymphoid series, whereas busulfan has predominant action against myeloid tissue.
- They damage other rapidly growing cells e.g., of cornea and the oral and intestinal mucosa causing ulceration; hair follicles causing alopecia; sperms causing infertility and can cause amenorrhoea and fetotoxicity in females.
- **Immunosuppressant action:** They suppress antibody production and encourage opportunistic infections.
- **Miscellaneous actions:** All the alkylating agents produce severe nausea and vomiting. **In general, they are mutagenic and leukemiogenic.**

Nitrogen mustards are also called ***radiomimetic drugs*** *as their actions resemble to some extent the biological effects of ionizing radiation. All alkylating agents, however, are not radiomimetic to the same extent.*

MECHLORETHAMINE: This first nitrogen mustard acts locally as a vesicant; the most susceptible tissues are skin, the eyes and the respiratory tract.

It was used earlier for cutaneous T-cell lymphoma as local application. However, being a very toxic drug, it is now replaced by other alkylating agents.

CYCLOPHOSPHAMIDE: It is a prodrug. It is not a local irritant and it can be given orally as well as parenterally.

Absorption, fate and excretion: Cyclophosphamide is well absorbed from the GI tract. It is converted in the liver to active metabolites, hydroxyphosphamide and aldophosphamide. They are metabolised further to inactive compounds. About 14% of the drug appears in the urine unchanged.

Adverse reactions: Toxicity of cyclophosphamide includes nephrotoxicity and urotoxicity because of its **toxic metabolite, acrolein.**

It can cause haemorrhagic cystitis. **Mesna** (sodium 2-mercaptoethane sulfonate), a synthetic sulphhydryl compound, given simultaneously with cyclophosphamide and again 4 and 8 h later, reacts with acrolein to prevent cystitis. The patient is advised to take plenty of fluids. In addition, cyclophosphamide can cause hepatic damage, myocardial necrosis, GI and pulmonary toxicities especially after the use of high doses.

Preparations and dosage: Cyclophosphamide is supplied as 50 mg tablets and in vials containing powder. Solution for injection is prepared by adding sterile water which remains stable for 3 h. The drug can be given intravenously, intrapleurally, intraperitoneally, intra-arterially and directly into the tumour. Cyclophosphamide can be administered as a single dose for low dose (2-6 mg/kg); moderate dose (10-15 mg/kg) or high dose (20-40 mg/kg) regimen every 10-20 days.

Indications: Cyclophosphamide is used as a part of a multiple-drug regimen to treat various malignancies such as chronic lymphatic leukaemia, lymphomas and solid tumours.

Its use as an immunosuppressing agent is discussed in Chapter 72.

Ifosamide is an analogue of cyclophosphamide with similar action and safety profile.

MELPHALAN: This drug has properties similar to the other alkylating agents. It is effective orally. It is less irritant locally and rarely causes alopecia. Other systemic toxic effects are similar to those of mechlorethamine. It is used to treat multiple myeloma.

CHLORAMBUCIL: This compound, (Fig. 59.3), is

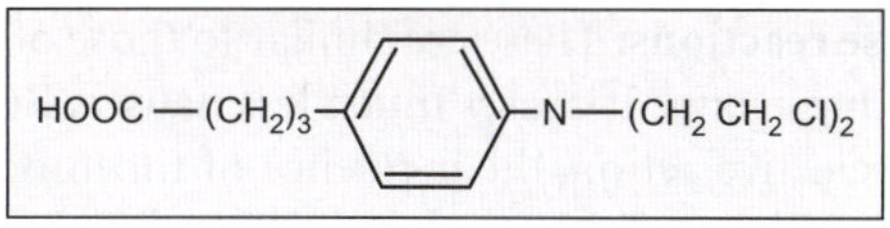

FIG. 59.3 Chlorambucil.

the shortest acting nitrogen mustard. **It is effective orally, predominantly against malignant cells of lymphoid series.** It is not a local irritant and is less likely to cause alopecia and is myelosuppressive which is dose dependent and usually reversible.

Chlorambucil is given orally, usually in the dose of 0.1–0.2 mg/kg of body weight daily for 3–6 weeks.

Indications: It was the drug of choice in the treatment of chronic lymphocytic leukaemia (CLL). But currently, B-cell antigen receptor signaling modulators are preferred. Chlorambucil is used when they are not available or not tolerated or for relapsed cases.

BENDAMUSTINE is used intravenously for CLL and non-Hodgkin lymphoma. Its toxicity is similar to other nitrogen mustards but myelosuppression and mucositis caused by it is rapidly reversible. It lacks cross resistance with other alkylating agents.

THIOTEPA: This ethylenimine is given intravenously. It is used by bladder instillation for superficial bladder tumours.

BUSULFAN: This drug (Fig. 59.4) differs from nitrogen mustards in its mechanism of action. **The drug causes a selective depression of granulocyte and platelet production;** it does not have a significant action on the intestinal epithelium or the lymphoid tissue. **It is more effective against cells of the myeloid series.**

Absorption, fate and excretion: Given orally it is well absorbed. It is excreted in the urine as methanesulfonic acid.

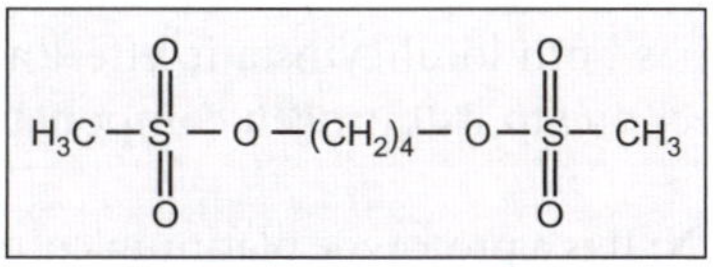

FIG. 59.4 Busulfan.

Adverse reactions: These are similar to those of other alkylating agents. It causes much less nausea. Because of its selective action, the incidence of thrombocytopenia is higher. Prolonged administration or high doses may cause amenorrhoea, wasting, pigmentation, gynaecomastia, anhidrosis, seizures, veno-occlusive disease of liver and pulmonary fibrosis.

Indications: It is used in combination in the treatment of chronic myeloid leukaemia. However, with the advent of tyrosine kinase inhibitor, imatinib mesylate, its use is restricted to patients who cannot tolerate imatinib or if imatinib is unavailable. Now it is used in high-dose as a preparation for stem cell transplants.

PROCARBAZINE HYDROCHLORIDE: This methylhydrazine derivative is activated in the liver. It is effective orally in the treatment of Hodgkin disease. The toxic effects reported are (a) CNS related – restlessness, drowsiness, nightmares and disorientation and (b) haematological: leucopoenia, thrombocytopenia and anaemia. It may cause disulfiram-like reaction following alcohol ingestion.

DACARBAZINE and **TEMOZOLOMIDE:** These traizene derivatives have properties similar to those of procarbazine. They kill cells in all the phases of the cell cycle. Dacarbazine is administered intravenously and most commonly used to treat malignant melanoma, Hodgkin lymphoma and soft tissue sarcomas, whereas temozolomide is given orally and used for the therapy of malignant glioma and astrocytoma.

NITROSOUREAS: This class includes drugs such as **lomustine** (given orally) and **carmustine** (given intravenously). They are lipid soluble and penetrate the BBB. Hence, they are preferred for the treatment of brain tumours (gliomas). They are also used for Hodgkin and non-Hodgkin lymphomas.

Estramustine is a stable combination of an estrogen and mustine, designed to deliver mustine to the estrogen receptor (ER) site of a tumour, e.g. prostate cancer. It has both local cytostatic effect and a hormonal effect due to its estrogen component.

CISPLATIN: It is a prototype platinum co-ordination complex given intravenously. In the cell, it gets converted into an active form, a potential mustard-like alkylating agent. It inhibits DNA biosynthesis and kills cells at any stage of cell cycle.

Adverse reactions: It commonly causes marked nausea, vomiting and anaemia. Prophylactic administration of an antiemetic is mandatory. Dose-related renal damage, ototoxicity, neuropathy and myelosuppresson can occur. Aggressive hydration with saline plus mannitol/furosemide is recommended to reduce the nephrotoxicity.

Carboplatin and **oxaliplatin** are newer analogues claimed to be less toxic. Myelosuppression remains as the dose limiting toxicity for carboplatin and peripheral neuropathy for oxaliplatin.

Indications: They are used in combination with other drugs such as vinblastine and bleomycin, to produce prolonged remissions in patients with germ cell, colorectal, ovarian, and testicular tumours. They are also useful in many solid tumours like oesophageal, gastric, lung, head and neck and breast cancers. Oxaliplatin is used for pancreatic cancer.

ANTIMETABOLITES

Chemical substances which take part in cellular metabolic reactions are called as metabolites. An antimetabolite is a chemical agent which, by virtue of its close structural similarity to the metabolite, blocks its actions. It can achieve this either by preventing the combination of the metabolite with its specific enzyme or by itself combining with the specific enzyme and thus getting transformed into a compound which is either metabolically inactive or harmful to the cell. They damage DNA indirectly.

Clinically useful antimetabolites are analogues of:

- **Substances essential for the synthesis of the nucleic acid bases, e.g. folic acid antagonist methotrexate**
- **Substances which get incorporated into the nucleic acid chains**, e.g. **purine and pyrimidine antagonists**

METHOTREXATE: This is a 4-amino substituted folic acid analogue which acts as a **folic acid antagonist.**

Mechanism of action: Folic acid is essential for the production of the coenzyme, tetrahydrofolic acid (THF). The conversion of folate to THF is carried out by an enzyme, folate reductase (Chapter 35). **Methotrexate competes with folic acid for this enzyme and binds to the folate reductase irreversibly, thus restricting the production of THF.** Lack of THF leads to inhibition of DNA synthesis, and thus cell replication. It is, therefore, more toxic to tissues with a high proportion of rapidly dividing cells, e.g. the bone marrow.

Pharmacological actions:

Cytotoxic actions: Methotrexate has a predominant action on the **bone marrow**. It inhibits erythropoiesis, myelopoiesis and finally may cause aplasia of the bone. This causes marked granulocytopenia, reticulocytopenia and moderate lymphopenia. The drug also causes ulceration of the oral and intestinal mucosa. It can cross the placental barrier and interfere with embryogenesis causing fetal abnormalities and death.

Immunosuppressive action: Methotrexate is a **potent immunosuppressant** and acts by preventing the clonal expansion of both, B and T lymphocytes.

Anti-inflammatory action: In small doses, it reduces lymphocyte proliferation, rheumatoid factor production, and interferes with the release of inflammatory cytokines like IL-2, IL-6, IL-8 and TNF-α. Thus, it acts as an **anti-inflammatory agent**. It is used as a disease modifying drug in RA (Chapter 73).

Absorption, fate and excretion: Methotrexate is well absorbed from the intestines. It remains in the tissue longer than folate causes a prolonged inhibitory effect. Its concentration in the CSF is poor. About 50%–90% of the dose is rapidly excreted via both, glomerular filtration and tubular secretion. Renal impairment or intake of probenecid and NSAID can augment its renal toxicity.

Adverse reactions: These are dose dependent and largely due to deficiency of THF and include megaloblastic anaemia, thrombocytopenia, leucopoenia, aplasia, oral and intestinal ulceration, nausea, vomiting and diarrhoea, alopecia, dermatitis, and liver damage. These cannot be reversed by giving folic acid as its conversion to THF is blocked. Ideally, THF should be administered to antagonise its toxicity. Since THF is too unstable, a related compound **folinic acid** (N5-formyl THF) is used as **calcium folinate** or **calcium levofolinate.** It is given in the dose of 120 mg (in divided doses) in the first 24 h, followed by 15 mg orally or by IM injection 6 hourly for the next 48 h.

Preparations and dosage: Methotrexate is supplied as 2.5, 5, 7.5, 10 and 15 mg tablets and as 2.5 mg, 7.5 mg, 15 mg, 20 mg, 25 mg, 50 mg and 100 mg/ml solution for injection. It can be given intrathecally, to treat meningeal infiltration in acute leukaemia.

Indications:

- **Acute lymphatic leukaemia** in children
- **Choriocarcinoma:** It is extremely useful in this condition where it has almost produced 'cure' in certain cases
- **Soft tissue sarcoma, breast cancer and acute myeloid leukaemia:** It has some place in the treatment of these conditions
- **Rheumatoid arthritis** (Chapter 73)
- **Psoriasis** (Chapter 69)
- **As an immunosuppressant** in steroid resistant asthma, Crohn disease and transplant rejection
- **For medical termination of pregnancy** (Chapter 66)

Pemetrexed is a pyrrolopyrimidine analogue which causes inhibition of DHFR and several other enzymes in purine and pyrimidine biosynthesis. Its main action is to inhibit thymidylate synthase. It is used in combination with cisplatin for non-small cell lung cancer and mesothelioma.

Pralatrexate is more effectively taken up by the target cell, wherein it undergoes polyglutamination. Thus it is retained by the cell better than methotrexate. Its mechanism of action is similar to methotrexate. It is used for treating relapsed or refractory cutaneous T-cell lymphoma (CTCL).

6-MERCAPTOPURINE: This purine analogue (Fig. 59.5) is converted in the cells to ribonucleotide of 6-mercaptopurine, which then suppresses the *de novo* biosynthesis of purines and hence of DNA. Like methotrexate, it is mainly toxic to the bone marrow and intestinal epithelium.

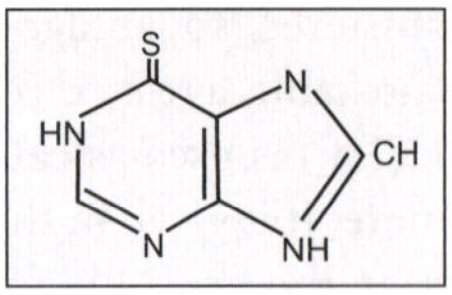

FIG. 59.5 **6-Mercaptopurine.**

Absorption, fate and excretion: The drug is well absorbed orally. It is metabolised rapidly by **xanthine oxidase,** which is also required to synthesise uric acid. Use of the xanthine oxidase inhibitor allopurinol decreases the inactivation of 6-mercaptopurine (Chapter 73). Mercaptopurine and its metabolites are rapidly excreted by the kidneys. Its penetration into the CSF is poor.

Adverse reactions: These are similar to those of methotrexate and are mainly related to bone marrow and GI tract. Sometimes, it causes hepatic necrosis.

It can cause hyperuricaemia with hyperuricosuria due to massive destruction of the cells of lymphoid tissues. Hence, urine should be maintained alkaline and its volume adequate.

Indications: Mercaptopurine is useful in the treatment of acute leukaemia, particularly in children. It is supplied as 50 mg tablets. Mercaptopurine is also effective in choriocarcinoma and chronic myelogenous leukaemia.

Other purine analogues which have selectivity for lymphoid tissue include **fludarabine phosphate, cladribine**; **clofarabine** and **nelarabine**.

Pentostatin (2′-deoxycoformycin) is an intermediate in adenosine deaminase reaction and inhibits the enzyme. This results in accumulation of intracellular purine nucleotides, adenosine and deoxyadenosine, which in turn block DNA synthesis. It is used to treat hairy cell leukemia and T-cell lymphomas. However, drug of choice remains cladribine, which is more potent and effective.

Azathioprine and **6-thioguanine** also possess cytotoxic actions. However, they have no distinct advantages over mercaptopurine. **Azathioprine** is **usually favoured as an immunosuppressive agent in organ transplantation and in certain autoimmune diseases** like haemolytic anaemias, glomerulonephritis and rheumatoid arthritis (see Chapter 73).

5-FLUOROURACIL (5-FU): This fluorinated analogue of pyrimidine (a) requires enzymatic conversion to nucleotide, **FU triphosphate**, which gets incorporated in RNA. (b) As an alternative, it also gets converted into **fluorodeoxyuridine monophosphate (FdUMP)**, which binds to thymidylate synthetase, thus preventing the production of thymine, the basic component of DNA. The derivative of FU, **fluorodeoxyuridine (floxuridine)** gets converted directly to FdUMP. Both have been used in the treatment of carcinoma of stomach, colon, rectum, breast, and ovaries. Both are relatively less toxic drugs but affect bone marrow, GI epithelium and CNS.

Capecitabine is a prodrug of 5FU but is administered orally. ADRs are similar to 5FU.

CYTOSINE ARABINOSIDE (Cytarabine): This pyrimidine analogue is considered to be the drug of choice in inducing remission in acute myeloid leukaemia, especially in adults. **It is an 'S' phase specific antimetabolite and acts by interfering with pyrimidine synthesis.** The toxic effects include nausea, vomiting, bone marrow depression and cerebellar ataxia.

GEMCITABINE, an antimetabolite, is an analogue of deoxycytidine and is **S phase specific**. It is metabolised intracellularly to the active diphosphate and triphosphate nucleosides, which inhibit DNA synthesis. It also inhibits the enzyme ribonucleotide reductase (RNR) irreversibly and blocks synthesis of deoxyribonucleotides required for DNA replication.

Gemcitabine is relatively well tolerated. Common ADR are flu-like symptoms, fever, fatigue, nausea, vomiting, hepatic damage and skin rash. The main dose-limiting toxicity is bone marrow suppression.

Indications: Gemcitabine is used to treat non-small cell lung cancer, bladder and breast cancer. It is currently used to treat pancreatic cancer.

RADIOACTIVE ISOTOPES

Radioactive isotopes act because of their physical property of emitting beta and gamma radiation. The radiations given out produce ionisation in the cells, thereby disrupting the cellular metabolism, and cell destruction. The therapeutically useful radio-isotopes are radioiodine ^{131}I, radiocobalt and radio-phosphorus.

RADIOIODINE (Sodium ^{131}I): Given orally, it is concentrated by the thyroid gland and causes acinar destruction. It acts by emitting beta radiation (Chapter 62). It is useful in those cases of thyroid carcinoma, which can concentrate enough radioiodine, e.g. thyroid follicular carcinoma. In thyroid carcinoma, surgery followed by radioiodine can achieve excellent results in selected cases. Usually, the patient is allowed to develop myxoedema before the administration of radioiodine. This ensures the maximum uptake by the left-over 'thyroid tissue'. Generally, 2–3 doses of 150 mCi, each at the interval of 2–3 months are considered adequate and the total dose should not exceed 500 mCi. *As it is highly selective, its systemic toxicity is minimal.* The patient must be isolated and arrangements made for the disposal of urine in order to reduce the possible radiation hazard to other people.

RADIOACTIVE PHOSPHORUS (Sodium phosphate ^{32}P): Radioactive phosphorus was used earlier in the treatment of polycythaemia vera. It is taken up rapidly by cells having high metabolic turnover of phosphorus. *Because of its wide distribution, it causes generalised body irradiation including that of lungs, GI tract and gonads.* It is **leukaemiogenic, and hence is now rarely used. Repeated phlebotomy is preferred for polycythaemia vera.**

The other drugs used to treat **polycythaemia vera** are **hydroxyurea** and **anagrelide** (see section, miscellaneous agents).

CYTOTOXIC ANTIBIOTICS

This group of antibiotics is derived from the *Streptomyces* species. They **bind to DNA directly and often generate free radicals leading to DNA damage. They also alter the topoisomerase function**. Their cytotoxic property and **ADR are similar to those of the alkylating agents including myelosuppression.**

ACTINOMYCIN-D (Dactinomycin): It is one of the first anticancer antibiotics. Given as IV injection, it gets excreted in both, bile and urine. Its t½ is 36 hrs. It does not cross the BBB. It is used for the treatment of Wilms' tumour, childhood rhabdomyosarcoma, Ewing's sarcoma and metastatic, nonseminomatous testicular cancer as a part of combination therapy.

DAUNORUBICIN (Dunomycin, rubidomycin): This antibiotic is obtained from a strain of *Streptomyces coeruleorubidus*. Used in combination with vincristine and prednisolone, it produces remission of acute leukaemia in children. It is also useful in acute myeloblastic leukaemia in adults. It causes bone marrow suppression and toxic cardiomyopathy.

BLEOMYCIN: This drug, derived from *Streptomyces verticillus*, is a mixture of glycopeptides. **In addition to binding to DNA, it forms complexes with iron, oxidation of which gives superoxide.** It is useful in epidermoid carcinomas of the skin, the upper respiratory passages, the oral cavity and the genitourinary tract and in lymphomas resistant to other drugs. It is not a vesicant and causes minimal myelosuppression. Its main toxicity is nausea, vomiting, anaphylaxis, dermographia, scleroderma like changes in the skin, pneumonitis, and occasionally pulmonary fibrosis. It is administered by IM/IV/SC routes.

MITOMYCIN C: This antibiotic, obtained from *Streptomyces caespitosus*, has been employed by intravenously or oral route in the treatment of chronic myeloid leukaemia and Hodgkin disease. Like alkylating agents, it may cause severe bone marrow depression, bleeding, toxic hepatitis, pulmonary fibrosis and haemolytic uremic syndrome. It is used intravesically to treat bladder cancer.

MITHRAMYCIN (Plicamycin): This drug, derived from *Streptomyces plicatus*, is useful in embryonal cell carcinoma of the testis and in hypercalcaemia due to malignant disease. It has high toxicity and causes myelosuppression, thrombocytopenia, liver and kidney damage and suppression of clotting factors.

DOXORUBICIN (Adriamycin): This antibiotic is obtained from *Streptomyces pneuceticus.* **It acts as a nonspecific inhibitor of topoisomerase II, thus interfering with DNA replication.** It produces remission in acute lymphoblastic leukaemia and lymphoblastic lymphosarcoma and its toxicity is similar to that of dounorubicin. It is used intravenously and by instillation into the bladder.

Epirubicin and **idarubicin** are other analogues of doxorubicin.

Ixabepilone is derived from apothiline, a cytotoxic macrolide. It has actions similar to those of taxane but can be used in taxane resistant cases. It is used in combination to treat advanced metastatic breast cancer. It is a CYP3A4 substrate. It causes peripheral sensory neuropathy.

ANTIMITOTIC NATURAL PRODUCTS

VINCA ALKALOIDS: From the various alkaloids isolated from periwinkle plant (*Vinca rosea; Catharanthus rosens*), three compounds, **vinblastine, vincristine** and **vindesine**, have been shown to be useful in the chemotherapy of malignancy. **Vinorelbine** is a semisynthetic derivative. They are substrates for p-glycoprotein efflux pump.

Mechanism of action: They bind to beta tubulin and prevent the formation of the mitotic spindle (**antimitotic spindle poison**). Thus, **they cause cell-cycle arrest in mitosis.**

Pharmacological actions: They have similar spectrum of cytotoxic activity. In spite of the close similarity, there is no cross resistance between these two agents.

Vinca alkaloids are not well absorbed orally. Being highly irritant, they are administered through a freely running IV infusion. They are excreted primarily by the liver into the biliary tract.

Adverse reactions: Toxic effects include nausea, anorexia, vomiting and constipation. Signs of intestinal obstruction due to **severe constipation** with paralytic ileus may occur.

Vinca alkaloids produce certain **neuropsychiatric effects.** They affect neuromuscular transmission and cause peripheral neuropathy. They may also cause mental depression, ataxia and tremors. The molecules of these alkaloids contain indole and dihydroindole groups, similar to psychotropic drugs like LSD.

Although these drugs are chemically related, their toxicity is relatively different. Thus, **vinblastine is more toxic to the bone marrow, whereas vincristine causes more neurotoxicity and alopecia.** They are teratogenic.

Indications:

Vinblastine sulphate is mainly useful in Hodgkin disease and other lymphomas, where it produces remission in 50%–60% of cases. It can also be used in methotrexate resistant choriocarcinoma and lymphosarcoma. It is used with doxorubicin as a part of ABVD combination (adriamycin, bleomycin, vinblastine and dacarbazine) for Hodgkin lymphoma.

Vinorelbine, a semisynthetic derivative of vinblastine is used for non-small cell lung cancer, breast cancer and ovarian cancer.

Vincristine is useful in the treatment of acute lymphatic leukaemia in children. It is a part of CHOP regimen (cyclophosphamide, doxorubicin, vincristine and prednisone) for non- Hodgkin lymphoma.

ERIBULIN: It is a synthetic macrocyclic ketone analogue of the natural product halichondrin B, isolated from Pacific marine sponge. Its mechanism of action is similar to vinca alkaloids but it is a poor substrate for P-glycoprotein pump. Therefore, it is used in drug-resistant metastatic breast cancer and liposarcoma.

TAXANES: Paclitaxel has been isolated initially from the bark of the Western yew tree and later on using semisynthetic approach from yew tree needles. **It binds to the beta subunit of tubulin and forms stable non-functioning microtubule bundle, thus interfering with mitosis.** This action differs from that of vinca alkaloids which inhibit microtubules. **It also induces apoptosis and has antiangiogenic property.** It is metabolised in the liver. It is administered by infusion.

It is a substrate for p-glycoprotein efflux pump. It is mainly used to treat breast and ovarian cancer.

Adverse reactions: Mainly, it affects the bone marrow. Commonly, it causes neutropenia and myalgias. Other ADR are asymptomatic bradycardia or episodes of silent ventricular tachycardia, alopecia, skin rashes, neuropathy and hypersensitivity reactions.

Docetaxel, an analogue of paclitaxel with similar properties but a longer half-life, is claimed to cause less neuropathy and neutropenia.

Camptothecin analogues: These have been isolated from the Chinese tree *Camptotheca acuminata* and include **irinotecan** (a prodrug) and **topotecan**. They inhibit nuclear topoisomerase I and thereby inhibit DNA replication. These drugs have been used in advanced colorectal, ovarian and small lung cell cancer. Their main adverse effects are neutropenia, diarrhoea, nausea and alopecia. Irinotecan inhibits acetylcholinesterase which results in a cholinergic syndrome within 24 h after its administration. It responds to atropine.

ETOPOSIDE: It is a semisynthetic compound prepared from podophyllotoxin obtained from *Podophyllum peltatum*. It inhibits topoisomerase II, leading to DNA damage. It is given orally or intravenously. The ADR include leukopenia, GI disturbances, hepatotoxicity. It may cause secondary leukemia. It is used in testicular and lung cancer, Hodgkin and non-Hodgkin lymphomas, acute myelogenous leukemia and for Kaposi sarcoma.

Teniposide is a related agent, for intravenous use. It can cause myelosuppression, nausea and vomiting. It is used to treat acute lymphoblastic leukemia in children, glioblastoma and neuroblastoma.

HORMONES AND ANTIHORMONAL DRUGS

Mechanism of action of hormones is different from the cytotoxic drugs and hence can be combined with them for synergistic effects. They may act by:

- **Inhibition of cell growth and differentiation**, e.g. androgens in breast cancer and estrogens in prostatic cancer
- **Stimulation of differentiation of cells which then regain their ability to respond to the body's controlling and inhibitory influence,** e.g. estrogens in breast cancer in postmenopausal women
- **Selective lysis of leukemic lymphocytes:** Glucocorticoids because of their direct lympholytic action are effective in acute lymphatic leukaemia
- **Inhibition of the circulating concentration of a substance which stimulates the malignant cells**, e.g. thyroxine suppresses certain thyroid cancers by inhibiting TSH secretion

Hormones do not directly kill the susceptible malignant cells, are slower in their effect and are less toxic.

ESTROGENS: Carcinoma of the prostate is androgen dependent; bilateral orchidectomy, in patients with prostatic carcinoma, can produce marked improvement. Similar beneficial effects are obtained by the administration of estrogens. The best results are obtained by combining estrogens with orchidectomy. Synthetic estrogens which are as effective as the natural ones but much cheaper are preferred. **Diethylstilbestrol** is used in the dose of 5 mg t.i.d. for several days and then reduced to 1 mg t.i.d. Adverse effects due to estrogen therapy are described in Chapter 65. In males, these mainly include sexual impotence and gynaecomastia.

AROMATASE INHIBITORS: These nonsteroidal drugs **inhibit the enzyme aromatase responsible for the conversion of the adrenal androgen androstenedione to oestrone** (Chapter 65). They markedly reduce the circulating estrogen levels. The currently used **nonsteroidal aromatase inhibitors** are **anastrozole** and **letrozole.**

The aromatisation occurs in the body fat. Such estrogen synthesis may be important in the pathogenesis of breast cancer growth in postmenopausal women. **Aromatase inhibitors are selective in action (selective medical adrenalectomy) and do not inhibit synthesis of adrenal glucocorticoids.** They are given orally and are generally well tolerated. Adverse reactions are mild and include nausea, headache, fatigue, hot flushes and arthralgia. The risk of vaginal bleeding and thromboembolic events is less.

They are now increasingly used as first line drugs in postmenopausal women to treat ER-positive breast cancer, including that which has progressed in spite of tamoxifen therapy. They can be combined with other drugs.

Exemestane, a steroidal hormonal compound, inhibits aromatase irreversibly. It is administered orally. It has comparable efficacy as that of nosteroidal aromatase inhibitors but shows specific ADR related to its androgenic structure.

TAMOXIFEN: This nonsteroidal **antiestrogen** is structurally related to diethylstilbestrol.

Mechanism of action: It acts by competing with the circulating estrogens for binding to the cytoplasmic ERs. The metabolites of tamoxifen have a much stronger affinity for the receptors and are not easily displaced by circulating oestradiol. At low concentrations, they have a cytostatic effect on ER-positive cells. Higher concentrations cause cell death of both, ER-positive and -negative cells.

Absorption, fate and excretion: Given orally, it is well absorbed. It is metabolised in liver to active metabolites and undergoes enterohepatic circulation. With a dose of 10 mg twice a day, a steady state serum concentration is achieved by 4 weeks of treatment. The approximate biological half-life of tamoxifen and its metabolite *N*-desmethyltamoxifen are 7 and 14 days, respectively. Hence, **the drug can be detected in the serum for 4 weeks after treatment is discontinued.** Approximately, 30% of the dose is excreted in faeces.

Adverse reactions: The adverse effects are usually minimal. The most frequent side effect has been hot flushes. About 10% of the patients may experience mild nausea and vomiting. It may also give rise to vaginal bleeding and ocular toxicity. Rarely, it causes bone pain associated with hypercalcaemia, particularly in patients with bone metastasis. Higher incidence of DVT and endometrial cancer has been reported in a few women on prolonged therapy.

Indications: Tamoxifen is well tolerated, reasonably safe and of proven efficacy in patients with breast cancer. It is the **adjuvant treatment of choice in the postoperative patients, irrespective of their age, menopausal status, the ER status of the tumour and whether the axillary lymph nodes are positive or negative; the results are better in patients with ER positivity.**

The dose is 10 mg orally twice daily. The optimum duration of treatment is uncertain; but it is usually for 2–5 years. *Larger doses are not more beneficial.* US FDA has approved the prophylatic use of tamoxifen and raloxifene for reduction of breast cancer in women with high risk.

The observation that there is less osteoporosis in women treated with tamoxifen led to the development of a new series of its analogues called **Selective Estrogen Receptor Modulators (SERM)** such as **raloxifene, which are used in osteoporosis** (Chapter 68).

FULVESTRANT: This selective antiestrogenic drug binds to estrogen receptors but repress their transactivation. It is termed as Selective Estrogen Receptor Downregulator **-SERD.** It increases proteolytic degradation of ERα but not of ERβ (see Chapter 65). This effect probably is responsible for its efficacy in tamoxifen resistant breast cancer. It is also used in metastatic breast cancer. It is given intramuscularly as a loading dose 500 mg biweekly in the first month and later monthly. It is generally well tolerated but may produce ADR such as nausea, vomiting, diarrhoea/constipation, hot flushes, rash, arthralgia, myalgia and abdominal or pelvic pain.

PROGESTINS: The endometrial carcinoma in humans is believed to be due to prolonged unopposed stimulation by estrogens. **Hydroxyprogesterone caproate** and **megestrol acetate** have been used with success in metastatic endometrial carcinoma. Medroxyprogesterone has also been used for this purpose in the dose of 100–500 mg per day orally (Chapter 65). Both agents have also been used to treat cachexia associated with cancer and AIDS.

FLUTAMIDE: This **nonsteroidal antiandrogen compound binds to androgen receptor and blocks the effects of testosterone.** It exerts substantial antitumour activity in patients with metastatic cancer of prostate.

Given orally, it is rapidly and completely absorbed. Its adverse effects are nausea, vomiting, loss of libido, sexual impotence, hot flushes and rarely serious hepatotoxicity.

It has been used in conjunction with a GnRH analogue in the **treatment of prostatic cancer**. The combination is as effective as but less toxic than stilbestrol. Flutamide, used as a single drug in the dose of 250 mg t.i.d., is also effective in the management of early prostatic cancer.

Nilutamide and **bicalutamide** are other antiandrogens (Chapter 67).

LH-RH AGONISTS: Leuprolide and **goserelin** have been used to treat metastatic cancer of the prostate (Chapter 65).

ABARELIX: This **GnRH antagonist causes suppression of LH and FSH and lowers the testosterone levels** and is used in advanced prostatic cancer.

SOMATOSTATIN ANALOGUES such as **octreotide** and **lanreotide** are sometimes used in the treatment of carcinoid tumours.

GLUCOCORTICOIDS: Glucocorticoids like hydrocortisone and prednisolone are useful in:

- **Acute lymphatic leukaemia** in children and in malignant lymphoma due to their **direct lympholytic effect**
- **Preventing the accelerated erythrocytic destruction** and thereby the occurrence of anaemia in disseminated cancer patients. They effectively counter the haemolytic and haemorrhagic complications (due to thrombocytopenia) accompanying chronic leukaemias, and malignant lymphomas.
- **Treating cerebral oedema** due to intracranial tumour metastases
- **Controlling the hypercalcaemia** following cancer chemotherapy
- **Critically ill patients** along with cytotoxic drugs to produce symptomatic relief and a sense of well-being
- **Preventing/treating vomiting** due to chemotherapy. Dexamethasone is useful as an adjunctive antiemetic

Prednisolone is generally started in doses of 60–100 mg daily in divided doses, and then, depending upon the response, reduced to a maintenance dose of 20–40 mg daily.

Follicular and papillary types of thyroid carcinomas are probably dependent on thyroid stimulating hormone (TSH). **The primary treatment of these conditions is surgical.** Papillary carcinoma is very slow growing and metastasises largely to cervical lymph nodes; postoperatively, it has been treated lifelong with thyroxine. Follicular carcinoma metastasises early and widely; postoperatively, it is best treated with radioactive iodine.

MISCELLANEOUS AGENTS

L-ASPARAGINASE: This enzyme, which deaminates asparagine to aspartic acid, is prepared from *E. coli*. **Asparagine is a nonessential amino acid normally synthesised by the mammalian tissue cells.** Certain malignant tumours, however, are unable to synthesise asparagine and consequently, are dependent on supplies from the host. **Asparaginase acts by depleting asparagine from the host, hydrolysing circulating L-aspargine to aspartic acid, thus denying the malignant cells the essential metabolite.** It is relatively nontoxic to normal cells. Given intravenously, it has produced relief in cases of lymphoblastic leukaemia and reticulum cell sarcoma. It may cause hypersensitivity, pyrogenic reactions and skin rashes.

HYDROXYUREA (hydroxycarbamide) is mainly used in the management of myeloproliferative disorders. It acts by inhibiting the enzyme ribonucleoside diphosphate reductase which is responsible for the conversion of ribonucleotides to deoxyribonucleotides (S-phase block). It inhibits myeloproliferation and normalises the platelet count. Hydroxyurea is almost 100% absorbed from the gut.

Adverse reactions: These include leukopenia, megaloblastic anaemia, thrombocytopenia, GI disturbances, skin reactions, stomatitis, alopecia, and neurological manifestations.

It is used in chronic granulocytic leukaemia, polycythaemia vera, thrombocytosis and sickle cell anaemia.

Anagrelide: This phosphodiesterase inhibitor given orally inhibits megakaryacytes maturation to platelets and causes lowering of platelets. Thus, **it helps to prevent thrombosis in primary thrombocythaemia and polycythaemia.** It also has been used in the treatment of chronic myeloid leukaemia. The drug may cause headache, palpitation, cardiac arrhythmia and fluid retention.

Mitotane: This drug, structurally related to the insecticide DDT, selectively concentrates in the adrenal cortex and acts as an adrenolytic. It has been used in the treatment of Cushing's syndrome due to adrenocortical carcinoma. The adverse effects include anorexia, nausea, diarrhoea, somnolence and lethargy.

Arsenic trioxide: It is used in acute promyelocytic leukaemia (APL). Arsenic trioxide, causes degradation of PML-RAR alpha in premature promyelocytes and promotes differentiation. It inhibits thioredoxin to generate reactive oxygen species. It also influences microenvironment of tumour cells leading to apoptosis and growth arrest. Low doses induce good clinical response in patients with relapsed APL.

Adverse reactions: It is well tolerated and ADR are reversible. These include fatigue, altered touch sensations, increased liver enzymes, hyperglycemia and leukocytosis. Leukocytosis may be observed in 50% patients. Rarely patients may develop leukocyte maturation syndrome, which is exhibited as fever, skin rash, oedema, pulmonary distress and effusion. It is relieved by glucocorticoids. The drug can produce QT prolongation.

Tretinoin: This is a synthetic analogue of vitamin A (Chapter 77). It is used to treat acute promyelocytic leukemia. In this leukemia there is a cytogenetic translocation of the retinoic acid receptor alpha (RARA) gene on chromosome 17 and the promyelocytic leukemia (PML) gene on chromosome 15. This results in a PML-RARA fusion gene, which is responsible for cellular transformation. Tretinoin promotes degradation of the PML-RARA fusion gene. The ADR include **leukocyte maturation syndrome** ("retinoic acid differentiation syndrome"), fever, dyspnea, pulmonary effusions, dry skin, cheilitis, hypercalcemia and renal failure.

MONOCLONAL ANTIBODIES (mAb)

Identification of the molecular and genetic changes that cause malignant transformation has proved useful in developing new anticancer drugs. The family of **Epidermal Growth Factor Receptor** (EGFR) – **tyrosine kinases on cell surface plays an important role in translating messages to the nucleus** and provides targets for chemotherapeutic agents. Many epithelial tumours, particularly breast cancer, express excess amounts of HER2, a member of the EGFR family and is associated with clinical resistance to cytotoxic and hormonal therapy. **The intracellular domain of HER2 encodes tyrosine kinase which inhibits apoptosis and promotes metastases.**

TRASTUZUMAB (Herceptin): This is a humanised, cDNA-derived antibody against HER2. Blocking this receptor prevents the tumour growth. It can cause nausea, vomiting, fever, hypersensitivity reactions, delayed bone marrow suppression and cardiomyopathy. It is used in patients with **breast cancer in combination with chemotherapy.**

Pertuzumab binds to HER2 receptors, inhibits dimerisation and blocks HER2 signalling, which leads to cell growth arrest. It is coadministered with trastuzumab for synergistic action.

Panitumumab and **cetuximab** are humanised monoclonal antibodies. They target EGFR. They are used in the treatment of metastatic colorectal cancer.

Rituximab targets CD20 and is used to treat non-Hodgkin lymphoma and leukaemia that express CD20. **Alemtuzumab** targets CD52 and is used to treat CD52 expressing lymphoid tumours and CLL; it depletes the leukemic and the normal lymphocytes by direct antibody-dependent lysis (see also Chapter 72).

BEVACIZUMAB: This is a recombinant, humanised, monoclonal anti-VEGF (Vascular endothelial growth factor) antibody, which prevents VEGF from binding to endothelial receptors. VEGF binding initiates angiogenesis (endothelial proliferation and the formation of new blood vessels). Bevacizumab **inhibits angiogenesis and thus retards further growth of all tissues including the metastases.** It is used for treating metastatic colorectal cancer, breast cancer, malignant mesothelioma and prostate cancer (off-label use). The ADR include proteinuria, hypertension and thromboembolism. It is administered by IV infusion. Intraocular injections are used to prevent angiogenesis and age-related macular degeneration (AMD).

^{131}**Iodine-Tositumomab** is a monoclonal antibody labelled with radioiodine. Given intravenously, it is taken up more specifically by the tumour cells than by normal tissues and gives selective radiation to targeted cells. It is used in refractory non-Hodgkin lymphoma.

TYROSINE KINASE INHIBITORS

IMATINIB Most of the patients with chronic myeloid leukaemia (CML) have a translocated, shortened chromosome 22, termed the Philadelphia chromosome. This translocation creates a tyrosine kinase fusion gene called BCR-ABL gene which phosphorylates effector proteins and drives cell proliferation. *Imatinib acts specifically by binding to the BCR-ABL gene and blocks the phosphorylation of the effector proteins.*

Imatinib mesylate is well absorbed orally and is highly protein bound. Its plasma t½ is 18 h and that of its active metabolite is about 40 h. It is metabolised in the liver.

Adverse reactions: These are usually mild and include nausea, vomiting, oedema, muscle cramps and diarrhoea, neutropenia, thrombocytopenia, and increased liver enzymes. Imatinib inhibits hepatic microsomal enzymes and may increase the serum concentration of warfarin, whereas the administration of itraconazole or erythromycin may increase its plasma concentration.

Indications: In patients with CML in the chronic phase, imatinib induces a complete haematological remission in almost 88% and a complete cytogenic remission in 30%. It is also useful in the acute phase, and to a smaller extent in blast crisis.

Nilotinib, and **dasatinib** are other tyrosine kinase inhibitors effective in CML. **Lapatinib** is an oral inhibitor of HER2 and EGFR1. It is used to treat metastatic breast cancer. **Ponatinib** is claimed to be useful in subjects resistant to above drugs.

Several other oral tyrosine kinase inhibitors such as **crizotinib, ceritinib, gefitinib, erlotinib, sunitinib, sorafinib, axitinib** and **pazopanib** are now available for therapy of various malignancies such as resistant metastatic melanoma, lymphoma, leukaemia, non-small cell lung cancer, pancreatic and renal cell cancer.

BIOLOGICAL RESPONSE MODIFIERS

For immunostimulants and other biological modifiers such as BCG, levamisole, interleukins and interferon alpha, see Chapters 57 and 72.

PROTEASOME INHIBITORS

Proteasome are large proteolytic complexes of the cell which play a role in the normal turnover of proteins. The proteins to be destroyed are delivered to proteasome which have 20S proteolytic core bearing active sites. Inhibition of these sites leads to intracellular aggregation of unwanted proteins in cells. This induces apoptosis and cell cycle arrest.

Bortezomib is the first **proteasome inhibitor** used in multiple myeloma. Multiple myeloma cells produce very large quantities of protein, which make them unusually susceptible to this drug. A selective irreversible proteasome inhibitor **carfilzomib** has been introduced, which is effective in myeloma refractory to bortezomib. ADR include fatigue, vomiting, diarrhoea, fever, dyspnoea, peripheral neuropathy and myelosuppression.

DRUG THERAPY OF MALIGNANT DISEASES

Chemotherapy has definitely improved the outlook of cancer therapy malady. In a few cases, long-term remissions (almost cure) can be obtained by chemotherapy e.g. acute myeloid and lymphoid leukaemia, Hodgkin lymphoma, choriocarcinoma, Wilms' tumour, disseminated testicular cancer, ovarian cancer and histiocytic lymphoma. **In majority of the conditions, however, it is purely suppressive and is used to improve quality of life.** In some, it improves the survival and almost cures, e.g. breast, ovarian and colorectal cancers.

Currently, anticancer drugs are used either as:

1. **Induction treatment** which is the initial treatment along with or after surgery and/or radiation to induce remission
2. **Consolidation therapy:** is given to kill any cancer cells remaining in the body after the induction treatment so as to sustain the remission
3. **Maintenance therapy:** is used in low doses to prevent reappearance of cancer in certain cases, e.g. ALL and APL
4. **Neo-adjuvant treatment** for localised cancer prior to surgery or radiation to reduce the size
5. **Adjuvant (adjunct) treatment** following surgery or radiation therapy, or both to destroy the leftover cancer cells
6. **Metronomic chemotherapy:** Use of small equally spaced doses (1/10–1/3 of the maximum tolerated dose) of chemotherapeutic agents without any drug-free interval results in the **sustained but low concentrations of drugs in tumour**. This therapeutic strategy is termed metronomic chemotherapy. It prevents angiogenesis and has other direct and indirect effects on the tumour cells and activated endothelial cells and their microenvironment, leading to induction of cell senescence, tumour dormancy and restoration of immune responses. Low doses are well tolerated without significant toxicity. It can be combined with other therapies. Usually orally administered drugs are preferred like cyclophosphamide, methotrexate, etoposide, capecitabine, prednisone and thalidomide. However, 5′-deoxy-5-fluorouridine, vinblastine/vincristine and paclitaxel have been used. It is used for recurrent or advanced cancers of breast, ovary, prostate, head and neck and also for multiple myeloma and non-Hodgkin's lymphoma.

PH 1.1

A detailed discussion of drug therapy in malignancy is beyond the scope of this book. **Certain principles, however, are outlined below:**

- **A physician should be aware of natural history of tumour growth.** Conditions like acute leukaemia, certain sarcomas and Hodgkin lymphoma which show rapid progression need prompt attention, whereas a condition like chronic lymphatic leukaemia, particularly in old people, may progress so slowly that patients may enjoy good health and can survive almost a normal span of life without any chemotherapy.
- **Aim of the chemotherapy should be to kill all the malignant cells** to stop progeny. But the total cell kill is difficult to achieve. Hence **relapse is the rule rather than exception.**
- Different forms of cancer differ in their sensitivity to drugs. It depends on the growth fraction i.e. the fraction of cells undergoing mitosis at any time. Thus, rapidly proliferating tumours are more responsive. For example, Burkitt's lymphoma, which has a growth fraction of 100% is very sensitive whereas carcinoma of colon, which has less than 5% growth fraction is refractory to drugs.
- By the time a tumour is clinically detectable, only about 10% of the cells are actively proliferating and therefore susceptible to the action of anticancer drugs. The remaining 90% are in the resting phase but are known to restart proliferating if the total tumour mass is reduced (by surgery or by radiotherapy) and become susceptible to the action of drugs.
- A single dose of a cytotoxic drug kills not a fixed number of cancer cells but a constant proportion of those present (**log cell kill hypothesis**). Hence, chemotherapy has the maximum chances of being curative when few tumour cells are present (small tumour volume). Once a clinical remission is obtained, continuation of chemotherapy (perhaps with a different drug) in the presence of inapparent, residual disease is highly effective.
- **Earlier the treatment, better the results.** Small tumors found at microscopic level have a high growth fraction, but large tumours have slower growth rate and are less amenable to treatment.
- **The drugs acting on specific molecular targets are to be preferred.**
  Cell cycle specific drugs act on a particular phase of the cycle. Their dose response curve (DRC) is initially exponential but at higher dose when maximum response is reached, it becomes flat. More rapid the turnover of the cells, more effective they will be.
  Cell cycle nonspecific drugs kill the cells exponentially as the doses go on increasing. They are effective against solid tumors with low proliferative activity
- Intermittently used high doses for short periods

are more effective than continuous low dose. Thus, **the treatment is administered in 'cycles'**. *At least six to eight cycles of therapy are required to get complete remission.* This allows bone marrow to regenerate in the intervals between treatment. Cancer cells recover slowly as their regrowth rate is less. *Such therapy is less immunosuppressive.*
If turnover of cancer cells is low, then continued low dose over long period is advocated (*metronomic chemotherapy*).

- **Generally the treatment is prolonged** because of the exponential nature of cell division and fractional kill achieved by the drug.
- **The drugs are always given in combination.** Different drugs acting through different mechanisms and at different stages of the cell cycle are used as combination therapy. Heterogeneous clones of cells in the tumour differ in their susceptibility to drugs. Combination therapy offers broader coverage against different clones, causing maximal log cell kill and prevents growing of resistant cells to a single drug.
  Similarly, timing and dosage scheduling of agents from different classes can be adjusted in such a way that one drug can modify the cell cycle to increase effectiveness of other drug e.g., vinca alkaloids can be followed by bleomycin. While using drug combination, care should be taken to use drugs with compatible ADR so as to reduce their intensity.
- Chemotherapy is used in conventional dose regimens unless there is well-documented indication for higher dose. **The dose response curve for many anticancer drugs is steep.** *Higher doses can precipitate marked and life threatening complications.* But in most cases, drugs have to be given in such doses that toxic effects are inevitable, which should be looked forand should be tackled.
  The most frequent adverse reactions are severe nausea, vomiting, infections and diarrhoea, mucositis and myelosuppression. Hyperuricaemia following the breakdown of large number of tumour cells can be prevented by using allopurinol, rasburicase or febuxostat.
  Use of bone marrow growth factor, e.g. G-CSF, GM-CSF erythropoietin and thrombopoietin may reduce the frequency and severity of anaemia, neutropenia and thrombocytopenia (Chapter 35).
- *Cytotoxic drugs are contraindicated during pregnancy as they cause abortions or fetal abnormalities.*
- Cancer cells may exhibit inherent or acquired resistance to drugs. The mechanisms of resistance can be
  i. loss of a necessary activating enzyme or
  ii. Over-expression of drug efflux pump.
  For example, multidrug resistance (MDR) is observed due to the overexpressed MDR_1 gene, which increases P-glycoprotein and reduces intracellular concentration of the anticancer drugs. P-glycoprotein inhibitors such as verapamil, quinidine, and cyclosporine are used to overcome the resistance.
- In choosing a drug regime one must always keep in mind its 'cost effectiveness' as chemotherapy in general is very expensive. These drugs should not be used **simply to prolong the 'act of dying' in terminal cases**.

Response to chemotherapy may be judged by:

1. Improvement of the sense of well-being of the patient
2. Decrease in tumour markers
3. Normalisation of organ function
4. Shrinkage of the tumour mass

In general, the possibility of cure is inversely related to tumour volume and directly to the dose of the drug.

Chemotherapy is only a part of the overall approach to the care of terminally ill cancer patient. When one can neither cure an illness nor prolong life, one must strive to **improve the quality of life** of the patient. Towards this end, **palliative therapy** to relieve the symptoms and reduce the suffering contributes significantly (Box 59.1). The measures taken are:

- **Maintenance of nutrition**
- **Treatment of anaemia and neutropenia** (Chapters 34 and 35) and **cachexia**
- **Protection from infection.** As chemotherapeutic agents, being immunosuppressants, reduce the body's resistance to infection
- **Control of symptoms** particularly pain on a day to day basis
- **Occupational and physiotherapy**
- **Adequate emotional and spiritual support** to

Box 59.1 Palliative Symptom Control in the Terminally Ill Cancer Patient

- Frequent re-evaluation is important as symptoms change often
- Enquiring daily about frequency of bowel movements is more important than monitoring pulse, temperature and BP
- **Never say 'nothing can be done'**. Consult or refer if the patient is uncomfortable.
- ***Pain:*** See Chapter 11
- ***Anorexia:*** Prednisolone 15–30 mg or dexamethasone 2–4 mg per day
- ***Nausea and vomiting:*** See Chapter 39. This may be morphine induced.
- ***Dyspnoea:*** It may respond to morphine, diazepam or a glucocorticoid
- ***Headache:*** If severe, it may be due to raised intracranial tension and may respond to dexamethasone 16 mg/day for a few days, followed by 4–6 mg/day
- ***Noisy upper respiratory secretions*** ('death rattle') are troubling to the family but not generally to the patient. They can be reduced by SC injection of atropine 200–400 mcg every 2–4 h, as needed.
- ***Convulsions:*** They are liable to occur in patients with cerebral tumours and should be treated with phenytoin or carbamazepine; when oral medication is no longer possible, rectal diazepam may be used. In very restless patients, midazolam may be used in the dose of 20–30 mg using syringe pump over 24 h subcutaneously.
- ***The treatment of other symptoms*** (constipation, cough, restlessness-confusion and pruritus) has been described elsewhere in the book
- ***Use of bone marrow growth factors*** can reduce the degree of neutropenia and protect against infection (Chapter 35)

the patient and the family. **This is very important particularly in a condition like incurable cancer** where the physician can hardly do anything specific but watch helplessly.

ANTI-CANCER DRUGS: CYTOTOXIC DRUGS

Alkylating agents

Nitrogen mustards
- Mechlorethamine
- Cyclophosphamide
- Melphalan
- Chlorambucil

Ethylenimines
- Triethylenethiophosphoramide (Thio-TEPA)

Alkyl sulphonates
- Busulfan

Methylhydrazine derivative
- Procarbazine

Triazenes
- Dacarbazine (DTIC)
- Temozolomide

Nitrosoureas
- Carmustine (BCNU)
- Bendamustine

Platinum coordination complexes
- Cisplatin
- Carboplatin
- Oxaliplatin

Antimetabolites

Folic acid antagonists
- Methotrexate

Purine antagonists
- 6-mercaptopurine
- Azathioprine

Pyrimidine antagonists
- Fluorouracil
- Fluorodeoxyuridine
- Cytosine arabinoside

Deoxycytidine analogues
- Cytarabine
- Gemcitabine

Radioactive isotopes
- Radioiodine
- Radiogold
- Radiophosphorus

Cytotoxic antibiotics
- Actinomycin-D
- Mitomycin-C
- Rubidomycin
- Doxorubicin
- Bleomycin
- Mithramycin

Antimitotic natural products
- Vinca alkaloids (vinblastine, vincristine, vindesin)
- Eribulin
- Taxanes (paclitaxel, docetaxel)
- Podophyllotoxin derivatives (etoposide, teniposide)
- Camptothecin analogues (irinotecan, topotecan)

Miscellaneous
- Hydroxyurea
- Mitotane,
- L-asparaginase
- Tretinoin
- Arsenic trioxide

ANTI-CANCER DRUGS: TARGETED CANCER THERAPIES

Hormones and antihormones

Glucocorticoids
- Prednisolone

Estrogens and progestins

Antiestrogens
- Tamoxifen
- Fulvestrant

Antiandrogens
- Flutamide
- Nilutamide
- Bicalutamide

Aromatase inhibitors
- Letrozole
- Anastrozole
- Exemestane

LHRH agonists
- Leuprolide
- Goserelin

GnRH antagonist
- Abarelix

Somatostatin analogues
- Octreotide
- Lanreotide

Signal transduction inhibitors

Tyrosine kinase inhibitors e.g.
- Imatinib
- Nilotinib
- Ponatinib
- Lapatinib
- Ceritinib
- Gefitinib
- Erlotinib

Immunotherapies

Monoclonal antibodies
- Trastuzumab
- Rituximab
- Panitumumab
- Cetuximab
- Alemtuzumab

Biological response modifiers
- Interferons
- Interleukins
- BCG
- Levamisole

Angiogenesis inhibitors

- Bevacizumab

Apoptosis inducers

- Proteasome inhibitors
- Bortezomib
- Carfilzomib

CHAPTER 60

PH 1.62

Antiseptics, Disinfectants and Insecticides

Learning Objectives

This chapter will enable the reader:

1. To classify antiseptics and disinfectants.
2. To state the factors that determine therapeutic efficacy of antiseptics.
3. To mention the mechanism of action, precautions, contraindications and indications for antiseptics, i.e. physical agents, acids, alkalies, alcohols, aldehydes, surfactants, phenols, halogenated compounds, oxidising agents, dyes, heavy metals and gases.
4. To enlist the selection criteria for choosing a particular method of sterilisation/disinfection.
5. To classify insecticides.
6. To state the adverse effects and uses of various insecticides, i.e. organochlorines, carbamates, organophosphorous compounds and botanical compounds.

KEY TERMS

antiseptic, disinfectant definition, p. 851
mechanism of action of antiseptics, p. 852
physical agents, p. 852
chemical disinfection, p. 853
surfactants, p. 854
zinc salts, p. 859
DDT, p. 861
pyrethroids, p. 863
limonoids, p. 863

Sterilisation can be defined as freeing an article, a surface or a medium, by *removing or killing all microorganisms including vegetative bacteria, spores, fungi and viruses.*

Disinfection (high-level disinfection) is the term used for *destruction of all pathogenic organisms* such as vegetative forms of bacteria, mycobacteria, fungi and viruses **but not spores**. If spores are killed during the process, only then it is equivalent to **sterilisation**.

A **disinfectant** or **germicide** is a chemical which *causes disinfection*. It may be bactericidal or bacteriostatic. *They are generally used to disinfect inanimate objects.* They are classified into the following:

- **Bactericides**
- **Viricides**
- **Fungicides**

Drugs toxic to the external parasites are called **ectoparasiticides.**

An **antiseptic** *is a chemical disinfectant* (**usually bacteriostatic** *in the concentration used) that can be diluted sufficiently for safe application to living tissues (intact skin, mucus membranes or wounds) while still retaining its antimicrobial property.* Antiseptics and disinfectants are often added to easily available daily utilities like soaps, toothpastes, mouth wash and after-shave lotions.

Classification

I. **Physical agents**, e.g. heat, filtration and radiation
II. **Chemical agents:** They are classified as:
   a. **Acids:**
      - ***Inorganic acids:*** Boric acid
      - ***Organic acids:*** Benzoic acid and salicylic acid
   b. **Alkalies:** Sodium and potassium hydroxide
   c. **Alcohols:** Ethanol and isopropyl alcohol
   d. **Aldehydes:** Formaldehyde and glutaraldehyde
   e. **Surfactants:**
      - ***Anionic:*** Soaps, sodium lauryl sulphate, sodium cetostearyl sulphate, dioctyl sodium sulphosuccinate, sodium tetradecyl sulphate
      - ***Ampholytic:*** Sodium *N*-dodecyl alanate, dodecyldi- (aminoethyl)-glycine hydrochloride

- *Cationic:* Benzalkonium, cetrimide, cetylpyridinium, dequalinium and triclobisonium
- *Nonionic:* Polysorbates

f. **Phenols and related compounds:** Phenol, cresol, chlorocresol, hexylresorcinol, bithionol, thymol, hexachlorophane and chlorhexidine
g. **Halogens and halogen-containing compounds:** Chlorine and chloramines; iodine and iodophors
h. **Oxidising agents:** Hydrogen peroxide and other peroxides, potassium and zinc permanganates
i. **Dyes:** Crystal violet, brilliant green, acriflavine and proflavine
j. **Heavy metals:** Silver nitrate, zinc compounds
k. **Gases:** Ethylene oxide

Mechanism of action: They may act by one or more of the mechanisms listed in Box 60.1.

Factors that determine the therapeutic efficacy of these agents are:

- **Drug concentration and its therapeutic index:** In general, the antiseptic effect increases with a rise in concentration. Alcohol, however, is an exception and shows maximum antiseptic activity in a 70% concentration. The potency of a particular concentration is meaningful only in relation to the tissue toxicity (*Therapeutic Index*). The presence of necrotic tissue reduces their penetration and lowers their effective concentration.
- **Species susceptibility:** Some forms, particularly spores and some species of bacteria, are resistant to many antiseptics. *Viruses are susceptible to alkalies but resistant to phenol.*
- **Temperature and duration of contact:** A limited rise in environmental temperature and prolonged contact can enhance sporicidal activity. A rise of temperature by 10°C generally doubles the antibacterial activity of chemical agents, whereas it increases that of moist heat a 100-fold.

Box 60.1 Mechanisms of Action of Disinfectants and Antiseptics

- Coagulation of the bacterial proteins
- An alteration in the properties of the bacterial cell wall
- Binding of free sulphhydryl (–SH) groups essential for enzyme action
- Competition with essential substrates for the important enzymes in the bacterial cell

PHYSICAL AGENTS

1. **Heat** applied at the right temperature and for optimum length of time is the best and most effective sterilising agent available. It may be applied either as **moist heat or dry heat**.
   a. ***Moist heat:*** Moist heat kills microorganisms by coagulating the proteins. It can be applied in several ways:
   - **Pasteurisation:** This is used to kill the pathogenic microorganisms in milk.
   - **Boiling:** Boiling in water for 20 min is an efficient method of *high-level disinfection*; spores are often resistant to boiling.
   - **Steam:** Steam is a very efficient means of *sterilization* because of its high penetrating capacity and because it gives up a large amount of heat (latent heat). By selecting the correct temperature and time cycle, a wide variety of materials can be sterilised.

   b. ***Dry heat:*** Dry heat kills the organisms by oxidising their cell constituents. It can be used in several ways.
   - **Hot air** in an oven is commonly used to dry *sterilise* glass syringes, instruments, and glassware. *Dry sterilisation must be carried at 160–180°C for 60–120 min.*
   - **Flaming**, i.e. direct heating in a Bunsen flame, is used in a bacteriology laboratory to sterilise inoculating wires, etc
   - **Incineration:** This is suitable for soiled dressings, pathological material, animal carcasses and heavily soiled bedding.

2. **Filtration** through different types of filters including the modern Millipore membrane filters is an efficient way of removing larger particles and bacteria from liquids that cannot be treated by other means, e.g. human serum albumin. It is also used to remove heat-resistant, pyrogenic cell-wall endotoxins from other solutions prior to autoclaving them.

3. **Radiation** used for sterilisation is of two types, nonionising and ionising:

a. ***Nonionising radiation:*** Two types of nonionising radiation are used for sterilisation:
- **Infra-red** radiation is another form of dry heat sterilisation
- **Ultra-violet** radiation is absorbed by the proteins and nucleic acids and kills microorganisms. It has low penetrating capacity and its main application is to reduce the bacteria in air, water and on contaminated surfaces. Care must be taken to protect the eyes while using UV radiation.

b. ***Ionising radiation:*** The lethal action of ionising radiation is due to its effect on the nuclear DNA and on the other vital cell components. High energy gamma rays from cobalt-60 are used to sterilise articles such as foods, syringes, swabs, culture plates, catheters and plastic material.

CHEMICAL AGENTS

1. Acids and alkalies

BORIC ACID: Boric acid and sodium borate (Borax) are weak **bacteriostatic and fungistatic** agents. Locally, boric acid is not an irritant. Aqueous solutions of boric acid (2%–4%) are used as mouth washes, eye and skin lotions. Mixed with starch, talc or zinc oxide, it is commonly used as a dusting powder (talcum powder).

Preparations:

i. Boric talc dusting powder contains 2.3 g of boric acid, 5 g of starch and 50 g of sterilised, purified talc
ii. Boric acid eye lotion contains 3.4 g of boric acid dissolved in 100 mL of freshly boiled and cooled purified water
iii. Borax glycerine (12% w/v) is used for painting throat and tongue

BENZOIC ACID: This organic acid has **antibacterial and antifungal properties**; in a concentration of 0.1%, it is used as a preservative. Its antimicrobial activity decreases, if the pH of the medium exceeds 5. Taken orally, benzoic acid is conjugated with glycine in the liver to form hippuric acid, which is excreted in the urine. Benzoic acid-salicylic acid ointment (Whitfield ointment) has been used to treat ringworm infection (see Chapter 69). Sodium benzoate is used as a food preservative.

SALICYLIC ACID: It is a mild antiseptic effect as it does not kill the existing bacteria but prevents the growth of bacteria wherever applied. In addition, the drug has **bacteriostatic, fungicidal and keratolytic properties** (Chapter 69).

Preparations:

i. Salicylic acid compound dusting powder contains 1.5 g of salicylic acid and 2.5 g of boric acid, made up to 50 g with sterilised, purified talc, with or without camphor

Alkalies like sodium hydroxide and potassium hydroxide are used for disinfecting excreta from patients with poliomyelitis.

2. Alcohols

ETHANOL: Ethyl alcohol in the concentration of 70% is a skin antiseptic. It acts by denaturation of the cellular protein. However, it exhibits poor activity against bacterial spores and hydrophilic viruses. As it evaporates quickly, it exerts a cooling effect but it lacks residual activity. *It should not be allowed to come in contact with cornea.*

ISOPROPYL ALCOHOL: This is an inflammable secondary alcohol with burning taste. It is about twice as toxic as ethyl alcohol. As a germicide, it is slightly more potent than ethyl alcohol and has a marked degreasing action. It is used in the concentration of 68%–72% v/v for disinfection of skin.

3. Aldehydes

FORMALDEHYDE: Formaldehyde, a gas at room temperature, is used as a fumigant or as a 40% w/v aqueous solution containing methanol (**Formalin**). It acts by alkylation of proteins and nucleic acids. The solution, in the concentration of 1:200, is a highly effective disinfectant against several bacteria, viruses and fungi; a higher concentration and prolonged exposure are necessary to eliminate spores.

Formaldehyde solution has a pungent odour and is extremely irritant to the mucous membranes. It hardens the epidermis, if applied to the unbroken skin.

Uses: A 10% solution is used for disinfection of excreta, sputa and brush bristles. It is sometimes used in dentistry as a mummifying agent for residual pulp tissue. A 3% solution is available for removal of warts on the palms and soles, and a 20%–30% solution to treat hyperhidrosis. A 4% solution in saline is a preservative for pathological specimens.

Formaldehyde gas, obtained by heating formaldehyde solution or formalin tablets, is used for sterilisation of those articles which cannot be wetted with solutions or subjected to high temperatures. It does not damage metal, plastics or fabrics.

GLUTARALDEHYDE: Glutaraldehyde is a saturated aldehyde which produces a slightly acid solution in water. It is a **potent bactericide, sporicide, viricide and fungicide**. The solution must be alkalinised to pH 7.4–8.5 for activation. The shelf life of activated solution is 14 days. A rise of pH above 8.5 causes polymerisation of glutaraldehyde with loss of activity. It is less irritant than formaldehyde to the eyes and the skin. Unlike formaldehyde, it does not damage lenses and cementing material in endoscopes and is superior to it for sterilising rubber, plastic and metal appliances. It can also be used to sterilise complicated apparatus like respirators. It is available as a 2% solution which is buffered to a pH of 7.5–8.5 with sodium bicarbonate before use. As 2% aqueous solution, it is used as a local application to treat idiopathic hyperhidrosis of palms and soles.

4. Surfactants

Surfactants are chemical compounds which lower the surface tension of solutions, usually aqueous ones. They are also termed **detergents.** They can be classified into:

I. ANIONIC SURFACTANTS: Soaps belong to this category. Anionic surfactants dissociate in aqueous solution to form a relatively large and complex anion, which is responsible for the **surface tension lowering activity**. Soaps are mainly effective against Gram-positive and acid-fast organisms. It is likely, however, that their cleansing action is secondary to emulsification of the lipoidal secretions in which the bacteria are embedded; the microorganisms are subsequently enmeshed in the lather and washed away with rinsing.

Soft soaps derived by combination of *unsaturated fatty acids* with potassium hydroxide or sodium hydroxide are more efficient germicidal agents than **hard soaps** formed by the treatment of *saturated fatty acids* with sodium or potassium hydroxide. The disadvantages of soaps are their:

- **Narrow antimicrobial spectrum**
- **Incompatibility with cationic surfactants**
- **Tendency to precipitate by hard water**
- **Ability to cause drying and cracking of the skin**

Preparations:

i. Sodium lauryl sulphate: **This is effective in hard water and is active in both acidic and alkaline media**. It is used in medicated shampoos and as a preoperative skin cleanser, usually along with another antiseptic.

ii. Sodium cetostearyl sulphate is used like sodium lauryl sulphate

iii. Soap water enema- Chapter 40

Other anionic surfactants include dioctyl sodium sulphosuccinate used as a faecal softening agent (Chapter 40), and sodium tetradecyl sulphate used as a sclerosing agent for varicose veins (Chapter 33).

II. CATIONIC SURFACTANTS: This group is the **most favoured of the antiseptics** at present. Cationic surfactants dissociate into a large and relatively complex cation, which is responsible for the activity and a smaller inactive anion. The cation usually contains pentavalent nitrogen atom, which is often present as a quaternary ammonium, pyridinium or piperidinium group. **In addition to emulsifying and detergent actions, the cationic surfactants have a marked bactericidal activity** against both Gram-positive and Gram-negative organisms. They are less effective against spores, viruses and fungi. They are most effective in neutral solution.

The mechanism of their antibacterial activity is not clear. It is postulated that by lowering surface tension, they damage the cell membrane. They may also inactivate certain enzymes.

They are incompatible with anionic surfactants like soaps. As these agents combine readily with proteins, their activity is greatly reduced in the presence of serum, pus and other organic matter. When applied to skin, they tend to form a film under which bacteria, particularly *Pseudomonas* *aeruginosa* and *Mycobacterium tuberculosis*, can remain viable.

The solutions of cationic surfactants are generally colourless, odourless, nonirritating and nontoxic in bactericidal concentrations. They remain stable for a long time and **do not deteriorate on boiling or autoclaving.**

Preparations:

i. **Benzalkonium chloride:** This occurs as a white or yellowish white powder or as gelatinous pieces. It has an aromatic odour, markedly bitter taste and is water soluble.
   a. A 1:1000 solution: for the preoperative disinfection of intact skin
   b. A 1:1000–1:4000 solution: for storing sterilised surgical instruments
   c. A 1:8000 solution: for soaking baby napkins to prevent napkin rash
   d. Contact lens solution
   Instruments and polythene tubes, treated with the drug must be thoroughly washed before use as the cationic surfactants have a deleterious effect on nerve tissue.
   It is used only as a disinfectant. **It is not recommended as an antiseptic** because resistant pseudomonas and other Gram-negative bacteria can grow in the antiseptic solution.

ii. **Cetrimide:** A concentration of 0.1%–1% in water is used for similar purposes as benzalkonium chloride. A 1:20,000 concentration is used as a preservative for eye drops. Cetrimide cream contains 5.0 g of cetrimide, 50.0 g of cetostearyl alcohol and 500 g of liquid paraffin made up to 1000 g with water. Cetrimide lotion contains 1% cetrimide in water.

iii. **Miscellaneous:** Other cationic surfactants available include cetylpyridinium chloride, dequalinium acetate and triclobisonium chloride

III. **AMPHOLYTIC SURFACTANTS:** They are derivatives of long chain N-substituted amino acids and can have anionic, nonionic or cationic properties depending on the pH. They are anionic at a pH above their isoelectric point and cationic at a pH below it. **They have the detergent properties of anionic surfactants and the antiseptic properties of cationic surfactants.** They, however, are incompatible with both anionic and cationic agents. The compounds available for use include sodium *N*-dodecyl alanate and dodecyldi-(aminoethyl)-glycine hydrochloride.

IV. **POLYSORBATES:** *They are devoid of antiseptic activity but serve as surfactants.* The elimination of one molecule of water from the hexahydric alcohol sorbitol results in the formation of compounds termed sorbitans, while elimination of another water molecule results in the formation of sorbides. By esterification of these with fatty acids, **nonionic surfactants are produced. These are termed polysorbates**. These substances are active water in oil emulsifying agents, while their polyoxyethylene derivatives are nonionic, oil in water emulsifying agents.

The polysorbates and their polyoxyethylene derivatives such as **Tween 80** are used:

- as surface active agents in insecticides and fruit spraying solutions
- as industrial detergents

5. Phenols and related compounds

PHENOL (Carbolic acid): Lord Lister introduced phenol (Fig. 60.1), into medicine in 1867. It is sparingly soluble in water but freely soluble in alcohol and has a typical odour.

- It is a potent bactericidal and fungicidal agent.
- It acts by denaturing the bacterial proteins and disrupting the cell wall.
- It is mainly effective **against nonsporulating pathogens.** *All spores and most viruses are resistant.*
- It penetrates the intact skin, the mucous membranes and other tissues and **acts as a corrosive.**
- It is extremely irritating to exposed tissues and may cause necrosis.
- It is carcinogenic.
- The antiseptic and corrosive properties are greatly

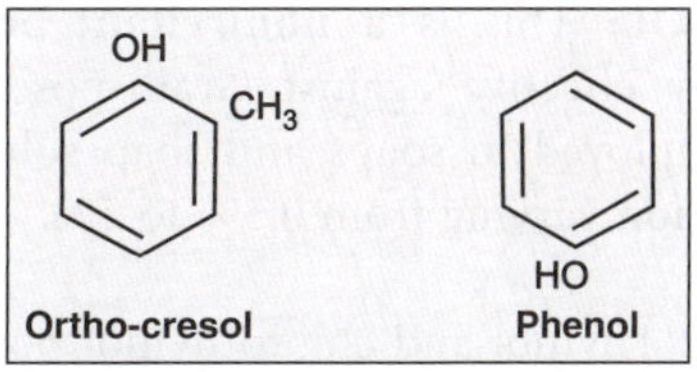

FIG. 60.1 Ortho-cresol and phenol.

reduced if it is dissolved in alcohol, glycerine or a fixed oil.

Ingestion of phenol results in severe GI corrosion, pain, vomiting and shock. Death is usually due to respiratory failure. Treatment is essentially symptomatic.

Uses: *Phenol is not used even as a disinfectant because of its corrosive properties.* It may, however be used as an in vitro deodorant. A 0.5% solution is occasionally used as antipruritic on the skin. It has been occasionally used as a 5% oily solution in almond oil for sclerosing unprolapsed haemorrhoids.

CRESOL: Cresol is a mixture of the ortho-, meta- and para-methyl derivatives of phenol. In the commercially available product, the meta-isomer is the major constituent. Cresol is 10 times as active as phenol and has a wider margin of safety. It is an almost colourless to pale brownish yellow liquid, becoming darker on keeping or on exposure to light, and with a characteristic phenolic odour. It is sparingly soluble in water and is used as 2% solution. It is irritant and can damage the skin and mucous membranes.

LYSOL (Cresol with soap solution): is prepared by saponification of a mixture of cresol with a vegetable oil or the mixed fatty acids derived therefrom. It contains 50% v/v of cresol. It has largely been replaced by safer preparations like iodophors.

CHLOROXYLENOL: It is a less toxic chlorinated phenol. It is supplied as a 4.8% solution. It is effective against Gram-positive and Gram-negative organisms. One of the commonly used preparations is **Dettol**. Surgical Dettol used for preoperative preparation of skin contains 1.44% of chloroxylenol; Dettol used for disinfection of surgical instruments contains 6.25% of the agent, whereas a 1%–3% concentration is employed in the antiseptic cream.

BITHIONOL: This is a **nonirritant bactericide,** particularly effective against Gram-positive cocci, usually employed in soaps and soap solution in a concentration varying from 0.5% to 5%.

THYMOL: Thymol and chlorothymol possess both antiseptic and antifungal properties. Both of these, however, are irritating to wounds, have a poor water solubility and lose their bactericidal power considerably in the presence of proteins. They are usually used in mouth washes and antiseptic solutions.

HEXACHLOROPHANE: This **chlorinated phenol** exhibits bacteriostatic activity against a wide variety of organisms. It retains its activity in the presence of soaps but not so much in the presence of serum or pus.

It can get absorbed from burnt or denuded skin and from mucous membrane and even from the unbroken skin in premature infants. Severe neurotoxicity in the form of a myelopathy and cerebral oedema has been reported in infants washed regularly with a 3% solution. Accidental ingestion or the application of high concentration (6%) to children has caused cardiovascular disturbances, convulsions and respiratory arrest.

Phenolic disinfectants are not to be used in the nursery.

CHLORHEXIDINE: It is a cationic biguanide with low water solubility. It:

- Acts against a wide range of Gram-positive and Gram-negative organisms and against fungi at pH 5.5–7.0
- Bacterial spores are prevented from germinating but are not killed
- It is effective even in the presence of blood or pus
- It is rapid acting, nonirritating and has residual activity
- It has low potential for producing contact dermatitis and photosensitivity. Oral toxicity is low because it is poorly absorbed

It is available as 5% aqueous concentrate or 1% water miscible cream. **Its activity is reduced in the presence of neutral soap, surfactants and anionic agents.** Chlorhexidine in alcohol is used for hand sanitisation.

6. Halogens and halogen-containing compounds

CHLORINE AND **CHLORAMINES:** Chlorine is the most commonly used halogen, largely for purification of water. **Chloramines**, which release chlorine slowly, are used for disinfection. Chlorine exerts a bactericidal action against a variety of Gram-positive and Gram-negative organisms in a concentration as low as 0.0002%. *The agent also kills protozoa and viruses including HIV.* The bactericidal action is significantly reduced in the presence of serum, faeces and other organic matters.

It is a strong oxidising agent and its antibacterial activity is due to the formation of hypochlorous acid (HOCl). *Interestingly, the killing of bacteria ingested by neutrophils in the animal body involves synthesis of HOCl by the intracellular action of the enzyme myeloperoxidase on H_2O_2 and halide.* Sodium hypochlorite 5.25% made up in tap water (pH 7.5) retains activity for months. An alkaline medium greatly reduces the antiseptic activity of hypochlorous acid by causing dissociation of the acid molecule.

Chlorine gas poisoning is characterised by severe irritation of the respiratory passage leading to pulmonary oedema, and by metabolic acidosis. Treatment is symptomatic.

Solutions of hypochlorous acid are corrosive to aluminium, stainless steel and silver.

Preparations:

i. Chlorinated lime and boric acid solution (**Eusol**) is prepared by dissolving 1.25 g of calcium hypochlorite and an equivalent quantity of boric acid and calcium hydroxide powder in 100 mL of water. *The solution is irritating and should, therefore, be diluted with saline before using on denuded surfaces.*
ii. Chloramine: This is an organic chloride. A 2% solution of the agent is used for irrigation of wounds, while a 0.2%–0.55% solution is recommended for mouth wash and for irrigation of bladder and urethra. The solution has to be freshly prepared for use.
iii. Chlorinated lime (**bleaching powder**) is extensively used for purification of water.

IODINE: Iodine being the oldest antiseptic is the most **potent bactericidal, sporicidal, fungicidal, amoebicidal agent with a moderate viricidal activity.** Its germicidal activity is less influenced than that of chlorine by pH, temperature and the time of contact. However, like chlorine, its activity is inhibited by reducing agents and organic material, whereas it is enhanced by alcohol.

Iodine stains the skin, is irritating, painful and may delay the healing. In rare cases, it causes severe reactions, such as bronchospasm, fever and skin eruptions. Elemental iodine, if ingested, can cause severe GI irritation and shock. Treatment consists of gastric lavage with a solution of soluble starch or 5% sodium thiosulphate, and correction of dehydration.

Iodism, may occur following prolonged systemic use of iodides (Chapter 62).

Preparations:

i. Strong iodine tincture contains 10% w/v of iodine, 6% w/v of potassium iodide, and 1% w/v of water in 90% alcohol.
ii. Weak iodine tincture contains 2% w/v of iodine and 2.5% w/v of potassium iodide in 50% alcohol.
iii. Iodine compound paint contains 0.31 g of iodine and 0.62 g of potassium iodide with mentha oil, water and 90% alcohol in glycerine base. A slightly different composition, containing peppermint oil instead of mentha oil is termed **Mandl's paint**.
iv. Nonstaining iodine ointment contains 5% iodine with arachis oil and yellow soft paraffin.
v. Aqueous iodine solution (**Lugol's solution**) is used in thyrotoxicosis (Chapter 62).

Uses: Iodine tincture may be employed for disinfection of skin prior to surgery. Iodine crystals have been used to sterilise water for drinking during hiking expeditions and in water for soaking fresh vegetables to disinfect them before consumption. *Iodine 1:20,000 solution is bactericidal in one minute and kills spores in 15 min.*

Iodine glycerine preparation (**Mandl's paint**) is applied to the mucous membranes in the treatment of follicular tonsillitis and pharyngitis. Iodine ointments are used as counterirritants and have also been used locally as fungicides in the treatment of ringworm. Iodinated hydroxyquinolines are used in amoebiasis (Chapter 55) and as topical antifungal agents (Chapter 69).

The use of iodides as expectorants (Chapter 26) and in the treatment of thyrotoxicosis (Chapter 62) is described elsewhere. *Unlike iodine, iodides have no antibacterial action.*

IODOPHORS: **Iodophors are developed by complexing iodine with surfactants** like nonionic detergents, quaternaries and macromolecules. The detergents act as solubilisers and carriers, combining detergent property with antibacterial activity. They owe their germicidal activity to the slowly released elemental iodine. They are sporicidal on prolonged contact.

Compared to aqueous/tincture iodine, **iodophors are nonirritating, nonstaining, water-miscible in all dilutions, less toxic and nonsensitising to the skin.**

The iodophors available are as follows:

i. **Povidone-iodine 5% (Betadine):** A complex of iodine with polyvinyl pyrrolidone, available as solution, ointment and eye-drops
ii. **Undecoylium chloride iodine:** A complex of iodine with the cationic surfactant undecoylium chloride

Uses: Iodophors are now extensively used as mouth and hand washes, for preoperative skin preparation, as local antiseptics, in ringworm and in oral and vaginal moniliasis. Iodophors may also be used for disinfection of operation rooms, wards, nurseries, etc.

Povidone eye drops (5%) are sometimes used for dry eye conditions.

7. Oxidising agents

HYDROGEN PEROXIDE: This colourless, odourless liquid is a potent oxidiser and owes its action to its ready release of nascent oxygen, when applied to tissues. It is used mainly as a disinfectant and an antiseptic. It has a broad spectrum of activity. Concentrations of 10%–25% are sporicidal. Vapour phase H_2O_2 is a cold gaseous sterilant and can be used as a substitute for formaldehyde.

Its application causes an effervescence which mechanically removes the tissue debris from otherwise inaccessible regions. It does not combine with tissue proteins and its degradation product is nontoxic. The action, however, is of short duration.

Hydrogen peroxide solution contains not less than 6.0% w/v of H_2O_2, corresponding to about 20 times its volume of available oxygen and, hence, is described as '20 volume'.

Peracetic acid prepared from H_2O_2 is a more potent bactericidal and sporicidal agent used in food processing industry.

Uses: It is used for:

- Cleansing wounds and abscesses
- Softening of ear wax and adhering dressings
- For irrigation and cleaning septic sockets and root canals in dentistry
- Gargling as mouth wash and as deodorant (when diluted with 3–8 parts of water)

Other peroxides: These include **magnesium peroxide** and the commonly used **zinc peroxide.** It releases nascent oxygen, leaving behind zinc oxide, which has a mild astringent action. It is applied locally as a 40% suspension for disinfecting, deodorising, and promoting healing of burns and wounds contaminated with anaerobic bacteria. A 25% suspension in water is used as a mouth wash to treat anaerobic infections.

POTASSIUM AND ZINC PERMANGANATES: These compounds possess oxidising and astringent properties. Zinc permanganate is more astringent than the potassium salt. The concentrated solutions and crystals of permanganates are caustic. Their ingestion may cause severe GI irritation and kidney damage.

Preparations:

i. Potassium permanganate occurs as dark purple crystals, with a metallic lustre. It is moderately soluble in water.
ii. Potassium permanganate gargle contains 25 mg of potassium permanganate in 100 mL of water (1 in 4000). It should be freshly prepared.
iii. Zinc permanganate occurs as brownish-black iridescent deliquescent crystals soluble 1 in 3 parts of water

Uses: It is used as a gargle, mouth wash or for vaginal irrigation. The concentrations of 1 in 5000 to 1 in 10,000 are used for urethral irrigation and as wet dressings and in baths for acute infective dermatoses. A 1% solution has been used locally in mycotic infections such as athlete's foot. **A 5% solution has a powerful styptic action.**

Because of its oxidising property, potassium permanganate as a crystalline insufflation has been employed topically to oxidise venom in case of snake and scorpion bite. A 0.02% solution in water is used for stomach wash in the treatment of alkaloidal poisoning.

Potassium permanganate is commonly employed to purify well water and to disinfect vegetables and fruits.

Zinc permanganate, because of its greater astringent activity, is preferred to the potassium salt for urethral irrigation.

8. Dyes

Natural dyes used since ancient times in foods, medicines and cosmetics, have been replaced by the more stable synthetic dyes. These are used as antiseptics, chemotherapeutic, diagnostic and colouring agents. They are nonirritant. They are sometimes used as aqueous solutions or ointments to be applied topically in the treatment of burns, impetigo and chronic ulcers of the skin and mucous membranes. They are claimed to promote healthy granulation tissue and thus help in healing of ulcers. Used locally, they are almost nontoxic. They cause local staining. The commonly used dyes are: **gentian violet** 0.1%, **briliant green** 0.5%–1.0% and **acriflavine** 2%.

9. Heavy metals

The pharmacology of heavy metals is discussed in Chapter 74. *Heavy metal salts used exclusively as antiseptics destroy the microorganisms in very low concentrations*. The antiseptic activity is due to precipitation of the bacterial proteins.

SILVER COMPOUNDS:

i. **Silver nitrate:** This occurs as colourless or white crystals, extremely soluble in water. Silver nitrate has antiseptic, astringent and caustic properties. If ingested, it produces severe GI irritation, vertigo, coma and convulsions. Applied to the skin, it stains the area.
   Aqueous solution containing **1% of silver nitrate** is used prophylactically as eye drops (two drops) for conjunctivitis and *ophthalmia neonatorum*. Aqueous solution of 0.5% is sometimes applied on second and third degree burns as prophylaxis against infection.
   Silver nitrate stick has been used to remove warts and other small skin growths and for cauterisation of wounds and trachoma follicles. The stick should be moistened before use.
ii. **Silver sulphadiazine** (Chapter 43)

ZINC SALTS: Zinc salts possess astringent, corrosive and weak antiseptic properties. The commonly used salts are:

i. **Zinc sulphate:** Zinc sulphate occurs as odourless, colourless, efflorescent crystals or as a white crystalline powder. It has an astringent metallic taste and is soluble in water.
   Externally, zinc sulphate is used as an astringent lotion for indolent ulcers and to assist granulation. Eye drops in the concentration of 0.1%–1% are sometimes used in angular conjunctivitis and in chronic inflammation of the cornea. The salt is the major ingredient of many commercially available deodorant anhidrotics.
ii. **Calamine** is a pink powder, almost odourless and tasteless and insoluble in water. Chemically, it is zinc carbonate (98%) with a small amount of ferric oxide which imparts the pink colour. It has mild astringent and antiseptic actions and is used as a **lotion and a dusting powder** in skin conditions like sunburns, eczema, insect bites, and urticaria, where it also acts as a soothing and protective agent.
   Calamine lotion usually contains 15% of calamine, 5% each of zinc oxide and glycerine, 3% of bentonite, 0.5% each of liquified phenol and sodium citrate, with rose water as the vehicle. It can also be used as oily lotion or cream (Chapter 69).
iii. **Zinc oxide** is a common constituent of several commercial preparations, used as powders and creams in cosmetics and dermatology
iv. **Zinc phosphate** is *toxic* and *used as rat poison*

10. Gases

Ethylene oxide, formaldehyde and betapropiolactone in the gaseous form are powerful agents used for sterilisation. Beta-propiolactone has been reported to have carcinogenic properties.

ETHYLENE OXIDE: *At normal room temperatures, it is a highly inflammable and highly explosive gas with a sweet ethereal smell.* The explosive tendency can be limited by keeping down the concentration of ethylene oxide to 10%. A relative humidity of about 30% is necessary for satisfactory sterilisation. It has powerful bactericidal, sporicidal and viricidal properties and a high penetrating capacity. It is an excellent agent for sterilising complicated equipment like heart–lung machines and respirators as well as suture material. **Its safe use necessitates special equipment**. It is mutagenic and carcinogenic.

CHOICE OF METHOD OF STERILISATION AND DISINFECTION

All instruments and apparatus to be sterilised should be first thoroughly cleaned by washing and scrubbing. The same applies to areas for fumigation **as the presence of organic matter reduces the efficacy of chemical disinfectants.**

Autoclaving is the method of choice for sterilising theatre appliances. Those which cannot withstand autoclaving are sterilised by chemical methods:

1. Lysol, chloroxylenol or iodophor for surgical blades and scissors
2. Formaldehyde or gluteraldehyde for endoscopes and specialised rubber equipment
3. Ethylene oxide for heart–lung machines
4. Syringes are sterilised by autoclaving, hot air sterilisation or gamma radiation. Diabetics are commonly advised to keep their nondisposable syringe and needle permanently immersed in spirit and to boil them once a week.
5. Gamma radiation is now increasingly used to sterilise disposable articles on a massive scale
6. Autogenous and some types of synthetic grafts used in cardiovascular surgery are sterilised with antibiotics

It is customary to sterilise the air in operation theatres with ultra-violet radiation or with iodophor spray. Ultra-violet radiation is also used to sterilise the air inside sterile dispensing cabinets. Solutions of biological materials such as sera and antibiotics which cannot be sterilised by heat are often 'sterilised' by filtration. Laboratory glassware is ordinarily sterilised in a hot air oven after thorough, preliminary cleansing.

Wards, theatres and sick rooms and the contaminated furniture can be swabbed with formalin or iodophor solution, fumigated with gaseous formaldehyde or sprayed with iodophor solution or with a commercial mixture containing glutaraldehyde, chemically bound formaldehyde and benzalkonium chloride. If facilities for incineration are not available, soiled dressings, pathological materials and animal carcasses are best disinfected with lysol or iodophor.

For preoperative preparation of the skin, the preferred antiseptics are tincture of iodine, aqueous iodophor (2%) solution and a 2% solution of hibitane in alcohol.

Acriflavine and **chloroxylenol** are useful as wound antiseptics. Although Condy lotion (a 0.1% aqueous solution of potassium permanganate) is still the favourite for bladder washes, 1% aqueous solutions of acetic acid and silver nitrate are far more effective for this purpose.

Chloroxylenol is a popular and effective disinfectant for hand-washing by attendants and for sick-room swabbing. Soiled bed linen and clothes of patients treated at home should be soaked in a disinfectant such as chloroxylenol and then washed.

Swimming pools and water supplies are generally disinfected by chlorination whereas **potassium permanganate** is a convenient domestic disinfectant for water, fruits and vegetables.

Table 60.1 summarises the chemical methods of high level disinfection.

Points to remember about utility of disinfectants are mentioned in Box 60.2.

Table 60.1 Some Chemical Methods of High Level Disinfection

Chemical	Concentration	Uses and Comments
Sodium hypochlorite	0.1%–1.0%	Efficient for disinfecting linen, clothing, spills, stainless steel instruments; syringes and needles before autoclaving/disposal; solution must be freshly prepared as it is unstable; cheapest disinfectant
Chloramine T	4%	Similar to above. More stable
Ethanol	70%	Useful for hand washing, spills, instruments and equipment
Cetrimide	Stock solution diluted 1:100	Useful for furniture, spills, fittings and equipment
Povidone-iodine	One part of 10% solution added to 3 parts of boiled water	Similar to ethanol. Immerse for 15 min
Formaldehyde	35%–40% solution diluted 1:10	Disinfection after 30 min immersion; sterilisation after several hours. Toxic
	Tablets releasing vapour	Requires special apparatus
Glutaraldehyde	2%	30 min immersion for disinfection, 10 h for sterilisation
Hydrogen peroxide	6%	Disinfection after 30 min of immersion

Box 60.2 Points to Remember About Disinfectants

- Most are highly active against Gram-positive bacteria
- Acid fast bacilli are less susceptible and need higher concentrations. They are resistant to chlorhexidine, oxidising agents and cresol.
- Aldehydes, sodium hypochlorite and povidone iodine have action against fungi too
- Spores are usually resistant to all except aldehydes, sodium hypochlorite and high concentrations of povidone iodine
- Hydrophilic viruses are usually resistant except to aldehydes and high concentrations of sodium hypochlorite
- Prions are resistant to most agents except high concentrations of sodium hypochlorite
- *Hand washing is the important method for preventing transmission of infection from person to person and is best done with soap and warm water, with or without a disinfectant,* as a disinfectant can cause irritation, dryness and sensitisation of the skin

INSECTICIDES

PH 1.51

These agents, primarily used to destroy insects, are important because of their toxicological properties.

Classification

I. **Organochlorines:**
   a. Chlorophenothane (DDT) and related compounds
   b. Cyclodienes, e.g. aldrin, endrin, diledrin, heptachlor, chlorolane, endosulphan and chlordecone
   c. Gamma benzene hexachloride (Gammexane)
   d. Toxaphene and related compounds

   All these compounds persist in the environment and can accumulate in the body tissues.

II. **Carbamate insecticides:** Carbaryl, dimetan, pyrolan, zectran and carbofuran.

III. **Organophosphorus compounds:** Malathion, parathion, TEPP and diazinon (Chapter 19).

IV. **Botanical compounds:** Pyrethrum, limonoids and rotenone

I. ORGANOCHLORINES

CHLOROPHENOTHANE (DDT, Dicophane), chemically dichloro-diphenyl-trichloroethane, (Fig. 60.2) occurs as a white powder, practically insoluble in water but slightly soluble in alcohol and kerosene.

DDT is lethal to many arthropods including fleas, body lice, houseflies and mosquitoes. It is absorbed through both the chitinous exoskeleton and the GI tract of the insect and thus **acts as a**

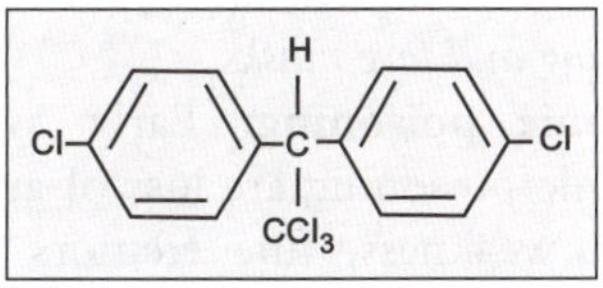

FIG. 60.2 **Dicophane (DDT).**

stomach and contact poison. It causes titanic convulsions and paralyses the CNS.

DDT, because of its low volatility, retains its insecticidal action for a long time (**residual effect**). The agent does not have an immediate lethal effect like pyrethrum and rotenone, but these may be combined to advantage with DDT.

Absorption, fate and excretion: DDT is slowly and incompletely absorbed from the GIT. Although it does not penetrate the intact skin in powder form, when dissolved in the various organic solvents, appreciable percutaneous absorption can occur. Absorption may also occur through inhalation. Slow poisoning can occur due to consumption of animal milk/meat containing DDT.

Following absorption, large amounts of **DDT are stored in body fat depots and in the liver.** The drug is excreted unchanged in milk to some extent but most of it is slowly degraded in the tissues and the products eliminated in urine.

DDT is a hepatic microsomal enzyme inducer.

Adverse reactions:

- **Acute poisoning:** This is characterised by vomiting, diarrhoea, paraesthesiae, giddiness and fatigue followed by tremors, convulsions and coma; associated solvents like kerosene can cause pulmonary oedema. Death occurs from respiratory arrest or from ventricular fibrillation as DDT sensitises the myocardium to adrenaline. The human lethal dose of the insecticide is estimated to be between 10 and 20 g.

  Treatment of acute poisoning is symptomatic and includes gastric lavage, saline purgation, diazepam for the treatment of convulsions, artificial respiration and oxygen. Treatment has to be continued for many days in view of the possible drug storage. *Workers engaged in spraying the insecticide should wear protective clothing and face masks.*
- **Chronic poisoning:** Early symptoms of chronic poisoning are loss of appetite, muscular weakness, fine tremors and mental apprehension. Rarely, it may cause motor neurone disease. Occasionally, anaemia, leucocytosis, liver and kidney damage may develop. It has been shown to be **carcinogenic** in animals (bladder cancer).

Uses: DDT is useful for eliminating fleas, bugs, mosquitoes, cockroaches and body lice. A 10% mixture of DDT with a suitable inert diluent like talc is employed. It is not ovicidal. The walls and furniture can be sprayed with a solution of DDT in kerosene; about 100 mg per square feet usually ensure effective control for about 6 weeks.

Its *value as an insecticide has diminished considerably due to the development of resistance in many strains of insect species. Furthermore, its storage in the body, its possible long-term neurotoxicity and its carcinogenicity are a matter of great concern which has led to a decrease in its use.*

ENDRIN AND **DIELDRIN:** These compounds are more toxic than DDT particularly to fish and birds. Endrin is 2–3 times more toxic than dieldrin. These agents are employed for residual spraying, usually as 0.6%–1.2% suspension for similar purpose as DDT.

GAMMA BENZENE HEXACHLORIDE (Gammexane): Chapter 69.

All organochlorine insecticides are CNS stimulants and can cause convulsions. As they are lipid soluble, they tend to concentrate in the tissues and have prolonged t½. They may also undergo enterohepatic circulation. **Endosulphan ingestion** causes prolonged convulsions, disseminated intravenous coagulation and myoglobinuria. Its treatment is mainly symptomatic: gastric lavage, activated charcoal and anticonvulsants like benzodiazepines. The patient may return after discharge for repeat convulsions a few days later, due to release of the compound from deposits in the fat.

II. CARBAMATE INSECTICIDES

These agents act **as acetylcholinesterase inhibitors and cause actions similar to the organophosphorus compounds** (see below). However, they have shorter duration of action and larger margin of safety. They are considered as nonpersistent insecticides (Chapter 19).

III. ORGANOPHOSPHORUS INSECTICIDES

The organophosphorus compounds such as malathion, chlorpyrifos and fenitrothion are effective against a variety of arthropods like lice, flies and mosquitoes. They cause irreversible cholinesterase inhibition. They act against both the larvae and the adult insects and are widely used as agricultural and horticultural pesticides (for toxicity and treatment, see Chapter 19).

IV. BOTANICAL COMPOUNDS

PYRETHRUM FLOWERS: These are the dried flower heads of *Chrysanthemum cineratiaefolium*. They owe their insecticidal activity to the two esters, **pyrethrin I and pyrethrin II**. Pyrethrum flower extract is rapidly lethal to the insects.

Pyrethrum **acts mainly by contact** and is **neurotoxic to the CNS of the insect.**

It has relatively low human toxicity. Excessive ingestion, however, may cause initial stimulation of the CNS followed by paralysis. The agent also produces contact dermatitis.

It is usually sprayed as solutions containing 0.4%–0.6% of total pyrethrins. Its applications are similar to those of DDT.

PYRETHROIDS: Synthetic pyrethroids include **allethrin, resmethrin, tetramethrin** and **permethrin**. They are chemically related to natural pyrethrins.

Mechanism of action: They act as neuropoisons by acting on sodium channels in the axons in the peripheral and CNS. A single dose produces toxic signs, which are reversible but at near–lethal doses, cause structural changes in the nervous system, such as axonal swelling and/or breaks and myelin degeneration. Such neurotoxicity is especially liable to occur in children.

Absorption, fate and excretion: Pyrethrum is absorbed following ingestion or inhalation but not significantly from the skin. *Hence, when they are being heated they should be kept away from infants and children.* Mats/coils containing pyrethroids, when heated, may cause irritation of the eyes, nose, throat and suffocation.

They are generally metabolised through ester hydrolysis, oxidation and conjugation. There is no tendency to accumulate in tissues.

In the environment, synthetic pyrethroids are fairly rapidly degraded in soil and in plants. There is little tendency for bioaccumulation in organisms.

Because of low application rates and rapid degradation in the environment, residue in food is generally low.

Uses: Because of their excellent activity against a wide range of insect pests and their nonpersistence in the environment, they are now extensively used as:

- **Agricultural insecticides** and **for control of household insects** (See section Mosquito repellents)
- **Ovicidal and pediculocidal agent** as a 1% cream-rinse permethrin preparation, for 10 min local application. **A single application eliminates head-lice infestation.**
- **Scabicidal agent** applied as 5% permethrin dermal cream (Chapter 69)

LIMONOIDS: Limonoids are derived from the ancient Indian plant, neem (*Azadirachta indica*). Several biological active compounds have been isolated from the oil, seeds, bark and leaves of neem. Neem oil or neem leaves have been used for centuries by households and farmers in India to protect the foodgrains.

The limonoid **azadirachtin** and other similar compounds are highly effective in minute quantities against a variety of insects. Since neem has multiple active ingredients, the development of resistance by insects is probably difficult. They appear to be harmless to humans and to useful insects such as honeybees. *Unlike the modern chemical insecticides, azadirachtin is not an instant killer but is a growth inhibitor, antifeedant and repellent.* Its biodegradability is an additional advantage. Neem oil also has spermicidal and antibacterial properties. A number of neem-based pesticides are now available.

ROTENONE: Rotenone is the principal active insecticidal constituent of *Derris or Tuba root.* Rotenone is a **stomach and contact insecticide**. Its action is more rapid but less persistent than that of DDT and less rapid but more persistent than that of the pyrethrum.

Rotenone may cause GI irritation, conjunctivitis,

pharyngitis and rarely, respiratory stimulation and convulsions. It is used either as a dusting powder diluted with talc or as an insecticidal wash.

Mosquito Repellents

Repellents are used on the skin to prevent mosquito bites. They also offer protection against ticks, which transmit Lyme disease. They do not kill mosquitoes but deter them from biting. *However, protection against the hungry Anopheles mosquitoes cannot be ensured.* They are sold as aerosols, creams, solids (sticks), pump sprays and liquids.

A simple remedy which acts as mosquito repellent by virtue of its fragrance has the following composition:

Cedar wood oil: 18 mL
Citronella oil: 42 mL
Spirit of camphor to: 100 mL

Citronella oil can also be applied in the form of vanishing cream. It is nonirritant, nontoxic, cheap and not so unpleasant. Citronella-based repellents, however, provide only a short term protection for about 1 h against mosquitoes and are not effective against ticks. Probably more effective is a 35% emulsion of **dimethyl phthalate** (DMP) which acts as an irritant to insect's feet. It must be rubbed into every part, *avoiding eyelids, lips and scrotum.*

Oil of lemon eucalyptus contains *p*-menthane 3,8-diol and offer protection up to 6 h, but it should be avoided in children below 3 years of age. Essential oils like clove, geraniol (from rose oil) and patchouli (from *pach*) in high concentrations may be used but can irritate the skin. Other agents used are ethohexadiol, butopyronoxyl, DEET, *n*-butyl acetanilide, and picaridin. These are also irritants and have an intensely bitter taste. They can cause allergic reactions and bronchial spasm.

DEET, *N, N* diethyl-*m*-toluamide, in concentrations of 5%–100% repels mosquitoes as well as ticks, fleas, gnats and some flies. However, *its efficacy does not increase above 50%.* DEET offers protection for 90 min to 12 h depending on the concentration. In concentration ,30%, it is probably safe in children and infants .2 months old. No effects have been reported on fetus when it is used by mothers during second and third trimester of pregnancy. However, it can damage synthetic fibre containing clothes and plastics on eyeglass frames and watch crystals.

Picaridin, 5%–20%, is used against mosquitoes, ticks, flies and chiggers. It appears to be as effective as equivalent concentrations of DEET but is better tolerated on skin and does not damage fabric or plastic.

Synthetic pyrethroids (see above) are used in antimosquito tablets and coils. **Permethrin**-treated clothing, shoes, bed nets, tents and sleeping bags provide protection against mosquitoes, ticks, and other arthropods by repelling and killing them. *It remains active for several weeks even after repeated laundering.* It is available in liquid and spray forms.

Highly effective, dependable and totally safe mosquito repellent is not yet available; nevertheless *use of long sleeve shirts and pants, DEET or picardin application on exposed skin and permethrin-treated bed nets are considered the most effective existing remedies.*

DISINFECTANT

Physical agents

- Heat
- Filtration
- Radiation

Chemical agents

Acids

Inorganic acids
- Boric acid

Organic acids
- Benzoic acid
- Salicylic acid

Alkalies

- Sodium
- Potassium hydroxide

Alcohols

- Ethanol
- Isopropyl alcohol

Aldehydes

- Formaldehyde
- Glutaraldehyde

Surfactants

Anionic
- Soaps
- Sodium lauryl sulphate
- Sodium cetostearyl sulphate
- Dioctyl sodium sulphosuccinate
- Sodium tetradecyl sulphate

Ampholytic
- Sodium *N*-dodecyl alanate
- Dodecyldi-(aminoethyl)-glycine hydrochloride

Cationic
- Benzalkonium
- Cetrimide
- Cetylpyridinium
- Dequalinium
- Triclobisonium

Nonionic
- Polysorbates

Phenols and related compounds

- Phenol
- Cresol
- Chlorocresol
- Hexylresorcinol
- Bithionol
- Thymol
- Hexachlorophane
- Chlorhexidine

Halogens and halogen-containing compounds

- Chlorine
- Chloramines
- Iodine
- Iodophors

Oxidising agents

- Hydrogen peroxide
- Other peroxides
- Potassium permanganate
- Zinc permanganate

Dyes

- Crystal violet
- Brilliant green
- Acriflavine
- Proflavine

Heavy metals

- Silver nitrate
- Zinc compounds

Gases

- Ethylene oxide

INSECTICIDES

Organochlorines

- Chlorophenothane (DDT)
- **Cyclodienes**
  - Aldrin
  - Endrin
  - Diledrin
  - Heptachlor
  - Chlorolane
  - Endosulphan
  - Chlordecone
- Gamma benzene hexachloride (Gammexane)
- Toxaphene

Carbamates

- Carbaryl
- Dimetan
- Pyrolan
- Zectran
- Carbofuran

Organophosphorus compounds

- Malathion
- Parathion
- TEPP
- Diazinon

Botanical compounds

- Pyrethrum
- Limonoids
- Rotenone

13
SECTION

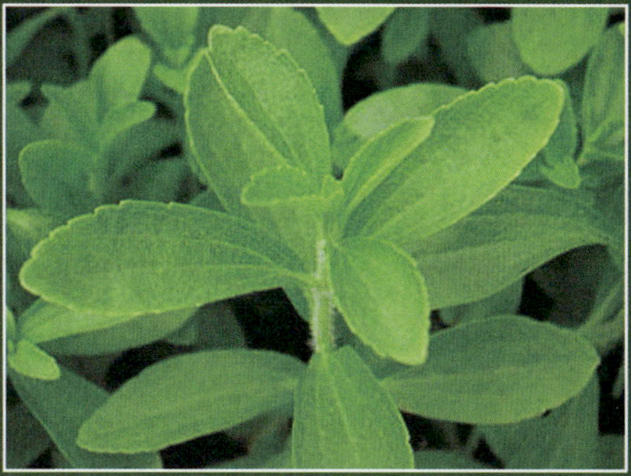

Stevia rebaudiana

Drugs Used in Endocrine Disorders

Section Outline

This section consists of the following chapters:

SECTION 13

Drugs Used in Endocrine Disorders

CHAPTER 61

Anterior Pituitary Hormones

Learning Objectives

This chapter will enable the reader:

1. To classify hormones.
2. To be aware of regulation of hormone synthesis and release.
3. To compare and contrast between peptide and steroid hormones.
4. To state the mechanism of action of hormones.
5. To enumerate pituitary hormones and state the hypothalamic releasing and inhibitory hormones controlling their secretion.
6. To be aware of the effects of hypopituitarism and hyperpituitarism.
7. To explain the pharmacological actions, salient pharmacokinetic features, ADR and indications for growth hormone (GH).
8. To enlist the indications for somatostatin analogues.
9. To enumerate GH-releasing hormone analogues.

KEY TERMS

The important functions of growth, self-preservation (homeostasis) and species preservation (reproduction) in a multicellular organism demand the highest degree of integration of the various body systems and adaptation to external environment. This integration is brought about by the **neuroendocrine complex** consisting of the CNS, the ANS and the endocrine system.

ENDOCRINE PHYSIOLOGY – INTRODUCTION

Hormone is defined as a substance secreted by specialised cells and transported to a distant site to exert its action upon specific tissues.

The endocrine glands, located at various sites in the body, consist of groups of highly specialised cells which synthesise and discharge their specialised secretions (hormones) directly into the circulation without the intervention of a duct. However, tissues like heart, kidneys, GIT and cells such as adipocytes, stem cells, and neurons, though not classical endocrine glands, synthesize and secrete hormones that play key physiological roles.

Hormones can be grouped into five major classes:

- **Amino acid derivatives**, e.g. Catecholamines, dopamine and thyroid hormones
- **Peptides**, e.g. hypothalamic regulatory hormones (TRH, GnRH, GHRH, CRH and others), somatostatin and vasopressin
- **Proteins**, e.g. insulin, GH and PTH
- **Steroids**, e.g. adrenocortical and gonadal steroids
- **Vitamin derived**, e.g. vitamin D derivatives and retinoids

Regulation and release of hormones: The synthesis and secretion of hormones is influenced by:

1. **Hypothalamic releasing and release-inhibiting hormones:** These act on the anterior pituitary to modify the synthesis and release of its trophic hormones. *They have an intrinsic diurnal rhythm* (Fig. 61.1).
2. **Anterior pituitary hormones:** These stimulate synthesis and release of hormones of the target glands – thyroid, adrenal cortex and gonads (**feed forward regulation**). They are called **trophic hormones**. Hormones produced by the target glands have a feedback effect on the hypothalamus–pituitary axis and alter the secretion of the respective trophic hormones, e.g. TSH, ACTH, FSH, LH (Fig. 61.1). Thus, in health, any change in the plasma concentration of a target gland

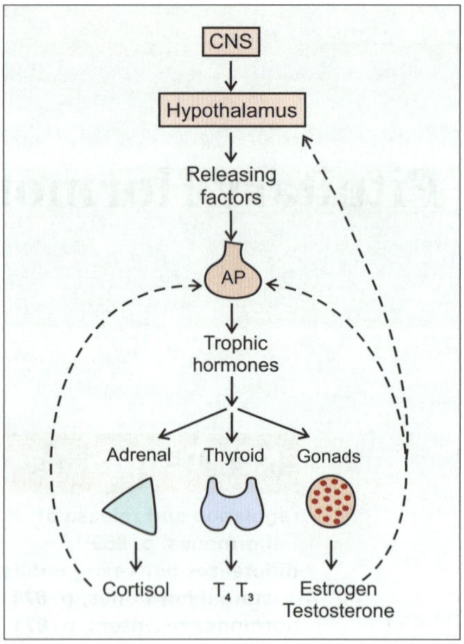

FIG. 61.1 Hormone release and feedback mechanisms. AP = Anterior pituitary; --- dotted lines indicate negative feedback

hormone tends to correct itself by altering the anterior pituitary function.

3. **Changes in the concentration of non-hormonal chemical substances in the plasma**: For example, hyperglycaemia stimulates the release of insulin but suppresses the release of GH
4. **Local regulatory systems:**
   - *Paracrine regulation* involves the release of a hormone by one type of cells that acts on adjacent cells in the same tissue, e.g. *somatostatin from the pancreatic islet D cells inhibits insulin secretion by the beta cells*
   - *Autocrine regulation* involves the action of a hormone on the same cells that produce it, e.g. **insulin-like growth factor 1 (IGF-1)** acts on many cells that produce it, including chondrocytes, gonadal cells and breast epithelial cells.
5. **Psychoneurogenic factors:** For example, acute stress increases the release of catecholamines from the adrenal medulla and cortisol from the cortex

Role of hypothalamus: The hypothalamus synthesises various *regulatory hormones* (Box 61.1). In response to appropriate stimuli, they are released in nanograms or smaller quantities into the portal circulation and travel to the pituitary (Fig. 61.1) to cause the synthesis and release of pituitary trophic hormones. In turn, the trophic hormones cause synthesis and release of target gland hormones.

Box 61.1 Hypothalamic Regulatory Hormones for Pituitary Hormones

Releasing hormone (RH) or factor (RF) for:
- Thyrotrophin: TRH
- Luteinising hormone and follicular stimulating hormone: LH/FSHRH or GnRH
- Growth hormone: GHRH
- Corticotrophin: CRH
- Melanocyte stimulating hormone: MSH-RF

Release inhibiting hormone (RIH) or factor (RIF) for:
- Growth hormone: GH-RIH, somatostatin
- Melanocyte stimulating hormone: MSH-RIF
- Prolactin: PIF-dopamine

The hypothalamic neurons which secrete the regulatory hormones are under the control of specialised monoaminergic, neurotransmitter neurons in the midbrain. Thus:

- **Dopamine** is involved in the release of GH and inhibition of release of PRL
- **Noradrenaline** is concerned in the release of GH, TSH, and gonadotrophins
- **Serotonin** (5-HT) causes the release of GH and PRL and inhibition of TSH release

Certain drugs (reserpine, chlorpromazine, 1-dopa, amphetamine, imipramine and bromergocriptine) act on the hypothalamus and influence the local monoamine concentration to bring about alterations in the secretion of anterior pituitary hormones particularly prolactin.

Transport and metabolism of hormones: The hormones are carried in the plasma partly protein bound and partly free. The metabolic degradation of free hormones occurs in the liver, in the target endocrine glands and in the tissues on which they act. With some hormones, metabolic transformation (e.g. thyroxine to tri-iodothyronine) renders the hormone biologically active. *Knowledge of the t½ of the circulating hormones helps to establish effective, physiological, hormonal replacement therapy as the time required to achieve a steady state plasma level is generally related to the t½ of the hormone(s). Most protein hormones such as insulin, ACTH and GH have very short t½ (minutes), whereas the steroids and the thyroid hormones have longer t½ (hours to days).*

Table 61.1 shows the important differences between the peptide hormones and the steroid hormones. In general, catecholamines behave like the peptide hormones and the iodothyronines (with important differences) behave like the steroid hormones.

Table 61.1 Important Differences between Peptide and Steroid Hormones

Parameter	Steroids	Peptides
Biosynthesis	Multiple enzymes	Single protein, prohormone
Storage in the gland	Minimal	Often substantial
Half-life	Long (h)	Short (min)
Binding proteins	Present	Less common
Peripheral transformations	Common	Do not occur
Initial binding site	Cytoplasmic receptor	Plasma membrane receptors
Principal site of action	Nucleus	Plasma membrane
Principal mechanism of action	Activation of genome	Activation of second messenger
Degradation products	Sometimes retain activity	Inactive
Administration	Oral, parenteral	Parenteral
Allergy	No	Yes

Mechanism of action: Hormones act through:

1. **Cell membrane receptors**
2. **Nuclear receptors**

Generally, amino acid derivatives and peptide hormones interact with cell-surface-membrane receptors; whereas steroidal and thyroidal hormones, vitamin D and its derivatives, and retinoids, which are lipid soluble, interact with nuclear receptors (Table 61.2). Nuclear receptors finally act to increase or decrease gene transcription.

A persistent increase in the concentration of a hormone brings about a *reduction* in the concentration of its specific receptors (**down regulation**). A hormone may bind to more than one class of receptors, e.g. insulin at high concentrations binds to somatomedin receptors and can have growth stimulating actions. Several clinical syndromes occur due to mutational abnormalities in the receptors, e.g. GH resistance, resistance to thyroid hormones.

Hormones as drugs: Hormones and their analogues, prepared synthetically, are now widely used as drugs. Synthetic analogues have the following advantage(s):

a. Abundant availability and are relatively cheap, e.g. prednisolone, thyroxine
b. Improved bioavailability because of resistance to metabolic degradation

Table 61.2 Different Types of Hormone Receptors

Receptor Type	Hormones
Membrane receptors	
a. GPCR	Catecholamines, LH, FSH, TSH, ACTH, hypothalamic releasing factors, somatostatin
b. Tyrosine kinases	Insulin, insulin-like growth factors, epidermal growth factor
c. Cytokine regulated kinases	GH, PRL
d. Serine kinases	Activin, transforming growth factor
Nuclear receptors[a]	
a. Type I (in cytoplasm[b])	Steroids, e.g. glucocorticoids, estrogens and progesterone
b. Type II (in nucleus)	Thyroid hormones, vitamin D, retinoids

[a]All nuclear receptors ultimately act to increase or decrease gene transcription.
[b]After ligand binding, the ligand–cytoplasmic–receptor complex translocates to the nucleus.

c. Longer or shorter duration of action as desired, e.g. rDNA analogues of human insulin
d. Greater specificity because of elimination of trace contaminants

Hormones are used:

- **For diagnostic purposes**, e.g. ACTH is used to diagnose Addison disease, and dexamethasone to diagnose Cushing disease
- **For therapeutic purposes,** either (a) as *replacement therapy* to supplement or replace a deficient natural hormone, e.g. thyroxine in hypothyroidism, or (b) as *pharmacotherapy*, e.g. glucocorticoids in asthma

THE PITUITARY GLAND

The pituitary gland, together with the hypothalamus, forms a neuroendocrine relay station for messages from the brain to the rest of the body. It consists of:

1. **Adenohypophysis**, which consists of the *anterior lobe*, the *pars tuberalis* and the *pars intermedia* and
2. **Neurohypophysis**, which consists of the posterior lobe and the infundibular stalk which connects it to the hypothalamus

The pituitary gland has a rich arterial blood supply and also has a '**portal system**' which connects it with the median eminence of the hypothalamus. The latter transmits the hypothalamic regulatory hormones released from mediobasal hypothalamus, including the paraventricular and the arcuate nuclei, to the pituitary via the portal system.

The anterior lobe of the pituitary secrete six adenohypophyseal hormones that have been definitely identified (Table 61.3). Of these, corticotropin (ACTH) and α-melanocyte–stimulating hormone (α-MSH) are pro-opiomelanocortin (POMC)-derived hormones. α-MSH exists in the pars intermedia of the anterior pituitary. Somatotropic hormones include growth hormone (GH), prolactin and placental lactogen, which are peptides in nature. TSH (thyrotropin or thyroid stimulating hormone), LH (lutropin or luteinizing hormone), and FSH (follitropin or follicle stimulating hormone) and placental human chorionic gonadotropin (hCG) are glycoprotein hormones. Vasopressin and oxytocin are present in the neurohypophysis.

Effects of hypopituitarism: Manifestations of hypopituitarism depend upon the age of the individual.

- **In children:** Retardation of linear growth and of bone age are the two important effects of GH deficiency (GHD). *They are due to IGF-1 deficiency secondary to GH deficiency.*

When GHD occurs as a part of panhypopituitarism, the associated deficiencies of ACTH and TSH make the clinical diagnosis easier. *In some cases, manifestations of GHD are due to GH resistance in the peripheral target tissues as in undernutrition.*

- **In adults:** Panhypopituitarism may be produced

Table 61.3 Hormones of the Anterior Pituitary — PH 1.37

Pituitary Cell	Hormone Produced	Stimulators	Inhibitors	Target Gland	Biologic Effects
Somatotrope	GH	GHRH	Somatostatin, IGF-1	Liver, bone, muscles and other tissues	Growth promotion, IGF-1 production, insulin antagonism
Corticotrope	ACTH	CRF, AVP	Glucocorticoids	Adrenal cortex	Glucocorticoid production
Thyrotrope	TSH[a]	TRH	T_4, T_3, dopamine, glucocorticoids	Thyroid	T_4, T_3 synthesis and release
Gonadotrope	FSH[a], LH[a]	GnRH	Sex steroids, inhibin	Testes, ovaries	Sex steroid production, follicular growth, germ cell maturation
Lactotrope	PRL	Estrogen, TRH	Dopamine	Breast, other tissues	Milk production, metabolic effects

Note: AVP, arginine vasopressin.
[a]Glycoproteins.

by destruction of the pituitary by a pituitary tumour, therapeutic hypophysectomy (for pituitary tumour) or postpartum pituitary necrosis (Sheehan syndrome)

The clinical manifestations are due to deficiency of:

1. **Gonadotropins**, such as infertility, impotence, amenorrhoea and total loss of sexual hair
2. **TSH**, giving rise to hypothyroidism
3. **ACTH**, causing hypotension and fasting hypoglycaemia; pigmentation of Addison disease is not seen, and aldosterone production is relatively unaffected
4. **GH:** These can be subtle and comprise of fatigue, lethargy, and impaired physical performance, accompanied by reduction in muscle and bone mass, increased adiposity and increased cardiovascular mortality, emotional liability and feelings of social isolation. Treatment with human growth hormone (hGH) reverses many of these manifestations.

The patients become moderately plump but not obese.

Effects of hyperpituitarism: Excessive production of anterior pituitary hormones may occur in the presence of anatomically demonstrable pituitary disease or its absence. Such excessive production is associated with gigantism, acromegaly, one form of Cushing syndrome, the galactorrhoea–amenorrhoea syndrome and rarely, hyperthyroidism.

High levels of plasma GH are seen in acromegaly, GH resistance, uncontrolled DM, anorexia nervosa and protein calorie malnutrition.

PH 1.37

GROWTH HORMONE (GH): Growth hormone is found in all vertebrates. In addition to its growth-promoting properties, it possesses several important metabolic effects which are essential for health. Earlier the source of GH, used in therapy, was human cadaver pituitaries but its availability was less and was associated with Creutzfeldt-Jakob disease. Now human GH (hGH) preparations are manufactured using recombinant DNA technology.

Source and chemistry: It is synthesised and stored by the (eosinophil) somatotrophic cells of the adenohypophysis. It is present at all ages. Human growth hormone (hGH) is a polypeptide consisting of a series of 191 amino acids.

The growth promoting effect of GH appears to be species specific. Thus, human beings respond only to human GH.

Plasma levels and regulation of GH secretion: Plasma level of hGH is undetectable between GH pulses in an adult. It rises (as high as 25 ng/mL or higher) several times in spikes during the day, mostly during exercise, deep sleep (especially in children), and several hours after a meal. Stimulated by the sex steroids, especially estrogen, GH levels rise during puberty.

GH secretion is profoundly influenced by nutritional factors and is stimulated by high protein diet. Other stimuli include DA, 5HT, and α_2 adrenergic receptor agonists, exercise, stress, emotional excitement and sex steroids.

Hypoglycaemia is the most consistent stimulus to GH secretion and insulin-induced hypoglycaemia is the gold standard for diagnosis of GHD.

The rate of release of GH by the pituitary is regulated by GH–RH and somatostatin (GH–RIH). *A substantial part of GH release occurs during the early hours of sleep and is probably important in the anabolic and repair processes of the body.* It is stimulated by **ghrelin**, a polypeptide, synthesised by the stomach, pituitary and hypothalamus. Hypothalamic ghrelin causes GH release by stimulating GHRH and also pituitary somatotropes. Ghrelin also causes increase in appetite and obesity. PH 1.37

GH release is inhibited by β adrenergic receptor agonists, free fatty acids, glucose, IGF-1, and GH itself.

Mechanism of action:

GH receptors belong to Class 1 cytokine receptor family. GH binds to two GH receptors to form a ternary complex. These receptors are linked to two molecules of JAK2, a cytoplasmic tyrosine kinase. GH binding induces transphosphorylation and autoactivation of JAK2, with consequent tyrosine phosphorylation of proteins. Amongst that are STAT proteins. STAT 5 is a gene that encodes IGF-1, which mediates many of the GH action (see under the section, Growth related effects).

Pharmacological actions: Endogenous GH circulates in the blood with a plasma t½ of about 20 minutes, though its metabolic effects last much longer. It exerts:

Metabolic effects including lipolysis and neoglucogenesis, directly, by acting on the tissue GH receptors which are widely distributed in the body:

- **Carbohydrate metabolism:** Effects on carbohydrate metabolism are complex. *Acute administration* of hGH to normal individuals and to nondiabetic, hypophysectomised individuals causes transient hypoglycaemia. On the other hand, its *chronic administration antagonizes insulin* and impairs glucose tolerance. Hypophysectomy ameliorates diabetic retinopathy; individuals so treated are prone to hypoglycaemia.
- **Protein metabolism:** GH has a **strong anabolic** action. It stimulates the transport of amino acids into the cells and accelerates intracellular protein synthesis. Retention of nitrogen, phosphate and potassium occurs. Blood urea falls and urinary excretion of hydroxyproline rises, indicating **increase in muscle mass and collagen synthesis.**
- **Fat metabolism:** GH **stimulates** differentiation of preadipocytes to adipocytes. It also shows anti-insulin action and stimulates **lipolysis** that causes a rise in the fasting plasma free fatty acid (FFA) level. Chronic administration, inhibits lipogenesis from glucose and acetate. The FFA thus released are utilised by the tissues. GH may, therefore, be of minor importance in lipolysis in man (Chapter 63).
- **Mineral metabolism:** It causes retention of potassium, sodium and phosphorus. **Calcium absorption is increased.** The hypercalciuric action of GH is not seen in the absence of endogenous parathyroid hormone activity.

Anabolic and growth-related effects: These occur predominantly **indirectly, through IGF-1 generated in the liver** and to a smaller extent by the direct actions of GH. *Seventy-five per cent of the circulating IGF-1 is synthesised by the liver in response to GH.* The rest comes from the spill-over of that produced for paracrine action by numerous tissues (bone, cartilage, erythroid precursors, myocytes and kidneys). It acts on specific IGF-1 receptors. **It has a negative feedback on GH release** through ts effect on the pituitary and hypothalamus. Unlike most other protein hormones, IGF-1 circulates in the blood, bound to IGF binding proteins (IGFBPs 1–5). The basic actions of IGF-1 are:

a. **Positive nitrogen and mineral balance; and synthesis and accretion of protein in most tissues (anabolic effect)**
b. **Cellular proliferation.**

Autocrine/paracrine IGF-1 can stimulate local, unbalanced growth such as wound healing at all ages and growth of the contralateral kidney after unilateral nephrectomy in childhood. This is independent of systemic GH.

The growth due to GH affects every tissue and organ in the body with the possible exception of the brain and the eye. *In children whose epiphyses have not yet closed, it promotes linear bone growth without accelerating skeletal or sexual maturation.* It acts on the epiphyseal growth plate but does not accelerate epiphyseal fusion. It increases bone mineral density if the epiphyses have closed. *The increase in body mass produced by GH mainly affects the lean body mass, and is due to retention of nitrogen, minerals and water but not of fat.*

The growth promoting effect is dramatic in young children with GHD. In most of such children, the effect continues during 8–10 years of hGH therapy. It is noteworthy that *hGH injected at intervals of 2–3 days will promote growth, although its metabolic effects are of short duration.*

The other actions of IGF-1 are:

- **Rise in GFR** (25%)
- **Hypoglycaemia** if sufficient amount is given
- **Marked increase in insulin sensitivity** in type 2 diabetics
- **Partial reversal of the catabolic effect induced by nutrient deprivation and glucocorticoids**

Miscellaneous: Excess of GH causes gigantism in children and acromegaly in adults. It induces visceromegaly as seen in patients with acromegaly.

Absorption, fate and excretion: Recombinant hGH is administered by SC route. The peak plasma level after SC administration occurs after 2–4 h, and the t½ is 20 min but biological effect is prolonged to have once a day administration. It is metabolised in the liver.

Adverse reactions: Recombinant hGH is well tolerated and safe, and causes a few adverse reactions in GH deficient children. There may be increase in T2DM and rarely headache, seizures and benign intracranial hypertension. Periodic blood glucose monitoring and fundoscopy is required. Too rapid growth can lead to scoliosis. It may cause hypothyroidism which must, therefore, be looked for. It may cause increase in blood glucose and lipid levels, especially in adults.

The other adverse reactions in elderly or obese adults, not seen in children, are peripheral oedema, carpal tunnel syndrome, myalgia and arthralgia. In diabetics, it may aggravate hyperglycaemia and cause ketosis. It may precipitate adrenal insufficiency in susceptible patients as it increases metabolic degradation of cortisol. It may decrease insulin sensitivity and dose adjustment is needed for insulin or oral antihyperglycemic drugs. Although antibodies to GH appear in about 30% patients on GH, they are present in low titre.

Preparations and dosage: *One milligram of hGH equals three units.* The preparations are:

i. Somatrem (methionyl hGH)
ii. Somatropin (nonmethionyl hGH): Available in various doses from 200-2000 micrograms as powder for injection. A long acting, encapsulated form for injection once or twice a month is also available.

Somatrem and **somatropin** are therapeutically equivalent. The dose in children with GHD is 25–50 mcg/kg/day, subcutaneously, given daily. The therapy is started with lower dose. If growth acceleration is considered inadequate at the end of the first year, larger doses may be used. In adults, the daily dose is 3–4 mcg/kg daily.

Indications:

- **GHD with short stature in children:** GH administration stimulates rapid linear growth and 5–10 cm of height may be added during the first year. Most patients continue to respond for several years. A few, however, become refractory; in some of these, the refractoriness is due to the development of antibodies. The advancement of bone age is not greater than the increase in linear growth with GH. Hypothyroidism may occur during hGH therapy.
- **Children with short stature associated with other conditions despite adequate GH production:** These include Turner syndrome, Noonan syndrome, Prader-Willi syndrome, chronic renal insufficiency, children born small for gestational age and children with idiopathic short stature. Results of GH therapy in idiopathic short stature are variable.
- **GH deficiency in adults:** *Since GH is prohibitively expensive it should not be recommended in short stature adults without confirming organic etiologies,* low GH level in response to standard stimulating tests or deficiency of other three pituitary hormones.
- **AIDS-associated wasting**
- **Malabsorption associated with the short-bowel syndrome**

The utility of GH in the following conditions is not proven: old age; osteoporosis; athletes; and cachexia and other catabolic states.

GH therapy is contraindicated in: (1) growth promotion in children with closed epiphyses; (2) acute critical illness and (3) patients with neoplasms (4) proliferative retinopathy or severe nonproliferative diabetic retinopathy.

SOMAPACITAN is a modified hGH analogue. It has a albumin-binding moiety, which prolongs its t½ by increasing its binding to plasma albumin (>99%). It is administered once weekly. Currently it is used only in adults with GH deficiency.

MECASERMIN (IGF-1): This recombinant human IGF-1, is given subcutaneously. It is metabolised in the liver and the kidney. Its actions and ADR are similar to those of GH. The common ADR is hypoglycaemia, occurring in over 40% of subjects. Overgrowth of fat, and lymphoid tissue with enlarged tonsils, facial bones and kidney can occur after prolonged treatment.

It is used to treat severe IGF-1 deficiency, growth failure and patients resistant to GH because of antibodies or in patients with IGF-1 gene defects. *It is not recommended for GH responsive GHD subjects.* It is very expensive.

A combination of mecasermin with its binding protein, IGFBP-3 (**mecasermin rinfabate**) is also available. It is mainly used in patients with severe insulin resistance, muscular dystrophy, and HIV associated lipodystrophy.

GH-RH AND ITS ANALOGUES PH 1.37

SOMATORELIN (GH-RH): This polypeptide with 40 amino acids acts on the somatotrophs (GH-RH receptor agonist). It is used to test the ability of the anterior pituitary to synthesise and release hGH (hGH reserve). Recombinant synthetic analogues of GH-RH, do not cause a down regulation of their own receptors.

Macimorelin is synthetic orally administered GH-RH analogue to diagnose GH deficiency.

Tesamorelin is a synthetic analogue with prolonged duration. It reduces visceral fat accumulation and is used in patients with HIV induced lipodystrophy. It is not recommended in GH deficiency.

GROWTH HORMONE SECRETAGOGUE RECEPTOR AGONISTS

The growth hormone secretagogue receptor (GHSR) is the natural receptor for Ghrelin.

Pralmorelin (GHRP 2, growth hormone-releasing peptide 2) is an orally active, synthetic growth hormone-releasing peptide,which acts on hypothalamus and pituitary. It increases growth hormone release from the pituitary and then through cascade of signaling events, hepatic production of IGF-1. It is used as a diagnostic agent for GH deficiency.

GROWTH HORMONE INHIBITORS

SOMATOSTATIN (GH-RIH): Somatostatin exists as two peptides, SST 28 and SST 14 based on the number of amino acids. *Somatostatin is secreted by the hypothalamus and the delta cells of the islets of Langerhans.* It is also found in the gut wall. There are 5 subtypes of somatostatin receptors (SSTR1-5). **It is widely distributed in the brain. It has a very short t½ and hence cannot be used clinically.** It:

- Inhibits the release of GH (through direct effect on somatotropes or indirectly through GHRH neuron inhibition), insulin and glucagon from pancreas, and of GI peptides
- Inhibits secretion of gastric acid independently of its action on the release of gastrin
- *Decreases the splanchnic blood flow and thus reduces portal pressure*

OCTREOTIDE: This longer acting **analogue of somatostatin** is used to control severe diarrhoea due to carcinoid syndrome and metastatic vasoactive intestinal polypeptide tumours (VIPomas), and to treat glucagonomas, malignant insulinomas and pituitary tumour causing acromegaly. It is given as IV bolus and subcutaneously.

Its other uses are dumping syndrome, acute pancreatitis, perioperative prophylaxis after pancreatic surgery, and oesophageal variceal bleeding. A long acting preparation with action for 30 days is available. Radiolabelled octreotide is used for localisation of neuroendocrine tumours. Octreotide associated with beta-emitter (90Y) is used for selective destruction of SST2 receptor-positive tumours.

Lanreotide is a long acting analogue of octeotride, which on deep SC injection every 4 weeks causes prolonged suppression of GH. Both, **octreotide and lanreotide promote rapid, symptomatic relief in acromegaly.**

Pasireotide is a selective centrally acting somatostatin analogue which inhibits secretion of ACTH. It is effective in Cushing disease (due to pituitary origin). Its long acting slow release formulation is also available.

Adverse effects:

The most common ADR of somatostatin analogues are nausea, diarrhoea and abdominal pain but tolerance develops to them without requiring any discontinuation. Gallstones, bradycardia and QT prolongation and rarely hypothyroidism may occur. Pasireotide can result in hypocortisolism. Patients receiving this drug often require antihyperglycemic treatment because it decreases secretion of incretins.

Pegvisomant, a genetically altered **GH antagonist,** is used weekly SC in the treatment of acromegaly. It binds to GH receptor and prevents its activation thus inhibiting IGF-1 production.

PROLACTIN: The lactotropes of pituitary gland secrete prolactin (PRL), the somatotropic hormone structurally related to growth hormone (23kDa, amino acids 199). **The secretion of prolactin is under control of a hypothalamic neurons, the major inhibitory regulator is dopamine.** *In the pituitary, D2 receptors are predominant and mediate the inhibition of PRL synthesis and release.* Serum PRL concentration starts increasing at 8 weeks of pregnancy and is maximum at term. It remains elevated during postpartum period if the mother breast feeds the infant. Breast manipulation and stimulation of nipple causes a reflex rise in serum PRL. Exercise, psychological and surgical stress, sleep, hypoglycemia, TRH and sex steroids can increase its level.

Endocrine actions: PRL acts on a receptor belonging to type-I cytokine receptor family. Physiologically, *the main actions of PRL are the preparation of the breasts for lactation, and the initiation and maintenance of lactation.* In addition to PRL, proliferation and differentiation of the ductal and lobuloalveolar epithelia of the breast is also influenced by hormones such as estrogens, progesterone, glucocorticoids and growth hormone.

Supraphysiological levels of prolactin:

1. **Inhibit GnRH and suppress reproductive function** and sex drive
2. **Impair gonadal steroid production** and block the development of the ovarian follicles, causing anovulation
3. **Cause direct luteolytic effect** leading to inadequate luteal phase
4. **Decrease plasma testosterone levels** in men thereby decreasing libido and spermatogenesis

Metabolic actions: PRL increases calcium absorption and mobilises calcium from the bone. *Hyperprolactinaemia is associated with increased bone loss and osteoporosis.* PRL receptors are present in the osteoblasts of developing bone. PRL also induces pancreatic beta cell growth. By acting centrally, it increases appetite and is probably involved in parenting behaviour.

Excessive prolactin can cause galactorrhoea, amenorrhoea and infertility in women, and sexual impotence in men. It can also be **drug induced** (Box 61.2). Primary hypothyroidism and pregnancy should be ruled out before confirming the hypothalamic or pituitary disease. Its rational therapy involves the use of drugs that decrease the PRL secretion. The drugs used are: **dopamine agonists – bromoergocriptine, lisuride, cabergoline and quinagolide.**

BROMOERGOCRIPTINE (Bromocriptine): This semisynthetic ergot alkaloid is a **selective D2 receptor agonist.** Since dopamine is a neurotransmitter or local hormone at various sites in the brain, bromocriptine can produce various motor, behavioural and endocrine effects.

Pharmacological actions:

Hormonal actions: Bromocriptine inhibits synthesis and release of prolactin and decreases the replication of the tumorous lactotrophs. Given to patients with hyperprolactinaemia, it causes a marked fall in serum prolactin levels and restores the normal cyclic release of gonadotropins.

Bromocriptine causes a **brief rise** in plasma GH in normal subjects but a **sustained fall** in patients with acromegaly.

It alters circadian neuronal activities by acting on the hypothalamic D2 receptors. This inhibits excessive sympathetic tone and serotonergic activity within CNS. This results in suppression of hepatic glucose output and exerts antidiabetic effect (Chapter 63).

Box 61.2 Drugs Causing Hyperprolactinaemia

Blockers of dopamine (D2)receptors: : Antipsychotic phenothiazines; haloperidol; metoclopramide; domperidone
Dopamine synthesis inhibitors:α-Methyldopa
Central dopamine depletors: Reserpine
Antidepressants: MAOI, imipramine, amitryptiline, fluoxetine
Hormones: TRH; oral contraceptives; antiandrogens
Miscellaneous: Cimetidine; verapamil; opiates

Motor effects: Bromocriptine causes a reduction in dopamine turnover with a decrease in concentration of the dopamine metabolites and an increase in dopamine content of the brain. It thus produces beneficial effects in Parkinson disease (Chapter 15). But the doses required are almost 10 times higher than those which suppress prolactin.

Behavioural effects: Prolonged treatment, can cause altered behaviour and awareness, sometimes accompanied by hallucinations.

CVS: These drugs cause vasodilatation (see adverse reactions below).

Absorption, fate and excretion: The drug is rapidly and almost completely absorbed from the gut and *readily crosses the BBB*. The drug exhibits extensive first-pass metabolism and only 6%–7% is excreted in the urine. The rest appears in the bile and faeces. Its t1/2 is 2-8 hrs and is administered in divided doses. Slow release formulation is available to avoid frequent dosing.

Adverse reactions: These include postural syncope, gastric upset like nausea, headache and drowsiness. Continuous high doses may cause constipation, nasal congestion, cramps in legs, digital vasospasm, hallucinations, nightmares, insomnia, dystonic reactions, arrhythmias and postural hypotension. Patients develop tolerance to these effects. They can be avoided by using small dose in the initial period and giving it at bedtime with food. The drug should be avoided in patients with a history of mental illness, IHD and peripheral vascular disease.

Preparations and dosage:

i. Bromocriptine mesylate 1, 1.25, 2.5 mg tablets and 5, 10 mg capsules
ii. Bromocriptine mesylate inj. 40 mg/mL. This is used intramuscularly in cases of prolactinomas compressing the optic chiasma (see below)
iii. Vaginal preparation may be useful in patients intolerant of oral bromocriptine

Indications:

- **Hyperprolactinaemia–galactorrhoea syndrome:** Given in the dose of 2.5–10 mg daily in divided doses, it restores serum prolactin levels to normal and stops galactorrhoea in patients with prolactinomas and those with functional hyperprolactinaemia. Amenorrhoea is corrected and fertility is restored in women. In patients with prolactinomas, it produces tumour regression and resolution of visual field defects. **It is considered a specific and safe primary treatment for prolactin-secreting adenomas.**
- **Prolactinoma with impotence in males:** It lowers serum prolactin levels and restores potency
- **Acromegaly:** Bromocriptine in the dose of 15–20 mg daily causes a sustained, dose-related decrease in plasma GH levels and clinical remission. However, complete remission is rare.
- **Parkinson disease:** See Chapter 15
- **Diabetes mellitus:** See Chapter 63

LISURIDE: This drug has properties and uses similar to those of bromocriptine. It is available as 0.2 mg tablets.

CABERGOLINE: This **long-acting analogue** (t½ 65 h) of bromocriptine, can be administered 500 mcg once a week, increased by 500 mcg increments, up to a maximum of 2 mg/week. It has more affinity and greater selectivity for D2 receptors. The adverse reactions to this drug are lesser. It can cause nausea, hypotension and dizziness. Some ADR different from those to bromocriptine include palpitation, epigastric and abdominal pain, epistaxis, hemianopia, syncope and hot flushes. It may cause valvular heart disease at high dose due to its effect at HT_{2B} receptors. Patients resistant to bromocriptine may respond to this drug. **Cabergoline is now preferred in clinical practice for the treatment of hyperprolactinemia.**

QUINAGOLIDE: This drug is a nonergot D2 receptor agonist. It has properties, ADR and uses similar to bromocriptine. Its t½ is 22 h. It should not be used when pregnancy is intended.

CHAPTER 62

Thyroid Hormones and Antithyroid Drugs

Learning Objectives

This chapter will enable the reader:

1. To explain the synthesis of thyroid hormone and relationship between pituitary gland and thyroid gland.
2. To explain the mechanism of action, physiological and pharmacological effects of thyroid hormone.
3. To state the differences between thyroxine and tri-iodothyronine.
4. To mention the salient pharmacokinetic features, ADR and indications for thyroid hormone.
5. To outline the pharmacotherapy of myxoedema coma.
6. To classify antithyroid drugs based on their mechanism of action.
7. To state the salient pharmacokinetic features, ADR and indications for thioamides, iodides and radioactive iodine.
8. To outline the management of hyperthyroidism.
9. To explain the indications, advantages and disadvantages of following treatment options, i.e. antithyroid drugs, radioactive iodine and surgery available for hyperthyroidism.
10. To mention the principles of treatment of thyrotoxic crisis.
11. To enumerate iodine-containing contrast media and state their adverse effects.

KEY TERMS

synthesis of thyroid hormones, p. 880
actions of thyroid hormones, p. 882
uses of thyroxine, p. 883
antithyroid drugs, p. 886
thioamides, p. 886
iodide, p. 887
radioactive iodine, p. 888
advantages and disadvantages of radioactive iodine, p. 889
treatment of thyrotoxic crisis, p. 890

Although the thyroid gland was discovered in 1656, the manifestations of thyroid deficiency were described by W.W. Gull in 1874. The isolation and crystallisation of the thyroxine (T_4) was achieved by E.C. Kendall in 1915 and its chemical structure was determined by Charles Harrington and George Barger in 1926. Tri-iodothyronine (T_3) was detected, isolated and synthesised by Rosalind Pitt-Rivers and her post-doctoral fellow Jack Gross in 1952.

The thyroid gland acini synthesise:

- **Thyroxine**
- **Tri-iodothyronine**

The third hormone, **thyrocalcitonin**, is secreted by the interstitial cells (Chapter 68). Chemically, T_4 is 3,5,3′,5′-tetra-iodothyronine (Fig. 62.1), and T_3 is 3,5,3′-triiodothyronine (Fig. 62.1).

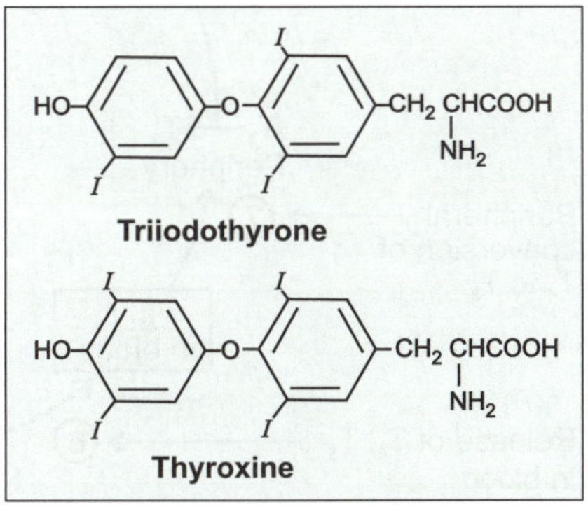

FIG. 62.1 Thyroid hormones.

Synthesis of Thyroid Hormones

Dietary iodide is absorbed from the upper GI tract and is carried in the plasma as inorganic iodide. The thyroid hormones are synthesised as follows (Fig 62.2):

- **Iodide trapping:** The thyroid gland actively transports iodide ion from the plasma into the thyroid follicular cells via the sodium iodine symporter. This active process is stimulated by thyroid stimulating hormone (TSH, thyrotropin). It is competitively inhibited by thiocyanate and perchlorate ions.
- **Organic binding of iodine:** Transport of iodine from the follicular cell to the colloid is facilitated by the apical transporter pendrin. The iodide is first oxidised by H_2O_2 and thyroid peroxidase to hypoiodate. Hypoiodate iodinates the tyrosyl residues in the thyroglobulin (TG) to form mono-and di-iodotyrosine (MIT and DIT) successively i.e. organification of iodine. These two reactions are extremely rapid and are stimulated by TSH. They may be defective in certain disease states and are inhibited by thioamides.
- **Coupling:** T_4 is formed by coupling of two molecules of DIT, and T_3 by coupling of one molecule of MIT and DIT each. They are oxidative reactions and need the same peroxidase involved in oxidation of iodide to hypoiodate. They are inhibited by thioamides.
- **Hormonal release:** TG, which contains T_4 and T_3, is stored within the thyroidal follicular lumen. It is resorped by the thyroid follicular cells by endocytosis. Under the influence of TSH, proteases release T_4, T_3, MIT and DIT from TG.
- **Fate of hormones:** MIT and DIT are deiodinated and the iodine is transported back into the follicular lumen for reutilization, whereas T_4 and T_3 directly enter the circulation. *About 40% of T_4 released by the thyroid is converted by peripheral tissues and also in thyroid to T_3* by deiodinases type 1 and 2; this accounts for almost 80% of the total T_3 formed in the body. Thus, T_4 acts not only as a hormone but also as a prohormone.

About 90% of the body iodine is in the thyroid gland, mainly as organic iodine. This large thyroidal pool of iodine (5–7 mg) turns over very slowly at the rate of 1% per day.

Plasma iodine: The plasma in health contains about 0.2–0.4 mcg of inorganic iodide and 4–15 mcg of hormonal iodine per 100 mL. The hormonal iodine

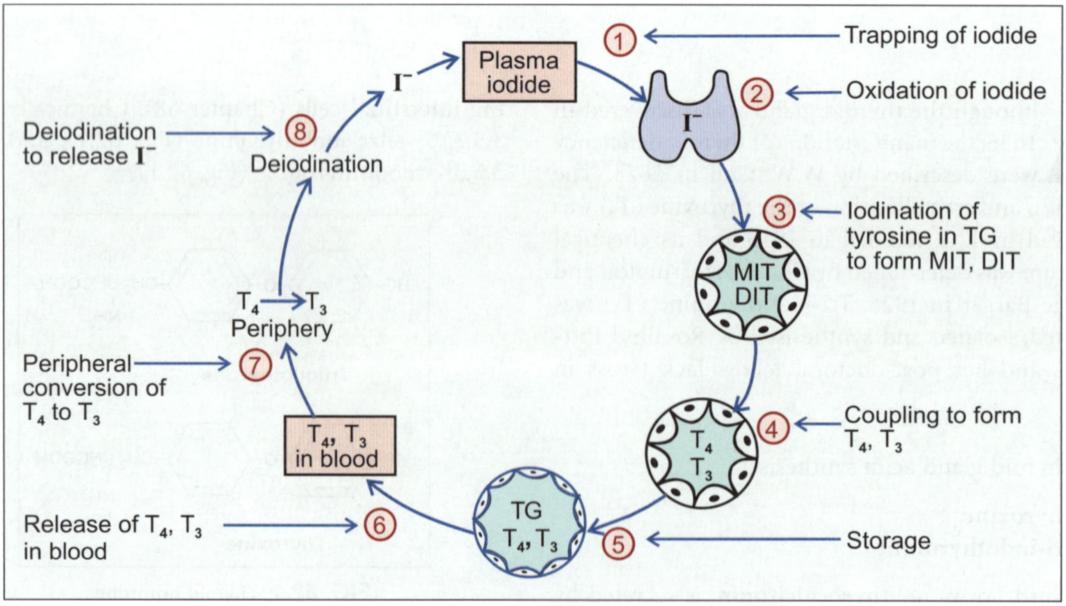

FIG. 62.2 Synthesis of thyroid hormone.

is made up mostly of **T_4 (4–13 mcg/dL) and a small quantity of T_3 (80–200 ng/dL).** T_4 and T_3 circulate in the plasma partly protein bound and partly as free hormones. The major binding protein is **thyroxine binding globulin** (TBG) which accounts for 60% of the binding capacity of the plasma. The level of TBG is influenced by estrogens and rises during pregnancy and oral contraceptive use. **The mean concentration of circulating *free* T_4 is 0.8–2 ng/dL** and of free T_3 145–348 pg/dL. The free hormones are physiologically active. *In states of iodine deficiency, the thyroid synthesises T_3 in preference to T_4.*

About 80% of the thyroid hormones (T_4 and T_3) are metabolised by deiodination by deiodinase type 3; the remaining 20% are excreted in stools. Liver is the major site of nondeiodinative degradation of thyroid hormones; **Although the thyroid normally forms more T_4 than T_3, the latter is the physiologically active hormone.** The peripheral conversion of T_4 to T_3 is inhibited by drugs such as propylthiouracil, glucocorticoids and propranolol; as well as during chronic (rheumatoid arthritis, tuberculosis) and acute (myocardial infarct, stroke, burns) illnesses.

Reverse T_3 (rT_3) is principally a byproduct of T_4 mono-deiodination in peripheral tissues. It is metabolically inactive.

PH 1.37

Pituitary thyroid relationship: Thyrotropic hormone (TSH), a glycoprotein, is synthesised and released by the thyrotropes in the anterior pituitary under stimulation by Thyrotropin Releasing Hormone (TRH) from the hypothalamus. The circulating T_3 (and to a smaller extent T_4) levels modulate the response of the pituitary to TRH. TSH acts on the TSH receptors in the follicular cell membrane and accelerates synthesis and release of thyroidal hormones. Its action on the thyroid is modulated by the thyroidal organic iodine content and is mediated by adenylyl cyclase-cyclic AMP mechanism. Repeated administration of TSH:

- **Increases the weight and vascularity of the thyroid gland**
- **Reduces its colloid and iodine content**
- **Increases the height of its acinar epithelium as seen histologically**

TSH secretion rises in the presence of low and falls in the presence of high levels of circulating T_4 and T_3. The **negative feedback** is believed to occur at the level of the pituitary rather than the hypothalamus. It has been implicated in the pathogenesis of some cases of simple goitre, a noninflammatory, nonmalignant enlargement of the thyroid gland. If, for any reason such as iodine deficiency, ingestion of goitrogens or genetic enzyme deficiency, thyroid hormone synthesis becomes impaired, the tendency of the plasma T_4 and T_3 level to fall is countered by an increase in TSH secretion. This leads to goitre formation.

Plasma level of TSH (measured by an immunoassay) is

1. **Undetectable or very low** in hypopituitarism and in hyperthyroidism
2. **Elevated** in **primary hypothyroidism.** Although TSH may be initially responsible for the development of some forms of nontoxic goitre, *plasma TSH levels are elevated only in goitrous patients who are hypothyroid.*

TRH: This synthetic substance is a tripeptide, (pyro) Glu-His-Pro (NH_2). Intravenous TRH results in a rapid rise in plasma TSH level and was used earlier to diagnose subclinical thyrotoxicosis. PH 1.37, IM 12.13

Mechanism of action: Thyroid hormones interact with the cells at **three thyroid receptor (TR) sites:**

1. **The nucleus** where they cause transcription of mRNA necessary for the synthesis of proteins (**Genomic action**). The affinity of T_3 for TRs is tenfold higher than for T_4.
   The thyroid hormone receptors are classified as **TRα and TRβ**. TRα are responsible for regulation of heart rate, body temperature, skeletal muscle function and bone and intestine development whereas TRβ are involved in liver metabolism, negative feedback mechanisms (at hypothalamus–pituitary–thyroid axis), retina and inner ear development.
2. The **non-genomic actions** of thyroid hormones at the **plasma membrane** and **mitochondria** occur early in the course of the exposure of cells to thyroid hormones. **T_3 acts on TRs involved in cellular metabolism.** It also stimulates NO

Table 62.1 Differences between T_4 and T_3

	Thyroxine (T_4)	Triiodothyronine (T_3)
Equipotent doses	100 mcg	25 mcg
Free hormone (% of total) in plasma	0.03	0.3
Onset of action	7–10 days	2–4 h
Absorption	70%–80%	>95%
Elimination t½	7 days	1 day
Dose titration	4–6 weeks	1–2 week
Wearing out of effect after cessation of therapy	Long	Short

production, which is responsible for vasodilation. **T_4 binds to plasma membrane receptors to activate MAP kinase.**

Difference between T_3 and T_4: The overall effects of T_4 and T_3 are qualitatively similar. Table 62.1 shows the important differences.

PH 1.36, IM 12.13

Physiological and pharmacological actions:

Calorigenic action: The thyroid hormones stimulate oxygen consumption and heat production in all tissues except the brain, gonads, lymph nodes, spleen, thymus and dermis. *Thus, they regulate the BMR.* The calorigenic response is most marked in the hypothyroid individual. However, there is a latent period of several hours or even days between the administration of the hormone and the response.

Growth: The thyroid hormones are **essential for intra-uterine tissue differentiation and as well as extrauterine growth:**

1. *Intrauterine thyroid deficiency causes defective brain development leading to cretinism with mental retardation*
2. Deficiency of thyroid hormones appearing after birth leads to retardation of physical growth, characterised by a marked delay in the bone maturation (**retarded bone age**). X-ray shows a characteristic **epiphyseal dysgenesis**, where calcification appears as multiple, small irregular foci causing stippled, porous, fluffy or fragmented appearance. It is associated with decrease in the serum alkaline phosphatase level.

Metabolic actions: In **physiological doses,** the thyroid hormones:

- **Promote growth and protein synthesis** and are, therefore, *anabolic in their effects.* In excessive amounts, as in thyrotoxicosis, their effect is *catabolic.*
- **Promote glucose absorption and its intracellular utilisation.** Larger doses may cause glucose intolerance. The liver may be depleted of glycogen in hyperthyroidism.
- **Enhance cholesterol synthesis by the liver, its biliary excretion, conversion to bile acids and faecal loss.** The preponderance of increased synthesis over metabolic degradation causes a rise in serum cholesterol in hypothyroidism. In hyperthyroidism, serum cholesterol is normal. They also enhance the lipolytic action of catecholamines on the fat cells.
- **Affect the water and electrolyte metabolism.** Thus, the hypothyroid subject retains water and sodium and cannot excrete an added load of water. Diuresis and natriuresis occur soon after starting thyroid medication.

Cardiovascular system: T_4 acts on the myocardium partly by a **direct genomic action and partly by sensitising it to the effects of catecholamines.** It stimulates the rate and increases the force of contraction of the myocardium and the cardiac output. This action is inhibited by beta blockers.

Central nervous system: T_4 is essential for myelination of the CNS. **Hence, its deficiency during fetal life leads to irreversible CNS damage.** A variety of neurological changes such as mental retardation and slow tendon reflexes are seen in hypothyroidism, whereas increased irritability, tremors and hyperkinesia are characteristic of hyperthyroidism. Psychosis may also be present in hypothyroidism.

Gastrointestinal tract: Diarrhoea and constipation are common in hyper and hypothyroidism, respectively. Achlorhydria is frequent in both these conditions.

Reproductive tract and the breast: Gonadal function is disturbed in males as well as in females in hypothyroidism; menorrhagia is seen in women and infertility in both the sexes. No specific changes are observed in hyperthyroidism.

Haemopoietic system: Anaemia, correctable only by thyroid medication, is seen in hypothyroidism.

Skin: T_4 deficiency causes deposition of a complex mucopolysaccharide material in the connective tissue of the skin, which makes it pale and rough.

Miscellaneous actions: Excess of T_4 impairs the conversion of creatine to creatinine leading to wasteful creatinuria. Various types of myopathies and periodic paralysis are seen in hyperthyroidism. Plasma level of creatine kinase (CPK), lactic dehydrogenase (LDH) and creatinine are increased in hypothyroidism. Conversion of carotene to vitamin A is defective in thyroid deficiency, whereas requirement of all vitamins is enhanced in thyrotoxicosis.

In some species, these hormones have special functions such as stimulation of oxygen consumption in fish, metamorphosis in amphibians and plumage growth in birds.

Absorption, fate and excretion: Both T_4 and T_3 are well absorbed when given orally (Table 62.1). **Food interferes with its absorption.** T_4 is concentrated mainly by the liver and the kidney, whereas T_3 gets distributed to a variety of organs and tissues. The hormones are deiodinated in the peripheral tissues and iodine thus liberated is returned to the extrathyroidal iodide pool for reutilisation. Plasma t½ of T_4 in health is 6–7 days and that of T_3 is 1–2 days. The hormones are conjugated with sulphuric acid in the liver and are excreted in the bile. Oxidative deamination and decarboxylation also occur. Sulphates are partly hydrolysed and reabsorbed in the intestines. About 20%–40% of the amount present in the bile is excreted in faeces.

Adverse reactions: Larger doses cause symptoms similar to that of thyrotoxicosis and include hyperkinesia, weight loss, palpitation, tremor, irritability, diarrhoea, and occasionally anginal pain; agitation and even psychosis may occur. Administration of large doses for prolonged periods can cause osteoporosis, left ventricular hypertrophy and pseudotumour cerebri. *If a patient with combined hypothyroidism and hypocortisolism is not pretreated with a glucocorticoid, T_4 can precipitate hypoadrenal crisis.*

Drug interactions: Several drugs such as antacids, ciprofloxacin, phenytoin, carbamazepine, amiodarone and certain cations like iron, calcium and foods such as fibres, coffee may interfere with T_4 absorption or its metabolism.

Preparations and dosage:

i. T_4 sodium available as tablets of different strengths, 12.5 - 200 mcg tablets. Dose: 0.05–0.2 mg.
ii. Levothyroxine sodium injection 200, 500 mcg. Dose in myxoedema coma: 200–500 mcg IV on first day; 100–200 mcg on second day.
iii. Liothyronine sodium (L-triiodothyronine sodium) 20 mcg tablets. Dose: 20 mcg 1–3 times a day.
iv. Liothyronine sodium injection, 10 mcg/mL. Dose in myxoedema coma: 25–50 mcg IV

T_3 is not used routinely because its rapid onset of action may precipitate angina or cardiac failure, especially in the elderly patients. Further, the longer half-life of T_4 maintains a substantial peripheral pool of T_4 from which T_3 is slowly formed. This provides a buffer against lapses in treatment. *For all therapeutic indications, T4 is preferred because it is not only as effective as T3 but also much cheaper than the other formulations.*

For replacement therapy, combinations of T_4 and T_3 are not superior to T_4 alone.

Table 62.2 summarises the thyroid function tests in health and disease.

Indications:

- **As substitution therapy:** In **cretinism,** therapy must be started as soon after birth, preferably within 4 weeks. With proper treatment, almost normal physical development and linear growth can be achieved. In cretins with goitres, the thyroid deficiency is milder.

Table 62.2 Thyroid Function Tests (Plasma Levels) in Health and Disease

	Normal[a]	Hypothyroidism, Primary	Hypothyroidism, Secondary	Thyrotoxicosis	Euthyroid, Sick Syndrome[b]	Pregnancy, OC Pill Use
Total T_4 (mcg/dL)	4–11	↓	↓	↑/N	N	↑
Free T_4 (ng/dL)	0.8–2.0	↓	↓	↑/N	N	N
Total T_3 (ng/dL)	60–180	N/↓	N/↓	↑	↓	N/↑
Free T_3 (pg/dL)	145–348	N/↓	N/↓	↑	↓	N
TSH (mcU/mL)	0.5–5.0	↑	N (inappropriately low)	↓	N/↓	N

[a]Normal values differ with different laboratories.
[b]Seen in chronic/severe acute, medical and surgical illness.

Table 62.3 Thyroxine Substitution Therapy in Hypothyroid Infants and Children

Age	Dose (mcg/kg)	Total (mcg/day)
Birth to 6 months	10–15	25–50
6–12 months	6–10	50–75
1–5 years	5–7	75–100
6–18 years	3–5	100–150

Therapy is started with a small dose (25 mcg) and is increased by 25 mcg only at fortnightly intervals. The entire daily dose is given once daily with a glass of water on an empty stomach in the morning followed by tea/breakfast ½ h later (Table 62.3). *Once started, thyroid medication must be continued lifelong.* This must be impressed upon the parents.

The dose of T_4 is adjusted to maintain normal free T_4 concentration (0.8 and 2 ng/dL). When such facilities are not available, the dose is adjusted clinically. *In the infant, the mental milestones are the crucial guide to adequacy of treatment. In older children, it can be monitored by the rate of linear growth and bone age.* Once the euthyroid state is achieved, follow up thyroid function test done at 6–12-month interval.

Overtreatment can result in symptoms and signs of hyperthyroidism; worse, it can lead to premature craniosynostosis of the skull.

IM 12.14

In **adult hypothyroidism**, a complete reversal of the physical and metabolic abnormalities can generally be achieved by adequate replacement therapy. However, this may not be possible in patients with coronary heart disease in whom angina or MI may be precipitated or aggravated by T_4. In the younger patients with no concomitant disease, therapy is started with 50–100 mcg (1.6 mcg/kg) of T_4 per day. The daily dose is increased by 25–50 mcg every 3–4 weeks until the plasma TSH becomes normal (1–5 mcU/mL). In most patients, the maintenance dose is 100–200 mcg (about 1.5–2 mcg/kg) of T_4 per day. After the maintenance dose is determined, therapy can be monitored clinically and by plasma TSH (6–12 monthly).

The dose is reduced in older patients (25–50 mcg/day). It is also about 50 mcg lesser in the hot summer months than during the cold winter months, in regions where the variations in ambient temperatures are marked, e.g. North India. *In patients with ischaemic heart disease, therapy is initiated with doses as low as 12.5 or 25 mcg per day and increased by 25 mcg every 3–4 weeks.*

Requirement of T_4 **during pregnancy** varies but on an average a **30% increase in the dose is required to maintain the TSH levels <3.0 mU/L.** This can be achieved by taking additional two tablets per week.

Therapy must be continued lifelong in most patients. In some situations, hypothyroidism is transient and thyroid replacement therapy may be omitted after a few months. In patients with secondary hypothyroidism, associated cortisol deficiency, if any, should be corrected.

Treatment of subclinical hypothyroidism (i.e. without symptoms and having normal free T_4 but higher TSH levels) remains controversial. *TSH is known to rise with age and many healthy elderly with normal free T4 may be wrongly diagnosed as hypothyroid*. Such asymptomatic individuals may not need any treatment unless their TSH levels are in the range of 5–10 mU/L.

- **Nontoxic goitres:** Normal plasma TSH levels are seen in most patients with nonendemic, simple goitres. Such goitre is thought to be due to locally generated growth factors. Hence, the mechanism of action of T_4 in these patients is obscure. T_4 also corrects any associated hormonal deficiency. It is used in the dose of 100–200 mcg per day. The goitre regresses in about 60% of the patients. Lifelong treatment is desirable except in puberty goitres, which require 2-3 years therapy. Similar dosage is used in the treatment of autoimmune thyroiditis (Hashimoto disease) with hypothyroidism.
- **Thyroid carcinoma:** Surgery is the treatment of choice in all cases of thyroid carcinoma. It is followed by radioiodine therapy in patients with papillary and follicular carcinoma. T_4 has been used instead of ^{131}I after surgery in patients with small, well-differentiated carcinomas as they are TSH dependent. The dose of T_4 is larger (>2 mcg/kg/day) than that customarily used in hypothyroidism and the plasma TSH is maintained at unmeasurable level.
- **Antithyroid drug treatment in hyperthyroidism:** T_4 (100–200 mcg per day) given concurrently prevents/reverses the enlargement and the increased vascularity brought about by thioamides.

  While treating hyperthyroidism **during pregnancy:** T_4 may be added to the antithyroid drug in a dose which maintains plasma T_4 in the upper range of the normal and TSH in the lower range of the normal to prevent hypothyroidism in the mother. *However, thyroid hormones do not cross the placenta significantly whereas the antithyroid drugs do*. Hence, it is necessary to keep the dose of the antithyroid drug to a minimum during pregnancy.

Thyroid hormone treatment does not appear to alter the course of the exophthalmos in Graves disease, nor that of obesity.

TREATMENT OF MYXOEDEMA COMA

Myxoedema coma is a serious complication of long standing, untreated hypothyroidism. It is characterised by coma, hypothermia, marked bradycardia and hypotension. It is most likely to occur in elderly people and during cold season. Inadequate treatment, exposure to cold, infection and trauma act as precipitating factors. The diagnosis is essentially clinical and can be confirmed by plasma free T_4 and TSH estimation. **Therapy should be started without waiting for the result of the tests.** The principles of treatment are given in Box 62.1.

Because of a 5%–10% incidence of coexisting, decreased adrenal reserve, IV administration of glucocorticoid should precede that of thyroid hormones in all cases. If available, T_4 sodium is given intravenously in a loading dose of 200–400 mcg, followed by 100 mcg IV every 24 h. If IV T_4 preparation is not available, 500 mcg can be given through a nasogastric tube as a loading dose. Some physicians prefer to add T_3 in the dose of 10 mcg IV every 8 h, for a few days, because the peripheral conversion of T_4 to T_3 is diminished in severely hypothyroid patients. *Over-aggressive treatment with T_4(>500 mcg/day) or T_3 (>75 mcg/day) is associated with increased mortality rate.* Prophylactic antibiotics are recommended in these patients.

Box 62.1 Principles of Treatment of Myxoedema Coma PH 1.1

- Hospitalise, preferably in an ICU
- Glucocorticoids
- Levothyroxine in large dose intravenously/orally
- Triiodothyronine intravenously, if available
- Antimicrobials
- Slow warming
- Management of hypoventilation, hyponatraemia and other electrolyte disturbances

Warming should be slow, with blankets. Ventilator should be used in case of hypoventilation and fluid restriction if hyponatremia. Fluid and electrolyte balance should be carefully monitored to avoid overhydration. Therapy of myxoedema coma remains unsatisfactory and mortality is high.

IODINE AND THE ENDEMIC GOITRE PH 1.36, PH 1.55, IM 12.13

Endemic goitre is a manifestation of iodine deficiency. The daily iodine requirement is 1–2 mcg/kg body weight and can be met with by ingestion of 200 g of sea fish 2–3 times a week. **Sea-fish and unpurified common salt obtained from sea water are important dietary sources of iodine.** Endemic goitre can be prevented by iodisation of the common salt by adding 50–80 mg of *sodium iodate* to 1 kg of common salt. This provides 30–50 ppm (parts per million) of iodine at the source of production. Considering the loss of iodine during storage to be about 50%, 10 g of salt, the usual daily consumption, provides about 150–250 mcg of iodine, which is the intended daily supplement. *Treatment of pre-existing simple goitre with iodine is generally unsuccessful. Therapy with T4 is more effective.*

Excess of iodine can cause goitre ± either hypothyroidism or hyperthyroidism (see section, Antithyroid drugs).

ANTITHYROID DRUGS PH 1.36, IM 12.13

The clinical manifestations of hyperthyroidism are due to an excess of circulating thyroid hormones. They can be ameliorated by using **antithyroid drugs**, which interfere with the synthesis, release or action of thyroid hormones.

Classification

I. **Drugs which interfere with hormonal synthesis:**
   a. **Ion inhibitors** which inhibit iodine trapping and binding, e.g. potassium perchlorate and Thiocyanate
   b. **Thioamides** which inhibit thyroid peroxidase and block the synthesis of MIT, DIT; and prevent the coupling reaction, e.g. propylthiouracil, carbimazole, methimazole

II. **Drugs that interfere with the hormonal release and promote its storage,** e.g. iodides, Lugol iodine

III. **Radioactive iodine** that destroys the acinii

Antithyroid drugs such as iodide and propylthiouracil may act by more than one mechanism.

Drugs interfering with hormonal synthesis (Class I) reduce the plasma T_4 and T_3 levels, which in turn stimulates TSH synthesis, Increased TSH stimulates the thyroid, which undergoes hypertrophy and hyperplasia, and increases thyroid vascularity. This causes enlargement of the thyroid gland, and hence these drugs are called **goitrogens**.

ION INHIBITORS: Potassium thiocyanate and **perchlorate** competitively inhibit the iodide trapping by the thyroid gland. Thiocyanate is not used in practice because of its toxicity but may be responsible for the goitrogenic action of certain staple foods (e.g. cassava).

Potassium perchlorate is not commonly used in the treatment of hyperthyroidism, as it not easily available in the market; it causes ADRs like gastric irritation, fever, skin rashes, lymphadenopathy, agranulocytosis and rarely aplastic anaemia It is a useful alternative in patients allergic to the thioamides.

THIOAMIDES: The important drugs belonging to this group are **methyl- and propyl-thiouracil, methimazole** and **carbimazole** (Fig. 62.3). They have similar modes of action but differ in pharmacokinetics, dosage and the incidence of adverse reactions.

Mechanism of action: These drugs bind to and inhibit the thyroid peroxidase; they thus **block thyroid hormone synthesis by inhibiting:**

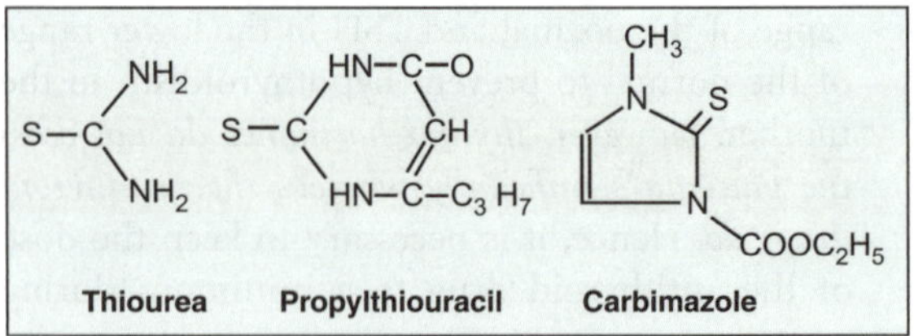

FIG. 62.3 Thioamides.

- **Coupling of iodotyrosines**
- **Formation of MIT**
- **Conversion of MIT to DIT**

Propylthiouracil (but not carbimazole) in addition inhibits the peripheral deiodinase and prevents conversion of T_4 to T_3. Carbimazole has also been claimed to encourage a remission in Graves disease by suppressing the autoimmune process in the thyroid; the anti-TSH receptor antibodies decrease and the circulating suppressor T cells increase.

Absorption, fate and excretion: These drugs are rapidly absorbed (20–30 min) after oral administration. They are concentrated by the thyroid gland. The duration of action of a single oral dose is less than 8 h. Usually, they are administered every 6–8 h. Some physicians, however, prescribe the entire daily dose of thioamides on a once a day basis.

They are partly metabolised in the liver and the thyroid and partly excreted in the urine unchanged. **Carbimazole is metabolised to the active metabolite methimazole.** The plasma t½ of propylthiouracil is about 75 min while that of carbimazole is 4–6 h. They cross the placental barrier and are secreted in milk.

Adverse reactions: The incidence of the adverse effects is reasonably small and does not probably exceed 5%. **The milder ADR** include drug fever, pruritus, urticaria, oedema of the feet, arthralgia, lymphadenopathy and hair loss. The **more serious effects** are leukopenia, thrombocytopenia, liver damage and rarely agranulocytosis. *The patient should be told to report any attack of sore throat, fever and oral ulceration during therapy.* Hypothyroidism is an extension of the pharmacological action of these drugs, which is reversible.

Preparations and dosage:

i. Propylthiouracil: 50 mg tablets. Dose: 150–450 mg daily in divided doses
ii. Methimazole 5 and 10 mg tablets. Dose: for control: 15–60 mg daily; for maintenance, 5–15 mg daily
iii. Carbimazole 5, 10 and 20 mg tablets; dose: for control 20–60 mg daily; for maintenance, 5–20 mg daily

Indications: In hyperthyroidism, see section, Pharmacotherapy of hyperthyroidism.

IODIDE: Iodide is the oldest remedy for thyroid disorders including hyperthyroidism. *It is the quickest acting drug in hyperthyroidism and its action becomes apparent within 24 h.* The acinar cells become smaller in size and the colloid content increases. The gland becomes less vascular and firm. The maximum clinical benefit is seen within 10–14 days. The hyperthyroid state is, however, only partially controlled by iodide and after some time, the beneficial effects seem to wear off.

Mechanism of action: It influences iodine metabolism as follows:

1. Iodide rapidly shuts off the release of the preformed thyroid hormones and promotes their storage (**thyroid constipation**; see section, Thyrotoxic crisis-treatment)
2. It inhibits synthesis of iodotyrosine and iodothyronine (**Wolff–Chaikoff effect**). This is due to high intracellular concentration of iodide. With time, there is an escape for this effect.
3. It limits its own transport resulting in low iodide levels
4. When given along with a thiourea compound, it prevents the increase in the size and vascularity of the goitre that can occur following antithyroid drugs

Adverse reactions: Chronic iodine intoxication (**iodism**) may occur in a susceptible individual, giving rise to skin rash, rhinorrhoea, lacrimation and increased salivation. Prolonged use of iodides (as in cough mixtures) has been reported to occasionally produce goitre and hypothyroidism. Iodides cross the placenta and may cause goitre in the fetus. *They must, be avoided during pregnancy.*

They may precipitate thyrotoxicosis (**Jod–Basedow effect**) occasionally. An iodine-containing organic dye and amiodarone can precipitate thyrotoxicosis.

Preparations and dosage: Preparations used are **Lugol iodine** and saturated solution of potassium iodide (SSKI). *The former is prepared by dissolving*

5 g of iodine in 100 mL of 10% solution of potassium iodide and it provides 150 mg of iodine per ml; the dose is 0.1–0.3 mL three times a day. SSKI is prepared by dissolving 30 g of KI in 21 mL of water to give 30 mL of SSKI and *it provides 1 g of KI per mL*. The dose of iodine needed to control hyperthyroidism is about 6 mg per day; however, much larger doses are used in thyrotoxic crisis.

Indications:

- **Prevention of endemic goitre** (see section, Iodine and the endemic goitre)
- **Preoperative preparation:** They are used in the preoperative preparation of a hyperthyroid patient to reduce the vascularity of the gland. It is given for 10–14 days preoperatively *in addition to a thiourea drug. T_4 given concurrently with antithyroid drugs can obviate the need for the preoperative addition of iodide to therapy.*
- **Rapid control of hyperthyroidism:** Iodides along with a thioamide are used to control hyperthyroidism very rapidly as in a patient with thyrotoxic crisis or with HF.
  Patients with hyperthyroidism tend to have little hormonal iodine stored in their glands. Iodide administration can increase the hormonal content of the gland. If such a patient is then given a thioamide drug, it fails to act quickly because thioamide blocks synthesis but not release of thyroid hormones. *Hence, iodide administration to a hyperthyroid patient should be commenced after first blocking thyroid hormone synthesis with a thioamide.*
- **Blocking the thyroidal uptake:** Iodide is used to block the thyroidal uptake before administration of a ^{131}I labelled compound for the localisation of a pheochromocytoma and in cases of a nuclear accident with possible release of ^{131}I into the environment.

RADIOACTIVE IODINE: Radioactive iodine, ^{131}I, is concentrated selectively by the thyroid gland. It emits gamma and beta radiations. Gamma radiation is used for measuring radioiodine uptake and for thyroid scan. **Beta radiation is particles that penetrate only up to 3–5 mm in the soft tissues.** Within this compass, they dissipate their energy and **act as ionising radiation**. They selectively destroy the thyroidal follicles, produce fibrosis and impair the ability of the remaining follicles to replicate.

Preparation and dosage: Radioiodine is available as a solution of Na ^{131}I. *It is administered orally in the dose of 3–10 mCi, on an empty stomach or after a light breakfast.* Patients can be treated on an out-patient basis but are instructed to dispose of their urine carefully into latrine. The effect of a dose becomes apparent within 3–4 weeks with maximum effect by 3–6 months. About 50% of the patients become euthyroid after a single dose. Others may need a second or even a third dose.

Adverse reactions:

- **Focal soreness in the neck** due to irradiation, and a transient **aggravation of the hyperthyroid state** are rare.
- **Hypothyroidism:** This occurs in 40%–60% of the patients in the long run. Hence, treated patients must be followed up for long periods.
- **Damage to the fetal thyroid:** *The fetal thyroid is extremely susceptible to radiation and may be quickly destroyed.*
- **Thyroid carcinoma:** Radiation is known to be carcinogenic and the possibility of development of thyroid cancer following radioiodine cannot be totally ruled out.
- **Genetic damage:** So far, this has not been demonstrated. PH 1.1, IM 12.15

PHARMACOTHERAPY OF HYPERTHYROIDISM

T_4 and T_3 assays are helpful in confirming the diagnosis of **thyrotoxicosis**. Thyrotoxicosis may be due to:

1. An excessive, ongoing production of thyroid hormones (**hyperthyroidism, with elevated ^{131}I uptake**) as in Graves disease or the nodular toxic goitre
2. May occur in its absence

Thyrotoxicosis *without hyperthyroidism* occurs in thyroiditis and during administration of excessive doses of T_4 as treatment. These patients need withdrawal of T_4 and supportive treatment such as propranolol and a benzodiazepine, *As the thyroiditis is self-limiting, destructive forms of treatment are not used in such patients.*

As the aetiology of **thyrotoxicosis with hyperthyroidism** is not known, the treatment is empirical and is aimed at reducing the production of the thyroid hormones or destroying the gland. There are three forms of treatment available for therapy of hyperthyroidism. They are as follows:

1. **Antithyroid drugs**
2. **Radioactive iodine**
3. **Surgery**

Choice of Therapy

Indications for various forms of therapy are outlined in Boxes 62.2–62.4. The treatment of thyrotoxicosis is essentially medical. In most instances, the choice rests between an antithyroid drug and radioactive iodine. Advantages and disadvantages of both are listed below.

Antithyroid Drugs IM 12.15

Advantages of thioamide drugs:

- They are well tolerated by most patients and are fairly rapidly effective; clinical benefits being apparent in about 2 weeks. The patient is rendered euthyroid in about 2–3 months. This state can be maintained as long as it is desired by the maintenance doses. If therapy is continued for 2 years, permanent remission is achieved in about 40%–50% of the cases.
- If hypothyroidism occurs, it is reversible.
- They do not generally aggravate the endocrine exophthalmos.
- They can be used safely in children.
- *They can also be used during pregnancy*. The lowest possible dose should be used.
- They can be used to perform a therapeutic test in patients with doubtful diagnosis.

Disadvantages of drug therapy:

- Prolonged treatment and follow up are essential.
- In spite of adequate treatment, recurrence occurs in 40%–60% of the cases.
- In patients with severe HF, their action is too slow. In such cases, iodide may be used along with a thiourea drug.
- *They rarely cause serious toxicity such as agranulocytosis.*

Radioactive Iodine IM 12.15

Advantages of radioiodine:

- The treatment is convenient, effective and can be carried out on an out-patient basis. It can be used with certainty of effects even in unintelligent or undependable patients.
- It is pleasant to take without any discomfort or fear and very acceptable to the patient. It avoids surgery and its attendant complications.
- There is generally no fear of recurrence once the patient becomes euthyroid.
- It is relatively inexpensive and safe. In many cases control can be achieved with a single dose.
- It can be offered to patients in whom surgery is not possible and to those who refuse surgery. It can be used routinely in all patients past the age of 35–40 years.

Disadvantages of radioiodine:

- Because of high incidence of hypothyroidism, it cannot be recommended for children.

Box 62.2 Indications for Antithyroid Drugs

- **Children**
- **Pregnant women:** Propylthiouracil is preferred to carbimazole because it is more protein bound and crosses the placenta to a smaller extent
- **Young adults with small goitres** and mild thyrotoxicosis of recent onset
- **Before thyroidectomy** in all cases
- **After radioiodine therapy**, for a few weeks, starting 7–10 days after ^{131}I dose

Box 62.3 Indications for Radioiodine

- **All patients above the age of 35 years;** in severe cases, the patient is first made euthyroid with a thioamide, before radioiodine administration
- **Recurrent hyperthyroidism after an adequate course of thioamide drugs or after surgery**
- **Allergy to thioamides**
- **In young patients in whom a severe, associated systemic disease contraindicates surgery and predicts shortening of the life expectancy**

Box 62.4 Indications for Surgery

- **Multinodular toxic goitre**
- **Solitary toxic nodule**
- **A large diffuse, toxic goitre,** especially when it fails to regress and disappear on thioamide treatment
- **Recurrence** after adequate treatment with a thioamide
- **When malignancy cannot be ruled out**

- *Pregnancy is an absolute contraindication for radioiodine. It cannot be given to a woman of the child bearing age without testing for pregnancy.*
- It is slow acting. However, the administration of radioiodine may be followed by a period of antithyroid drugs to achieve early clinical control.
- Follow up for several years is necessary in order to detect late onset hypothyroidism.
- There is a *very rare* possibility of late development of thyroid carcinoma.
- Special facilities for handling the radioactive material are necessary, so also for disposing the urine.

Supportive Measures

These comprise of:

1. A sedative/anxiolytic to allay anxiety
2. Administration of calcium orally (1000 mg/day) may be helpful in avoiding possible osteoporosis
3. **Propranolol** (30–120 mg/day) to control, palpitation, tachycardia and tremor. It does not correct the hyperthyroid metabolic state. Hence, propranolol alone should not be used for preoperative preparation of the patient. A CCB such as diltiazem (60–120 mg) can be used.
4. Treatment of CHF and AF; propranolol is the preferred drug
5. Vitamin supplements
6. Immunotherapy with B-lymphocyte–depleting agent rituximab, with methimazole, has been used for Graves hyperthyroidism and ophthalmopathy

THYROTOXIC CRISIS – TREATMENT

This is a manifestation of extreme hypermetabolism in a thyrotoxic patient and may occur:

Box 62.5 Principles of Treatment of Thyrotoxic Crisis PH 1.1

- **Hospitalisation,** preferably into an ICU
- **Treatment of the precipitating cause**
- **Large doses of an antithyroid drug** (propylthiouracil is preferred because it inhibits peripheral conversion of T_4 to T_3. 200 mg or carbimazole 20 mg every 4 h
- **Iodide,** started a couple of hours after the thioamide drug. It may be given intravenously (sodium iodide 1 g by infusion) or through a nasogastric tube (0.3 mL of SSKI every 8 h). These doses are in excess of that which controls hyperthyroidism
- **Propranolol** (intravenously) 2–10 mg repeated every 4 h, or labetalol (intramuscularly) every 4–6 h
- **Supportive measures** including dexamethasone 0.5–1 mg IM 8 hourly, oxygen, adequate intravenous fluids and glucose, B complex vitamins, antimicrobials, and treatment of hyperpyrexia with paracetamol and tepid sponging. Heart failure, if present, needs to be treated. Aspirin should be avoided as it can displace thyroid hormone from its binding proteins

1. After thyroidectomy in an inadequately prepared patient (**surgical storm**)
2. In the presence of an infection, injury or any surgical procedure other than thyroidectomy (**medical storm**)

The manifestations are hyperpyrexia, marked tachycardia, extreme irritability and delirium. Nausea, vomiting and diarrhoea may add to the dehydration. **It is a medical emergency and the treatment must be immediate** (Box 62.5). In spite of aggressive medical treatment, mortality is still high; hence, it is best be prevented.

Drug-Induced Thyroid Disease

Many compounds when used for other clinical purposes disturb the thyroid function as a side effect. They may interfere with the interpretation of the thyroid function tests. Sulphonamides, PAS, lithium and resorcinol interfere with thyroid hormone synthesis, whereas amiodarone, glucocorticoids and beta blockers block the conversion of T_4 to T_3. Hepatic enzyme inducers such as rifampicin, phenytoin and carbamazepine promote rapid inactivation of the thyroid hormones. Further, excessive iodide and the iodine-containing contrast media can also interfere with thyroid function. These changes however are usually reversible.

Amiodarone: This antiarrhythmic drug, which is structurally related to T_4, contains 37% of iodine by weight. Thus, patient taking 200 mg/day would receive nearly 75 mg of organic iodide daily. The drug is stored in the body fat and has a t½ of 54 days. During its metabolism substantial amount of free iodine gets into the circulation which can cause hypo- or hyperthyroidism in 10% of patients. Hypothyroidism is reversible after stoppage of the drug. Hyperthyroidism (Type 1), that is caused due to increased synthesis of hormone, needs large doses of thioamides; the recovery is slow.

Thyrotoxicosis (Type 2) that is caused by chemical thyroditis is due to release of the hormone from the gland and is difficult to treat; it responds only to prednisolone, 40–60 mg/day in divided doses for 1–3 months. If the mechanism is uncertain, combination of thioamide and prednisolone may be reasonable.

Glucocorticoids in thyroid disorders: Glucocorticoids are valuable in treating:

- **Myxoedema coma**
- **Thyrotoxic crisis**
- **Schmidt syndrome:** Concurrent Graves disease and hypoadrenalism, both due to autoimmune disease
- **de Quervain's subacute thyroiditis with low-uptake thyrotoxicosis**
- **Amiodarone-induced thyrotoxicosis**
- **Graves, opthalmopathy**

There is no evidence that the use of glucocorticoids benefits the average case of Graves disease or Hashimoto disease.

IODINE-CONTAINING CONTRAST MEDIA

Currently used nonionic iodinated low-osmolar (e.g. iopamidol, iopromide, iopentol, iomeprol) and iso-osmolar (e.g. iodixanol) contrast media have lower incidence of ADRs. The most common manifestations are dermatological such as transient warmth, flushing, pruritus, urticaria, which occur immediately within 1 hr of contrast media injection. Delayed manifestations (till 7 days) include exanthema, erythema multiforme, vasculitis and Stevens–Johnson syndrome. The other reactions are occasional and include nausea, vomiting, headache, bradycardia with hypotension, anaphylactoid reactions like facial and laryngeal edema, bronchospasm and shock.

The majority of these reactions are self-limiting. However, severe reactions need symptomatic treatment. Risk of contrast media induced nephropathy (CIN) in high risk patients like elderly, preexisting CKD and DM has been reduced with use of current agents and prior use of IV isotonic crystalloid solution.

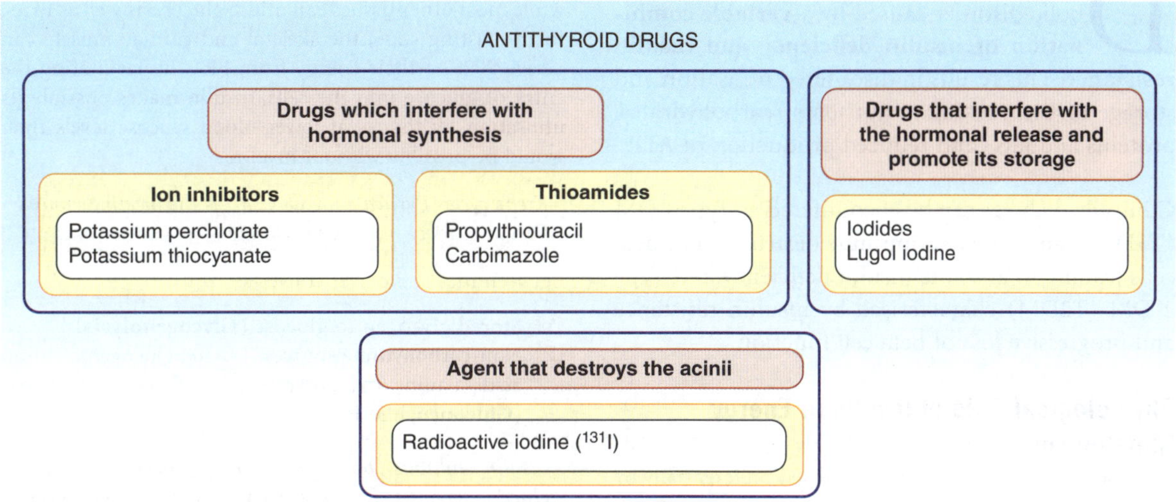

CHAPTER 63

Pancreatic Hormones, Antidiabetic Drugs and Pharmacotherapy of Diabetes Mellitus

Learning Objectives

This chapter will enable the reader:

1. To be aware of the physiology of energy metabolism.
2. To explain the factors controlling insulin release.
3. To describe the mechanism of action, pharmacological effects, ADR of insulin and state the precautions taken to prevent the ADR.
4. To enumerate human insulin preparations and insulin analogues along with their salient pharmacokinetic features.
5. To compare and contrast insulin and its analogues.
6. To classify noninsulin antidiabetic drugs and describe their mechanism of action, pharmacological effects, salient pharmacokinetic features, ADR and indications.
7. To discuss the factors determining the choice of an antidiabetic agent.
8. To explain the role of nonpharmacological therapy in diabetes mellitus (DM).
9. To outline the management of (a) Type 1 DM, (b) Type 2 DM without complications and (c) Type 2 DM with complications emphasising the principles.
10. To outline the management of diabetic emergencies.
11. To discuss the mechanism of action, pharmacological effects, salient pharmacokinetic features, ADR and indications for diazoxide.
12. To enumerate various sweetening agents.

KEY TERMS

Diabetes mellitus (DM) is a chronic metabolic disorder caused by a **variable combination of insulin deficiency and insulin resistance.** This results in disordered utilisation and storage of the proximate nutrients (carbohydrates, proteins and fats) and reduced production of ATP.

Clinically diabetes can be encountered as Type I DM (T1DM) caused by autoimmune destruction of beta cells leading to absolute insulin deficiency and Type 2 DM (T2DM) characterised by insulun resistance and progressive loss of beta cell function.

Physiological Role of Insulin in Energy Metabolism

Glucose absorbed after a meal, is utilised preferentially by all tissues for energy production and/or storage (Fig. 63.1). Tissues differ in their dependence on glucose and free fatty acids (FFA) for energy. The brain utilises only glucose while most other tissues can utilise glucose as well as FFAs. In the fasting state, the skeletal and cardiac muscle can derive 90% of their energy from FFA. By facilitating the entry of glucose into the cells, insulin makes possible its utilisation by tissues at lower blood glucose levels than would be possible without insulin.

Kreb's cycle (Pyruvate metabolism) is the meeting ground for the metabolism of carbohydrates, fats and proteins.

Between meals, the liver converts:

(1) Stored glycogen to glucose (**Glycogenolysis**)
(2) Non-carbohydrate sources (lactate; glucogenic amino acids-alanine and glutamine; and glycerol) to glucose (**Gluconeogenesis**)

Insulin inhibits both, hepatic glycogenolysis and gluconeogenesis; its deficiency in DM leads to exaggerated gluconeogenesis.

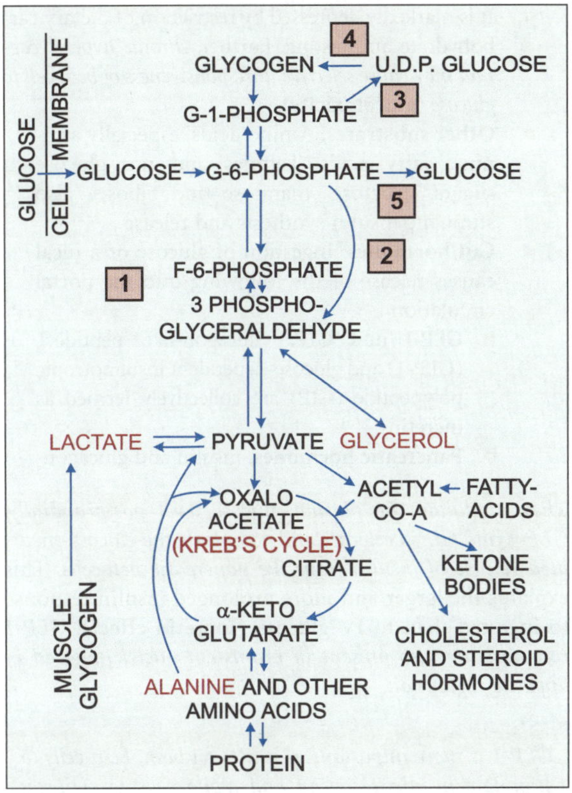

FIG. 63.1 Glucose metabolism G = Glucose; F = Fructose 1. Glycolysis; 2. Pentose-phosphate shunt; 3. Glucurunoic acid pathway; 4. Glycogenesis; 5. Conversion to glucose.

In the fasting state, the plasma glucose fluctuates between 60 and 100 mg/dL. After a meal, it rises to a maximum of 140–150 mg/dL and returns to the fasting level within 2–3 h. The arterial blood glucose is maintained so as to supply glucose to brain.

The main determinants of the variations in the blood glucose are (a) ingestion of food, (b) the plasma levels of insulin and (c) various hormones.

- **Ingestion of a mixed meal:** Absorption of food during the postprandial period results in elevation of blood glucose, amino acids and FFA, which cause insulin release. *Thus the overall effect is to* **increase the insulin/glucagon ratio in the portal circulation.** The liver plays a central role in regulation of the blood glucose level. **The enhanced insulin/glucagon ratio:**

a. Stimulates hepatic glucose uptake and glycogen formation
b. Inhibits glucose output

This curbs the rising blood glucose level.

The peripheral utilisation of glucose results in the production of substances such as pyruvate, NADPH, NADH and ATP. *Many of the biochemical consequences of insulin deficiency/resistance to its action can be explained by deficiency of these substances.* **Insulin is not necessary for glucose uptake by brain, leucocytes and RBCs, for its GI absorption or for its renal tubular reabsorption.**

- **In the post-absorptive state:** There is a reversal of insulin/glucagon release ratio in favour of glucagon, which increases the hepatic glucose output. **The relatively high levels of other counter-regulatory anti-insulin hormones lead to:**
  a. **Gluconeogenesis** by GH, corticosteroids, catecholamines and thyroid hormones
  b. **Glycogenolysis** by catecholamines
  c. **Lipolysis** with release of FFA into circulation
  d. **Availability of amino acids for gluconeogenesis** by the liver by anti-anabolic action of glucocorticoids

Thus, the carbohydrate, lipid and protein metabolisms are interlinked. **The central theme of these processes is to:**

a. *Promote storage of glucose and other metabolic fuels (fatty acids and amino acids), as well as their peripheral utilisation after a meal*
b. *Make glucose available to the brain by glycogenolysis and gluconeogenesis, and FFA to the other tissues, in the post-absorptive state*

During pregnancy, glucose is made available to the fetus by an excess of anti-insulin influences from mother's adrenal cortex as well as by insulin degradation. **Pregnancy is, therefore, a potentially diabetogenic state. During lactation,** extraction of glucose by the breast for milk production further affects blood glucose level.

INSULIN: The chemical structure of insulin was determined by Sanger in 1951. It is a polypeptide with a molecular weight of about 6000, consisting of two amino acid chains, A and B, linked by two disulphide bridges. The chains contain 21 and 30 amino acids, respectively (Fig. 63.2).

Synthesis and storage: The islets constitute 1% by weight of the pancreas. They contain:

- **Alpha or A cells which secrete glucagon**
- **Beta or B cells which secrete insulin**
- **Delta or D cells which secrete somatostatin**
- **PP or F cells which secrete pancreatic polypeptide (PP)**

Insulin is synthesised within the beta cells as a single

chain polypeptide precursor called *preproinsulin* which is converted to *proinsulin*. Proinsulin is biologically only one-eighth as active as insulin. It is cleaved by proteolytic enzymes to form the single chain C peptide and **double chain insulin, which is stored in the granules of beta cells.**

The pancreas of a normal human adult contains about 200 units (8 mg) of insulin. It secretes about 50 units of insulin in 24 h, which enters the portal vein and passes to the liver. Of this, about 50% gets degraded. The remaining enters the systemic circulation. **About half of the total daily insulin output is released at a slow rate, in repeated pulses, to provide a basal plasma insulin level;** the other half is secreted after meals. The plasma level of insulin fluctuates throughout the day with peaks after meals.

Factors determining insulin release:

As with other hormones, *insulin secretion is regulated by a feedback loop involving islet beta cells and insulin sensitive tissues, mainly liver, adipose tissue and muscle.* The released insulin promotes uptake of glucose, amino acids and fatty acids by the insulin sensitive tissues, which send feedback information to beta cells about their need for insulin. This mechanism helps to regulate glucose metabolism and to maintain plasma glucose concentration within normal range.

- **Glucose:** Glucose is the specific and the most potent stimulus for insulin synthesis and release. As the *plasma* glucose level rises, there is a progressive increase in insulin release which reaches its maximum at glucose level of 300–350 mg%.

It is markedly depressed by restriction of dietary carbohydrate and fasting. Further, *chronic hyperglycaemia may cause selective unresponsiveness of beta cell to glucose* (**glucotoxicity**).

- **Other substrates:** Amino acids, especially arginine, fatty acids, ketones and non-glucose sugars (fructose, mannose and ribose) also stimulate insulin synthesis and release
- **Gut hormones:** Ingestion of glucose or a meal causes release of the following into the portal circulation
  a. **GLP-1 and GIP:** Glucagon-like peptide-1 (GLP-1) and glucose-dependent insulinotropic polypeptide (GIP) are collectively termed as **incretins**
  b. **Pancreatic hormones,** insulin and glucagon

They modulate the plasma glucose level postprandially. GLP-1 and GIP accelerate and potentiate the glucose-mediated release of insulin from the pancreatic betacells. This explains the larger and more prolonged insulin response to ingested than to IV glucose (**Incretin effect**). *GLP-1 receptors are also present in brainstem nuclei involved in appetite regulation.*

GLP-1 is more important as it acts on both, beta cells to stimulate insulin secretion and alpha cells to suppress glucagon secretion.

- **Other hormones:** Glucagon, GH, thyroxine, ACTH, and glucocorticoids also stimulate insulin release, while somatostatin, adrenaline, noradrenaline and exogenously administered insulin inhibit it

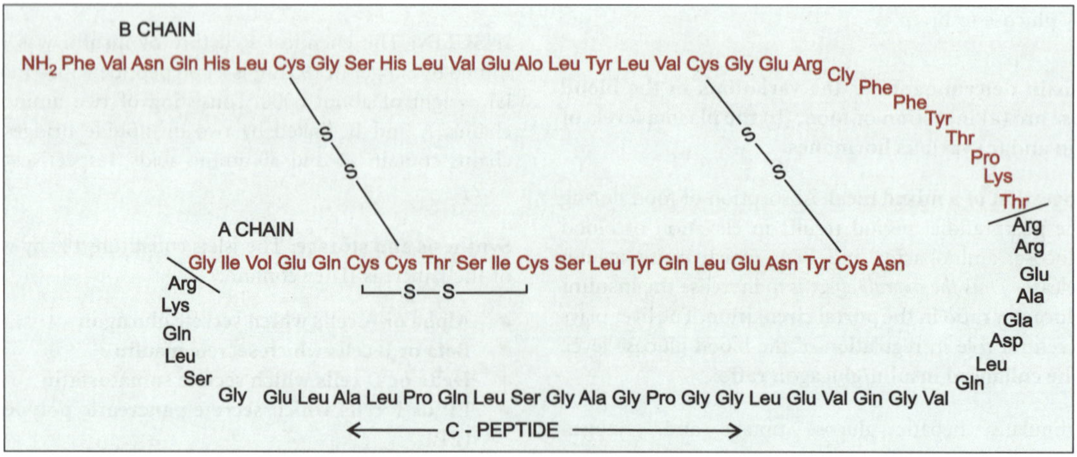

FIG. 63.2 **Human proinsulin, a precursor of insulin.**

- **Bile acids:** stimulate intestinal L-cells to secret GLP-1
- **Neurogenic:** Insulin release is enhanced by parasympathetic (vagal) stimulation and by beta-1 adrenergic stimulation. It is under tonic inhibition by pancreatic alpha-2 adrenoreceptors; *this is seen in conditions associated with increased sympathoadrenal discharge such as hypoxia, severe burns, surgery and MI with shock*. Hypothalamus acts as an integrator.
- **Hypokalaemia** inhibits insulin release
- **Drugs:** Glucose-induced insulin release is enhanced by xanthines. Sulphonylureas stimulate insulin release. It is inhibited by thiazides, diazoxide and phenytoin.

Mechanism of action: *Insulin affects all aspects of energy metabolism. It binds to specific insulin receptors present on the surface of target cells. The main target sites are the adipose tissue, the liver and the skeletal muscles.* The insulin receptor comprises two subunits:

1. **The extracellular alpha subunit** which serves as the recognition site
2. **The transmembrane beta subunit** which contains the **tyrosine kinase**

Binding of insulin to the receptors activates tyrosine kinase, which gets phosphorylated. Tyrosine kinase phosphorylates insulin receptor substrate 1 (IRS1). The IRS1 then phosphorylates other protein substrates in the cell, thus initiating a cascade effect. Such phosphorylation activates some enzymes while it inactivates others. The cascade is responsible for **multiple (pleotropic) effects** of insulin on intermediary metabolism:

a. **Immediate effects** on carbohydrate, lipid and protein metabolism
b. **Long-term effects: Mitogen-activated protein kinase (MAPK) pathway stimulates growth and mitogenic processes.** These include stimulation of DNA transcription, cell proliferation and differentiation. These effects are mediated by IGF-1 and local growth factors.

Number of insulin receptors varies inversely with the insulin concentration at the site of action.

- **With higher concentration,** the receptor number reduces (**downregulation**), so also the response to insulin (insulin resistance as seen in T2DM)
- **With low concentration,** the number of receptors at the site increases with resultant increase in insulin sensitivity (**upregulation**)

SYNTHETIC INSULIN PH 1.36, IM 11.16

Insulin was earlier obtained from bovine and porcine pancreas. 'Human' insulin biosynthesised by cultures of bacteria (*Escherichia coli*) and yeasts (**recombinant DNA or rDNA insulin**) is now commonly used in practice. Its primary structure (amino acid sequence) is identical with that of insulin derived from human pancreas. Synthetic, modified, human rDNA insulin analogues (lispro, aspart, glargine, etc.) have different pharmacokinetic but the same pharmacodynamic properties as the native human insulin.

Insulin is soluble in water but undergoes molecular aggregation to hexameric form at extremes of pH (3.2 and 10). Such aggregation is further enhanced by zinc which brings about its crystallisation. **Insulin is relatively insoluble at the pH range of 4–7.** The mechanism of action of all the synthetic insulins is identical to that of physiological insulin.

Pharmacological actions:

Immediate effects: The major actions of insulin on intermediary metabolism are summarised in Table 63.1.

Effects on carbohydrate metabolism and regulation of blood glucose level: Stimulation of insulin receptors causes **activation of**:

a. **Glucose carrier-mediated transport** by recruiting **glucose transporters** (GLUT-4) from the cytoplasm to the cell membrane. The liver cells are freely permeable to glucose which enters via glucose transporters. *Insulin stimulates the uptake and utilisation of glucose by the liver cells.*
b. **Glucokinase and Glucose-6-phosphatase**

The metabolic processes depicted in Table 63.1 are modified by insulin in a dose-dependent manner.

Long-term effects: Stimulation of synthesis of GLUT and the hexokinases

- **Vascular effects:** Insulin has vasodilatory properties, probably exerted via activation of endothelial NO production. Hyperglycaemia may impair endothelium-dependent vasodilatation. Hyperinsulinaemia of Type 2 DM may stimulate the proliferation of vascular smooth muscle cells.

Table 63.1 Actions of Insulin on the Major Target Organs

Metabolism	Adipose Tissue	Liver	Skeletal Muscle
Carbohydrate	Increased glucose uptake	Increased glycogen synthesis and storage. Decreased glycogenolysis and gluconeogenesis.	Increased glucose uptake and utilisation. Increased glycogen synthesis and deposition.
Fat	Decreased lipolysis (antilipolytic action). Increased formation of triglycerides (lipogenesis), weight gain Stimulates lipoprotein lipase and increased FFA uptake	Increased lipogenesis, weight gain, decreased ketogenesis	Decreased lipolysis
Protein		Decreased protein breakdown. Increased protein synthesis.	Increased amino acid transport into the cell and protein synthesis. Decreased protein breakdown.

- **Anti-inflammatory effects:** Insulin decreases the inflammatory process, especially in the vasculature.
- **Fibrinolysis:** Decreased fibrinolysis, associated with hyperinsulinaemia and hypertriglyceridemia in uncontrolled T2DM, has been implicated in atherogenesis.
- **Growth:** Insulin plays an important role in intra- and extra-uterine linear growth.

Factors modifying the actions of insulin:

- **Muscular Exercise:** Exercise training increases the sensitivity of muscles to insulin and lowers the blood glucose.
- **Other hormones:** Counter-regulatory hormones oppose the metabolic actions of insulin and elevate blood glucose.
- **Anti-insulin antibodies:** These are present in the plasma of all individuals who have received insulin. Their presence in high concentrations can cause 'insulin resistance'.

Plasma insulin: Plasma insulin can be measured by radioimmunoassay (IRI or immunoreactive insulin) and by bioassay (ILA or insulin like activity).

Immunoreactive insulin (IRI): The commercial kits measure both insulin and pro-insulin. In healthy individuals, the fasting level of IRI is 5–30 microunits/mL of plasma.

ILA: The term 'Insulin-like activity' indicates what is measured by the bioassay because the effect is the sum total of insulin itself, its potentiators and inhibitors.

Absorption, fate and excretion: Oral insulin is ineffective due to degradation in GI tract. It must be given parenterally. Addition of zinc and/or protein slows down its absorption and prolongs its duration of action. **Endogenous insulin** is in the monomeric form, which is highly diffusible and biologically active. On the contrary, **recombinant human regular insulin** contains insulin in *tetrameric or hexameric* form, which is minimally diffusible; thus delaying its onset of action. Amongst various synthetic insulins, VRA insulin analogues are absorbed very rapidly, and require no lag time. Further, the rate of their absorption is independent of the site of injection.

Synthetic insulin on injection directly enters systemic circulation and is distributed to the liver as well as other tissues. It circulates in the plasma in a free form and disappears rapidly with a t½ of 5–6 min. It is degraded by the liver, kidneys and skeletal muscles. *Sixty percent of exogenous insulin is degraded by the kidney* while the hepatic clearance accounts for 30%–40% of the dose. The reverse is true in the case of endogenous insulin which is secreted directly in the portal circulation. Only traces of free insulin appear in the urine. *In chronic kidney diseases, insulin degradation is retarded requiring dosage changes in these patients.*

Following SC insulin injection, *the absorption is fastest from the abdominal wall, less rapid from the arm and slowest from the thigh.* Exercising the limb into which short-acting insulin is injected speeds up the absorption and may even cause hypoglycaemia. Repeated injections at the same site can cause local fibrosis and delay absorption.

Classification of Insulin Formulations

These is listed in Box 63.1 and Table 63.2.

Injectable insulin

The human insulins are:

- **Pure and stable**
- **Neutral in pH and less likely to cause subcutaneous fat atrophy**
- **Less antigenic**

Insulin analogues: (Designer insulins): These are molecules that differ from human insulin in amino acid sequence but act like native insulin. They are:

1. **Lispro insulin:** This short-acting preparation exists as an insulin hexamer. On SC injection, it dissociates instantly into monomers. (Table 63.2). It is injected immediately before or within 5 min of commencing a meal. Its advantages are:
   - Rapid absorption
   - Effective in reducing the postprandial rise in blood glucose
   - Low incidence of hypoglycaemic reactions
   - No effect on absorption despite variation in the injection site

   It is very effective for use in continuous SC insulin infusion, and is particularly useful in intensive insulin regimens
2. **Aspart insulin** is short acting and has properties, uses and limitations similar to those of lispro, but with somewhat longer duration of action. It is injected SC twice a day within before or after 5 min of commencing the meals. A premixed preparation containing the rapid-acting and the long-acting aspart insulins (30:70) is available.
3. **Glulisine insulin:** See Table 63.2
4. **Glargine insulin** is a **long-acting analogue** (Table 63.2). It:
   - Provides a prolonged, continuous, low plasma insulin concentration (plateau; Fig 63.3)
   - Has more predictable effect
   - Has longer duration of action and require lesser frequency of injections
   - Does not cause hunger pangs due to hypoglycaemia between meals
   - Causes less or no weight gain

Box 63.1 Currently Available Human Insulins

1. **Recombinant insulins:**
   a. ***Rapid (short) acting:*** Regular Insulin
   b. ***Intermediate acting:*** NPH Insulin
   c. ***Premade mixture*** of (a) and (b) (Mixtard),
2. **Human Insulin analogues, recombinant:**
   a. ***Very Rapid (ultra short) Acting*** (**VRA**): Lispro, Aspart, Glulisine
   b. ***Intermediate acting*** Premade mixtures, Lispro-protamine + Lispro, Aspart-protamine + Aspart
   c. ***Long-acting insulins:*** Glargine, Detemir
   d. ***Ultra-long-acting insulin:*** Insulin Degludec

   - *Cannot be mixed with any of the SR insulins, because of its acid pH (pH 4.1).* **It is given SC once a day, and a very short-acting insulin is injected additionally before each major meal** (basal-bolus regimen). This mimics the delivery of endogenous insulin in non-diabetics except that it is into systemic and not portal circulation.
5. **Detemir insulin** has a fatty acid side chain that allows albumin binding, resulting in prolongation of its action. However, for most purposes it is shorter than that of insulin glargine, requiring twice daily injections in T1DM. Its efficacy is similar to that of NPH insulin (Table 63.2).
6. **Insulin degludec:** This insulin when injected SC forms soluble multihexamers locally, from which monomers slowly separate and get absorbed. It provides a stable and flat pharmacokinetic profile like glargine. However, it has a longer duration of action (more than 40 h; **ultra-long action**) so that **it can be given as three times a week** with weekend-off dosing regimen. It is usually given in the evening (not earlier than 1 h before last main meal).

Fig. 63.3 shows the time-action curves of various insulins.

Inhaled insulin: This new formulation, **'Afrezza'** when inhaled as dry powder is absorbed faster than injection of insulin lispro. It has a shorter duration of action but the dosing range is limited. It is moderately effective in reducing HbA1c. Commonly it causes cough and hypoglycaemia. Its long-term use is

Table 63.2 Properties of and Comparison among Available Insulins

	Short Acting	Ultra Short Acting	Intermediate Acting	Long Acting
	Regular Insulin	**VRA Analogues: Lispro, Aspart and Glulisine (Gl)**	**NPH and Analogue Mixtures**	**Glargine G) Detemir (D)**
Physical properties	Clear and neutral	Clear and neutral	Turbid and neutral	Clear G-acidic D-neutral
Route of Administration, timing	SC.; IM; IV ½ h AC	SC; IM; IV 0–5 min AC	SC Bed time or before breakfast & dinner	SC G-24 hourly D-12 hourly
Can be mixed with	NPH	NPH	Regular, Lispro, and Aspart	None
Premixed prep.	Regular+NPH	Lispro + Lispro protamine Aspart + Aspart protamine	Regular+NPH	None
Onset of action	30–60 minutes	5–15 min	2–4 h	2–4 h
Peak action	2–3 h	30–90 min;	4–10 h	No peak
Duration of action	8–10 h	Gl 1.5–5 h Others 2–6 h	18–24	G- ≈ 24 h D- ≈ 12 h
Hypoglycemia	Late during action	Early during action	4–10 h	Uncommon
Weight gain	Yes	Yes	Yes	Uncommon
Use during pregnancy	Yes	Lispro and aspart may be used	Yes	No

Control of HbA1c is similar with insulins and insulin analogues. Insulins are expensive; analogues are more expensive.
AC, ante cibum (before meal); NPH, Neutral Protamine Hagedorn

reported to decrease FEV1 and cause pulmonary symptoms. It needs further evaluation. Need for pulmonary function tests and uncertainties about the long-term safety has limited its use.

Delivery of insulin formulations:

Insulin preparations are available in vials or as prefilled single-use disposable pens or as insulin pens with replaceable cartridges. A needle-free system (Jet injection) for SC delivery of insulin is also available.

Route and time of administration of various formulations are depicted in Table 63.2.

i. **Regular insulin and short-acting analogues are injected:**
   a. SC premeal (½ h in the case of regular insulin, and immediately premeal in the case of analogues)
   b. SC for multiple, daily injections (Intensive Insulin Therapy)
   c. SC or (preferably) by IV infusion (Regular insulin, lispro, aspart and glulisine) in diabetic emergencies (see section on management of emergencies in the diabetic)
   d. SC by insulin pump (Regular insulin, lispro, aspart)

ii. **Intermediate acting insulin (NPH)** is used:
   a. Alone before dinner
   b. Together with day-time OHA, at bedtime (BIDS)
   c. It can also be mixed in the same syringe with regular insulin, lispro, aspart, glulisine for SC injection before breakfast and dinner (split-mixed therapy)
   d. Commercial pre-mixed preparations (Regular 1 NPH, i.e. Mixtard, lispro-protamine Mix and aspart-protamine Mix) can be used in a similar way as (c)

iii. **Long-acting preparations (Glargine** and **detemir)** are used SC either

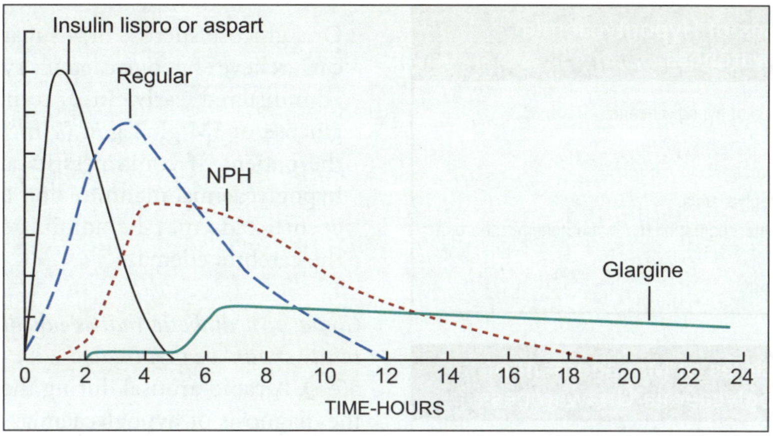

FIG. 63.3 Extent and duration of action of various types of insulin.

a. Once a day, but at the same time of the day (every 24 h); or
b. Every 12 h

Glargine and Detemir cannot be mixed with any other available insulin in the same syringe.

Adverse reactions:

- **Hypoglycaemia:** Hypoglycaemia is a common adverse effect of insulin. **It is less frequent with rapid and long-acting analogs than with regular insulin and NPH, respectively.** The common causes of hypoglycaemia are:
  a. Too large a dose
  b. Failure to eat
  c. Vigorous physical exercise
  d. Ingestion of alcohol

It is more common during 'intensive insulin regimens', in T1DM, aged diabetics and in diabetics with nephropathy. Box 63.2 gives the important symptoms of hypoglycaemia.

Prior ingestion of a non-selective β-blocker like propranolol can delay the recovery from hypoglycaemia (**hypoglycaemia unresponsiveness**). *Selective β1-blocking agents like atenolol or metoprolol are less liable to do so.*

Box 63.2 Symptoms of Hypoglycaemia

- ***Sympathetic*** (Adrenergic) due to adrenaline liberation: hunger, anxiety, cold limbs due to vasoconstriction, tachycardia, palpitation, tremulousness, pallor, sweating, piloerection and subjective feeling of impending disaster. The body temperature tends to be lowered in hypoglycaemic coma and this is of diagnostic importance.
- ***Cerebral*** (Neuroglycopenia) due to the brain being starved of glucose: confusion, bizarre behaviour, depression, coma, convulsions and focal lesions such as hemiplegia or visual disturbances. Cerebral oedema or organic damage may cause these symptoms to persist after correction of the low blood sugar level.
- ***Non-specific:*** Nausea, headache.

Repeated episodes of hypoglycaemia in patients with T1DM of long duration reduce the autonomic response to subsequent episodes because the threshold for activation of such response gets set to a lower level of glucose. Thus, the patient fails to recognise the symptoms of hypoglycaemia (**hypoglycaemia unawareness**). Box 63.3 lists differences in hypoglycaemic episodes that can be seen after short and intermediate acting insulin preparations and Box 63.4 outlines its management.

Hypoglycaemia must be prevented because:

a. *An unrecognised attack during night is followed by rebound hyperglycaemia with glycosuria next morning* (**Somogyi effect**): This is likely to lead to an increase in the dose of insulin with repetition of hypoglycaemia.

Box 63.3 Causes of Hypoglycaemia Unawareness

- Ignorance of symptoms of hypoglycaemia.
- T1DM
- Long duration of diabetes.
- Repeated severe hypoglycaemia.
- Impaired glucose counter-regulation (but not autonomic neuropathy)
- Strict glycaemic control

Box 63.4 Principles of Management of Hypoglycaemia Unawareness

Prevention:

- Educating the patient about symptoms of hypoglycaemia
- Strict avoidance of hypoglycaemia (blood glucose less than 70 mg/dL in this context) as even moderate hypoglycaemia causes transient impairment of glucose counter-regulation for as long as 24 h
- Between-meals and bedtime snacks
- Reduction in insulin dose before vigorous exercise
- Avoidance of glycated haemoglobin concentrations in the non-diabetic range
- Night-time insulin dose reduction after vigorous exercise
- Regular blood glucose monitoring

Treatment:

- Hospitalisation
- Blood glucose monitoring especially at 3 am, as hypoglycaemia at that hour often goes unrecognised
- At least three weeks of scrupulous avoidance of hypoglycaemia can restore hypoglycaemia awareness

b. *Hypoglycaemia can be followed by hypoglycaemia unawareness*
c. *Hypoglycaemia is harmful in patients with cardiovascular disease.* It can lead to the dead-in-bed syndrome via its pro-arrhythmogenic and pro-thrombotic effects, secondary to sympathoadrenal activation.
d. *Frequent attacks in childhood may cause permanent neurological damage*

Patients on insulin therapy should be explained the symptoms of hypoglycaemia. They should be warned about the dangers of missed meals, unplanned vigorous exercise and alcohol. They should carry sugar with them at all times and swallow it at the first symptom of hypoglycaemia. Finally, a patient started on insulin therapy should be forbidden to swim, to work near machines and to drive till the dose is stabilised.

Oral glucose/sucrose or, a sugar-containing food, can relieve hypoglycaemic symptoms if it is administered early. In a comatose patient, IV glucose or IM glucagon (1 mg) rapidly awakens the patient. If coma persists after correction of hypoglycaemia, mannitol and large doses of glucocorticoids may be administered IV to relieve the cerebral edema.

Coma in a diabetic that is not diagnosable with certainty should be first treated with IV glucose (50 mL of 50%). A rapid arousal during the injection confirms the diagnosis of hypoglycaemia.

- **Allergy:** Allergy to insulin is IgE-mediated. It may consist of local itching, redness, swelling and pain. Generalised urticaria is uncommon. Anaphylactic reactions are rare.
- **Lipodystrophy:** This occurs at the site of injection and is of two types:
  1. **Lipohypertrophy** presents as a spongy lump and is due to the lipogenic property of insulin injected repeatedly into the same area. It is advisable to rotate the site.
  2. **Lipoatrophy,** in which there is a loss of fat tissue, is probably of immunological origin. The treatment consists of injection of human insulin at the borders of the lipoatrophic area.
- **Obesity:** Insulin therapy without dietary restriction and exercise may increase the body weight (2–4 kg). This increases the insulin requirement.
- **Presbyopia:** When hyperglycaemia is rapidly controlled with insulin, the patient develops loss of visual accommodation due to alterations in the physical properties of the lens. It is reversible.
- **Neuropathy:** In an occasional patient, rapid control of hyperglycaemia with insulin either precipitates peripheral neuropathy or worsens a pre-existing on
- **Edema** may be seen in some patients on initiating insulin therapy. It can precipitate heart failure if used concomitantly with glitazones.

Indications:

- **Idiopathic diabetes mellitus:** discussed later in detail
- **Secondary diabetes mellitus:** Diabetes due to pancreatic diseases such as pancreatitis
- **Glucose–insulin IV drip** is used to treat hyperkalaemia

- **Glucose–insulin–potassium (GIP)** drip has been used to treat patients with MI complicated by arrhythmias due to **hypokalaemia**. The drip drives potassium into the cells.

PH 1.36, IM 11.16

NON-INSULIN ANTIDIABETIC DRUGS

The antidiabetic agents other than insulin can be classified according to their predominant mechanism of action (Fig. 63.4): and route of administration.

Classification of Non-Insulin Antidiabetic Drugs

A. **Oral:**
   I. **Inhibitors of hepatic gluconeogenesis, (AMPK activators),** e.g. Biguanides. (Metformin)
   II. **Stimulators of insulin release by beta cells (K^+_{ATP} channel modulators),** e.g. Sulphonylureas, Meglitinides
   III. **Inhibitors of intestinal α-glucosidases, (α-glucosidases inhibitors),** e.g. Acarbose, Miglitol
   IV. **Drugs which reduce insulin resistance, (PPAR activators),** e.g. Glitazones
   V. **Inhibitors of dipeptidyl dipeptidase-4 (DPP-4),** e.g. Sitagliptin, Linagliptin

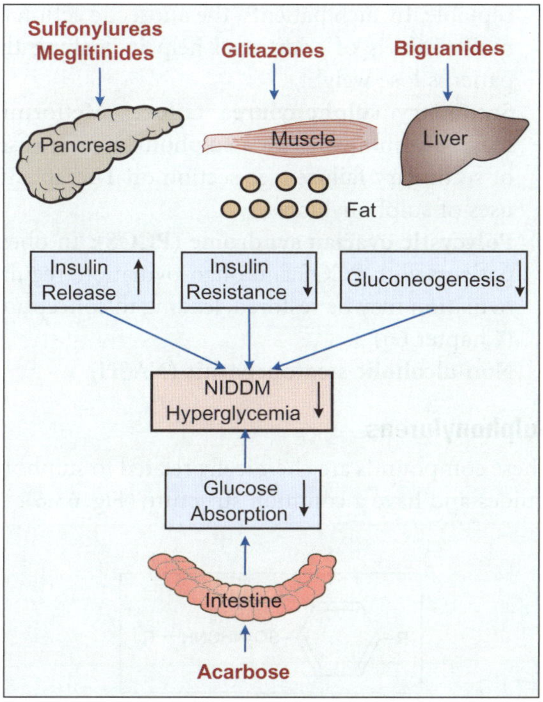

FIG. 63.4 Mechanism of action of oral antidiabetic drugs. (Ref. Classification)

   VI. **Inhibitors of SGLT2,** e.g. Dapagliflozin, Canagliflozin
   VII. **Others with novel mechanisms,** e.g. Bromocriptine, Hydroxychloroquine

B. **Parenteral:**
   I. **Amylinomimetics,** e.g. Pramlintide
   II. **GLP-1 agonists,** e.g. Exenatide, Liraglutide
   III. **GIP + GLP- 1 agonist:** Tirzepatide
   IV. **CD3-directed monoclonal antibody:** Teplizumab

An ideal non-insulin antidiabetic drug should:

a. Effectively correct the metabolic defects in a diabetic patient as insulin does
b. Be nontoxic
c. Be effective orally as a convenient route of drug administration

Although the drugs available at present do not meet all these requirements fully, they are very useful for controlling T2DM.

ORAL ANTIDIABETIC AGENTS

Biguanides

The general chemical structure of biguanides is shown in Fig. 63.5. A free guanidine radical is thought to be essential for the hypoglycaemic effect of biguanides.

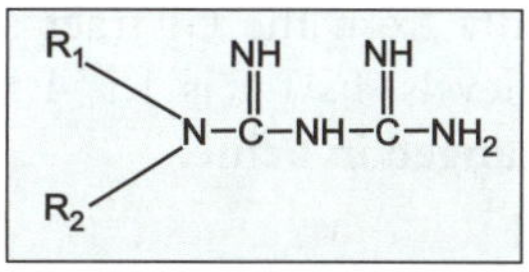

FIG. 63.5 General Structure of Biguanides.

METFORMIN: It is the biguanide currently used.

Mechanism of action: Presence of either exogenous or endogenous insulin is necessary for its action. Several mechanisms may be involved in the antidiabetic effect of metformin. It:

- **Inhibits hepatic gluconeogenesis and decreases hepatic and renal glucose output.** This is considered as its major action, which is mediated through the activation of the enzyme adenosine monophosphate-activated protein kinase (AMPK).
- **Increases the peripheral glucose utilisation** by enhancing anaerobic glycolysis, and increases the activity of glucose transporters (GLUT-4)

- **Delays glucose absorption**
- **Acts as insulin sensitiser in the muscle and adipose tissue, and reduces hyper-insulinaemia.** This action plays a relatively minor role.
- **Reduces the appetite,** which may be helpful in obese subjects. This is mediated through GLP1.

Pharmacological effects: *Metformin does not lower the blood sugar in normal subjects.*

- By itself, it does not produce hypoglycaemia in diabetics. However, it potentiates the hypoglycaemic effects of insulin, sulphonylureas, and other oral antidiabetic drugs.
- It reduces plasma total and LDL cholesterol and triglyceride levels. Lipolysis, FFA production and lipid oxidation are reduced. These effects reduce the risk of CVD.
- Weight loss is due to reduction in appetite. *Its main benefit is prevention of weight gain in contrast to sulphonylureas.*
- *It does not inhibit ketogenesis in the liver. Hence, diabetics on metformin may develop ketoacidosis with minimum hyperglycaemia and glycosuria.* Further, metformin decreases the glycogen content of the liver.

Metformin effect decreases when diabetes progresses due to beta cell failure.

Absorption, fate and excretion: Metformin is absorbed rapidly from the GI tract and gives adequate plasma levels. Its t½ is 1.5–4 h. **It is largely excreted unchanged in urine.**

Adverse reactions: Metformin is generally well tolerated.

- It produces bitter or metallic taste, anorexia, nausea, and abdominal discomfort. This can be minimised by starting with a small dose and giving it with, rather than before, meals and by using extended release preparations.
- It may produce lethargy and muscular weakness.
- **Lactic acidosis,** though reported rarely during metformin therapy, could be lethal during an acute illness such as a severe infection. **Before prescribing metformin to an elderly patient, serum creatinine should be measured to assess the renal function.** Patients undergoing a radiocontrast study (CT scan or coronary angiography) should be advised to omit metformin one day before and for 48 h after the procedure. **Metformin is considered safe in mild chronic kidney disease (CKD).** Its use is contraindicated in patients with liver disease, CKD (eGFR < 30 mL/min/1.73 m^2), COPD, HF and chronic alcoholism.
- The drug may *produce vitamin B_{12} and folic acid deficiency during long-term use,* especially in elderly.
- Severe allergic reactions are rare.

Preparations and dosage:

i. Metformin 500, 850 and 1000 mg. tablets. It is generally started in the dose of 250 mg 2–3 times a day with major meals, and the dose increased gradually up to 2000 mg per day. *Several FDCs of metformin with other oral antidiabetic drugs are available.*

ii. Metformin SR 500, 750 and 1000 mg tablet once a day

Indications:

- **Obese patients with T2DM,** who could be controlled with diet alone but find this therapy unacceptable. In such patients, the anorectic action of metformin is of additional help in making the patients lose weight.
- **Secondary sulphonylurea failure:** Metformin may be combined with a sulphonylurea in cases of secondary failure (see section on Therapeutic uses of sulphonylureas)
- **Polycystic ovarian syndrome (PCOS):** In obese patients with PCOS and oligo-ovulation, regular ovulation may be restored, leading to conception (Chapter 66)
- **Non-alcoholic steatohepatitis (NASH)**

Sulphonylureas

These compounds are chemically related to sulphonamides and have a common structure (Fig. 63.6).

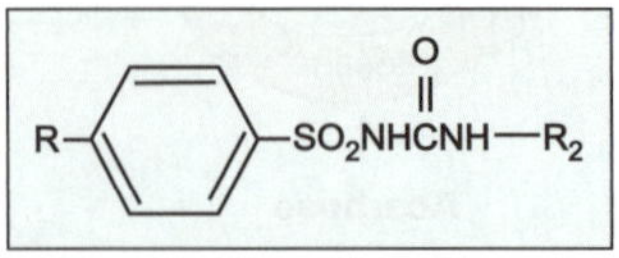

FIG. 63.6 General structure of sulphonylureas.

Mechanism of action:

- **Pancreatic beta cells:** They act on **sulphonylurea receptors (SUR)** linked to the ATP-sensitive K^+ channels (K_{ATP}) in the cell membrane of the islet beta cells. Activation of these receptors **closes the K_{ATP} channels and depolarises the cell membrane.** This results in a calcium influx into the cell, with **release of stored insulin.** *They are effective only in the presence of a functioning pancreas.*

Sulphonylureas release insulin slowly and for prolonged periods into the portal circulation; **its primary action is on the liver.**

- **Liver, muscle and adipose tissue:** They probably increase the sensitivity of liver, muscle and adipose tissue to insulin. The hepatic output of glucose is decreased while muscle uptake is increased. The hepatic glycogen stores are increased.

The basic action of all the sulphonylureas is identical. They differ in their pharmacokinetic properties. Their plasma t½ bear little relationship to the duration of their hypoglycaemic effect.

Pharmacological effects: These drugs:

- Lower the blood sugar in non-diabetics and selected diabetics
- Lower the elevated FFA levels even before they lower the blood sugar
- Normalise the metabolic state of the diabetic
- Promote weight gain

The beneficial effects of sulphonylureas on the serum lipids and lipoproteins are due to improved control of diabetes. They have not shown any beneficial effect on CV or renal outcome.

Compared to the first generation, the second generation agents (e.g. glibenclamide, gliclazide, glipizide, glimepiride) more potent, have early onset of effect, shorter t½ and lower risk of hypoglycaemia (Table 63.3). Hence, they are preferred.

Absorption, fate and excretion: Sulphonylureas are rapidly absorbed from the GI tract when *taken on empty stomach. Food reduces their absorption*. They are all extensively (>90%) protein bound and are mainly metabolised in the liver. Hence, **they are contraindicated in hepatic impairment.**

Adverse reactions: In general, their toxicity is remarkably low. The important adverse reactions are:

- **Weight gain:** There is a moderate weight gain of 2 kg in the 1st year of treatment.
- **Hypoglycaemia** can be precipitated by an excessive dose, decreased food intake, vomiting or by associated liver/kidney disease. Drugs like oral anticoagulants and salicylates, potentiate their hypoglycaemic effect by displacing them from protein binding. MAO inhibitors and propranolol produce a state of **hypoglycaemia unresponsiveness**. Alcohol also can produce dangerous hypoglycaemia.
- **Allergic reactions:** Sulphonylureas which are closely related to sulphonamides sometimes give rise to allergic skin rashes.
- **Liver:** Chlorpropamide can rarely cause cholestatic jaundice.
- **CVS:** These drugs act on SUR present on cardiac tissue and block ischaemic preconditioning via K^+ channel closure resulting in arrhythmia. This is seen mainly with glyburide.

Drug interactions: They sometimes potentiate and prolong the CNS effects of barbiturates and other sedative-hypnotics. Chlorpropamide, by potentiating the action of circulating ADH on the renal tubules, causes water retention and hyponatraemia.

Preparations and dosage: Table 63.3.

Indications:

- **T2DM:** Sulphonylureas are useful in treating patients with T2DM, who cannot be controlled by diet and exercise alone. Patients most eligible for sulphonylurea therapy have the profile shown in Box 63.5. About 70% show satisfactory response whereas the remaining are termed as **primary failures**.

Usually, it takes 1–2 weeks to achieve the maximum effect of a given dose; hence, the dose should not be increased more often than once in 1–2 weeks. In patients older than 60, with declining renal function, who are also liable to be forgetful about eating, a

Table 63.3 Commonly Used Sulfonylurea Compounds[a]

	Tolbutamide	Chlorpropamide	Glipizide[b]	Glibenclamide (Glyburide)	Gliclazide	Glimepiride[c]
Tablets	0.5 g	0.1 and 0.25 g	5 mg	2.5 and 5 mg	40 and 80 mg	1, 2, 3, 4 mg
Plasma half life (h)	4–5	35	4	12	8–12	3–4
Duration of action (h)	6–10	24–72	12–24	12–24	12–24	16–24
Doses per day	2–3	1	1–2	1–2	1–2	1
Relative frequency of severe hypoglycemia	<1	4–6	2–4	10–15	–	<1%
Use in renal impairment	At reduced dose	Contraindicated	At reduced dose	Contraindicated	Can be given safely in moderate-severe renal impairment	At reduced dose
Daily dose (mg/day)						
Average	1500	25	5	5	80	2
Max.	2000	50	20	20	320	8

[a]Sulphonylureas are best taken 15–30 min before meals; food may interfere with their absorption.
[b]Also available as a sustained release preparation. The tablets are swallowed intact.
[c]Rapid onset of action.

short-acting sulphonylurea like glipizide is preferred.

Of the patients who are initially well controlled with sulphonylureas, 5%–10% escape from control every year (**secondary failure**). The causes of secondary failure are dietary excess, intercurrent disease, inadequate dose, poor compliance and progressive deterioration of pancreatic function. This can be partly treated by:

Box 63.5 Profile of Sulphonylureas-Responsive Patients

- Over 40 years of age and obese (or at least not underweight) at the time of diagnosis
- Diabetes of recent onset
- No significant ketonuria
- Fasting blood sugar is less than 300 mg/dL
- If on insulin, the daily requirement is less than 40 units
- No acute complication likely to lead to ketoacidosis
- No serious cardiac, kidneys or liver disease
- Not candidates for surgery

- Improving compliance
- Changing over to another sulphonylurea
- Addition of metformin (if not given earlier), or glitazone; or addition of/change over to insulin

If a patient with T2DM, well controlled by less than 20 units of insulin, wishes to change over to oral therapy, insulin can be stopped abruptly and a sulphonylurea introduced. However, if the insulin requirement is between 20 and 40 units daily, the dose of insulin is progressively reduced while that of a sulphonylurea is progressively increased, till the latter completely takes over. *Such change over from insulin to oral drugs, if done repeatedly, can lead to the development of antibodies to insulin and insulin resistance because of intermittent insulin therapy.*

- ***Diabetes insipidus:*** Chlorpropamide has been used in diabetes insipidus (Chapter 37)

Limitations of sulphonylureas: Box 63.6.

Box 63.6 Limitations of Sulphonylureas

Sulphonylureas are ineffective in:
- IDDM
- Very long standing T2DM
- Diabetic coma
- Diabetes due to pancreatectomy or destruction of pancreas by disease
- Surgical diabetics
- The presence of infection and/or heavy ketonuria
- Further, they cannot be used in pregnant women and in patients with severe liver or kidney disease

Choice of the sulphonylurea preparation: Glipizide or **glimepiride** appears to be cost effective and relatively safe. **Glibenclamide** can cause a higher incidence of hypoglycaemia and therefore, is used in divided doses when dose requirement is more than 5 mg/day. *If good glycaemic control is not achieved with maximum doses of sulphonylureas, one should use combination oral drug therapy or change to insulin.*

Meglitinides (Glinides)

These drugs, chemically unrelated to sulphonylureas, have the same mechanism of action. They bind to a site adjacent to SUR but the binding is weaker and dissociation is faster, thus making them **short-acting insulin secretogogues.** But they are less effective than sulphonylureas. *Hence, patients on maximum dose of a sulphonylurea do not benefit if meglitinides are added.* They also cause hypoglycaemia. No beneficial effect has been seen on CV or renal outcome. They can be used in patients with decreased renal function.

REPAGLINIDE: It has a rapid onset and a short duration of action (t½ 1 h). It controls postprandial hyperglycaemia effectively. Because of its short duration of action, it is less likely than sulphonylureas to cause hypoglycaemic attacks. It is cleared primarily by the liver. It must be taken any time 30 min before each major meal to just at the start of a meal in the dose of 0.5–4.0 mg.

NATEGLINIDE is unrelated chemically to repaglinide. Its onset of action and duration of action (2–3 h) are shorter.

Alfa Glucosidase Inhibitors

Alpha glucosidases are the enzymes in the brush border of the jejunal enterocytes. They covert oligosaccharides derived from ingested polysaccharides into **monosaccharides** (glucose, fructose and galactose) which are promptly absorbed in the upper jejunum.

ACARBOSE is an oligosaccharide of microbial origin.

Mechanism of action: It binds competitively to carbohydrate binding sites of alpha glucosidases **and thus prevents the absorption of carbohydrates.** *It does not affect glucose absorption because it does not interact with the intestinal sodium dependent glucose transporter.*

Pharmacological actions: Given orally, acarbose *reduces postprandial hyperglycaemia*.

It is administered in the dose of 25–50 mg, chewed and swallowed during each meal. At least 3 doses are required per day. As acarbose interferes with the digestion of sucrose, *patients receiving insulin or a sulphonylureas as well as acarbose should carry* **glucose not sucrose.**

Adverse reactions: These include flatulence abdominal discomfort and loose stools due to undigested carbohydrates. Occasionally, liver enzymes may be elevated.

Indications: The drug is useful in patients on high carbohydrate diet and is generally used in combination with other drugs. However, low efficacy, frequent dosing and GI ADR limit its use.

Miglitol and **Voglibose** have similar actions.

Alph glucosidase inhibitors are contraindicated in patients with chronic intestinal disease, including IBD and intestinal obstruction.

Thiazolidinediones (Glitazones)

PIOGLITAZONE

Mechanism of action: It is a **potent agonist of the**

nuclear receptors Peroxisome Proliferator-Activated Receptors gamma (PPARγ), abundantly present in the adipose tissue and also present in the liver, heart and skeletal muscle. It modulates gene expression involved in glucose and lipid metabolism, insulin signal transduction, and adipocyte differentiation and proliferation. **Thus, pioglitazone reduces peripheral insulin resistance.**

Since its action is via genetic regulation, its maximum effect is seen after weeks or months. It synergises with sulphonylureas and metformin, as well as insulin in their antidiabetic effects.

Pharmacological effects: Pioglitazone:

- **Reduces peripheral resistance to insulin and increases the insulin sensitivity of the adipose tissue, liver and muscle (insulin sensitisers).** Thus, it counters hyperinsulinaemia and protects the body from *the damaging effects of chronic endogenous hyperinsulinaemia.*
- **Reduces the production of the pro-inflammatory cytokines by the visceral adipocytes and increase the adipose tissue production of adiponectin.** This further increases the insulin sensitivity of other insulin responsive tissues such as liver and muscle.
- **Increases the subcutaneous, small-adipocyte mass,** and diverts the triglyceride storage from the visceral adipocytes to the subcutaneous adipose tissue
- **Lowers the hepatic fat content** and ameliorates dyslipidaemia
- **Lowers the hepatic glucose production and increases glucose uptake by skeletal muscle.** *It does not cause hypoglycaemia.*
- **Preserves and enhances beta cell and vascular function** by reducing FFA and cytokine induced islet cell damage

Overall, it enhances insulin action (directly) and beta cell function (indirectly). It is classified as **insulin sensitiser**, and, by definition, requires the presence of endogenous insulin. *Hence, it can be used only in T2DM but not in T1DM.*

Absorption, fate and excretion: Pioglitazone is generally prescribed once daily. It is completely absorbed and is metabolised extensively by the liver. The metabolites of pioglitazone are active and are excreted in the bile.

Adverse reactions: These are:

- **Liver:** It can cause elevation of hepatic enzymes, which mandates periodic monitoring. **Fatal hepatotoxicity** was reported with earlier glitazone, troglitazone. Pioglitazone **induces hepatic drug metabolising enzymes** and can decrease the effectiveness of the drugs which are substrates of these enzymes, e.g. oral contraceptives.
- **Weight gain:** It causes weight gain (2–4 kg) in dose-dependent and time-dependent manner. The weight gain occurs due to proliferation of new adipocytes and redistribution of fat stores, increased appetite and fluid retention.
- **Fluid retention/HF:** It is more common with concomitant insulin therapy. Fluid retention may precipitate or worsen HF. In addition, macular oedema can occur and hence periodic eye examination is necessary.
- **Cardiovascular toxicity:** Cardiovascular safety is questionable. A meta-analysis has concluded that rosiglitazone (now withdrawn) was associated with a significant increase in the risk of death from myocardial infarction and stroke.
- **Miscellaneous:** It may cause unpleasant hunger sensation. It can decrease the BMD and increase risk of fractures.

  Retarded fetal development has been noted in animals; hence, it is not recommended during pregnancy.

Preparation and dosage:

i. Pioglitazone: 15–45 mg/day as a single or twice daily dose

Indications:

- **T2DM:** *As monotherapy, it is generally less effective than sulphonylurea or metformin.* Its use should be restricted to replacement for metformin or sulphonylurea in patients who for some reason cannot take these drugs. It may be used in combination with other oral antidiabetic drugs.

- **Other insulin resistant states** such as polycystic ovary syndrome
- **Non-alcoholic steatohepatitis** (NASH)

Recently, **Lobeglitazone** is introduced in India which is potent than pioglitazone, has favourable safety profile and demonstrated pleiotrophic effects in animal studies.

Incretinomimetics: Intestinal L-cells derived **GLP-1** and **GIP** (See section on Factors determining insulin release; gut hormones):

- Stimulate pancreatic beta cells and potentiate glucose-dependent insulin secretion
- Suppress glucose dependent inappropriate post-prandial hyperglucagonaemia
- Slow gastric emptying
- Promote satiety and cause weight loss

GLP-1 is degraded by the enzyme dipeptidyl peptidase-4 (DPP-4) and has a very short t½ of 2–5 min. Hence, drugs are now available as:

1. **GLP-1 agonists** (See later section on GLP-1 agonists) or
2. **DPP-4 inhibitors,** which increase the endogenous GLP-1

Fig 63.7 illustrates pharmacological effects of these agents.

DPP-4 Inhibitors

Sitagliptin, saxagliptin, vildagliptin, linagliptin, alogliptin and **teneligliptin:**

- Cause >80% inhibition of DPP-4 enzyme and thus prolong the t½ of endogenous GLP-1 and GIP thereby increasing insulin levels
- **If used alone are less effective than the established oral antidiabetic drugs.** They have not shown any beneficial effect on the risk of major adverse cardiovascular event, HF or CKD progression.
- Are used in combination with an oral antidiabetic drug (metformin, a sulphonylurea or a glitazone)

Absorption, fate and excretion: They are administered orally and get primarily excreted in the urine. *Hence, dose adjustment is necessary in the presence of kidney damage.* Linagliptin is eliminated by

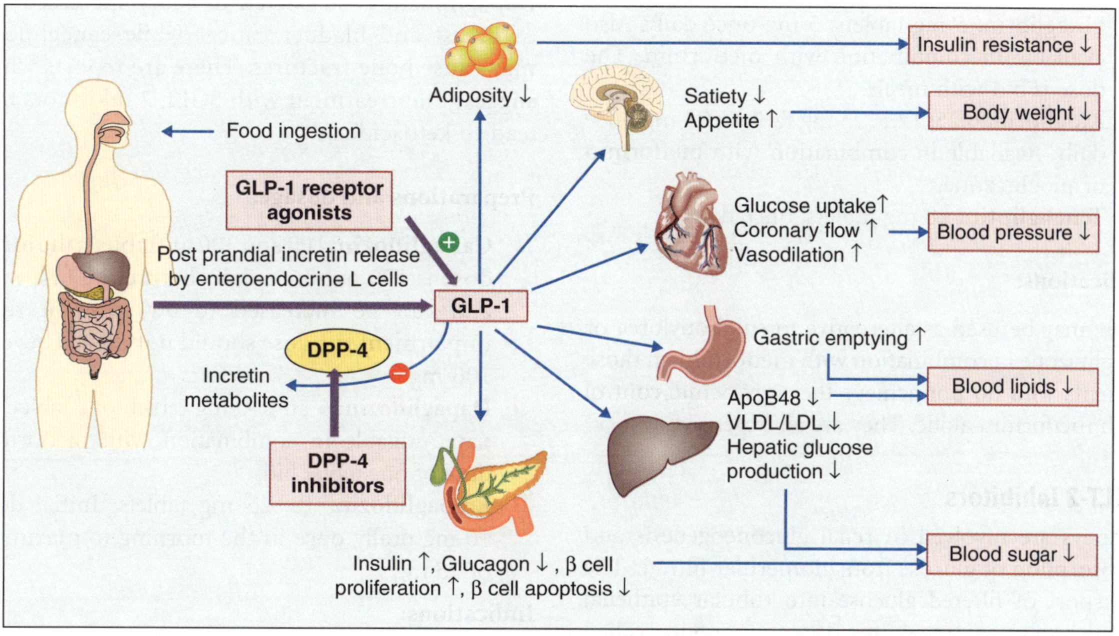

FIG. 63.7 Pharmacological Effects of GLP1-Receptor Agonists and DPP-4 Inhibitors

non-renal mechanisms and hence given safely in renal impairment.

Adverse reactions: Apart from mild GI upset, headache and nasopharyngitis, they sometimes cause severe hypersensitivity reactions including angioedema, anaphylaxis, exfoliative dermatitis, pancreatitis and hepatotoxicity. Severe joint pains can occur. Saxagliptin and alogliptin increase the risk of heart failure in those with heart or kidney disorder. Teneligliptin has a potential of QT prolongation. DPP-4 is involved in the regulation of immune functions and degradation of cytokines, hormones, neuropeptides and growth factors. *Hence, its inhibition may cause increased attacks of infections. Their long-term safety is not known.*

Preparations and dosage:

i. **Sitagliptin:** 25, 50, 100 mg tablets; 100 mg once daily. Dose is 25 mg if GFR < 30 mL/min. Available in combination with metformin. The dose is bid with meals.
ii. **Saxagliptin:** 2.5, 5 mg tablets; 2.5–5 mg once daily. The dose is 2.5 mg if GFR < 50 mL/min or patient is taking concomitant CYP3A4 inhibitors. Available in combination with metformin.
iii. **Linagliptin:** 5 mg tablets; 5 mg once daily. Also available in combination with metformin. The dose is bid with meals.
iv. **Alogliptin:** 6.25, 12.5, 25 mg tablets; 25 mg once daily. Available in combination with metformin or pioglitazone.
v. **Teneligliptin:** 20 mg tablets, once daily

Indications:

They may be used as alternative to sulphonylurea or pioglitazone in combination with metformin, in those patients who do not achieve their glycaemic control with metformin alone. They are all expensive.

SGLT-2 Inhibitors

Kidneys are involved in renal gluconeogenesis and reabsorption of glucose from glomerular filtrate. The transport of filtered glucose into tubular epithelial cells involve a renal membrane protein called '**Sodium-glucose co-transporter 2 (SGLT-2).**' It is a glucose transporter in the proximal tubule responsible for 90% of glucose reabsorption. In T2DM there is an overexpression of SGLT-2 leading to hyperglycaemia. **SGLT-2 inhibition reduces renal reabsorption of glucose by 30%–40% and increases its urinary excretion,** thus lowering the fasting and postpradial blood glucose without any action on metabolic dysfunction.

The currently available SGLT-2 inhibitors are **canagliflozin, dapagliflozin** and **empagliflozin.** They are given orally. They reduce blood glucose, body weight and HbA1c. They have shown to reduce major adverse cardiovascular events, hospitalization due to HF and progression to CKD. *They are usually combined with metformin.* The frequency of hypoglycaemia is claimed to be less.

Sotagliflozin is an inhibitor of SGLT-1 and SGLT-2. Inhibition of SGLT-1 present in the intestine reduces glucose absorption. This results in reduction and delay of post-prandial hyperglycaemia.

Adverse reactions: These include osmotic diuresis, increased genitourinary tract infections (including pyelonephritis), acute kidney injury, hyperkalaemia, hyperphosphataemia and hypermagnesaemia. Dapagliflozin is suspected to cause increased risk of breast and bladder cancer while canagliflozin may cause bone fractures. There are reports which suggest that treatment with SGLT-2 inhibitors may lead to ketoacidosis.

Preparations and dosage:

i. **Canagliflozin:** 100 and 300 mg tablets; the initial dose is 100 mg once daily before the first meal and can be increased to 300 mg. In renal impairment the dose should not exceed beyond 100 mg.
ii. **Dapagliflozin:** 5 and 10 mg tablet; one tablet per day. Available in combination with metformin; dose of one tablet bid.
iii. **Empagliflozin:** 10, 25 mg tablets; Initial dose: 10 mg orally once in the morning to maximum of 25 mg.

Indications:

- **T2DM:** They can be combined with any class of

drugs as their action is insulin independent and can be given at any stage of T2DM to improve glycaemic control. They can be used as monotherapy.

Bromocriptine

Bromocriptine mesylate, as quick released formulation, is US-FDA approved antidiabetic drug. It is not interchangeable with other bromocriptine products. It is a D_2 receptor agonist (Chapters 15, 61 and 65).

Mechanism of action: It acts on the hypothalamic D_2 receptors and alters circadian neuronal activities in the hypothalamus, which inhibits excessive sympathetic tone and serotonergic activity within CNS. This results in suppression of hepatic glucose output and therefore reduce plasma glucose, FFA and TG. It reduces HbA1c levels by 0.3-0.5 %.

The dose is 0.8 mg to be taken within two hours after waking in the morning (circadian-timed). It can be increased gradually weekly to maximum of 4.8 mg but pill burden is a concern. It is given with breakfast to minimize the GI adverse effects. The most common ADRs include transient mild to moderate nausea, headache and dizziness. At this dose hypoglycemia or weight gain are not observed.

It can be given alone but mainly used as an adjuvant drug in obese T2DM patients who are insulin resistant. Compared to other antidiabetic agents, it is less efficacious and long-term safety is not known. It is expensive.

Hydroxychloroquine

In T2DM increased release of mediators *viz.* TNF α, IL-1β, IL-6 etc. occurs from immune cells and adipocytes. The resultant chronic low grade inflammation contributes to insulin resistance. Hydroxychloroquine, an antimalarial drug (Chapter 54) has both, anti-inflammatory and immunomodulatory effects and hence it is already in use for the therapy of RA (Chapter73) and SLE. In T2DM patients who are uncontrolled on oral antidiabetic drugs or insulin, 400mg daily dose of hydroxychloroquine has been found to reduce HbA1c, improve glycemic control and decrease insulin requirement. It is well tolerated and may cause mild-moderate gastritis, constipation, and diarrhea.

PARENTERAL NON-INSULIN ANTIDIABETIC AGENTS

Amylinomimetics

The polypeptide, amylin, is co-secreted with insulin and is markedly reduced in diabetics. It controls postprandial hyperglycaemia by:

a. Suppressing endogenous glucagon production, especially postprandially
b. Slowing the gastric emptying rate
c. Inducing centrally mediated satiety, by opposing the action of ghrelin

Pramlintide, a synthetic amylin analogue, has been **used as an adjunct** in treating T1DM and T2DM patients in whom the post-prandial hyperglycaemia is difficult to control. It is injected subcutaneously. It is now replaced by the GLP-1 agonists.

GLP-1 Agonists

These long-acting synthetic analogues of GLP-1, bind to GLP-1 receptors in the brain stem, pancreatic islets and GI tract and have 3–4 times more activity than the endogenous GLP-1 (**incretinmimetic**). They:

- Augment glucose dependent insulin secretion
- Suppress postprandial glucagon
- Reduce hepatic glucose production
- Increase satiety, suppress appetite and cause weight loss
- Slow gastric emptying
- Decrease TG and increase HDL-C

By themselves, they do not cause hypoglycaemia. They decrease TG and increase HDL-C. They have shown to reduce the risk of major adverse cardiovascular events and microalbuminuria but not the hospitalization due to HF or progression of CKD. They are contraindicated in renal failure.

EXENATIDE: It lowers the postprandial blood glucose and HbA1c (0.9%) modestly but is not effective in lowering fasting blood glucose. It has t½ of 3.5 h. It is administered 5 mcg SC 60 min before lunch and dinner **as an add on treatment of T2DM with resistant postprandial hyperglycaemia.** Maximum dose is 10 mcg BID which is achieved over a month, if required. Extended release formulations are now available which can be given once a week. Another short-acting GLP1 agonist is **lixisenatide,** which is given once daily.

LIRAGLUTIDE is a longer acting exenatide analogue (t½ 13 h) with similar properties. It is however, useful in lowering fasting blood glucose as it causes suppression of overnight glucagon secretion. Chances of hypoglycaemia are less. Dose: 0.6 mg SC once a day, to be increased to 1.2–1.8 mg.

Other longer acting GLP-1 agonists are **dulaglutide, albiglutide** and **semaglutide** which are **injected subcutaneously once a week**. Longer acting analogues provide continuous GLP 1 receptor stimulation. The difference in efficacy of these agents is modest , semaglutide appears to be the most potent and exenatide and lixisenatide are the weakest. An oral preparation of semaglutide is available. Dose: 3 mg orally OD for 30 days and then 7 mg OD.

A fixed dose injectable combination of long acting insulin analogue and GLP-1 agonists, e.g. **Lixisenatide** with insulin glargine has synergistic effect and offers better compliance.

Tirzepatide is a dual incretinmimetic drug, which is both, GIP and GLP-1 agonist. The reduction in HbA1c is 2-2.5%. It causes significant weight loss (7-13 kg). The ADR are similar to those of GLP-1 agonists. It needs further evaluation.

GLP-1 agonists delay absorption of concomitant drugs and need to be given 1 h before or 3 h after the other medications. They undergo glomerular filtration followed by proteolytic degradation.

Adverse reactions of GLP-1 agonists:

- **GI disturbances:** such as nausea, vomiting and diarrhoea are common (40%–50%) and dose dependent. However, tolerance develops to them. Some of the patients with GI disturbances have been reported to develop acute renal damage. Hence, it is necessary to monitor renal function in patients with GI complaints.
- **Nasopharyngitis**
- **Injection site reactions**
- **Acute pancreatitis** may occur rarely. However no causal relationship to the drug is yet proven.
- **Hypersensitivity reactions**
- **Blunting of glycaemic control** may be observed with exenatide due to development of antibodies.
- **C-cell hyperplasia of thyroid** has been reported in rodents. Hence, they are avoided in patients with present/past or family history of medullary carcinoma of thyroid or multiple endocrine tumours.

Indications: Short-acting GLP-1 agonists are more useful in postprandial hyperglycaemia, while longer acting ones can also be useful in those having fasting hyperglycaemia. They may be used as an add-on drug with metformin or a sulphonylurea; but not with insulin. Liraglutide and semaglutide are used for treating resistant non-diabetic obesity (Chapter 38). They are expensive.

Teplizumab is recently approved to delay the onset of T1DM. In TDM, destruction of pancreatic β cells is mediated through T cells. Teplizumab, a humanized CD3-directed monoclonal antibody, deactivates pancreatic β cell autoreactive T lymphocytes. IV infusion of teplizumab in incremental doses for 14 days is advocated in T1DM patients who are yet to develop full blown T1DM. The ADR include serious infections, lymphopenia and cytokine release syndrome. It needs further evaluation for its efficacy and long term safety.

PHARMACOTHERAPY OF DIABETES MELLITUS

Diabetes mellitus is characterized by impaired ability of the body to produce or respond to insulin leading to elevated glucose levels in the blood. By the time diabetes is diagnosed (FBS > 126 mg/dL), 75% of the beta cells have been destroyed. Hyperglycaemia is its most easily measured laboratory marker and the liability to chronic degenerative disease in almost all body tissues is its hallmark. Untreated diabetes can lead to severe metabolic disturbances that can present as acute life threatening emergencies such as diabetic ketoacidosis and a hyperglycemic hyperosmolar state. Chronic end organ effects of diabetes are manifested as **microvascular and macrovascular complications.** The microvascular complications include retinopathy, nephropathy, and neuropathy. Macrovascular complications result in atherosclerosis and lead to myocardial infarction and stroke.

The etiology of DM is still obscure although it has a strong genetic basis. However, with proper management with diet, exercise and drugs a diabetic can enjoy an almost normal life.

Clinically, DM is classified as:

1. **Type 1 DM (T1DM):** This is **insulin dependent** (IDDM) and the patient's survival depends upon uninterrupted insulin therapy
2. **Type 2 DM (T2DM):** This is **not insulin dependent** (NIDDM) and the patient's survival (except in emergencies) does not depend upon insulin therapy. It has strong genetic predisposition.
3. **Gestational DM (GDM)**: This is diagnosed in the second or third trimester of pregnancy and must be treated with diet with or without insulin
4. **Specific types of DM** which is due to other hormonal disorders/drugs such as pancreatitis, genetic defects and acromegaly, and glucocorticoids; it may often respond to oral antidiabetic agents

T1DM occurs mostly in younger, underweight persons, in whom it often starts during childhood. T1DM accounts for 5-10% of total diabetic cases. The incidence in Asia is 15 in 1,00,000 population. It manifests acutely, commonly following a virus infection. In most (≥90%) patients, the destruction of the pancreatic islets is usually due to autoimmune 'insulitis'. **There is an absolute deficiency of insulin.** T1DM is labile and is often complicated by ketoacidosis.

T2DM, on the other hand, occurs in obese or normal weight adults, is stable and less likely to cause ketoacidosis than T1DM. It also occurs in adolescents and even preadolescents. **It is characterised by insulin resistance and relative insulin deficiency**, specifically loss of post-prandial insulin secretion. In India, 77 million people are estimated to be suffering from T2DM with the numbers increasing rapidly to make India the 'Diabetes' capital.

Other varieties usually lie in between these two extremes.

Symptoms such as polyuria, polydipsia and polyphagia along with a random plasma glucose of 200 mg% make the diagnosis of T2DM. In the absence of symptoms, American Diabetic Association defined criteria listed in Table 63.4 may be used.

In the early stages, T2DM subjects, especially the obese ones, have a relative excess of insulin in their plasma in response to a glucose load. This is due to peripheral insulin resistance.

- **Insulin resistance (IR):** The term insulin resistance indicates inadequate response to a given dose/level of insulin. Obesity is a major antecedent of IR. In obesity, increased intra-adipocyte triglyceride stores, especially in the visceral fat, promote the growth of large, intrinsically insulin-resistant, intra-abdominal adipocytes. The adipocytes release FFA and inflammatory cytokines (IL-1, IL-6 and TNFα) which contribute to IR in the skeletal muscle and the liver. *The current evidence indicates that hepatic insulin resistance is the key event in the pathogenesis of T2DM.*

Table 63.4 ADA Diagnostic Venous Plasma Glucose Values in T2DM

Plasma Venous Glucose (PVG) mg/dL	Fasting	2 h Post Glucose[a]	Random	HbA1c (%)
Normal	Less than 100	Less than 140	–	< 5.7
Impaired fasting glucose (IFG)	100–125	Less than 140	–	≥ 5.7– <6.5
Impaired glucose tolerance (IGT)	Less than 100	140–199	–	≥ 5.7– <6.5
Diabetes mellitus (DM)	126 or more	200 or more	200 or more[b]	≥ 6.5

IFG/IGT may occur independently of each other.
[a]75 g oral glucose load.
[b]Plus symptoms of DM.
ADA, American Diabetic Association.

The concentration of the adipose-specific **adiponectin**, which increases insulin sensitivity, diminishes in T2DM, adding to IR. Adiponectin acts via AMP kinase, an enzyme involved in various metabolic responses such as suppression of hepatic gluconeogenesis, glucose uptake in the exercising skeletal muscles, fatty acid oxidation and inhibition of lipolysis.

The normal pancreatic beta cells respond to IR by secreting more insulin (**hyperinsulinaemia**) and maintaining the plasma glucose at or just above the upper limit of normal. Over a period of time, the beta cells develop insulin secretory defect probably due to progressive elevation of plasma glucose (**glucotoxicity**) and elevated FFA levels (**lipotoxicity**). Failure of beta cells to increase insulin production leads to increased plasma concentration of glucose.

- **Insulin deficiency:** *In genetically predisposed individuals, an insulin secretory defect could be aggravated by obesity, acute illness or simple ageing leading to the onset of T2DM.*

One of the earliest defects in diabetes (before the abnormality of carbohydrate tolerance) is elevated plasma FFA in the overnight fasting state and after exercise. The oxidation of these FFA in the liver to acetyl CoA provides the energy necessary for gluconeogenesis. Acetyl CoA is converted by the liver (but not by other tissues) to ketone bodies (acetoacetate, beta hydroxybutyrate and acetone), which are utilised by peripheral tissues.

Thus, ketogenesis is a necessary accompaniment of gluconeogenesis. In the decompensated diabetic state, the greater availability of FFA from lipolysis leads to excess synthesis of ketone bodies by the liver. This causes ketoacidosis and possibly further resistance to insulin. *In a diabetic who is overeating, hyperglycaemia is unlikely to be accompanied by ketonuria; on the other hand, in a diabetic who is unable to eat due to an acute illness, hyperglycaemia due to gluconeogenesis from over-secretion of the counter-regulatory hormones, particularly glucagon is likely to be accompanied by ketonuria.*

Insulin deficiency results in:

- **Decreased peripheral utilisation of glucose**
- **Decreased production of ATP**
- **Decreased synthesis of glycogen in liver and muscle**
- **Increased protein catabolism and delivering the amino acids for gluconeogenesis**
- **Increased lipolysis with increased plasma levels of FFA; and decreased lipogenesis**
- **Increased gluconeogenesis with increased hepatic glucose output**
- **Increased ketogenesis**
- **Depressed cell mediated immunity (CMI)**

High fasting glucose levels indicate excessive hepatic glucose production due to either impaired insulin secretion or glucagon excess. Postprandial hyperglycaemia, on the other hand, reflects impaired peripheral utilisation of glucose which depends on sensitivity of the tissues to insulin.

Significance of HbA1c: A glycosylated haemoglobin (HbA1c) level of 6.5% or higher (to be confirmed by repeat test) is now considered to be an additional independent criteria for diagnosis of DM. HbA1c level is an index of the 'time averaged' blood sugar level over the previous 8–12 weeks (Blood Sugar Memory). *This parameter does not measure variations in glucose levels or hypoglycaemia and is not a substitute for fasting and. postprandial blood glucose estimation.*

The Aims of Therapy

The aims are given in Box 63.7.

An ideally controlled diabetic should:

- Be free from classical diabetic symptoms of polyuria, polyphagia and polydipsia.
- Have steady, ideal body weight
- Have venous plasma glucose levels as near normal (fasting less than 110 mg% and post-prandial less

Box 63.7 Aims of Therapy of Diabetes Mellitus

- To control symptoms with diet, exercise and drugs
- To avoid instability in blood glucose levels over time
- To maintain the optimum body weight
- To correct the metabolic disturbances
- To prevent or delay the degenerative vascular complications
- To maintain normal growth in children

than 140 mg%) as is possible without getting frequent/severe hypoglycaemia.
In insulin dependent patients (especially, long standing), elderly and those with organ dysfunction higher setting of target blood glucose level may be required to avoid repeated hypoglycaemia.

- Have less than 6.5% HbA1c level without risk of hypoglycaemia
- Have not developed ketoacidosis without severe provocation (T2DM only)
- Have normal plasma lipid levels

Diabetic children should have normal growth; and diabetic women should have normal pregnancies, and normal babies.

Table 63.5 summarises the venous plasma glucose and HbA1c criteria for judging the level of metabolic control. Capillary blood glucose values are higher than venous plasma glucose values.

In most of the patients HbA1c level of 7% is reasonable. Studies have demonstrated that *aggressive treatment of T1DM and probably T2DM to achieve tight control of hyperglycaemia reduces the microvascular complications of DM* **but not IHD.** Rigorous control of BP is more effective for the latter purpose. *However, such regimens demand intelligent, highly motivated and disciplined patients, which is difficult in practice.*

In patients with history of severe hypoglycaemia, advanced micro- or macro-vascular complications, comorbidities, dementia and limited life expectancy HbA1c levels (up to 8%) are acceptable. Same holds true for young children at risk and the elderly. In the latter age group, an attempt to achieve a tight control is associated with hypoglycaemia. In them, the *mantra* is 'Treat the patient and not the HbA1c. *Pay more attention to the risk factors such as hypertension, hyperlipidaemia and obesity'. It is wise to aim for a target HbA1c concentration up to 8% in patients older than 65 years with comorbidities.*

Education of the Patient

It is important and must include an understanding of his own disease, diet control, exercise, urine examination, insulin administration, adjustment of the insulin dosage, symptoms of hypoglycaemia, the danger of neglecting the disease and the rewards of adherence to the prescribed regimen. Self-monitoring of blood glucose (SMBG) helps to improve the control.

Diet and Physical Exercise

The **diet** should be adjusted to bring the weight down to optimum and to maintain it there. The total calories are generally divided as follows: protein calories 10%–20%, fat calories 10%–20% and carbohydrate calories 60%–80%. Sugar consumption must be limited to less than 5% of the total daily calories consumed; and most of the carbohydrates be derived from starchy foods (complex carbohydrates).

The total daily intake should be divided into three meals and two snacks. The distribution of calories among the meals should be constant from day to day; this is of critical importance in those on insulin. *Overeating and fasting must be avoided.*

Daily physical exercise reduces insulin requirement. Sudden, unaccustomed, vigorous exercise,

Table 63.5 Venous Plasma Glucose and HbA_{IC} Criteria for the Degree of Metabolic Control

	Good	Acceptable	Fair	Poor
Venous plasma glucose:				
Fasting (FPG)	<110	120–140	140–180	Above 180
Postprandial (PPG)	<140	140–180	180–235	Above 235
Hemoglobin A1c%	<6[a]	6–7.5[a]	7.5–9	>9

[a]Not to be attempted in T1DM. Good/excellent control mandatory during pregnancy.
FPG: Fasting plasma glucose; PPG: Postprondial plasma glucose.

however, may precipitate hypoglycaemia especially in patients on insulin and *ketoacidosis in the juvenile diabetic who has omitted insulin.* For adults, moderately intensive exercise should be at least 150 min per week or vigorous physical activity should be 75 min per week.

Diet control and weight reduction helps to normalise insulin sensitivity in peripheral tissues.

Pharmacological Therapy

The antidiabetic drugs includes insulin and non-insulin drugs. The choice of antidiabetic drugs depends on whether it is T1DM or T2DM. Many T2DM patients in addition to diet and exercise, need oral antidiabetic drugs to maintain glycaemic control. After a variable length of time, they may also need insulin. They may need insulin temporarily in the presence of a complication **(Insulin Requiring DM; IRDM)**. *T1DM patients need insulin lifelong for survival. Hence, phenotyping the patients into IDDM, NIDDM or IRDM can help in choosing the therapy, 'insulin' or 'no insulin'.*

Indications for insulin therapy: These are listed in Box 63.8. Every diabetic may require insulin at some time in his life and it is life-saving in some situations.

Choice of insulin preparation: Commonly, the **intermediate acting preparations** (NPH or long acting insulin analogues) and **short-acting preparations** (regular insulin and ultra short acting insulin analogues), (Table 63.2) are used.

Box 63.8 Indications for Insulin Therapy

- T1DM
- T2DM patients newly diagnosed with HbA1c >10% or FBG >260 mg%, who are under-weight, those who have a history of onset before 30–35 years and those whose diabetes is of long standing
- All diabetics with complications such as ketosis, infection, intractable pruritus, gangrene, congestive cardiac failure or progressive retinopathy
- During surgical procedures
- Diabetic pre-coma and coma
- Primary or secondary failure following oral antidiabetic therapy
- Pregnant diabetics

The merits of regular (also called plain or soluble) **insulin** are rapid onset and short duration of action. This makes it convenient in:

- Diabetic coma
- Intensive insulin treatment (see section on management of T1DM)
- Unstable diabetes
- Post-operative period. Ultra short acting insulin analogues are not administered IV and cannot replace regular insulin if clinical condition demands IV use.

For the same reason, it must be used when an illness such as infection, vomiting or diarrhoea prevents regular intake of meals and the patient is likely to get hypoglycaemia with longer acting insulins. When it is decided to change over from short to intermediate acting insulin, it is desirable to commence therapy with a dose of the latter only two-third of the total daily dose of the former.

The synthetic, human rDNA insulin analogues (lispro, aspart, glargine) have much to offer in terms of flexibility of the daily routine; but they are more expensive than the conventional and the SR insulins.

Insulin resistance: Clinically it is defined as the requirement of more than 2 units/kg/day. It may be acute or chronic.

a. **Acute insulin resistance** is associated with surgical or other trauma, emotional disturbance or infection. It is treated with elimination of its cause and administration of insulin as is required to attain normal blood sugar levels.
b. **Chronic insulin resistance** may be due to:
   - **Noncompliance**
   - **Associated medical/endocrine disorders** such as acromegaly or hypercortisolism
   - **Genetic, insulin-receptor abnormality**
   - **Insulin antibodies.** They develop in all persons who receive the available preparations of insulin. They are likely to develop in high titre in patients who have received insulin intermittently rather than continuously. Such resistance may respond to prednisolone (60–100 mg daily).
   - **Lipoatrophic type of diabetes**

I. Management of T1DM

In T1DM, glycaemic targets need to be individualised.

All insulin therapy protocols try to follow the patterns of endogenous insulin secretion, which include (1) Basal insulin secretion all throughout the day which is constant to take care of metabolic needs (0.6–0.7 U/kg/day; Range- 0.2–1 U/kg/day) and (2) The bolus secretion which occurs in short spurts after food intake. The bolus secretion has 2 phases, a rapid phase (10 min) which suppresses the hepatic glucose production and a delayed phase (120 min) which takes care of carbohydrate metabolism. **The daily insulin requirement is therefore split into 50% as basal and 50% to control postprandial hyperglycaemia.** *Long-acting insulins provide constant basal background insulin level whereas short-acting ones are given to cover the prandial peaks.*

Most patients need any one of the following regimens:

a. An injection of regular insulin before each major meal with or without an additional dose of NPH before dinner or at bed time
b. A mixture of regular with NPH insulin (50:50 rather than 30:70) before breakfast and before dinner (Split-mixed regimen). This method with a minimum of 2 blood tests (before breakfast and before dinner) is perhaps the simplest and the most convenient way to control blood glucose levels over 24 h.
c. An injection of glargine insulin at bed time + an injection of lispro, aspart or regular insulin before each major meal, which can offer the patient the maximum flexibility. This, however, is an expensive regimen.

The dose of basal insulin is relatively constant except in conditions such as illness and excessive exercise but requirement for bolus insulin may vary depending on carbohydrate intake. Three insulin regimens viz. basal, basal-bolus or premixed regimen can be used. Only bolus therapy (i.e. giving regular insulin 2–3 times a day) without giving basal insulin therapy is the least useful and may result in hypoglycaemic attacks.

In some unstable, poorly controlled patients, regular insulin has to be injected SC several times a day **(intensified insulin treatment)** using **SMBG.**

Continuous Subcutaneous Insulin Infusion (CSII) can be used to avoid repeated injections.

In overweight and obese individuals poorly controlled on insulin therapy, adding metformin or SGLT2 inhibitor to insulin therapy may reduce HbA1c and insulin requirements with improvement in metabolic control. However, such regimes need further evaluation. Moreover, SGLT2 inhibitor may precipitate euglycaemic ketoacidosis and monitoring for ketonaemia is essential.

II. Management of an Adult with T2DM without any Complication

It is an individualised approach. *In most such patients, diabetes is stable and relatively mild (HbA1c $\leq$ 7%). It can be controlled with diet, weight loss and exercise with or without oral antidiabetic drugs.*

Table 63.6 summarises various antidiabetic drugs used in T2DM.

Oral antidiabetic drug combinations: These can be used in T2 DM patients as they offer following advantages:

- **Additive effect because of different mechanisms of actions**
- **Lower incidence of ADR of individual drugs**
- **Effectiveness in patients showing resistance to monotherapy**
- **Convenience of administration**

These combinations target the primary defects in T2DM-insulin resistance and insulin deficiency, e.g. metformin, an insulin sensitiser is given with sulphonylurea, an insulin secretor or glitazone or incretin based therapy or exogenous insulin. However, fixed dose combinations lack the flexibility of dose adjustment of the individual drugs.

Selection of antidiabetic drugs: It depends on convenience of administration, ability of drug to

Table 63.6 Drugs Used in T2DM

Drug Class	Site of Action	FPG	PPG	HbA1c Reduction	ADR	Weight Effection	Remarks
Insulin	Several	Excellent	Excellent	1–2.5	Hypoglycaemia	Marked gain	**Adv:** 1. Useful in emergency situations 2. Long-term reduction in microvascular risk; **Disadv:** Available as injectable only
Metformin	Liver	Good	Good	1–2	Anorexia, nausea	weight neutral or loss	**Adv:** 1. Prevention of weight gain 2. No hypoglycaemia; 4. Prevention of CVD 4. Cost-effective **Disadv:** Causes GI intolerance
Sulphonylureas (Glipizide, glimepiride)	Beta cells	Good	Good	1–2	Hypoglycaemia	Moderate gain	**Adv:** 1. Inexpensive 2. Long-term reduction in microvascular risk; **Disadv:** Possible aggravation of myocardial ischaemia
Nonsulphonylureas (Repaglinide)	Beta cells	Fair	Good	0.5–1.5	Hypoglycaemia (occasional)	Moderate gain	**Adv:** Short acting **Disadv:** To be taken just before each meal
Alpha glucosidase inhibitors (Acarbose)	Intestine	Poor	Excellent	0.5–1.3	Bloating	Less gain	**Adv:** Reduces postprandial hyperglycaemia **Disadv:** GI intolerance
Glitazones (Pioglitazone)	Muscle adipocytes	Good	Good	0.5–2	Hepatotoxicity	Moderate gain	**Adv:** Increases insulin sensitivity **Disadv:** CVS safety doubtful and possible risk of bladder cancer

Continued

Table 63.6 Drugs Used in T2DM—Cont'd

Drug Class	Site of Action	FPG	PPG	HbA1c Reduction	ADR	Weight Effection	Remarks
DPP-4 inhibitors (Sitagliptin, Vildagliptin)	GIT	Fair	Good	0.5–1	Hypoglycaemia can occur when added to insulin or sulphonylureas, pancreatitis, hypersensitivity reactions, hepatic failure	Less gain or loss	**Adv:** No effect on weight **Disadv:** 1. Less effective than sulphonylureas or GLP analogs 2. ADRs can be fatal 3. Increase the risk of heart failure
SGLT2 inhibitors (Dapagliflozin, Canagliflozin)	Kidney	Good	Good	0.6	Genital mycotic infections, UTI, volume depletion	Loss by 2 kg	**Adv:** Low risk of hypoglycaemia **Disadv:** Frequent UTI
Amylinomimetics (Pramlintide)	GIT, central	Fair	Good	0.5	Hypoglycaemia, nausea vomiting, abdominal pain, decreased appetite, fatigue	Loss by 1–1.5 kg	**Adv:** 1. It is added to meal time insulin decreasing insulin dose 2. Reduces postprandial hyperglycaemia **Disadv:** Cannot be mixed with insulin in same syringe
GLP-1 agonists (Exenatide, Liraglutide)	Beta cells, GIT	Fair	Excellent	0.3–1.9	Nausea, vomiting, diarrhoea, URTI, pancreatitis, renal toxicity, hypersensitivity reactions	Loss by >2 kg	**Adv:** 1. Causes weight loss 2. Long acting **Disadv:** 1. Available as injectable only 2. ADRs can be fatal

FPG, Fasting glucose; PPG, Postprandial glucose; Adv, Advantage; Disadv, Disadvantage.

Box 63.9 Management of Uncomplicated T2DM

Initial treatment

Diet and exercise

If poor response or patient presents with HbA1c between 6.5%–7.5%

Monotherapy or	**Low dose combination therapy or**	**Insulin**[a]
Metformin	Metformin + Sulfonylureas	
Sulfonylureas, Pioglitazone	Metformin + Pioglitazone	
Alpha-glucosidase inhibitors, DPP-4 inhibitors, SGLT-2 inhibitor, GLP-1 receptor agonist		

If poor response to above or patient presents with HbA1c 7.5–9%

Combination therapy ± Insulin

Metformin + Sulfonylureas

Metformin + Pioglitazone

If poor response to above or asymptomatic patient presents with HbA1c >9%

Metformin + Sulfonylureas + Pioglitazone/DPP-4 inhibitors/SGLT-2 inhibitors } **± Insulin**

Metformin + Pioglitazone + GLP-1 agonist } **± Insulin**

If poor response or complications or Symptomatic patients with HbA1c levels >9 %

Insulin

[a]*Use of insulin from the diagnosis is now favoured by many authorities (see text) Combinations mentioned are the commonly used ones but may vary depending on factors listed in the text.*

influence HbA1c level, fasting/postprandial glucose level, its safety in comorbid conditions, weight of the patient, ADR and cost (Table 63.6).

Higher the HbA1c, higher is the reduction with antidiabetic drugs. At higher levels, majority of the contribution is from fasting plasma glucose and therefore, the primary target is to reduce it. *Metformin, sulphonylurea, repaglinide, glitazones and liraglutide reduce fasting blood glucose level.* If these levels are aggressively reduced early in the course, then benefits of glycaemic control on preventing the onset and progression of microvascular complications are better evident. This forms the rationale for early use of combination therapy or insulin for T2DM (see below). **At lower HbA1c**, the PPG also contributes and therefore, drugs are selected depending on abnormality in glucose levels, FPG or PPG or both. *Meglitinides, a-glucosidase inhibitors, DPP-4 inhibitors, exenatide/liraglutide reduce postprandial hyperglycaemia.*

The ability of an antidiabetic drug to sustain its action without the need for an additional agent (durability) needs to be taken into consideration. It indirectly indicates ability of a drug to preserve beta cell function. *Amongst the available agents, glitazones have the best durability, metformin intermediate and sulphonylureas the least.* Durability of newer agents is yet to be known.

Box 63.9 outlines a simplified plan for the management of uncomplicated T2DM.

For HbA1c between 6.5% and 7.5%, several oral drugs are used as monotherapy or their low dose combinations are used. Higher levels of HbA1c requires starting therapy with combination of oral antidiabetic agents or even insulin (see Box 63.9). *However, almost all guidelines support use of metformin as an initial choice, either alone or in combination irrespective of HbA1c levels.* It is preferred because it:

- Reduces HbA1c by 1%–2%
- Decreases LDL-C and TG
- Does not lead to weight gain or causes loss
- Decreases total mortality and CVD. This may be due to improvement in endothelial dysfunction, haemostasis, oxidative stress, insulin resistance and lipid profile.
- Has low risk of hypoglycaemia
- Has low cost

Effects of metformin may, however, be delayed by several weeks.

Sulphonylureas can also be an alternative and may be used initially at higher HbA1c levels. Both, metformin and sulphonylureas are in use for several years. They are effective, cheap with acceptable safety profile and help to correct the metabolic dysfunction; hence preferred in non-complicated T2DM with FPG levels 200–250 mg%. Those who do not respond to individual drugs can be treated with their combination.

Glitazones may be used as monotherapy but cause oedema, weight gain and possible cardiovascular toxicity. α-Glucosidase inhibitors, DPP-4 inhibitors like sitagliptin, SGLT-2 inhibitor or GLP-1 receptor agonist can also be given as monotherapy. However, for the newer drugs long-term safety data are lacking. DPP-4 inhibitors are less effective. Further, they are all expensive. However, these drugs or any other new agent may be useful as an adjunct to metformin in a few selected resistant cases to improve glycaemic control or if there is associated comorbidity (Table 63.7).

If patient fails to respond to monotherapy within 3 months, another antidiabetic agent is added to the first one. The first drug is discontinued only if there is an evidence of intolerance to it or if combination is incompatible or the patient develops a comorbid condition in which that drug is contraindicated. Accordingly, double or triple drug combinations can be used such as metformin and sulphonylureas (± glitazone/DPP-4 inhibitors/ SGLT-2 inhibitors) or metformin + glitazone (± GLP-1 agonist). All combination therapies containing metformin are superior to metformin alone.

For HbA1c 7.5%–9%, combination therapy with 2 drugs may be started from the beginning. They can reduce HbA1c more effectively but they are associated with more ADR. The increased cost of the combination, mainly when newer agents are added, may not justify the benefits one gets from the combination.

If glycaemic goal is not met within 3 months, then a third drug like glitazone/DPP-4 inhibitors/ SGLT-2 inhibitors can be added to metformin and sulphonylurea combination or GLP-1 agonist to metformin and glitazone combination. The third agent can be long-acting basal insulin.

For HbA1c >9% but without any symptoms, a triple drug therapy may be an initial choice. For HbA1c levels, close or above 9%, sulphonylurea should be one of the drugs in the combination. Insulin is added if the triple drug therapy fails.

For symptomatic patients with HbA1c levels >9% (or FPG > 260 mg%), insulin either alone or in combination with oral antidiabetic drugs is the best option.

Insulin therapy in T2DM: Many patients of T2DM well controlled in the initial period on oral antidiabetic drugs ultimately need insulin as the disease progresses (see earlier). Early insulin therapy is preferable to oral antidiabetic drugs in young patients as it may result in lower HbA1c levels and better long-term preservation of endogenous insulin secretion. It ameliorates glucotoxicity and gives rest to the beta cells. Insulin therapy in these patients is short term but the achieved normoglycaemia can be maintained by diet and exercise.

Three insulin regimens *viz.* basal, basal-bolus or pre-mixed regimen can be used. In case of high FPG, only basal insulin regimen suffices. Basal-bolus or pre-mixed regimen are useful if postprandial or both the plasma glucose components are high.

In **basal regimen,** a single injection of a long-acting insulin, either NPH, detemir, glargine or degludec is given before breakfast along with oral antidiabetic agents. Insulin controls hepatic glucose production (and therefore FPG) and oral antidiabetics control the postprandial hyperglycaemia.

Some physicians initiate therapy with a small (5–10 units) dose of NPH at bedtime, to normalise the fasting blood glucose. Some patients may be controlled by BIDS (Bedtime Insulin and Daytime Sulphonylurea) regimen.

In **basal-bolus regimen,** regular insulin (or lispro or aspart) is added to NPH insulin (or any other basal insulin) to mimic endogenous insulin secretory pattern as follows:

- The **intermediate acting NPH insulin** is started with 5–10 units SC daily ½ h before breakfast. Blood sugar is determined while fasting, before lunch, before dinner and at bed time (*day-profiling*)
- The dose of insulin is increased by 2–5 units once in 3–4 days till pre-dinner blood sugar is normal
- If the pre-lunch blood sugar is still high, a small dose (5–10 units) of **regular insulin** is added to the pre-breakfast dose of NPH
- Persistence of hyperglycaemia at bedtime is treated by giving an additional dose of regular insulin before dinner
- If the dose of NPH given before breakfast does not control next morning's fasting hyperglycaemia while normalising the blood sugar at other times, a small dose of NPH should be added before dinner or at bed time

In **pre-mixed regimen,** mixture of regular and NPH is used in various proportion; the commonest being 30:70. Analog mixtures (biphasic aspart with protaminated aspart) are also available. They are simple to use and improve compliance e.g. premixed of regular and NPH before breakfast and before dinner with or without regular insulin before lunch. In some of these, addition of an oral antidiabetic drug may improve the diabetic control.

Persistent elevations of PPG contribute in a major way to the occurrence of chronic degenerative complications of diabetes. Very short-acting insulin analogues, **lispro** and **aspart**, are effective in controlling postprandial hyperglycaemia even when injected immediately before or within 5 min of commencing a meal. This makes them easier to use than SR insulins.

The patients with renal, hepatic or coronary artery disease are also best managed with insulin. If HbA1c is above the desired target level but <8.5% then a single injection of long-acting insulin with largest meal or at bedtime suffices but with HbA1c ≥ 8.5%, intensive basal-bolus regimen is useful. These patients may also need GLP-1 agonist. The choice of antidiabetic drug based on presence of comorbidities is depicted in Table 63.7.

III. Management of an Adult with T2DM on Insulin and a Complication such as Acute Infection IM 11.18

Under these conditions, insulin requirements go up and ketoacidosis may develop. *If the patient can continue to take his normal meals, the insulin regimen need not be changed.* If unable to do so, then a liquid diet containing plenty of salt and about 200 g of carbohydrates per day (**Sick Day Dietary Regimen**) is recommended. Portions of this diet is given every 3–4 h **and regular insulin (10–50 units)** is given SC every 6 h after blood sugar determination. As soon as the patient can take solid food, the original insulin regimen is resumed.

Along with lifestyle modification, **prophylactic aspirin**, unless contraindicated, is recommended in all patients with T2DM. *A statin may be needed, regardless of the baseline lipid levels, in those who are at higher risk for CVD or have CVD, but not routinely.*

The important points in therapy of T2DM are summarized in the Box 63.10.

MANAGEMENT OF EMERGENCIES IN THE DIABETIC IM 11.18

Ketoacidotic Diabetic Coma

Ketoacidotic diabetic coma is a medical emergency which needs immediate treatment, preferably in ICU.

Box 63.10 Points to Remember

- Diet, exercise and changes in lifestyle are important
- Majority of T2DM patients respond to metformin and/or sulphonylurea. These drugs are well studied, effective in correcting metabolic dysfunction, relatively safe and cheap
- Long term safety of newer antidiabetics is not known and they are expensive
- Attention to treatment of comorbidity such as hypertension, obesity, dyslipidaemia, CVD needs to be given to prevent macrovascular complications
- Treat the patient and do not chase the blood sugar levels or HbA1c, particularly in the elderly. Strict glucose control may even be harmful for them.

Table 63.7 Symptom Profiling of Antihyperglycemic Drugs

Associated	Recommended	Not Recommended / Contraindicated
CAD or high risk for CAD	GLP-1 agonist, SGLT-2 inhibitor, insulin	Glitazone, glibenclamide
Heart failure	SGLT-2 inhibitors	Pioglitazone
Renal failure	Repaglinide, DPP-4 inhibitors or insulin	PMetformin (if GFR is <30 mL/min/1.73 m^2), sulfonylurea, GLP-1 agonist
CKD	Repaglinide, SGLT-2 inhibitors	–
Hepatic disease	Insulin	Metformin, sulphonylureas pioglitazone, alpha-glucosidase inhibitors
Obesity[a]	Metformin, SGLT-2 inhibitors, GLP-1 agonists, tirzepatide	Sulphonylureas, pioglitazone
Risk of hypoglycaemia	Metformin, DPP-4 inhibitors, GLP-1 agonists, SGLT-2 inhibitors, pioglitazone	Sulphonylureas
Needs substantial lowering of HbA1c	Sulphonylureas, GLP-1 agonists, SGLT-2 inhibitors, tirzepatide	
Cost concern	Metformin, sulphonylureas, insulin	DPP-4 inhibitors, GLP-1 agonists, SGLT-2 inhibitors
Pregnancy	Insulin (Metformin and glyburide relatively safe)	Data insufficient to recommend others
Breast feeding	Insulin, metformin	Data insufficient to recommend others

[a]DPP-4 inhibitors and alpha-glucosidase inhibitors are weight neutral and can be used in combination with recommended agents.

T1DM patients are ketosis prone and diabetic coma can be precipitated by merely omitting insulin. In T2DM, it is likely to be precipitated by a severe infection or acute MI.

Pathophysiology: The deficiency of effective insulin action under these circumstances brings about:

- **Failure of peripheral glucose utilisation, increased mobilisation of muscle protein and increased gluconeogenesis, leading to hyperglycaemia**
- **Impaired oxidation of glucose leading to non-availability of pyruvate**
- **Excessive mobilisation of FFAs (lipolysis) from the adipose tissue**
- **Excessive production of ketone bodies,** acetoacetic and beta-hydroxy butyric acids

These organic acids contribute to **metabolic acidosis, which causes a shift of potassium and phosphorus out of the cells.** *Their loss in the urine as salts of organic acids can result in severe potassium, sodium, phosphate, and water depletion.*

- **Depletion of liver glycogen due to increased hepatic glycogenolysis**
- **Dehydration due to solute diuresis** due to hyperglycaemia, glycosuria and ketoacidosis

The urine is loaded with sugar and ketone bodies and the breath smells of acetone. The blood sugar is commonly in the range of 600–800 mg%. Plasma bicarbonate is markedly reduced and the blood pH is lowered.

Management: The diagnosis must be confirmed before starting treatment. If hypoglycaemic coma cannot be ruled out, IV glucose (50%, 50 mL) should be tried first.

On admission, blood is withdrawn for the following estimations, which must be repeated every 2 h:

glucose, bicarbonate, serum potassium, sodium, creatinine and haematocrit.

The following clinical data are recorded on admission and one hourly after that: pulse rate, blood pressure, temperature, fluid intake and output, glycosuria, ketonuria and ketonaemia.

The principles of management of ketoacidotic diabetic coma are outlined in Box 63.11.

- **Correction of dehydration:** Normal saline is infused as follows: 1.5 L in the first hour; 1 L/h for the next 3–4 h; and 1 L every 4 h, thereafter. Half strength (0.45%) saline is used only if the initial plasma sodium is more than 150 mEq/L. *When blood glucose reaches 250 mg%, glucose and potassium should be added to the saline infusion.*
- **Insulin: Continuous, low dose, insulin infusion (CLDII)** is effective, physiological and safe. Administration of 5–10 units (generally 0.1 unit/kg) of regular insulin per hour by continuous IV infusion maintains the plasma insulin at about 100–200 microunits/mL, which is effective in correcting the ketoacidosis. In general, patients with infection show insulin resistance due to:
  a. Acidosis
  b. Mainly by infection itself. Advantages of CLDII are listed in Box 63.12

With minor modifications, the same regimen can be used to treat hyperglycaemic, hyperosmolar, nonketotic diabetic coma.

If blood glucose shows no response at the end of 2 h, double the rate of insulin infusion. When blood glucose comes down to 250 mg%, (i) decrease insulin to 3 units/h; and (ii) add 50 g of glucose and 20 mEq of potassium to each litre of infusion fluid.

Continue the infusion till the patient starts eating normally. Then, start SC insulin 30 min before discontinuing the infusion.

An excessively rapid reduction in blood glucose should be avoided as it can cause:

a. **Severe hypoglycaemia**
b. **Hypokalaemia**
c. **Cerebral oedema** as the plasma osmolality diminishes rapidly. This complication is abated by rapid correction of acidosis.

- **Correction of acidosis:** Acidosis, if severe (arterial blood pH less than 7.0), is corrected by 50 mEq IV sodium bicarbonate.
- **Treatment of the precipitating cause:** Infection is treated with antibiotics. Routine administration of antibiotics prophylactically is, however, not recommended.
- **Potassium and phosphorus:** As soon as urine output is satisfactory, 20 mEq of potassium per hour through the drip is started. It is generally given as potassium chloride (2 g = 26 mEq of K). If available, K_2HPO_4 (equivalent to 20 mEq of potassium) may be added to the drip instead of KCl. It gives not only potassium but also phosphorus which is depleted in such cases. *As soon as the patient can take orally, milk can be given as a rich source of phosphorus, and fruit juice and soups can provide potassium.*

Box 63.11 Principles of Management of Diabetic Ketoacidosis

- Rapid correction of dehydration
- Rapidly acting regular insulin intravenously, early and enough
- Correction of acidosis
- Treatment of precipitating cause, if found
- Correction of hypokalaemia and hypophosphatemia
- Nursing management
- Measure capillary glucose every 1–2 h and electrolytes every 4 h for 24 h

Box 63.12 Advantages of CLDII

- It provides a predictable fall of blood glucose, 60–100 mg%/h. In the presence of infection, the rate of fall is lower.
- It is safe and rarely causes hypoglycaemia, hypokalaemia or cerebral oedema. Stopping the insulin drip quickly corrects the hypoglycaemia, should it develop.
- Previous insulin therapy does not affect the response to it.
- It has sound pharmacokinetic basis
- It is simple to use and can be administered by trained nursing staff

- **Nursing care:** *Excellent nursing care is essential in the management of a patient in diabetic coma. Attention to skin, mouth, position and bladder are a must.* Catheterisation of bladder should be avoided.

After second day of the recovery, the patient should return to his normal food and insulin regimen.

Hyperglycaemic, Hyperosmolar, Nonketotic Coma

This is a less common form of metabolic coma which occurs in aged diabetics who have just enough (exogenous or endogenous) insulin to prevent ketosis but not hyperglycaemia. The blood sugar level may be in excess of 1000 mg%. Dehydration is severe. The treatment is similar to that of diabetic coma except that *0.45% sodium chloride solution is required in very large quantities.* Heparin is given to prevent clotting. Insulin should be omitted when the blood sugar reaches about 250 mg%.

Surgery in a Diabetic

Patients detected to be diabetic just before an emergency operation, T1DM patients, and patients with T2DM on insulin and on oral antidiabetic drug should be managed with low dose continuous insulin infusion during and after major surgery. Those on oral antidiabetic drug and undergoing minor surgical procedures such as cataract surgery (after which the meal pattern will not change) can be managed with drug alone. Those on diet alone should receive insulin as and when necessary after surgery.

HYPERGLYCAEMIC AGENTS

GLUCAGON: Glucagon is a single-chain polypeptide made up of 29 amino acids, with a molecular weight of 3485. It is **synthesised, stored and secreted by the alpha cells of the islets of Langerhans** in response to a fall in blood glucose and a rise of plasma amino acids.

Pharmacological actions: Glucagon is the **most potent glycogenolytic hormone.** It:

- Produces a rapid rise in blood glucose by activating the hepatic phosphorylase via cyclic AMP
- Is a defence against hypoglycaemia in healthy people
- Stimulates gluconeogenesis only in the presence of glucocorticoids
- Stimulates lipolysis in the peripheral tissues, which, in turn stimulates ketogenesis
- Is a significant **positive inotrope** on the heart as it stimulates adenylyl cyclase

Absorption, fate and excretion: Given orally, it is degraded by proteolytic enzymes. After parenteral administration, it is absorbed rapidly but has a short plasma half life (3–6 min). It is degraded mainly in the liver, kidneys and plasma.

Preparations and dosage: Injection glucagon hydrochloride, 1 mg Dose: 0.5–1 mg SC, IM or IV.

Indications:

- **For treating insulin hypoglycaemia.** Glucose IV is the treatment of choice. Glucagon is administered IM in the dose of 1 mg. If consciousness is not regained, 1 mg IM may be injected. In about 45 min from onset of coma, liver glycogen gets exhausted and use of glucagon thereafter is ineffective.
- **To diagnose the hepatic form of glycogen storage disease** wherein it fails to raise the blood sugar level on IV injection.
- **In beta-blocker toxicity with shock** (Chapter 32).
- **Bradycardia in cardiogenic shock unresponsive to atropine:** 2–10 mg IV in 5% glucose followed by an infusion 50 mcg/kg/h.

DIAZOXIDE: This benzothiadiazine analogue is a potent oral hyperglycaemic agent. Its effects are reversible.

- **It inhibits the insulin release from the beta cells of the pancreas by an alpha-adrenergic mechanism.**
- **It stimulates release of catecholamines from the adrenal medulla.** The latter also inhibit insulin release by beta cells.
- **It increases the hepatic glucose output,** through a beta-adrenergic mechanism
- **It is a direct vasodilator** when administered IV (Chapter 30)

Box 63.13 Drug-induced Hyperglycaemia and Hypoglycaemia

- ***Drugs which cause hyperglycaemia:*** **Hormones:** Glucagon, GH; glucocorticoids; thyroid hormones; estrogens; progestogens; adrenaline and noradrenaline
  Other drugs: Beta adrenergic receptor agonists; diazoxide; phenytoin; Atypical antipsychotics; Amphotericin B; thiazides; Calcineurin inhibitors; Protease inhibitors; nicotinic acid in large doses
- ***Drugs which cause hypoglycaemia:*** MAO inhibitors; beta adrenergic receptor blockers; disopyramide; alcohol; ACE inhibitors; quinine; lithium; large doses of salicylates; Ranolazine
- ***Drugs which cause hypoglycaemia unawareness:*** Nonselective beta adrenergic blockers, e.g. propranolol
- ***Drugs which cause hypoglycaemia/hyperglycaemia:*** Fluoroquinolones; Pentamidine

Adverse reactions: Water retention with oedema, hirsutism and with high doses nausea, vomiting and hypotension can occur.

The oral dose is 3–5 mg/kg/day in 2–3 divided doses. A thiazide diuretic is commonly given along with it to prevent oedema.

Indications:

- **In the treatment of resistant hypoglycaemias** such as those due to insulinoma, glycogen storage disease and leucine-sensitive hypoglycaemia
- **In hypertensive emergencies** (Chapter 30) as a vasodilator

Box 63.13 lists the drugs which affect the blood glucose level.

SWEETENING AGENTS

These are non-sugar substances (**NSS**) devoid of food value, used as substitute for free sugar in diet, prepackaged foods, beverages and personal care products (e.g. toothpaste, mouthwash). NSS include all synthetic and naturally occurring or modified non-nutritive sweeteners. Used in small amounts, they are considered harmless even in pregnancy. They are:

1. **Saccharin:** It is commonly employed as the sodium salt which is comparatively free from the unpleasant after-taste of saccharin. Saccharin tablet contains 12 mg of saccharin. One tablet is approximately equivalent to 1 teaspoonful of sugar (7.5 g sucrose).
2. **Aspartame** (Equal, Sugar-free Gold): Aspartame is a dipeptide formed by a synthetic combination of two natural amino acids, L-aspartic acid and the methyl ester of phenylalanine. It is 200 times sweeter than sucrose. *It decomposes at high temperatures as in cooking and loses its sweet taste.*
3. **Neotame:** This analogue of aspartame is water soluble and more heat stable at neutral pH. It is, therefore, suitable for use in cooked food. It is about 30–60 times sweeter than aspartame, and is claimed to have 'flavour enhancing' property. It increases the perception of flavours such as fruit flavours.
4. **Sucralose** (Splenda, Sugar-free Natura): This zero calorie trichlorinated sucrose is 600 times as sweet as the native sucrose. It is not absorbed, nor metabolised, and is excreted unchanged in the faeces. Currently it is perhaps the most favoured sweetening agent.
5. **Natural product:** *Stevia rebaudiana* is a natural sweetener and has been used by the Guaraní people of South America for more than 1500 years. Its extract is used as OTC product. It has 'sweetish' taste, but is not 'sweet' like other sweetening agents. Its long-term safety is not known. It is expensive.

NSS may exert short term beneficial effects on weight and body fat but there is no evidence of long-term effects. On the other hand, there exists a potential of increased risk of type 2 diabetes, CVD and mortality from their long-term use. Hence preferred alternatives to free sugars in the diet will be natural sweetners, such as fruits and dates, as well as use of minimally processed unsweetened foods and beverages. These help to improve dietary quality.

INSULIN FORMULATIONS

Recombinant insulins

Rapid (short) acting
- Regular

Intermediate acting
- NPH

Premade mixture
- Regular +NPH

Human Insulin analogues, recombinant

Very Rapid (ultra short) Acting (VRA)
- Lispro
- Aspart
- Glulisine

Intermediate acting
- NPH and its Premade mixtures
- Lispro-protamine + Lispro
- Aspart-protamine + Aspart

Long-acting insulins
- Glargine
- Detemir

Ultra-long-acting insulin
- Insulin Degludec

Inhaled insulin

NON-INSULIN ANTIDIABETIC DRUGS

Oral

Stimulators of insulin release by beta cells (K^+_{ATP} channel modulators)

- Sulphonylureas
  - Tolbutamide
  - Glipizide
  - Glyburide
  - Gliclazide
  - Glimepiride
- Meglitinides
  - Repaglinide
  - Nateglinide

Inhibitor of hepatic gluconeogenesis, (AMPK activators)

- Metformin

Inhibitors of intestinal α-glucosidases, (α-glucosidases inhibitors)

- Acarbose
- Miglitol
- Voglibose

Drugs which reduce insulin resistance, (PPAR activators)

- Glitazones (Thiazolidinediones)
  - Pioglitazone

Inhibitors of dipeptidyl dipeptidase-4 (DPP-4)

- Sitagliptin
- Linagliptin
- Saxagliptin
- Vildagliptin
- Alogliptin
- Teneligliptin

Inhibitors of SGLT2

- Dapagliflozin
- Canagliflozin
- Empagliflozin

Others with novel mechanisms

- Bromocriptine
- Hydroxychloroquine

Inhibitor of SGLT-1 and SGLT-2

- Sotagliflozin

Parenteral

Amylinomimetics

- Pramlintide

GLP-1 agonists

- Exenatide
- Liraglutide
- Dulaglutide
- Albiglutide
- Semaglutide
- Lixisenatide

GIP + GLP1 agonist

- Tirzepatide

CD3-directed monoclonal antibody

- Teplizumab

CHAPTER 64

Adrenal Cortical Steroids

Learning Objectives

This chapter will enable the reader:

1. To state the regulation, pharmacological actions and uses of ACTH.
2. To describe the synthesis, metabolism and regulation of various adrenocortical hormones.
3. To discuss the mechanism of action and pharmacological effects of glucocorticoids.
4. To classify glucocorticoid formulations.
5. To describe the salient pharmacokinetic features, ADR, drug interactions, precautions and indications for various glucocorticoids.
6. To outline the management of acute and chronic adrenal insufficiency.
7. To explain the pharmacological actions, ADR and indications for aldosterone.
8. To outline the treatment of hyperaldosteronism.
9. To state uses of fludrocortisone giving the rationale for the same.

KEY TERMS

The importance of the adrenal cortex attracted the attention of physiologists after 'the clinical picture of adrenal destruction' was published by Thomas Addison in 1855.

The adrenals consist of an outer cortex and an inner medulla, which are structurally and functionally different from each other. The adrenal cortex consists of three zones; from without inwards, they are **zona glomerulosa, zona fasciculata and zona reticularis**. It is the adrenal cortex and not the medulla that is essential for survival.

In mid-1930s. E.C. Kendall and Tadeus Reichstein isolated and analyzed various hormones from the adrenal cortex, which led to cortisone preparations. it was used for therapy of RA (1948) by Dr Philip Hench when he observed that symptoms of RA get ameliorated during pregnancy and all three were awarded Nobel prize in 1950.

Pituitary–adrenal relationship: The hypothalamus, pituitary and the adrenal cortex form the **HPA axis.** Adrenocorticotropin (ACTH) maintains the structure and regulates the function of the adrenal cortex. It is secreted by the pituitary basophil cells (corticotrophs) and is a polypeptide with 39 amino acids. Melanocyte stimulating hormone (MSH) from the anterior pituitary has a sequence of amino acids identical with that of the first 13 of ACTH.

ADRENOCORTICOTROPIN PH 1.37

Regulation of ACTH release: A corticotropin releasing hormone (CRH), formed by hypothalamus, is stored in the medial eminence, and from there reaches the anterior pituitary via the portal circulation. It stimulates the synthesis and release of ACTH. 5-HT probably plays an important role in the release of ACTH.

Diurnal fluctuations in the rate of release of ACTH regulate the rates of secretion of cortisol and corticosterone. The plasma level of cortisol modulates the rate of release of CRH and in turn that of ACTH by *negative feedback mechanism.* Thus, increased plasma level of cortisol inhibits ACTH release. Decreased plasma level of cortisol, as in Addison disease, stimulates ACTH secretion. This delicately balanced mechanism thus regulates the plasma level of cortisol within normal limits.

Under stressful situations, neuronal impulses from higher centres stimulate release of CRH which ultimately elevates the output of cortisol to meet the increased demands of the body. This important homeostatic mechanism is deranged in various disease states and in the functional suppression of the HPA complex by glucocorticoid administration.

The rate of secretion of cortisol is maximum in the early hours of the morning, declines during the day and reaches a minimum at about midnight. The plasma level is highest at about 6 am.

The term cortisol refers to the native hormone of the adrenal cortex present in the biological fluids, whereas the term **hydrocortisone** *is used to refer to the synthetic substance used therapeutically.*

Pharmacological actions: PH 1.37

On the adrenal cortex: ACTH stimulates the adrenal cortex to synthesise and **secrete cortisol and corticosterone, and weak androgens**. In hypophysectomised animals, the adrenal cortex undergoes atrophy and secretion of cortisol is markedly depressed. Such atrophy can be prevented by administration of ACTH.

ACTH acts on the cell membrane receptors, activating the adenylyl cyclase system and increasing intracellular cyclic AMP. Furthermore, it accelerates the intracellular conversion of cholesterol to pregnenolone, the rate limiting step in the synthesis of adrenocortical steroids.

Prolonged elevation of ACTH level causes hyperplasia and hypertrophy of the adrenal cortex with increased secretion of cortisol, corticosterone and weak androgens. *The pharmacological actions of ACTH are in fact the pharmacological actions of these hormones, mainly cortisol* (see section, Glucocorticoids; pharmacological actions).

Extra-adrenal effects: These are of less clinical importance and include cutaneous pigmentation, lipolysis in adipose tissue, ketosis and insulin resistance.

Absorption, fate and excretion: ACTH is administered intramuscularly/intravenously. It is well absorbed after IM injection with plasma t½ is about 15 min. It is rapidly metabolised and only a negligible amount appears in the urine. The quantitative response to a given dose of ACTH is greater when it is given **in the morning than in the evening.**

Adverse reactions: Apart from the rare allergy, all other adverse actions of ACTH are due to increased secretion of adrenocorticosteroids.

Preparations and dosage:

Synthetic ACTH: This contains the first 24 of the 39 amino acids of natural ACTH.

i. Cosyntropin solution, 250 mcg/ml for IM or IV

Indications:

ACTH is no more used in therapeutics.

Diagnostic: Short ACTH stimulation test is performed by injecting 250 mcg of cosyntropin intramuscularly or as an IV bolus and measuring plasma cortisol at 60 min; a level of 18 mcg/dL or higher indicates normal functioning of the HPA axis.

HORMONES OF THE ADRENAL CORTEX

The zones of adrenal cortex and their hormones are as follows:

- **Zona glomerulosa** which synthesises aldosterone and desoxycorticosterone (mineralocorticoids)
- **Zona fasciculata** which secretes cortisol (glucocorticoid) mainly
- **Zona reticularis** which forms dehydroepiandrosterone (DHEA) and androstenedione (androgens) and traces of estrogens

Chemistry and synthesis: The adrenal cortical hormones are steroids (Fig. 64.1) consisting of cyclopentanophenanthrene ring with various functional groups (–H, $-CH_3$, –OH, =O) attached to carbon atoms. All steroid hormones have similar basic structure with minor differences which, however, cause striking alteration in their biological activity. They are sparingly soluble in water and circulate in association with binding proteins.

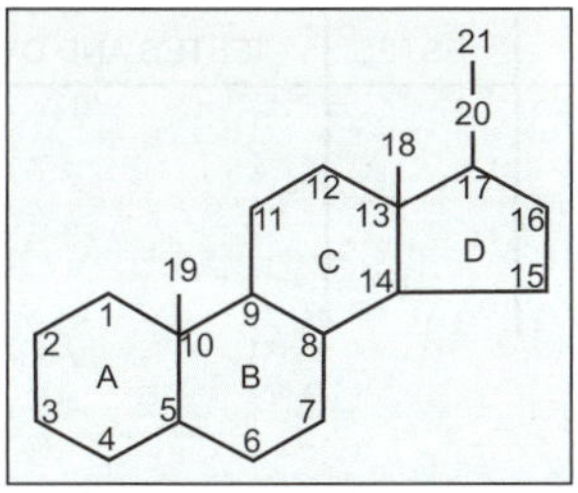

FIG. 64.1 **Cyclopentanophenanthrene ring.**

All the steroids can be synthesised basically from 2-carbon acetate chains via cholesterol. Cholesterol is converted through pregnenolone to progesterone. **Progesterone is an intermediary in the synthesis of other steroids and is not secreted by the adrenal cortex.** After progesterone, the synthetic pathways for the three groups of hormones separate out (Fig. 64.2). The enzymes in synthesis of cortisol, are sometimes congenitally deficient, leading to a deficiency of cortisol and an excess of ACTH and the adrenal androgens.

Secretory rate of cortisol is 10 mg/day and that of corticosterone is 2–4 mg/day.

Steroidal synthesis can be reduced by:

- **Metyrapone** which selectively inhibits synthesis of cortisol and corticosterone. It was used for testing adrenal function.
- **Aminoglutethimide** which acts by blocking the conversion of cholesterol to pregnenolone. It reduces the synthesis of all steroid hormones.
- **Ketoconazole,** an antifungal agent (Chapter 48), which is a nonselective inhibitor of adrenal and gonadal steroid synthesis. It is sometimes used in Cushing syndrome.
- **Mitotane,** an anticancer drug, which causes necrosis of the adrenal cortex (see Chapter 59)
- **Mifepristone,** an antiprogestin (Chapter 66) which in large doses blocks the glucocorticoid receptors. It has been used in Cushing syndrome due to adrenal carcinoma.
- **Cyproheptadine** and **etomidate** are steroidogenesis inhibitors which are useful in treating hypercorticism

Regulation of the secretion of adrenal cortical hormones: The rate of secretion of the glucocorticoids is regulated by the variations in the blood levels of ACTH. **Physiologically aldosterone output is independent of ACTH.** Aldosterone secretion is mainly regulated by angiotensin II, and serum potassium levels. A reduction in salt intake and a contraction of circulating blood volume are potent stimuli, acting via the RAAS pathway to aldosterone secretion (Chapters 25 and 31). Increase in the intake of potassium stimulates aldosterone synthesis and release.

Metabolism and excretion of adrenal corticoids: The adrenal corticoids are secreted into the blood as they are formed, and are not stored in the adrenal cortex in any significant quantities. They circulate partly free and mostly **bound to cortisol binding globulin (CBG).** The former is the biologically active form, the latter, a reserve form. These steroids are metabolised in the liver and the metabolites are excreted in the urine as conjugates with sulphuric and glucuronic acids. The corticosteroids, being water insoluble, are excreted in the urine only in traces. **The urinary metabolites can be estimated as neutral 17-ketosteroids and 17-ketogenic steroids** (Fig. 64.2). Aldosterone is excreted in urine partly as free aldosterone and partly as conjugates of tetrahydroaldosterone.

GLUCOCORTICOIDS AND MINERALOCORTICOIDS

Adrenocorticoids enable the organism to withstand 'stress'. In the absence of the adrenal cortex, survival is possible only under rigidly controlled and protected conditions wherein food and salt are available in plenty at all times and the environmental temperature is regulated. When exposed to 'stress', the adrenalectomised animal dies quickly unless pretreated with a glucocorticoid. Under optimum conditions, a small dose of hydrocortisone is sufficient to maintain such animal in a state of wellbeing, whereas under conditions of 'stress' larger doses of steroids are needed for survival.

A corticosteroid with predominantly sodium retaining effects is called a **mineralocorticoid**, e.g. aldosterone and desoxycorticosterone. A corticosteroid with predominantly liver glycogen depositing and neoglucogenetic actions is called a **glucocorticoid**, e.g. hydrocortisone, cortisone and most of the newer synthetic steroids. Corticosterone, a natural corticosteroid and 9-alpha fluorohydrocortisone, a synthetic steroid, have marked mineralocorticoid as well as some glucocorticoid activities.

PH 1.38

GLUCOCORTICOIDS: The important glucocorticoid secreted in man is cortisol. It has some

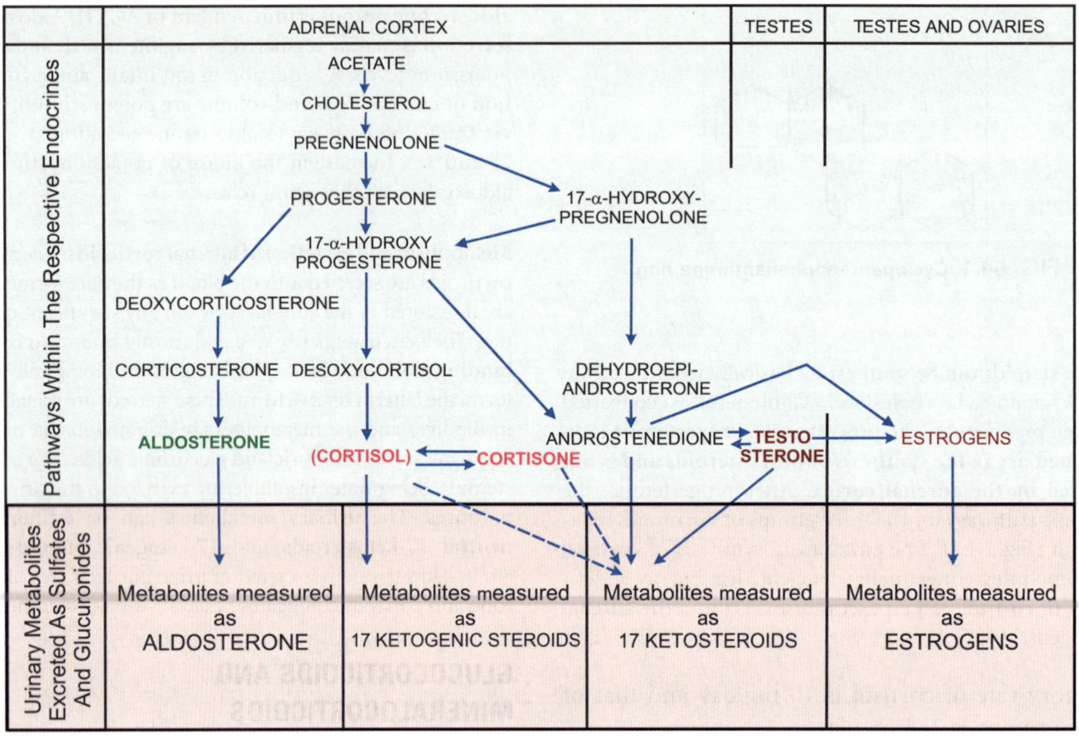

FIG. 64.2 Synthesis and metabolism of steroid hormones.

mineralocorticoid activity too. Since the pharmacological actions of **hydrocortisone** (**cortisol,** Fig. 64.3) are, in fact, its physiological actions, they are discussed together. The other synthetic glucocorticoids include **prednisone, prednisolone** (Fig. 64.4), **triamcinolone, paramethasone, dexamethasone** (Fig. 64.5)**, betamethasone** and **6-methyl prednisolone** (Table 64.1).The last four synthetic steroids show negligible or almost absent mineralocorticoid activity.

Mechanism of action: Synthetic glucocorticoids bound to CBG enter the cell as free molecules and bind to **cytosolic steroid receptors.** The complex translocates to the nucleus and the steroid binds to the glucocorticoid responsive element (GRE) in

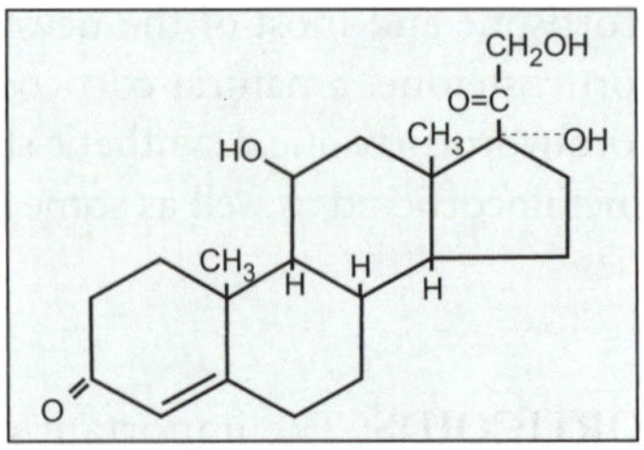

FIG. 64.3 Hydrocortisone.

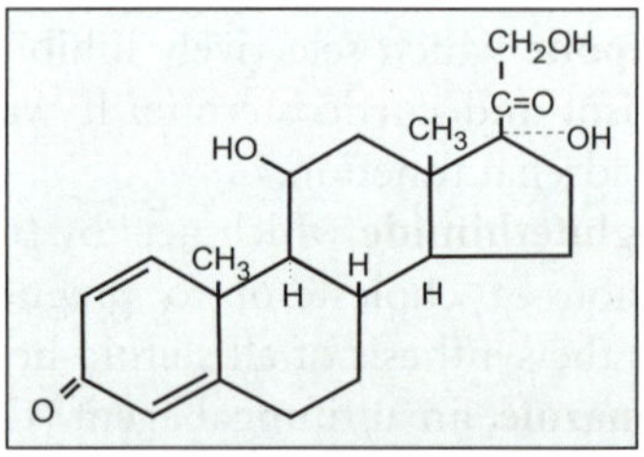

FIG. 64.4 Prednisolone.

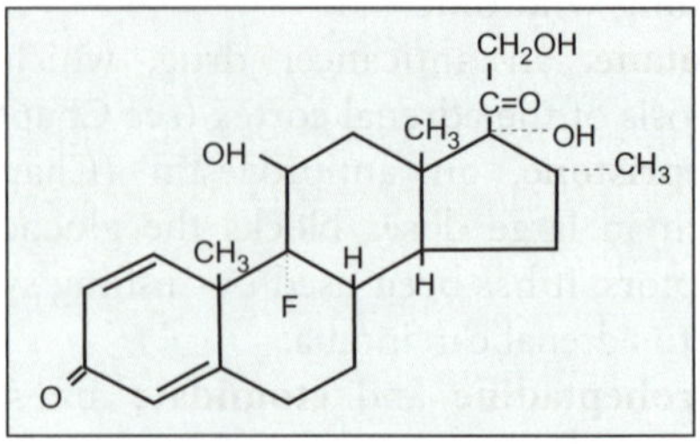

FIG. 64.5 Dexamethasone.

Table 64.1 Comparison of Various Glucocorticoids

Drug	Biological Half-life (h)	Glucocorticoid Activity	Mineralocorticoid Activity	Pituitary Suppression	Comparative Doses[a] (mg)	Affinity[b]
Short acting						
Cortisone	8–12	0.8	1	1	25	1
Hydrocortisone	8–12	1	1.25	2.5	20	100
Intermediate acting						
Prednisolone	18–36	4	0.5	5	5	220
Methylprednisolone	18–36	5	0	8	4	1350
Triamcinolone	18–36	5	0	–	4	–
Long acting						
Dexamethasone	36–54	25	0	100–200	0.75	540
Betamethasone	36–54	25	0	100–200	0.75	400

Notes: Therapeutic efficacy in inflammatory disorders is proportional to the glucocorticoid activity.
[a]These dose relationships apply to oral and intravenous administration of these compounds but not to intramuscular or intra-articular administration of these compounds or their derivatives.
[b]Affinity for human, intracellular, glucocorticoid receptor.

the regulatory region of the concerned gene. The interaction is responsible for the **genomic effects**, executed through activation or repression of DNA transcription. Repression of DNA transcription is believed to be responsible for anti-inflammatory actions of glucocorticoids whereas up-regulation of gene transcription which occurs with higher doses is believed to cause undesirable effects.

Pharmacological actions: Glucocorticoids **exert a variety of physiological effects and pharmacological actions with supra-physiological doses.** The physiological doses have beneficial effects while large pharmacological doses cause several adverse effects. The effects of corticosteroids that involve concerted actions with other regulatory hormones are termed *permissive.*

Metabolic effects: The glucocorticoids affect the metabolism of carbohydrates, proteins, fats, electrolytes, water and calcium.

- **Carbohydrate and protein metabolism:** Glucocorticoids:
  - i. **Inhibit the peripheral utilisation of glucose** by skeletal muscle and adipose tissue
  - ii. **Inhibit the incorporation of amino acids into protein** in the peripheral tissues (***anti-anabolic action***)
  - iii. **Promote the conversion of amino acids into glucose (*neoglucogenesis*) in the liver**

  All these help to maintain an adequate glucose supply to the brain. The plasma amino acid level rises significantly. Simultaneously, the plasma glucagon level also rises markedly during chronic but not acute administration.

  Chronic administration of glucocorticoids causes hyperglycaemia and glycosuria.

  In **physiological doses,** glucocorticoids stimulate protein and RNA synthesis in the liver; ***supra-physiological doses*** **cause catabolic and antianabolic effects** in the skin, muscles, lymphoid and connecting tissues. This leads to wasting of muscle, thinning of the skin and osteoporosis.
- **Fat metabolism:** Glucocorticoids play a 'permissive' role in the mobilisation of fat from the peripheral fat depots by adrenaline and GH. *Prolonged administration of large doses causes a redistribution of body fat,* with a loss from the extremities and a deposition in the neck (**buffalo hump**), supraclavicular area and face (**moon face**).
- **Electrolyte and water metabolism:** Hydrocortisone has a relatively weak salt retaining and

potassium wasting effect. However, when **large doses** (300 mg/24 h) are used, sufficient salt retention occurs to make the concurrent use of a mineralocorticoid unnecessary. Hydrocortisone, 25 mg has the same mineralocorticoid activity as 0.1 mg of fludrocortisone.

- **Calcium metabolism and bone:**
  a. In pharmacological doses, glucocorticoids **antagonise the action of vitamin D on the gut and reduce absorption of calcium**
  b. **Large doses for prolonged periods** may interfere with the development of cartilage and inhibit linear growth in children. Due to the protein catabolic action, glucocorticoids inhibit formation of new bony tissue.
  c. In chronic states of hypercorticism, the continuous resorption which occurs as a part of bone remodelling leads to severe osteoporosis

Cardiovascular system:

a. The cardiovascular changes in adrenal insufficiency are partly due to mineralocorticoid deficiency which affects electrolyte and water metabolism, and partly due to glucocorticoid deficiency. Usually, the blood volume and blood pressure diminish and blood viscosity increases. These defects are only partially corrected by administration of sodium chloride and/or a mineralocorticoid; addition of a glucocorticoid completely restores the circulation to normal.

b. Glucocorticoids potentiate the pressor response of blood vessels to adrenaline and NA by upregulating the adrenergic receptors in the vessel wall. The absence of glucocorticoids leads to increase in capillary permeability, inadequate vasomotor responses of smaller blood vessels and reduction in the cardiac output. **In pharmacological doses, they have a positive inotropic action on the heart.**

c. Hypertension is seen during chronic administration of glucocorticoids and in the patients with Cushing syndrome. In the latter condition, it is an important cause of death.

Muscles: Permissive concentration of cortisol is necessary for the normal functioning of the skeletal muscle. Muscular weakness is an important feature of Addison disease. It is largely due to inability of the circulatory system to respond to the stress of exercise. It is specifically corrected by a glucocorticoid. On the other hand, the muscle weakness of **hypercortisolism** is due to hypokalaemia and to muscle wasting (**steroid myopathy**) (see Adverse reactions).

Central nervous system: Patients with Addison disease show apathy, depression, irritability and sometimes psychosis. All these are corrected by a glucocorticoid.

Patients on pharmacological doses of glucocorticoids may show mood elevation, euphoria, nervousness, restlessness, depression and even psychosis. These are all reversible.

Haematological action: Glucocorticoids cause an increase in the number of circulating RBCs, platelets, neutrophils and a decrease in the number of lymphocytes, monocytes, eosinophils and basophils in the blood. This is brought about by a redistribution of the cells between the blood and other compartments; there is no lysis of lymphocytes in normal persons. However, *the pharmacological doses* in patients with acute lymphoblastic leukaemia, cause rapid destruction of the lymphocytes.

GI tract: Glucocorticoids inhibit the secretion of prostacyclin and increase both basal and nocturnal gastric acid secretion.

Anti-inflammatory action: Glucocorticoids prevent or suppress the symptoms and signs of inflammation such as local heat, redness, swelling and tenderness. They suppress the *early phenomena* namely, oedema, fibrin deposition, capillary dilatation and leucocyte migration into the inflamed area as well as the *late manifestations* such as capillary proliferation, fibroblastic proliferation, collagen deposition and cicatrisation. They interfere with wound healing. Fibrous tissue, once formed, is not affected.

The moderate doses of glucocorticoids suppress the inflammatory response so are useful in urticaria, allergic rhinitis and bronchial asthma. The mechanisms which possibly contribute to their **anti-inflammatory action** are as follows:

1. Inhibition of leucocyte migration into the inflamed tissue

2. Inhibition of the release of arachidonic acid from phospholipids by inhibiting the enzyme phospholipase-A_2 (see Fig. 25.4 in Chapter 25) and hence decrease in the production of proinflammatory cytokines, PGs, LTs, PAF and chemokines
3. Decrease capillary permeability by reducing the amount of histamine released by the basophils and mast cells
4. Diminution of chemotaxis and lysosomal enzyme synthesis by neutrophils and monocytes. This decreases the recruitment of neutrophils and macrophages into the affected area.
5. Stabilisation of lysosomal membranes, at high concentrations, thus preventing the spillage of hydrolytic enzymes

This anti-inflammatory effect of glucocorticoids forms the basis for their clinical use in many different conditions.

Earlier it was thought that the anti-inflammatory and immunosuppressive actions of glucocorticoids were limited to pharmacological doses. It is now realised that glucocorticoids produced, as a part of the response to stress, exert a beneficial anti-inflammatory-immunosuppressive effect and help to limit the damage caused by such reactions. Furthermore, they may prevent possible cardiovascular collapse due to the depressant action of released immune mediators on the vascular tone (physiological action).

Immunosuppressive and antiallergic actions: Glucocorticoids in **large therapeutic doses** (40–60 mg of prednisolone per day):

- *Inhibit the function of macrophages and reduce their ability to respond to antigens.* This affects phagocytosis and bactericidal action. Furthermore, production of TNF-α, some interleukins and interferons is reduced.
- *Inhibit the activation of cytotoxic T lymphocytes and their proliferation;* they cause transient peripheral lymphopenia.
- *Cause lysis of the T lymphocytes*
- *Inhibit the effects of the complement system,* but not the complement itself.
- *Suppress cell-mediated hypersensitivity reaction.* The glucocorticoid doses that modify CMI usually do not suppress the antibody production (humoral immunity).
- *Prevent homograft rejection*

Large doses (100–200 mg of prednisolone/day) diminish the effective concentration of specific IgG antibodies.

Clinically, glucocorticoids modify the course of many diseases involving the immune responses. They do not modify the basic disease process, but suppress the inflammatory response to injury and thus, protect the tissues. *However, they increase the susceptibility to a variety of bacterial, fungal, viral and parasitic superinfections.*

Miscellaneous actions: Glucocorticoids have **uricosuric and nonspecific antipyretic effects.** Glucocorticoids markedly increase the activity of phenyl-ethanolamine-*N*-methyltransferase, an enzyme located almost exclusively in the adrenal medulla and which catalyses the conversion of NA to adrenaline. They play an important role in the maturation of the fetal lung.

Inhibition of HPA axis: *Supraphysiological doses of glucocorticoids for longer than one week suppress the HPA axis and cause adrenocortical atrophy. This is most marked when the entire daily dose is given at bed time and is least when it is given on rising in the morning.* Such patients, during therapy, and for long periods (as long as 12 months) thereafter, are unable to increase the endogenous cortisol output in response to stress. It takes 4-6 mths for plasma ACTH to reach supranormal levels. Only then the atrophic adrenal cortex starts recovering its function. *But it can take the HPA axis as long as 8–12 months to be able to respond normally to stress. This recovery of the HPA axis is not accelerated by administration of exogenous ACTH. However, physiological doses of a glucocorticoid (20 mg of hydrocortisone or 5 mg of prednisolone, per day) may be used for prolonged periods after cessation of prolonged, large dose glucocorticoid therapy, without interfering with the recovery of HPA axis.*

Patients who are on **small doses** of any glucocorticoid (20 mg of hydrocortisone or equivalent doses of other glucocorticoids per day) and those who are on high doses of intermediate-acting glucocorticoids (see Table 64.1) **on alternate days** in the morning show little or no suppression of the HPA axis. The other advantage of the alternate day therapy is the minimisation of the nitrogen and calcium imbalance. It, therefore, permits safer administration of much larger total dosage of glucocorticoids. Hence, whenever possible, in patients requiring high-dose, prolonged glucocorticoid therapy, *the* **alternate day regimen** should be considered. *Because of their prolonged action, the long-acting glucocorticoids are not suitable for alternate day administration.*

All the patients on long-term glucocorticoid treatment should be considered to be suffering from adrenal insufficiency and during stress the dose of the glucocorticoid should be increased.

- The long-acting compounds such as dexamethasone, are eminently suited for uniform and continuous suppression of ACTH secretion in the syndrome of congenital, virilising, adrenocortical hyperplasia. *As the peak secretion of ACTH occurs at night (in this condition as in normal persons), the entire daily dose of the long-acting glucocorticoid should be given at bedtime.*
- **During minor stress,** such as a febrile illness, severe exercise, bouts of gastroenteritis with vomiting and diarrhoea, and minor surgery, the normal adrenals respond by secreting about 100 mg of hydrocortisone per day; this then is the requirement of hydrocortisone (or an equivalent dose of another glucocorticoid) during such situations. The dose can be abruptly reduced to the maintenance dose as soon as the stressful event is over.
- **During major stress,** such as major surgery, severe burns and MI, the daily requirement of 300–400 mg of cortisol can be met with by giving 100 mg by IV infusion every 6–8 h on the first day. From the next day onwards, the dose is halved every day till the physiological maintenance dose is reached, if the recovery is uneventful.

While withdrawing long-term glucocorticoid therapy, the reduction up to the physiological maintenance dose may be as rapid as the disease will permit. Too rapid a reduction can cause (a) a flare up of the disease under treatment and (b) nonspecific 'withdrawal symptoms' comprising of fever, malaise, myalgia and arthralgia.

After reaching the physiological maintenance dose, it should be continued up to 1 year in order to allow the HPA axis to recover its function fully. *Patients undergoing surgery should always be asked for history of glucocorticoid therapy during the past 1 year.*

Absorption, fate and excretion: *Administered cortisone is converted in the body to the active compound cortisol.* The oral bioavailability of hydrocortisone is about 96% and variable (30%–90%) on administration as an enema. The absorption from aqueous suspension of acetate given intramuscularly is slower than that of orally administered hydrocortisone and hence the effect lasts longer. **Absorption of prednisolone is almost complete (80%–100%) after both oral and rectal administration**. As much as 50% of intra-articular prednisolone, administered in patients with RA, is absorbed into systemic circulation. Dexamethasone is well absorbed (80%) orally. The bioavailability of oral methylprednisolone is variable (50%–80%).

Cortisone and prednisone act in the the body after being converted in the liver to hydrocortisone and prednisolone respectively. Hydrocortisone and prednisolone are highly protein bound. Dexamethasone is less protein bound than hydrocortisone. The pharmacokinetic parameters of methylprednisolone are similar to those of prednisolone.

The synthetic glucocorticoids are rapidly absorbed orally. Their long-acting esters used topically or administered via intra-articular injection are poorly absorbed. Like hydrocortisone, they are metabolised by the liver but more slowly. They are less extensively protein bound and hence diffuse more completely into the tissues.

Dexamethasone and betamethasone cross the placenta to achieve high concentrations in the fetal circulation and can suppress the fetal HPA axis. *Therefore, if a pregnant woman needs treatment with a glucocorticoid, prednisolone is preferred.*

The concentration of prednisolone in breast milk is about 10% that of plasma concentration, and no restriction on breast feeding is considered necessary in the mother who is receiving <20 mg of prednisolone/day.

The biological t½ of the glucocorticoids and their relative affinity for human, intracellular, glucocorticoid receptor are given in Table 64.1.

Adverse reactions: These are related to individual susceptibility, dosage and duration of therapy.

Single large doses of prednisolone 1–2 mg/kg or equivalent doses of other glucocorticoids, **are generally harmless and may, therefore, be used without hesitation in situations where life is threatened** by adrenocortical or pituitary insufficiency or by cerebral oedema. *Short-term therapy (generally 1–2 weeks) with moderate doses is unlikely to produce any serious harmful effects.*

Prolonged therapy with doses higher than 20–30 mg of hydrocortisone or equivalent doses of other steroids per day is likely to cause adverse effects. This is the generally recommended maximum maintenance dose in prolonged glucocorticoid therapy.

The ADR, other than sodium retention, are shared by all glucocorticoids. However, certain adverse effects seem to be unique to **triamcinolone;** these are anorexia, muscle wasting, weight loss, sedation and depression. *It should be avoided in renal disease.*

The important adverse effects are as follows:

- **Gastrointestinal tract:** Acute erosive gastritis with haemorrhage may occur during intensive therapy, and peptic ulceration may be troublesome during prolonged therapy. Intestinal perforation and pancreatitis are the other reported GI complications.
- **Endocrine system:** These are an extension of their pharmacological actions and comprise **hypercortisolism**
- **Metabolic effects:** Clinical manifestations (including, ketoacidosis) of idiopathic diabetes mellitus can be precipitated. *Pre-existing diabetes, however, is not an absolute contraindication to glucocorticoid therapy and development of hyperglycaemia during therapy in itself does not warrant cessation of treatment.* Some patients develop hyperlipidaemia and hypophosphatemia.

  Prolonged therapy causes central obesity with moon face and buffalo hump. Pink florid striae appear on the abdomen, hips and pectoral regions and the skin may become friable. The patient may get spontaneous ecchymosis and bruise easily (**Cushingoidism**).
- **Suppression of inflammation and immune responses:** Glucocorticoids may mask the clinical features of a serious illness, e.g. fever and abdominal rigidity may be absent when a patient on these drugs develops acute peritonitis, which may, therefore, be missed. Furthermore, pre-existing infections like tuberculosis can spread and **superinfection** with other organisms can occur.
- **Retardation of linear growth** occurs in children who receive high doses
- **Cardiovascular and renal system:** Hypertension, salt and water retention and rarely hypokalemic alkalosis can occur. They are uncommon with dexamethasone, betamethasone and triamcinolone.
- **CNS:** Glucocorticoids readily enter the brain and can influence mood, sleep patterns and EEG activity; patients may complain of insomnia. Acute psychotic reactions may occur especially during intensive therapy. Benign intracranial hypertension and aggravation of epilepsy particularly in children can occur.
- **Musculoskeletal effects:** Proximal myopathy and osteoporosis with compression fractures of the vertebrae are serious complications. Bisphosphonates are reported to prevent the osteoporosis. Occasionally, acute avascular necrosis of bone may occur.
- **Eyes:** Glaucoma occurs in some patients during local glucocorticoid therapy, and posterior subcapsular cataract has been reported during their long-term systemic use.
- **Inhibition of HPA axis:** Discussed earlier
- **Miscellaneous changes:** These include hypercoagulability of blood with thromboembolic complications, androgenic effects (acne, hirsutism, loss of scalp hair), subcutaneous atrophy and delayed wound healing.

Rapid IV injection of large pulse doses (see Pharmacological therapy) can cause vasoactive reaction.

The **Cushingoidism** produced by glucocorticoid therapy differs in certain respects from **Cushing syndrome** produced by endogenous hypercortisolism. Pseudotumour cerebri, glaucoma, cataract, pancreatitis, aseptic necrosis

Box 64.1 Adverse Skin Reactions to Topical Glucocorticoids

- Epidermal and dermal atrophy (thinning of the skin, striae, telangiectases superficial fissures and purpura)
- Acne, folliculitis, miliaria
- Hypertrichosis
- Hypopigmentation
- Allergic contact dermatitis (uncommon)
- Rebound of the lesion under treatment, on abrupt withdrawal especially of the potent steroids
- Masking or aggravation of dermatophytoses, impetigo or scabies

of bone, panniculitis and vasculitis are almost unique to the *iatrogenic form of Cushing syndrome.*

Box 64.1 shows the important adverse reactions to topical use of glucocorticoids on the skin. They are especially likely to occur:

1. In infants, children and the elderly
2. With the use of potent steroids, especially when used in large doses for prolonged periods
3. With the use of occlusive dressings
4. When used in areas with thin skin, e.g. face

Drug interactions: See Box 64.2.

The **synthetic steroids** have pharmacological actions and adverse effects identical with those of hydrocortisone except the mineralocorticoid actions. However, none is safer than prednisolone with respect to the peptic ulceration, osteoporosis and hyperglycaemia. *All of them are potent pituitary inhibitors.*

Triamcinolone has a greater propensity to cause myopathy, whereas the incidence of increased capillary fragility and ecchymosis is more with triamcinolone, dexamethasone and betamethasone. Hence they are not recommended for routine use.

Preparations and dosage:
For systemic use:

i. Cortisone acetate tablets, 25 mg dose: 12.5–37.5 mg (replacement therapy)
ii. Cortisone injection, a suspension of cortisone acetate (25 mg/mL). Dose: 50–200 mg daily intramuscularly in single or divided doses.
iii. Hydrocortisone tablet, 5 mg, 10 mg and 20 mg

Box 64.2 Drug Interactions of Glucocorticoids

- ***Glucocorticoid dosage is decreased:*** Antibiotics (erythromycin, trioleandomycin), cyclosporin, isoniazid and ketoconazole reduce the metabolic clearance of glucocorticoids. Estrogens increase the levels of corticosteroid binding protein and thus reduce the free fraction; they also reduce the clearance
- ***Glucocorticoid dosage is increased:*** Cholestyramine decreases the intestinal absorption. Antiepileptic drugs (barbiturates, phenytoin, carbamazepine), rifampicin, aminoglutethimide increase the metabolism by inducing hepatic microsomal enzymes
- ***Glucocorticoid dosage needs adjustment:*** Antianxiety and antipsychotic drugs: Recurrent or poor control of CNS symptoms due to inherent glucocorticoid effects
- ***Anticholinesterases:*** May precipitate myasthenic crisis
- ***Anticoagulants:*** Decreased effectiveness
- ***Antihypertensives:*** Decreased effectiveness
- ***Oral hypoglycemics:*** Decreased effectiveness
- ***Sympathomimetics:*** Increased effectiveness
- ***Salicylates:*** Increased clearance

iv. Hydrocortisone hemisuccinate being readily water soluble is administered intramuscularly, by IV infusion or as a retention enema. Hydrocortisone 100 mg by IV bolus lasts for 4 h only. A continuous infusion 4 mg/h provides adequate plasma levels (30–40 mcg/dL) for surgical cover. For retention enema, a dose equivalent to 100 mg of hydrocortisone, dissolved in 120 mL of normal saline is given each night.
v. Prednisone tablet, 5 mg and also as modified release tablet 1, 2 and 5 mg. Dose: 10–100 mg daily in divided doses.
vi. Prednisolone tablet in varied strengths 1–25 mg or an equivalent amount of prednisolone acetate. In addition, available as enteric coated tablets 2.5/5 mg and oral solution as 1 mg/ml. Dose: 10–100 mg daily in divided doses.
vii. Prednisolone acetate suspension, 25 mg/mL. It is administered by intramuscularly, intra-articular or peri-articular injection.
viii. Prednisolone sodium phosphate, in contrast to prednisolone acetate, is soluble in water. Approximately 27 mg of the salt are equivalent to 20 mg of prednisolone. Dose: equivalent to 20–100 mg of prednisolone intravenously and 20 mg by retention enema.
ix. Methylprednisolone, in various strengths 2–100 mg tablets. Dose: 2–40 mg daily in divided doses.

x. Methylprednisolone sodium succinate. Dose: equivalent to 40–120 mg of methyl-prednisolone base intramuscularly or intravenously, 40–120 mg as a retention enema; pulse dose 500–1000 mg by slow intravenously infusion.
xi. Methylprednisolone acetate 40 mg/ml IM injection
xii. Triamcinolone tablet, 4 mg. Dose: 2–24 mg daily in divided doses.
xiii. Triamcinolone diacetate injection available as 40 mg/ml for IM or intra-articular use. Dose: 5–40 mg.
xiv. Betamethasone tablet, 0.5 mg. Dose: 0.5–5 mg daily.
xv. Betamethasone sodium phosphate, a water soluble salt is available as tablets and for injection 4mg/ml; nearly 1.3 mg of the salt is equivalent to 1 mg of betamethasone. Dose: equivalent to 0.5–5 mg of betamethasone by mouth; for acute adrenal insufficiency, 10–20 mg by IV or IM injection daily in divided doses.
xvi. Dexamethasone tablet 0.5 and 2 mg. Doses similar to betamethasone tablets.
xvii. Dexamethasone 21-phosphate injection contains 4 mg of the salt per mL. Dose: 4–20 mg of the base by IM or IV

Choice of the glucocorticoid: *For routine systemic use, prednisolone is the drug of choice as it is effective orally, relatively safe and cheap.* When a potent glucocorticoid is indicated, dexamethasone/betamethasone is preferred; they do not cause sodium retention.

For topical use: Numerous preparations containing either the glucocorticoids alone or in combination with antibiotics are available for topical therapy. The *topical skin preparations* can be divided into four groups in increasing order of potency (Box 64.3). The potency of the topical preparations is proportional to their ability to cause vasoconstriction and cutaneous blanching on local application.

The skin preparations as creams or ointments and topical preparations for nasal, conjunctival and intra-articular use are available.

Beclomethasone dipropionate, budesonide and fluticasone as **inhaled steroids** in bronchial asthma are discussed in Chapter 27.

Box 64.3 Topical Glucocorticoid Preparations

Mild: Hydrocortisone 1%
Moderately potent: Clobetasone butyrate 0.05%; hydrocortisone 2.5%
Potent: Betamethasone valerate 0.1%; hydrocortisone butyrate 0.1%; fluocinolone acetonide 0.025%; triamcinolone acetonide 0.2%
Very potent: Clobetasol propionate 0.05%

Hydrocortisone oral paste 0.5% may be useful in treating painful, nonherpetic, oral ulcers.

Indications:

I. **Replacement therapy:** *This is used in the management of adrenocortical (AC) insufficiency* arising from adrenal disease (**Addison disease;** primary AC insufficiency) or hypopituitarism (secondary AC insufficiency). Either may be chronic or acute.

- **Chronic adrenal insufficiency** due to Addison disease is treated with replacement doses of a glucocorticoid. *Hydrocortisone with its moderate salt retaining property is preferred;* however, prednisolone in equivalent doses can also be used. The replacement dose of hydrocortisone in Addison disease may vary from 10 to 50 mg/day. Generally, it is given in the dose of 30 mg daily, divided into two doses, 20 mg in the morning and 10 mg in the evening.
  Once the patient is regulated on hydrocortisone, addition of 9-alpha-flurohydrocortisone (0.1–0.2 mg daily) helps to complete the replacement therapy. Alternatively, the same purpose may be achieved by prescribing additional intake of salt (2–4 g per day). *Additional quantities of salt must not be prescribed to patients taking mineralocorticoids.*

  It is essential to explain to the patient that treatment of this condition is lifelong and that it is dangerous to stop it abruptly. In times of stress, the dose must be rapidly increased three- to fourfold.
- **Acute adrenal insufficiency** may arise
  i. As a result of an acute infection, injury or surgery in a previously known as Addisonian patient
  ii. Following abrupt withdrawal of glucocorticoids from a patient taking large doses

Box 64.4 Principles of Treatment of Acute Adrenal Insufficiency PH 1.1

- Hydrocortisone hemisuccinate by IV infusion, 100 mg every 4–6 h
- Dextrose in normal saline in adequate amounts
- Vasopressor drugs to maintain blood pressure
- Antibiotics: when indicated

iii. In a fulminating meningococcal infection, *which is a medical emergency requiring energetic and immediate treatment.* The principles of therapy are shown in Box 64.4.

As large doses of hydrocortisone cause sufficient salt retention, mineralocorticoids are not needed at this stage. Following recovery, 4th–5th day onwards, hydrocortisone is given orally in maintenance doses, together with 9-alpha-fluorohydrocortisone.

- **Septic shock:** Chapter 32

II. **Pharmacological therapy:**

- **Pulse therapy:** Methylprednisolone intravenously, in dose of 150–300 mg, injected over ½ h, once daily, for three consecutive days, is useful in threatened acute rejection of a renal graft, vision-threatening Graves' exophthalmos and similar dire emergencies. Methylprednisolone in similar IV doses for 3–5 days can shorten the duration of relapse, and accelerate recovery from an acute exacerbation of multiple sclerosis. *Rapid IV administration of such large doses can cause cardiac arrhythmias.* High dose oral prednisolone is probably equally effective. It is usually combined with immunosuppressive drugs (Chapters 15 and 72).
- **Intensive short-term therapy** can save life and reduce morbidity in certain potentially lethal conditions in which the inflammatory or the metabolic response of the body itself threatens life. These conditions include: allergic emergencies such as anaphylactic shock; status asthmaticus; circulatory collapse unresponsive to pressor amines; acute necrotising vasculitis; central hyperthermia and acute hypercalcaemia following vitamin D intoxication or hormone therapy of metastatic breast cancer. In hypercalcaemic crisis (Chapter 68), glucocorticoids take several days to reduce the plasma calcium and must be used along with other quicker acting measures. Glucocorticoids used as adjuncts have been shown to be effective in preventing or minimising the long-term sequelae (such as deafness) of acute bacterial meningitis.
  In all these conditions, *large doses* such as 100–200 mg (1–2 mg/kg/day) of prednisolone per day may have to be used but therapy with such doses seldom lasts longer than 48–72 h. In such cases, the adverse effects mainly consist of burning and itching at the mucocutaneous junctions, and rarely of multifocal ventricular premature beats, precipitation of ketoacidotic coma in idiopathic diabetes, and acute erosive gastritis with haemorrhage.
  Cerebral oedema: Glucocorticoids are lifesaving in cerebral oedema due to neoplasms, either primary or metastatic. Also see Chapter 37.
  Neonatal respiratory distress syndrome (prevention): Lung maturation in the fetus is influenced by fetal cortisol secretion. This may be affected by prematurity. Betamethasone is administered to pregnant women in the dose of 12 mg, to be repeated after 18–24 h (Chapter 42), to prevent neonatal respiratory distress syndrome when delivery is anticipated before the 34th week of gestation (preterm).
- **Prolonged, high-dose, suppressive therapy** is indicated in severe acute rheumatic fever, severe ulcerative colitis, coeliac disease not responding to gluten-free diet, chronic active hepatitis, alcoholic hepatitis, autoimmune haemolytic anaemia, idiopathic thrombocytopenic purpura, acute lymphatic leukaemia, disseminated Hodgkin disease, nephrotic syndrome, transplant rejection, pemphigus and collagen diseases (vascultitis and SLE). In these diseases, the initial dose may be as high as 100–200 mg of prednisolone per day, the therapy continues longer than 7–10 days and the maintenance dose may be 15 mg of prednisolone or more per day. *The likelihood of adverse reactions is utmost in this group and the patients need close supervision.* A rapid reduction in the dose can cause an acute exacerbation of the disease being treated. The abrupt cessation is dangerous and can precipitate acute adrenocortical insufficiency; the patients must be warned about this possibility.

In order to minimise the suppression of the HPA axis during such prolonged, high-dose therapy, the **alternate day regime** should be tried once the clinical improvement has stabilised; if it is unable to maintain the clinical remission, the entire daily dose may be given in the morning with the same objective in mind.

- **Low-dose, chronic, palliative therapy** consists of the use of small doses of a glucocorticoid (2–10 mg of prednisolone per day) as an adjunct to some other drug, e.g. an NSAID in RA. *Such low-dose therapy should not be tried on alternate days as it is ineffective in controlling the disease adequately.* As the therapy is generally prolonged, the patients need close supervision. The dose of the glucocorticoid should be raised 2–4 times during such stress as surgery or a severe infection.
- **Chronic, suppression of ACTH secretion** is indicated in congenital, virilising, adrenocortical hyperplasia. This is achieved with the use of a long-acting compound such as **dexamethasone or betamethasone** in the dose of 0.5 mg at bedtime daily. *It must be impressed upon the parents of such a child that the therapy must continue lifelong.*
- **Topical application** is valuable in many dermatological, ocular and external ear conditions. Ocular conditions benefited by local therapy are interstitial keratitis, phlyctenular conjunctivitis, spring catarrh, iritis and iridocyclitis, whereas posterior uveitis and sympathetic ophthalmia need systemic medication.

  Local steroid therapy See Chapter 69. *They are not recommended for urticaria or infective skin lesions.*

  Glucocorticoids accelerate the opportunistic fungal growth, and cause local skin atrophy with resultant telangiectasia, purpura and striae. *Systemic toxicity including adrenal suppression can occur following local therapy, more so in infants*; and hence, *potent preparations like betamethasone valerate, triamcinolone acetonide, fluocinolone acetonide and clobetasol propionate should not be prescribed for treating infantile eczema.* Similarly, potent steroids should not be applied to facial skin as atrophy and telangiectasia occur more quickly on the face.
- **Intra-articular and intratendinous use:** Long-acting esters of glucocorticoids have been used locally by infiltration to treat painful osteoarthritis and painful tender fascial nodules. It has the advantage of minimum systemic absorption. Such injections should not be given more than three times a year.

III. Diagnostic use of glucocorticoids:

Dexamethasone suppression test: Plasma cortisol level is measured the morning after administration of 1 mg of dexamethasone orally at 10 pm. A level of less than 5 mcg% indicates normal suppression. This test is used to establish the diagnosis and cause of Cushing syndrome.

Precautions During Corticosteroid Therapy

These apply especially to the prolonged, high dose, suppressive therapy and are listed in Box 64.5. There are no absolute contraindications to glucocorticoid therapy other than Cushing syndrome and ocular herpes zoster. Proper precautions have to be taken while using them in patients suffering from diabetes mellitus, peptic ulcer, hypertension, CHF, osteoporosis; in debilitated or old patients; and in the presence of infection.

Box 64.5 Precautions during Glucocorticoid Therapy

Before starting therapy
- Enquire about and check for: peptic ulcer, diabetes mellitus, tuberculosis, any other infection (especially one not amenable to chemotherapy)

During therapy
- Prescribe the drug with food
- Advise diet low in calories and sodium, and high in potassium
- Check periodically for: weight gain, oedema, hyperglycaemia, hypertension, infection, GI bleeding, hypokalaemia, ocular changes
- Monitor growth in children
- Instruct the patient not to stop the drug abruptly
- Increase the dose in case of any stress (severe infection, major surgery)
- Prescribe oral calcium and vitamin D supplements; alendronate (Chapter 68); antacids; H_2 receptor blockers

While stopping therapy
- Taper therapy slowly (see text)

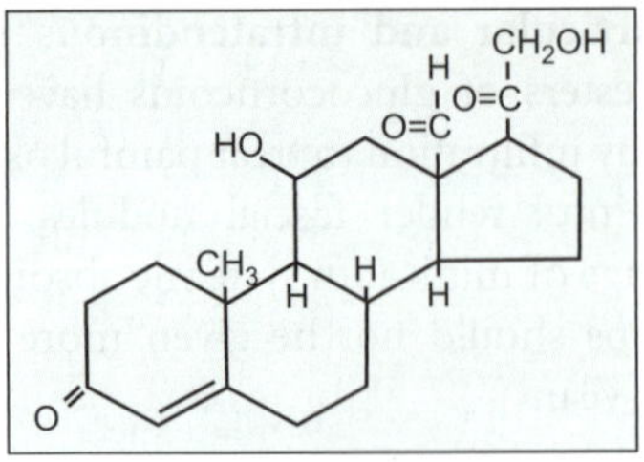

FIG. 64.6 **Aldosterone.**

PH 1.38

MINERALOCORTICOIDS: The important natural mineralocorticoids are **aldosterone** (Fig. 64.6) and **desoxycorticosterone**. They have identical effects on electrolyte and water metabolism and on cardiovascular system except that **aldosterone is 30 times more potent than desoxycorticosterone.**

Physiological and pharmacological actions:

Electrolyte and water metabolism: Physiologically, the major **stimulators of aldosterone production are angiotensin II and potassium**. Aldosterone secretion rises after consumption of foods rich in potassium and after vigorous exercise that causes release of potassium from the exercising muscle.

Aldosterone promote sodium resorption and increased excretion of potassium by the kidney, intestine and sweat and salivary glands. **On repeated administration** of aldosterone, and in patients suffering from an aldosterone producing adenoma (**primary hyperaldosteronism**) however, the subject escapes from the sodium retaining effect; potassium loss, however, continues.

The results of **aldosterone deficiency** are clearly seen in Addison disease. There is marked sodium loss with associated osmotic diuresis and a fall in plasma sodium. The extracellular fluid space contracts. Potassium excretion by the kidneys is impaired. Hyperkalaemia and acidosis add to the burden of metabolic disturbances. Increased intake of salt or administration of a mineralocorticoid corrects the above abnormalities, but the muscular weakness still remains and the patient is unable to withstand stress. *Addition of a glucocorticoid is necessary for complete correction of circulatory instability and muscular weakness in Addison disease.*

Aldosterone exerts similar effects on cellular sodium transport at other sites such as the intestines. *Furthermore, aldosterone is also produced locally by the endothelial cells and the vascular smooth muscle cells of the heart and the blood vessels.* Its production by the heart is regulated by angiotensin II (Fig. 64.7).

Cardiovascular effects: Along with angiotensin II, aldosterone also plays a role in blood coagulation, in contraction of systemic arterioles and in stimulating thirst. They are also involved in **regulating inflammatory and reparative processes** that follow tissue injury.

In congestive heart failure the excess of aldosterone (**secondary hyperaldosteronism**) can cause widespread damage. *The combination of hyperaldosteronism and an excess of sodium causes widespread periarterial fibrosis in the heart and the arterioles including the renal arterioles* (Fig. 64.7). This causes a progressive worsening of heart failure. It can be prevented by the **aldosterone antagonist spironolactone** in doses as small as 25 mg per day.

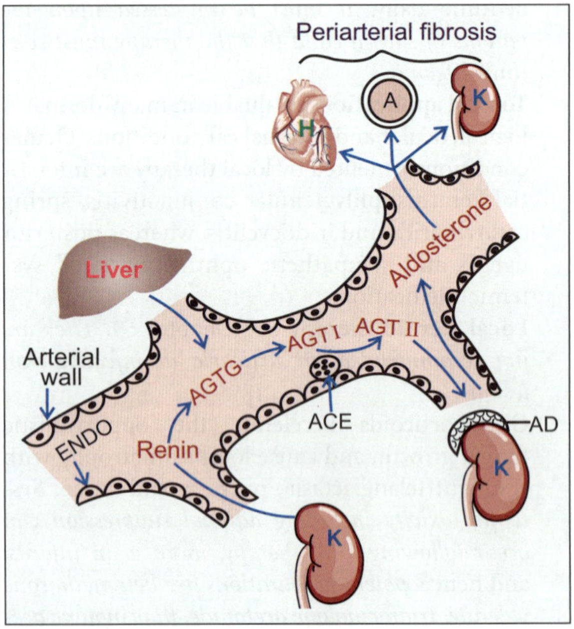

FIG. 64.7 **Pathogenesis and deleterious effects of secondary hyperaldosteronism in HF**

ENDO = Vascular endothelium K = Kidney
AGTG = Angiotensinogen AD = Adrenal gland
AGT I = Angiotensin I AGT II = Angiotensin II
ACE = Angiotensin converting enzyme H = Heart
A = Small arteries and arterioles.

Hypertension: Hypertension is a characteristic feature of primary hyperaldosteronism. Aldosterone is devoid of glucocorticoid effects.

Adverse reactions: These are related to the potent sodium retaining and potassium depleting actions and consist of weight gain, oedema, hypertension and hypokalaemia.

Preparations and dosage: Aldosterone has a transient action, so it is not used therapeutically. **9-α-Fluorohydrocortisone** (Fludrocortisone) is available as 0.1 mg. tablets. Dose: in adults: 0.05–0.30 mg daily; in children up to 12 years, 5 mcg/kg/day. The dose in patients with Addison disease is best adjusted to maintain plasma potassium (±plasma renin activity) within normal limits.

Indications: It is used in the treatment of:

- **Addison's disease** (see Therapeutic uses of glucocorticoids)
- **Salt losing congenital adrenal hyperplasia**
- **Hyporeninaemic hypoaldosteronism** as in chronic kidney disease due to diabetes mellitus and other causes
- **Severe postural hypotension from autonomic neuropathy of any aetiology**

Hyperaldosteronism

Aldosterone output may be raised in two entirely different groups of conditions:

1. **Primary hyperaldosteronism (Conn syndrome):** This is generally due to an adenoma of the adrenal cortex. The patient suffers from hypertension, hypokalaemia, polyuria, alkalosis, periodic paralysis and occasionally abnormal glucose tolerance. Oedema is rare. Serum sodium and total body sodium may remain within normal limits as the kidneys escape from the sodium retaining effects after few days.
   The treatment is essentially surgical. Spironolactone is used for preparing the patient for surgery.
2. **Secondary hyperaldosteronism:** This refers to:
   - An increased production of aldosterone in response to activation of the renin-angiotensin system or
   - Decreased metabolism of aldosterone by the damaged liver. It occurs in oedematous patients with hepatic cirrhosis, CHF and nephrotic syndrome.
     Spironolactone is used to treat these patients (Chapter 37).

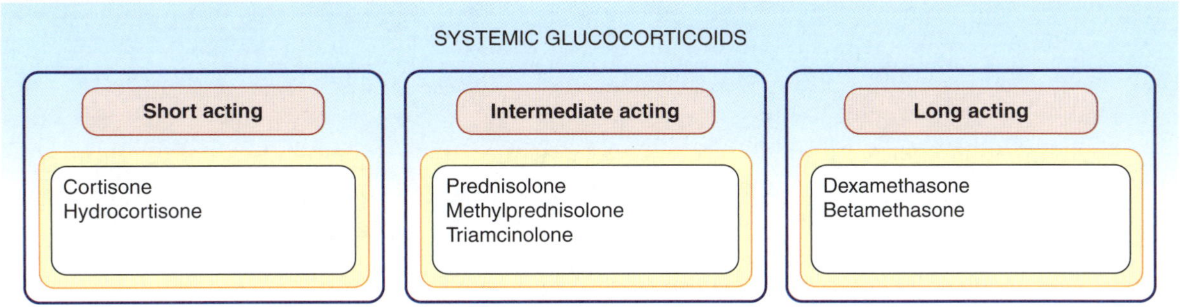

CLASSIFICATION OF TOPICAL GLUCOCORTICOIDS BASED ON POTENCY

Mild

Hydrocortisone 1%

Moderately potent

Clobetasone butyrate 0.05%
Hydrocortisone 2.5%

Potent

Betamethasone valerate 0.1%
Hydrocortisone butyrate 0.1%

Very potent

Clobetasol propionate 0.05%

CHAPTER 65

Gonadotropins, Estrogens and Progestins

Learning Objectives

This chapter will enable the reader:

1. To explain the physiology of pituitary gonadotropins.
2. To state the pharmacological actions, ADR and indications for GnRH and its analogues.
3. To mention the pharmacological actions, preparations, ADR and indications for gonadotropins.
4. To state the mechanism of action, pharmacological effects, salient pharmacokinetic features, ADR and indications for danazol.
5. To enlist the drugs causing hyperprolactinaemia.
6. To outline the pharmacotherapy of hyperprolactinaemia.
7. To be aware of the physiological actions of estrogens and progesterone.
8. To classify estrogens and progestins.
9. To describe the mechanism of action, pharmacological actions, preparations, ADR and indications for estrogens and progestins.
10. To enumerate selective estrogen receptor modulators and state their pharmacological actions and indications.
11. To state the indications, contraindications and regimens used in hormone replacement therapy.
12. To outline the management of dysfunctional uterine bleeding, dysmenorrhea, endometriosis.

KEY TERMS

Gonadotropes of the anterior pituitary secrete two distinct gonadotropic hormones *viz.*

1. **Follicle stimulating hormone** (FSH)
2. **Luteinising hormone** (LH), also known as interstitial cell stimulating hormone (ICSH)

Secretion of FSH and LH is regulated by a hypothalamic *gonadotropin releasing hormone-GnRH.*

Physiology of Pituitary Gonadotropins

The ovulation in women and spermatogenesis in men is regulated by complex interaction between the hypothalamus, the anterior pituitary and the gonadal sex steroids. This system is controlled by three feedback mechanisms:

- **Long feedback mechanism:** Gonadal sex hormones act on the hypothalamus by way of negative feedback mechanism (estrogen, progesterone, testosterone) or a positive feedback mechanism (preovulatory surge of estrogen)
- **Short feedback mechanism:** This involves a direct action of the sex hormones on the anterior pituitary, regulating the secretion of FSH and LH
- **Ultra-short negative feedback mechanism:** This comprises regulation of the hypothalamic GnRH by the pituitary FSH and LH

Dopamine formed in the nerve endings of hypothalamus is involved in the release of GnRH.

GnRH secreted in discrete pulses regulates the synthesis and secretion of both FSH and LH. Since it predominantly causes release of LH, **it is also known as LH–RH.**

The mode of action of GnRH is similar in both sexes but the secretory activities are modulated differently by estrogen, progesterone and testosterone.

The sequence of various hormonal changes that occur during a normal 28-day menstrual cycle in women is shown in Fig. 65.1. Day 1 is defined as the first day of menstrual flow. Generally, cycles between 21 and 35 days (average 28 days) are accepted as normal, the duration of menstrual flow being 2–7 days.

Pulsatile release of GnRH (LHRH) from the hypothalamus initiates a normal menstrual cycle. Ovarian follicular growth, once initiated by FSH, proceeds independently to the preovulatory phase. A rise of FSH early in the cycles is followed by a rise in blood estradiol. Under the influence of FSH alone, the follicle cells do not secrete estrogens unless a small amount of LH is also present. Most FSH-stimulated follicles undergo atresia whereas one follicle (the dominant follicle) per menstrual cycle becomes the graafian follicle. Theca and granulosa cells start expressing LH receptors under the influence of FSH. FSH stimulates the production of estradiol by granulosa cells by regulating aromatase. Various positive and negative feedback mechanisms regulate the integration of various hormones to produce the normal pattern of the menstrual cycle.

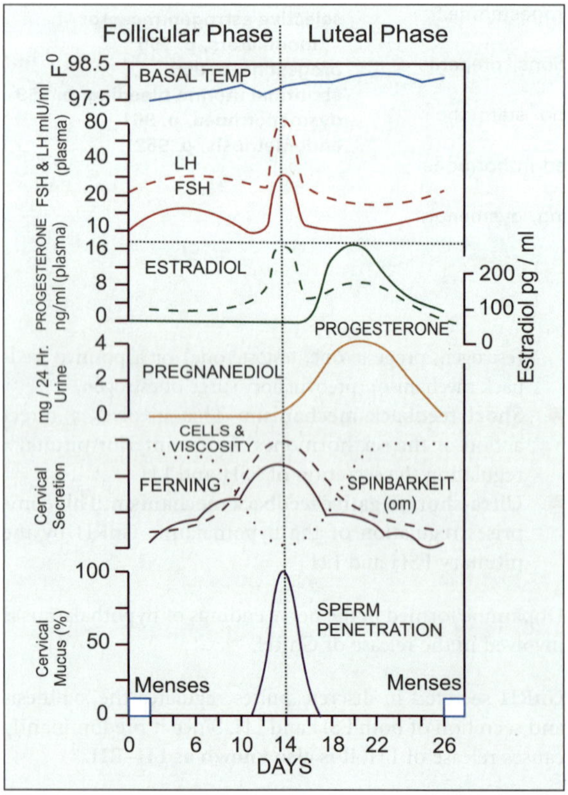

FIG. 65.1 Hormonal changes in blood and urine during the menstrual cycle in human female. Dotted line denotes the day of LH surge.

The **ovulatory peaks** of FSH and LH occur between days 11–23 of the menstrual cycle (Fig. 65.1). Abrupt increase in estradiol stimulates the pituitary gland to cause a sudden rise of LH (positive feedback). Following this large quantity of LH (**LH surge**), the follicle size increases resulting in follicular rupture and release of an ovum (**ovulation**) and the subsequent formation of **corpus luteum (CL)**.

Under the influence of FSH and LH ovary produces:

a. **estradiol, a potent estrogen, androstenedione and small amount of testosterone.** Androstenedione is the precursor of ovarian estrogens in premenopausal period. Testosterone is converted to dihydro derivative in skin and to estrogen in adipose tissue.
b. **secretes inhibin (A and B), which selectively inhibits FSH.** In addition to GnRH, the synthesis of FSH is also controlled by the gonadal peptides **inhibin** and **activin.** *Inhibition of GnRH secretion by estradiol and progesterone and selective inhibition of FSH by inhibin are critical for development of single mature oocyte.* Activin stimulates the synthesis of FSH.

LH surge suppresses the granulosa cell proliferation and triggers the release of mainly progesterone, estradiol, 17-α-hydroxy progesterone and also inhibin from CL. The lifespan of CL (supported by LH) during a nonpregnant cycle in humans averages about 11 days, whereas the functional lifespan of the CL of pregnancy is 9–10 weeks. Following conception, placental human chorionic gonadotropin (hCG) takes over the function of CL.

In case the cycle is nonpregnant, then the CL starts degenerating. Following degeneration of CL, estrogen and progesterone fall abruptly leading to menstruation. These hormonal changes before and after ovulation are associated with the characteristic **proliferative** and **secretory** changes, respectively, in the endometrium.

Although it is difficult to predict the day of ovulation in a given cycle, the reproductive cycle shows a remarkable regularity and in the majority, it is repeated every 26–30 days. What keeps the system cycling so regularly is not well understood. As progesterone is thermogenic, body temperature rises just after ovulation. However, the usual way of judging ovulation clinically by noting the rise in basal body temperature (BBT) is not so accurate.

Gonadotropic hormones stimulate the biosynthesis of sex steroids in the gonads. (Fig. 65.2). As seen in this figure progesterone is necessary for the synthesis of androgens, and androgens are obligatory precursors of estrogens.

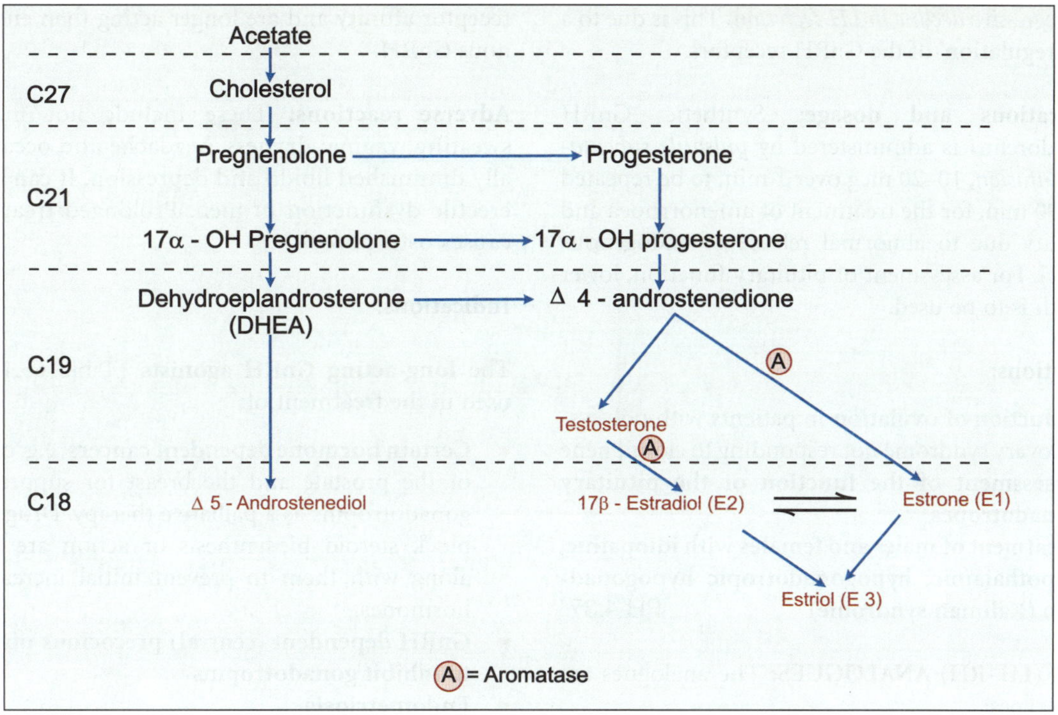

FIG. 65.2 **Biosynthesis of sex steroids in the gonads.**

The nonpregnant human female synthesises two biologically active estrogens – **estradiol (E2)** and **estrone (E1)** – and much larger amounts of prohormone estrone sulphate. The last is converted to estrone in the peripheral tissues. The third, weakly active estrogen, **estriol (E3)**, is synthesised by the placenta. The postmenopausal women have some circulating estrogen due to conversion of the adrenal androgens into estrogens in the peripheral adipose tissue.

Hypothalamo–pituitary–ovarian relationship: In addition to the **cyclical** release in relation to the menstrual cycle in women, LH is released in discrete bursts (**pulses**) every 1–2 h, separated by periods of little or no release. Similar pulsatile release is also seen in men. This is probably based on a similar, pulsatile release of GnRH from the hypothalamus. The intermittent release of a hormone permits the regeneration of its receptors in the end organ and maintenance of their sensitivity to the concerned hormone. The secretion of pituitary LH and FSH is regulated by the interaction between the sex steroids and hypothalamic GnRH.

Pharmacological doses of an estrogen exert only a negative feedback on the pituitary, causing inhibition of gonadotropin release in a dose dependent manner. PH 1.37

GnRH (LH–RH): GnRH is a decapeptide and is also found in human placenta. Placental GnRH may be involved in the synthesis and release of hCG. Its plasma t½ is 2–8 min.

The main function of GnRH is the promotion of synthesis and release of LH and FSH from the anterior pituitary. The relative amounts of FSH and LH released are related to the puberal status of the individual. *Prior to the onset of puberty, FSH is the predominantly released gonadotropin, whereas after puberty it is LH which is predominantly released.* Given in an intermittent, *pulsatile* manner, GnRH increases the responsiveness of the pituitary gonadotropes to GnRH itself. *This self-priming effect is not observed following a continuous GnRH infusion, which results in an initial increase for a short time, followed by a sustained and progressive decline in LH secretion.* This is due to a '**downregulation**' of the GnRH receptors.

Preparations and dosage: Synthetic GnRH (Gonadorelin) is administered by *pulsatile subcutaneous infusion*, 10–20 mcg over 1 min, to be repeated every 90 min, for the treatment of amenorrhoea and infertility due to abnormal release of endogenous LH–RH. For assessment of pituitary function, lower strength is to be used.

Indications:

- **Induction of ovulation** in patients with polycystic ovary syndrome not responding to clomiphene
- **Assessment of the function of the pituitary gonadotropes**
- **Treatment of males and females with idiopathic, hypothalamic, hypogonadotropic hypogonadism (Kallman syndrome)** PH 1.37

GnRH (LH–RH) ANALOGUES: The analogues are of two types:

I. **Agonists**
II. **Antagonists**

I. The **agonists** bind to the GnRH receptors on the pituitary gonadotropes. *Prolonged receptor occupation during their continuous use causes their down-regulation and reduces gonadal secretion.* The agonists enhance the release of gonadotropins initially; this is a disadvantage in the treatment of the hormone dependent cancers.

GnRH analogues are administered subcutaneously/intramuscularly and by nasal spray. They have higher receptor affinity and are longer acting than endogenous GnRH.

Adverse reactions: These include hot flushes, sweating, vaginal dryness, headache and occasionally diminished libido and depression. It can cause erectile dysfunction in men. Prolonged treatment causes osteoporosis.

Indications:

The **long-acting GnRH agonists** (Table 65.1) are used in the treatment of:

- **Certain hormone dependent cancers,** e.g. cancer of the prostate and the breast for suppressing gonadotropins as a palliative therapy. Drugs that block steroid biosynthesis or action are given along with them to prevent initial increase in hormones.
- **GnRH dependent (central) precocious puberty to inhibit gonadotropins**
- **Endometriosis**
- **Large uterine fibroids, priapism, acute intermittent porphyria:** These are steroid responsive conditions. GnRH analogues suppress steroid responses.
- **IVF regimens, as an adjunct to GnRH,** in order to inhibit untimely release of LH and ovulation

They are all very expensive.

II. The **GnRH antagonists** act by competitive inhibition of the binding of endogenous GnRH to the GnRH receptors and suppress the release of LH and FSH. Unlike agonists, they do not cause release of gonadotropins and sex steroidal

Table 65.1 Some Clinically Used GnRH Agonists

Name	Potency	Half-Life (min)	Dose and Mode of Administration
GnRH (gonadorelin)	1	5	See text
Leuprorelin acetate (Leuprolide)	15	180–220	3.75 mg SC/IM monthly
Buserelin acetate	20	75–85	300 mcg/day, in divided doses, intranasally; or 1 mg SC daily
Nafarelin	150	120–160	200–400 mcg intranasally
Triptorelin microspheres	144	480	3.75 mg deep IM monthly
Goserelin acetate polymer	100	120–240	3.6 mg SC monthly
Histrelin	150–200	240	50 mg SC implant per year

production. They are more expensive They often act as releasers of histamine.

Ganirelix and **cetrorelix** are GnRH antagonists, which are claimed to cause less histamine release than the other antagonists. Currently, they are used subcutaneously during IVF regimen to suppress LH surge and premature ovulation. **Elagolix** is an oral GnRH antagonist, approved for management of endometriosis.

Degarelix acetate suppresses testosterone and PSA and is used to treat advanced prostate cancer. It is injected subcutaneously on the abdomen, where it forms a depot gel. The release occurs from the site with t½ of 42 days.

GONADOTROPINS

PH 1.37

All the gonadotropins are glycoproteins. They have different plasma half-lives and undergo metabolic degradation by plasma proteases. The gonadotropins available for human therapy are as follows:

1. **Human chorionic gonadotropin (hCG)**
2. **Human menopausal urinary gonadotropin (hMG)**
3. **Purified gonadotropins**

HUMAN CHORIONIC GONADOTROPIN (hCG): This glycoprotein hormone of pregnancy is secreted by the trophoblasts and later by the placenta. *It can be detected in the maternal plasma several days before the first missed period.* Sufficient amounts of it is absorbed into the blood and interacts with LH receptors on CL to sustain the luteal function of steroid hormone synthesis until the placenta starts secreting estrogen and progesterone by the 3rd month of pregnancy.

Besides the placenta, certain tumours secrete hCG. Its serial estimation is valuable for monitoring therapy and detecting tumour recurrence.

Pharmacological actions: Like pituitary LH, *small doses of hCG can preserve the CL and prolong the secretory phase of the menstrual cycle.* This is associated with an increased urinary excretion of pregnanediol. The hCG can induce a decidual reaction in the endometrium even in the absence of conception (pseudo-pregnancy).

Injected into the males, hCG stimulates the interstitial cells of the testes to secrete androgen.

Adverse reactions: These include headache, oedema, gynaecomastia and occasionally depression. It may cause gynaecomstia in males due to induction of aromatase.

Preparation and dosage:

i. hCG 1500 IU, 5,000 IU, with 10 mL of diluent; intramuscularly or subcutaneously
ii. Choriogonadotropin alpha: is a recombinant hCG; 250 mcg/0.5 mL; subcutaneously depending on patient's response

Indications:

- **Ovulation induction:** hCG therapy can induce ovulation in an adequately developed follicle following endogenous FSH or exogenous hMG, leading to conception (see Chapter 66)

- **Cryptorchism:** Cryptorchism denotes failure of the testes to descend into the scrotum. hCG is used to promote this descent. It is given in doses of 3000–5000 IU / sq m body surface area every other day for 6 doses. If descent does not occur, orchidopexy is indicated. The treatment should be initiated as early as 1–2 years of age. The hormone should not be used if mechanical obstruction is present.

- **Delayed puberty in boys:** This is treated with 500–1000 IU of hCG 3 times a week for 4 weeks, repeated, if necessary, after several months. Once initiated, the puberty progresses without further treatment.

- **Testing the responsiveness of the immature testes to gonadotropins:** A level of 2 ng/mL of testosterone is considered a normal response following 5000 IU of hCG. It confirms the presence of testicular tissue when the testes are not palpable and detectable by imaging techniques.

- **Treatment of hypogonadotropic hypogonadism:** For this purpose, 2000 IU are injected 2–3 times a week for prolonged periods. Enlargement of the testes and development of secondary sex characters are stimulated. Addition of hMG or recombinant FSH (150 IU) may be necessary for inducing spermatogenesis.

- **Treatment of luteal phase defect:** hCG may be used to support the production of adequate amounts of progesterone in the luteal phase of the menstrual cycle in patients with luteal phase defect. Alternatively, progesterone has been used to supply the deficient hormone.

OTHER GONADOTROPINS: Human menopausal urinary gonadotropin (hMG, Menotropins) is prepared from the urine of menopausal women and is available in ampoules containing 75 IU of FSH and equal amounts of LH and is given intramuscularly. Purified gonadotropins include **urofollitropin**, which has low LH and **recombinant FSH** preparations. These are given subcutaneously.

Preparations:

i. Menotropins, purified preparation containing both FSH and LH and is injected intramuscularly
ii. *Purified* FSH preparation (**Metrodin** HP, devoid of LH activity) is injected intramuscularly or subcutaneously
iii. **Follitropin** α and **follitropin** β as rDNA monocomponent FSH products administered either intramuscularly or subcutaneously
iv. Recombinant LH preparation **lutropin** α is monocomponent, administered intramuscularly/subcutaneously

Adverse reactions: The main complication of this therapy is **hyperstimulation syndrome** after hCG injection. The ovaries become very large and friable due to maturation of many follicles. This causes abdominal pain, nausea and vomiting. If the friable ovary ruptures into the abdomen, the patient may develop ascites and shock.

Indications:

i. **Therapeutic uses**

- Gonadotropins are used, along with hCG to induce ovulation in women with anovulation due to
  a) *pituitary–hypothalamic disorders but with normal ovaries and*
  b) *polycystic ovaries*

Various regimens have been used with monitoring of the follicular growth by ultrasonography and plasma estradiol levels. Generally, the regimes involve daily injections of FSH and LH starting on day 2 or 3 of the menstrual cycle. When two or three follicles increase in diameter size by 16–18 mm as seen on transvaginal ultrasound, 5000–10,000 IU of hCG IM is administered to induce ovulation followed by intrauterine insemination and/or natural intercourse 24–36 h later. Ovulation can be successfully induced in 90% of selected cases, and pregnancy occurs in about 50%; of these, 20% end in abortion and multiple births may occur in 20%–30%. Such regimen can also be used in IVF technique. The growth and development of children so born have been normal.

- hMG has also been used with variable success in males with idiopathic oligospermia

ii. **Diagnostic Uses**

- **Detection of pregnancy:** Qualitative assay of hCG is done using antibodies specific for beta subunit of hCG as available in pregnancy kit. It detects pregnancy within a few days after the first missed menstrual period. Quantitative assay measures plasma hCG levels as used to detect the presence of an ectopic pregnancy, hydatidiform mole, or choriocarcinoma. It is also used to detect response to therapy of germ cell carcinoma, which secrets hCG.
- **Detection of ovulation:** To optimise conception, LH surge (and the ovulation) is detected by measuring urinary LH levels every 12-24 hrs starting from day 10-12 of menstrual cycle
- **Detection of endocrine diseases:** Hypogonadotropic hypogonadism is diagnosed if FSH and LH levels are low or undetectable whereas gonadal disorder is suspected with high levels. High FSH level is also used to confirm menopause.

PLACENTAL LACTOGEN

This somatotropic hormone has structural similarity to GH and PRL (190 amino acids). It is synthesized in placenta and levels are highest near term. It decreases insulin sensitivity in mothers and increases maternal blood glucose levels to facilitate the supply to the fetus. Its elevated levels are associated with gestational diabetes whereas low levels are associated with maternal obesity and fetal growth retardation.

ANTIGONADOTROPIC COMPOUNDS PH 1.37

DANAZOL: This is a synthetic derivative of ethisterone.

1. It has **antigonadotropic activity** but no estrogenic or progestational properties. Thus, in normal women it **eliminates the midcycle LH and FSH surge by acting as a selective pituitary gonadotropin inhibitor**; and in postmenopausal women it prevents the compensatory increase in FSH and LH.
2. Peripherally, it binds to androgen (partial agonist), progesterone and glucocorticoid receptors; thus it has some **androgenic and anabolic effects.**
3. It also directly inhibits the ovarian enzymes involved in the **estrogen synthesis**. Danazol, thus, induces a hypoestrogenic–hypoprogestational state. Complete ovarian suppression occurs only with doses of 600 mg or more per day; at lower doses its other actions may predominate.

Absorption, fate and excretion: It is well absorbed and is extensively metabolised in the liver; the metabolites are excreted in the urine. Its elimination t½ is about 4–5 h. **Therapeutic effect starts after 4 weeks.**

Adverse reactions: These are as follows:

- **Androgenic and anabolic**, such as weight gain, acne, hirsutism and voice change
- **Hypoestrogenic,** such as hot flushes, atrophic vaginitis and mental depression
- **Other effects:** Muscle cramps, rash, benign intracranial hypertension, altered hepatic and lipid metabolism

Indications:

- **Endometriosis:** See under the Section, Indications for Progestins
- **Benign fibrocystic breast disease:** See under the Section, Indications for Progestins
- **Gynaecomastia**
- **Menorrhagia** (See under the section, Indications for Progestins, Abnormal uterine bleeding)
- **Hereditary angioedema**
- **Idiopathic thrombocytopenic purpura**

Gestrinone is an analogue of danazol for the treatment of endometriosis.

ESTROGENS

Estrogens are produced mainly by the ovary and the placenta; small amounts may be produced by the adrenals and testes. Estrogens are also present in various plants and seeds. *The natural estrogens are steroids.* However, typical estrogenic activity is also shown by chemicals which are not steroids. Hence, the term 'estrogen' is used as a generic term to describe all the compounds having an estrogenic activity.

The pituitary gonadotropins regulate the production of the ovarian steroids. LH stimulates the production of *androstenedione and testosterone* by the theca cells of the ovarian follicles. These two androgens are taken up by the adjacent granulosa cells of the ovarian follicles. *Under the influence of FSH, the granulosa cells proliferate and express aromatase (CYP19A1) which converts the androgens into estrogens – estrone and estradiol.* The liver converts circulating estradiol to estrone. Both estradiol and estrone get converted to estriol (Fig. 65.2). The adipose tissue also contains aromatase which converts the circulating androgens (dehydroepiandrosterone secreted by the adrenals) into estrogens (estrone), and is the main source of estrogen in postmenopausal women. *Locally produced estrogens from androgens by aromatase or from estrogen conjugates by hydrolysis play a role in breast cancer.* Local production from androgen also occurs in brain, bone and placenta.

Physiological actions: It:

- **Promotes development of female reproductive tract** (uterus, fallopian tubes and vagina)
- **Promotes development of female secondary sex characters,** such as breasts (ductal growth), body contours, axillary and pubic hair, pigmentation of genital region, and voice. They are also responsible for the psychological and emotional get up typical of femininity.

- **Promotes the pubertal growth spurt and union of the epiphyses with the metaphyses** thus controlling the height. *The epiphyseal fusion is accelerated following the onset of menarche and once fused, no further increase in height can occur.*
- **Stimulates the proliferative or preovulatory phase of endometrium** and induces progesterone receptors. It increases proliferation and differentiation of Fallopian tube epithelium. It increases tubal muscle contractility and favours rhythmic contraction of myometrium. It increases cervical mucus and its water content.
- **Causes vasodilatation of capillaries** in general and those of the endometrium in particular by stimulating vascular endothelial growth factor and placental growth factor. It causes uterine artery remodelling in pregnancy.
- **Induces metabolic effects** such as retention of nitrogen, sodium and fluid in tissues
- **Exerts cardioprotection** in women of the reproductive age; this is mediated by maintenance of the LDL levels at a lower level than in males favouring higher HDL to LDL ratio. Menopausal women lose this protective influence, leading to increased incidence of IHD.
- **Maintains the integrity of the skeleton in women of reproductive age** and increases bone mass. Following menopause women suffer from osteoporosis.
- **Supports pregnancy and parturition** by inducing favourable changes in the endometrium, vaginal and cervical mucosa and uterine growth and contraction. It causes pigmentation of the nipples and areolae.
- **Role in male development:** Estrogen deficiency in men is associated with delayed skeletal maturation, epiphyseal closure, reduced pubertal growth spurts and macroorchidism

Classification of Estrogens PH 1.37

I. **Natural estrogens:** estradiol (Fig. 65.3), estrone and estriol and their esters
II. **Semisynthetic estrogens**, e.g. ethinylestradiol
III. **Synthetic estrogens:**
   a. **Those which are steroids**, e.g. mestranol
   b. **Those which are not steroids but derivatives of diphenylethylene** (stilbene), e.g. stilbestrol **and triphenylethylene**, e.g. chlorotrianisene (TACE) (Fig. 66.1)

Stilbestrol and chlorotrianisene are sometimes used only to treat carcinoma of the prostate (Chapter 59).

All the estrogenic compounds produce similar pharmacological actions and hence, are discussed together.

Mechanism of action: estrogens **bind to the nuclear estrogen receptors** in estrogen responsive tissues. The steroid–receptor complex undergoes conformational change and binds to the estrogen responsive element (ERE) located on the target gene, where it brings about changes in transcription. There are **two types of estrogen receptors:**

1. **ERα,** present in the female genital tract, ovarian theca cells, breasts, hypothalamus, endothelial cells and vascular smooth muscle
2. **ERβ,** present in bone, brain, prostate and ovarian granulosa cell

In addition there is a membrane localised G protein-coupled estrogen receptor, GPER, which is responsible for some physiological functions.

> *The vascular actions of estrogen do not require gene activation and are mediated by the membrane receptors.*

Pharmacological actions: These drugs, when used as **substitution therapy**, produce actions similar to the physiological actions of natural estrogens.

Endometrial effects: In women with deficient ovarian function, estrogens produce **proliferative changes** in the endometrium. Following these changes, withdrawal of estrogens causes menstrual flow known as *withdrawal bleeding.* This obviously cannot be compared with the natural menstruation where progesterone withdrawal plays an important

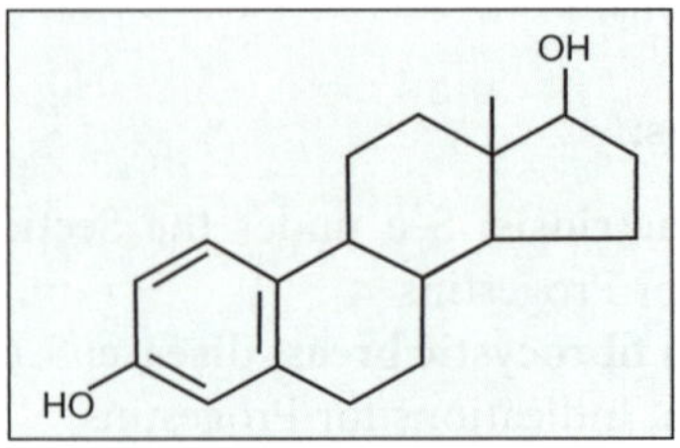

FIG. 65.3 **Estradiol.**

role. With very small doses irregular bleeding can occur even without the interruption of the drug (*breakthrough bleeding*).

Vaginal effects: Estrogens are responsible to maintain the vaginal lining integrity and flexibility. Vaginal secretions are increased having a lubricating effect. Estrogens also cause increase in vaginal pH.

Gonadotropin inhibition: Continuous administration of estrogens suppresses the secretion of FSH and also of midcycle LH surge resulting in inhibition of ovulation. In males, it inhibits spermatogenesis. The testes may undergo atrophic changes and the secretion of androgen is reduced.

Administration of estrogens, however, even in large doses, after the ovulation, does not alter the course of normal menstrual cycle.

Suppression of lactation: Estrogens suppress lactation without affecting prolactin levels.

Metabolic actions: They have a weak anabolic action. They may cause sodium and water retention. Estrogens reduce the level of plasma cholesterol but increase that of triglycerides. They promote urate reabsorption by the proximal renal tubule.

Large doses of estrogens given to children for long periods inhibit the growth of epiphyseal cartilage, and may cause epiphyseal fusion.

Effects on bones: Estrogens have a positive effect on the bone mass which is mediated by complex actions. Osteoblasts and osteoclasts express both ERα and ERβ. The former play a major role.

1. Estrogen directly **regulates the osteoblasts** and **brings about their differentiation**
2. It **increases the osteoblast and osteocyte survival** by inhibiting their apoptosis
3. The major effect is to **decrease the number and activity of the osteoclasts** either directly or through a cytokine osteoprotegerin (OPG). Estrogen prevents differentiation of osteoclast precursors into osteoclasts; and increases osteoclast apoptosis. This results in prevention of bone resorption by the osteoclasts.

Carcinogenic effects: Estrogens are carcinogenic in animals, and are implicated in the genesis of cancers of the breast, endometrium, liver and vagina in women (see Adverse reactions of estrogens and Chapter 66).

Antiandrogenic effects: Estrogens are beneficial in androgen-dependent prostatic cancer (Chapter 59).

Absorption, fate and excretion: Both the natural and synthetic estrogens can get absorbed through the skin and the mucous membranes and can cause systemic effects. Given orally, estrogens are well absorbed but the natural estrogens are not so effective as they are metabolised during their passage through the liver (first pass). Enterohepatic circulation of estrogens does occur.

Estradiol gets converted by 17β-hydroxysteroid dehydrogenase to estrone, which is further biotransformed to estriol, which is a major urinary metabolite. Ethinyl estradiol is slowly tmetabolised and its t½ is 13–27 h. About 10% of the dose is recoverable in faeces; the fate of the remaining is unknown. Liver plays an important role in the conjugation of steroidal estrogens. *Nonsteroidal estrogens such as diethylstilbestrol are not metabolised so easily and hence a large fraction of them is excreted in urine in free state.*

Estrogen esters, like valerate and cypionate when injected, are absorbed slowly and are effective for several days or weeks.

Adverse reactions: These are as follows:

1. Following **physiological doses** in hormone replacement therapy (HRT)
2. Following **pharmacological doses** as in oral contraceptives (see Chapter 66)

- **Small doses as in HRT** may cause nausea, vomiting and anorexia. These are similar to those occurring in pregnancy. They can be minimised by taking the drug with food or at bedtime. Sodium and water retention can cause oedema, and fullness and tenderness of the breasts. Intermittent vaginal bleeding may occur in some women on HRT. Any active ectopic endometrial tissue (endometriosis) and uterine fibroids can undergo deterioration during this therapy. Uncontrolled hypertension and migraine may worsen.

HRT does not cause a deterioration of glucose tolerance. It lowers the plasma levels of LDL and of total plasma cholesterol, while increasing those of plasma HDL. It causes only minimal elevation of the binding proteins (thyroxine binding protein, corticosteroid binding protein, sex hormone binding protein and renin substrate).

HRT is not contraindicated in women with diabetes mellitus, controlled hypertension or varicose veins. *It is unsafe in patients with CHD, TIA or stroke and in those with history of it.*

- **Prolonged, unopposed, estrogen therapy** *increases the risk of endometrial cancer by 5-15 fold. Progestin component in HRT increases the risk of breast cancer significantly. Estrogens promote coagulation and thromboembolic events. In older postmenopausal women treated with conjugated estrogens, increased risk of heart disease and stroke have been reported.* It has recently been suggested that HRT in postmenopausal woman can increase the incidence of ovarian cancer, in the female offspring of such women. *The use of 'synthetic' nonsteroidal estrogens for other purposes than prostate cancers is now obsolete.*
- **Pharmacological doses of estrogens administered to prepuberal girls** can cause:
  - a. Premature breast enlargement (thelarche): and precocious puberty
  - b. Stunting of linear growth of the long bones and hence of final height by accelerating the closure of the epiphysial plate

Preparations and dosage:

- **Natural estrogens and their esters:**
  - i. Estradiol 100 mcg, 650 mcg, 1 mg, 2 mg, 3 mg tablets tablets
  - ii. Estradiol, micronised, 0.5 mg, 1 mg, 2 mg tablets for oral use. For IM use, it is available as injection 1 mg/mL.
  - iii. Estradiol valerate, 1 and 2 mg tablets
  - iv. Estradiol patch: These are self-adhesive, estradiol patches, releasing 25, 37.5, 40, 50, 80 or 100 mcg of estradiol per 24 h for 3–4 days. They should not be applied near the breasts for fear of causing breast cancer.
  - v. Estradiol gel containing 500 mcg/g or 600 mcg/g, or 1 mg/g, to be applied to arms
  - vi. Estradiol topical emulsion 2.5 mg/g. Two foil pouches (3.48 grams daily) to be applied on the thigh and calf; provide systemic delivery of 0.05 mg of estradiol per day.
  - vii. Estradiol implant, 25 mg
  - viii. Estradiol vaginal tab 10 mcg, 25 mcg It is also available as softgel vaginal inserts - 4 mcg and 10 mcg
  - ix. Estriol succinate 2 mg tablets and *vaginal cream* (0.1%)
- **Semisynthetic steroidal estrogens:**
  - i. Ethinylestradiol tablets 0.002, 0.01, and 0.05 mg. In the treatment of prostatic cancer the dose recommended is 1–2 mg daily.
  - ii. Mestranol, the 3-methyl ether of ethinylestradiol, is a **prodrug,** converted to ethinylestradiol.
- **Conjugated equine estrogens:** This preparation is a mixture of numerous water soluble conjugated estrogens, mainly esters of estrone, equilin and other naturally occurring compounds, obtained from pregnant mares' urine. They are available as tablets, as an SC injection and as vaginal cream.
- **Synthetic conjugated estrogens:** Formulation containing mixture of estrogens produced from plants are available. They are water soluble, well absorbed in the GI tract and are metabolised in the liver. Their precautions, adverse effects and contraindications are similar to those of other estrogen preparations. It is used, for short-term treatment of vasomotor symptoms of menopause.
- **Synthetic nonsteroidal estrogens:** Diethylstilbestrol tablet contains 1, 5 and 25 mg. For prostate cancer: 1–3 mg/day and for breast cancer: 10–25 mg/day (Chapter 59).
- **Cosmetic preparations:** Topical preparations containing physiological amounts of estrogens or natural progesterone have been promoted as cosmetic, 'rejuvenating' creams. There is no evidence that the hormone creams are more effective than

simple emollients in relieving the dryness of the skin or in improving the facial appearance. Excessive use can cause systemic toxicity.

TIBOLONE: This synthetic steroid is a prodrug and *undergoes tissue-selective conversion to 3 metabolites that have estrogenic, progestogenic or mildly androgenic activity*. Its precautions and contraindications are similar to those of the standard estrogenic preparations. In the dose of 2.5 mg (one tablet) daily, it is used in the treatment of:

- **Vasomotor symptoms and prophylaxis of osteoporosis in menopausal women.** It is given continuously and concurrent administration of a progestin is not necessary.
- **Vasomotor symptoms in premenopausal women** who are being treated with a GnRH analogue

Its superiority over the standard estrogenic preparations is not established. It is expensive.

Indications for estrogen: The preparations commonly employed are as follows:

1. **For pharmacological therapy:** Ethinylestradiol and mestranol
2. **For replacement therapy:** Conjugated estrogens, estriol and estradiol.

Their therapeutically equipotent doses are shown in Box 65.1. Transdermal, nasal sprays and vaginal preparations are also available. Parenteral preparations are now rarely used.

- **Amenorrhoea:** Amenorrhoea may be (a) **primary** due to failure of establishment of menstruation or (b) **secondary,** which occurs after the menstruation is established.

Box 65.1 Therapeutically Equivalent Daily Doses of Estrogens

- Ethinylestradiol (oral) 5–10 mcg
- Conjugated estrogens (oral) 0.625 mg
- Micronised estradiol (oral) 1 mg
- Estradiol (oral) 2 mg
- Estradiol (transdermal) 50 mcg

a. ***Primary amenorrhoea (replacement therapy):*** Hypogonadism is diagnosed when a girl without any abnormality of the genital tract does not start menstruating by the age of 18 years. Such patients will need **hormone replacement therapy** (HRT).
The commonest cause of **primary hypogonadism** is gonadal dysgenesis (Turner syndrome) due to a sex chromosome abnormality. Most of such patients are short, in addition to being sexually infantile.
In *patients who are not short*, replacement treatment is started with low dose ethinyl estradiol 5 mcg or conjugated estrogens 0.3 mg per day. After 3-6 months the dose is increased (ethinyl estradiol 20 mcg/day or conjugated estrogen 0.9-1.25 mg/day). This is continued till the first vaginal bleeding (usually spotting) occurs; breasts start developing during that period. Progestin such as medroxyprogesterone 10mg/day is added for 12 days each cycle to optimise breast development and permit menses. Once this is achieved, the patient is prescribed either:
    i. A low-dose combined oral contraceptive pill (see Chapter 66), for 21 days every month; or
    ii. Conjugated estrogens 0.625 mg daily, without a break, plus a progestin (medroxyprogesterone 10 mg per day) for 10 days in every month.

The advantages of adding a progestin are:
a. Better breast development
b. More complete shedding of the stimulated endometrium every month
c. Prevention of endometrial cancer. However the protection is not complete.

In patients with **gonadal dysgenesis** *who are short*, treatment should begin with ethinylestradiol (100 ng/kg/day, uninterruptedly) at about the age of 12 years. *Therapy with larger, feminising doses (10 mcg and more) of ethinyl estradiol should be initiated only after the linear growth comes to a halt.* These patients may need initiation with growth hormone and androgen like oxandrolone, followed by estrogen.
Females with **secondary hypogonadism** are treated in an identical manner as those with

primary hypogonadism; but they may require replacement therapy with other hormones thyroxine and hydrocortisone.

b. ***Secondary amenorrhoea:*** The cause, if found, needs to be treated in addition to the hormone treatment. If the patient is **hypoestrogenic,** she needs hormone replacement as described above. If she desires to become pregnant, ovulation inducing drugs may have to be used.

- **Menopausal symptoms:** With age, the ovarian function decreases and finally ceases, resulting in menopause. The menstrual irregularity and sometimes excessive blood loss, observed just prior to the menopause, is due to anovulatory cycles and can be treated by cyclic administration of progestins. Menopausal changes include vasomotor disturbances, sweating, irritability, sleep disturbances, and atrophy of estrogen-dependent tissues such as vulva and vagina.

Mild cases with menopausal hot flushes (feeling of hot flashes and redness on face) and genitourinary symptoms need only proper explanation of the natural physiological process, reassurance and perhaps a tranquilliser for short term. Estrogen therapy is with minimum dose and for minimum duration. Hot flushes and genitourinary symptoms respond to oral estriol (in the dose of up to 3 mg/day), which has no other estrogenic effects. It can be used without concurrent administration of a progestin. Patients with symptoms due to urogenital atrophy without systemic symptoms of estrogen deficiency do well with **topical estrogen.** Local application includes the following:

i. Vaginal estrogen cream – 0.1 mg estradiol/g or 0.625 mg conjugated estrogens/g; or
ii. Vaginal tablet – 0.01/0.025 mg estradiol; or
iii. Vaginal ring – 0.0075/0.05/0.1 mg estradiol/day.
iv. **Prasterone** a steroid vaginal insert is used for moderate to severe dyspareunia. However, cervical Pap smears may show abnormality following its use.

They are expensive. Vaginal estrogens cause less systemic adverse effects. Oral therapy includes conjugated estrogens, E+P tablets or ospemifene.

Estrogen is absorbed from the vaginal mucosa and may rarely produce systemic effects. Gynaecomastia has been reported in the sexual partners of women using vaginal creams.

Patients with more troublesome symptoms need short term oral estrogen replacement treatment. *Patients with intact uterus who are on systemic estrogens should be given progestin so as to reduce the risk of possible endometrial carcinoma.* Antidepressants and vaginal lubricants are useful as adjunctive treatment.

If estrogen is contraindicated for any reason, medroxyprogesterone or clonidine may be used to relieve vasomotor symptoms.

- As **Hormone replacement therapy** (**HRT**) has been advocated to treat menopausal symptoms and to prevent the long term complications (e.g. osteoporosis, bone fractures, IHD, increased memory loss and cognitive decline), starting in the perimenopausal period.

HRT regimens in menopausal women refer Box 65.2.

Estrogens are potent inhibitors of osteoclastic bone resorption and are most efficacious for prevention of fractures rather than restoring bone loss. However, that they reduce fracture rate has not been established.

Long-term studies clearly indicate that HRT increases the risk of endometrial and breast cancer, venous thromboembolism, gall bladder disease and possibly that of coronary heart disease (CHD), stroke and dementia. Thus, its disadvantages outweigh whatever small benefits it offers. Hence, **HRT should not be used routinely to treat menopause, a natural phenomenon.** Its use is now restricted to women with severe menopausal symptoms and that too treated with smallest possible dose for limited period (5 years or less).

Before starting long term HRT, the patient should be examined for any contraindication to such therapy (Box 65.3). She should be told what to expect as a result of the treatment including a possible risk of developing breast cancer. She is advised to report any untoward symptoms,

Box 65.2 HRT Regimens for Menopausal Women

In women with intact uterus

- Conjugated estrogens 0.625 mg or an equivalent amount of another estrogen preparation (5-10mcg ethinyl estradiol) daily for 25 days out of every month plus medroxyprogesterone acetate (MPA) 10 mg daily for the last 10 days of the estrogen cycle[a] followed by no hormone therapy for 5-6 days
- Estrogen (as above) daily, uninterruptedly *plus* MPA (as above) 10 days every month.

  The above two regimens are associated with a return of monthly menstrual bleeding, which is unacceptable to most women
- Ethinylestradiol 20 mcg and norethisterone 350 mcg daily, both given without interruption. This regimen causes endometrial atrophy and may be associated with frequent breakthrough bleeding, especially during the first 6 months of therapy

In women who have had hysterectomy

- Estrogen as above, given continuously

[a]Norethisterone 1 mg, levonorgestrel 150–250 mcg, or dehydrogesterone 10–20 mg may be used in place of MPA. Combination preparations which may be used for the same purpose are: Estradiol valerate 2 mg plus levonorgestrel 75 mcg and conjugated estrogens 0.625 mg plus levonorgestrel 75 mcg.

especially vaginal bleeding. Regular, periodic monitoring, including breast examination, every 6–12 months, when on HRT is mandatory.

- **As contraceptives:** See Chapter 66
- **Vulvo-vaginitis in children:** In this condition, the infection persists because of alkaline vaginal pH at this age and the columnar epithelium both of which are not hostile to the growth of pathogens. Following estrogen therapy, the vaginal epithelium cornifies with the deposition of glycogen. The glycogen is converted into lactic acid by the *Doderlein bacilli,* resulting in acidic pH, which prevents growth of bacteria.
- **Acute severe dysfunctional uterine bleeding:** Conjugated, equine estrogen 20 mg given IV every 4 h for 4–6 doses are occasionally used in this condition. Bleeding usually ceases in 4–24 h.
- **Endometriosis:** in form of combined oral contraceptives
- **Prostatic cancer:** See Chapter 59
- **Hirsutism:** See Chapter 67
- **Miscellaneous uses:** Estrogens can be used for treatment of acne in women (Chapter 69)

Box 65.3 Contraindications to HRT in Menopausal Women

- Unexplained vaginal bleeding
- Endometrial or breast carcinoma
- Family history of carcinoma of breast
- Active endometriosis (unopposed estrogen)
- Chronic impairment of liver function
- Familial hypertriglyceridemia; serum triglyceride above 250 mg/dL
- Uncontrolled hypertension
- Any evidence of cardiovascular pathology
- Seizure disorder
- Recent thrombophlebitis
- Unreliable subject

Phytoestrogens

Phytoestrogens are nonsteroidal compounds such as isoflavones and lignans present in plants such as soy, flaxseeds, red clover and cohosh; they are converted in the intestines to compounds with 1/10,000th the estrogenic activity of estradiol. Some of them also have anti-estrogenic activity. Phytoestrogens have been commercially promoted for use in postmenopausal women for prevention of osteoporosis, breast cancer and IHD. The evidence in their favour is largely epidemiological in that women from certain Asian countries whose daily diet contains substantial quantities of soy have a lower prevalence of the above ailments. Current evidence suggests that commercial expensive supplements are inadequate in controlling vasomotor or other postmenopausal symptoms.

Selective Estrogen Receptor Modulators (SERMs) PH 1.37

Unlike the predominantly estrogenic compounds and the purely anti-estrogenic compound (clomiphene), SERMs exert pharmacological actions on binding to the two estrogen receptors (ERα and ERβ), and are **tissue-selective**. *They are partially estrogenic in some tissues (e.g. bone, brain and liver) with anti-estrogenic activity (e.g. in breast and endometrium) or no activity in others*, e.g. **tamoxifen** (Chapter 59) has anti-estrogenic action on the breast but estrogenic action on the bone and the endometrium. It is used to treat breast cancer. **Raloxifene** *is more selective and has estrogenic action on the bone, where it exerts antiresorptive activity. It has anti-estrogenic action on the breast and negligible action on the* *endometrium.* Hence it is used for prevention and treatment osteoporosis (Chapter 68).

Like Raloxifene, another SERM **Bazedoxifene** has estrogenic effects on bone and anti-estrogenic effect on the uterus. Bazedoxifene inhibits the stimulating effect of conjugated estrogens on endometrial and breast tissue but does not have the positive effects on vasomotor symptoms, vulvovaginal atrophy and bone mineral density. Thus SERM + conjugated estrogen combination can be used to treat hot flashes and vaginal dryness, and to prevent (but not treat) bone loss in menopausal woman with no effects ion endometrium and breast. It is devoid of ADR such as breast pain, vaginal bleeding seen with estrogen and progestin combination.

Toremifene is chemically related to tamoxifen and is used in the treatment of breast cancer (Chapter 59).

Ospemifene: Acts as **estrogen agonist** on vaginal epithelium, endometrium and bone. It has **anti-estrogenic action on breast**. It is used in the dose of 60 mg daily administered with food for the treatment of moderate to severe dyspareunia in postmenopausal women with vulvovaginal atrophy. The adverse effects include hot flushes, vaginal discharge, muscle spasms, hyperhidrosis, endometrial thickening, uterine polyps and DVT. The drug is contraindicated in thromboembolic disease.

For **anti-estrogenic agents** clomiphene, see Chapter 66, and for tamoxifen and fulvestrant, see Chapter 59.

PROGESTERONE AND OTHER PROGESTINS

Progesterone is naturally secreted by the ovaries, CL and placenta. LH stimulates its secretion. It is also synthesised by the adrenals and testes where it acts as a precursor of steroid hormones (Fig. 65.2).

Physiological functions: It:

- **Decreases the estrogen-driven, proliferation of the endometrium** (anti-estrogen action), and **promotes the development of secretory endometrium.** Its decline at the end of the cycle results in onset of menstruation.
- **Promotes the development of the alveolar (acinar) system of the breast**
- **Prepares the endometrium for the implantation of the fertilised ovum** and **induces decidual reaction**
- **Causes changes in the vaginal epithelium and secretion,** characteristic of progestational effect (see below)
- **Helps to maintain pregnancy**
- **Induces various metabolic changes** including the midcycle rise in BBT. This rise is correlated with ovulation and natriuresis.
- **Decreases GnRH pulse frequency** and reduces gonadotropin release to set the hypothalamic pituitary-gonadal axis back to the follicular phase in normal cycle.

Agents having progesterone-like biological activities are termed as progestins, progestational agents, progestagens, progestogens, gestagens, or gestogens.

Classification of Progestins — PH 1.37

I. **Progesterone**
II. **Derivatives of progesterone:**
   a. **Esters of 17-alpha hydroxyprogesterone** such as caproate or acetate
   b. **C6-substituted 17-alpha hydroxyprogesterone derivatives**, e.g. medroxyprogesterone acetate (MPA), megestrol and chlormadinone acetate
   c. **Dydrogesterone or dehydrogesterone**
III. **Derivatives of testosterone**, e.g. ethisterone and dimethisterone
IV. **Derivatives of 19-nortestosterone** (testosterone without the 19-methyl group Fig. 65.4), e.g. norethisterone (norethindrone), 19-norethisterone acetate, norethynodrel, ethynodiol diacetate, norgestrel, lynestrenol, desogestrel, etonogestrel, norgestimate, dienogest and gestodene

The progestational actions of the testosterone derivatives are, in general, similar to those of progesterone except that they are modified by the associated estrogenic and/or androgenic properties of these compounds. Hence, **progestins can also be classified as follows:**

I. **Pure progestins**, e.g. progesterone, dehydrogesterone, esters of 17-alpha hydroxyprogesterone, and C6-substituted 17-alpha hydroxyprogesterone derivatives

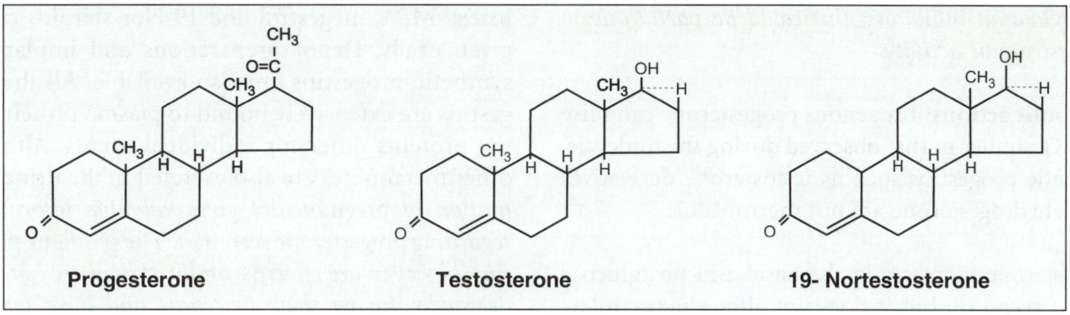

FIG. 65.4 Chemical structures of progestins.

II. **Progestins with less or negligible androgenic effects,** e.g. norgestrel, desogestrel, gestodene and norgestimate
III. **Progestins with androgenic effects,** e.g. norethisterone
IV. **Progestins with estrogenic effects,** e.g. norethynodrel
V. **Steroids of uncertain status,** e.g. ethynodiol diacetate
VI. **Spironolactone analogue:** Drospirenone having antimineralocorticoid and antiandrogenic properties

Mechanism of action:

Progesterone receptors are nuclear receptors and exist as PR-A and PR-B isoforms. On binding to progesterone, they get phosphorylated and form dimers that bind with high selectivity to progesterone responsive elements (PREs) located on target genes to cause transcriptional activation with the help of co-activators.

Stimulatory activities of progesterone are mediated through PR-B e.g. on mammary glands. PR-A inhibits stimulatory action of PR-B and is also a transcriptional inhibitor of other steroid receptors. PR-A may be associated with ovulation, decidualization and implantation.

Pharmacological actions:

Endometrium: Progesterone, administered to the **estrogen primed hypogonadal patients** *duplicates the changes of luteal phase* of the menstrual cycle. Its continuation prolongs the luteal phase and induces decidual changes, characteristic of early pregnancy. With testosterone derivatives and 19-nor compounds, however, the histological changes are not so classical. Progesterone suppresses menstruation and uterine contractility.

Vaginal epithelium and secretion: Progesterone prevents cornification of the vaginal epithelium and brings about increased glycogen deposition. The epithelial cells show increased folding and elongation of nuclei (Fig. 65.5). Thin, watery and profuse vaginal secretion, so characteristic of estrogenic action, becomes **thick, viscid and scanty.**

Mammary gland: Exogenous progesterone can promote acinar growth in estrogen primed mammary glands. Mitotic activity in the breast epithelium peaks under the influence of progesterone and progestin may be associated with increased risk of breast cancer observed with estrogen-progestin combination used in HRT.

Ovulation inhibition: Progesterone inhibits ovulation only in large doses. *The synthetic 19-nor testosterone derivatives however, are potent gonadotropin*

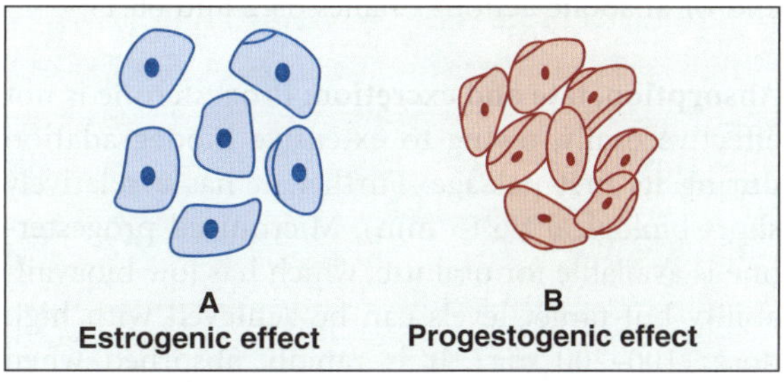

FIG. 65.5 Vaginal cytology.

and ovulation inhibitors; this could be partly due to their estrogenic activity.

Metabolic actions: Exogenous progesterone can raise the BBT similar to that observed during the midcycle. Synthetic progestins such as testosterone derivatives and dehydrogesterone are not thermogenic.

Progesterone increases in the basal and postglucose insulin secretion but it does not alter glucose tolerance. It promotes glycogen deposition and ketogenesis; stimulates lipoprotein lipase and causes fat deposition. Progesterone probably has some catabolic action and has been shown to promote nitrogen loss. It also promotes sodium and chloride loss (diuresis) by competing with aldosterone in the kidney.

Synthetic progestins, however, have no such consistent effects. In the doses used in HRT, levonorgestrel and MPA can cause insulin resistance and impairment of glucose tolerance. Norethisterone seems to be relatively inert in this respect. MPA and 19-norprogestins increase LDL and have no effect or reduce HDL levels.

Maintenance of pregnancy: Natural progesterone probably helps in the maintenance of pregnancy.

Antineoplastic action: There is some evidence to indicate that progesterone can suppress estrogen induced fibromyomata in animals. When added to estrogen as a part the HRT, progestins help to prevent possible development of endometrial carcinoma. Progestins have been used to treat advanced cancer of the breast (ER-positive and progesterone receptor [PR]-positive) and the endometrium.

Other actions: Progesterone causes mental depression and hypnotic effects. Some of the synthetic progestins have associated estrogenic, androgenic and/or anabolic actions (Tables 65.2 and 66.1).

Absorption, fate and excretion: Progesterone is not effective orally, owing to extensive biodegradation during its first passage. Further, it has a relatively short biological t½ (5 min). Micronized progesterone is available for oral use, which has low bioavailability but target levels can be achieved with high dose (100–200 mg). It is rapidly absorbed when injected in oily solution or from vaginal gel and insert. MPA, megestrol and 19 Nor-steroids can be given orally. Depot preparations and implants of synthetic progestins are also available. All the progestins are extensively bound to plasma proteins but the proteins differ for individual agents. Although other metabolites are also excreted in the urine, *estimation of pregnanediol gives valuable information regarding progesterone secretion. The synthetic progestins, however, are effective orally as they are not easily degraded during their first pass and have long t½ (MPA 24h; norethindrone 7h;, norgestrel 16 h; gestodene 12h)*. They are mainly metabolised in the liver.

Adverse reactions: Apart from their pharmacological actions which may modify the menstrual cycle (**spotting, breakthrough bleeding**) and decrease the flow, progestins, in general, are relatively safe drugs. Derivatives of testosterone and 19-nor testosterone can cause nausea, breast discomfort, headache, fatigue and rarely liver damage.

Some of the synthetic progestins such as norethisterone may cause **androgenic actions** on developing female fetus and hence, should be avoided during pregnancy. For the same reason, they may cause weight gain, acne and hirsutism.

Preparations and dosage: Table 65.2.

The newer progestins **desogestrel, gestodene** and **norgestimate** are derivatives of norgestrel. Desogestrel and norgestimate are prodrugs. As progestins:

a. In therapeutic doses they are extremely potent inhibitors of ovulation without any androgenic or anti-estrogenic effect.
b. They have a weaker androgenic and anti-estrogenic action than the earlier progestins.
c. They are more selective and cause fewer metabolic changes.

Dienogest is the only nortestosterone derivative with an antiandrogenic activity. It has very high progestogenic effects on the endometrium but causes only moderate suppression of estrogen levels. It has no significant mineralocorticoid or glucocorticoid activity. It is used in the treatment of endometriosis in daily dose of 2 mg.

Table 65.2 Progestins in Current Use

Preparation	Dosage[b]	Remarks
Progesterone	Functional uterine bleeding: 5–10 mg IM daily; habitual abortion: 1–2 mg daily; threatened abortion: 5–10 mg daily	Mildly catabolic
Derivatives of progesterone:		
Hydroxyprogesterone caproate	Threatened and habitual abortion: 125–500 mg weekly IM functional uterine bleeding: same dose	Mildly catabolic, long acting (8–14 days)
Medroxyprogesterone acetate[a]	Functional uterine bleeding: 5–10 mg daily; threatened and habitual abortion: 10–40 mg daily orally or 50–100 mg IM weekly	Mildly catabolic
Dydrogesterone	Dysmenorrhoea: 10–25 mg daily; same dose also used in threatened abortion and in functional uterine bleeding; in endometriosis: 30 mg daily	Does not inhibit ovulation. Mildly catabolic
Allylestrenol	5–10 mg daily	
Megestrol	Used in oral contraceptive combination pills.	
Derivatives of testosterone:		
Dimethisterone[a]	15 mg daily	Mildly estrogenic
Derivatives of 19 nor-testosterone:		
Norethisterone[a]	Primary and secondary amenorrhoea: 5–15 mg daily; functional uterine bleeding: 10–30 mg daily; endometriosis: 10–30 mg daily	Androgenic and anabolic actions
Norethisterone acetate[a]	2.5–15 mg daily. Indications similar as norethisterone	Mildly androgenic and anabolic
Norethynodrel[a]	Primary and secondary amenorrhoea: 5–10 mg daily; endometriosis: 20–30 mg daily	Estrogenic
Ethynodiol diacetate	Used in combination OC pills:	
Lynestrenol	5–10 mg daily	
Desogestrel	Used in combination OC pills	Prodrug (No androgenic or anti-estrogenic action)

[a]Also used as oral contraceptive.
[b]For various regimen details, see text. For Progestasert and Mirena IUCDs, see text.

Drospirenone is a spironolactone analogue with progestogenic, antimineralocorticoid and antiandrogenic activities. It is a constituent of a combined oral contraceptive pill, Yasmin (Chapter 66). It can cause hyperkalaemia.

Indications:

- **Abnormal uterine bleeding (AUB):** It is a common problem in women of reproductive age group wherein bleeding from the uterus deviates from the normal menstrual bleeding in volume, regularity, frequency or duration and the changes persist for 6 months or longer. AUB has many etiologies based on which it is classified using an acronym PALM-COEIN (the individual alphabets stand for Polyp, Adenomyosis, Leiomyoma [fibroid], Malignancy [hyperplasia], Coagulopathy, Ovulatory dysfunction, Endometrial, Iatrogenic[due to IUDs] and Not yet classified). Previously the term dysfunctional uterine bleeding (DUB) was used for AUB in absence of pregnancy, iatrogenic causes, systemic conditions, and genital tract pathology.

Ovulatory dysfunction (anovulation or oligo-ovulation) is the most common cause of AUB (AUB-O) and seen in more than 50% women in reproductive age and 20% adolescents. It is especially common at the beginning and the end of reproductive life. The other causes of AUB-O are polycystic ovary syndrome, primary ovarian insufficiency, systemic diseases such as liver or kidney disease, Cushing syndrome, hyperprolactinemia, hypothyroidism, and idiopathic (sometimes occurring when gonadotropin levels are normal). It is also observed in some patients with endometriosis.

AUB-E is the primary endometrial dysfunction with no detectable hormonal or structural abnormalities. The patient is ovulatory and bleeding is typically regular but heavy or prolonged.

During an anovulatory cycle, estrogen stimulates the endometrium unopposed, as the normal cyclical secretion of progesterone is absent (luteal phase dysfunction). The endometrial proliferation continues and outgrows its blood supply. This results in incomplete sloughing and irregular bleeding, sometimes profusely over many days. This is an estrogen breakthrough bleeding. If this occurs repeatedly, then the endometrium can become hyperplastic, sometimes with atypical or cancerous cells.

During perimenopause, AUB-O is observed because insufficient production of estrogen from follicles despite high levels of FSH. It may be an early sign of ovarian insufficiency.

AUB may occur in patients with ovulatory cycles. Here the progesterone secretion is prolonged but the estrogen levels are low (short follicular phase) and irregular shedding of the endometrium occurs. This is manifested as regular but heavy menstrual bleeding (menorrhagia). Blood loss of more than 80 mL/cycle is defined as criteria for menorrhagia. Human endometrium synthesises PGs locally and the endometrial dysfunction could be related to the excessive formation of PGE_2.

The main clinical manifestation, other than menstrual abnormalities, is iron deficiency anaemia and infertility in anovulatory women. A detailed history and physical examination help to establish the diagnosis and type (ovulatory or anovulatory) in most women. *Counselling of the patient is very helpful, so is correction of anaemia with oral iron.* Severe cases may require hospitalisation.

The **aim of therapy for AUB** is to:

- Control bleeding
- Correct iron deficiency anaemia, if present
- Treat structural lesions (e.g, hysteroscopic myomectomy, uterine fibroid embolization, hysterectomy) or correct the cause if possible

Table 65.3 summarises management of AUB.

Management of AUB

Nonhormonal medications: These are used intermittently when bleeding occurs. *They are the first line treatment of acute AUB, particularly in those who ovulate but bleed heavily*. They are used mainly when the patient desires pregnancy and wishes to avoid hormone therapy.

PG-synthetase inhibitors such as **mefenamic acid** and **ibuprofen** diminish menstrual bleeding in normal as well as AUB women by 25-35% and relive associated dysmenorrhea. These drugs are given for 3–4 days, starting with the onset of bleeding. Other nonhormonal agents used are: **tranexamic acid**, which reduces menstrual loss by 40-60% and **ethamsylate** **given for 3–4 days** (Chapter 33).

Hormonal therapy: It is preferred when contraception is desired or if women are

Table 65.3 Management of AUB

• ***Specific drug treatment*:**	
a. **Nonhormonal:**	NSAID; tranexamic acid; ethamsylate; ormeloxifene
b. **Hormonal**	Combined OC pill; norgestrel-releasing IUCD; progestin; danazol
• ***Correction of anaemia:***	Iron
• ***Treat structural lesions/ correct cause***	
• ***Nondrug treatment:***	Counselling

perimenopausal. Such therapy suppresses endometrial proliferation, establishes predictable bleeding pattern and decreases menstrual flow. In most patients hormonal disorder cannot be demonstrated.

A low-dose combination OC pill (Chapter 66), is most commonly given. It is administered in the dose of 1 pill 4 times a day for 5 days. The full course should be given even if the bleeding stops earlier. This is followed by cyclic administration of the same pill once daily from 5th to 25th day of the cycle for 3–6 cycles. COC control AUB-O as well as AUB due to fibroids or adenomyosis. They are useful in case of heavy bleeding as they decrease blood loss by 40 to 50%.

Norethisterone 5–10 mg 4–6 hourly will stop the bleeding within 24 h. It is usually continued in doses of 5 mg b.i.d. for 1–2 weeks. The patient should be warned that the first period which follows cessation of the progestin is likely to be heavy. It is continued later as 2.5 to 5 mg/day for 21 days a month for 3 more cycles. In patients with endometrial hyperplasia/anaplasia, it is advisable to continue daily progestin for 9–12 months.

Withdrawal bleeding is more predictable with cyclic progestin therapy. Progestins are preferred if estrogen is contraindicated. However, they do not control heavy bleeding.

Once the bleeding is controlled for a few months with hormonal therapy, patients may choose to continue hormone therapy for contraception or to stop it and check whether AUB still presents.

For the prevention of AUB, a combined OC pill or a progestin or a levonorgestrel releasing IUD may be used.

Depot medroxyprogesterone acetate: It provides contraception but may cause irregular spotting and reversible bone loss.

IUCDs **incorporating levonorgestrel (Mirena)** release the drug slowly. The serum levels achieved are low but adequate to suppress the ovarian function. In 90% of the subjects, the cycles are ovulatory. The locally released progestin causes endometrial thinning and atrophy; the cyclical changes related to the menstrual cycle are abolished. Thirty-five per cent of the women become amenorrhoeic at 1 year. *These changes are, however, reversible and normal menstruation is restored 1–2 months after removal of the device. They can be used to produce **endometrial ablation** in severe menorrhagia where hysterectomy is contraindicated.* They have also been used to control bleeding in uterine fibroids. They are highly effective (80%–90%), relatively safe and usually well tolerated. However in practice, many women desire to have normal cycle control and may not opt for this chemical ablation. They are expensive.

Patients in whom combination OCs (COC) are contraindicated may be prescribed **danazol** 200 mg daily on a continuous basis usually for 3 months. It reduces menstrual blood loss by causing endometrial atrophy. **Ormeloxifene**, the SERM, is also used in AUB because of its anti-estrogenic action (Chapter 66). It is given for 6 months.

Gonadotropin-releasing hormone (GnRH) agonists or antagonists: Suppression of ovarian hormone production by them results in amenorrhea and shrinkage of endometrium and fibroids. However, they cannot be given beyond 6 months as there is a possibility of bone loss. Usually low-dose estrogen and progestin therapy is used concurrently with them (add-back therapy).

Bleeding not controlled by medication or the structural lesion is treated with surgical procedure.

- **Dysmenorrhoea:** Some women complain of either discomfort or pain (either dull or colicky) in the lower abdomen before or during menstruation (dysmenorrhoea). **'Dysmenorrhoea' is only a symptom and not a diagnosis**. It is common in the teenagers but also occurs in the older women and **is usually associated with**

ovulatory cycles. *Before starting drug treatment, one should make certain that a local cause such as an IUCD is not responsible for the symptom.*

The **primary spasmodic dysmenorrhoea** of the teenager generally disappears with increasing age. It is probably **due to excess of PG production in the uterus.** Most girls with this symptom are helped by physical exercise, explanation, reassurance, and may not need drug therapy.

Drugs used are as follows:

a. **NSAID,** (e.g. **ibuprofen**) given alone or together with an antimuscarinic (antispasmodic) drug
b. Combination pill given daily from 5th to 25th day of the menstrual cycle for 4–6 cycles inhibits ovulation, when symptom are severe and incapacitating. *While dispensing such pills to unmarried girls, care should be taken not to label the container as 'contraceptive pills'*
c. **Oral dehydrogesterone** 5–10 mg twice daily from 8th to 25th day of the cycle if inhibition of ovulation is considered undesirable for some reason

Membranous dysmenorrhoea is rare and often familial. The menstrual endometrium is painfully shed in large strips or even as a complete cast. Although the COC can be used to treat these cases, the results are less rewarding; curettage is also unhelpful. **Norethisterone** 10 mg daily given for five, immediately premenstrual days may be beneficial in some patients.

- **Amenorrhoea:** If a woman presents with amenorrhoea, progestogen withdrawal test is helpful in distinguishing between patients with normal and low circulating estradiol levels. In the former case, administration of medroxyprogesterone or norethisterone (5 mg twice a day) for 5 days is followed by withdrawal bleeding within 7–10 days. Such bleeding, in patients with primary amenorrhoea, also establishes the patency of the lower genital tract. If there is no withdrawal bleeding, the possibilities are either very low estrogen levels or an abnormality of the uterus or vagina. This test is useful but *should be performed only after ruling out pregnancy in sexually active women of the reproductive age.* The same regimen may be used once in 1–2 months in patients with severe oligomenorrhoea due to chronic anovulation from polycystic ovary syndrome (PCOS).

- **Endometriosis:** It is a chronic, **estrogen dependent disorder** associated with pelvic pain and infertility. It is due to the presence of **extrauterine, endometrial deposits.** The aims of therapy are (1) relief of pain and (2) restoration of fertility by producing a relatively hypoestrogenic state. This is done by suppressing ovarian function and limiting growth and activity of the lesions. The drugs (Box 65.4) are used for a limited period (<6 months) because of unacceptable ADR.

Combination oral contraceptives serve as first-line therapy and act by suppressing gonadotropin release, thereby inhibiting estrogen biosynthesis.

Oral progestins, (e.g. norethisterone, medroxyprogesterone, dienogest) given continuously, are highly effective in this condition. They cause marked regression of the endometrium and ultimately cause endometrial atrophy. **Danazol** can be used to treat endometriosis. It causes atrophy of endometrial tissue including that at the ectopic sites, and amenorrhoea. Ovulation and menstruation are re-established promptly on cessation of therapy, and pregnancy may be achieved in the first cycle before menstruation occurs. It is administered orally in the dose of 200–800 mg daily for 3–9 months.

Antiprogestin gestrinone is also used instead of danazol. Oral GnRH receptor antagonist, elagolix, can be used but may cause estrogen withdrawal effects. In some patients suffering from estrogen withdrawal symptoms or significant reduction in bone density, addition of low dose of conjugated equine estrogens or high dose of progestin is essential (add-back therapy).

Box 65.4 Drugs Used in Endometriosis

- Combination oral contraceptives (Chapter 66)
- Oral progestins
- Danazol (See earlier)
- GnRH analogues (see earlier)

NSAIDs are prescribed for symptomatic relief of pain, if necessary.

- **Fibrocystic disease of the breast:** This condition in young women is believed to be associated with **excessive estrogen and/or prolactin** action on the breast tissue. **Danazol** though most effective is expensive and may cause side effects. A cheaper, less effective, alternative is one of the progestins given orally in divided, daily doses from 14th to 28th day of the menstrual cycle: medroxyprogesterone, 20 mg; norethisterone, 20 mg; or norethisterone acetate, 10 mg. In patients with elevated prolactin level, bromocriptine may be tried.
- **As oral contraceptives:** Chapter 66
- **Precocious puberty:** Medroxyprogesterone is useful in treating children with central precocious puberty. It acts by inhibiting the pituitary gonadotropin release and has to be used regularly for several years. Its use has been replaced by that of GnRH agonists (see earlier).
- **Postponement of menstruation:** Progestins can be used to prolong the luteal phase of the menstrual cycle and thus to postpone the onset of menstruation. **Norethisterone orally** 5 mg daily is adequate if the subject comes early in the second half of the menstrual cycle. If, however, she seeks advice only a few days before the due date, higher doses (5–10 mg t.i.d.) are needed. Hydroxyprogesterone caproate (250 mg IM) along with small oral doses of norethisterone can also be effective.
- **Endometrial carcinoma:** Chapter 59
- **Postmenopausal syndrome:** As a part of the HRT regimen (see Box 65.2)
- **Male sex offenders:** Large doses of medroxyprogesterone are used as an adjunct to psychosexual counselling
- **Miscellaneous:** Progesterone is used to treat short luteal phase. Progesterone inhibits the secretion of proinflammatory cytokines and delays cervical ripening and may prevent the preterm labour in women with previous history of preterm delivery. *Though intramuscular hydroxyprogesterone or vaginal progesterone has been used for this purpose, conclusive evidence is absent. Usefulness of progestins in the treatment of threatened and habitual abortion is doubtful.*

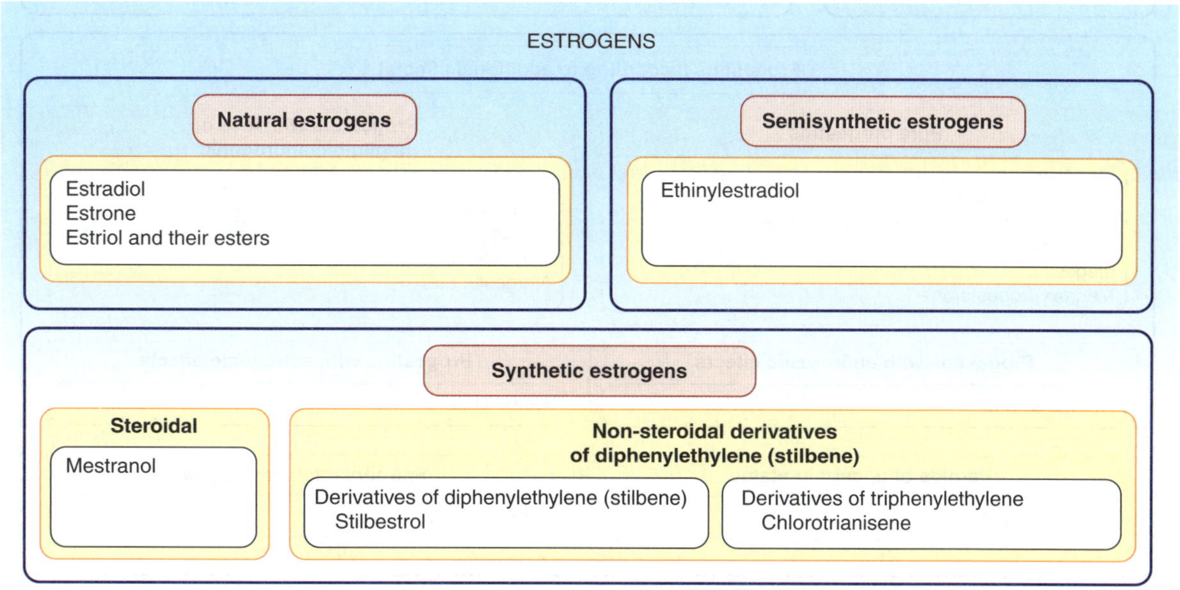

PROGESTINS

Progesterone

Derivatives of progesterone

Esters of 17-alpha hydroxyprogesterone
- Hydroxyprogesterone caproate
- Hydroxyprogesterone acetate

C6-substituted 17-alpha hydroxyprogesterone derivatives
- Medroxy progesterone acetate (MPA)
- Megestrol
- Chlormadinone acetate

Dydrogesterone or dehydrogesterone

Derivatives of testosterone
- Ethisterone
- Dimethisterone

Derivatives of 19-nortestosterone
- Norethisterone (norethindrone)
- Norethisterone acetate
- Norethynodrel
- Ethynodiol diacetate
- Norgestrel
- Lynestrenol
- Desogestrel
- Etonogestrel
- Norgestimate
- Dienogest
- Gestodene

Progestins (according to additional effects)

Pure progestins
- Progesterone
- Dehydrogesterone
- Esters of 17-alpha hydroxyprogesterone
- Chlormadinone
- Megestrol
- Medroxyprogesterone

Progestins with less or negligible androgenic effects
- Norgestrel
- Desogestrel
- Gestodene
- Norgestimate

Progestins with androgenic effects
- Norethisterone

Progestins with estrogenic effects
- Norethynodrel

Steroids of uncertain status
- Ethynodiol diacetate

Spironolactone analogue
- Drospirenone

CHAPTER 66

Antifertility Agents and Ovulation-Inducing Drugs

Learning Objectives

This chapter will enable the reader:

1. To be aware of the physiology of human reproduction.
2. To enlist the fertility control measures.
3. To explain the mechanism of action, pharmacological effects, methods of administration, ADR, drug interactions, contraindications and indications for combination oral contraceptive (COC).
4. To explain the mechanism of action, methods of administration, ADR of progestin-only pills.
5. To enumerate injectable contraceptives, their ADR, contraindications and dosage schedule.
6. To enumerate hormonal contraceptives administered as implants and intrauterine contraceptive devices and state their adverse effects.
7. To explain the mechanism of action, pharmacological effects, salient pharmacokinetic features, ADR and indications for antiprogestins.
8. To enumerate various regimens used for postcoital contraception and medical termination of pregnancy.
9. To classify ovulation-inducing agents.
10. To explain the mechanism of action, pharmacological effects, salient pharmacokinetic features, ADR and indications for clomiphene.

KEY TERMS

combination oral contraceptive (COC), p. 966
contraindications to COC, p. 969
progestin-only pills, p. 972
parenteral contraceptives, p. 973
intrauterine contraceptive devices, p. 974
postcoital contraception, p. 975
mifepristone, p. 976
clomiphene citrate, p. 979
medical termination of pregnancy, p. 977

Global human population growth amounts to around 83 million annually, or 1.1% per year. The global population has crossed 8 million in 2023 with India population accounting for a whooping 1.4 billion. The expected estimates of the total population are 9.4–10.0 billion in 2050 and upto12.4 billion in 2100. Considering the world resources, such a growth in population can create major problems unless fertility is controlled.

Fertility control is very essential for maintaining satisfactory standards of living and for raising the existing standards in developing countries. Furthermore, it is equally important for family planning which is defined as 'the limitation and spacing of births in the best interests of the mother, the child and the rest of the family'. The use of drugs for this purpose is but one aspect of the whole programme.

Physiology of human reproduction: The reproductive cycle in the human, in whom ovulation is a key event, is the result of the interplay of the hypothalamus, the pituitary and the ovaries.

Under the influence of pituitary FSH, the ovarian follicle matures and considerable amounts of estrogen are produced. The sudden midcycle spurt of LH is followed by ovulation, releasing the ovum. Ovulation usually occurs on day 14 (±2) of a 28 day cycle (Fig. 65.1). The oocyte enters the fallopian tube and when it reaches the ampullary region it can be fertilised by the sperm. By 18th day of the cycle, the fertilised ovum is converted into a blastocyst which reaches the cavity of the uterus and gets implanted beneath the endometrium by the 21st–23rd day of the cycle, This stage is completed by the 35th day when the fetal placental circulation starts developing. Thus pregnancy may be considered as existing only 5 weeks after the onset of last menstrual cycle.

Ovulation can be judged by noting:

- **Changes in the cervical mucus**
- **Vaginal cytology** (Fig. 65.5)
- **Serum progesterone level**
- **Endometrial biopsy**
- **Rise in basal body temperature**

All these changes reflect the production of progesterone by the corpus luteum.

The **cervical mucus** is an alkaline gel, rich in protein and fructose. During the follicular phase it is clear, thin, copious, acellular and elastic. This property permits the mucus to be stretched into threads from 5 to 15 cm in length. The mucus assumes a characteristic fern-like pattern when dried on a glass slide. *Clinically, ferning and 'thread test' (spinnbarkeit) are utilised to judge the estrogen influence.* Just before the ovulation, its consistency is considered to be the most ideal for the transport of sperms into the uterus. Soon after the ovulation, under the influence of progesterone, the cervical mucus becomes tough, viscous and translucent and the sperms may find it difficult to penetrate it. Some women experience unilateral low abdominal pain near midcycle which is attributed to the occurrence of ovulation.

However, the only definite evidence of ovulation is either recovery of the ovum or pregnancy.

The exact duration of survival of sperms in the vagina is not known but is believed to be about 1–2 h while they can remain active in the cervix and uterine cavity for about 45–50 h.

CONTRACEPTION

Apart from *coitus interruptus*, fertility control can be achieved by:

- **Modifying physiological mechanisms of reproduction**
- **Preventing the union of sperm with ovum** by using physical or chemical barriers

The conception is delayed in women who breastfeed their babies exclusively probably because of elevated levels of prolactin. It is believed that more births are prevented by breastfeeding than by all other forms of contraception put together!

Classification of Pharmacological Contraceptives

A. **Oral:**
   I. **Combination Oral Contraceptives (COC) containing estrogen and progestin component**
      - Fixed dose (monophasic) COC
      - Biphasic and triphasic COC, which have variable amount of ingredients
      - Extended cycle COC
   II. **Progestin alone as contraceptive (minipill)**
   III. **Anti-estrogenic agents** e.g. ormeloxifene

B. **Parenteral:**
   I. **Injectables** e.g. depot-medroxyprogesterone acetate (DMPA), norethisterone enanthate (NET-EN)
   II. **Implants** e.g. levonorgestrel implant
   III. **Transdermal contraceptive system**

C. **Medicated Uterine/ Vaginal devices:**
   I. **Vaginal contraceptive rings**
   II. **Intrauterine contraceptive medicated devices (medicated IUCD)**

Drugs used for contraception act by: PH 1.39

- **Inhibiting ovulation**
- **Modifying the cervical mucus**
- **Interfering with the implantation**
- **Slowing down the rate of transport**
- **Preventing the ovum maturation and sperm capacitation**
- **Immunological methods (vaccine)**
- **Inhibiting spermatogenesis in males**

The drugs which are currently in use act mainly by the first three mechanisms and are discussed below.

Oral contraception is a highly effective and acceptable method. In this method, either an estrogen–progestin combination or a progestin alone is used.

ESTROGEN–PROGESTIN COMBINATION PILL

Since the first clinical demonstration of usefulness of such an oral combination for contraception by Pincus (1955), several commercial preparations have been available. Though commonly termed as pills, the available preparations are tablets and not the pills. The following attributes have made these oral combination pills popular among the educated, higher and middle class women:

- *Remarkable efficacy*
- *Relative safety*
- *Ease of administration*
- *Cost-effectiveness*

Combination oral contraceptive (**COC**) pill contain:

1. Ethinyl estradiol (EE) or its 3-methyl ether (mestranol) as the estrogen
2. A progestin belonging to 19-nortestosterone group or (norethisterone, norgestrel), one derived from progesterone (megestrol acetate) or a derivative of norgestrel (desogestrel)

Mechanism of action: The mechanism of the contraceptive action of these agents is complex. The **combination type suppresses both FSH rise (due to the estrogen component) and LH peak** (due to the progestin component) observed during the normal menstrual cycle. *Thus, follicular growth is not initiated and ovulation does not occur.* Although estrogen alone can be effective it is not suitable as it may cause profuse, irregular bleeding. The progestin in the pills:

- *Increases the certainty of the contraceptive effect. In fact, it plays the major role in ovulation inhibition.*
- *Modifies the cervical mucus, making it thick, tenacious and hostile to the sperms*
- *Prevents breakthrough bleeding*
- *Ensures predictable withdrawal bleeding after each cycle of treatment*
- *Reduces the menstrual blood loss*

Pharmacological actions of COC pills:

Endometrium: The effect produced by the COC pills is similar to that of 'luteal phase'. The full **secretory activity of the endometrial glands is achieved within 3–4 days of starting these pills,** leading to predecidual changes. Later, the endometrium becomes thin and hypoplastic. The changes are reversed 2–3 months after stoppage of treatment.

Cervical mucus: Continuous administration of a progestin increases the thick cervical mucus, causing a 'cervical barrier' hostile to sperm penetration.

Pituitary–ovarian axis: Prolonged administration of these *drugs does not cause any permanent structural changes in the pituitary or ovary,* although during therapy ovaries may appear smaller and their secretion may practically cease. *The conception may be delayed but there is no permanent infertility.*

Metabolic effects:

- Hyperglycaemia, glycosuria and mildly impaired glucose tolerance along with a rise in the postabsorptive serum immunoreactive insulin levels have been reported. The incidence of abnormal GTT is related to the dose and potency of progestin. *The newer progestins such as desogestrel have less effect on carbohydrate metabolism.*
- Increase in cholesterol and LDL and lowering of HDL has been observed following the progestins. Because the estrogen component has an effect opposite to that of the progestin, no significant alterations in the cholesterol level have been observed. *The data indicate that the use of COC with EE ≤50 mcg by healthy, nonsmoking women up to the age of 35 is not associated with an increased risk of serious cardiovascular disease.*
  The pill also causes a slight increase in plasma triglycerides in some women.
- Acceleration of platelet aggregation and adhesion and reduction of the activity of the fibrinolytic system. The estrogen component is thought to be responsible for these changes.

Other endocrine glands: As in pregnancy, all COCs increase levels of thyroxine, cortisol as well as thyroxine and steroid hormone binding proteins. The latter cause decrease in free testosterone concentration, which may help to improve acne and hirsutism.

Adverse reactions: *The earlier preparations (in 1970s) contained higher doses of both estrogen (> 50 mcg) and progestin; some of the adverse effects described with those pills may not be relevant to the lower dose pills (estrogen < 30 mcg) that are currently in use.*

- **General:** Nausea, anorexia and vomiting are

common and are due to the estrogen component. The pill should be taken at bedtime on a full stomach, to minimise them. The estrogen may also be responsible for other effects like breast engorgement, mastalgia, chloasma and increased vaginal secretion (leucorrhoea).

In certain individuals, the anabolic action of these compounds causes **weight gain**. In others, the weight gain is due to sodium retention and oedema, mostly due to estrogens. There is a rare chance of masculinisation of a female fetus, if preparations containing 19-norsteroids are used.

Blurring of vision and **mental depression** has also been rarely reported. The risk of depression is greater in women with past history of depression. It appears to be related to estrogen-induced alteration in vitamin B_6 metabolism and may respond to pyridoxine 20 mg twice a day.

Oral contraceptive use increases significantly, though to a small extent, the risk of **vaginal infection**, particularly candidiasis.

The 'pill' may decrease serum levels of pyridoxine, folic acid, vitamin C, calcium and zinc, whereas those of vitamin A, copper and iron are elevated.

- **Bleeding irregularities:** Cycle control is usually excellent. A large proportion of women experience regular cycles and **relief from dysmenorrhoea, premenstrual tension and excessive menstrual blood loss**. This is beneficial. Occasionally, however, bleeding similar to that of a normal menstrual period occurs during the course of medication (**breakthrough bleeding**). In such cases, the tablets are stopped and a new course started five days later with a preparation containing larger quantity of progestin. **Spotting** is characterised by unexpected, intermittent blood-stained trickling during the therapy. *Its incidence appears to be higher with low estrogen, extended cycle COCs, continuous regimes and progestin-only pills (POPs).*

  The return of menstruation following stoppage of the 'pill' may be delayed for 6–8 weeks. Informing the patient about this temporary amenorrhoea in advance can spare her many anxious days. *Conception may be delayed for 3–12 months after stopping the 'pills'.*

- **Thromboembolic phenomena:** There is a definite relationship between the use of COC pill and the incidence of venous thromboembolism (VTE), cerebral thrombosis and pulmonary embolism. Persistent headache may be a warning of an impending cerebrovascular accident. The risk is more in women > 35 years of age, especially in smokers. It is related to the concentration of the estrogen component. *A dose of 50 mcg of EE seems to be the safe upper limit beyond which the risk increases. The currently used low ethinyl estradiol (30 mcg) pills have considerably reduced this risk.*

  COC containing EE with desogestrelor drospirenon are associated with higher risk of VTE than those with levonorgestrel or norgestrel.

- **Migraine:** Majority experience no change in their migraine and a few show improvement especially if they were having migraine attacks associated with menstrual cycles. But in some migraine may worsen.

  There may be increased stroke risk in patients with migraine given COC, especially in those having aura, or having stroke risk factors such as increased age, smoking, and hypertension.

- **Hypertension:** The reported incidence of hypertension has been as high as 15%. It is reversible within about 3 months of its discontinuation. It is probably due to the estrogen-induced increase in plasma angiotensinogen. *Before treating the hypertension in a female patient, the 'COC pill' as a cause should be ruled out.*

- **Liver:** The hepatic abnormalities induced and changes in liver function tests are usually reversible and are basically alterations in the bile-secreting function of the hepatocytes (cholestatic). Usually, the 'pill' produces no clinical problem, only a few develop cholestatic jaundice.

- **Uterine fibroids:** They can undergo enlargement during therapy with pills, and hence the presence of fibroids is a relative contraindication.

- **Carcinogenicity:** Although estrogens are carcinogenic, the evidence regarding breast cancer following COC pill use is controversial. However, they are absolutely contraindicated in the presence of estrogen dependent malignancies such as breast cancer, in Hodgkin disease and in malignant melanoma. *Furthermore, it is a wise precaution to examine the breasts and the cervical smear for malignancy before starting the treatment and then periodically during the therapy.*

Box 66.1 lists the absolute contraindications to the use of combined COCs.

COC has **protective effect** against **endometrial and epithelial ovarian cancers.** They cause lower incidence of benign breast disease. Women who use COC for at least a year show a significant protection which persists for at least 15 years after the use of COC ceases.

Currently used low dose OC pills carry very small risk to undiagnosed pregnancy/fetus.

Drug interactions: See Box 66.2.

Preparations: Tables 66.1 and 66.2. (Groups A-D)

Methods of administration:

- **Fixed dose combination pills (monophasic pills)**: Commonly one pill containing both, an estrogen (<20 mcg EE) and progestin is administered daily, at bed time, for 21 days, from 5th to 25th day of a 28 day cycle. The next course is started 7 days after the last dose. If the patient forgets to take a 'pill', and she remembers it within 12 h, she should take the forgotten pill immediately, and then return to the usual schedule. If more than 36 h have passed between that last (regular) 'pill' taken and the delayed consumption of the missed 'pill', the course should be continued but along with the use of barrier method or abstinence for 7–10 days to prevent conception. *If more than one pill is forgotten, the woman should consider herself similarly unprotected and take other measures to prevent conception.*
- **Biphasic and triphasic combination pills:** These are combination pills containing varying proportions of an estrogen and a progestin and are designed to simulate the hormonal profile of the normal menstrual cycle. This allows lower doses of both synthetic steroids in the early part of the cycle. Slightly higher doses later in the cycle help

Box 66.1 Absolute Contraindications to Combination OC Pills

- Pregnancy
- Estrogen-dependent cancers (breast, endometrium)
- Cardiovascular (HF, ischaemic heart disease, severe uncontrolled hypertension, cardiomyopathy, most types of valvular heart diseases, pulmonary hypertension, cerebral vascular disease, arterial thrombosis, VTE or known proneness to it Hypercoagulopathy)
- Migraine with focal neurological symptoms or migraine of any type if women age > 35 years
- Diabetes for 20 years or diabetes with end organ disease
- Hyperlipidaemia
- Active liver disease
- Smoker (>15 cigarettes per day)

Table 66.1 Comparative Biologic Properties of Synthetic Progestins[a]

Properties	Norethisterone	Norethisterone acetate	Norgestrel	Lynestrenol	Norethynodrel	Ethynodiol diacetate	Desogestrel[b]
Progestogenic	++	++	++++	++	++	+++	++++
Estrogenic	–	–	–	+	++	+	–
Anti-estrogenic	+	+	++	–	–	+	–
Androgenic	+	++	++	+	–	+	–
Anabolic	+	+	+	+	–	–	–

[a]Experimental study data

[b]Prototype of third-generation progestins (the others being gestodene and norgestimate) which are derivatives of norgestrel.

Box 66.2 Drug Interactions of Combination OC Pills

- ***Decreased efficacy of the other drug:*** Coumarin anticoagulants; thyroid hormone and oral hypoglycaemics
- ***Increased efficacy/toxicity of the other drug:*** Theophylline; imipramine; cyclosporine and glucocorticoids (pharmacological doses)
- ***Decreased efficacy of OC pills:*** Barbiturates; antiepileptic drugs; rifampicin; griseofulvin; ampicillin and tetracyclines
- ***Increased efficacy of OC pills:*** Ascorbic acid 1 g daily
- ***Hypercoagulable state:*** Aminocaproic acid

to prevent breakthrough bleeding. They are, however, more complex to use, offer little, if any, advantage over the monophasic pills.

- **Extended cycle COC:**
  a. A COC pill containing 30 mcg of ethinyl estradiol and 150 mcg of levonorgestrel (Seasonale) is taken daily for 84 days, followed by a placebo pill for 7 days. **This allows withdrawal bleeding once in 3 months**, *i.e. four times a year compared to 13 times during the use of conventional, monthly, COC pills.* Spotting may occur more frequently with this method. **The major advantage is that it reduces the number of menses and hence appears to be acceptable to many women.**
  b. Low dose COC containing 20 mcg ethinyl estradiol + 100 mcg levonorgestrel administered daily for 84 days followed by 10 mcg ethinyl estradiol tablet for 7 days.
  c. COC containing varying doses of ethinyl estradiol with 150 mcg of levonorgestrel is administered daily. Estrogen is used in increasing doses e.g. 20 mcg ethinyl estradiol for 42 days followed by 25mcg for 21 days and then 30 mcg for next 21 days. Lastly 10 mcg ethinyl estradiol is given for 7 days.
  d. Another pill available contains EE 20 mcg and levonorgestrel 90 mcg. It is taken daily, uninterruptedly, for 365 days a year. **About 60% of the women develop amenorrhoea within a year.** Breakthrough bleeding and spotting are common initially, but decrease subsequently. After stopping the drug, menses resume within 2–3 months in over 90 % of women. The potential long-term ADR are not known.

Table 66.2 Some Commercial Combination Oral Contraceptive Pills

Name	Progestin	(mg)
A. With EE 0.02 mg		
Loestrin 1/20	Norethisterone acetate	1.0
Femilon	Desogestrel	0.15
B. With EE 0.03 mg		
Eugynon 30	Levonorgestrel	0.25
Microgynon, Ovral L, Triquilar[a] (Varying EE and levonorgestrel) Primovlar 30, Mala D	Levonorgestrel	0.15
Choice	Norgestrel	0.30
Novelon	Desogestrel	0.15
Yasmin[b]	Drospirenone	3.0
C. With EE 0.05 mg (high dose) and less progestogenic		
Eugynon 50, Duoluton, Ovral G Ovral, Primovlar 50	Norgestrel	0.5
Minovlar ED	Levonorgestrel	0.25
Orlest	Norethisterone acetate	1.0
Orthonovin 1/50[c]	Norethisterone acetate	1.0
D. With EE 0.05 mg (high dose) and more progestogenic		
Orgalutin	Lynestrenol	2.5
Norlestrin 2.5/50	Norethisterone acetate	2.5
Gynovlar 21	Norethisterone acetate	3.0
Anovlar 21	Norethisterone acetate	4.0

[a]Triphasic pill.
[b]Can cause hyperkalaemia (Chapter 65).
[c]Contains mestranol 0.05 mg and not EE. Most progestins are derivatives of 19-nortestosterone.

Although extended COCs, in general, cause fewer adverse symptoms such as headache, bloating sensation and menstrual pain, traditional 21/7 day OC pills used continuously skipping placebo pills or without giving pill free period can produce similar extended effects. The latter is far more cost effective.

Extended COC may be useful forwomen with dysmenorrhoea, pre-menstrual syndrome, or menstrual dysphoric syndrome.

Indications:

- **As oral contraceptives**
- **Postcoital contraception** (see Box 66.5)
- **Polycystic ovary syndrome**
- **Abnormal uterine bleeding** (Chapter 65)
- **Premature menopause** (Chapter 65)
- **Turner syndrome:** This is characterised by primary amenorrhoea, lack of secondary sex characters and short stature, with or without certain dysmorphic abnormalities due to a chromosomal defect. After initial treatment with small doses of an estrogen (Chapter 65), the patient may be treated with a COC pill.

- **ORAL CONTRACEPTIVES: USE IN THERAPY:** In practice, the net pharmacological effect produced by a 'combination pill' probably depends upon the relative progestogenic, estrogenic and androgenic properties of its individual constituents (Table 66.1). The COC can be grouped into those which are **strongly progestogenic** and those which are **weakly progestogenic** in action. The newer progestins, desogestrel and norgestimate have only progestogenic effects and are less androgenic. However, the efficacy of COC containing these appears to be similar to the other COC as contraceptives and in the treatment of acne. Since the same combinations are also useful in controlling certain menstrual disorders in a woman with an associated menstrual irregularity, a proper combination can be selected. Thus, *in women with normal menstrual cycles, a combination containing 0.03 mg or less of ethinyl estradiol with the minimum effective dose of a progestin* (Group A/B) is to be preferred. In patients receiving hepatic microsomal enzyme-inducing drugs, pills with 50 mcg ethinyl estradiol are recommended. A patient with excessive acne, hirsutism, abdominal and leg cramps, and scanty vaginal secretions may benefit from a less progestogenic combination (Group C). Drosperinone has some antiandrogenic and antimineralocorticoid activity and may help in premenstrual dysphoric disorder, hirsutism and acne. But it is expensive. Premenstrual tension, oedema, cyclic weight gain, irregular bleeding and heavy periods suggest an estrogen excess which can be countered by the strongly progestogenic pill (Group D) (Table 66.2).

In general, these pills appear to be safe, highly effective (>99%) and acceptable. Usually, they do not affect the libido; in fact, the removal of the fear of pregnancy may greatly improve the sexual as well as the marital relationship. Subsequent fertility is not affected. They can be used by women of all ages from menarche to menopause. They also provide some noncontraceptive health benefits (Box 66.3).

Before starting the pill, it is essential to go through the personal history and to carry out a detailed examination to exclude any medical contraindication especially cardiovascular risk factors. *Women older than 35 years who smoke* should be encouraged to seek alternative methods of contraception.

After the start of oral contraceptive, the woman should be initially seen during the second or third cycle of medication in order to check that all is well and that she really understands how to take the drug. Thereafter, she may be called after 6 months and still later annually. The observations should include:

a. Blood pressure and weight
b. Liver function and glycosuria
c. Cervical and breast abnormalities

Box 66.3 Noncontraceptive Benefits of Combination OC Pills

- Menstrual benefits such as less menstrual blood loss, less iron-deficiency, lower incidence of menorrhagia, dysmenorrhoea and premenstrual syndrome
- Lowered incidence of benign breast disease, uterine myoma, endometrial and epithelial ovarian cancer, ovarian cyst, ovarian cancer and osteopenia
- Protection against pelvic inflammatory disease, colon cancer
- Abolition of the risk of tubal (ectopic) pregnancy because of anovulation

d. Evidence for thrombophlebitis
e. Changes in the retinal blood vessels
f. Psychological changes

It is advisable to stop the pill for 1 month before any elective surgery, since it increases the vascularity and causes oedema of the tissues and elevates the plasma concentration of some clotting factors. As a result, deep vein thrombosis is more common in postoperative period.

The pill should be avoided in breastfeeding women, as it interferes with lactation. If the woman is exclusively breastfeeding the baby at regular intervals, including night time (full breastfeeding), the pill may be started in the third postpartum month.

Since the pill is capable of causing various systemic effects, *a history of taking the pills should form a part of the routine medical history in women of the childbearing age* and should be communicated to any other doctor to whom they may be referred.

PROGESTINS ALONE AS CONTRACEPTIVES

LEVONORGESTREL: This 19, nortestosterone compound possesses very potent progestational activity. In the daily oral dose of 30 mcg (Microval) continuously, it prevents conception. **The drug reduces the sperm penetrability of the cervical mucus and impairs luteal function.** **Norgestrel**, *a racemic dl mixture, is only half as potent as* **levonorgestrel** *as the latter alone is active.*

The other **progestin only pills (POP; minipills)** are **norgestrel 75 mcg, norethisterone 350 mcg** and **ethynodiol diacetate 500 mcg**.

Advantages of 'minipills' are as follows:

a. *The usual estrogen-induced adverse effects* such as alterations in coagulation factors, suppression of lactation and rise in triglyceride metabolism are low
b. There is no delay in conception following cessation of POP
c. They can be used during breastfeeding

Disadvantages are:

a. *All of them cause irregular and generally short bleeding intervals and spotting in a high proportion of cases.*
b. *Concurrent use of enzyme-inducing drugs such as rifampicin can render POP ineffective*

Furthermore, even one pill is forgotten or is delayed by 3 h or longer by a woman who is not breastfeeding, intercourse should be considered as unprotected and an alternative method (condom) should be used.

The use of progestin alone for contraception is much less reliable than that of COCs. Hence, they are used only if there is specific contraindication to estrogen, in breastfeeding mothers and in those who find other contraceptive measures unacceptable. The progestin-only pill should be started by a breastfeeding mother 6 weeks after childbirth.

ANTI-ESTROGENIC AGENTS

ORMELOXIFENE (Centchroman, Saheli): This chroman derivative is a SERM (Chapter 65). It shows weak estrogenicity (in bone), potent anti-estrogenicity (in uterus, breasts), and is devoid of progestogenic or androgenic activity. It causes asynchrony in the menstrual cycle between ovulation and development of the uterine lining.

Given orally, it is well absorbed and is metabolised in the liver. The plasma t½ after a single 60 mg dose is 169 h. It is given twice weekly for 3 months followed by 30–60 mg once a week. However, it is less effective than COC pill and has high failure rate.

The drug appears to be well tolerated. The main side effect is prolongation of the menstrual cycle. It may cause enlargement of ovaries. It should be avoided in polycystic ovarian disease, renal and hepatic disorders, tuberculosis and lactating mothers.

Box 66.4 Contraindications to Injectable Progestin Contraceptives

- The patient has one of the following medical conditions:
  - Likely pregnancy
  - Unexplained vaginal bleeding
  - Past or current breast cancer
  - Severe high blood pressure
  - Coronary heart disease
  - Diabetes mellitus with vascular complications
  - H/O thrombosis, past stroke
  - Severe liver disease
- The patient wants to conceive in the next 6 months
- The patient does not want weight gain or changes in the pattern of vaginal bleeding

PARENTERAL CONTRACEPTIVES

IM progestational preparations, **depot-medroxy-progesterone acetate** (DMPA) and **norethisterone enanthate** (NET-EN), are highly effective, long acting and produce reversible effects. They enter the circulation directly without passing through the liver. They may lower the sex drive in less than 5% of women; they do not cause any birth defects. To get the best results the woman must return in time for the next injection. However, they have certain disadvantages (Box 66.4).

MEDROXYPROGESTERONE ACETATE (MPA) is a potent progestational compound, which is effective both orally and parenterally. The long acting, slowly absorbed, depot preparation DMPA is given intramuscularly once every 3 months. It exerts its effect primarily by inhibition of pituitary LH, leading to suppression of ovulation. Its action on the endometrium, the fallopian tubes and the cervical mucus may also contribute to the contraceptive effect. It is excreted in the breast milk but **does not suppress lactation.**

Repeated injections of DMPA cause prolonged inhibition of ovulation for several months, even after discontinuation.

Adverse reactions: The major drawback is the **disruption of the normal menstrual cycle** that occurs in two-thirds of the recipients. It causes bleeding **irregularities, spotting and prolonged amenorrhoea.** Return of fertility is delayed by 6–12 months. Weight gain is common. It decreases bone mineral density. **Large doses** used to treat cancer or precocious puberty can cause adrenal suppression.

NET-EN: This C-18 progestin has properties and mechanism of action similar to DMPA; it, however, has to get hydrolysed to become biologically active. It has a relatively short duration of action. It also causes menstrual disturbances similar to DMPA.

DMPA and NET-EN therapy may be initiated:

- Any time the physician is reasonably certain that the patient is not pregnant, e.g. within the first 7 days of the menstrual bleeding.
- Immediately after an abortion or after a childbirth *if the mother chooses not to breastfeed the baby;* it should be delayed by 6 weeks in those planning to breastfeed.

Table 66.3 lists the available injectable contraceptives. Preparations containing EE are probably more effective and cause regular vaginal bleeding pattern. Fertility returns sooner after stopping them.

Table 66.3 Injectable Contraceptives and Their Doses

Formulation	Brand Name	Injection Schedule
DMPA 150 mg IM	Depo-Provera	Every 3 months
DMPA 104 mg SC	DMPA–SC	Every 3 months
NET-EN 200 mg IM	Noristerat	Every 2 months
DMPA 25 mg + estradiol cypionate 5 mg IM	Cyclofem	Every month
NET-EN 50 mg + estradiol valerate 5 mg IM	Mesigyna	Every month

LEVONORGESTREL AND ETONOGESTREL IMPLANTS:

These two small, flexible, match-stick sized plastic rod implants release progestin, either levonorgestrel (Jadelle) or etonogestrel (Nexplanon) slowly. Etonogestrel is an active netabolite of desogestrel. Jadelle is a two rod system, whereas nexplanon has a single rod. The rods are inserted under the skin, usually on the inside of the woman's upper arm. They do not interrupt an existing pregnancy and **can be removed any time as per the woman's wish**, following which the fertility is restored immediately. **They provide long term protection against pregnancy** (5 years with Jadelle and 3 years with Nexplanon).

Adverse reactions: Local infection may occur if the implant is inserted without proper asepsis. *About 70% of the users experience irregular bleeding or amenorrhoea.* Users have few pregnancies; many of them are likely to be ectopic. Other adverse effects are similar to that of oral progestins.

It is an invasive procedure and needs trained personnel and monitoring.

Transdermal contraceptive system (TCS): This three-layer patch contains **norelgestromin** and **ethinyl estradiol**. Norelgestromin is the active metabolite of norgestimate. It is applied once a week for 3 successive weeks in a month. It delivers a daily dose of 20 mcg EE and 0.15 mg norelgestromin and allows withdrawal bleeding in the patch-free week. ADRs are similar to COC pills. It is as effective as the COC except in very obese women. It is convenient but expensive.

Vaginal contraceptive ring: This intravaginal device delivers a daily dose of 15 mcg of EE and 0.12 mg of etonogestrel. It is kept for 3–4 weeks following a ring-free week. It offers excellent cycle control and fertility returns rapidly after its removal. It may cause local discomfort, headache and vaginal discharge. Its efficacy is similar to that of COC pills. It is very expensive.

Intrauterine contraceptive devices (IUCDs) *are highly cost effective and satisfactory reversible method of contraception*. It is the most commonly used method with high continuation rate. **Copper containing IUCDs** are small, flexible plastic frames containing coiled copper impregnated with barium sulfate (T shaped device-CuT380A and an inverted U shaped device- Cu 375).

Copper containing IUCD release copper ions which alters the uterine and tubal fluid environment, thereby hampering sperm motility and function. In addition the device induces foreign body reaction in the endometrium which prevents implantation. They are the cheaper alternatives. CuT 380 A remains effective till 10 years and IUCD 375 for 5 years from insertion. *Vaginal and pelvic examination is mandatory before insertion to rule out pregnancy, any pelvic infection, fibroids, cervicitis, vaginitis, STI or HIV.* It can be inserted during interval period (any time during the menstrual cycle or after 6 weeks of delivery) or postpartum period (within 48 hours of delivery or within 12 days of completion of abortion.

The ADR include discomfort or cramps during menstruation, backache, spotting or light bleeding for initial period after insertion. Severe abdominal pain and heavy, irregular bleeding may require its removal. There can be expulsion from uterine cavity or complaints of missing threads. Moreover, *adequate counselling of the woman is necessary to allay her anxiety and to train her how to check the IUCD thread regularly.* This is to confirm that IUCD is in place and not expelled without her knowledge. Follow-up with physician is also needed.

For details of IUCD insertion, removal and patient counselling, 'Reference manual of IUCD services' by Family Planning Division Ministry of Health and Family Welfare Government of India can be referred to (https://nhm.gov.in/New_Updates_2018/NHM_Components/RMNCHA/Family_planning/Schemes_&_Guidelines/IUCD/IUCD_Manual_English.pdf).

Levonorgestrel releasing IUCDs depending upon their rate of release of levonorgestrel remain effective for 3–7 years. **They are useful for treating heavy menstrual bleeding and dysmenorrhoea.** They may reduce the risk of endometrial and cervical cancer.

The **complications of IUCD** are as follows:

- *Initial increase in menstrual blood loss and dysmenorrhoea with copper IUCD*
- *Increased risk of upper genital infection and pelvic inflammatory disease which can lead to ectopic pregnancy or infertility*
- *Irregular bleeding in first 3–6 months*
- *Rarely, perforation of the uterus*

BARRIER CONTRACEPTIVE METHODS

Various non-medicated or medicated **physical barriers** include condoms, pessaries, vaginal rings, diaphragms or intrauterine contraceptive devices (IUCD).

Chemical barriers are in the form of vaginal gels containing lactic acid, citric acid and potassium bitartrate which maintains vaginal pH between 3.5–4.5. This pH hampers the sperm motility. Gel should be used no more than one hour prior to intercourse. It can cause vaginal burning, pruritus, fungal infection and UTI. Spermicidal gels and foam tablets are also available, which are simple to use and involve little genital manipulation. Most of the spermicides contain the surfactant **nonoxynol 9**, which interferes with sperm motility.

Barrier methods though have less ADR compared to COC, are not very reliable and often inconvenient to practise.

Tubal ligation and vasectomy are the surgical approaches.

Box 66.5 Various Regimens for Postcoital Contraception

- One **levonorgestrel** 0.75 mg tablet, as soon as possible (certainly within 72 h), repeated 12 h later or 2 tab once
- Two **COC pills** containing 50 mcg of EE each (Table 66.4) as soon as possible (certainly within 72 h) after intercourse, and the same dose 12 h later
- **Ulipristal** 30 mg as soon as possible (within 5 days)
- **Copper-containing IUCD** within 5 days (see text)
- **Mifepristone** 10 mg once within 72–120 h (see text)

Choice of contraceptive: All contraceptives have advantages and disadvantages. In a given lady/situation, one method may be considered better than the others. Hence, it is better to have a 'cafeteria type' approach, where the woman concerned is allowed to choose the method after being adequately informed about the advantages and disadvantages of various procedures. 'A happy, knowledgeable and communicating couple, especially if they have a sense of humour, can get along with almost any method'. Women who cannot be relied upon to take pills regularly should be advised methods such as IUCD or etonogestrel implant which are the most effective reversible contraceptive methods or surgical sterilisation.

Chlorpromazine and reserpine can modify the menstrual cycle in women; and suppresses menses to cause amenorrhoea (Chapter 13). This is an ADR of these drugs and is not used therapeutically.

EMERGENCY POSTCOITAL CONTRACEPTION

A possible method of contraception by preventing implantation of the fertilised ovum; **however so far, an ideal anti-implantation drug is not available.**

The emergency oral contraceptives, probably act by interfering with tubal transport, preventing implantation, or by causing regression of the corpus luteum. As these drugs are administered within hours of intercourse and implantation occurs only about 7 days after ovulation, their use is not equivalent to therapeutic abortion. *It does not disrupt an existing pregnancy.*

The various postcoital contraceptives recommended are given in Box 66.5.

Although postcoital contraception is safe to use more than once, this method should not be used in place of standard methods of contraception because it is less effective. *It should be used only as an emergency method, e.g. following rape, in case of unprotected sex, if there is concern about possible contraceptive failure or its incorrect use (condom breakage, 3 or more consecutively missed COC).* There is no age bar to using this technique.

The regimen may cause nausea and vomiting and the treatment may fail if the drug is not retained. There may be light irregular vaginal bleeding (spotting), fatigue, headache, dizziness, tenderness in breast. Repeated use results in menstrual irregularities. Chances of contraception failure are more if levonorgestrel pill is taken after 72 h and in that case resultant pregnancy is more likely to be ectopic as with other progesterone -only contraceptive pills, A possible explanation is that progesterone modifies tubal function, reduces contractility and thus slows the rate of ovum or blastocyst transport. *A pre-existing pregnancy must be ruled out before such treatment is initiated.* If such hormonal form of postcoital treatment fails, there is no evidence that the embryo gets affected to result in adverse fetal outcome. Hence if the woman desires the pregnancy can be continued. This should be explained to the subject before such therapy. If she is not willing to continue, then, the pregnancy should be terminated by other methods after counselling for MTP.

Ulipristal acetate, a selective progesterone receptor modulator (SPRM) **blocks or delays ovulation and also delays the maturation of the endometrium.** It is the most effective method and can be taken within 5 days. It should not be taken in the presence of severe liver diseases. Breastfeed should be avoided within 36 h of taking the drug. Common ADR include abdominal pain and menstrual disorder.

Copper-containing IUCD or the levonorgestrel 52-mg IUCD inserted within 5 days from the day of sexual intercourse is the most effective postcoital contraceptive agent and is to be preferred if hormonal treatment is contraindicated. **COCs** are less effective than ulipristal and IUCD.

Box 66.6 depicts the points that one should remember while prescribing contraceptives.

ANTIPROGESTIN

MIFEPRISTONE (RU 486): This derivative of norethisterone has antiprogestin activity.

Box 66.6 Points to remember while prescribing contraception

- Method of contraception should be cost-effective, durable, convenient, reversible with least adverse effects.
- Its selection should be individualised based on the contraceptive needs of the woman, her reproductive age group, patient specific factors and patient preference. Adequate counselling for how to use a contraceptive, how long to use and its adverse effects aids selection. This should be followed by sufficient training to ensure proper use. Informed consent should be sought.
- A physician practising in rural area must remember that resource limitation may hamper the choice of a woman. In addition, there can be technological, social and administrative issues which pose barriers for selection and use. Lack of or inadequate or improper counselling also leads to failure of contraception. This perceived efficacy of any method may vary depending on the local setting.
- For family planning i.e. for spacing between childbirths, commonly used contraceptive methods include COC, IUCD and condoms. Ideally for family planning, COC can be used for 1–2 years, they are effective and have noncontraceptive benefits. After the desired number of children either IUCD or tubal ligation or vasectomy can be opted for.
- Women may find use of COC cumbersome because of misconceptions, inconvenience of daily administration and adverse effects like nausea. At times they are not available at the family planning centre. Their irregular intake disturbs the menstrual cycle. In addition, their prolonged use has adverse effects on the fertility.
- Use of condoms and IUCD have definite points in their favour:
  - they are cheap, safe and readily available,
  - they require no planned schedule as is necessary in the case of oral contraceptives and
  - condoms offer protection against STD/HIV.

  However, high failure rates, allergic reactions, and poor acceptability are the disadvantages with condoms. IUCD remains the most effective reversible method for woman who wish to have contraception for $\geq$ 1 year, but screening for IUCD eligibility is required. Adequate emphasis should be given on self-monitoring and regular follow -ups.
- Though tubal ligation or vasectomy are permanent contraceptive methods, failures have been reported if the procedures are not performed properly; main reason being inadequate training of the performing physicians.
- Beware of adverse effects of depot preparation of MPA. Its prolonged use can result in irreversible contraception.
- Use of emergency post-coital contraceptive should be restricted only to its indication. It is inferior to the standard methods of contraception; if used repeatedly it can affect fertility; it is not a method to terminate pregnancy and it cannot protect against STI.

Mechanism of action: It acts as a **potent competitive antagonist of progesterone receptors in the presence of progesterone**, and also of glucocorticoid receptors. In the absence of progesterone, it is an agonist.

Pharmacological actions:

Administered to women in early and late luteal phases of the menstrual cycle, it:

a. Shows luteolytic property
b. Causes inhibition of the uterine glandular secretory activity
c. Accelerates degenerative vascular changes, leading to menstrual bleeding within 72 h (**progesterone withdrawal bleeding**)

Hence, it can be used as an emergency contraceptive. Larger doses, however, block the proliferative action of estradiol on the endometrium, and causes endometrial atrophy, suggesting a progestin-like property.

Administered during pregnancy, it:

a. Binds to the progesterone receptor with high affinity and causes decidual necrosis and detachment of the products of conception.
b. Damages the endometrial blood vessels
c. Inhibits PG dehydrogenase activity thereby increasing the PGE_2 level which stimulates uterine contractility
d. Causes cervical dilatation

Doses higher than those needed to produce antiprogestin effects block the effects of glucocorticoids at the level of the tissues. Thus, it ameliorates the manifestations of hypercortisolism in patients with Cushing's syndrome.

Absorption, fate, excretion: Mifepristone is administered orally or parenterally. Given orally, its plasma level peaks at 1–2 h. It is metabolised slowly by the liver and is excreted in the bile with an elimination plasma t½ of 20 h. *The plasma level is lower but is sustained longer after intravaginal than after oral administration.* The metabolites also have antiprogestin and antiglucocorticoid activity.

Adverse reactions: Single doses may cause nausea, vomiting, abdominal pain (in >60% subjects), and sometimes heavy prolonged bleeding. Long term use of mifepristone can cause fatigue, anaemia, weight loss, thinning of hair, menstrual disturbances, decrease in libido and gynaecomastia. Mifepristone-PG combination should be used cautiously in subjects with heart disease.

Indications:

- **Postcoital contraception:** Mifepristone in a **single dose of 10–50 mg** given within 5 days of unprotected intercourse is as effective as a combination of 100 mcg of ethinyl estradiol and 0.5 mg of levonorgestrel given twice in a day.
- **Induction of abortion** (see section, Medical termination of pregnancy): For this purpose, mifepristone is used in a **large single dose of 600 mg** followed by a vaginal suppository of gemeprost 48 h later.
- **Cervical dilatation:** It is useful for preoperative preparation of women for surgical abortion. It is as effective as PGs and has fewer side effects.
- **Induction of labour** after intrauterine fetal death.

MALE CONTRACEPTION

In males, spermatogenesis can be inhibited by androgens, estrogens and progestins. Although steroid combinations can inhibit spermatogenesis, such therapy has adverse effects. *Vasectomy, carried out in properly selected cases, would be the most economical, reliable and relatively safe procedure for the males. It does not affect the libido.* The other alternative is to use a condom.

GOSSYPOL, a compound obtained from the cotton seed is an effective male antifertility agent. However, its major ADR include decreased libido, occasional hypokalaemic paralysis, and atrophy of seminiferous tubules, which are not acceptable.

MEDICAL TERMINATION OF PREGNANCY (MTP)

Although termination of pregnancy has been legalised in many countries it is estimated that 20 million pregnancies are terminated illegally often by quacks, with more than 78,000 deaths, each year. Use of drugs for emergency postcoital contraception is described earlier. Drugs used for MTP during the **early part of the first trimester** can be classified as follows.

Classification

I. **Progesterone synthesis inhibitors:** Epostane and trilostane They are under investigation.
II. **Antiprogestins,** e.g., mifepristone (see section, Antiprogestins)
III. **Anti-estrogen**, e.g. tamoxifen (see Chapter 59)
IV. **Trophoblast inhibitors**, e.g. methotrexate
V. **Oxytocics**, e.g. **prostaglandins** and oxytocin (Chapter 42)
VI. **Miscellaneous**, e.g. ethacridine, hypertonic saline (Chapter 42)

Although **PGs** can be given alone to terminate pregnancy with a success rate of 90%, the high doses needed cause a high incidence of adverse effects such as nausea, vomiting, diarrhoea, pain and dizziness. Hence, *PGs in low dose are combined with mifepristone or methotrexate.* The synthetic PGE compounds **misoprostol** and **gemeprost** (Chapter 25) are generally preferred. Misoprostol can be stored at room temperature and is relatively inexpensive. It is administered orally or vaginally. Gemeprost is more expensive and thermolabile. It is given as vaginal pessary.

Mifepristone – misoprostol combination is highly effective in almost 98% of the pregnant women. *Mifepristone is given orally as a single dose of 400–600 mg, (in contrast to 10 mg for emergency contraception), followed 48 h later by misoprostol 400 mcg or gemeprost 0.5–1.0 mg vaginally.* Oral misoprostol is less effective. The common ADR include backache, headache and uterine cramps. They are not dose-related. *Severe side effects include prolonged and sometimes excessive vaginal bleeding.* Women with severe asthma, adrenal insufficiency and those on long-term glucocorticoid therapy should not be given this combination because of its antiglucocorticoid action. It should be used cautiously in women with DM, severe anaemia, haemorrhagic disorders and those on anticoagulants.

Methotrexate (Chapter 59), 25–50 mg given orally and followed 3–7 days later by **misoprostol** 800 mcg vaginally, is effective in 85%–95% of women with **pregnancy of less than 8 weeks duration**. The combination may cause nausea, vomiting, pain (due to misoprostol) and stomatitis and oral ulcers (due to methotrexate). It is contraindicated in women over 35 years of age and in those with cardiac risk factors, as it can precipitate heart failure.

The **advantages** of above combinations are as follows:

- **The termination can be carried out on outpatient basis** - first dose is given in the clinic and misoprostol is self-administered at home.
- **Relatively safe, do not require anaesthesia and hence highly acceptable.**
- **Effective in 98% of women with less than 8 weeks' pregnancy.** The treatment failure rate rises with menstrual delay of 35 days or more.

The disadvantages are that they are not 100% effective; further they can sometimes cause prolonged and severe bleeding.

Tamoxifen 20 mg once daily for 4 days, followed by **vaginal misoprostol** 800 mcg, is also reported to be effective in 90% of women.

Ethacridine: This acridine compound has been used **extra-amniotically** for **second trimester abortion.** GI adverse effects and bleeding may occur but serious toxicity is claimed to be rare. On an average, it takes 30 h to effect abortion.

Medical termination, however, is more painful and less effective in women with pregnancy of more than 8 weeks duration. In such cases, vacuum extraction is more acceptable and safer.

OVULATION-INDUCING DRUGS

It is estimated that infertility occurs in about 15%–20% of couples. Both the partners need detailed examination. One-third of these problems are due to female factors, another one-third is due to male factors and for the remaining third, the cause is unknown.

Unexplained infertility in women with advanced reproductive age is probably due to diminished quality and quantity of oocytes. It should be remembered that 20%–30% of infertile but otherwise normal women ovulate spontaneously.

Deficiency of the thyroid hormone is an uncommon cause probably responsible in less than 3% of anovulatory cycles.

As mentioned in Chapter 65, estrogens may be responsible in triggering an ovarian signal for midcycle LH release. Low dose estrogen may be useful in cases where some follicular activity is present but midcycle LH peak is lacking or corpus luteum is inadequate. An estrogen can be tried along with ovulation inducing drugs.

Generally, in **women with anovulatory cycles** and normal hypothalamic–pituitary–ovarian function, fertility can be induced by ovulation inducing agents. In **women with hypothalamic amenorrhea,** administration of FSH–LH combination is used from the beginning.

PH 1.40

Classification of Ovulation-Inducing Drugs

I. **Synthetic GnRH:** (Chapter 65)
II. **Human menopausal and chorionic gonadotropins** (Chapter 65)
III. **Bromergocriptine** (Chapter 65)
IV. **Anti-estrogenic compound:** Clomiphene citrate, letrozole

ANTI-ESTROGENIC DRUGS

CLOMIPHENE CITRATE: This is a triphenylethylene compound, with structural resemblance to stilbestrol and chlorotrianisene (Fig. 66.1). It is effective in inducing ovulation in women with anovulation.

Mechanism of action: Clomiphene **acts by competing with the circulating estrogen for receptor sites in the hypothalamus and the pituitary.** It is a partial agonist of estrogen. On binding to the estrogen receptor, it prevents binding of native estrogen to the receptors and exhibits estrogen antagonist action. This blocks the negative feedback of native estrogen on the hypothalamo-pituitary axis leading to release of pituitary FSH and LH and ovulation.

Pharmacological actions:

Induction of ovulation: See indications of clomiphene.

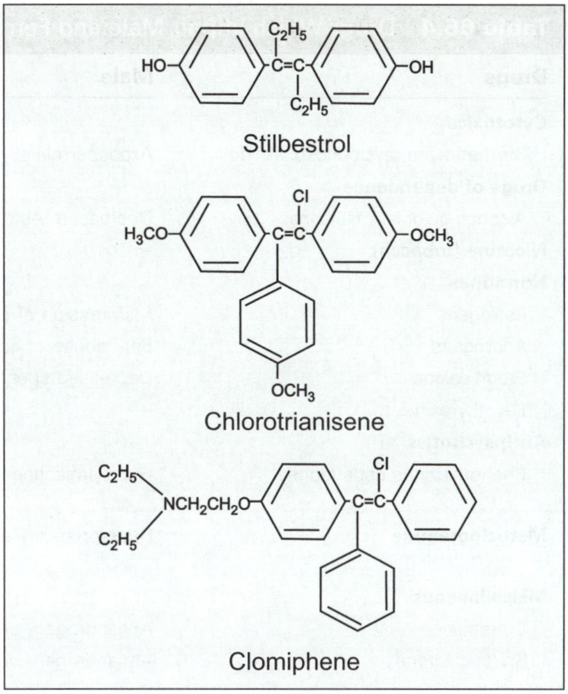

FIG. 66.1 Structural resemblance between nonsteroidal estrogens and the anti-estrogen clomiphene.

Anti-estrogenic action: Clomiphene causes regression of estrogen induced proliferative endometrium and counters the keratinisation of vaginal epithelium. It can prolong the luteal phase in normally menstruating women and nullify the ovulatory inhibition produced by OC pills.

Miscellaneous actions: It has a weak estrogenic action, on the bone and endometrium. Given to premenopausal women, it causes hot flushes.

Absorption, fate and excretion: The drug is well absorbed orally. It is concentrated in the bile and excreted in the intestines, from where it is reabsorbed (enterohepatic circulation). It is mainly excreted in the faeces and only a small amount appears in the urine. Half of the dose is excreted within 5 days.

Adverse reactions: It causes hot flushes, GI disturbances, breast discomfort, blurring of vision, abnormal uterine bleeding and alopecia. The important drawback is that it causes:

- **Ovarian enlargement** (and *ovarian hyperstimu-*

Table 66.4 Drugs Which Impair Male and Female Fertility

Drugs	Male	Female
Cytotoxics		
Methotrexate, cyclophosphamide	Azoospermia	Ovarian failure
Drugs of dependence		
Alcohol, opioids, marijuana	Decreased testosterone and sperm abnormalities	Menstrual irregularities
Nicotine (tobacco)	–	Premature ovarian failure
Hormones		
Estrogens	Suppression of pituitary and hypothalamus	Menstrual irregularities
Androgens	See 'abuse of anabolic steroids by athletes'	Anovulation
Prednisolone	Decreased sperm count	–
Levothyroxine	–	Anovulation with large doses
Antipsychotics		
Phenothiazines risperidone	Hyperprolactinaemia, impotence	Hyperprolactinaemia, menstrual irregularities
Metoclopramide	Hyperprolactinaemia, impotence	Hyperprolactinaemia, menstrual irregularities
Miscellaneous		
Cimetidine	Antiandrogen, azoospermia	Menstrual irregularities
Spironolactone	Antiandrogen, decreased testosterone	Menstrual irregularities
Sulphasalazine	Decreased sperm count	–
Phenytoin	Decreased sperm count	–

lation) and cyst formation, which may rarely lead to rupture and internal haemorrhage

- **Multiple ovulation**, resulting in multiple pregnancies and fetal wastage

Indications:

- **Ovulation induction:** Clomiphene is **indicated in the treatment of anovulatory infertility, with adequate endogenous estrogenic activity.** Clomiphene is given orally in doses of 50–200 mg at bed-time for 5–7 days. It is started between day 2 and 5 of the menstrual cycle. Nearly 70%–80% anovulatory patients ovulate, of which 30%–40% will become pregnant. *Most of these pregnancies occur after 3–6 consecutive cycles.*

  Ovulation usually occurs 2–12 days after completion of the treatment. **In case of an amenorrhoeic patient,** the drug can be given at any time but it is customary to start it on the 5th day of withdrawal bleeding after a course of medroxyprogesterone (5 mg b.i.d. for 5 days).

  Compared to human pituitary gonadotropin, clomiphene is less effective but less hazardous, and is much less expensive. It is claimed that the incidence of abortions can be reduced by using progesterone (micronised 100 mg b.i.d. for 14 days) soon after the existence of conception is confirmed.

  Treatment in an individual patient should be limited to 12 cycles in the lifetime because of the reported increase in the incidence of ovarian cancer following longer treatment.

- **Polycystic ovary syndrome (PCOS):** This is characterised by polycystic ovaries associated with anovulation, hyperandrogenism, and infertility. It has a familial basis and many patients show insulin resistance and DM. The current management of PCOS includes:

  1. Lifestyle modification; diet control and exercise for weight reduction in obese patients; and cessation of smoking; this treatment often can induce ovulation.

2. **Metformin** can improve insulin resistance, regulate the menstrual cycles and cause ovulation in patients with glucose intolerance. It is administered in the dose of 500 mg o.d. and increased to 500 mg t.i.d.
3. If metformin is not effective in 3–5 months, **clomiphene may be added** for further 6 months. Metformin should be stopped when pregnancy is confirmed.
4. If the treatment fails after 12 cycles, **gonadotropin therapy** may be considered.
5. **Dexamethasone** in small doses (0.25–0.5 mg daily) induces ovulation in some **patients with PCOS,** by suppressing the adrenal androgen contribution.

Cauterisation of the ovarian cysts may be done only as a last resort.

- **Oligospermia:** Clomiphene has also been used in this condition with variable results.

CYCLOFENIL: This compound has a structure similar to clomiphene and is used for similar purposes. It does not exert a peripheral anti-estrogenic effect.

Letrozole, is an aromatase inhibitor that blocks estrogen synthesis by inhibiting the final step of the estrogen biosynthetic pathway. This increases the secretion of pituitary FSH as a feedback to stimulate ovulation. Letrozole causes temporary accumulation of intra-ovarian androgens, which may increase follicular sensitivity to FSH by amplifying FSH receptor gene expression. In addition, androgens accumulation in the follicle may stimulate IGF-1 and other factors, which may synergize with FSH to promote folliculogenesis.

The adverse effects are headache, hot flushes, abdominal cramps, bloating, mood disturbances, somnolence, anxiety, fatigue, and cognitive dysfunction.

Indications:

- **As an ovulation inducer:** It is extensively used in anovulatory infertility patients with PCOS or unexplained infertility. For this letrozole is prescribed as 2.5 to 7.5 mg daily for 5 days during Day 3 to Day 7 of menstruation.
- **Adjunct in intrauterine insemination and *in vitro* fertilization techniques.**
- **For fertility preservation in women with estrogen-sensitive cancers.**
- **Treatment of estrogen dependent breast cancer** (See chapter 59)

Table 66.4 lists some drugs which may impair fertility in males and females.

DRUGS USED FOR MEDICAL TERMINATION OF PREGNANCY (MTP)

Progesterone synthesis inhibitors
- Epostane
- Trilostane

Antiprogestins
- Mifepristone

Anti-estrogen
- Tamoxifen

Trophoblast inhibitors
- Methotrexate

Oxytocics
- Prostaglandins (Misoprostol, Gemeprost)
- Oxytocin

Miscellaneous
- Ethacridine
- Hypertonic saline

OVULATION-INDUCING DRUGS

Synthetic GnRH

- GnRH
- Leuprorelin acetate
- Buserelin acetate
- Nafarelin
- Goserelin acetate

Human menopausal and chorionic gonadotropins

Bromergocriptine

Anti-estrogenics

- Clomiphene citrate

PHARMACOLOGICAL CONTRACEPTIVES

Oral

Combination Oral Contraceptives (COC) containing estrogen and progestin component

- Fixed dose (monophasic) COC
- Biphasic and triphasic COC
- Extended cycle COC

Progestin alone as contraceptive (minipill)

Anti-estrogenic agents

- Ormeloxifene

Parenteral

Injectables

- Depot-medroxyprogesterone acetate (DMPA)
- Norethisterone enanthate (NET-EN)

Implants

- Levonorgestrel implant

Transdermal contraceptive system

Medicated Uterine/ Vaginal devices

Vaginal contraceptive rings

Intrauterine contraceptive medicated devices (medicated IUCD)

CHAPTER 67

Androgens, Anabolic Steroids, Antiandrogens and Treatment of Sexual Dysfunction

Learning Objectives

This chapter will enable the reader:

1. To be aware of the physiological actions of androgens.
2. To describe the mechanism of action, pharmacological effects, salient pharmacokinetic features, ADR, preparations and indications for testosterone.
3. To enlist anabolic steroids and describe the pharmacological effects, ADR and indications.
4. To classify antiandrogens.
5. To state the salient features of antiandrogens, i.e. finasteride, cyproterone acetate, flutamide, spironolactone.
6. To discuss the management of hirsutism.
7. To outline the pharmacotherapy of benign prostatic hyperplasia.
8. To outline the treatment of erectile dysfunction.

KEY TERMS

testosterone, p. 984
anabolic steroids, p. 986
cyproterone acetate, p. 988
hirsutism, management, p. 988
benign prostatic hyperplasia, p. 989
finasteride, p. 990
erectile dysfunction, p. 991
sildenafil, p. 992

The first pure hormone with androgenic activity – *androsterone* – was isolated from the male urine by Adolf Butenandt in 1931. The hormone secreted by testes, *testosterone*, was isolated in pure form in 1935. Androgens in smaller amounts are also produced in the ovary, the adrenal cortex and the placenta.

Physiological actions of androgens: Androgens determine the differentiation of the fetal external genitals in the male direction. In males they prevent the development of the hypothalamic cyclic release of LH. At puberty, hypothalamic GnRH release in discrete pulses increases the pituitary FSH and LH.

Increased LH acts on Leydig cells to stimulate synthesis and secretion of testosterone markedly, which is responsible to convert a boy into a man. It is associated with:

1. A marked **rise in intratesticular testosterone** which is essential for spermatogenesis
2. Elevated *plasma testosterone* which promotes the development of external genitalia and secondary sexual characters

FSH acts on the seminiferous tubules. It promotes the growth of the testes and **spermatogenesis** as well as stimulates the Sertoli cells. **It is thus gametogenic in action.** Sertoli cells also secrete inhibin beta, which selectively suppresses FSH. Thus, both FSH and LH play an important role in initiating and maintaining the normal testicular functions. These are as follows:

- **Development of male external genitals** (penis and scrotum), and **secondary sex characters** (pubic hair and beard) and **change in voice**
- **Development of the male internal genitals:** seminal vesicles, prostate and epididymis
- **Maintenance of spermatogenesis**
- **Development of skeletal musculature and emotional make up of male type**
- **Anabolic and growth promoting effects**

Failure of the testicular function causes male hypogonadism.

The daily testosterone plasma concentration is 4–10 ng/mL. A small proportion of the circulating testosterone arises from the extra-adrenal conversion of the weak adrenal androgens dehydroepiandrosterone and androstenedione. *In the female, the latter is an important source of plasma testosterone, which measures 30–50 ng/mL.*

Testosterone is converted in androgen-responsive tissues to the active metabolites, 5α-dihydrotestosterone and small amount of estradiol. It circulates in the blood, mainly bound to albumin and partly to sex hormone binding globulin; small amount is present in free form. In men, nearly 80% of circulating estradiol is derived from testosterone.

Male hypogonadism: Failure of testicular function can be either:

a. Primary, due to testicular failure, or
b. Secondary, due to failure of the HP (hypothalamic–pituitary) complex

In primary testicular failure, gonadotropin secretion is increased, producing **hypergonadotropic hypogonadism**, whereas in HP failure, the gonadotropin secretion does not increase, causing **hypogonadotropic hypogonadism**.

The testicular deficiency could be selectively gametogenic or both gameto- and androgenic. In the former, the individual is sterile but has normal secondary sex characters; in the second case both the functions are impaired.

Failure of the testes before puberty (prepuberal hypogonadism) causes infantile penis, feminine distribution of fat (more on buttocks, breast and hips) and arrest of laryngeal and sexual hair growth. The muscles remain soft; skin becomes smooth and there is a lack of sex drive. Intelligence is not affected.

In a patient with **postpuberal hypogonadism**, the general body proportions and size of the penis are not altered. But the body hair become sparse and silky, voice becomes high pitched and libido is greatly reduced. Skeletal muscles become flabby and there is a tendency to develop obesity. The semen volume is less and emotional weakness is seen. However, the life expectancy is not shortened nor is premature senility produced. PH 1.37

TESTOSTERONE, its synthetic analogues and **dihydrotestosterone** bind to a cytoplasmic androgen receptor protein before acting on the nucleus in a similar manner as estrogen.

Mechanism of action:

1. **Direct:** Testosterone and its most potent metabolite, **dihydrotestosterone** produced by 5-alpha reductase, activate the androgenic receptors. They bring about the development of male sexual organs, prostate, increase in muscle mass and strength and promote erythropoiesis.
2. **Indirect:** effects are through other active metabolite, **estradiol** produced by its aromatisation, which acts on both the estrogen receptors. This causes regulation of body fat and prevention of bone loss.
3. Both, testosterone and estrogen regulate the sexual function maintain normal libido and erectile function.

Pharmacological actions: These are dose related. There appears to be a variation in tissue sensitivity to androgens.

Androgenic action: Administration of testosterone in prepuberal hypogonadism reverses most of the changes of hypogonadism. The secondary sex characters develop, muscle strength increases and sex desire and erections occur normally. The testes do not enlarge and spermatogenesis does not occur.

In females, testosterone causes increased libido as well as masculinisation, e.g. hirsutism, growth of clitoris and change in voice (male type). The development of proliferative phase of the endometrium may be inhibited and large doses suppress the ovulation and lactation. Administered during pregnancy, androgenic compounds can masculinise the external genitals of the female fetus.

Anabolic actions: Protein synthesis (**anabolism**) and protein breakdown (**catabolism**) are the important functions of a cell. Adequate supply of nutrient material is necessary for protein synthesis. Testosterone promotes nitrogen retention and increases the appetite, muscle mass and body weight especially in eunuchoid men, in prepuberal boys and in women. It is insignificant in normal healthy male adults. Along with nitrogen, potassium, sulphur and phosphorus are also retained, whereas the urinary excretion of calcium and creatinine is decreased.

Bones and epiphyses: Testosterone in small doses can promote growth of epiphyseal cartilage, particularly in boys with short stature due to hypogonadism. *However, large doses bring about early epiphyseal fusion and reduce the final adult height.*

Androgens may reduce bone resorption and cause beneficial effects in senile osteoporosis. This effect is probably due to estradiol.

Effect on pituitary: Testosterone exerts a negative feedback effect on LH and a smaller one on FSH. The LH inhibiting action could be due to the small quantities of estrogen to which testosterone is converted in the pituitary. Mesterolone, a testosterone analogue, which is not converted into estrogen, lacks this property.

Haemopoietic action: They stimulate renal erythropoietin secretion, and directly stimulate haem synthesis in the bone marrow.

Miscellaneous actions: Androgens increase appetite and cause a feeling of well-being. They can cause sodium retention. They also cause growth and increased secretion of the sebaceous glands, clinically manifested as acne.

In females, these compounds generally antagonise many actions of estrogen.

Absorption, fate and excretion: Testosterone is well absorbed orally but is largely inactivated by the liver (first pass) and hence, is therapeutically ineffective. Its 17-methyl derivatives methyltestosterone and fluoxymesterone are much less degraded by the liver and are orally effective.

Ninety-eight per cent of plasma testosterone is in bound form. Its plasma t½ is about 10–20 min. It is largely metabolised in the liver, and in small amount in prostrate and skin. It is excreted in the urine, mostly as androsterone and etiocholanolone, as sulphates and glucuronides. *The plasma testosterone levels are a useful indicator of androgen production in the male.*

Esters of testosterone with weak organic acids like propionic acid, when injected, produce prolonged action for 2–3 days, whereas cypionate and enanthate are effective for 1–2 weeks. Testosterone pellets implanted under the skin are slowly absorbed; their therapeutic effect lasts for 6–8 months.

Assay: For clinical purposes, androgens are measured by radioimmunoassay. The androgenic activity of a compound can be bioassayed by the measurement of growth of the seminal vesicles or the prostate in castrated rats.

Adverse reactions:

- In large doses, testosterone can cause precocious puberty in boys, and masculinisation (deepening of voice, hirsutism, acne, baldness and clitoromegaly) in girls and women. Some of these changes may be irreversible.
- In young children, prolonged use of these drugs may bring about early closure of the epiphyses and thus stop the growth.
- In pubertal boys, androgens can cause gynaecomastia.
- **Large doses** can suppress spermatogenesis and may even cause degeneration of seminiferous tubules.
- **Androgens aggravate a pre-existing cancer of the prostate.** They can also aggravate bladder neck obstruction in patients with benign prostatic hypertrophy.
- Large doses can cause retention of sodium and oedema.
- Methyl testosterone, fluoxymesterone and many anabolic steroids are potentially hepatotoxic and can cause cholestatic jaundice.

Preparations and dosage:

- **Testosterone esters:** Parenteral forms are all 17 β OH ester derivatives of testosterone.
    - i. Testosterone propionate injection available as 25,50 and 100 mg/ml. Dose: 10–50 mg IM three times a week.
    - ii. Testosterone phenylpropionate 40–60 mg IM every 3 weeks, usually combined with other testosterone esters.
    - iii. Testosterone cypionate 50–400 mg IM every 2–4 weeks

iv. Testosterone enanthate injection as 100 or 250 mg/ml. Dose: Initially 250 mg IM every 2-3 weeks followed by 250 mg every 3-6 weeks.
v. Testosterone undecanoate in tea seed oil or castor oil 250 mg/mL depot IM injections. Dose: 1 g every 10-14 weeks; if necessary, second dose after 6 weeks and then every 10-14 weeks

- **Oral preparations:** Testosterone undecanoate 40 mg per capsule. Dose 120–160 mg/day in divided doses. Buccal tablet 30 mg is also available and given twice daily.
- **Transdermal preparations:** Testoderm patch (300 mcg for 24 h) and androgel (50 mg/5 g tube) for rubbing are available for application to the scrotal skin daily.
- **Testosterone implants** 100–200 mg. Dose: 100–600 mg doses every 4 months.

Indications: It is used either for its androgenic and antiestrogenic actions or for its anabolic effects. The uses are:

I. **For replacement therapy:**
- **Hypogonadism:** In primary testicular failure, the treatment should be started at puberty. For sustained effect, the long-acting esters are preferred to the shorter acting ones. Oral preparations are not very effective in initiating sexual development but are often adequate for maintenance therapy.
  The diagnosis of hypogonadism in young children should be made cautiously because of marked variations in age of maturation in different individuals. *Testosterone should not be used routinely to hasten the onset of puberty and sexual maturation in otherwise normal boys.*
  In postpuberal hypogonadism, only replacement therapy is needed and long-acting testosterone preparation is given in the dose of 200 mg every 2 weeks; some patients need 'low dose' replacement therapy in the form of 50–100 mg of the same preparation(s) intramuscularly once every 2 weeks. Oral preparations need to be given daily.
- **Male climacteric** (Andropause): Testicular function declines as the age advances. This is manifested as muscular weakness and tendency to obesity. In such cases small doses of testosterone may be useful. However, the criteria for such diagnosis are very vague.

II. **For pharmacological therapy:**
- **As anabolic steroid:** It is replaced by anabolic steroids.
- **Impotence:** Sexual impotence may be defined as inability for a man to have satisfactory sexual intercourse. This can be due to:
  i. Lack of sexual desire (libido)
  ii. Inability to achieve or maintain an erection (erectile dysfunction, ED)
  iii. Failure of ejaculation
- **Refractory anaemias, particularly aplastic anaemia**

Testosterone and anabolic steroids are absolutely contraindicated in carcinoma of prostrate and breast in males.

ANABOLIC STEROIDS PH 1.37

Although testosterone has potent anabolic activity, it cannot be used freely for this purpose because of its androgenic action. Hence, various steroids were synthesised with anabolic actions but reduced virilising effects. The clinically used anabolic steroids are given in Table 67.1. Chemically, they are derivatives of testosterone or methyl testosterone. *None of the presently available compounds, however, is selectively anabolic, without an androgenic ADR.*

Table 67.1 Anabolic Steroids

Name	Recommended Adult Dose
Nandrolone decanoate[a,c]	25–100 mg every 3 weeks
Methenolone acetate	10–20 mg daily
Oxymetholone	5–15 mg daily
Methandienone	2.5–15 mg daily
Ethylestrenol	2–4 mg daily
Norethandrolone	10–40 mg daily
Oxandrolone[b]	2.5–20 mg daily
Stanozolol[c]	2.5–10 mg daily

[a]These are given intramuscularly; the rest are given orally. The first three are derivatives of testosterone, the rest of methyltestosterone.
[b]Not converted to estrogen.
[c]Available in the market; the rest of the preparations are not freely available currently.

Pharmacological actions:

Anabolic effects: In therapeutic doses, the anabolic action is predominant. Anabolic steroids promote protein anabolism, as manifested by increase in the muscle mass and the body weight.

The androgenic effect becomes more apparent during prolonged therapy, particularly in females.

Anticatabolic effects: In short-term studies, anabolic steroids have been shown to produce positive nitrogen balance in individuals on prolonged glucocorticoid therapy. However, their routine use in combination with glucocorticoids may be dangerous as ADR due to glucocorticoids such as hypertension, acne, hirsutism and sodium retention may be potentiated.

Progestational effects: Some of the anabolic steroids like norethandrolone have significant progestational activity.

Miscellaneous actions: Like testosterone, anabolic steroids may reduce bone resorption and thus may prevent osteoporosis.

Adverse reactions: These are due to their **androgenic action** and are similar to those produced by testosterone. They are most likely to occur in children and females and need monitoring. The use of anabolic steroids in pregnancy has led to virilisation of the fetus and advanced bone age. In addition, the orally active anabolic steroids which have a substituted alkyl group at C17 can cause **cholestatic jaundice, and liver damage**. Prolonged treatment may cause sodium and water retention.

Preparations: See Table 67.1. The paediatric doses of these drugs are: methandienone 0.04 mg/kg/day; ethylestrenol 0.1–0.2 mg/kg/day; oxandrolone 0.1 mg/kg/day.

Indications:

- **Chronic illness:**. Protein catabolism or negative nitrogen balance is observed in various chronic conditions such as protein-energy malnutrition, fever, infections, all forms of stress, prolonged immobilisation and following broad-spectrum antibiotics. In majority of these conditions, correction of the cause and providing adequate calories and nutrients including proteins will accelerate anabolism. *Anabolic steroids are certainly not effective during the acute phase of the illness or continuing stress.* Used during recovery from such conditions, they may stimulate appetite and the sense of well-being nonspecifically, and promote weight gain. They have been used during chronic illness especially HIV cachexia to improve appetite and the sense of well-being.
- **Growth:** They are used to **promote growth in hypogonadal children.** If available, oral oxandrolone is the preferred drug. Their place in the treatment of short stature from other causes is very limited. *They should not be used in girls.*
- **Renal failure:** They are sometimes used in acute or chronic renal failure, along with protein restriction, to reduce blood urea and thus to decrease the nitrogen load on the kidneys.
- **Anaemias:** They are claimed to be effective in certain refractory anaemias associated with bone marrow hypoplasia or aplasia.

Anabolic steroids are not tonics and should not be used to treat nonspecific symptoms like anorexia and loss of weight without investigating the cause. They are not useful in the absence of adequate protein-calorie intake.

Abuse of anabolic steroids by athletes: Anabolic steroids in large doses are commonly misused by athletes in order to improve their athletic performance. When large doses of these drugs are combined with intense athletic training and proper diet, muscles increase in size and strength; the muscle fibres are, however, structurally abnormal. The other perceived benefit is a heightened aggressive tendency ('killer instinct'). The adverse reactions are the well-known hepatotoxicity of the orally administered 17 alpha methylated steroids; virilisation in women athletes; diminution in LH and testosterone levels in male athletes; decreased spermatogenesis and testicular size; gynaecomastia; insulin resistance and glucose intolerance. Hallucinations, delusions and manic episodes have been reported in athletes who self-administer large doses of anabolic steroids. Puberty may be induced in young boys whose final adult height may be compromised. Hypertension can occur as a result of salt and water retention. Finally, abnormalities of lipid and lipoprotein metabolism, which are potentially atherogenic, can occur. **Such misuse of anabolic steroids is harmful, illegal and is to be deprecated medically.**

ANTIANDROGENS PH 1.37

Any compound which antagonises or interferes with the action of androgens at the tissue level is referred to as an antiandrogen. **Estrogens** and **potent progestins** such as medroxyprogesterone **block the synthesis of androgens** by their central gonadotropin inhibiting action and thus act as antiandrogen (Chapter 65).

Classifiation of antiandrogens

I. **Steroid synthesis inhibitors:** Ketoconazole; relatively toxic in the doses needed and hence not used
II. **5-Alpha-reductase inhibitors:** Finasteride (see section, Benign prostatic hyperplasia)
III. **Noncompetitive androgen receptor antagonists:** Cyproterone
IV. **Competitive androgen receptor antagonists:** Flutamide and spironolactone

FINASTERIDE: See section, Benign prostatic hyperplasia.

CYPROTERONE ACETATE: This drug has **potent progestogenic, moderately potent antiandrogenic and mild glucocorticoid actions.** Its **antiandrogenic action is due to competitive antagonism of dihydrotestosterone in the target cells.** By its marked progestogenic effect, it reduces the plasma level of gonadotropin and testosterone. Cyproterone, unlike cyproterone acetate, exerts only the peripheral antiandrogenic action.

Absorption, fate and excretion: Cyproterone acetate is lipophilic with t½ of 40 h. Cyproterone acetate is metabolised by CYP3A4, to an active metabolite, which has similar antiandrogen activity, but only 10% progestogenic activity. Coadministration with CYP3A4 inhibitors may increase its potency. It is further metabolised by hydrolysis into cyproterone and acetic acid.

Adverse reactions: Cyproterone acetate produces physical demasculinisation, gynaecomastia, galactorrhoea, sexual dysfunction (including loss of libido and ED), impaired spermatogenesis, and reversible infertility in males. It has been associated with an increased rate of depression. It also decreases serum vitamin B_{12} levels and its supplementation is necessary. The most serious ADR of cyproterone acetate is hepatotoxicity. Therefore, LFT monitoring is necessary. Sudden withdrawal can cause adrenal insufficiency and androgenic effects.

Indications: Cyproterone acetate is used orally in the dose of 50–100 mg per day. It is used in:

- Deviant hypersexuality in males to reduce libido and sexual potency
- Precocious puberty in boys
- Hirsutism in females
- Carcinoma of the prostate as an adjunct to GnRH analogues (Chapter 59)

FLUTAMIDE: This nonsteroidal antiandrogen, given orally, is converted to its active metabolite 2-hydroxyflutamide which acts as a **competitive antagonist at the androgen receptor.** It is used to treat prostatic cancer (Chapter 59). Its use in hirsutism is discussed below.

Bicalutamide nilutamide, enzalutamide, apalutamide and **darolutamide** are newer analogues of flutamide, used for prostate cancer.

SPIRONOLACTONE: This aldosterone antagonist (Chapter 37) **blocks the binding of androgens to the androgen receptor competitively** at the level of hair follicle; in larger doses it also inhibits the synthesis of androgen in the ovaries. It is used in the treatment of hirsutism (see below).

Indications:

- Hirsutism (see below)
- Benign prostatic hyperplasia (BPH) e.g. Finasteride (See section, Benign prostatic hyperplasia)
- Prostate cancer e.g. Flutamide (Chapter 59)
- Acne (Chapter 69)
- Androgenetic alopecia (Chapter 69)

MANAGEMENT OF HIRSUTISM

The physiology of hair growth is discussed in Chapter 69. **Hirsutism** implies the excessive growth of androgen dependent (male pattern) hair in children and adult women due to either inappropriately elevated plasma androgen levels or increased sensitivity of the hair follicles to their normal levels. It occurs mostly in the back and lateral aspects of face. Hirsutism is commonly accompanied by the occurrence of acne. By contrast, **hypertrichosis** is increase in terminal hair density mainly located on forehead and the temporal region and may be accompanied by growth of hair in nonandrogen-dependent areas. Hypertrichosis can be due to: drugs (phenytoin, diazoxide, glucocorticoids, danazol and minoxidil); hypothyroidism; acromegaly; multiple sclerosis; encephalitis and metabolic disorders such as porphyria; or it may accompany congenital conditions such as Hurler syndrome and trisomy 18.

Hirsutism **in childhood** *is always due to inappropriate androgen production or administration, and needs to be investigated thoroughly.* The treatment is specific and depends on the cause. The majority of cases in adult women are either idiopathic or due to polycystic ovarian syndrome (PCOS).

Patients with idiopathic hirsutism need treatment with local cosmetic measures, and sometimes with an antiandrogen. If a woman with PCOS desires to conceive, the treatment is ovulation induction with drugs (Chapter 66). If she does not wish to become pregnant, her treatment depends on the degree of hirsutism.

Management: Box 67.1 summarises the principles of management of hirsutism.

- **In mild cases** not accompanied by menstrual dysfunction, cosmetic treatment such as shaving, waxing, bleaching, chemical depilation, electrolysis or laser therapy is sufficient and no specific drugs are needed.
  Eflornithine: This antitrypanosomal drug (Chapter 56) inhibits the synthesis of the hair cuticle and is effective in inhibiting the growth of hair as long as it is used. It is massaged locally as a cream twice a day, 5 min after hair removal from the hirsute (hairy) area, and is washed 3–4 h later. It needs to be applied for several weeks before the result is seen. Hair removal is continued throughout its use. It is well tolerated generally, but may cause local irritation in some patients.
- **In moderate cases**, especially when the menses are irregular and acne is troublesome, the treatment of choice is a **COC pill** taken from day 5 to day 25 of the menstrual cycle, for at least one year. *A pill containing norgestrel, levonorgestrel, norethisterone or norethisterone acetate should not be used as these drugs have androgenic action* and reduce the plasma level of sex hormone binding protein. A pill containing desogestrel (see Chapter 66), would be preferable. **Spironolactone**, in the dose of 100–200 mg per day may be used to supplement therapy of PCOS with the COC pill.
- **Severe cases** need treatment with *cyproterone acetate.* **Bromocriptine** is useful when hirsutism is a part of hyperprolactinaemia – amenorrhoea syndrome. **Flutamide, finasteride** and **GnRH analogues** are reserved for resistant cases.

Box 67.1 Management of Hirsutism

- Rule out drugs and neoplasm as cause
- Reassurance
- Cosmetic treatment
- Combined oral contraceptives
- Glucocorticoids
- Spironolactone
- Bromocriptine
- Cyproterone acetate (reverse sequential regimen)
- Flutamide
- Finasteride
- GnRH analogues

BENIGN PROSTATIC HYPERPLASIA (BPH)

BPH, a common condition in men ≥ 60 years, has two components:

- **A static component** that is related to the enlargement of the prostate **(obstructing urethra)**.
- **A dynamic component** that represents the tone or the degree of contraction of *the smooth muscle within the prostate.* It is mediated by α_1 **adrenergic receptors** (and is increased in BPH due to increase in muscle mass). This resists urine outflow.

The therapeutic aim is to:

- Relieve symptoms

Box 67.2 Drugs Used in BPH

Nonselective Alpha$_1$ adrenergic antagonists:
a. *Short acting* – Prazosin; alfuzosin
b. *Long acting* – Terazosin; doxazosin; alfuzosin
Selective alpha$_{1A}$ adrenergic antagonists: Tamsulosin; silodosin
Androgen antagonists: (a) GnRH agonists; (b) antiandrogens; 5-alpha reductase inhibitor, e.g. finasteride; dutasteride
Miscellaneous: Tadalafil

- Prevent disease progression and complications, e.g. recurrent UTI

Nonpharmacological measures like fluid restriction, frequent bladder emptying, use of bladder emptying techniques and exercises, pelvic floor muscle strengthening and avoidance of drugs/ items precipitating symptoms (oral decongestants, first generation antihistaminics, anticholinergics, caffeine, alcohol, carbonated beverages and very spicy food) remains the management for mild BPH and should be continued in patients with moderate to severe BPH along with pharmacotherapy.

The drugs used in treating BPH are listed in Box 67.2. Of these, GnRH agonists decrease libido, may cause impotence and are rarely used.

The alpha$_1$ adrenergic antagonists are more effective and less toxic; further, their action is immediate. They act on the dynamic component and relax smooth muscles in prostatic capsules, bladder neck (trigone) and urethra. Thus they reduce the bladder neck resistance to the urine outflow and decrease the risk of retention. They also have additional antihypertensive effect (Chapter 18).

Alpha blockers are also used in patients with acute urinary retention due to BPH. Patients should receive alpha blockers at least 3 days before undergoing an initial trial without catheter. Later a combination therapy with alpha blocker and finasteride is given to reduce recurrence.

BPH treatment.

Selective alpha$_{1A}$ (and alpha$_{1D}$) antagonists: Tamsulosin and **silodosin** are usually preferred because they have less risk of causing hypotension and syncope; though the efficacy is similar to that of nonselective agents. Both may, however, cause diminished or retrograde ejaculation.

Alpha$_1$-blockers remain effective for long period of time as tolerance does not develop easily. However, they do not reduce the prostate size or slow disease progression. They are also available as extended release preparation given once daily. They may cause blurred vision and amblyopia. They increase the risk of intraoperative floppy iris syndrome during cataract surgery and therefore, should be withheld or not be started unless the surgical procedure is completed.

Other Uses: As α_1 adrenergic blockers cause relaxation of the ureteric muscle and may allow the passage of a small stone, **tamsulosin has been used to treat patients with ureteral stones** measuring less than 1 cm, especially those in the distal ureter.

FINASTERIDE: This drug is **an inhibitor of the enzyme 5-alpha reductase and blocks the conversion of testosterone to dihydrotestosterone** especially in male external genitalia. It decreases the prostate size and thereby improves urinary flow. It is effective only in patients with palpably enlarged prostate, in contrast to alpha$_1$ adrenergic antagonists which are effective in patients with and without such enlargement.

However, decrease in prostate size following 5-alpha reductase inhibitor therapy occurs over several months and maximal symptom relief may not occur till 6 months of therapy. *Hence, it is combined with alpha1 blocker to treat moderate to severe BPH.*

Absorption, fate and excretion: Finasteride given orally gets 60%–70% absorbed, which is not affected by food. It is 90% plasma protein bound. It is extensively metabolised by CYP3A4 with t½ of 6 h.

Adverse reactions: It can cause occasional decreased libido, diminution in semen volume and impotence. It may be combined with PDE-5 inhibitor (e.g. tadalafil, see later) to reduce these sexual adverse effects. Other ADR include breast enlargement or tenderness and rash. It is teratogenic to male foetus if mother comes in contact with it through semen of male partner or through handling of crushed tablets as it gets easily absorbed through vagina and skin. *It is contraindicated in patients with obstructive uropathy or cancer of the prostate.* Their use decreases prostate specific antigen (PSA) levels by 50% so any increase in PSA level (even though within normal range) signals prostate cancer.

Indications:

- **Benign prostatic hyperplasia:** The dose is 5 mg daily orally
- **Androgenetic alopecia in men:** 1 mg/day

Dutasteride, an analogue, has similar properties as finasteride. Dose 0.5 mg o.d.

Tadalafil, a phosphodisterase-5 (PDE-5) inhibitor 5 mg o.d., has been reported to relieve some urinary symptoms of BPH within a month by decreasing smooth muscle tone and proliferation in the prostate, bladder neck and urethra but does not significantly improve the urinary flow rate (see below). It does not decrease prostate size or slow disease progression. Its use with alpha1 adrenergic blockers may produce additive effects on BPH symptoms and mitigate sexual adverse effects of alpha1 adrenergic blockers.

Anticholinergics and beta-3 agonists (mirabegron and vibegron), which are used to treat overactive bladder, may be used in combination with alpha blockers if the bladder irritation is suspected. They improve symptoms and and quality of life but do not slow down the disease progression or relieve symptoms related to bladder outlet obstruction. Risk of urinary retention with anticholinergics is less when combined with alpha blockers.

Though there is a promotion of dietary supplements and herbal products such as saw palmetto extract for BPH management, there is no evidence to support their use.

Patients with BPH having kidney dysfunction or haematuria, recurrent UTI, bladder stones are advised surgical removal of prostate.

SEXUAL DYSFUNCTION

Sexual dysfunctions are classified as follows:

I. **Erectile dysfunction (in males):** The normal erectile response is mediated by a combination of **psychogenic** (central) and **reflexogenic** (peripheral) stimuli. The CNS plays an important role by either stimulating or inhibiting the spinal pathways that mediate erectile function and ejaculation.

Physiological Mechanism of Erection

It involves release of nitric oxide (NO) from the vascular endothelium and the nitrergic nerves into the corpora cavernosa of the penis during sexual stimulation. NO then activates the enzyme guanylate cyclase, which results in increased levels of cyclic guanosine monophosphate (cGMP), producing smooth muscle relaxation in the corpora cavernosa and penile arteries, and allowing inflow of blood. The cGMP is metabolically degraded by the enzyme PDE-5 present in the corpora cavernosa. In addition to NO, locally synthesised PGF2α and PGE2 also contribute to the relaxation of the cavernosal smooth muscle cells.

The **parasympathetic** (cholinergic) **input to the penis is proerectile,** whereas the sympathetic (adrenergic) **input is antierectile**. Emission, which is the deposition of the seminal fluid into the posterior urethra, is regulated by activation of the sympathetic system. The proerectile afferent stimuli from the perineum and the lower urinary tract to the penis and the efferent ejaculatory stimuli to the levatorani muscles (which cause rhythmic ejaculation of the semen out of the penile urethra) are carried through **somatic** sacral **reflex arc**.

The basic mechanisms involved in ED are as follows:

a. **Failure to initiate,** due to psychological, endocrinological or neurogenic causes
b. **Failure to fill blood into cavernosa,** due to arteriogenic vascular causes
c. **Failure to hold adequate blood volume in the cavernosa** (vaso-occlusive dysfunction)

An organic cause can be found in about 50% of the cases of ED; the rest are either psychogenic or are due to a psychiatric illness such as depression. Systemic disease, such as chronic liver or kidney disease, and drug addiction are other important causes. *Only a few cases are due to androgen deficiency, and they alone benefit from treatment with testosterone.*

Management

PH 1.40

Drugs used in the treatment of sexual impotence are listed in Box 67.3.

The adult replacement dose is 200 mg of a long-acting ester of testosterone such as cypionate or enanthate once in 2 weeks or 300 mg once in 3 weeks. *Testosterone improves the libido, but not erectile failure in patients with normal libido.*

Almost 25%–30% of the patients with ED may have drug-induced ED. Hence, before starting such treatment, **drug-induced sexual dysfunction** *should be ruled out* (Box 67.4).

In many instances, sexual impotence is temporary and situational; and in these patients, expectant waiting is as good a treatment as any drug. *Counselling and change of environment are often beneficial.*

Box 67.3 Drugs Used in the Treatment of Sexual Impotence

Oral: Sildenafil; tadalafil; trazodone; bromocriptine; yohimbine

Intramuscular injection: Testosterone

Intracavernosal injection[a]: Papaverine; phentolamine; PGE_1 (alprostadil)

Transurethral injection: PGE_1

[a]Act as local vasodilators.

Box 67.4 Some Drugs Causing Sexual Dysfunction

- **Drugs acting on CNS:**
  Sedative-hypnotics, antipsychotics
  Antidepressants, anti-Parkinson drugs
  Antihistaminics, opioids
- **Anticholinergics**
- **Antihypertensives**, including beta-adrenergic blockers
- **Diuretics**
- **H_1 and H_2 receptor antagonists**
- **Hormonal agents:**
  Estrogens, Antiandrogens, Spironolactone, GnRH agonists
- **Fibrates**
- **Cytotoxic drugs**, e.g. methotrexate
- **Recreational drugs**, e.g. alcohol, cocaine, cannabis

SILDENAFIL: This methylpiperazine compound **inhibits the enzyme PDE-5 in the corpora cavernosa of the penis, thereby prolonging the life of cGMP at that site.** This causes relaxation of the smooth muscle of the corpora cavernosa **permitting inflow of blood into the sinuses resulting in better erection. The presence of NO is essential for this action.** *It does not improve sex desire (libido), orgasm or ejaculation. By itself, it does not bring about erection but it improves the quality and duration of erection in response to sexual stimulation.*

It is not of much value in subject with loss of erection due to spinal or other damage to innervation, and in those who lack libido.

Sildenafil has also been found effective in reducing clinical symptoms as well as pulmonary artery pressure in patients with primary pulmonary hypertension.

Absorption, fate and excretion: After a single oral dose, peak plasma level is reached in 30–120 min with 40% bioavailability. High fat meal delays its absorption. The plasma t½ is 2–4 h and its clinical effectiveness lasts for 4 h. It is metabolised in the liver by CYP3A4. **It is administered on empty stomach in the dose of 25–100 mg 1 h before the intended coitus.**

Adverse reactions: Sildenafil causes headache, dyspepsia, nasal congestion back pain, myalgia and rarely, priapism with irreversible erectile tissue damage. *The drug potentiates the hypotensive effects of nitrates, and hence, its administration to persons who are using nitrates in any form is dangerous.* Furthermore, there is some cardiac risk associated with sexual activity, especially in the elderly. As many users of drugs for impotence are likely to be elderly, although such therapy may increase the patients' 'vigour' and make them feel 'younger', it can also increase the risk of morbidity and mortality during sexual activity. It can potentiate the hypotensive effects of antihypertensives, alpha blockers and guanylate cyclase stimulators (riociguat, vericiguat).

It occasionally imparts bluish tinge to vision due to its effect on the PDE-6 in the retina. It may cause retinal detachment and retinal vascular occlusion. It is contraindicated in persons with retinal degenerative disorders. The drug has been reported to cause Nonarteritic-Ischaemic Optic Neuritis (NAION), leading to acute loss of vision. A sudden loss of hearing is reported.

Vardenafil, chemically related to sildenafil, has properties and duration of action similar to those of sildenafil. Its bioavailability is 15%.

TADALAFIL: This **long-acting drug** is chemically unrelated to sildenafil. Like sildenafil, it selectively inhibits PDE-5; it has less affinity for PDE-6 present in the retina, but greater affinity for PDE-11 present in the skeletal muscle, heart, prostate and kidney. It is claimed to cause less ocular toxicity.

Food does not interfere with its absorption. It **has a t½ of 17.5 h, with clinical effect lasting for almost 36 h.** When given in the dose of 10–20 mg twice a week, its effect is almost continuous and the patient can attempt intercourse any time at will, without planning. Adverse reactions are similar to those of sildenafil.

Avanafil is a short acting PDE – 5 inhibitor with duration of action for 6 hours.

All PDE-5 inhibitors can potentiate hypotension, especially when used concurrently with α blockers such as doxazosin or tamsulosin which are often prescribed in BPH.

II. **Premenopausal hypoactive sexual desire disorder (HSDD) (in females):** Deficiency or lack of sexual thoughts can occur in some premenopausal women leading to personal distress. It can be due to psychiatric/medical/drug-related causes or simply relation difficulties.

FLIBANSERIN: This drug given orally, daily is claimed to be helpful in some women with HSDD. Its mechanism of action is not known. It has $5HT_{1A}$ agonist and $5HT_{2A}$ receptor antagonistic action. In animal models it increases, noradrenaline and dopamine levels and decreases 5HT levels in prefrontal cortex.

Adverse reactions: These include hypotension, depression and rarely syncope. Alcohol and CYP3A4 inhibitors increase the risk of its toxicity. Its long-term safety is not known.

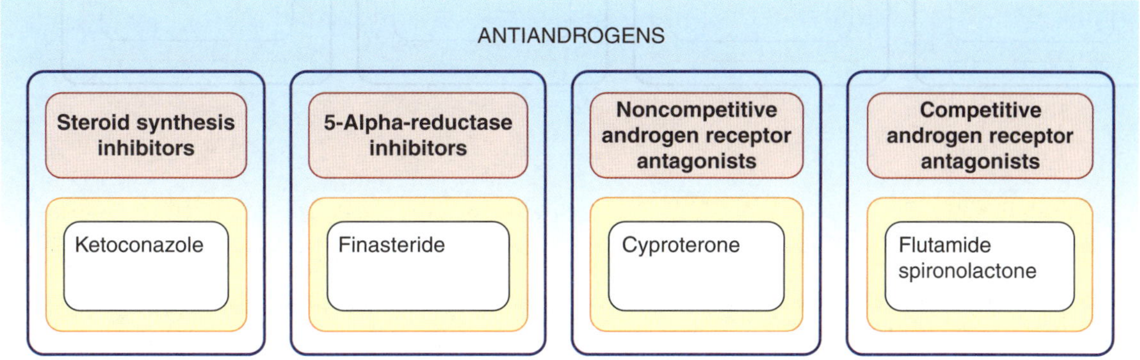

DRUGS USED IN THE TREATMENT OF BPH

Nonselective alpha$_1$ adrenergic antagonists

- *Short acting*
  - Prazosin
  - Alfuzosin
- *Long acting*
  - Terazosin
  - Doxazosin

Androgen antagonists

- GnRH agonists
- *5-alpha reductase inhibitors*
  - Finasteride
  - Dutasteride

Selective alpha$_1$ adrenergic antagonists

- Tamsulosin
- Silodosin

Miscellaneous

- Tadalafil

DRUGS USED IN THE TREATMENT OF SEXUAL IMPOTENCE

Oral

- Sildenafil
- Tadalafil
- Trazodone
- Bromocriptine
- Yohimbine

Intramuscular injection

- Testosterone

Intracavernosal injection

- Papaverine
- Phentolamine
- PGE_1

Transurethral injection

- PGE_1

CHAPTER 68

Calcium, Phosphorus, Fluoride and Magnesium Metabolism; Parathyroid Hormone and Vitamin D; Treatment of Osteoporosis

Learning Objectives

This chapter will enable the reader:

1. To be aware of the body distribution and physiological functions of calcium and phosphorous.
2. To enlist the oral and parenteral calcium preparations.
3. To explain the ADR and indications for calcium and phosphorous.
4. To outline the treatment of hypercalcaemia.
5. To describe the mechanism of action, pharmacological actions and indications for parathormone and calcitonin.
6. To be aware of the steps in activation of vitamin D, its mechanism of action and physiological effects.
7. To enumerate vitamin D preparations and describe their salient pharmacokinetic features, ADR and indications.
8. To describe the mechanism of action, salient pharmacokinetic features, ADR and indications for bisphosphonates.
9. To explain the management of osteoporosis.
10. To state the pharmacological action, salient pharmacokinetic features, ADR and indications for fluoride.
11. To state the indications for various magnesium salts giving pharmacological basis for the same.

KEY TERMS

The human skeleton undergoes remodelling throughout life, which involves both, bone resorption and bone formation in a linked manner. The process involves:

- **Activity of osteoblasts and osteoclasts.** Osteoblasts are bone forming cells and secrete bone matrix (Osteoid) on which Ca^{++} and $PO4^{3-}$ precipitate and mineralize the bone. Osteoclasts are large multinucleated cells derived from macrophage-monocytes and are involved in bone resorption.
- **Actions of various cytokines** e.g. insulin-like growth factor (IGF-1), and transforming growth factor (TGF)-β family and interleukins.
- **Turnover of bone minerals,** such as calcium and phosphate. More than 99% of calcium in our body exists in the skeleton mostly in the form crystalline hydroxyapatite (hard bone matrix) and as non-crystalline phosphates and carbonates.
- **Actions of several hormones:** parathyroid hormone (PTH), the vitamin D family, calcitonin, estrogens, growth hormone, steroids.

Bone remodelling starts with recruitment of osteoclast precursor cells to the bone surface. Their activation is regulated by osteoblast-derived cytokines (e.g., IL-1 and IL-6).

The osteoblasts secrete a protein called **Receptor Activator of Nf-Kappa B Ligand (RANKL).** The RANK ligand initiates osteoclastogenesis by binding to **RANK**, its receptor, on the surface of bone mesenchymal osteoclast precursors.

Osteoblasts also secrete **osteoprotegerin (OPG)**. This serves as a decoy receptor for RANKL. It neutralizes RANKL and prevents RANKL from binding to RANK, thereby inhibiting osteoclastogenesis. Thus, OPG is a physiological inhibitor of RANKL. RANKL/OPG ratio is an important determinant of bone mass and skeletal integrity. It is regulated by various cytokines and hormones. For example, estrogens inhibit RANKL that recruit osteoclasts. They oppose the bone-resorbing, calcium mobilising action of PTH. They increase osteoblast proliferation, augment production of TGF-β and bone morphogenic proteins, and inhibit apoptosis. During estrogen deprivation as in postmenopausal period, OPG is suppressed. This allows RANKL to interact with RANK, and thus osteoclast production increases.

During the process of resorption, cytokines such as IGF-1 and TGF-β which are already embedded in the osteoid get liberated. They recruit and activate successive teams of osteoblasts. Thus, the osteoblasts start invading the site. They secrete new bone matrix constituents which synthesise osteoid. Some osteoblasts become embedded in the osteoid, forming osteocytes. They sense mechanical strain and trigger remodelling at later stage.

PTH is one of the important hormone which activates osteoblast precursors lining the bone surface to proliferate and differentiate into osteoblasts *via* release of growth factors FGF-2, TGF-β and IGF-1. It also delays the apoptosis of mature, matrix-secreting osteoblasts. The osteoids then undergo mineralization to complete one remodelling cycle. It may take nearly 6 months. Various factors such as dietary sufficiency, exercise, hormones, and drugs affect this bone resorption and formation balance.

Bone mass peaks during the third decade, remains stable until the age of 50 and then decreases progressively. The loss during the menopause is due to increased osteoclast activity and affects mainly trabecular bone while the loss with increasing age is due to decreased osteoblast numbers and affects mainly cortical bone. Maintenance of bone mass density (BMD) needs optimal amount of physical activity, reproductive endocrine status, and calcium intake. If any one of them is inadequate then the BMD suffers.

Calcium, apart from forming an essential constituent of bones, plays an important role in body homeostasis. Disturbances in calcium metabolism are associated with derangement of various cellular functions. Food is the only important source of calcium. Milk and milk products are an excellent source of completely assimilable calcium. Green leafy vegetables and cereals are rich in calcium but their calcium is less well utilised because of the concurrent presence of oxalates and phytates, respectively. *Ragi* is especially rich and rice (especially highly polished one) very poor in calcium. In certain areas, drinking water contains calcium.

The recommended daily calcium intake is 200–250 mg in infants; 1000 mg in children of age 4–10 years; 1300 mg in children 10–18 years; 1 g in adults including pregnant and lactating women; and 1000–1200 mg in adults over 50 years of age. *Mature fetus* contains about 30 g of calcium which constitutes 3%–4% of the total calcium in the mother. Most of it is deposited during the last trimester of pregnancy; loss of maternal calcium during lactation is even larger, which needs correction by consumption of 1 g of calcium supplement daily. **A 1-year-old baby contains about 100 g of calcium, a gain of 70 g over the total calcium content at birth; most of this increment is supplied by milk.**

Normal dietary intake of calcium in Americans varies between 400 and 1500 mg/day. The average daily diet of Indians, which is based mainly on milled rice and very little milk, may contain as little as 200–500 mg of calcium.

Body distribution: An adult human body weighing 70 kg contains about 1.0–1.3 kg of calcium. Ninety-nine per cent of it is present in bones; 1% in the soft tissues, and 0.1% in the body fluids. The bone mineral exists in the form of a complex salt containing calcium, phosphate and carbonate, and it constantly contributes to the maintenance of extracellular levels of calcium and phosphorus by two processes:

- **Exchange between the newly deposited bone mineral and the extracellular ionic calcium**
- **Constant and concurrent resorption and formation of bone (remodelling),** controlled by parathyroid hormone (PTH), calcitonin and vitamin D

Blood calcium: *Calcium is essentially distributed extracellularly*, its concentration being maintained within narrow limits.

Most of the calcium in the blood is present in the plasma. The human plasma contains 9–11 mg%. It is present as follows:

- **Ionised calcium (50% of total)**
- **Protein bound calcium (40%)**
- **Calcium bound to citrate and other organic acids (10%)**

The **ionic fraction**, 4.5–5.4 mg/100 mL, is diffusible, physiologically active, and exchanges with the bone calcium; it is also the fraction which is affected by bone formation and resorption and which regulates the rates of secretion of the PTH and calcitonin. *It is the ionic calcium that plays a critical role in variety of cellular functions involved in neuromuscular activity, secretions and signal transduction.*

Intracellular (cytoplasmic) calcium content is very low, 0.4–4.0 mcg%. Most of this is sequestered in the mitochondria and (in the muscles) in the sarcoplasmic reticulum. *Although very low in concentration, it is important in regulating the functions and metabolic processes of cells*, such as stimulus-contraction coupling in the muscles and stimulus-secretion coupling in most exocrine and endocrine glands.

Absorption of calcium: Ingested calcium must be dissolved before it is absorbed. Calcium is absorbed passively, primarily from the distal small bowel, whereas it is **absorbed actively from the proximal small bowel** under the influence of 1,25-$(OH)_2$D (**calcitriol**), the active metabolite of vitamin D. The active absorption is stimulated by low calcium intake (Box 68.1). On the other hand adequate or high intake of calcium promotes passive absorption and reduces synthesis of 1,25-$(OH)_2$D and thus decreases its own absorption.

The net calcium absorption on a daily diet containing 1 g of calcium is about 200–300 mg. *However, by virtue of an adaptive mechanism, comprising PTH and calcitriol even in the presence of lower calcium intake of less than 1 g, net absorption remains within normal limits. Taking calcium in doses of 500 mg or less with food increases its absorption, particularly in patients with diminished gastric acidity. Calcium absorption declines after puberty, especially in old age*. Box 68.2 enumerates substances and conditions that interfere with calcium absorption.

Human milk contains proportionately less phosphorus (Ca:P = 2.2:1) than cow's milk with a Ca:P ratio of 1.1:1. Hence, in infants the calcium absorption from human milk is more efficient than from cow's milk. Mean calcium content of cow's milk, however, is 125 mg% as against 33 mg% in human milk.

Excretion of calcium: Calcium is excreted in faeces, urine and sweat. The total amount of calcium secreted into the intestinal tract is about 200 mg daily, of which 130–150 mg is excreted in faeces. **Zero dietary calcium intake (as in starvation) and lack of vitamin D will thus cause marked calcium deficiency as the faecal loss continues.**

Ninety-nine per cent of the calcium filtered by the glomeruli (about 9 g/day) is reabsorbed by the proximal tubules. The absorption of the rest in the distal tubule is under the influence of vitamin D and PTH. ***Calcitonin*** *inhibits proximal tubular reabsorption of calcium and increases its urinary excretion while* ***PTH*** *promotes calcium absorption.* The urine contains 2–4 mg of calcium per kg body weight per 24 h. A rise in plasma ionic sodium or calcium from any cause (refer Box 68.5) increases its urinary excretion. Frusemide increases calcium excretion but thiazide decreases the same.

The factors which prevent the precipitation of calcium in normal urine are known incompletely; low calcium concentration and adequate citrate concentration in the urine are two important factors. **In alkaline urine, calcium is precipitated as calcium phosphate.**

Excretion of calcium in the sweat is negligible in the temperate climate but may be significant in the tropics because of excessive sweating.

Box 68.1 Agents and Conditions that Stimulate the Absorption of Calcium

- Low calcium intake
- Vitamin D
- PTH (indirectly)
- Negative calcium balance
- Acid residue in the intestines

Box 68.2 Agents and Conditions that Interfere with Calcium Absorption

- Excess of phosphate, oxalate (from vegetables), phytate (from cereals) and fatty acids[a] (in malabsorption) in the intestines
- Deficiency of vitamin D
- Deficiency of PTH
- Glucocorticoids

[a]Fat does not interfere with calcium absorption in normal subjects.

If intestinal absorption and renal tubular reabsorption of calcium are insufficient to maintain the plasma calcium within the normal range, it is mobilised from the bone, following the increased levels of 1,25-$(OH)_2$D and PTH.

PH 1.36

Physiological and Pharmacological Actions

Excitability: Calcium is an important component of the cell membrane and controls its permeability and electrical properties. Calcium ions compete with sodium ions for sites on the membrane. **An excess of extracellular calcium reduces the permeability of the membrane to sodium** and raises the critical level of depolarisation at which sodium permeability is increased and at which the action potential is fired off. This stabilises the membrane and reduces its excitability. **Hypercalcaemia thus reduces the excitability of nerves and muscles. Hypocalcaemia increases membrane permeability to sodium and reduces its excitation threshold, leading to tetany.**

Coupling between excitation and response (second messenger): Calcium is essential as a coupling agent between excitation and contraction in all forms of muscle and between stimulus and secretion in certain endocrine glands, e.g. release of ADH by nerve impulses to the posterior pituitary and of catecholamines from the adrenal medulla by acetylcholine. In mediating these responses, calcium enters the cytoplasm to activate the contractile processes or to cause release of stored hormone from the granules. Further, certain drugs acting on the heart owe their action to promotion (digoxin) or inhibition (CCB) of entry of calcium ions into the cell.

In the visceral smooth muscle, the acetylcholine released following stimulation of the cholinergic nerves binds to muscarinic receptors, resulting in increased influx of Ca^{++} into the myocytes and their contraction.

Automaticity: The automaticity of the cardiac pacemaker tissues (nodal and conducting) is dependent predominantly upon the slow, inward calcium current (Chapter 28). Thus calcium plays important role in:

- **Various metabolic processes** and serves as **second messenger** in various cells
- **Functioning of neuromuscular and cardiovascular system.**
- **Integrity of mucosal membrane and cell adhesion.**
- **Formation of bone and teeth:** Calcium is essential for proper formation of bone and teeth; calcium deficiency during intra-uterine life and extrauterine growth period leads to delayed and defective dentition and to poor bone formation.
- **Coagulation of blood:** Plasma ionic calcium is essential for the conversion of prothrombin to thrombin (see Chapter 33).
- **Renal concentrating mechanism:** Ability to concentrate the urine maximally is impaired in hypercalcaemia and in hypokalaemia.
- **Functioning of many enzymes** where it acts as cofactor.

Hypocalcaemia

Box 68.3 lists the causes of hypocalcaemia. Mild hypocalcaemia (8–8.5 mg%) is usually asymptomatic. Acute hypocalcaemia is characterised by increased neuromuscular irritability with paraesthesiae, tetany, seizures, and laryngeal spasm. Teeth show hypoplasia. Skin and nails may show atrophy. Hair loss is present. There may be associated psychological symptoms such as anxiety, emotional lability etc. Most of these effects are reversible on treatment.

Chronic negative calcium balance leads to:

1. **Osteoporosis**, in which the bones are normal in chemical composition but the **total bone mass is reduced.**
2. Stimulation of the parathyroid glands with consequent secondary hyperparathyroidism. Excess

Box 68.3 Common Causes of Hypocalcaemia

- Vitamin D deficiency
- Abnormal vitamin D metabolism
- Vitamin D resistance
- Chronic renal failure
- Severe hyperphosphataemia
- Hypoparathyroidism
- Pseudohypoparathyroidism
- Malabsorption syndrome

PTH, increases the hepatic degradation of 25-(OH)D (see section, Vitamin D); this seems to be an important mechanism of the occurrence of **osteomalacia and rickets in sunny countries** such as India. Other mechanisms are deficient intake of vitamin D, vitamin D resistance and hypophosphataemia.

Preparations and dosage: The **oral preparations** are given in Table 68.1. **Calcium carbonate** has the highest calcium content (about 40%). It is tasteless and is generally preferred for clinical use. **Calcium lactate** has a sour taste and is sparingly soluble in water. **Calcium citrate** is tasteless and water soluble.

Parenteral calcium preparations are as follows:

i. Calcium gluconate 1 g in 10 mL dose: 1–2 g IV
ii. Calcium laevulinate (10% solution) IM/IV: Its calcium content is 13%.
iii. Calcium chloride is an ingredient of Ringer-lactate infusion. It is given diluted with saline as a slow infusion. Inj. calcium chloride as 10 % w/v is also available. It contains 27% Ca^{++}.

The points to remember while prescribing calcium are listed in Box 68.4.

Adverse reactions: Oral calcium supplements are generally well tolerated but may produce constipation and abdominal bloating. Calcium chloride solution is irritating by all routes. It causes vasodilatation and cutaneous burning sensation. *Extravasation of calcium salts during IV administration may cause local sloughing. Rapid IV calcium can cause nausea, tingling, sweating, hypotension, cardiac arrhythmia, shortening of QT interval and cardiac arrest. Potassium counters cardiac effects of excess of calcium. Prolonged excessive consumption of calcium has been claimed to cause hypercalcaemia and increased risk of CAD.* Calcium should not be injected intramuscularly as it can cause abscess.

Table 68.1 Calcium Content of Various Calcium Salts PH 1.36

Calcium Salts	Ca Content mg per g of Salt	Grams Required to Provide 1 g of Ca
Carbonate	400	2.5
Phosphate (dibasic)	230	4.4
Citrate	211	4.7
Glycerophosphate	162	6.2
Lactate	130	7.7
Gluconate	89	11
Heptagluconate	82	12

Box 68.4 Calcium Supplements: Points to Remember PH 1.1

- It should be taken in doses ≤500 mg at a time. At higher doses absorption of calcium is proportionately less.
- It is the elemental calcium contents of the salt that is important; not its weight.
- All calcium salts are poorly absorbed and their elemental calcium content (per g of salt) varies. But there is little evidence that any of them is therapeutically superior to other.
- Calcium carbonate is well tolerated and relatively inexpensive. It is best absorbed with food as it requires acidic medium for solubility.
- Calcium deficiency causes vitamin D deficiency and vitamin D is necessary for calcium absorption. Hence, vitamin D supplementation with calcium is useful.
- Overdosing with calcium and vitamin D must be avoided as excessive doses can cause hypercalcaemia and cardiac toxicity.

Indications:

- **To prevent or correct calcium deficiency**, oral supplements of calcium are used in:
  a. Growing children, pregnant women and lactating mothers
  b. Individuals with dietary deficiency
  c. Postmenopausal osteoporosis, and osteoporosis due to Cushing syndrome and long-term glucocorticoid therapy
  d. Patients with vitamin D deficiency rickets and osteomalacia, who are prescribed vitamin D
  e. Following removal of a parathyroid adenoma

The oral dose of calcium salts depends on the condition under treatment. Salts, containing about *1 g of elemental calcium per day, in divided doses, with meals*, are needed for the prevention and treatment of osteoporosis and in the treatment of osteomalacia due to vitamin D deficiency, whereas higher doses of *2–3 g/day*, are used in malabsorption, and in hypocalcaemia due to hypoparathyroidism.

- **In the treatment of hypocalcaemic tetany:** Calcium gluconate (10%) 10–20 mL IV very slowly, followed by IV infusion 40 mL in 1 L saline over 4–8 h.

- **Osteoporosis:** See section, Osteoporosis – management
- **As an antacid** (Chapter 41)
- **As phosphate binders in chronic kidney disease (CKD):** Chronic renal failure is associated with hypocalcaemia, hyperphosphataemia and secondary hyperparathyroidism. Serum calcitriol level is low. Main treatment is replacement of vitamin D. It corrects secondary hyperparathyroidism and normalises serum calcium. As the hyperphosphataemia of CKD causes secondary hyperparathyroidism leading to renal osteodystrophy, restraining the former is important. In addition to dietary phosphate restriction, the commonly used drugs are calcium carbonate and acetate. Both are effective but sometimes cause hypercalcaemia. In resistant cases and in those with hypercalcaemia, **sevelamer** may be used (see section, Phosphorous metabolism).
- **Lead colic** (Chapter 74)
- **Hypermagnasaemia** (See section, Magnesium metabolism)
- **Hyperkalemia:** Calcium gluconate is life saving in patients having serum K^+ >7 mEq/L
- **Cardiac arrest:** Intracardiac injection of calcium in cardiac arrest is for the specialist and **should not be attempted outside ICCU**
- **Black widow spider poisoning**
- **Placebo:** Calcium gluconate intravenously produces a feeling of warmth which spreads as a wave all over the body, and is often used as placebo. However, in view of its adverse cardiac effects, it is no longer recommended.

Hypercalcaemia

Box 68.5 lists the common causes of hypercalcaemia. The effects of hypercalcaemia include:

a. **Gastrointestinal:** Lethargy, anorexia, nausea, vomiting and severe constipation

Box 68.5 Common Causes of Hypercalcaemia

- Hyperparathyroidism (primary or tertiary)
- Malignancy with or without bone metastases
- Hypervitaminosis D

b. **Musculoskeletal:** Weakness, muscular hypotonia
c. **Renal:** Inability to concentrate the urine leading to polyuria and dehydration
d. **Cardiac:** Rhythm irregularities

Excess calcium gets deposited in tissues (**metastatic calcification**) such as arteries, cornea, muscles and kidneys. Dehydration is caused by hypercalcemia due to impaired renal concentrating mechanisms. *The development of mental changes indicates severe hypercalcaemia (over 15 mg%) and is a medical emergency.* IM 22.3

Hypercalcaemia management: Mild to moderate, asymptomatic hypercalcaemia can be treated by:

- *Control of the underlying causative factors*
- *Hydration*
- *Reduction of GI calcium absorption by restriction of calcium intake, oral neutral phosphate mixture and cellulose phosphate. For glucocorticoids, see below.*

Severe hypercalcaemia with serum calcium 14 mg/dL or higher requires *emergency intensive management* (Box 68.6). It is started with:

1. **Isotonic saline IV infusion** (2–4 L in the first 24 h, sometimes even 6-8 L in a day) to correct

Box 68.6 Principles of Treatment of Severe Hypercalcaemia PH 1.1

Correct dehydration: Isotonic saline intravenously
Increase the renal excretion of calcium: Isotonic saline with or without furosemide
Inhibit bone resorption: Bisphosphonates; calcitonin
Reduce the GI absorption of calcium: Reduction in calcium intake; oral phosphate; corticosteroids; cellulose phosphate
Promote uptake of calcium by bones and other tissues: Phosphate

the dehydration and establish adequate urine output (100–150 mL/h). The calcium is coexcreted in the urine along with sodium. Overloading of the circulation should be watched during the infusion. Once diuresis is established (*but not earlier*), **furosemide** 20–40 mg IM 6–12 hourly can lower serum calcium by inhibiting its resorption in the distal renal tubules. However, it may cause electrolyte disturbances and can worsen hypercalcaemia.

2. **Bisphosphonates:** Pamidronate or zolendronic acid or ibandronate are the drugs of choice and are given by **IV infusion**. Their effect persists for longer time. They inhibit osteoclastic bone resorption. They are particularly useful in hypercalcaemia of malignancy. *Oral biphosphonate is not useful in acute severe hypercalcaemia.*
3. **Calcitonin SC** inhibits the osteoclastic bone resorption and directly increases the urinary calcium excretion. Its action is rapid (hours) but short lived (days). The dose is 4 units/kg 12 hourly, which is titrated based on the response and increased to a maximum of 8 units/kg every 6 h. It can lower serum calcium by 1 to 2 mg/dL.
   All the above three agents must be started concurrently for optimum result.
4. **Neutral phosphate mixture** orally helps by binding calcium in the GI lumen. It is appropriate in patients with serum phosphate less than 2.5 mg/dL.
5. **Glucocorticoids** (e.g. prednisolone 20–40 mg/day) lower serum calcium in vitamin D intoxication, granulomatous disease, sarcoidosis, lymphoma and myelomatosis, *but not in primary hyperparathyroidism, and in most malignant solid tumours.* They cannot be relied upon in acute, severe hypercalcaemia, as it may take 1-2 weeks to lower the serum calcium due to their slow action.
6. **Mithramycin (Plicamycin)** is a cytotoxic antibiotic used in malignancy to decrease serum calcium by inhibiting bone resorption. This can be achieved rapidly within 1-2 days but ADR are unacceptable and hence is not preferred (Chapter 59).

Patients with life-threatening hypercalcaemia or severe renal insufficiency may need **haemodialysis** or **peritoneal dialysis** to reduce serum calcium.

Long-term treatment of hypercalcaemia involves use of an oral ion-exchange agent, sodium cellulose phosphate. It has selective affinity for calcium in the gut. The complex is excreted in the faeces. It is useful for patients who overabsorb dietary calcium. In patients with primary hyperparathyroidism, gland should be removed.

CINACALCET: This *calcimimetic* **drug inhibits PTH secretion by binding to and stimulating the calcium sensing receptor (CaSR) on the parathyroid cells**; the latter is rendered more sensitive to serum calcium. Orally, it is well absorbed and is metabolised by the liver and excreted in the faeces. The adverse reactions are nausea, vomiting and diarrhoea. Hypocalcaemia can occur and can precipitate seizures. The drug has been used **to treat hypercalcaemia secondary to CKD and parathyroid carcinoma.**

Secondary hyperparathyroidism is common in CKD. This is often associated with hypercalcaemia and hyperphosphatemia. Cinacalcet reduces PTH and also lowers serum calcium and phosphorus levels in such patients.

Etelcalcetide is another calcimimetic with similar safety profile as cinacalcet, but is administered intravenously.

Sevelamer is a cationic polymer that binds phosphate through ion exchange. Thus, **it acts as an effective phosphate binder and lowers plasma phosphate in CKD patients with secondary hyperparathyroidism.** It is a non-calcium containing phosphate binder and hence the risk of hypercalcaemia is less. **Its use is reserved for resistant cases.**

PHOSPHORUS METABOLISM

Phosphorus is abundantly present in almost all foods: milk, meat, fish, cereals, pulses and nuts. A part of the phosphorus in cereals is present as phytate and is unassimilable. Its daily intake varies with the diet and is about 500–1000 mg/day.

Dietary requirements: It is estimated at about 0.9 g in adults. It is higher in growing children, pregnant women and lactating mothers.

Body distribution: The total phosphorus content of the average adult human body is about 500–600 g, 75% of which is in bones and 25% in other tissues. Most of the body phosphorus is in the organic form.

The RBCs contain far more phosphorus than the plasma; hence, even slight haemolysis gives fallaciously high plasma phosphorus values. The plasma phosphorus is present as:

- **Inorganic phosphorus** 3–5 mg%
- **Ester phosphorus** 0.1–1.7 mg%
- **Lipid phosphorus** 7–15 mg%

The term 'plasma phosphate' usually means the plasma inorganic phosphate measured as phosphorus. Its plasma concentration varies with age, dietary intake and in relation to meals.

Absorption, fate and excretion: Absorption of phosphorus is more complete than that of calcium. About 70% of the dietary phosphorus is absorbed in the small bowel. **Vitamin D stimulates** the GI absorption of calcium and phosphorus. **A high calcium intake** and aluminium hydroxide in large doses **interferes with its absorption.** Like calcium, phosphorus filtered by glomeruli is largely reabsorbed by proximal tubules. Its urinary excretion varies directly with dietary intake, whereas its reabsorption is affected by hypocalcaemia, hypomagnesaemia and severe hypophosphataemia. Low serum level directly stimulates tubular synthesis of 1,25-$(OH)_2$D.

Physiological and pharmacological actions:

- **Formation of bone and teeth:** Along with calcium, phosphorus is essential for the formation of bones and teeth.
- **Phosphorylation:** Phosphorylation of a chemical compound is the transfer to it of a phosphate group from an inorganic or organic phosphate. *It is an essential preliminary step in the metabolism of almost all substances in the body including enzyme regulation, energy transformation and storage, and in the regulation of the delivery of oxygen to the tissues.*
- **Modification of Ca^{++} concentration in tissues**
- **Act as buffer:** Phosphates are important intra- and extracellular buffers in the body and regulate the renal excretion of H ions.
- **Miscellaneous:** Phosphorus forms an integral part of the structure of the nuclei and cytoplasm. Further, chemical energy is stored in the form of 'high energy phosphate bonds'. It is a major component of several organic phosphate compounds.

Hypophosphatemia can occur due to dietary deficiency or sustained use of antacids. **Mild to moderate hypophosphataemia** interferes with calcification of the osseous matrix, leading to rickets or osteomalacia. Malaise and muscle weakness also accompanies.

Severe hypophosphataemia (serum inorganic phosphorus less than 1 mg%) *is a life threatening condition and* can cause haemolysis, muscular weakness, mental changes, decreased myocardial contractility and respiratory failure.

Preparation:

i. Neutral phosphate solution: Its composition is: disodium hydrogen phosphate 3.66 g, sodium dihydrogen phosphate 1 g, orange syrup 16 mL, water to make 60 mL. Sixty mL of this solution gives 1 g of phosphorus.

Indications:

- **Hypophosphataemia:** Neutral phosphate solution is used orally to treat familial hypophosphataemic rickets. Therapy is commenced with 5 mL thrice daily and increased slowly to tolerance but not exceeding 60 mL t.i.d. Larger doses can cause diarrhoea and hyperparathyroidism. **Severe hypophosphataemia** may be treated by IV neutral phosphate solution.
- **Hypercalcaemia:** Oral neutral phosphate may be used to treat chronic hypercalcaemia except in the presence of concurrent hyperphosphataemia. **Burosumab** is a human mAB against fibroblast growth factor 23 (FGF23), which promotes urinary excretion of phosphate. It is approved for X-linked hypophosphatemia (XLH) and tumour induced osteomalacia.

PARATHORMONE (PTH): This hormone is secreted by the chief cells of the parathyroid glands. It is secreted as an 84 amino acid polypeptide but is cleaved in the plasma.

The secretion of PTH **is directly stimulated by a fall (Ca^{++} levels < 3.5 mg%) and is inhibited by a rise in the plasma ionic calcium level** via the calcium sensing G protein coupled receptor (CaSR) in the chief cells.

Mechanism of action: PTH acts on the cell membrane to:

1. Stimulate the formation of cyclic AMP
2. Increase its permeability to calcium ions which then move intracellularly
3. In the bone, it stimulates the conversion of mesenchymal cells to osteoclasts and regulates the activity of osteoclasts and osteoblasts during bone remodelling. It also inhibits the osteoblasts and hence collagen synthesis.

Physiological and pharmacological actions:

All the actions of PTH are directed towards maintaining the ionic calcium of the plasma and ECF. It probably influences ion movements in other tissues.

Gastrointestinal tract: It enhances the synthesis of 1,25-$(OH)_2$ vitamin D (calcitriol) in the kidneys and thus indirectly **promotes the active absorption of calcium and phosphorus from the gut.**

Bones: In physiological doses PTH causes mobilisation of calcium from the bone in 2 phases, rapid and slow.

In the rapid phase the serum calcium levels increase in minutes when PTH binds to receptors on osteocytic membrane overlying the bone matrix. The membrane pumps the calcium ions from bone fluid into ECF. Slow phase occurs over several days during which PTH binds to receptors on the osteoblasts which then secrete a protein, RANKL, that:

- activates the osteoclasts to cause bone resorption
- differentiaties mesenchymal cells to osteoclasts
- prolongs half-life of osteoclasts
- with prolonged effect, increases osteoblasts

This increases bone turnover and remodelling i.e. minute zones of osteoclastic resorption followed by osteoblastic bone formation. Such remodelling cycles repeat themselves all over the bone tissue throughout life. After the age of 20, bone formation slightly falls short of bone resorption in each cycle; this is the basis of age-related bone loss in adult life.

Clinically, **administration of small intermittent doses** of PTH **(1–2 h/day) stimulates bone formation** (anabolic action; see teriparatide later). This process requires a normal vitamin D intake to permit calcification of the matrix laid down during bone formation.

Continuous high plasma levels of PTH as in hyperparathyroidism cause excessive bone loss due to increase activity of osteoclasts.

Kidney: The effect on the kidney is of more rapid onset than that on the bone, and is exerted at multiple sites.

1. **PTH promotes the calcium reabsorption** (distal tubules), increases excretion of phosphate (by decreasing reabsorption at all segments) and **stimulates the conversion of calcifediol to calcitriol, the active metabolite of vitamin D**, by stimulating 1α-hydroxylase in the proximal renal tubules.
2. It increases the urinary excretion of sodium, potassium, bicarbonate and citrate; and decreases the excretion of hydrogen and magnesium.

Absorption, fate and excretion: Given subcutaneously, its peak effect is seen in 18 h and the response lasts up to 36 h. It is partly degraded by liver and partly excreted in urine. Its t½ is 1 h.

Adverse reactions: Higher doses can cause orthostatic hypotension, hypercalcaemia and anaphylactic reactions. It should not be given for more than 2 years and also not to patients who are at increased risk for osteosarcoma.

Preparation and dosage:

i. rDNA synthetic PTH (hPTH (1-34); Teriparatide as 250 mcg/ml, 20–40 mcg SC o.d.
ii. **Abaloparatide:** This analogue PTHrP(1-34) of PTH is available as injector pen with daily doses for 30 days to be given subcutaneously. Its t½ is

1.7 h. The binding sites are different for teriparatide and abaloparatide on PTH receptors, which permit the use of the higher dose.

Indications: Both are used **to treat postmenopausal osteoporosis** with fractures. See section, Osteoporosis – management.

CALCITONIN: Calcitonin, a 32 amino acid polypeptide is a **hypocalcaemic hormone** produced by C cells in the mammalian thyroid.

C cells are also present in the parathyroids and thymus. Hence, thyroidectomy has no effect on plasma calcium level. **Calcitonin is secreted continuously but its levels increase in response to increased plasma levels of ionic calcium. It acts on the calcitonin receptors present on the osteoclasts and the renal tubules.** The receptors are also present in brain, GIT and immune system.

Pharmacological actions: In humans, salmon calcitonin has the most potent pharmacological action. It is given by SC/IM route. Its action of lowering plasma calcium level is rapid and of short duration.

Bone: It blocks bone resorption by **direct anti-osteoclastic action.** Calcium from the circulation is shunted to bone. It stimulates osteoblasts.

Kidney: It increases excretion of calcium, and phosphorus.

Central action: it alleviates osteoclastic bone pain.

It has no effect on GIT.

Antibodies can develop to calcitonin particularly that from pork.

Preparations and dosage:

i. Salcalcitonin (Salmon calcitonin): available as 50 IU/ml, 100 IU/ml, 200 IU/ml. Dose: subcutaneously/intramuscularly 100 IU daily; 50–150 IU thrice a week.
ii. Salcalcitonin nasal spray. Dose 200 IU once daily.

Indications:

- **Hypercalcaemia: Salcalcitonin** in a*dults:* 4 IU/kg IM or SC b.i.d. It can be administered as 2–16 IU/kg IV infusion b.i.d.
- **Paget disease:** To relieve bone pains or nerve compression, SC injections are used as nasal spray has limited bioavailability.
- **Postmenopausal osteoporosis with unremitting bone pain:** 100 IU calcitonin IM/SC daily, or 200 IU (one spray) daily in alternating nostrils, **together with calcium and vitamin D, till pain subsides or maximum of 4 weeks.**
- **Osteogenesis imperfecta***:* 2 IU/kg calcitonin IM/SC three times weekly, with daily oral calcium supplementation.
- **Bone pain in metastatic cancer.**

VITAMIN D: The term vitamin D is applied to a group of related sterols which have the common property of preventing and curing rickets and osteomalacia.

Chemistry and source: Many sterols develop the antirachitic property on ultraviolet (UV) irradiation. They are fat soluble and have the same general structure (Fig. 68.1).

Solar UV-B irradiation of 7-dehydro-cholesterol present in the secretion of sebaceous glands converts it to **Vitamin D3 (cholecalciferol)**. Vitamin D of animal origin as from fish oil and irradiated milk is D3. Irradiation of ergosterol present in yeast produces **Vitamin D2 (ergocalciferol)**.

In human beings D2 and D3 have similar actions, qualitatively and quantitatively and hence, both are referred to as vitamin D for discussion.

In the liver, vitamin D is hydroxylated to yield **25-hydroxy vitamin D** [25-OHD or 25 cholecalciferol D or **calcefediol**). **In the kidney tubule**, the enzyme 25-OHD-1-alpha-hydroxylase causes further

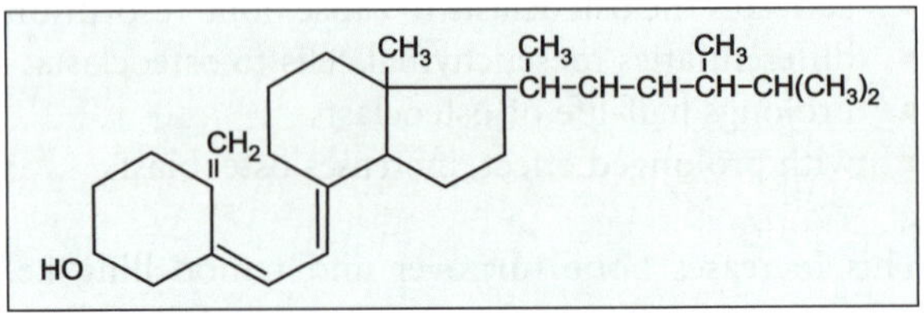

FIG. 68.1 **Calciferol (D2).**

hydroxylation to produce the *active metabolite* **l-alpha, 25-(OH)2D (calcitriol) with biological activity 500–1000 fold higher than that of the precursor 25-OHD** (Fig. 68.2). Its production is regulated by PTH, and serum calcium and phosphorus levels. Both the active products of vitamin D are metabolised by 24-hydroxylase to inactive water soluble products.

Vitamin D may be looked upon both as a vitamin and as a hormone. **As a vitamin, it prevents:**

- **Rickets and osteomalacia**, by maintaining plasma calcium and inorganic phosphate levels above a certain threshold
- **Hypocalcaemic tetany**, by maintaining plasma calcium above a certain critical level
- **Osteoporosis**, by promoting GI calcium absorption
- **Muscle weakness** PH 1.36

Physiological and pharmacological actions: *Vitamin D receptors are widely distributed in many body tissues and cells*, many of which can convert circulating 25-OHD into 1α–25-$(OH)_2$D. Calcitriol acts by binding to specific nuclear receptor-VDR (vitamin D receptor). It gets translocated to the nucleus to cause gene transcription. Along with PTH and calcitonin, **it exerts actions on the classic target tissues: bone, kidney and intestine (Fig. 68.2) and regulates calcium homeostasis and bone mineralisation.**

1. Regulation of calcium metabolism:

- **Bone:** Bone tissue undergoes constant remodelling in that the osteoclast-mediated bone resorption is in equilibrium with osteoblast-mediated reformation of new bone material. *Calcitriol, in physiological amounts acts as a hormone for the*

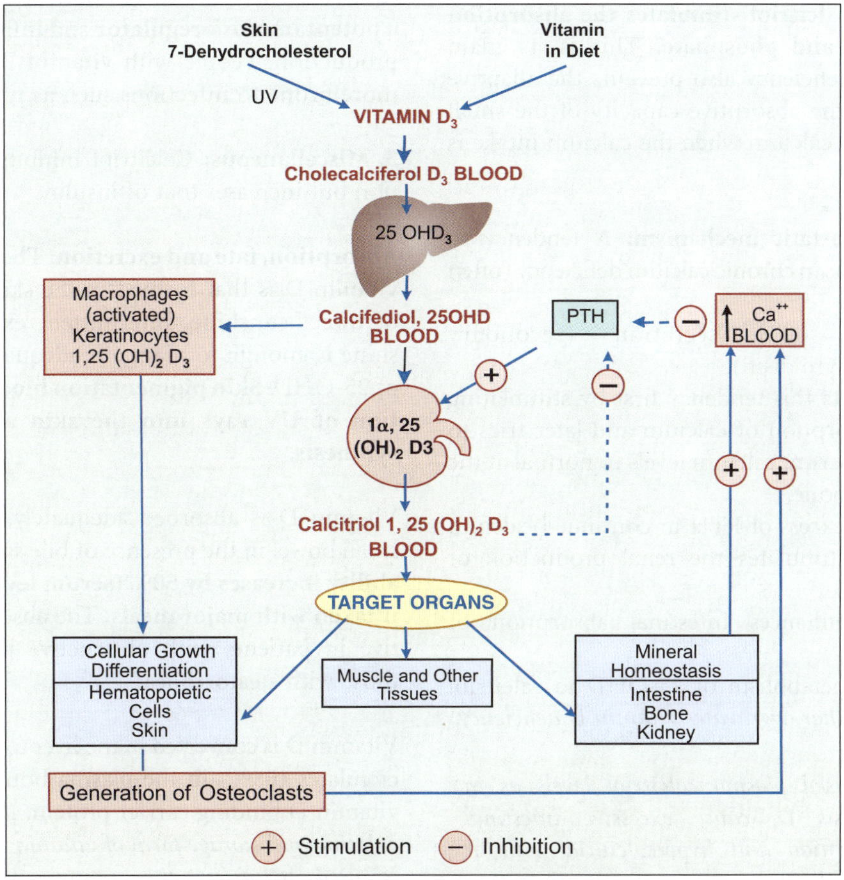

FIG. 68.2 Vitamin D activation and actions.

mineralisation of new bone. It stimulates bone mineralisation by:

a. **Providing mineral for incorporation** into bone matrix through increased intestinal absorption of calcium and phosphorus.
b. **Regulating the function of osteoblasts,** which possess calcitriol receptors.
   However in large doses, it is a potent bone resorptive agent. It increases the differentiation of myeloid precurssor cells to osteoclasts and thus increases their number. It also increases secretion from osteoblasts (osteocalcin) which stimulates osteoclasts and IL-1 which promotes bone resporption.

- **Kidney:** Calcitriol
  a. **Stimulates the proximal tubular reabsorption** of calcium and phosphorus.
  b. **Inhibits the tubular renal formation of calcitriol by negative feedback.**
- **Intestine: Calcitriol stimulates the absorption of calcium and phosphate.** This is its main action. Its deficiency also prevents the adaptive increase in the absorptive capacity of the small intestine for calcium when the calcium intake is low.

Calcium homeostatic mechanism: A tendency to hypocalcaemia, as in chronic calcium deficiency (often nutritional):

i. Stimulates PTH secretion (secondary hyperparathyroidism).
ii. PTH corrects this tendency first by stimulating renal reabsorption of calcium and later tries to restore the serum calcium levels to normal at the expense of bone.
iii. Continued excess of PTH in continued calcium deficiency stimulates the renal production of calcitriol.
iv. Calcitriol enhances intestinal absorption of calcium.
v. Increased metabolism of 25-OHD to calcitriol by *PTH further aggravates vitamin D deficiency.*

Persistently raised plasma calcitriol levels as in hypervitaminosis D, cause excessive intestinal calcium absorption and hypercalciuria with or without hypercalcaemia.

2. Muscle: The uptake of radiocalcium by the sarcoplasmic reticulum is subnormal in vitamin D deficiency; it can be corrected by its administration. *Clinically, muscle weakness is a prominent feature of deficiency; and may be the only manifestation in old persons.*

3. Cellular growth and differentiation: Calcitriol inhibits the proliferation and promotes the differentiation of several tissues. Under certain conditions, keratinocyte-derived calcitriol may induce epidermal differentiation locally and inhibit the proliferation of epithelial cells. The **active analogues of vitamin D are used topically in the treatment of psoriasis** (Chapter 69).

4. Immunoregulatory properties: Receptors for calcitriol are expressed in activated, proliferating human B lymphocytes and T lymphocytes, but they cannot be detected in quiescent lymphocytes. **It is a potent immunoregulator** and influences cytokine production. People with vitamin D deficiency are more prone to infections such as tuberculosis.

5. Miscellaneous: Calcitriol inhibits renin production but increases that of insulin.

Absorption, fate and excretion: The main source of vitamin D is that formed in the skin by the action of direct sunshine. Intermittent exposure to sunshine is enough to maintain adequate plasma levels of 25-OHD. **Skin pigmentation blocks the penetration of UV rays into the skin and reduces its synthesis.**

Vitamin D is absorbed adequately from the distal small bowel in the presence of bile salts. **Its bioavailability increases by 50% (serum levels of 25-OHD) if taken with major meals.** The absorption is defective in patients with obstructive jaundice and in those with steatorrhoea.

Vitamin D is converted in the liver to **25-OHD** which circulates (88%) in the plasma bound to a specific vitamin D binding carrier protein. *It is the main circulating and storage form of vitamin D. Its estimation is used to assess the vitamin D status of an individual.*

Vitamin D absorbed from the gut is presented to the liver in relatively larger quantities at a time; as a protective mechanism, the liver degrades it and excretes the metabolites in the bile. *Hence, adequate exposure to natural or artificial sunlight wherein conversion occurs in the skin, is far more efficient in maintaining plasma 25-OHD levels than oral administration of vitamin D.*

In the proximal renal tubules only small quantities of 25-OHD is converted to the active metabolite 1,25-$(OH)_2D$, while a large fraction is converted to another inactive metabolite 24,25-$(OH)_2D$. The production of calcitriol is strictly regulated by the demands of the organism. The renal production of calcitriol requires the presence of PTH.

The metabolic degradation of 25-OHD in the liver is increased with resultant depletion of vitamin D in:

1. Hyperparathyroidism, primary or secondary.
2. Patients on anticonvulsants, phenobarbitone and phenytoin. These drugs *accelerate metabolism of vitamin D and increase the resistance of target organs (intestine and bone) to vitamin D.* Phenytoin also inhibits calcium absorption from GI tract.

The renal production of calcitriol is stimulated by a diet poor in calcium or phosphorus, and is inhibited by a phosphorus rich diet. Low calcium diet acts through stimulation of PTH release; low phosphorus diet acts directly.

Excess of vitamin D is stored in the body fat. The mammalian liver contains limited amount of vitamin D. Very little vitamin D is found in the urine.

Assay: The plasma levels of 25-OHD and 1,25-$(OH)_2D$; are 30–80 ng/mL and 15–60 pg/mL, respectively.

Significance of serum vitamin D levels: There are several factors that determine serum total 25-OHD levels. Apart from deficient Vitamin D and calcium intake, genetic polymorphism can cause low levels of vitamin D. Thus, total 25-OHD levels are consistently lower in black Americans than in white Americans, which would qualify them as vitamin D deficient. However, they possess higher BMD, higher calcium levels and only slightly higher PTH levels than their white counterparts. This is because of lower levels of vitamin D binding protein in the black due to genetic polymorphism. The levels of bioavailable 25-OHD in black are equivalent to those in white Americans. Giving them vitamin D, simply on the basis of low levels of total 25-OHD would invite vitamin D toxicity. Thus, **low levels of 25-OHD itself do not always indicate vitamin D deficiency unless accompanied by hypocalcaemia, hyperparathyroidism and low BMD.** Too high levels of vitamin D have been associated with increased risk of 'stroke and coronary occlusion'.

Currently a person is considered as vitamin D deficient if serum concentration is <20 ng/mL. Levels between 20–29 ng/ml indicate vit D insufficiency whereas optimal level is believed to be >30–35 ng/mL. However, **supplementation of vitamin D only on the basis of serum level of 25-OHD is not justified.** Rickets or other bone diseases (with lower bone density) are not expected till the 25-OHD levels reach <15 ng/mL (<37 nmol/L).

Adverse reactions: Hypervitaminosis D is likely to occur in an individual with normal vitamin D sensitivity receiving 50,000 IU or more per day for weeks to months. It gives rise to generalised decalcification of bones, hypercalcaemia, hyperphosphataemia, hypercalciuria and metastatic calcification. *It does not occur following excessive exposure to sunlight.*

Preparations and dosage:

i. Calciferol (Vitamin D2) is derived from yeast by UV irradiation. It contains 40,000 IU of antirachitic activity per mg.
ii. Cholecalciferol (Vitamin D3): It is derived by UV irradiation of 7-dehydrocholesterol from lanolin. It is available as 60,000 IU powder in a sachet, 1000 IU in oil based capsules and as an oily injections containing 300,000 and 600,000 IU of vitamin D3. The same preparation may be given orally and will be cheaper.
iii. Shark liver oil contains 6000 IU of vitamin A activity and 1000 IU of antirachitic activity per millilitre. Dose: 0.5–1.5 mL daily orally.
iv. For other preparations containing both vitamins A and D, see Chapter 76

Indications:

- **Supplementation of vitamin D:** It is needed to prevent vitamin D deficiency in certain group of individuals as mentioned below.

Current evidence suggests that daily requirement of vitamin D is 400 IU/day for subject less than 1 year of age and 600 IU/day for subjects in the age range of 1–70 years. *All breast fed infants are considered to have a higher risk of insufficient vitamin D because often the vitamin D status of mother is unknown*, more so in developing countries. *Unfortified cow's milk is a poor source of vitamin D (about 1 mcg of activity per litre);* so is human milk. *Premature infants are more susceptible to rickets because fetal storage of calcium takes place in 3rd trimester. and may require supplemental vitamin D and calcium.* Hence supplementation with 400 IU is recommended and is not a bad idea to give vitamin D to all children. One teaspoonful (5 mL) of cod liver oil gives about 650 IU (85 IU/g), whereas 5 mL halibut liver oil contains 3000 IU of vitamin D. **Excess vitamin D, however, may cause more harm than good.** This must be remembered while prescribing vitamin D supplements to infants and children whose 'vitaminised' food may already be supplying their daily requirement.

As vitamin D is stored in body fat for several months, unwittingly administered supraphysiological doses of vitamin D for prolonged period to make baby's bone strong can end up in toxicity.

It is necessary to supplement elementary calcium (1 g per day) while repleting vitamin deficiency.

Vitamin D supplementation of the pregnant mother is superior to supplementation of the lactating mother because some vitamin D is transferred across the placenta and is stored in the fetus, to be utilised in the first few months of extrauterine life.

Vitamin D supplementation is essential in the elderly in whom both skin synthesis and GI absorption are impaired. Daily vitamin D requirement is about 800 IU for subjects aged more than 70 years.

- **For prevention and treatment of vitamin D deficiency:** *The commonest cause of vitamin D deficiency is a deficient intake or absorption of calcium (because of high phytate and oxalate content of a cereal–vegetables-based diet);* this explains why vitamin D deficiency is common even in the tropical countries with abundant sunlight. Further, unlike in the rich western countries, the foods are not fortified with vitamin D. It must be noted that the sun rays which induce vitamin D activity in the skin are in the UV range and can get absorbed by atmosphere, by glass and by buildings. *Generally, a serum level of 25-OHD below 20 ng/mL is considered diagnostic of vitamin D deficiency.*

In children with vitamin D deficiency, newly formed bone and cartilage matrix fail to mineralize, which results in defective growth or rickets. In adults the deficiency causes generalized accumulation of undermineralized bone matrix, termed as osteomalacia. *Unlike osteoporosis, osteomalacia is accompanied by localised or generalised bone pains, and tenderness on pressing the sternum or the anterior tibia.*

For the prevention and treatment of nutritional vitamin D deficiency, the preparation of choice is cholecalciferol (D3). *Alfacalcidol and calcitriol which are more expensive are not appropriate for that purpose* (see section, Synthetic vitamin D analogues). **Calcitriol** inhibits PTH function directly and reduces bone turnover. Higher doses of calcitriol may increase BMD, but **often causes hypercalciuria and less frequently hypercalcaemia.** Restriction of dietary calcium may reduce this toxicity.

Unless the pregnant women receive vitamin D supplements, there is hardly any store of vitamin D in the newborn, and its administration is recommended from the first month especially in breast fed infants. If the diet is deficient in older children, the daily requirement can be easily supplied by a teaspoon of cod liver oil. *Excessive administration must be avoided.*

Rickets in children and osteomalacia in adults are best treated with a single oral or IM dose of 300,000–600,000 IU (7.5–15 mg) of *calciferol.* It may be repeated 4–6 weeks later, if the blood chemistry so indicates. Simultaneously, calcium must also be prescribed in order to facilitate the calcification of the osteoid.

Administration of a single IM dose of 600,000 IU is desirable in patients with chronic obstructive jaundice and also once in 6 months in patients on long-term therapy with anticonvulsants and glucocorticoids and in elderly people.

- **Vitamin D 'resistant' rickets and osteomalacia:** This term is applied to rickets and osteomalacia due to chronic renal insufficiency, hereditary hypophosphataemic rickets and hypophosphatasia. Large doses of vitamin D in such patients (up to 50,000 IU, 1.25 mg, daily) are required to bring about healing of bone lesions. *Alfacalcidiol and calcitriol are preferred in these conditions.*
- **In hypoparathyroidism:** Oral vitamin D (0.5–2.5 lac IU Cholecalciferol) together with oral calcium is used to treat hypoparathyroidism. *Alfacalcidol or calcitriol may be preferred because of their rapid action.*
- **Osteoporosis:** For prevention and treatment. (See section, Management of osteoporosis).

There is a considerable confusion regarding the supplementation with vitamin D. The latter has been projected as a panacea that can prevent various chronic disorders. This assumption also leads to increasing requests for vitamin D measurement in the blood – an expensive test for routine use. *The effectiveness of vitamin D supplementation has been definitely proved only in rickets and osteomalacia.* There is at present no evidence that vitamin D supplements in normal subjects reduce the risk of cardiovascular diseases, DM or cancer.

SYNTHETIC VITAMIN D ANALOGUES

25-(OH)D3 (**Calcifediol**, Calcidiol), 1-alpha-(OH) D3 (**Alfacalcidol**) and 1,25-$(OH)_2$D3 (**Calcitriol**) are the synthetic vitamin D analogues used in therapeutics (Table 68.2).

Unlike cholecalciferol, calcifediol is absorbed from the gut even in patients with fat malabsorption. It is the drug of choice in liver disease with vitamin D deficiency. It has a long t½ (19 days). In contrast to cholecalciferol, which is recommended in treating nutritional rickets and osteomalacia, **calcitriol** and **alfacalcidol** are indicated primarily in the treatment of:

- **Hypoparathyroidism**
- **Renal osteodystrophy due to chronic renal failure**
- **Renal tubular defect with vitamin D 'resistant' rickets and osteomalacia**
- **Vitamin D 'dependent' rickets**

Doxercalciferol is 1-alpha-(OH) D2 and is used to treat secondary hyperparathyroidism with CKD.

Calcipotriol, an analogue of calcitriol suppresses cell proliferation and promotes cell differentiation to the same degree as calcitriol but is 200 times weaker than the latter compound in its action on calcium metabolism. It is used **topically to treat of psoriasis** (Chapter 69).

Table 68.2 Commonly Used Compounds with Vitamin D Activity

Property	Ergocalciferol and Cholecalciferol	Calcifediol	Calcitriol	Alfacalcidol
Physiological dose (mcg/day)[a]	10	5	0.5–1.0	0.5–1.0
Pharmacological dose (mcg/day)[b]	1200	50	0.5–3.0[c]	0.5–3.0
Onset of maximum effect (days)	30	15	2–3	2–3
Duration of toxicity (if it occurs) after cessation of therapy (weeks)	6–18	4–12	0.5–1.0	0.5–1.0
Available as	In variable strengths	20, 50 mcg capsules	0.25, 0.5 mcg tablets	0.5–1.0 mcg tablets

[a]Will cure nutritional rickets and osteomalacia.
[b]Used in other conditions listed above.
[c]Dose may be as high as 10 mcg in vitamin D 'dependent' rickets

Paricalcitol is a synthetic calcitriol derivative which reduces PTH release without producing hypercalcaemia except in overdoses.

22-Oxacalcitriol (Maxacalcitol) is another calcitriol derivative which is a potent suppressor of PTH gene, with limited activity on the intestine and the bone. This it has no calcemic activity It is used in patients with secondary hyperparathyroidism with CKD.

Dihydrotachysterol (DHT): Action of reduced form of calciferol is faster and shorter lived than that of vitamin D. It gets activated in liver and does not require renal hydroxylation. *Its antirachitic property is negligible.*

Table 68.3 summarises the actions of the 'calcitropic' hormones, calcitriol, PTH and calcitonin. PH 1.36

BISPHOSPHONATES: These synthetic nonhydrolysable pyrophosphate analogues were developed initially as water softeners. They are characterised by phosphorus–carbon–phosphorus (P–C–P) bonds (Fig. 68.3). Their potency depends on the length and the structure of the side chain.

Classification:

I. **First Generation:** Etidronate, Tiludronate – No longer used
II. **Second Generation:** Alendronate (oral), Pamidronate (IV)

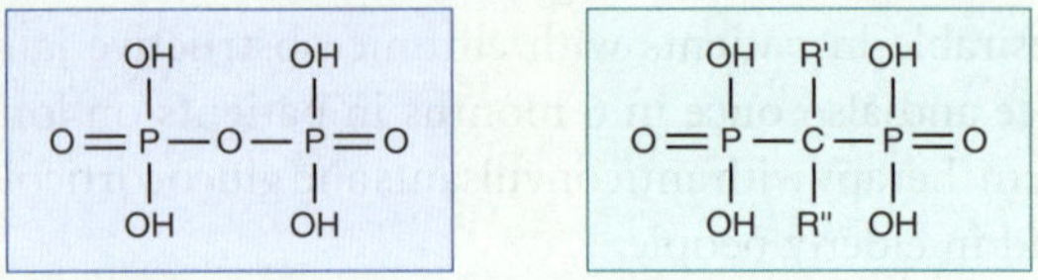

Pyrophosphate: Tissue fluid constituent in bone

Bisphosphonate: Synthetic pyrophosphate analogue

FIG. 68.3 **Pyrophosphate and bisphosphonate**

III. **Third Generation:** Risendronate (oral), Zolendronate (IV)

Mechanism of action: Bisphosphonates have a strong affinity for the bone hydroxyapatite, they:

- **Are effective calcium chelators** and **get deposited in the bone mineral selectively.** They are released slowly on bone resorption by osteoclasts, so the cells get exposed to local high concentration of bisphosphonates.
- The first generation compounds are similar to pyrophosphate. **After ingestion by the osteoclasts,** they get incorporated into ATP analogues that accumulate within the osteoclasts and **impair their functions** and **hasten their death by apoptosis.**
- Newer bisphosphonates have N-containing side chain and are potent. They **inhibit multiple steps in the pathway from mevalonate to cholesterol and isoprenoid lipids required for the prenylation of proteins.** Prenylation reaction is required for

Table 68.3 Actions of Calcitropic Hormones

	Calcitriol	PTH	Calcitonin
Intestinal absorption	Ca and PO_4 ↑	Ca and PO_4 ↑ (via calcitriol)	—
Kidney	Ca and PO_4 reabsorption ↑	Ca reabsorption ↑ PO_4 reabsorption ↓, PO_4 excretion ↑ Calcitriol synthesis ↑	Ca and PO_4 reabsorption ↓
Bone	Calcification of osteoid[a]; resorption of bone ↑ in toxic doses	Bone formation > bone resorption on acute administration; bone resorption > bone formation[b]	Osteoclastic bone resorption ↓
Plasma levels	Ca and PO_4 ↑	Hypercalcaemia; low to normal PO_4	Ca ↓[c]; hypophosphataemia
Urinary excretion	Ca normalises[a]; hypercalciuria in toxic doses	Ca ↑ due to hypercalcaemia; PO_4 ↑ by direct tubular action	Ca and PO_4 ↑

Notes: Ca, calcium; PO_4, phosphates.
[a]In physiological doses.
[b]In chronic high concentration.
[c]Only in the presence of hypercalcaemia.

membrane surface proteins to anchor osteoclasts. In absence of prenylation, attachment of osteoclasts to bone is prevented.

- They may stimulate osteoblasts to release OPG, which neutralizes RANKL and thus prevents interaction between RANKL and RANK. This prevents osteoclast differentiation and their activity (Fig. 68.4).

Thus biphosphonates slow the rate of bone thinning and can lead to increase bone density.

They are useful for preventing bone resorption and helping to reduce the vertebral and hip fractures in osteoporosis; and in treating life-threatening hypercalcaemia.

It is necessary to correct the disturbances of calcium and mineral metabolism before starting the therapy.

Absorption, fate and excretion: Given orally, their bioavailability is low, 1%–3% of the ingested dose. Food, iron, calcium, aluminium, magnesium, milk, tea, coffee and fruit juices interfere with their absorption. They are rapidly cleared from the plasma, with 50% deposited in the bone, and the remaining excreted unchanged in the urine. They cross the placenta and get deposited in the fetal bone.

Adverse reactions: Bisphosphonates in the doses used are generally well tolerated. The ADR include:

- **General:** Headache. IV injection releases cytokines resulting in fever, joint pains, myalgia and ocular inflammation.
- **Gastrointestinal:** Nausea, abdominal pain and diarrhoea. These are relatively common. Occasionally, they (particularly alendronate) may cause heartburn, oesophagitis and oesophageal ulcers.
- **Renal:** Renal failure and electrolyte abnormalities have been reported following IV use. Zolendronate is nephrotoxic. It can cause severe hypocalcemia.
- **Miscellaneous:** *Excessive doses* cause demineralisation of bones. Fractures of the jaw at the sites of pre-existing infection can occur during the IV use, of bisphosphonates. These are secondary to osteonecrosis as a result of suppression of bone remodelling. Atypical femoral fractures have been observed after long term use. These are rare with new biphosphonates.

Biphosphonates are contraindicated in GERD, peptic ulcer disease and renal impairment.

Preparations and dosage: Table 68.4.

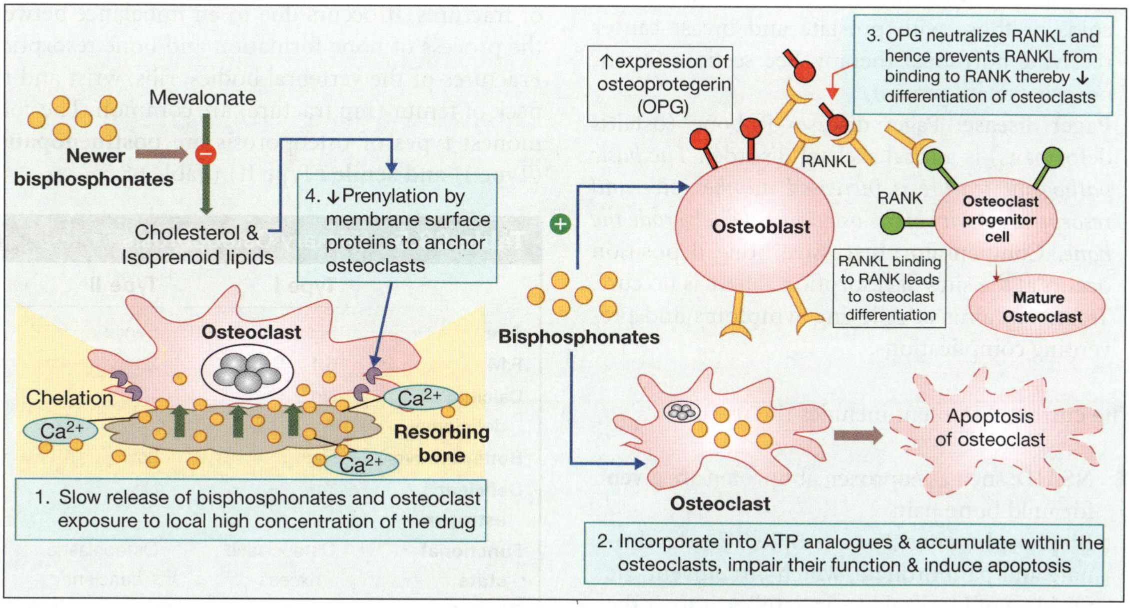

FIG. 68.4 Mechanism of action of bisphosphonates

Table 68.4 Bisphosphonate Preparations

Drug	Dose
Alendronate[a]	70 mg once a week
Risendronate	35 mg once a week; 75 mg/day for 2 consecutive days once a month
Ibandronate	2.5 mg daily or 150 mg once a month; 3 mg IV bolus every 3 months
Zolendronate	4 mg, 5 min slow IV infusion once a year
Pamidronate	60–90 mg IV infusion over 2–24 h

Notes: Doses are oral unless specified.
Clodronate, etidronate and tiludronate are other bisphosphonates.
[a]Preventive dose 35 mg/week.

To prevent oesophageal ADR, *the patient should be instructed to take the drug on empty stomach in the morning with 250 mL (a glass) of water, in the erect posture; not to lie down for at least ½ to 1 h after that; and not to eat or drink anything except water for a similar period.* In practice, these reactions can occur even after following these instructions. *A patient with upper GI symptoms should not be prescribed an oral bisphosphonate.*

Indications:

- **Osteoporosis:** They are used for primary prevention of osteoporosis in patients with multiple risk factors or for secondary prevention e.g. postmenopausal women, patients taking glucocorticoids or those with prostate and breast cancer receiving hormonal therapy. See section, Osteoporosis – management.
- **Paget disease:** Paget disease of bone (osteitis deformans) is a focal skeletal disorder. *The basic pathogenic feature is increased number, size and resorptive activity of the osteoclasts which erode the bone.* Compensatory excessive bone deposition occurs at the sites of resorption. There is no cure. Treatment aims at relieving symptoms and preventing complications.

The current treatment includes the use of:

1. **NSAID:** such as naproxen, ibuprofen are given for mild bone pain
2. **Bisphosphonates:** For example, IV zolendronate and pamidronate, which circumvent the problem of low oral bioavailability, impair the activity of osteoclasts and prevent bone resorption. It can provide long term remission. Oral bisphosphonates can also be given daily or weekly for 6 months.
3. **Calcitonin,** also has shown to decrease bone turnover. But it needs parenteral administration and is expensive. It is more antigenic.

Administered parenterally, these drugs have prolonged action (months to years after a course of therapy). They induce remission, relieve bone pains and prevent fractures. *They do not cure the disease, and recurrence can occur.*

- **Avascular necrosis of femur:** Several noncontrolled studies have reported the beneficial effects of bisphosphonates in patients with avascular necrosis of femur. They have been found to decrease pain, lower articular collapse and improve mobility.
- **In malignancy:** Clodronate orally and pamidronate, ibandronate and zoledronic acid are administered by slow IV infusion to treat hypercalcaemia and to prevent or shrink osteolytic bone metastasis in breast cancer and multiple myeloma.

OSTEOPOROSIS – MANAGEMENT

Osteoporosis is a multifactorial disease in which, there is a diminution in the quantity of trabecular and cortical bone mass, that increases the frequency of fractures. It occurs due to an imbalance between the process of bone formation and bone resorption. Fractures of the vertebral bodies, ribs, wrist and the neck of femur (hip fracture) are common. The commonest types of osteoporosis are **postmenopausal** (Type I) and **senile** (Type II) (Table 68.5).

Table 68.5 Primary Osteoporosis

	Type I	Type II
Age	Postmenopausal	Senile
F:M	6:1	2:1
Calcium deficiency	No	Yes
Bone turnover	High	Low
Deficient estrogen	Yes	No
Functional state	Osteoclastic excess	Osteoblastic deficiency
Type of fracture	Vertebral crush	Vertebral wedge; long bones

The bone mass normally increases up to the age of 30 years, after which there is a gradual but progressive diminution, faster in women than in men, accelerated after menopause.

The bone mass is best **estimated** by bone densitometry, which measures **Bone mineral density (BMD)** expressed as *T* **score** which stands for its difference in standard deviation from the said mean. *A T score from –2.0 to –2.5 mandates* **antiresorptive drug treatment** *in the presence of risk factors.*

Osteoporosis is diagnosed when the individual has a *nontraumatic, nonpathological fracture* of the spine or when the T score is lower than –2.5 in the hip or the spine. PH 1.36

The treatment aims at:

- Restoration of the bone strength
- Prevention of fractures

Management: Box 68.7 outlines the principles of management of postmenopausal osteoporosis.

The dietary modifications advised are reduction in the consumption of:

a. Common salt as calcium is coexcreted with sodium in increased quantities in the urine
b. Animal foods (except milk) as they are acid-ash producing and increase calciuria
c. Alcohol and to stop smoking

A daily calcium intake of 1200–1500 mg with a vitamin D intake of 800 IU/day and regular physical exercise are recommended in adolescents and in all postmenopausal women. The exercises recommended are walking and resistance exercise (weight lifting), under supervision.

In patients *with severe vitamin D deficiency* (25-OHD < 37 nmol/L) and/or low calcium intake, supplementation of vitamin D along with calcium is necessary.

Classification of drugs for osteoporosis

1. **Antiresorptive drugs:** Bisphosphonate, raloxifene, calcitonin,, denosumab
2. **Anabolic drugs** (stimulating bone formation): Teriparatide and abaloparatide
3. **Having both the effects:** Strontium ranolate

Antiresorptive drugs slow the rate of bone loss and and show increase in BMD in first few years. But as bone resorption and bone formation are linked processes, later on the bone formation also decreases and there will not be true increase in the BMD.

Box 68.7 Principles of Management of Postmenopausal Osteoporosis PH 1.1

- Risk factor control
- BMD determination
- Lifestyle changes, diet, exercise
- Analgesics as needed
- Short period of bed rest following a fracture of the spine
- Calcium and vitamin D
- Antiresorptive and anabolic drugs (See text)

Bisphosphonates *are the first drug of choice for treating postmenopausal osteoporosis.* They suppress bone resorption at doses that do not inhibit mineralization. **Alendronate, risendronate** and others have been used in combination with calcium and vitamin D. Alendronate 70 mg once a week is usually preferred (see Table 68.4).

Estrogens are antiresorptive. They:

- Inhibit the cytokines that recruit osteoclasts and oppose the bone-resorbing, Ca++-mobilising action of PTH.
- Increase osteoblast proliferation, augments production of TGF-β and bone morphogenic proteins, and inhibit apoptosis.
  They prevent osteoporosis if given to postmenopausal woman or any one with estrogen deficiency but risks associated with HRT (heart disease and breast cancer) precludes its use (Chapter 65).

RALOXIFENE: This analogue of tamoxifen is a 'selective estrogen receptor modulator' (SERM) and has beneficial effects on the bone and CVS. It may be preferred in middle and late post-menopause. **It causes dose-dependent increase in the osteoblastic activity.** It prevents bone loss and increases BMD by 1–3%. It has been shown to decrease vertebral fracture risk by 50%. Unlike estrogen it reduces the risk of breast cancer but not of postmenopausal vasomotor symptoms. Given orally, it undergoes extensive hepatic first-pass metabolism and has low bio-availability. It has an active metabolite. It is used in the dose of 60 mg o.d. in the prophylaxis of menopausal osteoporosis. Usually it is well tolerated. ADR include hot flushes, leg cramps and rarely, thromboembolic disease.

Raloxifene is less efficacious then bisphosphonates in preventing fractures and serves as a second line drug in the prevention and treatment of osteoporosis in postmenopausal women.

Calcitonin (SC/IM/intranasal), in general, is less effective and more expensive for prevention of bone loss in women 5 years beyond menopause. However, it is more effective in relieving severe bone pain.

Parathyroid hormone (PTH, teriparatide): Intermittent (i.e. 20 mcg once daily) subcutaneously, h-PTH-1–34 **increases BMD, bone mass and bone strength by stimulating periosteal and endosteal bone formation.** Its effect is faster and more marked than that of biphosphonates or estrogens. *It is the first drug available with* **anabolic action** *on the bone.* It reduces the fracture rate. However it is expensive.

Abaloparatide (80 mcg SC) has also shown to reduce the risk of new vertebral and nonvertebral fractures.

Combination therapy of alendronate and PTH has shown decrease in anabolic effect of PTH.

Strontium ranelate is claimed to stimulate bone formation and reduction of bone resorption. Its mechanism of action is unknown but it inhibits bone resorption and stimulates bone formation. It is a reserved drug for elderly women >75 years who have suffered fractures and are unable to tolerate biphosphonates.

Denosumab is a monoclonal antibody that binds with high affinity to RANKL. The resultant effect is similar to that of OPG. Thus it Inhibits osteoclast differentiation and function. Given subcutaneously in a dose of 60 mg every 6 months, it increases BMD and decreases markers for bone turnover. Osteonecrosis and fracture femur may occur following its use. It is a treatment option when no other drug can be given.

Drug-Induced Osteoporosis

Many drugs can cause/worsen osteoporosis. These include heparin, warfarin, cyclosporine, glucocorticoids, medroxyprogesterone acetate, antiepileptic drugs such as phenobarbitone, phenytoin and carbamazepine, anticancer drugs and thyroid hormones. Caution should be exercised and perhaps BMD monitored during their long-term use. Calcium and vitamin D supplements should be prescribed during prolonged use of such drugs.

In contrast, thiazide diuretics and perhaps statins can minimise bone loss. *Hence, a thiazide may be the preferred drug if an osteoporotic patient also has hypertension or nephrolithiasis.*

FLUORIDE

The fluoride ion is widely distributed in nature. It is of medical interest mainly because of its toxicity. It can enter the human body through edible plants, drinking water, fluorine containing pesticides, contaminated food additives and by inhalation of fluoride dust and gases.

Pharmacological actions: Children who drink water containing fluorine (1 part per million) have been shown to develop permanent teeth which are resistant to the development of caries. Topical application of fluoride solution to the teeth after eruption is claimed to reduce the decay. With the exception of its actions on the teeth *in very low concentrations*, the actions of fluoride are toxic (see below).

Fluoride inhibits several enzymes and diminishes tissue respiration and anaerobic glycolysis in excised organs. It is a useful *in vitro* anticoagulant.

Absorption, fate and excretion: Fluoride is absorbed from the GI tract, the lungs and the skin. In the body, fluoride can be detected in all tissues but *is preferentially deposited in bones and teeth*. It is excreted mainly by the kidneys and in small amounts by the sweat glands, the lactating breast and the GI tract.

Adverse reactions:

- **Acute poisoning:** Acute poisoning results from ingestion of insecticides containing fluoride salts. The symptoms are due to:
  a. Irritation of the GI tract: nausea, vomiting, abdominal pain and diarrhoea
  b. Hypocalcaemia caused by binding of plasma calcium (increased irritability of the central nervous system)
  c. Medullary depression leading to fall in BP and respiratory paralysis

  Treatment is symptomatic and consists of stomach wash with lime water, IV fluids, IV calcium and treatment of respiratory and cardiac failure.
- **Chronic poisoning** (Fluorosis): Chronic fluoride poisoning is usually reported following drinking contaminated water. It causes two main changes:
  a. **Osteosclerosis**
  b. **Mottled enamel of the teeth**

Osteosclerosis consists of an increase in density and calcification of bones and varies greatly in severity. It results in various body deformities. Mottling affects only the developing teeth, teeth which have already erupted being spared.

Indications:

- **Dental caries** can be defined as '*the localised destruction of susceptible dental hard tissue by acidic byproducts from bacterial fermentation of dietary carbohydrates*'. It is the most common but preventable disease in children. Treated in early stages, the pathological changes can be reversed.

Endogenous microorganisms, mostly mutant streptococci and lactobacillus species present in the biofilms (colonising the tooth surface) produce weak acid, following fermentation of residual food carbohydrates. The decreased pH leads to demineralisation of tooth tissues. **This is naturally prevented by saliva which acts as a buffer and raises the biofilm pH.** It can also be reversed by uptake of Ca, P and fluoride. Once the tooth is destroyed, its treatment becomes difficult.

The fluoride ion is one of the micronutrients that has been demonstrated to have a clear effect on dental caries. The use of fluoride tooth paste or gel is highly effective, safe and acceptable. Frequent sipping of sugar containing drinks and eating sugar containing foods such as chocolate, sweets and pastries should be avoided.

Further, rinsing the mouth after eating and regular brushing of the teeth at least twice a day *after meals* is advisable. Decrease or lack of saliva helps the pathological process. Chewing of clove/cardamom may be beneficial. It also helps to prevents bad breath.

The best way to prevent caries is maintaining optimal oral hygiene so as to reduce the causative microbial agents. The teeth should be brushed with a tooth paste and flossed twice a day. Pregnant women should be urged to have all open lesions restored and to follow good dietary practices to reduce the transmission of cariogenic microbes to the fetus.

MAGNESIUM METABOLISM

Magnesium is an important constituent of the human body. The average amount of body magnesium in an adult weighing 70 kg is about 2000 mEq (25 g). Of this, approximately 50%–70% is in bones, 1% is in the ECF and the remaining is intracellular. **It is a major intracellular cation and is concentrated mainly in the mitochondria.** Bone acts as a magnesium reservoir during depletion. The plasma magnesium levels vary from 1.5 to 2.0 mEq/L; nearly

33% of this is bound to plasma proteins. Cardiac and skeletal muscles, liver, brain and kidneys contain appreciable amounts of magnesium.

Physiological and pharmacological actions: In general, magnesium causes depression of both, CNS and CVS.

CNS: Low magnesium level may evoke increased irritability, muscle weakness, tremors, ataxia, depression and psychosis. It may cause convulsions.

Magnesium also possesses local anaesthetic activity and depresses myoneural transmission by reducing the quantal release of acetylcholine and by antagonising its depolarising effect at the motor end plates, and by reducing the excitability of muscle cell membrane. The CNS and the myoneural junction depression produced by magnesium can be antagonised by calcium.

CVS: Heart block, prolonged PR interval and widening of QRS complex may result if the plasma level exceeds 10 mEq/L. Magnesium causes peripheral vasodilatation and may cause hypotension.

Miscellaneous: Magnesium is a cofactor of many vital enzymes like membrane ATPase, transporters and nucleic acid.

Absorption, fate and excretion: Magnesium and calcium probably have common transport mechanisms across the gut and the renal tubules. The daily intake of magnesium in Americans is 150–350 mg/day and of this, nearly 1/3rd is absorbed from the GI tract. Vitamin D stimulates its absorption. Magnesium is excreted by the kidney by glomerular filtration. Most of it is reabsorbed, only 3%–5% of filtered magnesium appears in urine. Renal impairment may cause magnesium retention and toxicity even with oral magnesium salts.

Magnesium deficiency: Box 68.8 gives the common causes of hypomagnesaemia.

Clinically, magnesium deficiency is characterised by weakness and mental disturbances like restlessness, and aggressiveness. Involuntary movements, and rarely tetany may develop. Ventricular arrhythmias have been reported. Magnesium deficiency is usually associated with low level of intracellular potassium, particularly in the skeletal muscle. The plasma potassium levels are usually normal.

Box 68.8 Common causes of Hypomagnesaemia

- Severe and continued diarrhoea or fistulous discharge
- Chronic alcoholism
- Diabetic ketoacidosis (DKA)
- Hyperthyroidism
- Drug induced: Thiazide/loop diuretic therapy, amphotericin, cyclosporin, aminoglycosides
- Intestinal malabsorption
- Hyperparathyroidism
- Impaired renal tubular absorption, renal tubular acidosis
- Hyperaldosteronism, SIADH
- During recovery from acute tubular necrosis and DKA
- Pregnancy (third trimester), lactation

Indications for magnesium salts:

- **Hypocalcaemia resistant to treatment:** It may respond only after administering magnesium.
- **In magnesium deficiency:** Magnesium deficiency can be treated by daily administration of approximately 300 mEq of magnesium given as magnesium hydroxide mixture.
- **As antacids and osmotic purgatives:** See Chapters 40 and 41, respectively.
- **As anticonvulsant:** Magnesium sulphate is used to control seizures in toxaemia of pregnancy. It is given during labour and for 24 h afterwards. A 20% solution is usually administered intramuscularly/intravenously for this purpose. It also achieves a moderate reduction in BP. *Care must be taken to keep a calcium preparation handy to counter excessive central depression with magnesium.*
- **In cardiac arrhythmias:** Hypomagnesaemia is known to occur in the immediate post-MI period and may be associated with cardiac arrhythmias. This responds to IV magnesium sulphate, 4 mL, 50% given over 15 min.
- **To lower raised intracranial tension: Hypertonic solution** of magnesium sulphate is sometimes used rectally to reduce increased intracranial tension.
- **Local uses:** Magnesium sulphate, 25%–50% in glycerine is used topically for alleviation of inflammation. It acts by exerting an osmotic effect.

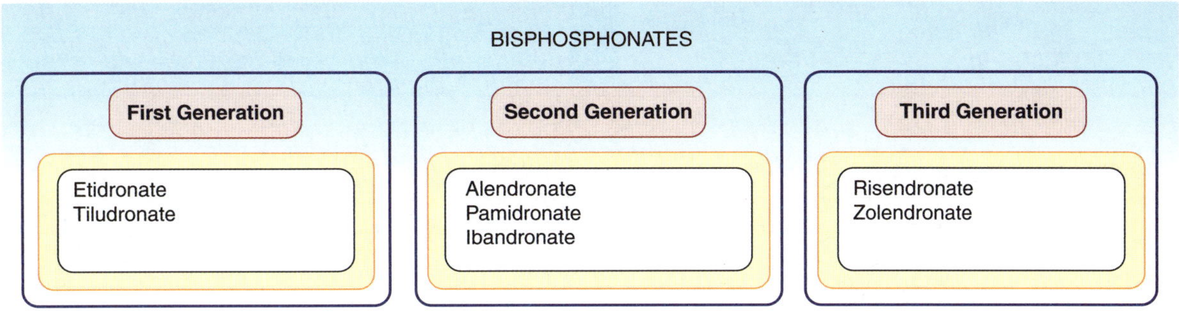
BISPHOSPHONATES
First Generation
Etidronate
Tiludronate
Second Generation
Alendronate
Pamidronate
Ibandronate
Third Generation
Risendronate
Zolendronate

14

SECTION

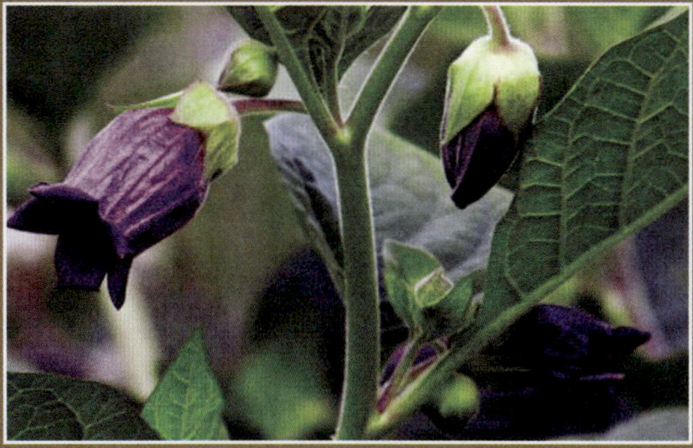

Atropa belladonna

Drugs Used in Common Skin and Eye Disorders

Section Outline

This section consists of the following chapters:

CHAPTER 69

PH 1.57

Pharmacotherapy of Common Skin Disorders and Skin Protectives

Learning Objectives

This chapter will enable the reader:

1. To be aware of the structure of normal skin and enumerate the different types of skin lesions.
2. To state the factors influencing cutaneous drug absorption.
3. To enumerate the different dermatological formulations.
4. To state the role played by a vehicle in dermatological formulations emphasizing the factors that determine its choice.
5. To state the factors for selection of a topical formulation for a given dermatological condition.
6. To outline the management of pruritus.
7. To state the different keratolytic agents with their adverse effects and indications.
8. To state the drugs used for common bacterial, viral and fungal skin infections giving rationale.
9. To outline the therapy of seborrhoeic dermatitis, scabies and pediculosis.
10. To discuss the management of acne vulgaris.
11. To outline the drug therapy of allergic skin disorders.
12. To discuss pharmacotherapy of psoriasis.
13. To state the drug therapy of alopecia.
14. To enumerate various demelanising and melanising agents with their indications and adverse effects.
15. To classify sunscreens and state their uses.
16. To enumerate common pharmacological ingredients of cosmetic preparations like dusting powders, shampoos, cold cream, tooth powders, dermal fillers, anhidrotics and deodorants.
17. To state the drugs causing different types of drug-induced skin disorders and outline their treatment.

KEY TERMS

keratolytics, p. 1023
azoles, p. 1026
permethrin, p. 1029
gamma benzene hexachloride, 1029
comedolytics, p. 1031
isotretinoin, p. 1032
etretinate, p. 1036
minoxidil, p. 1038
hydroquinone, p. 1038
psoralens, p. 1037
sunscreens, p. 1039
anhidrotics, p. 1041
drug induced skin disorders, p. 1041

Skin diseases are common in clinical practice, more so in the warm and humid tropical countries. The skin, the target tissue of drug treatment, is also a route of drug administration. It can act as a drug reservoir and is also a site for drug metabolism. It is important in regulation of body temperature and water loss. Application of drugs to the skin can affect the function(s) of internal organs.

Anatomy and physiology of the skin: Anatomically, the skin consists of three distinct layers (Fig. 69.1):

- **The epidermis**
- **The dermis**
- **The subcutaneous tissue**

The **epidermis** consists of a multilayered, keratinising, stratified, squamous epithelium. The outermost part of the epidermis is the lipid-rich **stratum corneum** which prevents water loss from the body. It also protects against noxious agents in the environment.

The **dermis** is a thick, highly vascular layer made up of ground substance, fibroblasts and collagen fibres, together with the appendages of the skin, sweat glands and pilosebaceous follicles, embedded in it. It is metabolically active.

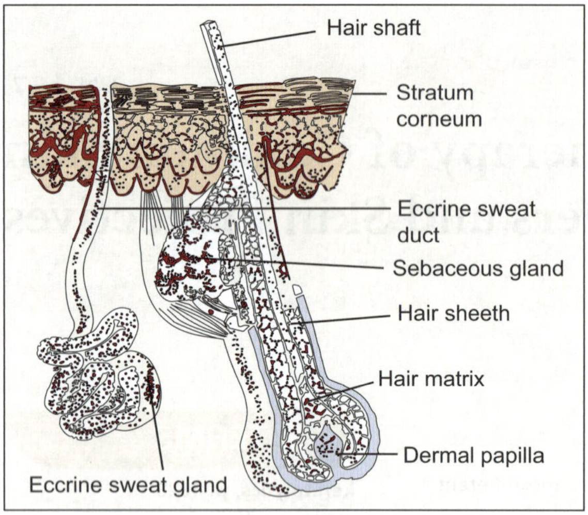

FIG. 69.1. Structure of normal hairy skin.

PRINCIPLES OF TOPICAL DRUG APPLICATION

PH 1.1

Topical drug treatment aims at providing high concentration of the drug at the site of application with minimal systemic absorption, to avoid systemic adverse effects. To be effective, a drug must enter the skin in adequate concentration.

Drugs are applied to the skin in various formulations in pharmacologically inactive *vehicles.* **However, the therapeutic effects depend not only on the properties of the drug but also on those of the vehicle.**

The **absorption of drugs into the skin** is slow and incomplete. It depends on:

- **The lipid solubility of the preparation**
- **The state of hydration of the stratum corneum** – increased hydration increases the drug penetration
- **Drug concentration in the vehicle**
- **Thickness of the skin**: Thicker the skin lower is the drug penetration. The skin of neonates is highly permeable to drugs; on the other hand, the ageing skin is relatively less permeable to drugs.
- **Quantity of the preparation applied**, which varies with the extent of the skin lesion. Large amounts of 'very potent' glucocorticoids (Chapter 64) can cause serious systemic toxicity.
- **The presence of inflamed skin** which allows higher penetration of a drug.
- **The use of an occlusive dressing** which increases the drug penetration into the skin.

An absorbed drug may be stored in the skin for prolonged periods, e.g. a topical glucocorticoid applied to the skin under occlusion for 24 h can establish a reservoir lasting for up to 2 weeks.

Intradermal and transdermal drug administration: This is discussed in Chapter 1.

VEHICLES

Vehicles: Topical preparations consist of two parts: (1) the base or vehicle and (2) the active ingredient(s). The important vehicles are liquids, powders, oils and ointment/cream bases. Such vehicles have several important functions:

- *They provide a reasonably safe infrastructure for practical application.*
- *They form a reservoir for the active ingredient.*
- *They allow local release of suitable amounts of the active drug.*
- *Many vehicles are also useful for their physical actions* such as soothing, lubricating, cooling, drying, moisturising, softening, hydrating or protecting effects.

The factors which influence the choice of a vehicle are listed in Box 69.1.

FORMULATIONS

PH 1.3

- **Powders** act by their physical property of absorbing moisture. They contain ingredients such as talc, starch, chalk, cellulose, menthol and zinc or magnesium stearate. They can produce a cooling effect. They protect the skin by reducing friction, especially in the intertriginous areas such as axillae and groins and in the skin folds under the female breasts.

Box 69.1 Factors Determining the Choice of a Vehicle

- Its hydrating or drying property
- Its ability to assist in the absorption of the active ingredient
- Its physical and chemical interactions with the stratum corneum
- The stability of the final formulation

- **Wet dressings** are soft dressing materials soaked in aqueous solutions containing ingredients such as isotonic saline, aluminium acetate and potassium permanganate (0.01%–0.05%). They are used in acute exudative inflammation with marked oozing. They cause local cooling.
- **Lotions** are liquid preparations with a viscosity a little higher than that of water and alcohol, e.g. the calamine lotion. **Lotions are used to treat subacute inflammation, after the marked exudation has stopped.** Evaporation of water from the lotion has a cooling effect, whereas the residual dry powder acts as a protective. However, lotions sometimes cause excessive drying. But, those containing glycerol or propylene glycol, help to retain water in the epidermis. Addition of alcohol (15%) and menthol (0.25%–2.0%) enhances the cooling effect. Phenol (0.5%–1.0%), camphor (1%–3%), salicylic acid (1%–2%) and coal tar (1%–3%) impart an antipruritic and keratolytic action to the lotion.
- **Lubricating preparations (emollients)** include plain oil, liniment, gel, water-in-oil emulsion *(most but not all ointments)*, oil-in-water emulsion *(most cosmetic, washable, vanishing creams)* and paste. Water-in-oil creams behave like oils and are suitable vehicle for lipid-soluble agents. Vegetable oils, liquid, soft and hard paraffin, lard, lanolin and beeswax are important ingredients of lubricating preparations. Emollients soothe, smoothen and hydrate the skin and are indicated for dry or scaling disorders.
- **Pastes** are stiffer and more adhesive than other lubricating preparations, and are made of a finely divided insoluble powder such as zinc oxide, incorporated into an ointment base. They protect the skin from external irritants, sunlight and friction caused by clothing/bandages.

CHOICE OF THE PREPARATION BASED ON THE SKIN LESION

From the therapeutic viewpoint, the skin lesions are divided into (a) oozing and (b) dry types.

- **An oozing dermatosis** is associated with dilatation of subepidermal capillaries (erythema), oedema and disruption of the epidermis by formation of vesicles. When oozing is copious, folded muslin soaked in a lotion such as an aqueous solution of potassium permanganate (1:5000 or 1:10,000) is applied half-hourly. Evaporation of water produces surface cooling, capillary constriction and reduces oozing. At that stage, an aqueous suspension such as calamine lotion is substituted and applied every hour. In addition to producing surface cooling, it forms an adsorbing layer on the lesion. Lesions with little oozing are best treated with a liniment or a cream, e.g. zinc cream which produces an emollient effect. When oozing ceases but the lesion still appears moist, a paste is applied. It acts as an adsorbing, protective and splinting agent.

  Some dermatoses may be associated with infection as indicated by a seropurulent discharge. In such instances, an appropriate antimicrobial agent such as povidone, bacitracin or neomycin is incorporated into the formulation. Judicious incorporation of a glucocorticoid hastens the subsidence of inflammatory phenomenon. The dangers of local glucocorticoid therapy are discussed in Chapter 64.
- **Dry skin lesions** are best treated with an ointment or a paste.

In cases of urticaria and acne vulgaris, a lotion is generally preferred to other forms of applications though the skin lesions are dry.

In general, the desired penetration of medicaments is better from an aqueous base than from an oily base. Furthermore, raising the local temperature of the skin and its hydration, for example by a polyethylene occlusive dressing, enhances penetration of the active drug such as a glucocorticoid.

KERATOLYTIC AGENTS

Keratolytics are the drugs which, when applied locally, cause a mild peeling of the superficial layers of the skin.

SALICYLIC ACID: It is an irritant and **causes peeling and comedolysis;** 0.5%–2% is used to treat acne vulgaris. A 6% ointment is useful in the treatment of dandruff, seborrhoeic dermatitis and psoriasis. A thicker preparation in the form of a collodion is used locally to treat warts and thick calluses. It also has an **antifungal action.**

PROPYLENE GLYCOL: Its 2% aqueous solution is used as a vehicle. Higher concentrations (up to 70%) affect the keratin and soften the skin, leading to desquamation. It is used in combination with salicylic acid to treat ichthyosis.

UREA: Urea, in the form of cream or ointment, **softens the skin** and is used in the treatment of psoriasis and atopic dermatitis. *It has hydrating, keratolytic and antipruritic actions on the skin.* It increases the absorption of hydrocortisone when used in combination.

BENZOYL PEROXIDE: It is mainly keratolytic, but also has moderate bacteriostatic properties against acne bacilli. In the form of 5%–10% cream or lotion, it is used for mild to moderate acne (see section, Drug therapy of acne vulgaris).

TRETINOIN: It acts on the nuclear retinoid receptors and normalises follicular keratinisation. It is used topically to treat acne vulgaris and other disorders of keratin. (See section, Drug therapy of acne vulgaris and Chapter 77).

PHARMACOTHERAPY OF SKIN LESIONS

PH 1.1

The description of various skin lesions is beyond the scope of this book. However, the pharmacotherapy of some selected, common, dermatological conditions seen in general practice is described below.

The various descriptive terms used to characterise skin lesions are listed in Box 69.2. They aid in defining the skin lesions of a given patient and formulating a differential diagnosis.

Box 69.2 Definitions of Various Skin Lesions

1. **Macule:** A flat, coloured lesion, less than 2 cm in diameter, not raised above the skin surface
2. **Patch:** A macule larger than 2 cm
3. **Papule:** A small solid lesion with diameter <1 cm, raised above the skin surface and hence palpable
4. **Nodule:** A raised lesion >1 cm, firm and easily palpable. It differs from a papule in size, palpability and depth
5. **Vesicle:** A small fluid-filled lesion <1 cm in diameter, often translucent
6. **Pustule:** A vesicle filled with leucocytes
7. **Bulla:** A raised fluid-filled lesion >1 cm in diameter
8. **Cyst:** A soft, raised, encapsulated lesion containing semisolid or liquid material
9. **Wheal:** A raised erythematous papule, usually due to short-lived dermal oedema

In the examination of the skin, one must consider:

- *The type(s) of primary lesion(s)*
- *The shape of the individual lesions(s)*
- *Their arrangement*
- *The distribution of the eruption*
- *Presence of itching*

In cases where the diagnosis is not immediately obvious, the prescription of a bland local application such as oily cream (while awaiting specialist opinion) is better than the indiscriminate use of a blunderbuss commercial preparation containing multiple agents, in the hope that 'something will work'. The use of such an irrational preparation can change the morphology of the lesions and make the subsequent diagnosis difficult.

The next step is to choose between local and systemic therapy. Whenever such a choice exists, local treatment is always preferable to systemic. However, the local use of some drugs such as antihistaminics and (most) antibiotics is best avoided because of the possibility of inducing allergic reactions. *While selecting drugs, one should consider the physical properties of the formulations and morphology of the skin lesions rather than the aetiologic diagnosis.*

MANAGEMENT OF PRURITUS

The exact mechanism of itch/pruritus is not clear but it probably involves both central and peripheral components. **Generally, it is associated with local liberation of histamine and other autacoids.**

Adequate treatment of **pruritus** depends upon recognition of the local and/or systemic factor(s) responsible for it and their rectification. For example, adequate treatment of scabies would generally relieve the itching in this condition.

In cases of pruritus ani, presence of piles, local candidiasis or oxyuriasis should be looked for and treated.

The itching in elderly patients, which is *due to dryness of the skin*, is best treated by moisturising the skin by applying a little edible oil or moisturising cream to the affected area immediately after bath and by minimising the use of soap for washing and bathing. Dry skin during cold season often causes itching in dependent part and needs only application of moisturising and hydrating agents such as calamine lotion and/or 2% menthol in aqueous cream. Emollients or urea cream may be useful when pruritus is associated with dry skin.

Itching due to inflammatory skin conditions can be relieved by a combination of a weak corticosteroid applied locally and a systemically administered antihistaminic. Topical antihistaminics and local anaesthetics are generally partially effective. Anxiolytics such as **doxepin** or **hydroxyzine** are also beneficial.

Pruritus due to neuropathy (diabetes, vitamin deficiency) may respond to carbamazepine, gabapentin and local anaesthetics.

DRUG THERAPY OF BACTERIAL AND VIRAL SKIN INFECTIONS

Impetigo: This is a common skin condition, characterised by superficial infection by *Staphylococcus aureus* or streptococci (Group A beta hemolytic). Generally, it is a mixed infection. The primary lesion is a superficial pustule that ruptures and forms a typical yellow brown crust. The lesion may occur on normal skin or may be superimposed upon another skin disease such as pediculosis.

After gentle cleaning and debridement of the adherent crusts, application of an ointment containing povidone-iodine 5%, chlorhexidine 1%, neomycin 1%, framycetin 1.5%, bacitracin 1% can be used. Mupirocin 2%, retapamulin 1% ointment or ozenoxacin 1% cream are also recommended. *Topical use of antibiotics such as tetracycline and gentamicin should be avoided for fear of sensitisation and development of drug resistance*. Topical bacitracin or neomycin may cause contact dermatitis.

Since glomerulonephritis can develop in children following streptococcal infections of the skin, systemic antibacterial therapy must be considered for impetigo in children between 1 and 11 years of age. Systemic therapy is also recommended in patients with renal and heart disease, with coexisting eczema and in those on immunosuppressive drugs. In such circumstances, a penicillinase-resistant penicillin like cloxacillin, erythromycin or cotrimoxazole should be given in full doses for 10–12 days.

Improvement of personal hygiene is recommended and is more important.

DR 15.3

Furuncle or boil: This is an acute infection of the hair follicle commonly caused by staphylococci. In healthy individuals, it responds to fomentation and the use of local antiseptics like povidone-iodine and chlorhexidine (Chapter 60). In severe cases and in those with persistent lesions, a cream containing neomycin, framycetin or mupirocin may be applied. Patients who develop boils frequently may require long-term treatment with an appropriate antibiotic. *In such cases, an underlying systemic disease, like diabetes mellitus, uraemia should be excluded.* DR 8.7

Herpes simplex and herpes zoster: Herpes simplex (HSV) can be treated by topical application of 5% acylovir or of 1% penciclovir. Both these drugs are applied 4–5 times a day. Topical acyclovir is, however, less effective than systemic acyclovir (Chapter 57), and it offers no significant clinical advantage in recurrent genital herpes. Docosanol is used for orolabial HSV.

Infections due to herpes zoster also respond to oral acyclovir, but to a lesser extent than herpes simplex. In severe cases of herpes zoster, acyclovir is administered orally 800 mg 5 times a day for 7 days. It can be also given intravenously in dose of 10 mg/kg every 8 h for 5 days in immunocompromised patients. Alternatively, vidarabine can be infused intravenously in the dose of 15 mg/kg once daily, over 12 h, at a concentration of 0.5 mg/mL. *Use of glucocorticoids in herpes zoster is contraindicated.*

Postherpetic neuralgia may respond to local application of 2% capsaicin, and to analgesics. Drugs like amitriptyline, carbamazepine and gabapentin also may be beneficial (Chapter 11).

Warts: Warts are human papillomavirus-induced benign proliferation of the skin and mucosa. Most of the patients do not need any treatment as warts are known to undergo spontaneous regression within 1–2 years. Several methods are used to treat warts. These range from cryotherapy and electrodesiccation to carbon dioxide laser ablation. Warts can also be treated by local application of keratolytic agents like **salicylic acid** in flexible collodion. Other topical drugs include **podophyllin** 15%–25% solution, **trichloracetic acid** and **phenol**. **Formaldehyde** (5% solution) and podophyllin are particularly useful in the management of plantar warts. **Silver nitrate** in the form of pencil may be used to cauterise the warts (see Chapter 51).

DRUG THERAPY OF FUNGAL SKIN INFECTIONS DR 8.7

For therapeutic purposes, fungus infections (mycoses) have been classified as superficial (affecting the skin, and its appendages – hair and nails), subcutaneous and deep.

The common fungi which cause superficial skin infection are as follows:

- **Dermatophytes** (trichophyton, microsporon and epidermophyton) which cause ringworm (dermatophytosis)
- **Candida species** which cause mucocutaneous candidiasis
- ***Pityrosporon orbiculare, also known as Malassezia furfur***, which causes tinea versicolor

Majority of superficial fungal infections can be treated by local antifungal agents, and azoles are preferred because of their wide spectrum and safety. Only chronic, resistant infections may need systemic antifungal therapy.

AZOLES: Various azoles used to treat skin fungal infections are listed in Box 69.3. Their mechanism of action is described in detail in Chapter 48.

Azoles are used locally as creams, powders, lotions, and as vaginal tablets or suppositories. They are generally used topically to treat superficial mycoses, and cutaneous and vaginal candidiasis. Generally, they are safe and do not stain the skin or clothing.

CLOTRIMAZOLE: It is an imidazole, used as 1% cream or 100-mg tablets in **vaginal candidiasis** and mild to moderate, localised tinea pedis/cruris infection. *This drug is not used for systemic infections because of its toxicity.*

Other azoles for topical use (Box 69.3) have similar actions and uses as clotrimazole.

MICONAZOLE: Good results are reported in infections caused by Candida, Cryptococcus and Aspergillus. It is used as a 2%–4% cream in mixed skin infections. The drug may cause fever, chills, nausea and allergic reactions and rarely, leucopenia and thrombocytopenia.

Efinaconazole topical solution (10%) is available for toenail onychomycosis.

Systemic therapy with itraconazole or fluconazole is indicated in patients with chronic, extensive infection, scalp and nails infection resistant to local therapy and in immunocompromised patients. In all fungal infections, therapy has to be carried out for a few weeks to 3–4 months, depending on the severity of infection (for griseofulvin, see Chapter 48).

BENZOIC ACID AND SALICYLIC ACID: Salicylic acid is a weak antifungal agent but has keratolytic properties. Benzoic acid compound ointment (**Whitfield's ointment**) contains 6% of benzoic acid and 3% of salicylic acid. It is effective in treating dermatophytosis. It is relatively safe, cheap and is in use for ages. Sometimes it may cause local irritation.

Box 69.3 Azoles for Dermal Skin Infections

- ***For topical use:***
  Clotrimazole, miconazole, econazole, butoconazole, oxiconazole, sulconazole, tioconazole, sertaconazole, luliconazole, isoconazole, fenticonazole
- ***For systemic use:***
  Ketoconazole, itraconazole, fluconazole, voriconazole (These can also be used locally)

TERBINAFINE is an allylamine. Applied as 1% cream or solution daily for 1–2 weeks, it is effective in tinea corporis and onychomycosis. It can also be used orally. **Naftifine** 1% has similar activity (Chapter 48).

Butenafine, a benzylamine (1%) is also available for tinea pedis infection.

TOLNAFTATE: This drug, used as 1% solution/ cream, is effective in the treatment of superficial fungal infections of the skin caused by trichophyton and epidermophyton. *It is not effective against fungal infection of nails and hair, and relapses are frequent when it is employed in the treatment of Trichophyton rubrum of the trunk.* It is nonirritating, nonstaining and odourless.

UNDECYLENIC ACID: This drug is applied to the skin in the concentrations of 2%–15%, sometimes in combination with zinc undecylenate in the treatment of dermatophytoses, particularly tinea pedis.

CICLOPIROX OLAMINE: This drug is as effective as the imidazoles in the treatment of cutaneous candidiasis and dermatophytoses, as well as in tinea versicolor. It causes minor local but no systemic adverse effects. Its use should be avoided in pregnant and lactating women. It is available as 1% cream.

SELENIUM SULPHIDE: This drug has been used in the treatment of tinea versicolor. It is also effective in the treatment of dandruff. It has mild toxicity but possesses an unpleasant odour. It is irritant to the eyes. The drug is commonly used as a 2.5% suspension; the preparation is applied once daily for 5 days to the wet skin, lathered in place for 15–20 min and then washed thoroughly. After that, one application once a month is continued to prevent re-infection.

TAVABOROLE: This antifungal drug, used as 5% solution topically, is effective against **onychomycosis** due to *T. rubrum* or *T. mentagrophytes.* It blocks fungal protein synthesis and has a broad spectrum of activity against yeast, moulds and dermatophytes. Systemic absorption is minimal. It is applied once daily for 48 weeks. **Ciclopirox** 8% used similarly is probably equally effective and much cheaper. Other drugs used for toenail onychomycosis are terbinafine and itraconazole, which are given orally for 3 months; but the cure rate with these drugs is less and relapses are common.

Other topical fungicidal agents include tincture iodine, iodophors, haloprogin, phenol, oxidising agents, e.g. potassium permanganate and dyes like gentian violet. Fungicidal actions of iodochlorhydroxyquinoline 3% and nystatin are discussed earlier.

Choice of antifungal therapy: It depends on the site involved and the type of infection. Small localised lesions are best treated with keratolytic agents like salicylic acid (Whitfield's ointment) or topical application of an azole. Systemic antifungal therapy with an azole or griseofulvin is required for extensive lesions, very chronic lesions, tinea capitis and fungal infections of the nails (Chapter 48).

Tinea versicolor is caused by the fungus *Malassezia furfur*, also known as *Pityrosporon orbiculare.* It causes patches of lesions on the chest, shoulder and back. These patches often appear as hypopigmented areas particularly on a dark skin.

> Many topical fungicides are effective, but preparations containing salicylic acid 1%, sodium thiosulphate 10% or selenium sulphide 2.5% are preferred. *Repeated infection from the infected clothing must be prevented by properly disinfecting the clothing.*

It must be emphasised that fungal skin infections and scabies are common among the population from warm and humid climates, particularly in those with unhygienic habits. Simple preventive measures such as cleanliness and mass education are far more important than any drug.

DANDRUFF AND SEBORRHOEIC DERMATITIS

Dandruff is scaling and moderate itching of the scalp without inflammation of the skin; the scales are white, dry and loose. **Seborrhoeic dermatitis** is an acute, subacute or chronic scaly dermatitis

Seborrhoeic dermatitis affects areas of sebaceous activity such as the scalp, hairline, forehead, face (especially the nasolabial folds), retroauricular areas, the external ear canals, the presternal and the interscapular areas. The scales are either dry, grey and flaky or yellowish and greasy. In severe cases, there may be **seborrhoeic eczema** with or without oozing of the skin.

These conditions are the manifestations of an abnormal immune response to *Pityrosporum ovale*, a constituent of the normal skin flora. The lipase in these organisms splits triglycerides into fatty acids, which are thought to be responsible for the dermal irritation. There is often an atopic background. There are several predisposing factors: e.g., excessive sweating and sebum production, alkalinity of the skin and emotional component.

The drugs effective in dandruff and seborrhoea are listed in Box 69.4. They are usually applied to the scalp as shampoos. The common action of all these drugs is an **antipityrosporal action**, though other actions such as cytostatic, anti-inflammatory and antiseptic may also be contributory.

Topical azoles or **ciclopirox** are the most effective treatment in these conditions. Their high affinity for the keratin of the skin and the hair leaves a prolonged residual antipityrosporal activity at the site of application. If failure then a 4-week course with a weak-to-moderately potent corticosteroid can be given.

Topical corticosteroid treatment (hydrocortisone 1% liniment and solution, 0.1% lotion or Alclometasone 0.05% ointment or Desonide 0.05%

Box 69.4 Drugs Effective in Dandruff and Seborrhoeic Dermatitis

- ***Antipityrosporal:***
  Imidazoles (ketoconazole / Efinaconazole 2% shampoo, 2% scalp foaming gel 20 mg/g hydrogel or cream)
  Salicylic acid (2% aqueous cream)
  Ciclopirox (1–1.5% shampoo, gel, suspension)
- ***Anti-inflammatory:***
  Mild corticosteroid topically
- ***Cytostatic:***
  Selenium sulphide (2.5% shampoo)[a]
  Zinc pyrithione (1–2% shampoo weekly)[a]
  Salicylic acid (3% shampoo)
  Sulphur (2% aqueous cream)
  Tar (1–2% shampoo)

[a]Also have antipityrosporal action

cream once daily) is almost as effective as topical azoles but recurrence is common after stopping the therapy. *In view of the chronic and recurrent nature of the illness in adults, the treatment has to continue for a long time and as a combination of antifungal and topical steroids. For resistant cases, potent corticosteroids such as fluocinolone acetonide 0.01% or clobetasol propionate 0.05% may be used twice weekly, applied for 5 min, for 2 weeks. In the most resistant cases systemic antifungals (itraconazole, fluconazole or terbinafine) are used.*

In addition to drug therapy, the predisposing causes such as mental stress, excessive sweating and skin alkalinity need treatment; the last factor can be taken care of by application of lemon juice to the affected areas of the skin. **Comb of other user should be avoided.**

DRUG THERAPY OF SCABIES AND PEDICULOSIS

Scabies

Scabies is caused by the itch mite *Sarcoptes scabiei* var. *hominis*

The female mite burrows into the superficial layers of the skin to form tortuous channels in which the eggs are deposited. Transmission of the mites occurs by close body contact. Unhygienic conditions and crowded housing favour the spread of the infection, which is characterised by intense itching, usually worse at night. It is important to note that *scabies can give rise to urticarial rash and eczematous lesions, which can be mistaken and wrongly treated with local and even oral steroid therapy.* DR 5.3

The principles of treatment are as follows:

- All members of the household must receive the treatment simultaneously.
- The medicament should be applied to the whole body surface below the lower jaw. Contact with the eyes and the urethral meatus should be avoided carefully for fear of irritation.
- The drug should be applied after bathing ,left on for 8-12 hours and then rinsed off.

- Secondary infections often require treatment with antimicrobials and should be prescribed based on culture and sensitivity data. They can be treated either simultaneously or after the basic treatment is over.
- Intimate clothing and bedding used during the previous 48 h should be disinfected by boiling or by steam
- The patient must be educated regarding personal hygiene.

Drugs used in the treatment of scabies are as follows:

SULPHUR: The scabicidal effects of sulphur, the oldest remedy, is probably due to its conversion into hydrogen sulphide and parathionic acid. It is irritant and stains the clothes and has an unpleasant odour. Hence, though cheap, it is not preferred. It is considered safe in pregnancy and infants.

BENZYL BENZOATE: Benzyl benzoate is a **highly efficient scabicide.** It is usually applied in the form of benzyl benzoate 25% emulsion. Even after cure of infection, the itching may persist for a few weeks but usually responds to calamine liniment. Children are treated with the application of 12.5% emulsion. Secondary bacterial infection can be successfully treated only after the primary infestation is eradicated. The drug is slightly irritant and has an unpleasant smell.

GAMMA BENZENE HEXACHLORIDE (GBH/Gamma BHC/gammaxene/lindane): This gamma isomer of hexachlorocyclohexane (Fig. 69.2) is an insecticide, larvicide and acaricide. It binds to $GABA_A$ receptor at the picrotoxin binding site and blocks ion flow through $GABA_A$ regulated chloride channels. This causes neuronal hyperstimulation and parasite paralysis. The drug is excreted slowly from the body. Applied externally, it is not so toxic; but *if absorbed/ingested, it can cause neurotoxicity, e.g. convulsions.* The other serious but rare toxic manifestation is aplastic anaemia (Chapter 60).

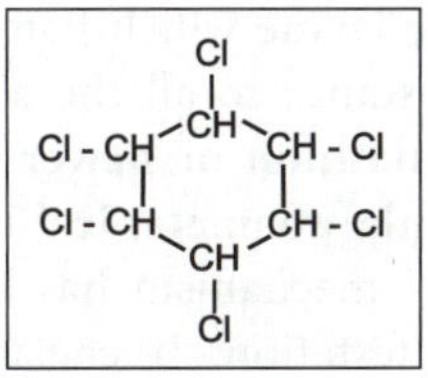

FIG. 69.2. Gamma benzene hexachloride.

A vanishing cream containing 1% of the drug, applied to properly dried skin all over the body below the neck in the form of a thin film without preliminary bathing, results in total eradication of scabies. The film is left over for a period of 12 h following which the patient is given a bath. An average adult requires 25 g of the cream per treatment. *Unlike benzyl benzoate, the agent is odourless and nonirritant and can, therefore, be applied safely to the face but care should be taken to prevent contact with eyes and mucus membranes. The treatment may be repeated after a week. Not more than two applications should be used during pregnancy.*

Because of enhanced skin absorption and the risk of CNS toxicity, gammaxene should be avoided in infants and children.

It is also useful in pediculosis.

As an insecticide 0.1%–0.5% solution in kerosene is lethal to flies and mosquitoes. It may be combined with other insecticides, such as a pyrethroid (permethrin) to obtain a rapid, lethal effect.

PERMETHRIN: This is a synthetic pyrethroid, available as 5% cream or lotion. It causes neurotoxicity and paralysis in parasites by interfering its Na+ transport. It is left on for 12 h after application and then rinsed off. Unlike gammaxene, only a small quantity is absorbed which is rapidly metabolised to inactive compounds and excreted in the urine. It can be used even in 2 monh old infant. It may cause local reactions and cross reacts with sunflower family plants to cause allergic contact dermatitis.

IVERMECTIN: This antifilarial drug, given orally in a **single dose** of 200 mcg/kg (Chapter 58), is reported to be highly effective in clearing up scabies. It causes nerve or muscle cell hyperpolarisation by activating glutamate-gated chloride channels of the parasites. Repetition of the dose after 2 weeks gives almost 95% cure.

MONOSULPHIRAM: It is an effective scabicide and is used as 25% solution diluted with 2–3 parts of water. It is also incorporated in soap, recommended for the prophylaxis of scabies. The drug may cause mild irritation.

CROTAMITON: Though less effective than other agents, it exerts antipruritic effect.

Pediculosis

Pediculosis, a common condition in tropical countries, is caused by the louse *Pediculus humanus* and usually affects the scalp (capitis), the body (corporis) and pubic area (pubis).

It is responsible for intense itching and may cause impetigo and eczematous lesions. Furthermore, during famine and natural calamities, the body louse can act as a vector for typhus, relapsing and trench fevers. Finding of nits or the lice on hair clinches the diagnosis.

The drugs used in the treatment of pediculosis are given in Box 69.5.

PERMETHRIN: A 1% cream or lotion is applied to clean damp hair, left on for 10 min and then rinsed off. It is an effective pediculocide with a residual effect for two weeks. (see Chapter 60).

MALATHION: This organophosphorus compound applied as 0.5% lotion causes NM paralysis and is **rapidly acting pediculocidal and ovicidal drug** in the treatment of head lice, even in patients resistant to permethrin. The drug is well tolerated and no systemic adverse effects have been reported. It is usually applied and left in place for 8–12 h, and the application is repeated 7–9 days later. It is inflammable because of the alcohol base. Care should be taken to keep the lotion away from heat and open flame, and to avoid its contact with the eyes.

Box 69.5 Drugs Used in Pediculosis

- Permethrin 1%
- Malathion 0.5%
- Dicophane (DDT) 2% (Chapter 60)
- Gamma benzene hexachloride 1% cream, 2% shampoo
- Kerosene oil
- Ivermectin

DICOPHANE (DDT): Used as a 10% dusting powder, it is an effective pediculocide. Its prolonged residual effect makes it lethal to the larvae which hatch out later (see Chapter 60).

Topical suspension (0.9%) of **spinosad**, an organic insecticide, is also a pediculoside and ovicide. Single application induces neurotoxicity in lice but it is safe for humans.

For **pediculosis capitis, permethrin** cream/lotion is preferred for initial treatment. For failures, **malathion,** the fastest-acting and the most ovicidal pediculocide, is recommended. However, it has an objectionable odour. *Because it is inflammable, a hair dryer and a curling iron should not be used during the treatment.*

In resistant cases, **ivermectin** is safe and highly effective when used as two doses of 200–400 mcg/kg each, a week apart; the second dose is required as the drug is not ovicidal.

The other drugs used are **Gamma BHC, DDT** and **kerosene.** Gamma BHC (lotion, cream 1% or shampoo 2%) and DDT (2% dusting powder) are generally used as two applications, 7–10 days apart. The application of kerosene, though not very pleasant, is the cheapest and effective treatment for head lice. It destroys lice and suffocates nits by covering them with an impervious film. Usually, one tablespoonful of kerosene is rubbed into the whole scalp and the head wrapped in a piece of cloth. Two hours later, it is washed thoroughly with soap and water. Kerosene does not cause irritation and usually, a single application is all that is necessary. *Of course, the individual must keep away from fire.*

In patients with **pediculosis corporis or pubis,** DDT used as 10% dusting powder is highly effective. A single application can give an adequate residual effect against the larvae which hatch out later. Lice can develop resistance to all the above-mentioned drugs, hence **malathion** or **newer pyrethroids** are preferred. Recently **abametapir** (0.74% lotion),an agent with novel mechanism has been introduced for head lice infestation. It chelates heavy metal cations and inhibits metalloproteinases critical to louse ova development, hatching, and adult survival. It is well tolerated and can be used in 6 month old infants. *The clothing should be disinfected with heat and all the contacts are treated simultaneously.*

DRUG THERAPY OF ACNE VULGARIS

Acne vulgaris (pimples) is a common, chronic skin disorder, particularly in teenagers, and it generally regresses with time. However, it can persist for a long time and in some individuals, can cause disfigurement and permanent scarring.

It usually affects the face but can also spread to the trunk. Acne is known to develop frequently in patients with androgen excess. Most patients with acne probably have sebaceous glands that are hyper-responsive to androgens.

Pathophysiology: The important features are as follows:

- *Increased sebum production by the sebaceous glands.*
- *Hyperkeratinisation and excessive desquamation of epithelial cells* from the walls of the hair follicle, leading to *blockade of the follicular openings.*
- *Formation of comedone,* a fleshy, hyperkeratotic plug blocking the opening of the pilosebaceous follicle ('black' and 'white' heads).
- *Proliferation of locally present Propionibacterium acnes and a few staphylococci.*
- These bacteria split the sebaceous fat to form irritant fatty acids leading to *local inflammation*

The therapy of acne is, therefore, directed to:

- **Counteract the excessive production of sebum**
- **Prevent the abnormal desquamation of epithelial cells in sebaceous follicles**
- **Treat and control the growth of *P. acnes***

Drugs used in the treatment of acne are given in Box 69.6. *Dietary modifications have not been shown to modify the course of acne vulgaris and undue diet restrictions are unnecessary.* However, the application of cosmetic oils and greases to the affected area should be avoided. Prolonged and vigorous washing will not resolve the lesions. On the contrary, scrubbing may damage the delicate openings of the hair follicles, and block the flow of sebum, thus worsening the acne.

Box 69.6 Drugs Used in the Treatment of Acne

- ***Cleansers:*** Soaps (gentle)
- ***Comedolytics:*** Local tretinoin, adapalene
- ***Exfoliants*** (peeling agents): Salicylic acid
- ***Sebostatics,*** e.g. oral isotretinoin
- ***Hormones:*** Cyproterone acetate, estrogen
- ***Antibacterial drugs:***
  Local: Erythromycin, clindamycin, azelaic acid, benzoyl peroxide
  Systemic: Tetracyclines, erythromycin, minocycline, cotrimoxazole

1. **Comedolytics and exfoliants:**

   TRETINOIN (Trans-retinoic acid, Retin-A) **used topically** is an effective local comedolytic. It enhances the penetration of other anti-acne agents into the epidermis. Frequent application of this agent, however, produces redness and peeling of the skin. Improved appearance may take as long as 2 months. It is applied as 0.01%–0.025% gel, 0.025% lotion or as 0.025% cream. Gels are preferred in hot and humid climate and cream in cold and dry climate. *People using retinoic acid should avoid exposure to sun because of increased susceptibility to sunburns. It should be avoided in pregnancy.*
   Tretinoin is also useful in treating acanthosis nigricans and skin striae such as those of Cushing syndrome.
   ADAPALENE: This third-generation retinoid selectively binds to retinoid receptors. Used as 0.1% cream, it acts like tretinoin but is claimed to be less irritant. **It is stable in sunlight.**
   Tazarotene is yet another retinoid which also remains stable in sunlight.
   Salicylic acid has a keratolytic property and is used as 0.5%–2% hydroalcoholic formulation.
   All these drugs can be combined with local or systemic antimicrobial agents.

2. **Sebostatics:** Sebaceous glands are androgen dependent and therefore, estrogens and antiandrogenic drugs are useful in therapy of acne. Estrogens are usually prescribed as COC containing ethinyl estradiol 50 mcg and a nonandrogenic progestin such as desogestrel or cyproterone acetate 2 mg. The COC must be given for 3–4 months before substantial improvement is observed. More prolonged therapy is needed to avoid relapse.

Box 69.7 Drug Therapy of Acne Vulgaris

- ***Mild cases without inflammation:*** Topical – tretinoin cream/gel; adapalene 0.1% gel; salicylic acid, benzoyl peroxide
- ***Mild cases with inflammation:*** Topical antibiotics, benzoyl peroxide or combination of erythromycin and benzoyl peroxide for 4–6 weeks
- ***Severe cases with inflammation:*** Topical tretinoin plus systemic antibiotic therapy; if response is unsatisfactory, particularly in multinodular cystic lesions, add oral isotretinoin; in women of reproductive age, use COC or cyproterone acetate

Cyproterone acetate, a potent antiandrogen, can be used in place of oral contraceptives but is more expensive (Chapter 67). **Spironolactone** in the dose of 50–200 mg/day reduces sebum production, but again several months of therapy are required to get maximal benefit. Combination OC pills containing cyproterone acetate 2 mg (Diane, Ginette) are also effective. For obvious reasons, *only women should receive the antiandrogen therapy.*

ISOTRETINOIN (13-cis-retinoic acid): This vitamin A metabolite, **given orally, as well as applied topically**, can cause prolonged remission, permanent in 40%, It:

a. Causes marked atrophy of sebaceous glands, and inhibits sebaceous secretion (**sebostatic action**).
b. Normalises keratinisation of the hair follicle, thus reducing the formation of comedones.
c. Suppresses inflammation by inhibiting growth of *P. acnes.*

It is usually prescribed at a dose of 0.5–1 mg/kg body weight daily for 3–4 months. Its bioavailability is increased if it is taken during or after meals. A dramatic reduction in the oiliness of the skin is apparent within a month of starting treatment. The improvement persists even after its stoppage.

Adverse reactions: Common effects include dryness of the skin and itching. Less commonly, it can cause hyperlipidaemia, hypercalcaemia, photosensitivity, hair loss, arthralgia, myalgia, epistaxis intracranial hypertension, premature fusion of epiphyses, depression and psychosis. *The drug is* ***highly teratogenic*** *and if it is used in women of child-bearing age, pregnancy should be ruled out and two methods of contraception should be continued for one month after stopping the treatment.* There is no risk to male patients treated with this drug. Anyone taking this drug should not donate blood for 1 month after stopping it. Due to its toxicity and high cost, the drug should be reserved for severe pustular acne not responding to other medications. *This drug is not useful in the treatment of psoriasis.*

3. **Antimicrobial drugs for *P. acnes:*** Antibiotics used against *P. acnes* are listed in Box 69.6. **Applied locally** once or twice daily, they exert a beneficial effect both by killing *P. acnes* and indirectly, by inhibiting the production of proinflammatory mediators by the organisms. Combination of **erythromycin** 3% with **benzoyl peroxide** 5% appears to be highly effective. Clindamycin is also effective.

Benzoyl peroxide (2.5%–10%) as gel or lotion is lipophilic and suppresses effectively the growth of *P. acnes.* It is also keratolytic. Drug resistance does not develop. It has no anti-inflammatory property. It can cause local irritation and allergy.

Antibiotics used for the systemic therapy of acne include **doxycycline** (100–200 mg daily), **minocycline, erythromycin** (500–1000 mg daily) and **co-trimoxazole**. Generally, **doxycycline** is preferred. These drugs need to be given for 4–6 weeks and then tapered off gradually by 10–12 weeks. This is followed by topical treatment with tretinoin and benzyl peroxide for 6 months.

The suggested therapeutic approach for treating acne is outlined in the Box 69.7. To prevent recurrence, topical treatment must be continued for 6 months.

Agents that predispose to the formation of comedones include topical agents such as lanolin, butyl stearate, lauryl alcohol and paraffin in commercial cosmetic and hair preparations. Industrial compounds that contain impure paraffin oil, halogenated hydrocarbons, coal tar and its derivatives can also precipitate or worsen the condition. *Local or systemic glucocorticoids used for long periods can also cause acne.*

DRUG THERAPY OF ALLERGIC SKIN DISORDERS

Allergic skin reactions occur when an allergen triggers an immune system response in the skin.

Urticaria: See Chapter 23 and Section on Management of Pruritus.

Atopic dermatitis: Atopy is defined as a genetically determined tendency to hyper-react to common environmental allergens with the production of IgE and immediate hypersensitivity/allergic (type I) reaction. Majority of the patients have a family history of asthma or hay fever. Atopic dermatitis, a chronic condition, is a cutaneous expression of the atopic state. The clinical presentation differs according to the age of the patient. Itching is prominent. Secondary infection may be present.

Atopic dermatitis in infants often resolves spontaneously. The treatment includes:

- **Avoidance of cutaneous irritants** like soaps, detergents and hot water
- **Adequate cutaneous hydration**
- **Judicious use of mild topical glucocorticoids** to control itching and inflammation (Chapter 64)

Infection should be treated with systemic antibiotics. Oral sedative H_1-antihistaminics may be useful to control the itching. The role of dietary allergens in atopic dermatitis is controversial. However, if such an allergen can be identified, particularly in children, it should be avoided.

For local application low-potency steroids are to be preferred and used for consecutive 2 weeks. Severe exacerbations need to be treated with high-potency topical steroids and/or systemic glucocorticoid therapy. Although such treatment will generally clear the skin, the lesions may return after stoppage of therapy.

An antidepressant, **doxepin,** (Chapter 14), 5% cream exhibits significant antipruritic activity in atopic dermatitis, due to its antihistaminic property. It can get absorbed from the skin and may cause drowsiness and anticholinergic effects. **Crisaborole**, 2% topical ointment is a PDE4B inhibitor, which is applied twice daily topically for the treatment of mild-to-moderate atopic dermatitis. The most common ADR is burning or stinging at the application site.

Immunomodulating agents such as calcineurin inhibitor, tacrolimus have been used orally but are toxic. Tacrolimus ointment is also claimed to be effective (Chapter 72). Several biologicals including IL-4/IL-13 inhibitors (e.g. Dupilumab and Tralokinumab) and JAK inhibitors (e.g. Baricitinib and Upadacitinib) have been developed for atopic dermatitis.

Allergic contact dermatitis: This condition is caused by contact of the skin with some offending agents.

The most common type is plant dermatitis caused by members of the Rhus family. It is characterised by erythema, vesiculation and severe itching at the areas of contact. The other common sensitisers include preservatives in topical preparations, cosmetic sprays, formaldehyde, potassium dichromate, detergent, rubber curing agents, synthetic paints, plastic/synthetic bed and pillows and drugs. Chronic and excessive exposure to water and detergents can initiate or aggravate hand dermatitis. The condition is common in housewives and food handlers. However, many times, the offending agent is difficult to identify.

The ideal treatment is to avoid the offending agent. Symptomatic relief can be achieved *by local calamine lotion or with topical glucocorticoids for about 2 weeks.*

Eczema: Eczema is a common form of inflammation of the skin (dermatitis), with variable clinical and histological features.

It may be the common final expression of allergic conditions, such as atopic dermatitis, contact dermatitis, or may accompany seborrhoeic dermatitis (see section, dandruff and seborrhoeic dermatitis). Initial lesions occur as erythematous macules, papules or vesicles which later coalesce to form patches and plaques. Eczema is associated with itching and is of two types:

- **Weeping (oozing)**
- **Dry**

As in other allergic disorders, attempts should be made to identify the offending agents and eliminate them. These are commonly found in food stuff (dairy products, eggs, nuts, wheat, soy products, etc.) and additives, perfumes, cosmetics, insecticides, mosquito repellents, environmental chemicals, synthetic fibres often in clothing, plants, flowers, pollen, etc.

Most of the cases of localised eczemas respond well to **calamine lotion/liniment or to a mild topical glucocorticoid preparation** such as 1%–2% hydrocortisone (Chapter 64).

Due to adverse effects of long-term administration of glucocorticoids on the skin, some physicians prefer **tar preparations**. Other topical preparations which are useful in eczema are potassium permanganate solution used for bringing about drying of weeping lesions; and **zinc containing creams, pastes, calamine liniment to counteract excessive dry lesions.** A simple emulsifying ointment like rose ointment or a cream containing urea, which acts by increasing the hydration, is often useful for dry lesions.

- *Systemic glucocorticoid therapy has no place in routine treatment of chronic eczema,* but it can be beneficial in the acute form of the disease.
- *Antihistaminics should not be used topically because of their propensity to cause contact dermatitis.*
- Antibacterial agents should be used only in severe infections.

Infants of allergic parents kept on 'allergen avoidance regimen' (avoidance of exposure to cow's milk, dairy products, eggs, house dust and pets) for first six months of life may have strikingly low incidence of eczema.

Angioedema: This acute allergic condition induced by drugs or food involves swelling without itching in the deep layers of the skin. It may be associated with urticaria. It often involves soft tissues like eyelids, mouth or genitals. NSAIDs and ACEI cause angioedema without urticaria. There may be chronic recurrent angioedema without an identifiable cause and each recurrence lasts for hours to several days.

The condition may require emergency management with attention to patency of airway. Treatment should be as early as possible with antihistaminics, glucocorticoids and epinephrine as the clinical condition demands. The triggers like offending drug should be stopped (chapter 23).

DRUG THERAPY OF PSORIASIS

Psoriasis is a common, chronic, immune-mediated inflammatory genetic disease.

Of the various subtypes reported, **plaque-type dermatosis is common.** It is characterised by erythematous, well-demarcated plaques and rounded scales, which look like silvery mica. Pruritus may be present. Lesions are usually symmetrical and occur on the extensor surfaces such as the elbows and knees, and on the scalp. About 50% of the patients have involvement of the fingernails and some have psoriatic arthritis. Furthermore, drug-induced flares of psoriasis can occur (Box 69.8).

Pathogenesis: The commonest variety of psoriasis is characterised by plaques, which consist of greatly thickened horny layer of the skin (**hyperkeratosis**). They are characterised by hyperproliferation of the epidermal keratinocytes and inflammation of both the epidermis and the dermis, along with angiogenesis. These changes are due to cytokines released by T-lymphocyte, which initiate autoimmune dermal response to unidentified antigenic stimuli (keratinocyte proteins).

TNF-α is the primary activator of the T-lymphocytes and it also contributes to the maintenance of a complex inflammatory reaction.

The current therapy only suppresses the disease and recurrence is common. However, the disease may undergo spontaneous remission.

Drug therapy of psoriasis: It depends on the type, the location and the extent of the lesions. The patients are advised to avoid known exacerbating factors (Box 69.8).

Box 69.8 Possible Risk Factors in Psoriasis

- Skin injury/sunburns/chemical irritant
- Infection, particularly Streptococcal
- Some systemic drugs (beta blockers, ACE inhibitors, lithium, NSAID, chloroquine)
- Psychological stress

Mild cases of psoriasis are harmless and may not warrant any drug therapy. Indications for drug treatment are as follows:

- *Marked local symptoms* such as pain and itching
- *Prominent hand, leg or facial lesions*
- *Diminished mobility*

Drugs used in the treatment of psoriasis are listed in Box 69.9. These drugs either cause keratolysis and/or inhibit cell division. They do not cure the disease.

1. **Topical therapy:**
   Emollients: These act by hydrating and softening the scales. The commonly used emollients are yellow, soft paraffin and aqueous cream. Although greasy emollients are sometimes preferred, they are less well accepted by the patients.

   Salicylic acid: This is the most widely used keratolytic agent, used either alone or with coal tar. It is an irritant, and care should be taken to avoid contact with the eyes (see section, Keratolytic agents).

Box 69.9 Drugs Used in Psoriasis

Topical therapy
- Emollients
- Keratolytic agents: Salicylic acid 2%–10%
- Cytostatic agents: Coal tar, dithranol
- Glucocorticoids
- Calcipotriol, tacalcitol
- Retinoids: Tazarotene
- Roflumilast
- Calcineurin inhibitors: Pimecrolimus and tacrolimus
- Aryl hydrocarbon receptor (AhR) agonist: Tapinarof

Systemic therapy
- Etretinate, acitretin
- Apremilast
- Immunosuppressants: Methotrexate, cyclosporine, mycophenolate mofetil
- JAK inhibitors: Upadacitinib, tofacitinib, deucravacitinib
- Biological agents
  a. T cell activation inhibitors: Alefacept
  b. TNF-α inhibitors: Etanercept, infliximab
  c. IL-12 and IL-23 blocker: Ustekinumab
  d. IL-17A blockers: Secukinumab
  e. IL-23 blockers: Guselkumab
- Systemic glucocorticoids

Phototherapy
- Ultraviolet B irradiation with or without coal tar application
- Ultraviolet therapy with psoralens

Cytostatic agents (dithranol and coal tar): They are used, along with ultraviolet (UV)B phototherapy, in the treatment of psoriasis and other hyperplastic skin disorders. In these conditions they restore a normal rate of epidermal proliferation. In severe cases, systemic therapy with either **etretinate** or **methotrexate** (see later), both of which act as cytostatic agents in the skin may be needed.

a. **Crude coal tar** (3% ointment): This is a distillation product of coal and has been used to treat chronic, lichenified lesions. Coal tar, even in low concentration, has an unpleasant odour, and can cause irritation and acneform eruption. Hence, it is less acceptable.

b. **DITHRANOL** (anthralin): It **reduces the epidermal cell DNA synthesis and mitotic activity** (antimitotic) of the hyperplastic epidermis. It is an irritant and should not be applied to the face, scalp and to tender skin.It stains the skin and fabric brown and is not suitable for treatment of lesions on the face. Skin patch test is necessary prior to its use as hypersensitivity reactions can occur. All these limit its use.

A commercial preparation, Derobin, contains dithranol 1.15% with salicylic acid and coal tar.

GLUCOCORTICOIDS: Topical glucocorticoid preparations of the mild and potent varieties (Chapter 64) are preferred because of their efficacy, high degree of acceptability to the patients and low cost. They act mainly as **anti-inflammatory agents.** However, the relapse rate is higher than with other forms of therapy. *The use of potent and very potent, topical, glucocorticoid preparations should be reserved for the specialist.* They can be used in combination with phototherapy or systemic therapy.

CALCIPOTRIOL (calcipotriene): This vitamin D derivative (Chapter 68) is applied locally to mild to moderate psoriatic lesions. It has minimal effect on calcium metabolism. The drug is as effective as topical, medium-potency glucocorticoids but is much less toxic. It is applied daily as an ointment containing 50 mcg/g for about 8 weeks. The ointment is colourless, does not stain clothes and does not have unpleasant smell. **Calcitriol** and **tacalcitol** are vitamin D analogues which are effective. *Combination of a topical vitamin D analogue and betamethasone/phototherapy is a well-accepted regimen for psoriasis.*

TAZAROTENE: This retinoid is effective for topical treatment of psoriasis. Its effect remains sustained for 4 weeks after stopping the treatment. ADR include erythema, burning, pruritus, peeling, and an increased risk of sunburn. It is tetratogenic and contraindicated during pregnancy.

ROFLUMILAST: This is the first topical PDE4 inhibitor available to treat plaque psoriasis. By inhibiting PDE-4, it leads to accumulation of intracellular cAMP and reduces expression of pro-inflammatory cytokines.

CALCINEURIN INHIBITORS: Pimecrolimus and tacrolimus are used topically and decrease T cell activation. they do not cause skin atrophy. They are shown to be effective for psoriasis involving the face and intertriginous areas. The application site reaction disappear after continued use.

TAPINAROF: It is a aryl hydrocarbon receptor (AhR) agonist. The AhR is a ligand-dependent transcription factor, which regulates gene expression in various cells, including immune and epithelial cells. AhR signaling is dysregulated in psoriasis. This affects the skin barrier. Tapinarof binds to AhR and activates it to decrease proinflammatory cytokine production and normalise the skin barrier. It is available as a 1% cream for treatment of plaque psoriasis.

2. **Systemic therapy**: Although most patients with psoriasis respond to local therapy, about 20% may require systemic therapy, which is expensive and more toxic. The drugs used are discussed as follows.

ETRETINATE: This second-generation **retinoid** is also known as methoxsalen. **It inhibits keratinisation and proliferation,** and normalises differentiation of epithelial tissues. It is administered orally in the dose of 0.5–1.0 mg/kg per day. It is usually combined with psoralen and UVA phototherapy in chronic plaque psoriasis with moderate to severe disease. The drug accumulates in the adipose tissue and the liver.

Adverse reactions: These include dryness, scaly erythema and tenderness. *It is teratogenic and should not be used in woman of the reproductive age until pregnancy is excluded. Furthermore, the patient must avoid pregnancy during treatment and for at least 3 years after the treatment is over because of its long half-life (about 120 days).* Similarly, anyone taking this drug should not donate blood for 3 years after stopping it. *The drug has no sebostatic action and is of no use in acne.*
Acitretin, a metabolite of etretinate, is now preferred to etretinate in therapy. Its limitations are similar to those of etretinate.

APREMILAST: This PDE- 4 inhibitor is used to treat moderate to severe plaque psoriasis. with continued therapy the remission can be maintained for 2 years. Its ADR include diarrhea, nausea, upper respiratory infection, and headache. but tolerance develops to them. Weight loss (5–10% of b.w.) and depression have been reported.

Immunosuppressants:

METHOTREXATE: This folic acid antagonist **acts by blocking DNA synthesis and inhibiting cell proliferation.** Methotrexate may also act as an immunosuppressant. It is given orally in three doses, usually 7.5–25 mg orally/ IM/SC every week. It is preferred in severe case with arthritis, where coal tar–UV therapy has failed. It should be used only in patients with normal haematological, renal and hepatic status. The drug is usually well tolerated in the doses recommended. The main long-term toxicity is hepatic cirrhosis (Chapter 59).
CYCLOSPORINE: This drug is used in low doses (3–5 mg/kg/day) as an immunosuppressant and acts by inhibiting the production of IL-2, a cytokine necessary for proliferation of activated T cells and other T cell cytokines (Chapters 25 and 72). The important adverse effects are hypertension and renal toxicity which may be irreversible. It is reserved for patients with severe refractory psoriasis.
MYCOPHENOLATE MOFETIL: This immunosuppressant (chapter 72) has been reported to be useful in the treatment of psoriasis. Adverse effects reported are mild and dose dependent. The drug has also been used to treat pyoderma

gangrenosum, pemphigus vulgaris and systemic vasculitis.

JAK inhibitors: Janus kinases (JAKs) are non–receptor tyrosine kinases involved in cytokine receptor signaling. They activate the transcription of genes and produce many effects including inflammation. JAK inhibitors are used for treating chronic and progressive inflammatory conditions. **Upadacitinib** and **tofacitinib** are the JAK inhibitors approved for treatment of psoriatic arthritis.

Deucravacitinib is a selective TYK2 inhibitor. TYK2 is a protein in the JAK family. It is used for treating plaque psoriasis. **Serious infections can occur with the use of JAK inhibitors and they are very expensive.**

Biological agents: Recently, biological agents have been introduced in the treatment of psoriasis (Box 69.9). They do not cause cumulative toxicity or drug interactions like conventional drugs. Given parenterally, they are effective in about 30%–70% of patients with moderate to severe psoriasis but they lose efficacy over time. These agents include:

1. **Alefacept,** which binds to CD_2 on activated T cells and impairs the costimulatory signals of leucocyte-function-associated antigen-3 (LFA-3). This decreases the number of T cells.
2. **Infliximab,** which inihibits TNF-α functionally.
3. **Etanercept,** a recombinant human TNF receptor antagonist (Chapter 73).
4. **Adalimumab,** a humanised IgG_1mAb, which blocks TNF-α. Chances of development of neutralising antibody are less compared to infliximab.
   Golimumab, a human IgG1 mAB also acts similarly and is used in psoriatic arthritis.
   Certolizumab pegol, a humanized antigen-binding fragment (Fab') of a monoclonal antibody, that has been conjugated to polyethylene glycol. It is the only pegylated anti-TNFα agent. It is used in psoriatic arthritis. the other uses are rheumatoid arthritis and Crohn disease.
   Methotrexate can be used with TNF inhibitors to improve efficacy and reduce the risk of anti-drug antibody formation.
5. **Ustekinumab,** a human monoclonal antibody, which reduces skin inflammation by blocking the activity of IL-12 and IL-23.
6. **Secukinumab,** which acts by blocking IL-17A, a key effector cytokine. **Ixekizumab** and **brodalumab** are the other two IL-17A antagonists. They can increase the risk of mucocutaneous candidiasis.
7. **Guselkumab,** a humanized IgG1 mAB, selectively binds to the p19 subunit of IL-23, and prevents it from binding to the IL-23 receptor. This blocks downstream release of pro-inflammatory cytokines. Other IL-23 antagonists are **tildrakizumab** and **risankizumab**. They are more effective than ustekinumab or adalimumab.

However, they are all very expensive and should be reserved only for resistant cases. Such patients can be prescribed biologic agent with phototherapy or systemic therapy to improve response.

Systemic glucocorticoids: Systemic glucocorticoid therapy, though very effective, needs high doses to suppress the disease, and therefore causes ADR. Furthermore, the relapse rate is high. Hence, **it should be reserved for acutely ill patients with erythrodermic psoriasis.**

UV phototherapy can be used for widespread disease or if topical agents fail. Narrow-band UVB is preferred because it is safer. It is a choice in pregnant or breastfeeding woman suffering from psoriasis.

UVA may be combined with oral or topical psoralens (PUVA) but may increase risk of skin cancer.

Excimer or laser therapy is also safe and effective for localized disease and can be used in pregnancy.

DRUG THERAPY OF ALOPECIA

Alopecia is loss of hair in any region of the body.

Alopecia of the scalp can be:

1. **Scarring** which is associated with inflammation, fibrosis and destruction of the hair follicles due to primary skin disorders such as lichen planus or systemic diseases such as lupus erythematosus. Such alopecia is permanent.
2. **Nonscarring** in which the hair follicles are preserved, and the alopecia is **temporary and reversible**

following correction of cause. Dandruff is perhaps the most common cause. The other causes of nonscarring alopecia are crash dieting, physical trauma, iron deficiency, hypothyroidism, chronic malnutrition, chronic illness, androgen excess and androgenetic alopecia. It can also be caused by drugs.

The forms of alopecia of the scalp are as follows:

- *Androgenic alopecia*
- *Androgenetic alopecia* (male pattern)
- *Alopecia areata*
- *Drug induced* (see Table 69.1)

Androgenic alopecia occurs in women and is due to elevated plasma levels of androgens. They may have other manifestations of hyperandrogenism such as menstrual abnormalities, hirsutism, acne and infertility. The treatment is that of hyperandrogenism (Chapter 67).

Androgenetic alopecia is a hereditary disorder due to excessive conversion of testosterone to DHT in the scalp skin in genetically susceptible men and women.

Treatment: This comprises topical **minoxidil** (see below) in both sexes and oral **finasteride in men** (Chapter 67). The response to finasteride is better in the frontal region of the scalp, which has higher levels of 5-alpha reductase, than in the occipital region (which has higher levels of aromatase).

It must be remembered that androgens cause:

a. The vellus hair follicles to be replaced by terminal hair follicles in the region of ambisexual and sexual hair
b. Miniaturisation of the terminal hair follicles of the scalp

As these changes are irreversible, complete reversal of hirsutism (Chapter 67) *and of androgenic/androgenetic alopecia is not to be expected.*

Alopecia areata (which is nonscarring) causes *patches of complete baldness*, varying in size, in any region of the body including the scalp. The treatment comprises **topical minoxidil** and a **topically injected glucocorticoid.**

Minoxidil, an antihypertensive agent (see Chapter 30), when applied locally as a 2%–5% solution twice a day over a prolonged period, may produce some hair growth in a few patients. The results are best in mild cases and good to excellent results are seldom seen in more than 30% of patients even after prolonged use. Minoxidil increases the dermal blood flow which causes an elongation and normalisation of the hair follicles. *New hair follicles are not formed. Cosmetically acceptable hair growth is uncommon, and the beneficial effect ceases when the treatment is discontinued.* One millilitre of 2% solution is applied to dry scalp twice daily. The dose of 2 mL per day should not be exceeded. The therapy is prolonged, expensive and results are unpredictable.

There is no reliable and safe treatment for irreversible alopecia. Had there been one, many dermatologists themselves would not have been bald! It would be better and perhaps cheaper to use a wig!

DRUGS AFFECTING SKIN PIGMENTATION

Drugs can be used:

- **To decrease localised hyperpigmentation** such as freckles and postinflammatory pigmentation
- **To increase pigmentation** in acquired, localised, skin disorders with hypopigmentation such as vitiligo
- **To treat acanthosis nigricans** (see later)

These drugs are not recommended below the age of 12 years.

1. **Demelanising/skin bleaching agents**

HYDROQUINONE: This drug **inhibits tyrosinase and hence melanin synthesis** in the melanocytes of the skin. It is also toxic to the melanocytes. It is commonly used in the form of a 2%–4% cream or lotion in the treatment of freckles, postinflammatory pigmentation and melasma of pregnancy and that due to oral contraceptives. Its effect is reversed by sunlight and hence it is used in combination with an opaque sunscreen.

MONOBENZONE: This is a monobenzyl ether

of hydroquinone and has similar properties. However, **it causes total, irreversible depigmentation.** The incidence of skin allergy to this drug is high.

GLUTATHIONE: This antioxidant agent, given orally or intravenously, is reported to cause lightening of the skin. The results are variable and unpredictable. Fairness of 2–3 shades may be achieved after repeated use for 2–3 months. The fairness is not suntan proof and is not permanent. ADR include allergic reactions including shock and Stevens–Johnson syndrome. The treatment is very expansive with limited benefits.

Commercial 'fairness products' are heavily promoted for both men and women with tall claims of converting 'black' to 'white'. Such lightening creams may alter the chemical structure of the skin by inhibiting synthesis of melanin. The common basic ingredients in these creams are hydroquinone, mercury and highly potent fluorinated steroids along with chemicals of unknown safety. Constant use of these agents can give rise to skin rashes, dirty greyish brown waxy pigmentation, colloid milium, superficial fungal infection, viral warts, severe acne vulgaris, folliculitis and striae formation. The skin becomes thinner and wound healing is delayed. Percutaneous absorption may cause renal damage.

2. **Melanising agents**

Vitiligo is probably an autoimmune disorder. It may be localised or generalised. The drug treatment is unsatisfactory. The affected skin can be painted by artificial tanning preparations or with 1%–2% dihydroxyacetone in 50:50 water and acetone. The concentration should be adjusted to suit the patient.

TRIOXSALEN (Trisoralen): Given orally, it may be effective in the treatment of vitiligo. By increasing the skin pigmentation, it increases the tolerance of the skin to UV light. For large lesions of vitiligo, it is given in the dose of 0.6 mg/kg/day 2–3 times a week 2 h before exposure to 5–10 min of direct, mid-day sunlight. Exposure is increased by 2 min per day until erythema sets in. If the desired effect is not obtained after 90 min of exposure, the dose is increased gradually up to a maximum of 80 mg daily. Repigmentation is usually evident after 3–4 months of treatment. Blue-grey, plastic sunglasses, opaque to UV rays, and a light-screening lipstick should be used during UV exposure in order to protect the eyes and the lips. The drug sometimes causes cutaneous reaction. *It is contraindicated in patients with diseases associated with photosensitivity such as porphyria and systemic lupus erythematosus, and should not be given concurrently with other photosensitising drugs.*

METHOXSALEN (Oxsoralen): This psoralen compound is used topically 0.1%–1% lotion to treat small vitiliginous lesions. Topical application is followed by exposure to sunlight or a UV lamp. This causes erythematous reaction and activation of melanocytes. Topical use can cause acute, vesicular, cutaneous photosensitivity reaction. The drug can also be given orally in the dose of 20 mg/day (single dose), 2–4 h before exposure to UV light. Commonly, it causes gastric discomfort. Long-term therapy can accelerate skin ageing and has an increased risk of severe sunburn, skin wrinkling, cataract and skin cancer.

Treatment of acanthosis nigricans: This is hyperpigmented, velvety thickening of the skin occurring most commonly on the neck, in the axillae and in the groins. It is believed to be a manifestation of hyperinsulinaemia due to insulin resistance. The drugs used locally are tretinoin 0.025% cream; adapalene 0.1% gel; and calcipotriene 0.005% cream, ointment or gel.

SUNSCREENS AND BARRIER PREPARATIONS

Solar UV radiation that can damage the skin is of three types according to wavelengths: UVA1, UVA2 and UVB. Of these, UVA forms 15% of the total radiation and is mainly responsible for photo-ageing and photo-toxicity. UVB is mostly absorbed in the epidermis and causes sunburn and tanning. UVA2 is also erythemogenic. *Chronic exposure to both, UVA and UVB can damage the DNA, suppress immune mechanisms and can cause skin ageing and cancer in animals.*

Skin can be protected from solar UV radiation by:

1. **Inorganic** preparations such as zinc oxide, calamine and titanium dioxide which are opaque to

all wavelengths of light and reflect them (**reflectant sunscreens**); thus they are physical barriers.

2. **Organic chemicals** that absorb UVA and UVB at the skin surface (**absorbent sunscreens**). Examples are aminobenzoates, benzophosphophenones-3 (oxybenzone), methoxycinnamate (octinoxate), a salicylate (octisalate), octocrylone and a dibenzylmethane (avobenzene) (Box 69.10).

Since none of these agents give complete protection from solar UV radiation, they are usually combined to increase photostability and to broaden their spectrum. A newer agent, **ecamsule,** has broad protective spectrum.

Barrier preparations: They are used as water repellents to protect the skin against nappy rash. They contain a water repellent such as **dimethicone** along with **zinc oxide.** They are used as creams or ointments.

Dihydroxyacetone (DHA), a pigment agent, is commonly used for sunless tanning. It binds to stratum corneum and changes the skin colour from white to orange-brown.

COSMETICS, TOOTH POWDERS AND DERMAL FILLERS

Various preparations of cosmetic dusting powders contain mainly talc (native magnesium silicate with small amounts of aluminium silicate) which acts as an adsorbent and provides 'slip'. Another substance which also acts as an adsorbent and a mild antiseptic, added to such powders, is zinc stearate, a light, impalpable, amorphous powder. Zinc oxide is commonly used to cover the 'shine', whereas chalk acts as a colour carrier. However, starch is a better absorbent of moisture than the above-mentioned substances. Addition of phenol, menthol and camphor exert a local antipruritic and cooling action. Various antiseptics like boric acid and salicylic acid may be added to these powders. The powder has absorbent, mild antiseptic, antipruritic and cooling properties; it may be applied to the axillae and the groins three to four times daily, with benefit. Application of such powders may cause blocking of the sweat gland pores and hence, after-cleansing is essential. Use of talc on surgical gloves is known to cause granulomatous reaction in wounds.

Box 69.10 Types of Sunscreens

I. **Inorganic (reflectant) sunscreens:**
- ***UVB, UVA2/1***
  Zinc oxide, calamine, titanium dioxide

II. ***Organic (absorbent) sunscreens:***
- ***UVB***
  PABA and PABA derivatives: Octyldimethyl PABA (Padimat O)
  Cinnamates: Octyl methoxycinnamate, cinoxate
  Salicylates: Octyl salycilates (octisalate), homosalate, trolamine salycilates,
  Octocrylene, phenylbenzimidazole sulphonic acid (ensulizole)
- ***UVB, UVA1***
  Benzophenones: Oxybenzone, dioxybenzone, sulisobenzone,
  Terephthalydine dicamphor sulphonic acid (ecamsule)
- ***UVA1***
  Butyl methoxydibenzoyl methane (avobenzone)
- ***UVA2***
  Methyl anthranilate (merdimate)

Baby powder generally contains zinc stearate and talc in the proportion of 1:2. There is no evidence that they are superior to good quality regular talc powder. In general, it is better to avoid such medicated powders in babies as they tend to form cake in skin fold causing dermatitis and may also get into the lungs. Similarly there appears to be no need for special 'baby soap' or 'baby oil'. Any nonperfumed quality soft soap and good quality oil (e.g. coconut oil) is equally effective.

There is no evidence to suggest that medicated cosmetic powders are any better than nonmedicated ones for routine use in individuals with healthy skin. Medicated powders are costly, liable to produce skin sensitisation and rashes.

Tooth powders contain simple chalk as the basic ingredient, with added white soap, surfactants, saccharin, colour and flavour. **Toothpaste** or gels contain abrasives (calcium salts, silica), fluoride and detergents. Various antiseptics and deodorants like clove oil, peppermint oil and lemon oil are added to these basic ingredients. Evidence suggests that nonmedicated toothpastes are as effective as medicated ones and possess the additional advantage of being cheaper and more acceptable. No toothpaste or powder can, however, act as a substitute for simple and repeated cleansing of mouth immediately after eating.

Shampoos are liquid soaps or detergents used to wash the hair and clean the scalp of scales or dandruff. *They are expensive cleansers.* Toilet soap can be used for the same purposes at a much lower cost. Shampoos are also used as vehicles for applying medicaments to the scalp. Medicated shampoos usually contain various antimicrobial agents such as selenium sulphide, ketoconazole, povidone and cetrimide.

Most of the commercial cold creams are modifications of a popular emollient preparation, rose water ointment, which contains spermaceti (a waxy substance obtained from the head of the sperm whale), bleached beeswax, almond or prussic oil, rose water and rose oil. Such creams are useful for their soothing and moisturising effect.

Dermal fillers given by injection are used for soft tissue augmentation of facial wrinkles and folds to give a young look. They are used in conjunction with botulinum toxin A. Majority of them consist of **hyaluronic acid** derived from bacteria or human/bovine collagen. Some contain a biodegradable synthetic polymer. They are used to remove facial wrinkles and lipoatrophy. Their effect lasts for 6–24 months. Usually, they are well tolerated, but occasionally may cause local bleeding, infection or skin discoloration; and rarely necrosis and nodule/granuloma formation. *Prior skin testing for allergy is essential.*

ANHIDROTICS AND DEODORANTS

Sweating is common in the tropics and no drug should be used to block this normal physiological response. It could, however, become excessive **(hyperhidrosis).** The eccrine sweat glands, although anatomically innervated by sympathetic nerves, are physiologically cholinergic. *Anhidrotics (antiperspirants) are the drugs used for controlling hyperhidrosis.* They are as follows:

- **Systemic anhidrotics,** e.g. agents such as synthetic atropine substitutes like methantheline. None of the available systemic anhidrotics, however, are safe and reliable.
- **Local anhidrotics,** e.g. aluminium salts like aluminium chlorhydrate, formalin, glutaraldehyde and esters of hyoscine.

Aluminium chlorhydrate acts by local astringent action and blocks the sweat ducts at the skin surface. **Formalin** acts by forming keratin plugs in the orifices of sweat ducts. **Glutaraldehyde** is a tanning agent with antibacterial and deodorant activity. Anticholinergic drugs like propantheline bromide and esters of hyoscine are also effective when applied locally in the form of lotions.

Mild hyperhidrosis of the feet is easily managed by foot baths with **potassium permanganate,** 1:10,000, and simple talcum powder. Individuals should be instructed to avoid nylon socks and rubber footwear and to use open sandals. Where an emotional factor is suspected, counselling and small doses of an anxiolytic agent may help.

Undesirable body odour results from the action of bacteria on the organic substances in the apocrine sweat. Excess eccrine sweat promotes this process by increasing wetness, which encourages bacterial growth. Anhidrotics, by virtue of their drying action, also act as *deodorants*. The other drugs used are as follows:

- **Cleansers,** e.g. sodium carbonate 20% in talc
- **Aluminium salts,** e.g. aluminium chloride hexahydrate
- **Antibacterials** which retard bacterial decomposition of the apocrine sweat, e.g. hexachlorophane, tetrachlorosalicylanilide, trichlocarbon, thiram and bithionol
- **Masking perfumes**

Some of these agents can cause irritation, allergy, contact dermatitis and photosensitivity reactions.

It may be noted that there is a great demand for deodorants in today's society and it is estimated that an affluent country like the USA spends more than half a billion dollars a year on being 'nice to be near'. They are popular more because of fragrance (exotic) than anything else! Most of us do not really smell as much as we are made to believe by the advertisers, and *simple measures like personal cleanliness, shaving of axillae, daily bath with ordinary soft soap, and applying, if required, a simple adsorbent like talcum powder will provide similar good results as any expensive spray without risk of 'deodorant allergy'.*

DRUG-INDUCED SKIN DISORDERS

Adverse skin reactions to drugs are frequent in clinical practice (Table 69.1). The most common are exanthematous reactions (rashes) and urticaria. Other relatively rare reactions are erythema multiforme, Stevens–Johnson syndrome, exfoliative dermatitis and toxic epidermal necrolysis. Some reactions have an immunological basis.

Urticaria can be produced by allergic mechanism by several drugs such as ampicillin and antisera; and by drugs which liberate autacoids such as histamine. Urticaria can be dangerous if accompanied by angioedema of the larynx (Chapter 23).

Table 69.1 Some Dermatological Reactions to Drugs Used Systemically and Topically

Skin Reaction	Examples of Implicated Drugs
Urticaria	Penicillin, NSAID, sulphonamides, captopril, enalapril
Acne or aggravation of existing acne	Corticosteroids, androgenic and anabolic steroids, phenytoin, OC-containing androgenic progestogens, iodides, cytotoxic therapy, lithium, danazol, barbiturates, isoniazid
Exfoliative dermatitis	NSAID, sulphonamides, gold salts
Contact dermatitis	Topical antimicrobials like penicillin, chloramphenicol, neomycin; sulphonamides; topical antihistaminics; cream and lotion preservatives; lanolin cosmetics
Purpura	Corticosteroids, anticoagulants, aspirin, barbiturates, thiazides, sulphonamides, sulphonylureas, cytotoxic drugs
Stevens–Johnson syndrome	Sulphonamides, barbiturates, NSAID, phenytoin, allopurinol
SLE-like reaction	Hydralazine, procainamide, phenytoin, isoniazid, alpha-methyldopa
Fixed drug eruption	Phenolphthalein, barbiturates, aspirin, sulphonamides, quinine, tetracyclines
Photosensitivity	Demeclocycline, phenothiazines, griseofulvin, nalidixic acid, sulphonamides, sulphonylureas, thiazides, piroxicam
Alopecia	Cytotoxic drugs, heparin, androgens, OC, carbimazole, vitamin A (large doses), beta blockers, levodopa, thallium
Hirsutism	See Chapter 67

Photosensitivity disorders of the skin can occur following topical as well as systemic administration of drugs. They are either phototoxic or photoallergic in nature.

Phototoxicity is a nonimmunologic reaction, usually occurring as erythema that desquamates or 'peels' within several days; oedema and vesicles may appear.

Photoallergy is an immunologic cell-mediated process and usually manifests as intensely pruritic, eczematous dermatitis, which later leads to local, thickened, 'leathery' changes in sun-exposed areas.

The treatment of drug-induced skin reactions includes:

- *Withdrawing the offending agent*
- *Systemic antihistaminic therapy*
- *Use of glucocorticoids and SC adrenaline in severe cases.*

Exfoliative dermatitis, Stevens–Johnson syndrome and allergic vasculitis are serious drug reactions and will need systemic glucocorticoid therapy.

With the first occurrence of an allergic drug reaction, the patient should be informed that he/she is allergic to the particular drug, and its future administration should be avoided.

AZOLE ANTIFUNGAL DRUGS

For topical use

- Clotrimazole
- Miconazole
- Econazole
- Butoconazole
- Oxiconazole
- Sulconazole
- Tioconazole
- Sertaconazole
- Luliconazole

For systemic use

- Ketoconazole
- Itraconazole
- Fluconazole
- Voriconazole

DRUGS EFFECTIVE IN SEBORRHIC DERMATITIS

Antipityrosporal

- Topical ketoconazole/ Efinaconazole
- Salicylic acid
- Ciclopirox

Anti-inflammatory

- Topical corticosteroids

Cytostatic

- Selenium sulphide
- Zinc pyrithione
- Sulphur
- Tar
- Salicylic acid

ANTI- ACNE DRUGS

Cleansers

- Soaps

Comedolytics

- Local tretinoin
- Adapalene

Exfoliants

- Salicylic acid

Sebostatics

- Oral isotretinoin

Hormones

- Cyproterone acetate
- Estrogen

Antibacterial drugs

Local

- Erythromycin
- Clindamycin
- Azelaic acid
- Benzoyl peroxide

Systemic

- Tetracyclines
- Erythromycin
- Minocycline
- Cotrimoxazole

DRUGS USED IN THE TREATMENT OF PSORIASIS

Topical therapy

Emollients

Keratolytic agents
- Salicylic acid 2%–10%

Cytostatic agents
- Coal tar
- Dithranol

Glucocorticoids

Calcipotriol
Tacalcitol

Retinoids
- Tazarotene

Roflumilast

Calcineurin inhibitors
- Pimecrolimus
- Tacrolimus

Aryl hydrocarbon receptor (AhR) agonist
- Tapinarof

Systemic therapy

Etretinate
Acitretin

Apremilast

Immunosuppressants
- Methotrexate
- Cyclosporine
- Mycophenolate mofetil

JAK inhibitors
- Upadacitinib
- Tofacitinib
- Deucravacitinib

Biological agents
- *T cell activation inhibitors*
  - Alefacept
- *TNF-α inhibitors*
  - Etanercept
  - Infliximab
- *IL-12 and IL-23 blocker*
  - Ustekinumab
- *IL-17A blockers*
  - Secukinumab
- *IL-23 blockers*
  - Guselkumab

Systemic glucocorticoids

Phototherapy

Ultraviolet B irradiation with or without coal tar application

Ultraviolet therapy with psoralens

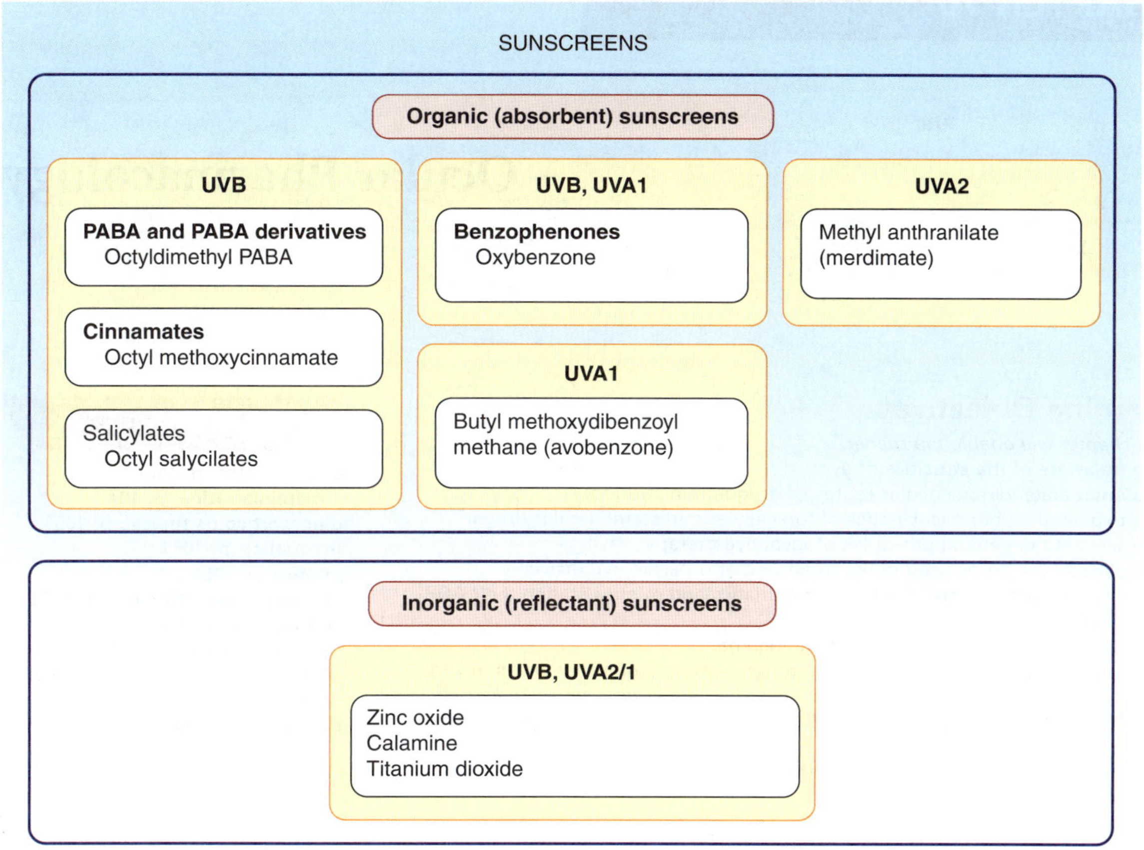
SUNSCREENS
Organic (absorbent) sunscreens
UVB
PABA and PABA derivatives
Octyldimethyl PABA
Cinnamates
Octyl methoxycinnamate
Salicylates
Octyl salycilates
UVB, UVA1
Benzophenones
Oxybenzone
UVA1
Butyl methoxydibenzoyl methane (avobenzone)
UVA2
Methyl anthranilate (merdimate)
Inorganic (reflectant) sunscreens
UVB, UVA2/1
Zinc oxide
Calamine
Titanium dioxide

CHAPTER 70

Ocular Pharmacology

Learning Objectives

This chapter will enable the reader:

1. To be aware of the structure of eye.
2. To enumerate various ocular routes of drug administration.
3. To explain the pharmacokinetics of topically administered ocular drugs.
4. To discuss the general principles of local eye therapy.
5. To classify the drugs used in the treatment of different eye diseases.
6. To explain mechanisms of action of mydriatics and miotics stating their ADR and uses.
7. To discuss the pharmacotherapy of glaucoma.
8. To enumerate different antimicrobial drugs, anti-inflammatory drugs including glucocorticoids, antihistaminics, mast cell stabilizers, immunosuppressives, antimitotic drugs, local anaesthetics, diagnostic agents, wetting agents and tear substitutes stating their indications.
9. To mention the drugs causing ocular toxicity giving type of lesions induced by them.

KEY TERMS

ocular routes of drug administration, p. 1047
glucocorticoids topical, p. 1051
mydriatics, p. 1051
miotics, p. 1051
glaucoma, drug therapy, p. 1052
latanoprost, p. 1053
VEGF inhibitors, p. 1054
ocular local anaesthetics, p. 1055
diagnostic agents, p. 1055
drug-induced ocular toxicity, p. 1056

Eye complaints are common in general practice and some of them, if neglected, can lead to blindness. The eye is readily accessible to observation, and the diagnosis of several eye diseases can be made easily. The drug treatment of majority of ocular diseases is largely concerned with alleviation of inflammation, control of infection and reduction in intraocular pressure.

Anatomy and Physiology of the Eye

Fig. 70.1 depicts the various parts of the eyeball. The human eyeball is composed of three concentric layers from outwards: (a) the cornea and sclera; (b) the iris, ciliary body and choroid, and the lens; and (c) the retina.

The **cornea** is an almost avascular, transparent structure which acts as an important barrier to foreign matter, including drugs. Drug absorption across the cornea involves penetration through its multiple layers. The **sclera** is the outermost, dense, imperfectly elastic, opaque, supporting coat of the eyeball; its forward continuation is the cornea.

The **conjunctiva** is a modified mucous membrane that lines the outer surface of the anterior most part of the sclera and

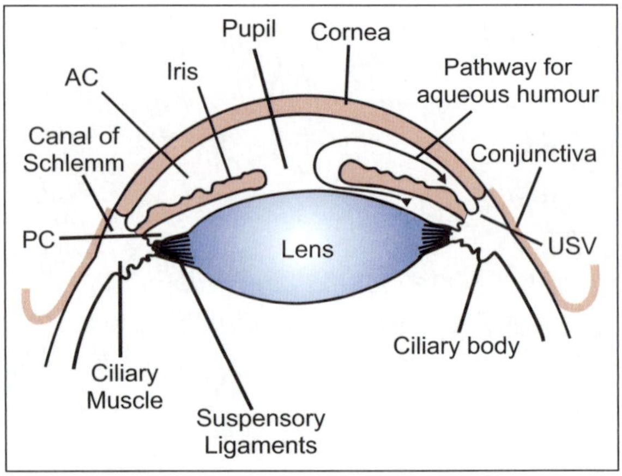

FIG. 70.1 Anatomy of the eye and pathway for secretion and drainage of aqueous humour in the anterior chamber. AC, anterior chamber; PC, posterior chamber; USV, uveoscleral vasculature.

the inner surface of the eyelids. The conjunctival epithelium is continuous with the corneal epithelium.

The **iris, ciliary body and choroid** form the uveal tract. The pupillary size is controlled by two types of muscle fibres:

1. *Radial,* innervated by the sympathetic nerve fibres, causing dilatation of the pupil (**mydriasis**)
2. *Circular,* innervated by the parasympathetic nerve fibres, causing constriction of the pupil (**miosis**)

The **ciliary body** is made up of unstriated muscle fibres (ciliary muscle) and epithelial cells; the latter secrete aqueous humour into the posterior chamber; that fluid passes through the pupil into the anterior chamber, and from there drains into the *canal of Schlemm.* When the ciliary muscle contracts, the zonules which suspend the lens relax, and the lens becomes more convex and is drawn slightly forward. This process is known as accommodation and allows to focus on near objects.

Ocular Routes of Drug Administration PH 1.11

Ocular routes can be classified as topical, systemic and periocular. **Topically applied** drugs (such as eye drops/ointment) target cornea, conjunctiva, sclera, iris and ciliary body and hence used to treat anterior segment diseases. Topically administered solutions get washed away within 15–30 s after instillation, resulting in less contact time with the absorptive membranes and hence <5% of the applied dose reaches the intraocular tissues.

Drugs when administered **systemically** (i.e. orally or parenterally) to target ocular tissues have to cross the blood–aqueous barrier and blood–retinal barrier to reach the anterior segment and posterior segment, respectively. The drug particle size and lipophilicity play an important role in determining the intraocular concentration of the drug. Usually only 1%–5% reaches the vitreous humour.

To overcome the inefficiency of topical and systemic routes and to deliver therapeutic drug concentrations to the posterior segment, the drug can be administered via the **periocular routes** (periphery of the eye). The drug administered by periocular injections can reach the posterior segment by three different pathways: trans-scleral pathway; systemic circulation through the choroid plexus; and the anterior pathway through the tear film, cornea, aqueous humour and the vitreous humour.

Periocular injections are as follows:

a. **Subconjunctival injection** involves introduction of the drug (e.g. anaesthetic drugs, triamcinolone) beneath the conjunctiva.
b. **Subtenon injection** involves injecting the drug (e.g. lignocaine) into the Tenon's capsule located around the upper portion of the eye and into the superior rectus muscle.
c. **Retrobulbar injection**, drug is injected into the conical compartment within the rectus muscles and intramuscular septa. This route provides high local concentration of drug with no influence on the IOP.
d. **Peribulbar injection** involves injecting the drug in the extracellular spaces surrounding the rectus muscle. This route is safe but less effective. Anaesthetic drugs are administered via retrobulbar and peribulbar routes.
e. **Posterior juxtascleral injection** involves injecting the drug using blunt tipped curved cannula into the outer surface of the sclera. This route allows sustained drug delivery to the macula.

Among all the periocular routes, retrobulbar route is most efficient but is associated with complications like retrobulbar haemorrhage, globe perforation and respiratory arrest.

In addition, direct injection of drug (e.g. anaesthetics, antibiotics) can be given into anterior or posterior chamber of the eye, usually during surgery. This is termed as **intracameral route.**

Intravitreal injections are used to deliver drugs (e.g. ranibizumab, bevacizumab) directly into the vitreous humour to reach the retina and other structures in the back of the eye. This route is used to deliver drugs without causing systemic toxicity.

Pharmacokinetics of topically administered ocular drugs: Most drugs in ophthalmic practice are administered topically in the form of eye drops or ointments. The time course of drug delivery from eye drops into the eyeball follows first-order kinetics (Chapter 1). For majority of drugs, 1% or less of an applied dose is absorbed across the cornea to reach the anterior chamber. Box 70.1 summarises

Box 70.1 Factors Influencing Penetration of Ocular Drugs

- ***Drug-related:*** Chemical nature, lipid solubility, dissociation constant and route of administration
- ***Vehicle-related:*** Chemical nature, physical state (liquid or solid) and viscosity
- ***Formulation-related:*** Drug concentration, osmolality, tonicity and pH

the factors affecting the penetration of ocular drugs. PH 1.1

1. **Drug-related factors:** These are similar to those that govern the classical pharmacokinetics. Topically administered drugs can be absorbed through the cornea, conjunctiva and sclera. Drugs injected subconjunctivally and under the Tenon's capsule as well those injected into the retrobulbar space diffuse through the sclera and the cornea into the anterior and posterior chambers and into the vitreous humour. In order to enter the eye, systemically administered drugs have to cross the **blood–eye barrier**, which resembles the blood–brain barrier (Chapter 1). Hence drugs like chloramphenicol, which are highly lipid soluble, can penetrate through the normal uninflamed eye unlike drugs with a large molecular size such as penicillin, which when administered systemically can penetrate only if the eye is severely inflamed. Lipid-soluble drugs pass readily through the corneal epithelium and endothelium, whereas the water-soluble agents penetrate through the stroma.
2. **Vehicle and ocular drug delivery:** Most of the ophthalmic drugs are administered in aqueous solution. Since the **aqueous solutions** are liable to be carried away by the tears, their repeated administration is necessary to maintain their local concentration. **Ointment bases act as reservoir** for drugs, release them slowly and ensure higher penetration as well as prolonged action. Petrolatum and lanolin are viscous vehicles commonly used as bases in ophthalmic ointments. Other bases used to enhance drug penetration into the eye are a gel-forming base for timolol, and 0.5% hydroxycellulose for dorzolamide. Polymers are also used to increase the penetration of drugs; these are cellulose ether, polyvinyl alcohol, carbopol, polyacrylamide and poloxamer-407. Solid inserts such as pilocarpine **ocusert** provide a constant rate of release of drugs (zero-order kinetics). **Liposomes** can also serve as drug reservoir and maintain better drug concentration of ocular drugs. **Applicaps** are yet another form of ophthalmic formulation. *Sterility of all commercially available ophthalmic products is of utmost importance to prevent ocular infection.*
3. **Formulation-related factors:** Drug concentration as well as tonicity and pH of the formulation can be adjusted to obtain the desired speed and duration of action of a drug.

After penetration into the eye, the drug may be washed out rapidly from the inflamed eye because of hyperaemia or it may accumulate in an ocular tissue, e.g. α-adrenergic receptor agonists bind to and accumulate in the melanin pigment in the iris. This has therapeutic and toxicological implications. Sometimes, the drug may be biotransformed locally into an active compound. Thus, **dipivefrine** is a prodrug for adrenaline.

Since all ophthalmic medications are liable to be absorbed into the systemic circulation, they can cause systemic toxicity. This is particularly true for drugs reaching the nasal cavity through the nasolacrimal duct; it is more likely to happen with eye drops than with ointments. The final disposal of the ocular drugs may often take place after absorption into systemic circulation.

Systemic administration of drugs: Certain ocular disorders require systemic drug therapy, e.g. carbonic anhydrase inhibitors in glaucoma; glucocorticoids in uveitis; and analgesics for ocular pain; antibiotics for deep ocular infections; and antihistaminics for ocular allergy.

General Principles of Local Eye Therapy PH 1.1

The selection of the drug(s) depends upon accurate diagnosis, although symptomatic treatment is often necessary.

1. **Nonpharmacological modalities:** These include eye rest; bed rest; proper lighting; protection from strong light, infection and trauma; hot or cold

compresses; eye exercises; and nutritional management.

2. **Pharmacological treatment:**
   - Apart from the diagnosis, choice of the drug depends upon (a) assessment of the potential/actual threat to vision and (b) presence of a local condition or a systemic disease. For example, beta-adrenergic receptor blocker eye drops can aggravate bronchial asthma. Persons with a family history of open angle glaucoma are more likely to develop glaucoma during glucocorticoid therapy.
   - The health care giver and the patient should strictly observe hygienic and aseptic practices while applying the medication to the eye.
   - The ophthalmic formulation should be used as purchased and no attempt should be made to dilute it or otherwise modify it.
   - The remnant after the patient gets well should not be stored for future use.
   - Eye drops are convenient for ambulatory patients who are well enough to continue working. Their main disadvantage is their short duration of action and hence the necessity of frequent instillation. *Only one drop should be instilled into an eye at one time because that is the capacity of the conjunctival sac.* The patient should then lie down with the eye(s) closed. If a drop of another medication needs to be instilled at the same time, then 5 min should be allowed to elapse before adding the second drop. Ointments act as reservoir of the drug and have a prolonged action. However, apart from being messy, they may cause blurring of vision.
   - Associated conditions such as diabetes mellitus and hypertension should be treated.
   - Systemic drug therapy may have to be employed in serious ocular conditions and in those conditions, which have failed to respond to topical drug therapy.
   - Corneal ulcers and keratitis require treatment by an opthalmologist. PH 1.58

Classification of Drugs Used in the Eye

I. **Antimicrobials:** Antibacterials, antivirals, antifungals, antiprotozoals
II. **Anti-inflammatory agents** such as NSAIDs
III. **Glucocorticoids**
IV. **Antihistaminics** and **mast cell stabilisers**
V. **Mydriatics and miotics**
VI. **Drugs for glaucoma**
VII. **Immunomodulatory drugs** such as immunosuppressives, vascular endothelial growth factor (VEGF) antibodies and antimitotic agents
VIII. **Local anaesthetics**
IX. **Diagnostic agents** such as fluorescin and rose bengal
X. **Miscellaneous drugs** such as tear substitutes and zinc preparations

ANTIMICROBIAL AGENTS

Eye infections can be caused by bacteria, viruses, fungi and protozoa. Many antimicrobial agents are used topically. Drugs with limited solubility are administered as suspensions, whereas ointments are preferred for a prolonged contact with the medication. The choice of the appropriate antibiotic depends on the suspected infective agent and its predicted antibiotic sensitivity.

The common eye infections are blepharitis, hordeolum, acute conjunctivitis, infective corneal ulcers, ophthalmia neonatorum, and iridocyclitis. Box 70.2 lists the anti-infective preparations used in eye infections. All **fluoroquinolones** are active against most Gram-negative organisms associated with conjunctivitis. They are, however, not effective against methicillin resistant Staphylococcus aureus (MRSA). **Trimethoprim** has a broad spectrum of activity including against ocular MRSA.

Antibacterial agents:

Acute blepharitis may be caused by staphylococci or by parasites such as the head lice. Since eye drops do not penetrate well into the eyelids, ointments are the mainstay of treatment, accompanied by removal of the crusts. Staphylococcal infection is best treated with topical erythromycin or sulphacetamide. Recurrent disease may need additional treatment with a topical glucocorticoid. **Chronic blepharitis** is due to a combination of staphylococcal infection and seborrhoea. It requires additional antiseborrhoeic treatment (Chapter 69). Angular blepharitis is mainly caused by the Gram-negative *Morax–Axenfeld* bacilli. It responds to the topical application

Box 70.2 Anti-Infective Drugs Used in the Eye

Antibacterial:
- Chloramphenicol 0.5% S, 1% O
- Ciprofloxacin 0.3% S
- Norfloxacin 0.3% S,O/ofloxacin 0.3% S/Levofloxacin 0.5%, 1.5% S,/ Moxifloxacin 0.5%S
- Besifloxacin 0.6% S
- Gatifloxacin 0.3% S,O
- Erythromycin 0.5% O/Azithromycin 1% S
- Gentamicin/tobramycin 0.3% S,O
- Sulphacetamide 10% S
- Tetracycline 1% S

Combinations:
- Bacitracin + Polymyxin B (500U–10,000 U/g)
- Trimethoprim (1mg/ml) + Polymyxin B (10,000 U/ml)

Antiviral:
- Acyclovir 3% O; 400–800 mg tab oral
- Ganciclovir 0.15% gel
- Valacyclovir 500–1000mg tab oral, Famciclovir 125-500 mg oral tab
- Valganciclovir 450 mg oral tab
- Foscarnet IV, intravitreal/Cidofovir IV
- Idoxuridine 0.1% S
- Vidarabine 3% O
- Trifluridine 1% S

Antifungal:
- Amphotericin B 0.1%–0.5% S; 0.8–1.0 mg subconjunctival; 5 mcg intravitreal, 2–10 μg intracorneal and intracameral,
- Natamycin 5% S
- Fluconazole oral
- Ketoconazole oral
- Miconazole 5–10 mg subconjunctival
- Voriconazole 50 μg intracorneal and intracameral, oral, IV

Notes: S, solution as eye drops; O, ointment.

of sulphacetamide, gentamicin or zinc sulphate. For allergic blepharitis, anti-inflammatory drugs or antihistaminics are needed. Head lice, if present, must be treated (Chapter 69).

Hordeolum (stye) is a staphylococcal infection of sebaceous glands of the eyelids and is usually self-limiting. The treatment comprises of hot moist compresses, removal of the eyelashes to facilitate the drainage and antibacterial ointments. Repeated styes possibly indicate uncorrected refractive error.

Acute conjunctivitis and **bacterial corneal ulcers** can be treated with one of the preparations shown in Box 70.2. The bacteria commonly encountered are staphylococci, streptococci, pneumococci and *Haemophilus* species. **Ophthalmia neonatorum**, caused by *Chlamydia*, gonococci or other organisms, needs more aggressive treatment. Gonococcal illness needs systemic as well as local therapy (Chapter 51). Chlamydial infection (trachoma) is best treated with topical tetracycline *plus* oral azithromycin. For **herpetic ophthalmia neonatorum**, see below.

Antiviral agents: The common viral infections of the eye are conjunctivitis, keratitis, iridocyclitis and retinitis. They are due to herpes simplex virus, herpes zoster virus and cytomegalovirus. Box 70.2 lists the antiviral preparations commonly used in the eye. **Viral keratitis** is either (a) epithelial which responds to topical treatment with antiviral drugs or (b) stromal and requires administration of the same drugs orally. **Herpes zoster ophthalmicus** is more serious and needs systemic acyclovir in addition to local antiviral therapy. **Viral retinitis** requires prolonged treatment with antiviral drugs, by either intravitreal or IV route.

Antifungal agents: Fungal infections of the eye are rare. The important ones are keratitis, scleritis, endophthalmitis and canaliculitis. The antifungal agents commonly used in ocular fungal infections are shown in Box 70.2.

Antiprotozoal agents: The protozoa causing eye infections are *Toxoplasma gondii* and *Acanthamoeba*. Ocular toxoplasmosis is the ocular manifestation of a systemic infection (Chapter 56). *Acanthamoeba* causes deep eye infections which occur more commonly in contact lens users. They require a combination of topical and systemic multidrug therapy.

***Onchocerciasis** caused by Onchocerca volvulus is one of the major causes of blindness.* Its treatment is described in Chapter 58.

ANTI-INFLAMMATORY DRUGS

The drugs belonging to this group are the NSAIDs such as **diclofenac** (0.1% eye drops), **nepafenac** (0.1% and 0.3% eye drops) **flurbiprofen** (0.03% eye drops) and **ketorolac** (0.5% eye drops). Nepafenac is a prodrug,

Box 70.3 Glucocorticoid Ocular Preparations

- Betamethasone 0.1% S,O
- Dexamethasone 0.1% S,O
- Hydrocortisone 1% S, 0.5% O
- Prednisolone 1% S
- Triamcinolone intravitreal
- Dexamethasone intravitreal
- Flluocinolone intravitreal

Notes: S, solution as eye drops; O, ointment.

which readily penetrates cornea and gets converted to an active moiety, amfenac. They are commonly used topically during and following ocular surgery such as cataract extraction, for prevention of intraoperative miosis and postoperative inflammation (Chapter 11).

GLUCOCORTICOIDS IN THE EYE PH 1.38

Topical glucocorticoids (Box 70.3) are used for treating anterior uveitis and for reducing postoperative inflammation following eye operations. Posterior uveitis needs to be treated with oral or parenteral glucocorticoids or with subtenon capsular injections of a glucocorticoid. Optic neuritis needs initial parenteral administration, followed by tapering oral doses of glucocorticoids.

The main ocular adverse effects of glucocorticoids are posterior subcapsular cataract (*steroid cataract*), open angle glaucoma (*steroid glaucoma*) and secondary infection. *Undiagnosed red eye may be due to herpes simplex infection and glucocorticoids may aggravate the condition, leading to corneal ulceration and loss vision. Hence, routine use of a combination of a glucocorticoid with an anti-infective agent is not justified.*

Topical glucocorticoids are **contraindicated** in herpetic epithelial keratitis due to active viral replication, fungal disease of the eye, other viral diseases of the cornea and conjunctiva, ocular tuberculosis, hypersensitivity and after removal of a superficial corneal foreign body.

ANTIHISTAMINICS AND MAST CELL STABILISERS PH 1.16

Allergic conjunctivitis can be treated with topical antihistaminics such as antazoline 0.05%, emedastine 0.05% and levocabastine 0.05%. Mast cell stabilisers such as cromolyn sodium 4%, ketotifen 0.025%, nedocromil 2% and epinastin 0.05% can also be used to treat allergic and vernal conjunctivitis.

MYDRIATICS AND MIOTICS PH 1.13, PH 1.14

Mydriatics are the drugs which produce pupillary dilatation. They are of two types:

- **Muscarinic receptor antagonists,** atropine and atropine substitutes, which also cause paralysis of the iris and ciliary body and lead to **cycloplegia** (paralysis of accommodation) by blocking the muscarinic receptors.
  The main drawback of atropine is its long duration of action so that the cycloplegia lasts for 7–10 days. Atropine substitutes which have a shorter duration of action causing minimal cycloplegia are preferred.
- **α-Adrenergic receptor agonists** (sympathomimetic agents) which directly stimulate the adrenergic receptors in the radial muscle fibres of the iris, and do not lead to cycloplegia.

Mydriasis is required for:

a. Determination of refractive error.
b. Fundoscopic examination of the eyes.
c. Treatment of iridocyclitis, an inflammation of the iris and the ciliary body in which there is severe pain due to spasm of these muscles; atropine paralyses these muscles and relieves the pain.
d. Breaking the adhesions between the lens and the ciliary body, by alternating mydriatics with miotics.

Miotics are the drugs that produce constriction of the pupils by acting as:

- **Muscarinic receptor agonists (pilocarpine)**
- **Anticholinesterases (physostigmine)**

They act on the circular fibres of the iris. They also constrict the ciliary muscle, thus improving trabecular pathway. They are used in the treatment of glaucoma (see below). Their ADR include headache, brow ache, vascular congestion, conjunctival congestion, burning and blurred vision. Prolonged use may cause myopia and vitreous haemorrhage.

Box 70.4 Mydriatics and Miotics

Mydriatics:

Antimuscarinic

- Atropine 0.5%–2% drops
- Homatropine 2%–5% drops
- Eucatropine 2%–5% drops
- Cyclopentolate 0.5%–2% drops
- Tropicamide 0.5%–2% drops

Sympathomimetic

- Phenylephrine 2.5%–10% drops

Miotics:

Cholinomimetic

- Pilocarpine 0.5% drops; ocusert
- Acetyl choline 1% Solution, Carbachol 0.01% solution

Cholinesterase inhibitors

- Physostigmine 1% drops

Miotics are contraindicated in acute iritis and acute uveitis. They should be avoided in acute inflammatory diseases of the anterior segment.

Box 70.4 lists the mydriatics and miotics in common use (see Chapters 19 and 20).

DRUG THERAPY OF GLAUCOMA

Glaucoma, the second most frequent cause of blindness in the world, is a disease of unknown origin. It is:

1. Characterised by progressive degeneration of retinal ganglion cells and optic nerve fibres,
2. Usually accompanied by, but not always, increased intraocular pressure (IOP).

If untreated, it leads to optic neuropathy with loss of optic nerve tissue and excavation or 'cupping' of the ophthalmoscopically visible optic nerve head. This may be accompanied by loss of vision. *Most forms of glaucoma are painless initially and the loss of vision is insidious. If diagnosed and treated early, most patients retain good vision.*

Glaucoma is classified into (a) open-angle, (b) closed-angle, (c) congenital and (d) drug-induced glaucoma. The condition may be either primary or secondary. The aetiology of **primary glaucoma** is not known. The common causes of **secondary glaucoma** include inflammation, neovascularisation, pigment dispersion syndrome and drugs.

Fig. 70.1 shows the pathways for secretion and drainage of aqueous humour in the anterior chamber of the eye.

Classification of antiglaucoma drugs: refer in Box 70.5. *Before starting the treatment, drugs (e.g. atropine like) as a cause of increased IOP should be ruled out.*

Elevated IOP may be reduced by:

- *Increasing the outflow of aqueous humour* through:
  a. The trabecular meshwork (cholinergic agonists and cholinesterase inhibitors)
  b. The uveoscleral pathway (PG analogues)
  c. A surgically created pathway
- *Decreasing the production of aqueous humour by the ciliary body* (Box 70.5)

In acute (narrow angle) congestive glaucoma, the iris probably blocks the entrance to the trabecular space at the canal of Schlemm. This blockade causes a precipitous increase in IOP and severe pain, headache, nausea and often loss of vision due to optic atrophy. *The reversible anticholinesterases are invaluable for reducing the increased IOP.* The contraction of sphincter of iris induced by the anticholinesterases removes the iris blockade and facilitates the drainage of the intraocular fluid. Acute congestive glaucoma is a medical emergency and **a combination of pilocarpine nitrate (4%), timolol and apraclonidine** is the preferred treatment. Adjuvants such as acetazolamide, preferably sustained release capsules (a carbonic anhydrase inhibitor) are also employed (Chapter 37). In an emergency, 20% mannitol (maximum 500 mL) may be infused intravenously to lower the IOP. Once the acute attack is controlled, definitive surgery is advised. Even after surgery, continuation of drug therapy may be required.

***Chronic open angle glaucoma** has an insidious onset and needs lifelong drug therapy.* The cause of raised IOP is not known. Because the decline in vision is gradual, the diagnosis is often delayed. The mechanism of reduction of tension in this condition by drugs is not definitely understood; there is no physical obstruction.

Box 70.5 Drugs Used in Glaucoma

1. **Those which increase the outflow of aqueous humour**
   - ***Cholinergic agonists (miotics)***
     Pilocarpine drops 0.25%–4.0%[a]
     Pilocarpine ocusert
   - ***Cholinesterase inhibitors (miotics)***[b]
     Physostigmine 0.25% ointment[b]
     Demecarium 0.125%–0.25% drops
     Echothiophate 0.03%–0.25% drops
   - ***Prostaglandin analogues***
     Latanoprost 0.005% drops
     Bimatoprost 0.01%
     Unoprostone 0.15%
     Travoprost 0.004%
     Tafluprost 0.0015%
     Latanoprostene bunod 0.024%
   - ***Rho kinase inhibitor***
     Netarsudil 0.02% solution, Ripasudil 0.4% solution
2. **Those which decrease the production of aqueous humour by the ciliary body**
   - ***Nonselective beta-adrenergic blockers:***
     Timolol 0.25%–0.5 % drops
     Levobunolol 0.5%
     Carteolol 1%
   - ***Selective beta1-adrenergic blocking agents***
     Betaxolol 0.5% drops
     Metipranolol 0.3%
   - ***Nonselective adrenergic agonists***
     Adrenaline hydrochloride 0.1%–2.0% drops
   - ***Selective alpha2-adrenergic agonists***
     Apraclonidine 0.5%–1% drops
     Brimonidine 0.2% drops
   - ***Carbonic anhydrase inhibitors***
     a. *Topical:* Brinzolamide 1% suspension, dorzolamide 2%
     b. Systemic: Acetazolamide 250 mg q.i.d.; methazolamide 25 mg b.i.d.
   - ***Combinations of above agents***
     Brinzolamide + brimonidine
     Timolol + brimonidine
     Timolol +dorzolamide
     Latanoprost + timolol
     Latanoprost + netasurdil

[a]For details, see Chapter 19.
[b]Now used rarely.
All eye drops except PG analogues are generally used twice daily; PG analogues are used once daily in the evening.

The **major goals of therapy** are:

a. To maintain an IOP below which further optic nerve damage is unlikely to occur.
b. To reset the IOP to a lower level if deterioration occurs.
c. To minimise the local and systemic side effects of the drugs, and to improve the quality of life.
d. To educate the patient about his/her disease and emphasise the importance of compliance.

In general, the initial aim is to achieve a 20%–50% reduction in the IOP at diagnosis, with the least amount of medication. The PG analogues, e.g. **latanoprost** are usually the drugs of choice to start with because of their once-a-day dosage, fewer systemic effects and good therapeutic efficacy. Prostaglandin analogues increase uveoscleral flow through their action on FP receptors (for $PGF_{2\alpha}$) but precise mechanism is still unknown. The recently introduced **Latanoprostene bunod** contains a NO donating moiety, which relaxes cytoskeleton in trabecular meshwork along with usual increase in uveoscleral flow. However, *they are expensive.*

Alternatively, a beta-adrenergic blocker **timolol** may be used. Selective beta blockers are less effective as the beta receptors of the eye (ciliary epithelial) and vessels are beta-2. Beta blockers decrease the aqueous humor production by decreasing cAMP generated through adrenergic activation. They decrease ocular blood flow, and thereby decrease the ultrafiltration.

The α_2 adrenergic agonists appear to be less effective than the above two and are used if there is any intolerance or contraindications to beta blockers or prostaglandin analogues. They stimulate presynaptic α_2 receptors and decrease NE flow and through postsynaptic α_2 receptors they stimulate Gi pathway and decrease cAMP. Both these mechanisms lead to decrease in aqueous humour production. They may also increase uveoscleral flow. **Apraclonidine** is ionised at physiological pH and therefore cannot cross biological barriers to cause adverse effects. **Brimonidine** is lipophilic and can easily penetrate cornea and other biological barriers to cause adverse effects. It should be avoided in children for fear of respiratory arrest.

Netarsudil inhibits the NA transporter. It is also a potent Rho-associated kinase (ROCK) inhibitor. Rho kinase is involved in maintaining the patency of trabecular meshwork. Both the mechanisms together, increase trabecular outflow, decrease aqueous humour production and reduce episcleral venous pressure. It is available as a 0.02% ophthalmic solution for once-daily topical application. It is as effective as timolol but is very expensive.

Ripasudil is another Rho-kinase inhibitor.

Topical carbonic anhydrase inhibitor preparations, **dorzolamide** and **brinzolamide,** cause less systemic toxicity and are preferred to oral acetazolamide. Inhibition of carbonic anhydrase in the ciliary body epithelium reduces the bicarbonate ions and therefore aqueous humor production. The latter is used in resistant cases in the dose of 0.25–1.0 g daily, in 3–4 divided doses.

All the above-mentioned agents are available also in combination e.g. beta blockers and prostaglandin analogs or carbonic anhydrase inhibitors and α_2 agonists. Such combinations decrease the instillation burden and is more acceptable.

Reversible anticholinesterases give fairly satisfactory results in glaucoma following cataract surgery. They are avoided in patients with cataract because they may impair vision further; the long-acting miotics may exacerbate cataract and increase the risk of complications (retinal detachment) during and after cataract surgery. *Sufficient transconjunctival absorption of anti-ChE drugs can occur following their repeated instillation and can cause systemic adverse effects.* Absorption can be minimised by digital compression of the inner canthus of the eye during and after instillation.

If topical therapy fails then systemic therapy with a carbonic anhydrase inhibitor may be used. Sustained release acetazolamide formulations are better tolerated. The other options are laser or incisional surgery.

Pilocarpine is now less often used because of its short duration of action and ADR. The ADR are because of myopia and refraction changes due to spasm of ciliary muscles.

Beta-adrenergic blockers may cause cardiovascular and respiratory adverse effects. PG agonists may cause increase in growth of eyelashes, irreversible darkening of the iris and rarely macular oedema.

Finally, it is important to remember that lowering of IOP may not necessarily halt the progression of the disease and damage to the optic nerve in all cases of glaucoma.

IMMUNOSUPPRESSIVES AND ANTIMITOTIC DRUGS — PH 1.50

5-Fluorouracil and **mitomycin-C** are used in ophthalmic practice (a) to limit scarring after certain types of surgical procedures and (b) in certain systemic diseases such as Wegener granulomatosis and Behçet disease with life threatening ocular manifestations.

The mediator of neovascularisation in wet age-related macular degeneration (AMD) is believed to be VEGF. It causes angiogenesis and increased vascular permeability.

VEGF inhibitors act by binding to VEGF receptors. They are as follows:

BEVACIZUMAB: This humanised mAb, an angiogenesis inhibitor (Chapter 59), is reported to prevent further loss of vision in AMD and diabetic macular oedema. It is administered *intravitreally,* once a month for 3 months initially, and then as required.

RANIBIZUMAB: This derivative of bevacizumab, specially tailored for intraocular use, is also an angiogenesis inhibitor. It does the same thing as the parent drug in AMD, but at a very high cost.

Pegatenib: A selective VEGF antagonist and **verteporfin,** an inhibitor of choroidal neovascularisation are the recently approved drugs for AMD.

Aflibercept: This is a fusion protein. It is claimed to be as effective as ranibizumab.

All these agents are administered intravitreally. They can cause pain, conjunctival haemorrhage and endophthalmitis.

Vitreomacular adhesion, a progressive ageing disorder, causes vitreomacular traction, retinal distortion and macular oedema. It can be managed with intravitreal injection of **ocriplasmin,** a recombinant selective proteolytic enzyme, which cleaves extracellular matrix proteins resulting in their dissolution.

Lifitegrast (*5% solution*) inhibits an integrin, lymphocyte function– associated antigen 1 (LFA-1), from binding to intercellular adhesion molecule 1 (ICAM-1), which downregulate inflammation mediated by T lymphocytes and used in dry eye.

LOCAL ANAESTHETICS PH 1.17

These agents are used topically to anaesthetise the ocular surface:

1. To remove foreign bodies from the cornea and conjunctiva.
2. Prior to tonometry.
3. For pre-operative preparation. Usually, **proparacaine** and **tetracaine** are used.
4. In the manipulation of the nasolacrimal system (**tetracaine** or **lignocaine**)
5. During the use of excimer laser for surgery for refractive errors (**tetracaine**)
6. For infiltration and retrobulbar block anaesthesia (**lignocaine** and **bupivacaine;** Chapter 16)

Local anaesthetics should never be used for management of ocular pain.

DIAGNOSTIC AGENTS

The dyes fluorescein and rose bengal are the most commonly used diagnostic agents for anterior and external lesions of the eye. Both are available as 2% alkaline solutions and as impregnated paper strips.

Fluorescein is preferred for detecting epithelial defects (due to foreign body) in the cornea and the conjunctiva, and leakage of aqueous humour that may occur after trauma or surgery. It is also used to test the patency of the nasolacrimal system.

Rose bengal stains devitalised tissue of the cornea and the conjunctiva, and helps to detect tears in those structures.

In the posterior segment of the eye, fluorescein and **indocyanine green** are used for retinal angiography. They may cause nausea and may precipitate allergic reactions.

MISCELLANEOUS AGENTS

Wetting agents and tear substitutes: Many systemic and local diseases damage/disrupt the precorneal tear film, leading to 'dry eyes'. The discomfort may be relieved symptomatically by using either:

a. Artificial tears which are aqueous, hypotonic or isotonic solutions containing **sodium chloride** and **hydroxymethyl cellulose;** or
b. Ophthalmic lubricants which are complex, viscous formulations, including ointments. Appropriate treatment of any systemic, causative disease is important.

Table 70.1 Some Drugs Causing Ocular Toxicity

Drug	Ocular Toxicity
Ethambutol	Optic neuritis
Chloroquine	Retinopathy
Chlorpromazine	Retinal pigmentation
Chloramphenicol	Retinal pigmentation
Aminoglycosides	Optic neuritis
Sildenafil	Blue vision
Antimuscarinics	Glaucoma
Vigabatrin	Visual field constriction
Tamoxifen	Visual field constriction, cataract
Digoxin	Scotoma
Alendronate	Conjunctivitis, iritis
Glucocorticoids	Posterior subcapsular cataract

DRUG-INDUCED OCULAR TOXICITY

Some drugs used in therapeutics (Table 70.1) can cause ocular toxicity.

It must be remembered that the three major causes of blindness in developing countries are vitamin A deficiency, trachoma and onchocerciasis, all of which are preventable. They are discussed elsewhere.

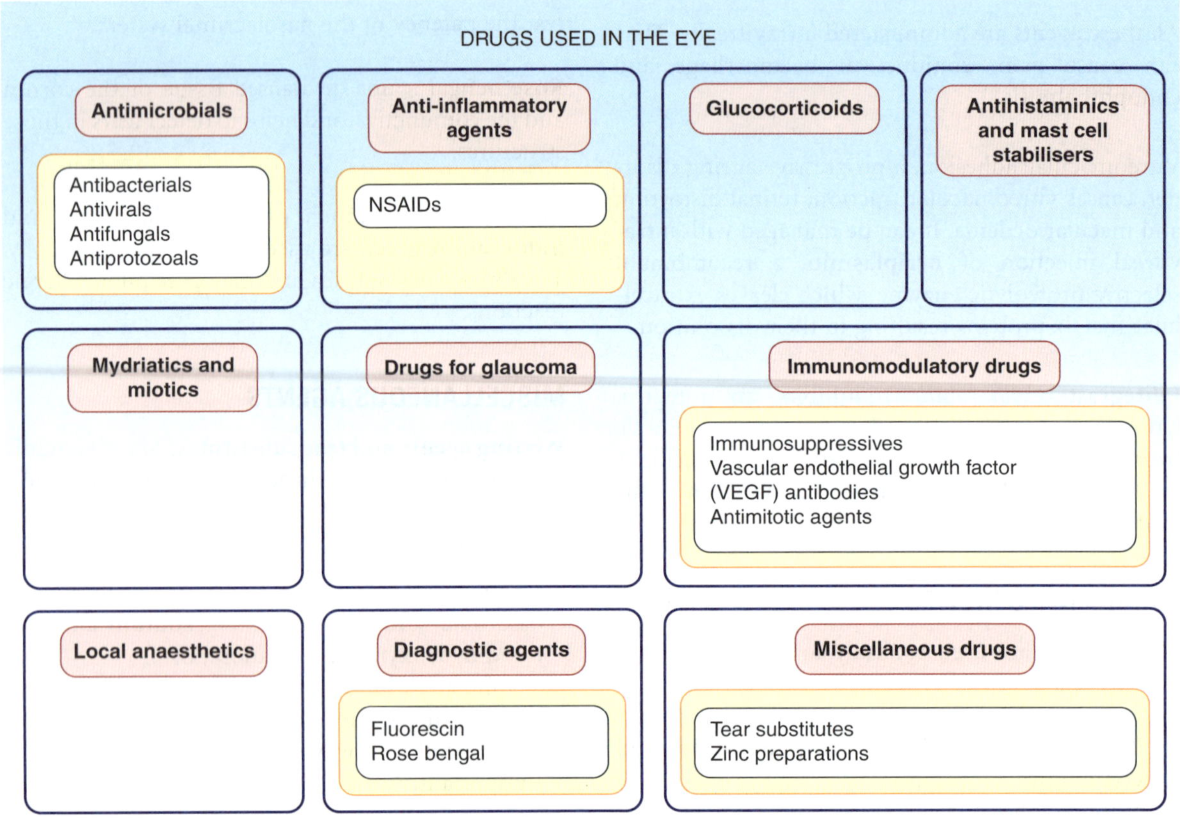

ANTI-INFECTIVE DRUGS USED IN THE EYE

Antibacterials as single agents

Chloramphenicol 0.5% S, 1% O
Ciprofloxacin 0.3% S
Norfloxacin 0.3% S,O
Ofloxacin 0.3% S
Levofloxacin 0.5%, 1.5% S
Moxifloxacin 0.5%S
Besifloxacin 0.6% S
Gatifloxacin 0.3% S,O
Erythromycin 0.5% O
Azithromycin 1% S
Gentamicin/tobramycin 0.3% S,O
Sulphacetamide 10% S
Tetracycline 1% S

Antibacterial combinations

Bacitracin + Polymyxin B (500U–10,000 U/g)
Trimethoprim (1mg/ml) + Polymyxin B (10,000 U/ml)

Antiviral

Acyclovir 3% O; 400–800 mg tab oral
Ganciclovir 0.15% gel
Valacyclovir 500–1000mg tab oral,
Famciclovir 125-500 mg oral tab
Valganciclovir 450 mg oral tab
Foscarnet IV, intravitreal
Cidofovir IV
Idoxuridine 0.1% S
Vidarabine 3% O
Trifluridine 1% S

Antifungal

Amphotericin B 0.1%–0.5% S; 0.8–1.0 mg subconjunctival; 5 mcg intravitreal/intracorneal/intracameral
Natamycin 5% S
Fluconazole oral
Ketoconazole oral
Miconazole 5–10 mg subconjunctival
Voriconazole 50 μg intracorneal and intracameral, oral, IV

S: solution; O: Ointment

MYDRIATICS AND MIOTICS

Mydriatics

Antimuscarinic
Atropine 0.5%–2% drops
Homatropine 2%–5% drops
Eucatropine 2%–5% drops
Cyclopentolate 0.5%–2% drops
Tropicamide 0.5%–2% drops

Sympathomimetic
Phenylephrine 0.12%–10% drops

Miotics

Cholinomimetic
Pilocarpine 0.5% drops; ocusert
Acetyl choline 1% Solution,
Carbachol 0.01% solution

Cholinesterase inhibitors
Physostigmine 1% drops

DRUGS USED IN THE TREATMENT OF GLAUCOMA

Those which increase the outflow of aqueous humour

Cholinergic agonists (miotics)
- Pilocarpine drops 0.25%–4.0%
- Pilocarpine ocusert

Cholinesterase inhibitors (miotics)
- Physostigmine 0.25% ointment
- Demecarium 0.125%–0.25% drops
- Echothiophate 0.03%–0.25% drops

Prostaglandin analogues
- Latanoprost 0.005% drops
- Bimatoprost 0.01%
- Unoprostone 0.15%
- Travoprost 0.004%
- Tafluprost 0.0015%
- Latanoprostene bunod 0.024%

Rho kinase inhibitor
- Netarsudil 0.02% solution
- Ripasudil 0.4% solution

Those which decrease the production of aqueous humour by the ciliary body

Nonselective beta-adrenergic blockers
- Timolol 0.25%–0.5 % drops
- Levobunolol 0.5%
- Carteolol 1%

Selective beta1-adrenergic blocking agents
- Betaxolol 0.5% drops
- Metipranolol 0.3%

Nonselective adrenergic agonists
- Adrenaline hydrochloride 0.1%–2.0% drops

Selective alpha2-adrenergic agonists
- Apraclonidine 0.5%–1% drops
- Brimonidine 0.2% drops

Carbonic anhydrase inhibitors
- *Topical*
  - Brinzolamide 1% suspension
  - Dorzolamide 2%
- *Systemic*
  - Acetazolamide 250 mg q.i.d.
  - Methazolamide 25 mg b.i.d.

Combinations of above agents
- Brinzolamide + brimonidine
- Timolol + brimonidine
- Timolol + dorzolamide
- Latanoprost + timolol
- Latanoprost + netasurdil

15
SECTION

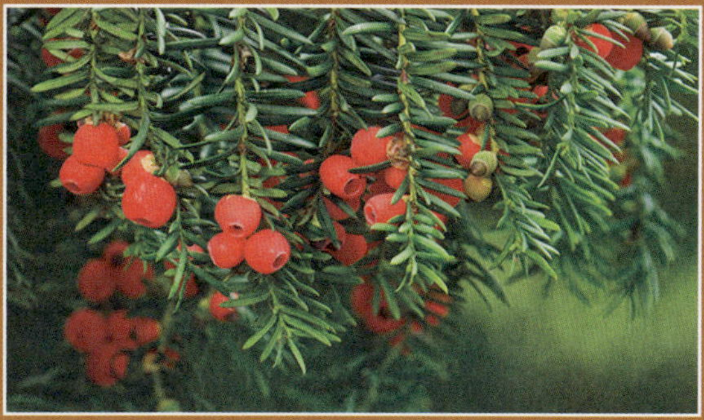

Taxus brevifolia

Immunopharmacology

Section Outline

This section consists of the following chapters:

CHAPTER 71

General Considerations: Vaccines and Antisera

Learning Objectives

This chapter will enable the reader:

1. To be aware of functions of different components of the immune system.
2. To differentiate between active and passive immunity.
3. To enumerate the various immunological agents used to induce/bolster immunity.
4. To compare and contrast vaccines and sera.
5. To explain the terms, toxoids, nucleic acid vaccines, immunoglobulin (Ig).
6. To enlist various vaccines and toxoids with their immunisation schedule.
7. To state the different formulations, indications, ADR and dosage schedule of commonly used bacterial, viral and rickettsia vaccines and toxoids.
8. To state the National Immunisation Schedule.
9. To enlist the principles of active immunisation.
10. To state the commonly used sera and immunoglobulin preparations with their indications and ADR.
11. To outline the drug therapy of snake bite and scorpion sting.

KEY TERMS

pneumococcal vaccine, p. 1069
Sabin vaccine, p. 1067
human diploid cell inactivated vaccine, p. 1071
COVID-19 vaccines, p. 1072
tetanus toxoid, p. 1074
tetanus immunoglobulin, p. 1077
rabies immunoglobulin, p. 1077
anti-D immunoglobulin, p. 1078
anti-snake venom serum, p. 1079
anti-scorpion venom serum, p. 1080

The 'fight or flight' response by an animal to external danger preserves its integrity at the macrolevel but its safety from bodily invasion (external, by microbes; or internal, by errant native cells) at the microlevel and survival depends upon an efficient **immune system**. This is a complex system with genetic, cellular and molecular arms, which decide the immune response, commonly inflammation. Such responses are usually beneficial as they protect the body, but occasionally they can be detrimental to the host, e.g. allergy (Chapter 2).

Normal immune system has three main components:

1. Antigen receptors that recognise infinite range of organisms
2. Immune memory
3. Immunological tolerance that helps to avoid immune damage to normal tissue

Antigens may be classified as 'self' and 'nonself or foreign' molecules that trigger the immune cells to produce a response. Antigens in 'dysregulated' tissues (tumours) can also be regarded as foreign. **Immunity** may be defined as the ability of an animal's body to react to a foreign antigen and eliminate it, in the interest of safety of the animal.

The **immune system** consists of two divisions:

- **The innate immune system**, which is a primitive immune recognition system.
- **The adaptive immune system**, which is a recently evolved system of immune responses. It is found only in vertebrates.

Cells of the **innate immune system** include natural killer (NK) cells, macrophages, dendritic cells, neutrophils, basophils, eosinophils, tissue mast cells and epithelial cells. *They recognise and destroy foreign antigens and pathogens without prior exposure.* The recognition of pathogen molecules by the cells leads to activation of the complement cascade, and production of cytokines, and antimicrobial peptides as effector molecules that lead to slowing of infection. It has low affinity.

In contrast, the **adaptive immune system** is characterised by *antigen-specific responses* to a foreign antigen or pathogen. Unlike innate (immediate) immunity, it generally takes several days to develop. An important feature of this system is immunological memory for the antigen so that a subsequent exposure to the same antigen causes a rapid and vigorous immune response. It has high affinity.

The adaptive immune system consists of dual limbs of cellular and humoral immunity (Fig. 71.1). The main effectors of this immunity are lymphocytes which get activated after they recognise a specific antigenic determinant (**epitope**). These lymphocytes are of two types:

1. **T lymphocytes,** with several subtypes
2. **B lymphocytes**

T lymphocytes (thymus-derived) are called so because, after they arise in the bone marrow, are processed in the thymus. B lymphocytes are called so because of their relation to the bursa of Fabricius, a lymphoid organ similar to thymus, present in chicken.

When a foreign antigen enters the body, the following responses may occur (Fig. 71.1):

- *It may be recognised as foreign by the innate immune system and be destroyed.*
- *The antigen may be taken up by macrophages as well as dendritic cells and presented to a T cell,* which can recognise an epitope on the antigen. The T cell then proliferates into a cluster of T cells identical with the parent T cell (**clone of T cells**). These clones may be of several types:
  a. **Cytotoxic** (directly destructive of the antigen as well of tissue cells)
  b. **Helper** (which enhance immune response)
  c. **Suppressor** (which inhibit immune response)

The activated T cells secrete a variety of cytokines (Chapter 25) which regulate the inflammatory response as well as T cell function. Furthermore, the cytokines lead to a more effective activation of B lymphocytes (see below) by antigens. Several cytokines and cytokine receptors have been identified.

The various subtypes of T lymphocytes (cytotoxic, helper and suppressor) and their responses collectively constitute **cell-mediated immunity** (CMI). Furthermore, as mentioned above, the T cells **regulate humoral immunity,**

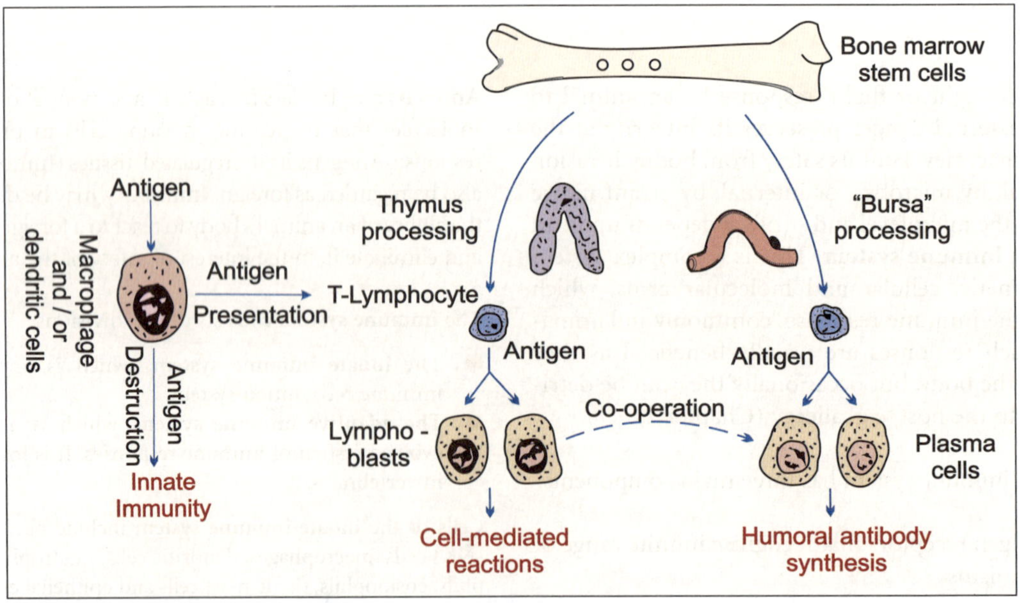

FIG. 71.1 Innate immunity and processing of bone marrow cells by thymus and gut-associated central lymphoid tissue to become immunocompetent T and B lymphocytes, respectively. Proliferation and transformation to cells of the lymphoblast and plasma cell series occurs on antigenic stimulation. Modified from *Essential Immunology* by Ivan Roitt. Courtesy of Blackwell Scientific Publications and author.

primarily a B lymphocyte function, though they themselves do not secrete antibodies.

The antigen may be recognised by a specific receptor on the surface of a B lymphocyte: The B lymphocytes are concerned with the synthesis of circulating antibodies and hence with the **humoral immunity**.

Antibodies are **B cell–produced molecules** (encoded by genes) in response to the presence of foreign substances (**antigens or immunogens**; antigens which stimulate IgE production are called **allergens**). The antibodies exist on B lymphocyte surface as antigen-recognition molecules or as secreted molecules in the plasma and body secretions. They are globulins, designated as **immunoglobulins** or Ig. Five major groups have been defined in man. They are IgG, IgA, IgM, IgD and IgE. IgG is the main immunoglobulin class (Table 71.1). Apart from their role in body's defence mechanism, certain antibodies (IgE) also have other properties such as fixing to basophils and mast cells (**homocytotropic or reaginic antibodies**), which can cause unpleasant and dangerous ADR.

The two important features of the immunological responses are as follows:

- **Specificity** that is the ability to recognise and respond to a particular antigen
- **Memory** that is the ability to recognise and respond more vigorously to an antigen encountered for the second or subsequent time

Immunity is subdivided into (1) *active immunity* and (2) *passive immunity*.

Active immunity: This type of immunity is due to the development of antibodies by the individual himself. It can be natural and species specific, e.g. the relative immunity of horses, dogs and rats to tuberculosis, or it can be acquired by introduction of an antigen.

Passive immunity: Immunity **acquired by the transfer of antibodies from a donor to a recipient**, is called passive immunity. It can be acquired naturally, e.g. by a fetus receiving maternal antibodies across the placenta, or artificially by the administration of antisera containing Ig antibodies.

The immune cells learn at an early stage in fetal life how to discriminate between self and foreign antigens, and do not attack the former. Serious consequences may follow if that ability is impaired or lost at any time in life so that the immune cells attack and damage the host's own

Table 71.1 Biological Properties of Human Immunoglobulin Classes

Property	IgG	IgA	IgM	IgD	IgE
Molecular weight	46,000	160,000	970,000	184,000	188,000
Serum concentration (mg%)	1250	280	120	0.3–30	0.002–0.2
Plasma half-life (days)	23	6	5	3	3
Found in	Internal body fluids	Seromucosal secretions, colostrum, saliva, tears, GI tract	Serum	On lymphocyte surface	On the surface of mast cells and basophils
Physiological role	Main Ab against infection; immunity against microbes in tissues and extravascular spaces	Mucosal immunity	Main intravascular Ab, important role in immunity in circulation	Role in B cell maturation	Immunity against helminthic infection
Injurious	Arthus reaction, serum sickness	Impaired mucosal immunity, autoimmune disorders	Arthus reaction, serum sickness	Anti-D antibodies in Rhesus incompatibility	Local and systemic anaphylatic reaction

Notes: Ab, antibody. IgG alone crosses the placenta.

tissues (**autoimmune disease**) e.g. rheumatoid arthritis, type I diabetes mellitus, systemic lupus erythematosus (SLE), multiple sclerosis (MS); however, immune system is actively and beneficially suppressed during pregnancy.

Clinically, when a foreign agent invades the body, it reacts with immune system in the form of inflammation. The inflammatory response is characterised by pain, swelling, redness and warmth at the site of tissue damage/infection. It is accompanied by the recruitment of various cells, and release of cytokine and mediators of inflammation (Chapter 25), resulting in fever, body ache, malaise and loss of appetite. Usually such immune responses act as body defence, and rapidly counter the causative agent (e.g. pathogens), preventing the tissue damage and promoting repair. *Occasionally the immune response is abnormal, not beneficial, giving rise to phenomena such as allergy, autoimmune disease or graft rejection.* In case of infection, it can become chronic.

In practice immunological agents are used to induce/bolster immunity. The various preparations employed for conferring immunity are as follows:

1. **Vaccines:** They are employed prophylactically to stimulate the immune system of the recipient. This results in primary immune response in form of CMI, e.g. BCG vaccine or humoral immunity from protective antibodies, e.g. typhoid vaccine. The antibody response occurs after 7–10 days. Initially, antibodies are of IgM type, followed later by IgG antibodies, which are produced in high concentrations, and are mainly responsible for resistance to infection. When the individual gets exposed to a pathogen, a rapid secondary immune response is generated. This results in rapid elimination of the organism and protection from the clinical disease. **Thus, they confer active immunity.** *Vaccines are of no value if administered during the incubation period or in the active stage of a disease.*

Classification of Vaccines

PH 1.54

I. **First generation:**
   a. **Inactivated vaccine:** These are suspensions of killed microorganisms. The bacteria or viruses, which are grown in culture are killed using either heat or formaldehyde. However, their membrane/wall antigens or the virus capsid proteins remain intact enough to be recognised by the immune system and evoke a response. These vaccines cannot generate specific killer T cell responses. There is a need to give periodic booster doses to reinforce the immune response. e.g. killed bacterial vaccines are typhoid vaccine, cholera vaccine, and killed viral vaccines are rabies vaccine, Salk polio vaccine.
   b. **Live attenuated vaccines:** These are suspensions of attenuated but live microorganisms, which have low disease-causing ability but comparable antigenicity. They engage specific tissue for site of action, e.g. intestinal mucosa by oral polio vaccine and induce cytotoxic T cell responses, T_H responses and humoral responses. Hence, **they are antigenically superior to the inactivated vaccines.** A single dose is usually sufficient to achieve almost lifelong immunity; the exception is polio vaccine, which requires three or more doses. Some examples of live attenuated vaccines are typhoid oral vaccine, BCG vaccine, oral polio vaccine, measles vaccine, and epidemic typhus vaccine.

II. **Second generation:** These are products or derivatives of microorganisms and include toxoids and cellular fractions of microorganisms. They are also termed as **subunit vaccines.**
   a. **Toxoids:** Toxoids are manufactured by addition of formalin to the toxins of microbes and incubating them at 37°C for 3–4 weeks. **This results in loss of toxicity without reduction of the antigenicity.** The antibodies produced against these antigens then act against specific toxins. The examples are diphtheria and tetanus toxoids.
   b. **Cellular fractions:** These contain purified pieces of a pathogen. They are specifically selected because they are most capable of stimulating immune system. Use polysaccharide antigen of cell wall, e.g. meningococcal vaccine, or of capsule, e.g. pneumococcal vaccine, *Haemophilus influenzae* type b (Hib) vaccine, or polypeptide of surface antigen, e.g. hepatitis B vaccine. Recombinant protein components used for these vaccines induce T_H and antibody responses, but not cytotoxic T cell responses. The purified fragments are not capable of inducing disease and hence

these vaccines are safer but they are complex to manufacture.

III. **Third generation:** These are nucleic acid-based vaccines, including DNA (as plasmids) and RNA [as messenger RNA (mRNA)] vaccines. DNA vaccines are genetically engineered by inserting a gene encoding antigens into a bacteria-derived plasmid. They induce both humoral immunity and CMI including cytotoxic T cell response, e.g. ZyCoV-D, covid vaccine.
They produce the antigen over long periods, and exhibit sustained immune response. They do not require adjuvants. mRNA vaccines use a synthetic version of viral mRNA. When delivered to the cells, it is translated to produce some viral proteins. These proteins do not assemble to form virus but the immune system recognises them to produce antibodies e.g. the Covid vaccines – Comirnaty, Moderna.
mRNA vaccines are non-infectious, undergo cellular degradation and are safe. They are highly efficacious. They are synthetic and their manufacturing does not take time.
To ensure the safe delivery of mRNA vaccine nanoparticle based system has been used. One of the Covid vaccines (Covovax) is a nanoparticle based vaccine, in which a strand of genetic code (mRNA) that can produce spike protein is enclosed in nanoparticles. This protects it from early lysis and controls its release and uptake offering targeted delivery. The genetic material remains stable long enough to reach the target site to produce proteins. The immunogenicity of such vaccines is higher (Table 71.5).

2. **Sera and Igs:** They **provide passive immunity**, which is short lasting as memory response is not generated. However, they **provide immediate protection.**
   I. **Immune animal serum (antiserum):** This is the serum obtained from animals like horse and rabbit which have been injected with a vaccine, toxin or a toxoid. The sera of such animals contain antibodies either against the microorganisms or their toxins, e.g. antisera against the toxins of *C. diphtheriae, C. tetani, C. welchii* and against snake venom or scorpion venom. There is a risk of hypersensitivity, and therefore sensitivity testing is a must regardless of previous exposure.
   II. **Immune human serum:** This is derived from convalescent, immune or hyperimmunised adults, e.g. human hyperimmune anti-Ebola virus serum.
   III. **Ig (human):** This is a refined product prepared from pooled human plasma having a high antibody titre and termed as normal human Ig. One of the leading products obtained by fractionation of plasma is IVIG. It can cross the placental barrier. **Specific Igs (human-specific Ig)** are procured from the donors who have high titres of the desired antibodies (see Chapter 72).
3. **Immunostimulants:** Levamisole, thalidomide, lenalidomide (Chapter 72), interferons (Chapter 57), human recombinant interleukin-2 (Aldesleukin, Chapter 25), BCG (Chapter 52).
4. **Monoclonal antibodies:** These are antibodies produced by a single clone of B cells. They target various proteins present on the surface of normal and cancer cells that influence cell activity (see Chapter 72). Of these, ipilimumab binds to cytotoxic T lymphocyte-associated antigen 4 (CTLA-4) and blocks its inhibitory effect on CLTs. Thus, it activates the immune system against cancer, especially advanced melanoma.

ACTIVE IMMUNISATION

This may be primary or secondary.

- **Primary immunisation** is commonly carried out in infants and in children to induce primary immunity and consists of administering two or more doses of the vaccine or the toxoid at suitable intervals. Combinations of multiple vaccines/toxoids are now available for primary immunisation.
- **Secondary immunisation** is carried out **to reinforce the primary immunity** by giving a single 'booster' or 'recall' dose of the antigen.

All vaccines and antisera should be stored at temperature recommended by the manufacturer. Usually the storage temperature is 2–8°C. Polio and measles vaccines must be stored in freezer.

Multidose vials without any preservative, once opened, should be used within 1 h and those with a preservative within 3 h.

Adverse reactions to vaccines are generally mild and are as follows:

- Local/general reactions related to injection: consist of local pain, tenderness, erythema, induration, fever, arthralgia and malaise.

In adolescents fainting/syncope is commonly observed, which is triggered by anxiety or pain. It is advisable to observe the recipient for at least 15 min after vaccination.

- **Allergic reactions**: may occur. Any vaccine produced from the organisms grown in chick embryo culture is contraindicated in patients allergic to eggs, chicken or chicken feathers. Allergic reactions can also occur due to other components such as preservatives, antibiotics and stabilisers like gelatin used during vaccine manufacturing.

Many viral vaccines contain traces of antibiotics, e.g. neomycin in MMR, trivalent IPV, and varicella vaccine. They have to be withheld from individuals known to be allergic to the antibiotic concerned.

- Vaccines should be avoided in individuals on corticosteroid therapy or immunosuppressive drugs and in those with impaired immune responses.

Corticosteroids induce immunosuppression that reduces the ability to respond to a killed vaccine or enhance the susceptibility to live vaccines which could result in disseminated disease. **Live virus vaccines are usually avoided during pregnancy for fear of infecting the fetus;** however, such risk has not been substantiated.

- **Specific reaction:** There may be reactions specific to vaccines, though they are rare.

Generally, vaccines (particularly those containing live organisms) are not administered in individuals with:

- Severe acute illness
- Debilitating diseases
- Agammaglobulinaemia
- Immunocompromisation (leukaemia, lymphoma, malignancy)
- Immunosuppressive therapy or radiotherapy

Although vaccination may be avoided during severe acute illnesses, mild upper and lower respiratory tract infections and other mild illnesses are no more considered as contraindications. In fact, it is now recommended that children with minor illnesses should be vaccinated regardless of the degree of fever. Prematurity does not increase the incidence of vaccine-induced adverse reactions. No dose reduction/delayed vaccination is needed for premature babies.

VACCINE ADJUVANTS: In order to increase the immunogenicity and duration of protective effects of vaccines, certain substances are added to the vaccine preparations, which are termed as vaccine adjuvants. They stimulate the innate immune system. Aluminium hydroxide or aluminium phosphate, monophosphoryl lipid A, MF59 (an oil-in-water emulsion of squalene oil), AS03 (α-tocopherol and squalene in an oil-in-water emulsion) are some of the vaccine adjuvants. Subunit vaccines need such adjuvants as they are immunogenically weaker.

VACCINE PRESERVATIVES: Agents like 2-phenoxyethanol, benzethonium chloride, phenol or thimerosal are used to kill or inhibit the growth of bacteria and fungi that could contaminate a vaccine vial, especially of multidose vial. Reactions to vaccines can be due to its preservatives.

The vaccines and toxoids employed for active immunisation are listed in Tables 71.2 and 71.3. **Dosage schedules recommended by the manufacturer should be followed.** The vaccines used in the National Immunisation Schedule are described below.

BCG VACCINE: Discussed in Chapter 52.

POLIOMYELITIS VACCINES: The **Salk vaccine** (IPV with trivalent fully inactivated virus) induces serum immunity on IM or SC administration but does not offer intestinal immunity. Thus, the recipient of IPV is protected from polio but serves as a

Table 71.2 Bacterial Vaccines, Toxoids and Rickettsial Vaccines

Vaccine/Toxoid	Immunising Agent	Route	Adverse Reactions	Efficacy and Remarks
		Bacterial vaccines		
BCG	Live attenuated *M. bovis*	ID	Fever; regional adenitis	75%–80% against miliary and meningeal TB; controversial in other forms
Pertussis	a. Inactivated bacterial antigen b. Acellular	IM	Local reaction	80%–90%; combined with diphtheria and tetanus vaccines – DPT
Typhoid oral (typhoral)	Live mutant bacilli Ty2IA	Oral	Mild GI disturbance; fever	50%–70%
Typhoid (Vi)	Vi capsular polysaccharide	IM; SC	Local reaction	70%–75%; single dose per course
Typhoid conjugate	Polysaccharide of Ty2 conjugated to TT	IM	Local reaction, fever, allergic reaction	T-dependent antibody responses, for infants and children ≤2 years, 98.05% seroconversion
Cholera (oral)	Whole cell killed (El tor strain)	Oral	None	Two doses, 2 weeks apart; 50%; protection 3 years
Plague	Inactivated bacteria	IM	Fever; swelling	90% antibody response; efficacy variable
Anthrax	Inactivated, avirulent bacteria	SC	No serious reaction	90% antibody response; efficacy variable
***H. influenzae* type B (Hib)**	Bacterial poly-saccharide	IM; SC	Local reactions	90%; not beyond 6th birthday
Meningococci A, C, Y, W135	Bacterial polysaccharide alone/conjugated with proteins	SC; IM	Local reactions	90%; given after 2nd birthday
MenB	Inactivated four components of meningococcal group B bacteria	IM	Fever, loss of appetite, sleepiness	For children ≥10 years and adults with risk of developing meningitis
Pneumococci PPSV23	Capsular polysaccharide, unconjugated	IM; SC	Local reactions	60%–80%
PCV13	Conjugated	IM	Local reactions	>90%
		Bacterial toxoids		
Diphtheria	Inactivated toxins	IM	Local reactions	95%–98% } Can be avoided
Tetanus	Inactivated toxins	IM	Local reactions	95%–98% } Can be avoided
		Rickettsial vaccine		
Typhus vaccine	Killed organisms	SC	Allergic reactions	High

Notes: ID, intradermal; SC, subcutaneous; IM, intramuscular.

reservoir for the excretion of live virus in faeces. Adverse effects are usually mild and consist of local pain, induration and fever.

The **Sabin vaccine** (oral poliomyelitis vaccine with attenuated strain [OPV]), given orally provides systemic immunity as well as a local resistance (intestinal immunity) to reinfection by the poliovirus by inducing mucosal secretion of IgA antibodies. This leads to stoppage of faecal excretion of the virus and consequent elimination of the carrier state. It is effective and inexpensive.

It is important to complete the primary immunisation before the age for greatest risk of poliomyelitis. *Hence, the recommendation is to give the first dose of*

Table 71.3 Viral Vaccines

Vaccine/Toxoid	Immunising Agent	Route	Adverse Reactions	Efficacy and Remarks
Viral vaccines				
Varicella (chickenpox)	Live attenuated virus	IM	Local reaction	95%; CMI lasts longer
Measles	Live attenuated virus	SC	? Encephalopathy	95% } Given as MMR or MR
Mumps	Live attenuated virus	SC	Parotitis	90% } Given as MMR or MR
Rubella	Live attenuated virus	SC	Arthralgia	95% } Given as MMR or MR
Poliomyelitis:				
Sabin (trivalent, oral OPV)	Live attenuated virus	Oral	Rare, vaccine associated polio	95%; may eliminate carrier state
Salk (IPV)	Inactivated virus	SC	Local reaction	95%; does not affect carrier state
Hepatitis A	Inactivated virus Live attenuated (H2 and L-A-1 strains)	IM	Fever; arthralgia Hypersensitivity	95%, two doses of inactivated hepatitis A vaccine given 6 months apart provides better seroprotection than one dose live attenuated vaccine in children and adults; it lasts for 10 years
Hepatitis B rDNA	rDNA antigen	IM	None	80%–95%
Yellow fever	Live attenuated virus	SC	Neurological	High; life long
Japanese B encephalitis	Live attenuated SA14-14-2 virus Inactivated (killed) Vero cell–derived using an Indian strain of JE virus Purified inactivated SA14-14-2 virus	SC	Allergic reactions	Seroprotection rate 67.2% after 1 month, 43.1% after 1 year.
Influenza (Trivalent/Quadrivalent)*	Inactivated virus; or virus component	IM	? Neurological	40%–60%; efficacy varies due to changes in the infective strain
Rotavirus	Live attenuated vaccine	Oral	Diarrhoea	95% BRV-PV is thermostable
HPV	Bivalent, quadrivalent and multivalent	IM	Syncope, injection site pain and reactions	Equieffective for anogenital cancers Protection lasts for 5–10 years
Rabies	See text and Table 71.4			
Herpes zoster	– Live, attenuated zoster vaccine (LZV) – Recombinant vaccine (RZV)	SC SC	Redness, soreness, swelling, or itching at the site of the injection; headache and rarely, the live vaccine can cause herpes-like rashes	Indicated in all adults age > 50 years LZV: Single dose of 0.65 ml RZV : Two doses at 0 and 2-6 months. RZV is preferred as it can be administered to individuals with past history of Herpes or administration of LZV

Notes: ID, intradermal; HPV, human papilloma virus.
*Also available as ID and nasal spray.

OPV (along with BCG) at birth, followed by three more doses at 6, 10 and 14 weeks of age. A booster dose of OPV is given at 16–24 months. Repeated **mass vaccination with OPV** up to the age of 5 years is also recommended (**Pulse Polio Immunisation**). As a result of such programme, India has been declared as polio-free nation.

Due to eradication of type-2 polio virus, the trivalent polio vaccine (tOPV, containing types 1, 2 and 3 of polio virus) has been switched to bivalent OPV (bOPV containing types 1 and 3) since April 2016.

WHO recommends combined protocol of using OPV with IPV. It has been shown that IPV at fractional dose (one-fifth the usual dose, fIPV) given intradermally is cost-effective. The National Immunisation Programme uses the combined approach using two doses of fIPV, which offers higher immunogenicity than one full IM dose of IPV.

HEPATITIS B VACCINE: This vaccine contains hepatitis B virus surface antigen (HBsAg) produced by recombinant DNA technology. Adequate immunity against the infection develops after 6 months and lasts 5–7 years. The dose delivered at birth prevents perinatal transmission of HBV and subsequent doses to infants are expected to provide long-lasting immunity. It is available as monovalent or in combination with other vaccines (pentavalent or with hepatitis A vaccine).

PNEUMOCOCCAL VACCINE: Pneumococcal disease among children below 5 years accounts for nearly 20% of global pneumonia deaths. Vaccines can prevent death and illness. These are available as unconjugated pneumococcal polysaccharide vaccine (PPSV23) and conjugate vaccine (PCV13). The former is a capsular polysaccharide of 23 serotypes, whereas the latter is of 13 serotypes. PPSV23 has expanded spectrum but its efficacy is limited, whereas PCV13 shows robust immune response and memory. PCV, though expensive, has been introduced in immunisation schedule since 2017 in certain selected states. For individuals with high risk to invasive pneumococcal disease, both should be given one year apart.

ROTAVIRUS VACCINE: Rotavirus infects the intestines of virtually all children by the age of 3 years. A pentavalent, human–bovine reassortant rotavirus vaccine (BRV-PV) is now available. It is effective and safe. The oral vaccine is administered in three, monthly doses from the age of 6–12 weeks to the age of 32 weeks. It may cause mild diarrhoea or vomiting in some children. It can be given concurrently with other vaccines.

TYPHOID VACCINE: Several effective and safe typhoid vaccines are now available. Live attenuated vaccine (TY21a, mutant strain of *Salmonella enterica* serovar Typhi) is available as gelatin capsule, **to be taken orally** every other day as a single capsule 1 h before eating, for a total of four doses. Capsules are to be refrigerated. It provides protection for 5 years. Generally, it is well tolerated. Sachets are also available.

Parenteral vaccines include monovalent typhoid vaccine (Vi polysaccharide as a single dose), capsular polysaccharide vaccine (Vi antigen prepared from the surface polysaccharide of *Salmonella* Typhi strain Ty2, ViCPS, as a single dose), conjugate vaccines (TCV wherein Vi antigen is coupled to a carrier protein like TT). TCV has better immunogenicity and provides protection for 5 years after a 0.5 mL of single dose. It can be used for infants from 6 months of age. **Subsequent booster dose of typhoid is not recommended.**

MMR VACCINE: The contraindications to MMR vaccine (Table 71.3) include children with altered immunity and those on high doses of corticosteroids or immunosuppressants. It is avoided in children who have received another live virus by injection within the past 3 weeks. If it is given to an adult woman, pregnancy should be avoided for a month; the vaccine should not be given within 3 months of an Ig injection.

It is advocated in immunisation schedule in private sector.

JAPANESE ENCEPHALITIS (JE) VACCINE: JE is caused by a flavivirus transmitted by *Culex* mosquitoes and is characterised by brain inflammation with high fever. It is the leading cause of acute encephalitis syndrome (AES). The available vaccines are (1) **inactivated (killed) Vero cell–derived vaccine** prepared from an Indian strain of JE virus, (2) **purified**

inactivated (killed) vaccine that uses the SA 14-14-2 strain of JE virus, (3) **cell culture–derived** (Vero cells as well as primary hamster kidney) live, attenuated vaccine using SA 14-14-2 strain. Recently, a recombinant attenuated chimeric virus vaccine has been developed, which is safer for use as a booster dose in children.

HAEMOPHILUS INFLUENZAE TYPE B (Hib) VACCINE: Vaccination against Hib bacteria prevents over one-third cases of pneumonia and 90% cases of meningitis and reduces incidences of bacteraemia, epiglottitis, septic arthritis, etc. Hib vaccine is a part of National Immunisation Schedule, wherein it is administered as three doses, a month apart (6, 10 and 14 weeks) as a combination pentavalent vaccine with DTwP and hepatitis B. There is no booster dose recommended.

INFLUENZA VACCINE: In India there is round the year circulation of influenza serotype B virus that peaks during rainy season and winter, which accounts for high morbidity and mortality in high-risk groups. These include elderly (($\geq$65 years of age), children below 5 years, persons with comorbid conditions, immunocompromised patients, medical practitioners and pregnant women irrespective of duration of pregnancy. Both **trivalent** (two A subtype viruses, H1N1 and H3N2, and only one of the B subtype virus, Victoria lineage) and **quadrivalent** (two A virus strains and two B virus strains, Victoria and Yamagata) vaccines are available. Influenza vaccination is most effective when circulating viruses are well-matched with vaccine viruses and that time efficacy is 70%–80%. It takes 2–3 weeks to develop immunity. Annual dose of vaccine is needed.

HUMAN PAPILLOMA VIRUS (HPV) VACCINE: HPV group of viruses are responsible for **anogenital cancers** (uterine cervix, anus, penis, vulva, vagina and oropharynx) and **genital warts**. HPV vaccines now available have virus-like particles (VLP) having resemblance to HPV cuspid proteins, which are immunogenic. All are equieffective and are considered to be safe. Bivalent and quadrivalent vaccines are available in India. Both protect against anogenital cancers and precancerous lesions, while quadrivalent vaccine offers protection against genital warts. They are administered intramuscularly to girls/women between the ages of 9 and 26 years in three doses, the second and the third being given 2 and 6 months after the first dose. Multivalent vaccine protects against 7 HPV types causing cancer and 2 HPV types causing genital warts. All the vaccines are prohibitively expensive.

RABIES VACCINES: Rabies occurs commonly after the bite of an infected animal such as a dog. Rabies virus can be found in the animal saliva for up to 7 days before the appearance of signs of illness. Rabies infection can also occur without direct animal contact, by inhalation of the virus in bat-infested caves or in the laboratory. Although the usual incubation period is 4–6 weeks, a range of 5 days to more than 1 year has been reported.

In endemic areas, it must be emphasised that a bite is not necessary for transmission of the virus and that children must be guarded against contact with unknown animals.

In unvaccinated patients, the mortality from rabies is almost 100%. PH 1.52

Pre-exposure prophylaxis is required for those handling rabies virus and animals and working in wildlife areas, and also for those living in or travelling to endemic/high-risk regions. Hospital staff attending a patient who is highly suspected of, or known to be suffering from, rabies should be offered pre-exposure prophylaxis. **Post-exposure prophylactic treatment is started immediately in all cases with suspected bite or scratch of an animal.** *The course may be discontinued if it is proven that the animal is still alive and healthy 10 days after the bite or is negative for rabies by laboratory technique.*

It has been demonstrated that immediate thorough washing of the wound with soap/detergent and water alone increases the survival by almost 50%. Local dressing with povidone-iodine, ethyl alcohol/methylated spirit is recommended. **Passive immunisation with antiserum/Igs should be done along with vaccination** (see under the section, Rabies Antiserum and Immunoglobulins).

Table 71.4 Suggested Regimens for Various Rabies Vaccines PH 1.52

Vaccine Type	Pre-Exposure Treatment	Post-Exposure Treatment
1 HDCV 1 mL vial	Three, 1 mL doses intramuscularly in deltoid on days 0, 7 and 21 or 28 Booster dose only if neutralising antibody titre at 6 months is <0.5 IU/mL	Five doses intramuscularly in deltoid on days 0, 3, 7, 14 and 28 Or Two sites IM on day 0 and one site IM on days 7 and 21
2. PCECV 1 mL vial	IM doses as above Or 0.1 mL intradermally on 0, 7, and 21 or 28 days	IM doses as above Or 0.1 mL per ID site and on two sites per visit (one on each deltoid area, an inch above the insertion of deltoid muscle) on days 0, 3, 7 and 28
3. PVRV 0.5 mL and 1 mL vial	Doses similar to PCECV	Doses similar to PCECV
4 PDEV 0.5 mL vial	IM doses as above	IM doses as above

Notes: HDCV, human diploid cell vaccine; PCECV, purified chicken embryo cell vaccine; PVRV, purified Vero-cell vaccine; PDEV, purified duck embryo vaccine; ID, intradermal.
For infants and young children, anterolateral area of the thigh is used as vaccination site.
Rabies vaccine should never be administered in the gluteal area as lower neutralising antibody titres are observed following injection at this site.

The rabies vaccine produced using brain tissue (Semple vaccine) is no longer used due to neurological complications. The current rabies vaccines available are cell culture or embryonated-egg origin. They provide better antibody response with longer lasting immunity. They are more effective (>95% protection) and are well tolerated. The ADR are mild and include local pain, erythema, swelling and pruritus. Occasionally, systemic reactions like malaise, generalised aches and headaches are reported. The available vaccines are:

1. **Cell culture vaccines (CCV)**
   a. **Purified chick embryo cell vaccine** (PCECV): This vaccine (e.g. Rabipur, Vaxirab-N) is obtained by growing the virus in primary cultures of chick fibroblasts.
   b. **Human diploid cell inactivated vaccine** (HDCV): This is obtained from human fibroblast culture (e.g. Rabivax).
   c. **Purified Vero-cell vaccine** (PVRV) is grown in Vero-cell line (e.g. Verorab, Indirab, Abhayrab).
2. **Embryonated egg-based vaccines (EEV)**
   a. **Purified duck embryo vaccine (PDEV):** This vaccine (e.g.Vaxirab) uses duck embryo cells as substrate.

Various vaccine regimens recommended are given in Table 71.4. The vaccines are given by IM or ID route. **Currently, in India only PCECV and PVRV have been approved for ID administration.** It is essential to refer to vaccine package leaflet to confirm the route for pre- or post-exposure prophylaxis.

Rabies Ig is not required for persons who have previously received a complete pre- or post-exposure vaccination. They should be administered two booster doses of vaccine, one on the day of exposure and the other 3 days later.

SARS-CoV-2 Vaccines

A number of COVID-19 vaccines have been developed globally. These include viral-vectored, protein subunit, nucleic acid (DNA, RNA), live attenuated and inactivated vaccines. The initial focus of these vaccines was on providing acquired immunity against severe acute respiratory syndrome corona virus 2 (SARS-CoV-2) and thereby preventing symptomatic, often severe illness and decreasing mortality. However, immunity from the vaccines has been found to wane over time, requiring people to

Table 71.5 COVID-19 vaccines

Vaccine	Type	Age group & Dosing	Adverse effects	Protective Efficacy
Covaxin	Whole-Virion Inactivated SARS-CoV-2 Vaccine	Age > 6 years, Two doses,0.5 mL each on day 0 and day 28 IM.	Local Pain/Swelling, Fever, Headache, Irritability.	79% in adults less than 60 years, and in those above 60 years it is 68%. Efficacy against severe disease is 93%.
Covishield	Recombinant, replication-deficient chimpanzee adenovirus vector vaccine encoding the spike glycoprotein	Age ≥ 18 years, Two doses 0.5 mL each 4-6 weeks apart, IM.	Fever, Local Pain/ Swelling, headache, Irritability.	67% against symptomatic COVID & nearly 100% against severe disease, beginning 21 days after 2nd dose.
Sputnik V	Combined viral vector with Component I and II – Component I: Recombinant adenovirus serotype 26 particles containing the SARS-CoV-2 protein S gene – Component II: Recombinant adenovirus serotype 5 particles containing the SARS-CoV-2 protein S gene	Age ≥ 18 years, Two doses, 0.5 mL each on Day 0 (component I), Day 21 (component II), IM.	Nausea, dyspepsia, loss of appetite. Very rare – enlarged regional lymph nodes , Allergic reactions, Elevated LFT, CPK, Creatinine Vertigo, sore throat, sleep disorder; decreased Hematocrit, Neutrophil count, MCV also reported	Efficacy of 97.6%
Spikevax (Moderna)	mRNA	Age ≥ 18 years, Two doses, Day 0 and day 28, IM	Local pain/swelling, fever, loss of appetite.	94.5% efficacy Approved but not purchased by Indian Government
Jcovden (Janssen)	Non-replicating viral vector	Age ≥ 18 years Single dose, 0.5mL, IM.	Local Pain, fever, headache, fatigue, very rarely risk of blood clot (e.g. cerebral venous sinus thrombosis, splanchnic vein thrombosis, arterial thrombosis)	Single dose efficacy 72%. Efficacy of 94% with two doses, 2 months apart.
ZyCoV-D	Recombinant DNA-plasmid-based vaccine	For ≥ 12 years, Each dose has 3 shots 0.1 mL on day 0 and day 28 ID; to be used with Pharmajet device only.	Local Pain/swelling, headache, nausea, fever, fatigue, myalgia.	66.6% Efficacy against symptomatic COVID. 100% protection against moderate or severe disease.

Table 71.5 COVID-19 vaccines

Vaccine	Type	Age group & Dosing	Adverse effects	Protective Efficacy
Corbevax	Recombinant receptor-binding domain protein subunit (part of the spike protein)vaccine	For ≥ 5 years, Two doses, 0.5 mL day 0 and day 28, IM	Local pain/swelling, fever, headache, myalgia, fatigue, arthralgia, urticaria.	Over 90% efficacy – Can be used in immuno-compromised patients – Approved for a COVID-19 heterologous booster shot. To be administered 6 months after two doses of Covisheild or Covaxin for all adults
Covovax	Recombinant spike protein Nanoparticle	Age ≥ 7 years, Two doses, 0.5 mL each on day 0 and day 28, IM.	Local pain/swelling, fatigue, headache, myalgia, arthralgia, and nausea, vomiting	89% efficacy
Sputnik Light	Viral vector First component (recombinant human adenovirus serotype number 26 – rAd26) of Sputnik V	For ≥ 18 years Single Dose 0.5 mL IM	Local pain, oropharyngeal pain, nasal congestion, rhinorrhoea, sore throat, fatigue, headache, myalgia, fever.	80% efficacy against COVID-19 (all variant) 70% efficacy against Delta variant.
Gemcovac-19 (HGCO-19)	mRNA Self-amplifying RNA (or "saRNA")	Age ≥ 18 years Two doses, 0.5 mL each on day 0 and day 28, IM	Local site reactions, fatigue, headache, fever, myalgia, rarely, Influenza like illness	Efficacy data unavailable – First RNA vaccine from India – SaRNA replicates itself on administration and therefore very small dose is required. – Stable at refrigerator temperature
iNCOVACC	Recombinant replication deficient adenovirus vectored vaccine	Age ≥ 18 years Intranasal, Two doses, 0.5mL (8 drops, 4 drops in each nostril) each on day 0 and day 28	Systemic: Headache, fever, myalgia, fatigue, nausea and vomiting Local: Rhinitis, sore throat, lacrimation	Efficacy data unavailable – T cell response + IgG and mucosal IgA – Multi-Dose vials to be used within 6 hours and stored at 2 to 8ºC – Satisfactory response against several variants (Delta, Beta, Omicron and BA.5) – Suitable for mass immunisation
Vaxzevria	Non-replicating viral vector	Age ≥ 18 years, Two doses 4-6 weeks apart, IM.	Injection-site pain, headache, nausea	76.0% efficacy 22days after the first dose, and 81.3% after the second dose 61% against the Delta variant

get booster doses of the vaccine to maintain protection against COVID-19. Similarly the original virus has undergone mutations and some of the mutants are also virulent e.g. Omicron variant. Hence attempts have also made to develop bivalent vaccines to protect against the original strain and its mutants. Many countries implemented phased distribution plans that prioritized those at highest risk of complications, such as the elderly, and those at high risk of exposure and transmission, such as healthcare workers. Common adverse effects of COVID-19 vaccines include soreness, redness, rash, inflammation at the injection site, fatigue, headache, myalgia and arthralgia.

The first vaccine developed against COVID-19 was Comirnaty (by Pfizer Ltd), which was a mRNA vaccine. Its protective efficacy is 95% but it is expensive. Being a mRNA vaccine it requires ultra-cold storage. Its use in India for mass vaccination was difficult and it was not made available in our country. However, Indian Government extended support to Indian pharmaceutical companies to develop vaccines and first two vaccines that made available to Indians were Covishield (Oxford-AstraZeneca vaccine, manufactured under license by Serum Institute of India) and Covaxin (first indigenously developed by Bharat Biotech in collaboration with the Indian Council of Medical Research [ICMR] and the National Institute of Virology [NIV]). The former uses adenovirus vector while latter uses inactivated virus. Since then 11 vaccines are available in Indian market. Their details are presented in Table 71.5. All these vaccines were made available to the public through emergency authorizations / conditional approval during the COVID pandemic.

TETANUS TOXOID: After the full course of seven doses (Table 71.6), booster doses are given every 10 years. Td (TT with reduced dose of diphtheria) can replace TT.

Hypersensitivity reactions are known to occur due to high concentrations of the antibody in persons given too frequent booster doses.

During pregnancy, two doses of TT or Td (0.5 mL IM upper arm) are administered at 4 weeks' interval, at first contact or as early as possible, **to women not previously immunised; this prevents neonatal tetanus.** The third dose is given 6 months later. If there is a history of receiving TT in previous 3 years, then one dose is enough. If immunisation history is unknown, at least two doses of TT or Td are given in second or third trimester. Tdap should preferably be given between 27 and 36 weeks of pregnancy **to protect the newborn against pertussis through maternal antibodies.** A dose of TT or Td may be replaced by Tdap. It may be given regardless of last dose of TT or Td.

DIPTHERIA, TETANUS AND PERTUSSIS VACCINES

These are available as those containing whole cell pertussis vaccine (DTwP) or acellular pertussis (DTaP). Efficacy of both the vaccines in preventing pertussis in the first year is similar. But after this period, immunity wanes rapidly and impact on transmission is inferior with DTaP. Though DTwP is superior in terms of immunogenicity and duration of protection, it is more reactogenic. When used in the immunisation schedule, after three primary doses and a booster dose after a year, both vaccines confer protection for 6–12 years and hence either can be used.

DTwP, hepatitis B and Hib are available in combination as pentavalent vaccine; the latter is used in the National Immunisation Schedule. PH 1.55

Universal Immunisation Programme of India

The recommended National Immunisation Schedule is given in Table 71.6. In this schedule, in addition to vaccines, vitamin A has been introduced (see Chapter 77).

The neonate is naturally immune to a majority of infections because of maternal antibodies; such immunity, however, may last for only the first 6–10 months. The newborn does not have any immunity against tuberculosis. Immunoprophylaxis is recommended right from birth so as to build up a substantial active immunity against a number of viral and bacterial infections, within the first few months of life. **Ideally, the aim should be to achieve the goal of >90% vaccination coverage by the 2 years of age.** Subsequently, the antibody titre can be maintained/augmented by the 'booster doses' of

Table 71.6 Immunisation Schedule of Universal Immunisation Programme PH 1.55

Age	Vaccine
Birth	BCG (0.05 mL ID, left upper arm), OPV$_0$ (2 drops oral), hepatitis B$_0$ (0.5 mL IM anterolateral side of left mid thigh)
6 weeks	OPV$_1$, fractional IPV$_1$ (0.1 mL ID on right upper arm), Pentavalent vaccine$_1$ (0.5 mL IM, anterolateral side of left mid thigh), PCV$_1$ (0.5 mL IM anterolateral side of right mid thigh), Rotavirus$_1$[a] (5 drops oral)
10 weeks	OPV$_2$, Pentavalent vaccine$_2$, Rotavirus$_2$[a]
14 weeks	OPV$_3$, fractional IPV$_2$, Pentavalent vaccine$_3$, PCV$_2$, Rotavirus$_3$[a]
6 months	**Typhoid$_1$**[b] (0.5 mL IM upper arm/ anterolateral side of mid thigh, 6 months onwards)
9–12 months	Measles/MR$_1$ (0.5 mL SC right upper arm or **MMR**$_1$), JE$_1$[c] (0.5 mL SC left upper arm), PCV-B, **MCV$_1$, hepatitis A$_1$** (at 12 month; 0.5 mL IM)
15 months	**Varicella$_1$**[d] (0.5 mL SC)
16–24 months	DTwP-B$_1$ (0.5 mL IM, anterolateral side of left mid thigh), OPV B, **MR 2** or **MMR$_2$**, JE$_2$[b], **Hib B$_1$, fractional IPV B**
18 months	**Hepatitis A$_2$**
2–3 years	**MCV**
5 years	DTwP B$_2$, **OPV$_5$B, Varicella$_2$, MMR**
10 years	TT/**Tdap/Td**, **HPV (to girls)**[e], **PCV**
16 years	TT/**Tdap/Td**

Source: National Immunisation Schedule 2017 and Indian Academy of Paediatrics Immunisation Timetable 2018.

Notes: Vaccines in bold – additional vaccines recommended by IAP. Tdap preferable to TT/Td.

BCG if not given at birth, then up to 1 year, 0.1 mL after 1 month; hepatitis B within 24 h of birth; OPV, oral polio vaccine; OPV$_0$ can be given up to 15 days after birth; IPV, inactivated polio vaccine; PCV, pneumococcal conjugate vaccine in select states; MR, measles – rubella. IAP recommends use of MMR, mumps, measles, rubella; JE, Japanese encephalitis; MCV, meningococcal vaccine, second dose to be given after 3 months; Second dose of varicella vaccine can be given 3 months later; TT, tetanus toxoid; Tdap, TT, reduced dose diphtheria, acellular pertussis; Td, TT, reduced dose diphtheria; MMR, mumps, measles, rubella; HPV, human papilloma virus vaccine; *B*, booster.

[a]2–3 doses based on brand at 4–8 weeks' interval, phased introduction in selected states.

[b]Typhoid conjugate vaccine (Typbar-TCV, 25 mcg); can be given with MR.

[c] Introduced in 230 selected endemic districts.

[d]If started above 13 years, give two doses 4–8 weeks apart.

[e]0, 1–2 and 6 months.

Box 71.1 Principles of Active Immunisation PH 1.1

- Use only a properly stored vaccine.
- A vaccine should be injected intramuscularly into the lateral aspect of the thigh in infants.
- Killed or live vaccines do not affect the safety of breastfeeding.
- In infants, immunisation should not be postponed because of mild respiratory infections, diarrhoea or low-grade fever.
- In premature infants, vaccination should be carried out as per the usual schedule.
- Many vaccines can be safely and effectively given simultaneously, e.g. pneumococcal polysaccharide vaccine with whole virus influenza vaccine. But, two different vaccines should not be mixed in a syringe for administration. Use premixed vaccine, if available.
- *Avoid all vaccines* in the first trimester.
- *Avoid live virus vaccines* in women who are pregnant or are likely to become pregnant within 3 months.
- *Avoid live vaccines* in immunocompromised persons also. They may be administered 3 months after stopping corticosteroids and 6 months after stopping cancer chemotherapy.
- If a vaccine and Ig are to be administered concurrently, each should be administered at a separate site. Live vaccine avoided with Igs; Igs given 2 weeks after live vaccine; Live vaccine 12 weeks after Igs.
- If two live virus vaccines are to be given, they should be given on the same day at two separate sites, or at least 30 days apart. The response to tuberculin test may be hampered by live virus vaccines and therefore, a gap of 4–6 weeks should be maintained.
- Health care workers should be immunised against hepatitis B, measles, rubella, influenza and varicella.

antigens at regular intervals. The principles of active immunisation are given in Box 71.1.

Simultaneous active and passive immunisation may be necessary because of imminent exposure to disease. There is little interaction between IgG and inactivated or nonlive vaccines, e.g. HIV and hepatitis B IgG. *With* **live virus vaccines,** *e.g. measles vaccine immunity may be compromised by IgG administration;* so vaccination should be repeated after 3 months, unless specific antibodies are demonstrable on serological testing. However, OPV and yellow fever vaccines are not affected by IgG administration at any time.

PASSIVE IMMUNISATION

The first Nobel Prize in Medicine was awarded to immunologist Emil von Behring in 1901, for his work on serum therapy against diphtheria. This passive immunisation showed a new mode of treating diseases apart from drugs.

Passive immunisation involves the administration of antibodies in the form of serum, plasma or Ig to a person who is exposed to infection but in whom the disease has not yet developed.

It provides readymade antibodies against the organisms; such immunity, however, is short lived. Passive immunisation is often associated with allergic reactions including fatal anaphylaxis. Some authorities use adrenaline, glucocorticoids and an antihistaminic prophylactically with the hope of preventing such serious reactions. **The current trend, however, is to use homologous antibody preparations and concentrated Igs.**

It is advisable to determine if the patient is allergic to the antiserum before giving an injection of an antiserum regardless of whether or not he has received it previously.

The **intradermal test** dose is 0.01 mL of a 1:100 dilution of the serum, injected intradermally. **In subjects with a history of allergy, it should be reduced to 0.02 mL of a 1:1000 dilution.** The test is considered as positive if a wheal develops within 30 min. In the **scratch test**, one drop of a 1:100 dilution of the test serum in saline is applied to a superficial scratch on the skin. A positive reaction consists of erythema and wheal formation. For the **conjunctival (eye) test**, one drop of a 1:10 dilution of serum in normal saline solution is put into one eye; one drop of normal saline alone is instilled into the other eye as a control. The patient is considered allergic, if the treated eye shows lacrimation and conjunctivitis within 30 min. The **intradermal skin test** is performed if the conjunctival or scratch test is negative.

A patient **who is allergic** but needs the antiserum can be desensitised by injecting small, graded doses of the antiserum. Thus, the following doses are injected either subcutaneously or intramuscularly generally at 15 min intervals under supervision; **the next dose is injected if there is no reaction to the previous one:**

- 0.05 mL of 1:20 dilution, subcutaneously
- 0.1 mL of 1:10 dilution, subcutaneously
- 0.3 mL of 1:10 dilution, subcutaneously
- 0.1 mL of undiluted serum, subcutaneously
- 0.2 mL of undiluted serum, intramuscularly
- 0.5 mL of undiluted serum, intramuscularly

Finally, the entire remaining dose is injected intramuscularly. In case of anaphylaxis 0.5 mL of adrenaline 1:1000 is injected intramuscularly (less dose in children) and repeated if necessary (see Chapter 22).

The important antisera available are as follows:

DIPHTHERIA ANTITOXIN (DAT): This is a serum preparation from the horse, actively immunised against *C. diphtheriae.* It contains the antitoxin globulins, which neutralise the diphtheria toxin at the site of infection and that circulating in the blood. However, it is probably ineffective in neutralising the toxin fixed to the tissues.

It forms mainstay of treatment of diphtheria. Clinically diagnosed mild to moderately severe cases should be administered 10,000–30,000 units intramuscularly. *In all severe cases, doses up to 100,000 units are recommended, of which a portion is given intramuscularly, and the rest intravenously 1.5–2 h later.* The IM injection should be given in the lateral aspect of the thigh. *In no case should the IV dose precede the IM dose,* and it should not be resorted to in individuals with an allergic diathesis or a family history of allergic disorders.

The use of **penicillin** and **erythromycin** in diphtheria is discussed in Chapter 44.

TETANUS ANTITOXIN: This is a serum preparation from the horse, actively immunised against the toxins of *C. tetani.* It contains the antitoxin globulins.

In areas where tetanus is almost endemic, severely contaminated or deep penetrating wounds should be treated with wound toilet, antitetanus serum (ATS) and a course of an antibiotic to give the maximum protection. ATS is also given when the person having contaminated wound is not immunised or his/her immune status is not known. **Clean wounds or small abrasions or lacerations may be treated without**

ATS. *A second dose of ATS, in a patient who has received ATS once before, is very rapidly eliminated and hence, is ineffective.* In such cases, active immunisation should be started at once.

A single large IV dose of ATS is used in the treatment of proven or suspected tetanus, **if human tetanus immunoglobulin (TIG) is not available.** *Ideally TIG is preferred to ATS.*

The ideal thing to do is to immunise everyone in the country with pre-exposure tetanus toxoid injections. In such individuals, post-exposure prophylaxis is also with tetanus toxoid. This is safer and economical.

HUMAN TETANUS IMMUNOGLOBULIN (TIG): This preparation contains specific gamma globulin prepared from human plasma having a high titre of tetanus antitoxin. Such plasma is obtained from blood of hyperimmunised subjects or from placentas of mothers who have received tetanus booster inoculations a few weeks before delivery.

The half-life of human immune globulin is 3–4 weeks. Its **prophylactic dose** for wounds of average severity is 250–500 IU, IM Active immunisation with tetanus toxoid should be carried out simultaneously. It is also used in proven or suspected cases in the dose of 500–10000 units given intravenously. Serious adverse effects are rare.

BOTULINUM ANTITOXIN (BAT): This is a heptavalent horse serum preparation, containing the antitoxin globulin fragments [Fab and $F(ab')_2$], which neutralises the neurotoxins formed by *Clostridium botulinum,* types A, B, C, D, E, F and G (HBAT).

It is indicated for the treatment of symptomatic foodborne or wound botulism or suspected exposure to botulinum serotypes.

For effective treatment, it must be administered in the very early stage of botulism (within 24 h after onset of symptoms) as a single dose. Following a test dose, HBAT 10–20 mL (amount in one vial diluted as 1:10 in normal saline) is administered **by slow IV infusion** at a rate of 0.5 mL/min. Infusion rate is doubled every 30 min, if BAT is tolerated to the maximum of 2 mL/min. The ADR include infusion-related reactions (e.g. chills, fever, difficulty breathing, headache, nausea, vomiting, arthralgia, myalgia, fatigue), acute hypersensitivity reactions (e.g. urticaria, erythema, angioedema, anaphylaxis) and delayed hypersensitivity reactions like serum sickness.

RABIES ANTISERUM AND IMMUNOGLOBILINS: All persons, having single or multiple transdermal bites, scratches or licks on the broken skin, contamination of mucous membrane with saliva and exposure to bats should also receive rabies antiserum/equine rabies Ig (ERIG)/$F(ab')_2$ products/**human rabies Ig (HRIG) before or immediately after the first dose of vaccine.** This passive immunisation with immunoglobulins neutralises the virus at the site of the bite and blocks its progression into the uninfected cells, especially CNS. It also promotes antibody-directed cell-mediated cytotoxicity (ADCC) of infected cells by natural killer cells. The protection starts immediately and lasts till 7–10 days, by the time active immunity develops to rabies vaccine.

If passive immunisation is not possible on the same day due to non-availability, then it can be done until the 7th day of initiation of post-exposure vaccination.

Rabies antiserum is a hyperimmune, horse serum containing the globulins. *Due to possible severe allergic reactions to the rabies horse antiserum, ERIG or HRIG is now preferred.*

ERIG is a highly purified Ig prepared from plasma of hyperimmunised horses. Currently available ERIGs are highly purified **$F(ab')_2$ fragments**. They are likely to cause less ADR than the whole IgG. The dose of ERIG/$F(ab')_2$ products is 40 IU/kg.

HRIG is prepared from plasma of donors hyperimmunised with the rabies vaccine and contains 150 IU/mL. It has longer half-life than ERIG, and therefore its dose is 20 IU/kg IM

The full dose of rabies Ig should be administered into and around the wound site as far as possible. Any remainder should be injected intramuscularly at a site distant from the site of vaccine administration. Dilution of the dose with physiological buffer saline may be needed to cover wound area, if it is too large.

Recently **Rabies Human Monoclonal Antibody (Rabishield)** has been prepared using recombinant DNA technology. It is indicated for post-exposure prophylaxis to prevent rabies infection in people suspected of exposure to the virus. This IgG1 human monoclonal antibody binds to the extracellular G glycoprotein and neutralizes a wide variety of rabies viruses.

The side effects include injection site reactions (such as pain, redness, and swelling), headache, muscle pain, and upper respiratory tract infection. The safety profile is better than other antirabies products which contain blood / serum.

The recommended dose of Rabishield is 3.33 IU/kg . If feasible, the full dose of Rabishield is infiltrated in the wound area if any amount is remaining it is further injected intramuscularly at a site distant from vaccine administration. It is available as 40 IU or 100 IU / ml

HEPATITIS B GLOBULIN: This is immune globulin prepared from the pooled plasma of donors with high titres of antibody to the surface antigen. It is indicated as an IM injection for post-exposure prophylaxis in susceptible individuals who did not receive prior vaccination, or when the hepatitis B antibody level is inadequate (<10 IU/L), e.g. neonates born to mothers who are positive for HBsAg, people having percutaneous or permucosal exposure to contaminated blood, needle stick, sexual contact with an infected patient. It is also used to prevent hepatitis B in people undergoing liver transplant and in haemodialysed patients. The ADR consist of local pain, erythema and tenderness, headache and angioedema. The antibodies persist for 3 months. It has been shown that it does not interfere with immunogenicity of hepatitis B vaccine. Administration of HBIG and hepatitis B vaccine together can produce immediate and sustained high levels of protective antibody against HBsAg.

HUMAN ANTI-D (Rh) Ig (human RhIG): This is prepared from pooled plasma of naturally immunised women with high titre of anti-D antibodies or from the serum of suitably immunised males.

In an Rh-negative woman with an Rh-positive husband, if the fetus is Rh-positive, the fetal erythrocytes may escape into the maternal circulation across the placenta during delivery, and even, rarely during pregnancy. In order to neutralise this antigen before it causes maternal rhesus immunisation and to prevent erythroblastosis fetalis in subsequent pregnancies, it is necessary to give a dose of RhIG, 300 mcg IM preferably within 72 h of delivery. It can be given up to 28 days following delivery. ***Antepartum prophylaxis** may be offered as 2 doses, at 28 and 34 weeks of pregnancy. There are IV preparations of RhIG. The doses of RhIG vary with preparations.*

RhIG is contraindicated in Rh-positive women and in Rh-negative women who develop Rh antibodies because of a previous conception or transfusion of Rh-positive blood.

ADR to RhIG are usually mild and include nausea, headache, dizziness, injection site reactions, rash, malaise and fever.

PH 1.52, IM 20.7

DRUG THERAPY OF SNAKE BITE

Snake bite is common in rural areas of tropical countries. The poisonous snakes belong to three families: (1) **Viperidae** (phoorsa, rattle snake, daboia), (2) **Elapidae** (cobra, krait, mamba) and (3) **Hydrophiidae** (sea snakes).

Venom is injected by the snake using fangs, which are hollow and are connected with the venom glands. Based on the length and characteristics of fangs (long and foldable for viperids and short and fixed for elapids), venom reaches subcutaneous or intramuscular tissues. The **viper venom** commonly kills by its action on the cardiovascular system, though some venoms contain a neurotoxin as well. The **elapid venom** contains mainly a **neurotoxin** which causes muscle paralysis by its neuromuscular blocking action. **Such paralysis is not always reversible with the antivenom, particularly in case of krait bite. However, it is spontaneously reversible after about 2 days.** *Hence, management involves general support such as artificial respiration, intragastric feeding and maintaining vital parameters.* A 20-minute whole blood clotting test (20 WBCT) to detect coagulopathy.

Avoid aspirin or NSAIDs to relieve pain as they may exacerbate bleeding diathesis.

The dangers of poisonous snakebite in human victims appear to be greatly exaggerated. Nearly half of the people bitten by poisonous snakes such as cobra and vipers develop no significant systemic poisoning because of very low dose of the venom injected. Obviously, such patients need no antivenom therapy. *Hence, in doubtful cases it is better to wait and watch the patient carefully for clear clinical evidence of systemic poisoning such as ptosis, limb and neck muscle paresis, blood-stained sputum and failure of the blood to clot, before giving antivenom.* A 20-minute whole blood clotting test (20 WBCT) to detect coagulopathy.

Avoid aspirin or NSAIDs to relieve pain as they may exacerbate bleeding diathesis.

A patient with snake bite must be reassured of prompt medical help and carried to the hospital immediately. He should not be allowed to walk. The affected part is immobilised with splint and bandages to slow venom spread. No tourniquet or cutting or pressure is allowed. Eyes are irrigated with ample water if eyes are exposed to venom. *Continuous monitoring at 10–15 min intervals is needed* for a minimum of 24 hours. One should remember that there may be delayed onset of symptoms, which can worsen rapidly. Attention should be paid to maintenance of airway patency, management of shock and respiratory paralysis and if required, assisted ventilation and intravenous fluids.

Since antivenom can sometimes cause severe reactions, e.g. anaphylaxis, it should be administered only if there are definite signs of envenomation.

Polyvalent, anti-snake venom serum (**ASV, antivenin**) obtained from immunised horses contains the purified antitoxin globulins that have the power of **neutralising the venom of cobra, krait, Russell's viper and saw-scaled viper.** ASV neutralises unbound, free venom and not the toxin fixed to the tissues. Thus, it cannot reverse the damage already caused by the toxin.

No test dose is recommended for ASV because it cannot reliably predict early or late hypersensitivity reactions. Total dose of ASV usually varies between 10 and 30 vials and it remains the same in children or pregnant women. Initially 10 vials are dissolved in 100 mL distilled water or normal saline and then added to 400 mL normal saline or 5% dextrose to be **administered as an IV infusion over 1 h.** Another method is to give slow IV injection (not more than 2 mL/min) Any new symptoms during this period should be considered as reaction to ASV.

Allergic reactions and anaphylaxis are treated by the conventional methods. In high-risk patients (having history of allergic reactions or severe asthma), it is advisable to use prophylactic SC adrenaline (0.1% solution, 1 in 1000, 1 mg/mL), IV antihistaminic and a glucocorticoid simultaneously, and repeat them later, if needed, to protect the patient against allergic reactions. Other ADR include pyrogenic reactions and serum sickness syndrome. The latter can be treated with 5 days course with antihistaminics and if they fail, then with glucocorticoids.

If there is a deterioration of neurotoxicity or cardiovascular signs after ASV, then repeat 10 vials after 1–2 h. In case of haematotoxicity, coagulation test should be done after 6 h; if defect persists, repeat dose should be administered. The repeat doses are given 6 hourly till haemostasis is restored.

For the use of **cholinesterase inhibitor, edrophonium** or neostigmine with atropine, for antagonising neuromuscular blockade in the treatment of snake bite, see Chapter 19.

DRUG THERAPY OF SCORPION STING PH 1.52, IM 20.8

Two types of poisonous species of scorpions are found in India: black scorpion (*Palamneus gravimanus*) and red scorpion (*Mesobuthus tamulus*). The latter is more poisonous and is responsible for a hazardous and potentially lethal condition due to stinging. **The scorpion toxins target sodium, potassium and calcium channels** and cause:

1. **Neuronal excitation and ANS stimulation**
2. **Massive release of adrenaline, NA, vasoactive peptides (endothelins) and neuropeptide Y**

In addition to intense pain at the site of the sting, there is **initially transient cholinergic stimulation followed by a prolonged sympathetic storm due to the sympathetic discharge.** The initial manifestations are vomiting, profuse sweating, excessive salivation, transient hypertension followed by hypotension, bradycardia, priapism and ventricular ectopy. These are followed by hyperglycaemia, tingling and numbness, restlessness, tachypnoea, tachycardia, arrhythmias, pulmonary oedema, and cardiogenic shock.

The treatment depends on observed clinical effects.

- Temporary relief of local pain can be obtained by application of ice packs over the affected part.
- Severe pain is relieved by infiltrating with a local anaesthetic agent (lignocaine *without adrenaline*) and/or with oral analgesic like ibuprofen.
- In case of severe neuromuscular excitation and agitation, oral **benzodiazepines** (diazepam or, if required, midazolam, 0.05–0.1 mg/kg IV bolus followed by 0.1 mg/kg/h infusion) are used.
- **Prazosin** (conventional tablet form and not SR) in the dose of 0.25–0.5 mg (adult dose) orally, repeated 6 hourly till improvement occurs (Chapter 30). The dose for children is 30 mcg/kg). The drug can also be administered through nasogastric tube. Prazosin reduces the mortality markedly (Chapter 18).
- In life-threatening pulmonary oedema, glyceryl trinitrate (10 mcg/min for adults and 1–4 mcg/kg/h for children) by IV infusion under careful monitoring has been recommended.
- Aminophylline IV can also help in management of pulmonary oedema.
- If there is hypotension due to cardiogenic shock, dobutamine (5–15 mcg/kg/min) is a drug of choice.

Anti-scorpion venom serum (AScVS) **against the venom of Indian red scorpion,** manufactured by Haffkine Biopharmaceuticals, Mumbai, is available and has been shown to be effective. It binds to the toxin and prevents them from reaching target sites. It can be administered intravenously. No test dose is required due to high circulating levels of catecholamines which reduces the risk of anaphylaxis. The dose varies from 40 to 80 mL based on the severity of envenomation (as judged clinically). Combination therapy of prazosin with AScVS further improves the survival rate.

The following drugs should be used with caution or avoided in victims of scorpion sting as they are likely to worsen the clinical condition: atropine (used only if there is severe bradycardia associated with hypotension or cardiac decompensation), antihistamines, glucocorticoids, captopril, sodium nitroprusside, digoxin, diuretics and dopamine. Tachyarrhythmias are treated with IV metoprolol or esmolol.

VACCINES

First generation

Inactivated vaccine
- Typhoid vaccine
- Cholera vaccine
- Rabies vaccine
- Salk polio vaccine

Live attenuated vaccines
- Typhoid oral vaccine
- BCG vaccine
- Oral polio vaccine
- Measles vaccine
- Epidemic typhus vaccine

Second generation

Toxoids
- Diphtheria toxoid
- Tetanus toxoid

Cellular fractions
- Meningococcal vaccine
- Pneumococcal vaccine
- *Haemophilus influenzae type b (Hib) vaccine*
- Hepatitis B vaccine

Third generation

Nucleic acid vaccines (Under development)

AGENTS CONFERRING PASSIVE IMMUNITY

Sera and Igs

Immune animal serum (antiserum)
Against the toxins of
- *C. diphtheriae*
- *C. tetani*
- *C. welchii*
- Anti-snake venom
- Anti-scorpion venom

Immune human sera
- Human hyperimmune anti-Ebola virus serum

Immunoglobulin (human) IVIG

Immunostimulants
- Levamisole
- Thalidomide
- Lenalidomide
- Interferons
- Human recombinant interleukin-2 (Aldesleukin)
- BCG

Monoclonal antibodies
- Ipilimumab

RABIES VACCINE

Cell culture vaccines (CCV)

- **Purified chick embryo cell vaccine (PCECV)**
  - Rabipur
  - Vaxirab-N
- **Human diploid cell inactivated vaccine (HDCV)**
  - Rabivax
- **Purified Vero-cell vaccine (PVRV)**
  - Verorab
  - Indirab
  - Abhayrab

Embryonated egg-based vaccines (EEV)

- **Purified duck embryo vaccine (PDEV)**
  - Vaxirab

CHAPTER 72

Immunoglobulins, Monoclonal Antibodies, Immunosuppressants and Immunomodulators

Learning Objectives

This chapter will enable the reader:

1. To be aware of the structure of immunoglobulin.
2. To state the ADR and indications for human normal immunoglobulin and immunoglobulin G.
3. To explain the nomenclature of monoclonal antibodies giving examples and stating their indications.
4. To explain mechanism of action of monoclonal antibodies, their advantages and limitations.
5. To classify immunosuppressants.
6. To describe mechanism of action, ADR and indications for calcineurin inhibitors, glucocorticoids, antiproliferative agents and monoclonal antibodies.
7. To enumerate various immunostimulants/immunomodulators used in clinical practice stating indications for their use.
8. To state the mechanism of action, ADR and indications for thalidomide.

KEY TERMS

IV immunoglobulin-G, p. 1084
monoclonal antibodies, p. 1086
calcineurin inhibitors, p. 1089
sirolimus, p. 1091
mycophenolate mofetil, p. 1092
antithymocytic globulin, p. 1093
thalidomide, p. 1097

Immunoglobulin (Ig) and antibody, the component proteins of immune system, have similar regions in the structure. Immunoglobulins are attached on the plasma membrane of B cells and possess a transmembrane domain while antibodies are found in circulation and are devoid of transmembrane domain. Antibody molecule or immunoglobulin consists of two light and two heavy chains composed of different domains (1) Fab fragment and (2) Fc fragment (Fig. 72.1).

The **Fab fraction of Y shaped structure serves as the antigen-binding site.** The specific antigen-binding properties are conferred by the three dimensional stearic arrangement inherent in the amino acid sequence of the variable region of the light and the heavy chains of the molecule. This portion is called the **idiotypic determinant.** Only one antigenic determinant can have a 'best fit' with this arrangement. Apart from the idiotypic region, the remainder of the molecule, i.e. **the Fc fragment is relatively constant and determines the effector function of the antibody.**

Normally, the total gamma globulins in the plasma vary between 600 and 1500 mg per 100 mL. Total serum gamma globulins in normal Indians are much higher than those in Western people. Patients with **serum gamma globulin concentration of 200 mg or less are considered to be suffering from hypogammaglobulinaemia.**

IgG appears to be involved in the regulation of both allergic and autoimmune reactions, i.e. disease-inducing reactions to foreignness and self, respectively. Although allergy is commonly equated with **IgE-mediated immediate hypersensitivity reaction** (Chapter 2), there is increasing recognition that the undisciplined and even chronic release of cytokines represents a form of allergy that may produce disease. Cytokines such as IL-1, IL-6, interferons alpha and beta and TNF-alpha have an effect both, on the cells of the immune system and on many other cells and body systems from the CNS to the liver.

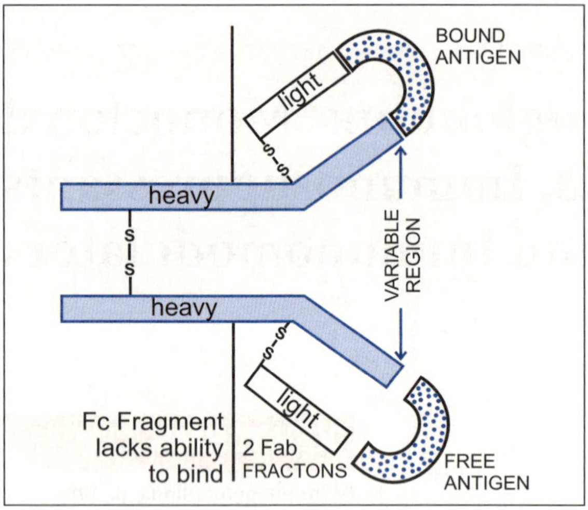

FIG. 72.1 **Basic structure of an immunoglobulin molecule. Two heavy and two light chains of amino acids are linked by disulphide (S–S) bridges. At one end of the molecule, the three dimensional stearic configuration (idiotypic determinant) of each arm allows only one antigenic determinant to have best fit status. The Fab fractions are variable and have antibody activity; and the other fraction is relatively constant (Fc). The amino acid sequence of the Fc fraction determines the main functional activity of the molecule.**

PH 1.50

HUMAN NORMAL IMMUNOGLOBULIN (HNIg) or IMMUNOGLOBULIN (Ig):

It is a sterile serum protein solution (15%–18%) containing **antibodies from human blood**, which is derived from pooled human serum. They are available in lyophilised form or in stabilised solution.

These antibodies are not specific to a particular infection. There are several immunoglobulin preparations available for intramuscular (IMIg), subcutaneous (SCIg) and intravenous (IVIg) routes, which differ with respect to manufacturing, protein content and tolerance. Most of these preparations contain more than 95% IgG with intact Fc-dependent effector functions (Chapter 1). The highly concentrated IgG preparations contain a vast 'library of antibodies' capable of reacting with thousands of determinants because of the diversity of the experience of the thousands of donors contributing to the pool. Among such antibodies will be many with anti-idiotypic specificities. Ig can be used both for prophylactic and therapeutic purposes.

Currently available IVIg formulations are sorbitol-based formulations, which can cause less reactions on i.v. administration.

Mechanism of action: Ig are immunomodulators. They:

- Neutralise toxins and viruses
- Opsonise bacteria.
- Modulate complement activation
- Strengthen nonspecific defence mechanisms
- Bind to Fc receptors on antigen presenting cells and cause temporary blockade
- Suppress various inflammatory mediators (cytokines, chemokines)
- Enhance anti-idiotype regulation of autoantibodies

Absorption, fate and excretion: Injection of IVIg results in steep increase in concentration of Ig which reduce to half within 6–12 h due to distribution to EC spaces and subsequently get slowly metabolised to reach the basal level over 3–4 weeks. Hence repeat doses at regular interval are required. IMIg shows peak rise in Ig after 20 min whereas SCIg shows peak rise after 4 days.

Adverse reactions: Ig can cause pain at the site of injection. Allergic reactions can occur. IVIg can cause headache, nausea, flushing, low grade fever, myalgia or arthralgia. They can be reduced by keeping the infusion rate slow or giving NSAIDs. The patients who get ADR with IVIg may be benefitted by changing to SCIg as usually the doses used are smaller and absorption by this route is slower.

Severe bronchospasm, hypotension and collapse, however, are rare with Ig and occur mostly following IVIg. Rarely anaphylaxis, aseptic meningitis, thromboembolic events, renal tubular necrosis, eczematous cutaneous reactions can also occur.

A period of 2 weeks should be maintained between injections of Ig and attenuated live vaccines to avoid interference with active antibody formation.

It is very expensive.

Indications:

Ig, especially IVIg is used:

a. as replacement therapy for antibody deficiency
b. to treat various autoimmune, infectious, and idiopathic diseases.

SCIg (given on the abdomen and/or thigh) serves as an alternative to IVIg, if the latter is not tolerated.

- **Primary immunodeficiency diseases:** These conditions are associated with absent or deficient antibody production and are associated with recurrent or unusually severe infections (due to group A *Streptococcus, Streptococcus pneumoniae, Haemophilus influenzae* type b, and to a lesser extent *Neisseria meningitides)*. IVIg therapy is advocated to reduce incidences of severe infections and their sequelae. It is administered as 0.4–0.8 g/kg initially and then the dose is adjusted for serum IgG concentrations and the clinical picture. These maintenance doses vary as 0.4–0.6 g/kg given at 2- to 10-week intervals.
- **Secondary immunodeficiency diseases:** IVIg is **not recommended routinely** in these patients. Patients who are chronically immunosuppressed, patients after stem cell transplantation, common variable immunodeficiency (CVID), chronic lymphocytic leukemia (CLL), multiple myeloma and other malignancies having a secondary antibody deficiency syndrome and susceptibility to infections are given IVIg therapy. In HIV-1 infected infants and children, it is indicated if the patients show increased susceptibility to bacterial infections and an antibody deficiency.
- **Autoimmune diseases and diseases of unknown etiology:** In these cases high dose IVIg is recommended.
- **Idiopathic thrombocytopenic purpura (ITP):** IVIg is administered prior to invasive treatment (e.g. surgery, tooth extraction). The response rate of IVIg therapy in cases of ITP is 90% in children and 70–80% in adults.
- **Guillain–Barré syndrome (GBS):** IVIg (0.4 g/kg for 3–7 days) has been shown either equivalent to or rather better and more cost-effective than plasma exchange therapy.
- **Kawasaki syndrome:** During acute phase, along with aspirin.
- **Bacterial sepsis and septic shock:** IVIg (especially enriched for IgM) along with antibiotic therapy has shown promising results in treatment of sepsis or septic shock in adults, children and neonates.
  However, IVIg should not be used as a prophylaxis of infection in preterm infants. They also have cellular immune defects, which cannot be corrected by IVIg.
- **Chronic inflammatory demyelinating polyneuropathy (CIDP)**
- **Multifocal motor neuropathy with conduction blocks**

Apart from the above indications, IVIg has been used in many clinical conditions with varying success rates as an off-label use e.g. rapidly progressing relapsing multiple sclerosis, aplastic anaemia; myasthenia gravis; heparin-induced thrombocytopenia type II; doses vary according to the diseases.

- **Miscellaneous:** HNI/IVIg can be used as **post-exposure prophylaxis for measles and hepatitis A**, both vaccine-preventable diseases, only if the exposed person is not already immune. It will attenuate or prevent the symptoms if given early in the incubation period. Ig can also be used for **pre-exposure immunoprophylaxis** wherein it will offer protection for 3 months.

HUMAN SPECIFIC IMMUNOGLOBULIN (HYPERIMMUNOGLOBULINS)

More selective type of gamma globulin against a particular infection can be obtained from the blood of individuals convalescing from that disease or from the blood of subjects recently immunised against that disease. They have concentrations of the specific antibody that are many times higher than normal immunoglobulin preparations, e.g. specific immune globulin preparations for hepatitis B, rabies, tetanus, diptheria, varicella zoster, cytomegalovirus, botulism and anti-D immunoglobulin (Chapter 71). Hyperimmune immunoglobulins are not routinely recommended to pregnant women but susceptible pregnant women can receive post-exposure immunoglobulins if exposed to above mentioned organisms or antigen.

MONOCLONAL ANTIBODIES (mAb) IN THERAPEUTICS

The greatest impetus for immunotherapy came from the discovery of the **hybridoma technique** for producing **monoclonal antibodies** (mAb) by George Kohler and Cesar Milstein in 1975. Both shared the Nobel Prize in Medicine/Physiology with Niels Kaj Jerne in 1984.

Monoclonal antibodies (mAb) are **single type of antibodies that are identical and are directed against a specific epitope.** They are produced by clones of a single parent cells or single hybridoma cell line. Compared to polyclonal antibodies, mAb are **monospecific** and **homogenous.** Such antibodies are now used for diagnostic and therapeutic purposes.

Structure of the mAb is same as described earlier (Fig. 72.1). There are 4 types of mAb.

1. **Murine monoclonal antibodies**: Anti-CD3 mAb of murine origin (OKT-3) was the first therapeutic mAb developed in 1986, known as Muromonab. **It has a limited use now** as it has short t½ and its effects are mild. ADRs can be serious and there can be treatment failures.
2. **Chimeric monoclonal antibodies:** These are developed through fusion of murine Fab domain with human constant regions and thus **has about 65% human genetic component.** This minimises risk of unwanted reactions to foreign antibodies. It also increases the *t*½ by almost 5 fold, which improves the functionality of the antibody, e.g. infliximab, rituximab, abciximab.
3. **Humanised monoclonal antibodies** are available in which murine hypervariable amino domain is grafted into human antibody and **thus of 95% human origin**. Hence, they are less immunogenic. However, sometimes they are weaker than the parent murine mAb in terms of binding with antigens. They remain in circulation for a longer time and are preferred. The examples include daclizumab, omalizumab, alemtuzumab.
4. **Fully human monoclonal antibodies**: These are prepared by transferring human IgG gene into murine gene, followed by vaccination in transgenic mouse or using phage display technique. The immunogenicity risk gets reduced further. Adalimumab and panitumumab are the examples.

Mechanism of action: They specifically **block the characteristic of the targeted antigen, its function, its cell surface density and tissue distribution.** Their action is directed against targets like T lymphocytes, B lymphocytes, TNF, interleukins and epithelial growth factor receptors. Addition of active compounds to mAb to produce immunoconjugates can provide targeting specificity to cytotoxic actions. **Thus, mAb can be conjugated with catalytic toxins, radioisotopes and chemotherapeutic agents, and can be used as therapeutic guided missiles to target-specific tissues with cytotoxic payload (e.g. arcitumomab and capromab).**

Epidermal growth factor receptor (EGFR) is a cell surface receptor involved in regulation of cell proliferation and survival. Selective antibodies have now been produced which act as **EGFR inhibitor** and are used to treat cancer, e.g. cetuximab in colorectal cancer.

Some of the currently available mAb, their targets and indications are listed in Table 72.1.

Absorption fate and excretion: mAb are used intravenously and they remain essentially intravascular, the volume of distribution is small and tissue penetration is limited. Depending on their nature, they remain in human circulation for 2 days to 2 weeks.

Adverse reactions: These vary according to antibody used.

- **Hypersensitivity reactions** are rare. However, sometimes the first injection may induce an influenza-like syndrome causing fever, headache, chills, tachycardia, vomiting, diarrhoea, arthralgia and hypotension. The reaction is reversible. It is believed to be due to massive systemic release of cytokines, following activation of T lymphocytes. These can be controlled by glucocorticoids and/or antihistaminics.
- **Suppression of physiological function** may occur depending on specificity of tissues targeted; thus, antilymphocytic mAb causes immunosuppression.
- **Activation of inflammatory cells.**
- **Increased risk of infection**
- **Bleeding with poor wound healing, proteinuria and hypertension may occur with** bevacizumab.
- **Trastuzumab can depress cardiac activity.**

Table 72.1 Monoclonal Antibodies for Clinical Use

Generic Name	Target/Receptor	Indications
	Cancer Chemotherapy	
Trastuzumab	HER2/neu	Breast cancer
Rituximab	CD20 (B cell)	Lymphoma; CLLRA
Gemtuzumab	CD33	AML
Cetuximab, panitumumab	EGFR	Colorectal cancer; NSCLC
Daratumumab	EGFR	NSCLC
Elotuzumab	SLAMF7	Multiple myeloma
Pembrolizumab, Nivolumab	Programmed cell death-1 protein	Melanoma, NSCLC, head and neck squamous cell carcinoma
Ipilimumab	CTLA4	Malignant melanoma
Bevacizumab	VEGF	Colorectal, lung cancer; neovascular AMD
Olaratumab	PDGF R alpha	Soft tissue sarcoma
	Autoimmune Disease and Transplant Rejection	
Muromonab	CD3 (T cell)	Graft rejection
Basiliximab	CD25 (IL-2 receptor)	Prophylaxis of renal transplant rejection
Alemtuzumab	CD52	Graft rejection; CLL
Infliximab, adalimumab, golimumab	TNF-alpha	RA; Crohn disease; plaque psoriasis
Tocilizumab, Sarilumab, Satralizumab	IL-6	RA, severe or life-threatening CRS
Efalizumab	$CD11_a$ (LFA-1)	Psoriasis
Ustekinumab	IL-12 and 23	Psoriasis
Secukinumab, ixekizumab	Il-17 A	Psoriasis
Brodalumab	Il-17	Psoriasis
Guselkumab, Risankizumab	IL-23	Psoriasis
Belimumab	CD2	SLE, lupus nephritis
Certolizumab	TNF-alpha	Crohn disease
Vedolizumab	Integrin alpha 4 beta 7	Crohn disease; UC
Natalizumab	Integrin	Crohn disease; MS
Alemtuzumab	CD52	MS
Daclizumab	CD25 (IL-2 receptor)	MS
Ocrelizumab	CD20	RA; MS
	Metabolic, Degenerative and Other Diseases	
Alirocumab, evolocumab	PCSK9	Primary hyperlipidaemia
Denosumab	RANKL	Osteoporosis
Ranibizumab	VEGF	Neovascular AMD
Eculizumab	Complement protein C5	Paroxysmal nocturnal haemoglobinuria; haemolytic uremic syndrome
Abciximab	GpIIb/IIIa	Unstable angina (Antiplatelet)
Idarucizumab	Dabigatran	Reversal of dabigatran effect
Omalizumab	IgE receptor	Bronchial asthma
Mepolizumab, reslizumab	IL-5	Asthma
Benralizumab	IL-5Rα	Asthma
Dupilumab	IL-4 and IL -13	Atopic dermatitis
	Infection	
Palivizumab	Fusion protein	Respiratory syncytial virus infection
Raxibacumab, obiltoxaximab	Protective antigen of *Bacillus anthracis*	Inhalation Anthrax
Bezlotoxumab	*Clostridium difficile* toxin B	*C. difficile* infection

Notes: AMD, age-related macular degeneration; BAFF, B cell activating factor; CRS, cytokine release syndrome; MS, multiple sclerosis; NSCLC, non-small cell lung carcinoma; PCSK9, proprotein convertase subtilisin-kexin type 9; PDGF R alpha, platelet-derived growth factor receptor alpha; RANKL, receptor activator of nuclear factor Kappa-B ligand, SLAMF7, signalling lymphocytic activation molecule F7; UC, ulcerative colitis; VEGF, vascular endothelial growth factor.

Indications: They are used in:

- **Cancer chemotherapy,** usually combined with conventional cytotoxic agents (Chapter 59).
- **Autoimmune disease and transplant rejection,** e.g. infliximab in RA (Chapter 73) or natalizumab against Integrin in multiple sclerosis (Chapter 15). To prevent the acute rejection of renal transplant, basiliximab and daclizumab targeted against IL-2 are used.
- **Metabolic, degenerative and other diseases:** Evolocumab and alirocumab have been reported to reduce LDL-C level by over 50% and increase HDL-C in patients with hyperlipidaemia. Ranibizumab is used to treat neovascular AMD (age-related macular degeneration). In asthma, omalizumab, targeted against IgE receptors is used. Abciximab, a GpIIb/IIIa antagonist serves as antiplatelet agent (Chapter 33).
- **Infection**, e.g. Palivizumab to treat respiratory syncytial virus infection in infants.

Diagnostic uses of mAb: They are extensively used in immunoassay and other procedures in the laboratory for identification, location and targeting neoplasms, infections (e.g. herpes, hepatitis, influenza, streptococcal and chlamydial), diagnosis of pregnancy and for purification of hormones.

They are all very expensive and unaffordable to many.

In addition to monoclonal antibodies, **fusion proteins** are available for therapeutic use. Fc fragment of immunoglobulin is linked to ligand-binding portion of receptor to form fusion receptor protein, which serves as decoy receptor. They bind to specific growth factors or cytokines, which prevents them from activating the receptor. They have longer t½. The examples are **abatacept** and **etanercept** (Chapter 73). Alefacept is a human LAF-IgG1 fusion protein, which reduces T effector memory cells. It is used in psoriasis. **Belatacept** prevents T cell activation and used as immunosuppressant in transplant (See under the Section Immunosuppressants for Solid Organ Transplant).

IMMUNOSUPPRESSANTS SU 13.2

Drugs which are used to suppress the immunity are called immunosuppressants. Since immunity confers resistance to disease, the use of drugs for deliberately suppressing it appears odd at first sight. However, Immunosuppressive drugs (Table 72.2) are useful in:

a. Treating autoimmune diseases
b. Prventing immunorejection of organ transplants.

a. The ability of the body to recognise self from non-self or foreign, which is the basis of immunity, is liable to cause disorders due to failure to recognise and tolerate antigens produced by its own tissues. This may cause exacerbation of an existing disease process or even produce new ones called **autoimmune diseases.** Several autoimmune diseases have been recognised, e.g. SLE, RA, systemic vasculitis, psoriasis, multiple sclerosis, autoimmune hepatitis, Crohn disease, cardiomyopathy, dermatomyositis, etc.

b. Solid organ transplant is a definitive therapy for patients with end-organ dysfunction. Advances

Table 72.2 Classification of Immunosuppressants

1. Calcineurin inhibitors (CNI)	Cyclosporine Tacrolimus
2. Glucocorticoids	Prednisolone
3. Cytotoxic/ antiproliferative agents	Azathioprine, cyclophosphamide, Methotrexate, Mycophenolate, Sirolimus
4. Sphingosine-1-phosphate (S1P) receptor modulators	Fingolimod, siponimod, ozanimod, ponesimod
5. Biologicals	
Polyclonal antibodies:	Antilymphocyte globulin (ALG), anti-thymocyte globulin (ATG)
Monoclonal antibodies:	
• T cell–depleting antibodies	Muromonab
• IL–2 receptor (anti-CD25) antibodies	Basiliximab, daclizumab
• Anti-CD 52 antibody	Alemtuzumab
Fusion protein:	Belatacept
Cytokine signalling inhibitors (Janus Kinase Inhibitors)	Ruxolitinib, baricitinib , tofacitinib

in surgical techniques have allowed transplants for a variety of solid organs—liver, kidney, pancreas, heart, and lung. Procurement of donor organs is done in a refined way and the transplant procedure is carried out with minimal complications and decreased ischemic injury events. Addition to the pool of immunosuppressant therapy has resulted in dampening the host immune response and improving short and long-term graft survival.

All the immunosuppressants are likely to increase the susceptibility of individuals to infection. PH 1.50

Classification of Immunosuppressants

See Table 72.2. Their mechanism of action is illustrated in Fig. 72.2.

1. CALCINEURIN INHIBITORS (CNI)

CYCLOSPORINE: The drug, formerly known as cyclosporin A, is a cyclic undecapeptide (11 amino acid) produced by the fungus *Beauveria nivea*. It has now been synthesised.

Mechanism of action: Cyclosporine acts as a selective immunosuppressant; it targets intracellular signalling pathway induced during the activation process of T cell receptor after interacting with an antigen. Within the T lymphocytes, it binds to an intracellular protein, immunophilins (cyclophilin) and forms a complex. This complex binds the Ca^{++} dependent phosphatase, calcineurin and inhibits it. This prevents dephosphorylation of nuclear factor of activated T cells (NFAT) complexes, which is required to make them active.

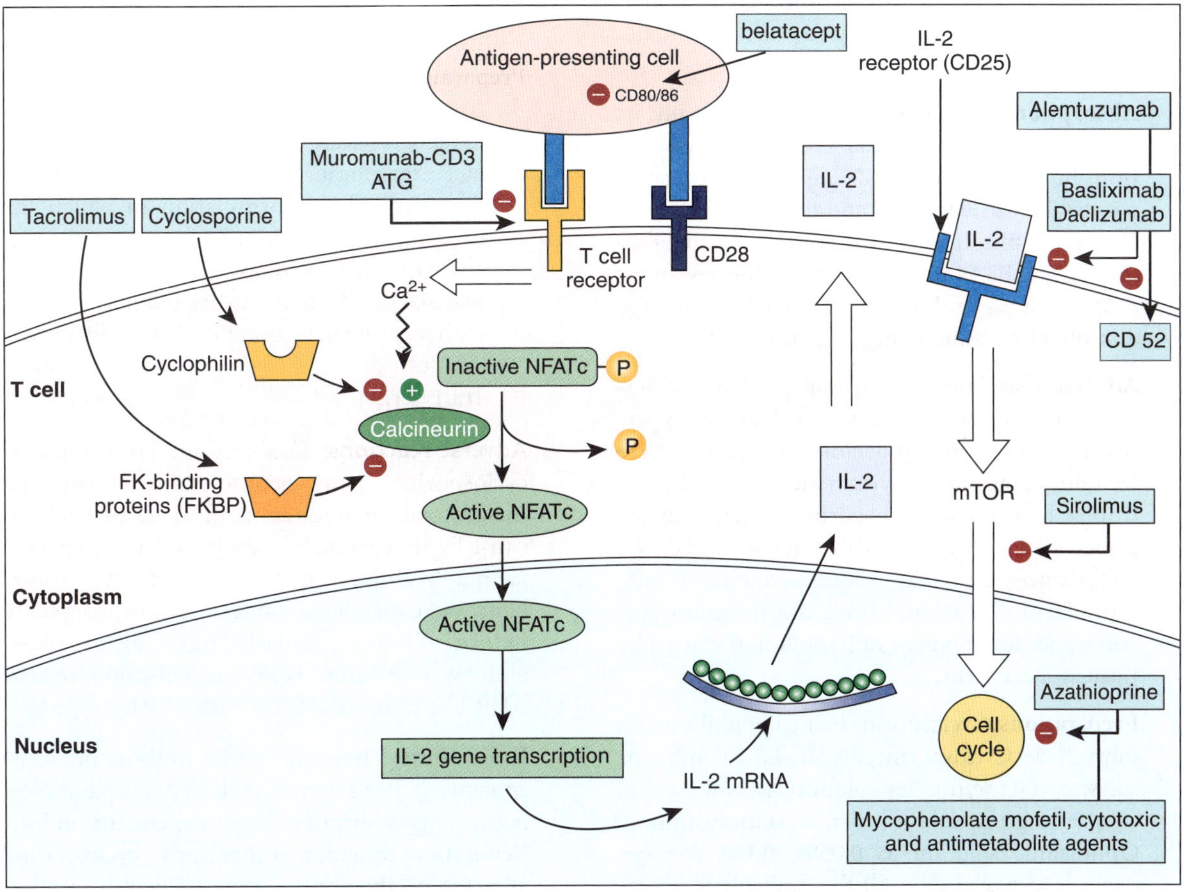

FIG. 72.2 A T cell showing target sites for action of various immunosuppressant drugs.

Only active NFAT complexes move to the nucleus and interact with nuclear components leading to transcription of IL-2, IL-15 and lymphokine genes. The IL-2 thus formed is released from the T cell and binds to CD25 (also known as the IL-2 receptor) on the surface of other T cells to activate mammalian target of rapamycin (mTOR), which results in T-cell proliferation (Fig. 72.2).

Thus cyclosporine inhibits T cell–dependent immune mechanisms to exert following effects. It:

- Prevents complete activation of T cells following specific antigenic stimulation
- Blunts expression of many lymphokines, including IL-2 and antiapoptotic proteins
- Increases expression of transforming growth factor β (TGF β), a potent inhibitor of IL-2 stimulated T cell proliferation and generation of cytotoxic cells

However, this immunosuppression is not associated with anti-inflammatory response, cytotoxicity or bone marrow suppression.

Absorption, fate and excretion: Given orally, its bioavailability is 20%–50%. Food delays absorption. In the circulation, 50% is bound to erythrocytes, 10% to leucocytes and 40% to lipoproteins in the plasma. It is almost completely metabolised, by CYP3A4 in liver, intestine, kidney and is excreted in faeces. Intersubject variability is large and therefore monitoring is required.

Adverse reactions: The major toxic manifestations of cyclosporine are nephrotoxicity, hypertension and hyperlipidaemia; the others are tremors, paraesthesia, hypertrichosis, gum hypertrophy, hepatotoxicity, hyperuricaemia, diabetogenic state if given with steroids and GI disturbances especially, anorexia, increased susceptibility to infection, leucopenia, thrombocytopenia and development of lymphomas caused by Epstein–Barr virus.

Preparations: Cyclosporine being lipophilic needs oily vehicle. Cyclosporine, 25, 50 and 100 mg capsules; as 100 mg/mL oily solution for oral use and as a 50 mg/mL solution for i.v. administration. Ophthalmic solution as 0.05%, 0.1%, 5% eye drops is also available. All the available formulations are not bioequivalent.

Indications: It is mainly used for prophylaxis and treatment of organ rejection in transplantation surgery. It is combined with a glucocorticoid. Its other indications are in the treatment of autoimmune diseases such as RA, psoriasis, xerophthalmia and uveitis, IBD and nephrotic syndrome.

TACROLIMUS: It is a macrolide antibiotic isolated from *Streptomyces tsukubaensis*. It binds to an immunophilin (FK-binding protein); the complex inhibits calcineurin, thereby affects the T cell activation and production of IL-2 (Fig. 72.2). **Tacrolimus is 100 times more potent than cyclosporine** as an immunosuppressant. It has greater efficacy, less variability in absorption and its TDM is easy.

Absorption, fate and excretion: Given orally, its bioavailability is variable and is reduced by food. It is highly protein bound (75%–99%). It is extensively metabolised in the liver. It can also be given intravenously.

Preparations:

i. Immediate release tacrolimus: twice daily
ii. Extended release tacrolimus: Once daily
iii. LCP tacrolimus(LCPT): This is a novel extended release formulation in which the drug particle is reduced to single molecules and is then bound to a matrix that slowly releases the drug. It has better bioavailability with less diurnal variability. The daily dose is also less.
iv. Transdermal gel

Adverse reactions: These are similar to those of cyclosporine, with nephrotoxicity being the major toxic manifestation. It is more likely to cause hypertension, hypomagnesaemia, hyperkalaemia, hyperglycaemia and diabetes, GI disturbances like diarrhoea, alopecia and neurotoxicity in form of tremor, headache, motor disturbances, and even seizures. Peak concentration related ADR like tremors are less with LCPT.

Indications: These are similar to those of cyclosporine. It is preferred in liver transplantation because its absorption is not dependent on bile. Being more potent, it is superior to cyclosporine as a rescue therapy to suppress acute rejection episodes and for allograft survival. Once daily, extended-release formulations of tacrolimus are as efficacious as immediate release formulations. Other indications are severe atopic eczema and other inflammatory diseases of the skin.

2. GLUCOCORTICOIDS

The two glucocorticosteroids used in transplant recipients are methylprednisolone and prednisone. The glucocorticoids are potent immunosuppressants having multiple mechanisms to influence all the immune system cells. They are used to prevent and treat organ transplant rejection along with other immunosuppressants. They are useful in graft-versus-host disease (GVHD) in bone-marrow transplantation. They prevent or limit allergic reactions that occur with other immunosuppressive agents. The other use as immunosuppressive is to treat autoimmune diseases like RA, SLE, dermatomyositis, psoriasis, IBD, auto-immune haematological disorders and acute exacerbations of MS. They also possess anti-inflammatory action (Chapter 64).

3. CYTOTOXIC/ANTIPROLIFERATIVE AGENTS

These are cytotoxic drugs which act on the dividing cells. An immune response is associated with division of lymphoid cells and these drugs act by interfering with the dividing lymphoid cells in the body. They, however, are nonspecific and produce toxicity as they also affect the other rapidly dividing cells (Chapter 59). Continuous, prolonged immunosuppression with cytotoxic agents is associated with increased susceptibility to infection. These drugs include:

- **Sirolimus, everolimus**
- **Azathioprine, cyclophosphamide, methotrexate, leflunomide**
- **Mycophenolate mofetil**

SIROLIMUS: Although structurally related to tacrolimus, its mechanism of action is different. Sirolimus (rapamycin) acts on the late stage of T cell activation. In this stage, the released IL-2 from the activated T cells binds to IL-2 receptors (CD 25) on the cell surface of other T cells, which in turn activates a protein kinase, termed as mTOR (mammalian target of rapamycin). This is a key enzyme in cell-cycle progression and leads to T cell proliferation. Sirolimus after entry into the T cells forms a complex with immunophilin, FKBP-12 (FK506 binding protein 12). This complex binds to and **inhibits mTOR** (Fig. 72.2) and causes arrest of cell cycle in G1 phase. Hence, it is also termed as **proliferation signal inhibitor (PSI).**

Absorption, fate and excretion: It can be given orally but its bioavailability is 15%. It is bound to albumin and has a long *t*½ (62 h). It is a substrate for CYP3A4 and is transported by p-glycoprotein, so drug interactions can occur. Excretion is through faeces.

Adverse reactions: Its main ADR include profound myelosuppression, especially thrombocytopenia, hepatotoxicity, diarrhoea, mouth ulcers, hypokalemia, increase in LDL-C and triglyceride levels and pneumonitis, delayed wound healing, Proteinuria and renal impairment may occur.

Indications: It is used alone or in combination with CNI, MPA with or without glucocorticoids to prevent and treat rejection of solid organ transplant. This also allows use of low dose of CNI to prevent renal damage. Although sirolimus alone is not nephrotoxic, its combination with CNI has shown to cause renal impairment. Hence sirolimus alone is often preferred to avoid nephrotoxicity seen with CNI. It has shown to prevent and reduce progression of chronic allograft vasculopathy (CAV). It is not recommended for lung transplant. Topically, it is used for uveoretinitis and skin cancer. Sirolimus-eluting intracoronary stents are used in CAD (Chapter 1) as it inhibits cell proliferation in the endothelium, decreases neointimal hyperplasia and reduces the risk of in-stent stenosis.

Everolimus is a new PSI which acts like sirolimus but has shorter t½ and reaches steady state concentrations faster. It is used for the prophylaxis of kidney and liver transplant rejection. It is used for treatment of variety of cancers except skin cancer.

Temsirolimus is specifically approved for renal cancer.

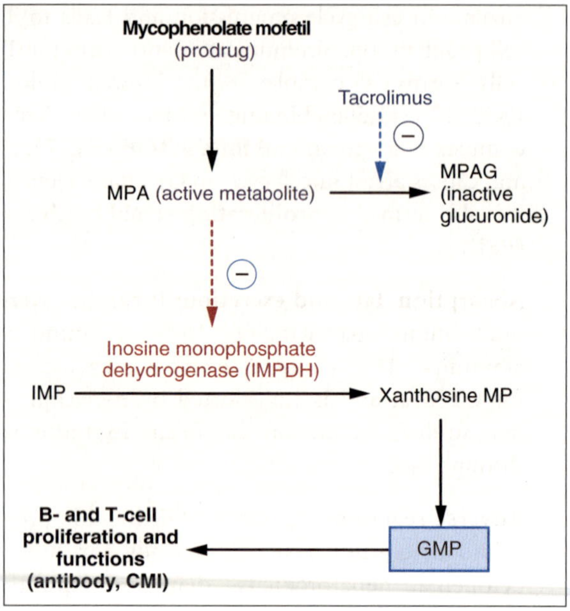

FIG. 72.3 Mechanism of action of mycophenolate mofetil.

PACLITAXEL, a cancer chemotherapy drug, has potent anti-proliferative effects. It is used in drug-eluting intracoronary stents to prevent restenosis.

AZATHIOPRINE, CYCLOPHOSPHAMIDE and **METHOTREXATE:** These agents are used in cancer chemotherapy (Chapter 59). They are also used as immunosuppressants (Table 72.2). Azathioprine is used as an adjunct for prevention of organ transplant rejection. It is the antimetabolite of choice for all transplant recipients who are or wish to become pregnant. It is also used for the treatment of autoimmune diseases like progressive RA. Cyclophosphamide is used as immunosuppressant for nephrotic syndrome, SLE and MS. Methotrexate and leflunomide are also used to treat autoimmune disease like RA (Chapter 73).

MYCOPHENOLATE MOFETIL (MMF): This prodrug, given orally or intravenously, is rapidly hydrolysed to the active compound, **mycophenolic acid** (MPA). It is also available as enteric coated mycophenolate sodium (EC-MPS), a safe and effective alternative. MPA is a potent, selective, reversible, **noncompetitive inhibitor** of inosine monophosphate dehydrogenase (enzyme involved in purine nucleotide biosynthesis). It prevents formation of guanosine monophosphate (GMP), required by proliferating T and B cells (Fig. 72.3). Thus lymphocyte proliferation is inhibited (Fig. 72.2) along with diminished CMI and antibody formation against allografts.

MPA is metabolised in the liver, intestine and kidney. Concurrent administration of tacrolimus impairs the conversion of MPA to glucuronide, making MPA available for long time but this may enhance GI toxicity.

Adverse reactions: These include GI disturbances, (diarrhoea, vomiting, abdominal pain) headache, hypercholesterolemia, hypertension and neutropenia and red cell aplasia, which are predominantly dose dependent. Reduction in MMF doses in transplant recipients having GI adverse effects may increase the chances of rejection. Such patients are benefited from EC-MPS. It may increase risk of infections. Skin cancers are frequent in patients treated with MMF. It should never be used with azathioprine as both are potential myelosuppressants.

Indications: The drug is used for the prophylaxis of solid organ transplant rejection in combination with other CNI and/or glucocorticoid. It has also shown to prevent or decrease progression of coronary artery vasculopathy in cardiac transplant recipients and is preferred for cardiac transplant. It is used to prevent or treat GVH reaction. In addition, it is used in the treatment of autoimmune diseases like MS, sarcoidosis, psoriasis, SLE, pemphigus vulgaris, systemic vasculitis and nephrotic syndrome.

4. SPHINGOSINE-1-PHOSPHATE RECEPTOR MODULATORS

Sphingosine-1-phosphate (S1P) is derived from sphingolipid. It regulates the egress of lymphocytes from thymus and peripheral lymphoid tissues into circulatory fluid. This movement of lymphocytes is required for immunological activities and to reach the site of inflammation. Thus SIP is involved in inflammation and immunity.

S1P acts intracellularly as well as extracellularly. It interacts with transmembrane receptors on the cell surface via G-protein coupled receptors, termed as S1P receptors. There are 5 S1PR. Of these, S1P1R are found on B and T lymphocytes and S1P4R are located in the immune system.

S1PR modulators viz. **fingolimod, siponimod, ozanimod,** and **ponesimod** are indicated in the therapy of various conditions such as CNS degenerative diseases, IBD, psoriasis. They are the irreversible agonists at S1P1R and cause their downregulation. The receptors undergo internalization and subsequent degradation. Hence the T cells cannot exit the lymphoid tissue and remain sequestered in lymph nodes and Peyer patches. This reduces inflammation and protects the tissues/sites from lymphocyte attacks.

All are given orally. Fingolimod is a prodrug and acts through an active metabolite, fingolimod phosphate.

They cause a variety of ADR including increased risk of infections, bradyarrhythmias and impaired AV conduction, hypertension, hepatic transaminase elevation, macular edema and dyspnea. The risk of skin and breast cancer increases.

They are used in the therapy of multiple sclerosis (Chapter 15). Ozanimod is approved for ulcerative colitis.

5. BIOLOGICALS

Both polyclonal and monoclonal antibodies against lymphocyte cell-surface antigens are widely used for prevention and treatment of organ transplant rejection.

Polyclonal Antibodies

Polyclonal antisera are generated by repeated injections of human lymphocytes, lymph node and spleen cells (lymphoid tissue) or thymus into animals such as horses, rabbits, sheep, or goats and is termed as **Antilymphocytic serum (ALS).** If thymocytes are used then it is called as **Antithymocytic serum (ATS).** The T lymphocytes are more vulnerable to ALS, which depletes the thymus-dependent areas of lymphoid tissue, the lymphocytes being replaced by histiocytes.

Antilymphocytic globulin (**ALG**) or **antithymocytic globulin** (**ATG**) serve as immunosuppressants to prevent or treat acute rejections of organ transplant. They are also used in patients with acute graft versus host reactions following bone marrow transplantation.

ANTITHYMOCYTIC GLOBULIN (ATG): It is composed of purified gamma globulin containing primarily IgG against human thymus lymphocytes. Various ATG products differ in the source of inoculated animal (rabbit or horse) and in the type of antigen product used to produce immunoglobulin (thymocytes, peripheral T cells, etc.). These cytotoxic antibodies bind to a variety of immune system proteins on the surface of T cells and block their function (Fig. 72.2), induce apoptosis and thus T-cell lymphopenia.

Adverse reactions: These include infusion reactions like fever with chills, headache, pain and hypotension. The other effects include GI disturbances like nausea, diarrhoea, abdominal pain, leukopenia and thrombocytopenia. Immune-mediated reactions, including anaphylaxis or cytokine release syndrome have been reported Classic Serum sickness can be induced by ATG.

Indications: ATG is useful in the prevention and treatment of acute rejection of transplant. When used as a suppressant with other immunosuppressants, it enables reduction of their doses. It is used as a rescue treatment in steroid resistant cases. It is also used in the treatment of aplastic anaemia.

Monoclonal Antibodies (see Table 72.2)

MUROMONAB- CD 3: It is a specific T cell–depleting antibody. It binds to CD3, a component of the T cell receptor complex (Fig. 72.2) and leads to internalisation of these receptors, followed by rapid depletion of T cells from blood and lymphoid organs. It is used in acute rejection episodes resistant to glucocorticoids.

The major adverse effect of anti-CD3 therapy is potentially life threatening cytokine release syndrome, which is worst after the infusion of first dose. Muromonab can also cause pulmonary oedema, ARDS, arrhythmias, cardiovascular collapse, and cardiac arrest.

ANTI-CD25 ANTIBODIES: Basiliximab and **daclizumab** specifically inhibit activated T cells by blocking CD25 (IL-2) receptors on the activated T cells (Fig. 72.2). They do not cause significant depletion of T cells or cytokine-release, but anaphylactic reactions can occur. Rarely they can cause pulmonary oedema or circulatory collapse. Both are used for prophylaxis of renal transplant rejection. Daclizumab is also used in the treatment of MS.

ANTI CD 52 ANTIBODY: Alemtuzumab is a humanized monoclonal antibody targeting CD52 which is located on T and B cells, NK cells, and to a lesser degree monocytes and macrophages. The resultant antibody dependent cellular lysis results in profound depletion of T cells and to a lesser degree B cells and monocytes. It may last for more than a year. Its main ADR is thus neutropenia. Thrombocytopenia and anaemia may occur in 50% patients. The ADR of concern are autoimmune hemolytic anemia and other autoimmune diseases, which may occur due to immune reconstitution in response to T cell depletion. It is used for induction of immunosuppressive therapy (See below). It thus avoids the use of early high dose of glucocorticoids.

JANUS KINASE INHIBITORS PH 1.50

These small molecular weight agents interact with various isoforms of janus kinase and inhibit the intracellular signaling, which may be generated by multiple cytokines from different pathways. This results in inhibition of cellular functioning. JAK inhibitors either interact with ATP binding site of JAK tyrosine domain or at allosteric site. JAK isoforms include JAK1, JAK2, JAK3, and tyrosine kinase 2 (TYK2). Some of the inhibitors are selective for specific JAK isoform. They are administered orally. JAK inhibitors do not produce any antibodies and therefore immunogenicity is not a concern. Table 72.3 presents some of the JAK inhibitors currently in practice with their target isoform, indications and ADR.

IMMUNOSUPPRESSANTS FOR SOLID ORGAN TRANSPLANT

Various immunosuppression regimens exist which include appropriate combination of immunosuppressants with different mechanism of action. The therapeutic objective of these regimens is to prevent the proliferation and cytotoxic actions of T cells. This is associated with suppression of antibody production from B cells. Selection of drugs and their doses depend on type of organ transplant, recipient characteristics (age, comorbidity, concomitant drugs,

Table 72.3 Target, indications and Adverse effects of JAK inhibitors

JAK Inhibitor	JAK isoorm	Indications	Adverse effects
Tofacitinib	JAK1, JAK2, JAK 3	RA, psoriasis, ulcerative colitis	Risk of infection, leukopenia, neutron- and lympho-penia, anemia, thrombocytopenia, diarrhea hyperlipidaemia, hypertension,
Peficitinib, delgocitinib	Pan-JAK [JAK1/JAK2/JAK3/ TYK2]	RA	
Upadacitinib, filgotinib,	JAK1	RA, Psoriatic arthritis, ulcerative colitis	
Abrocitinib	JAK1	Atopic dermatitis	Sudden death, myocardial infarction, stroke
Ruxolitinib, baricitinib	JAK1 and JAK2	RA, GVHD (See under Section Haemopoietic Stem cell transplant), myelofibrosis, polycythemia vera	Thromboembolism (more with Baricitinib, tofacitinib, and upadacitinib)
Fedratinib, pacritinib	JAK2	Myelofibrosis	Cancer

immunological risk factors), drug characteristics (mechanism of action, pharmacokinetics, ADR, their availability and cost) and clinician's preferences and hospital's policy.

Though this is a specialized area, these regimens are classified as 1. Induction regimens 2. Maintenance regimens and 3. Rejection regimens.

1. **Induction regimens** are initiated prior to or immediately during the transplant operation. Not all transplant institutions routinely use induction regimens e.g.in liver transplant patients maintenance therapy is started within 24 hours of transplantation.

   Induction regimens include **high-dose glucocorticoids, anti-T cell agents (rabbit antithymocyte globulin-rATG, alemtuzumab, teplizumab-CD3 mAb) or IL-2 receptor antagonists (basiliximab).**

   Other biologic drugs, such as eculizumab, belatacept, and rituximab, are used in specific clinical conditions.

2. **Maintenance regimens** include a combination of two to three immunosuppressants from different classes e.g. combination of CNI, antiproliferative drugs (azathioprine), and a glucocorticoid (prednisone). The various maintenance immunosuppressants preferred in different transplants are presented in Table 72.4.
   - The preferred CNI is tacrolimus. If there is an intolerance to CNI or in patients with renal injury post-transplant or those with coronary artery vasculopathy, mTOR inhibitors (sirolimus or everolimus) can be used. However, they should not to be used in the liver transplant patients in the first 4 weeks as it may impair healing and result in hepatic artery thrombosis. Everolimus is preferred to sirolimus in liver and lung transplant.
   - Antimetabolite drug such as MMF is preferred to antiproliferative agents as it has shown better outcomes.
   - Since long-term glucocorticoid use is associated with many adverse effects, in liver and heart transplant patients glucocorticoids are tapered- between 3 to 6 months and are often weaned off by 12 months post –transplant. They are continued if there is associated renal impairment or in renal transplant patients.
   - The patients with stable renal transplant can be switched over from a CNI- to a belatacept –based regimen 6–60 months after transplantation. Belatacept, a fusion protein, selectively blocks the CD28 mediated co-stimulation of T- lymphocytes by binding to CD80 and CD86 on antigen-presenting cells (Fig. 72. 2). It improves renal function and metabolic outcomes including hypertension, diabetes, and hyperlipidemia. There may be an increase in early rejection, for which a short concomitant course of tacrolimus can be given. But in the long run belatacept has been found to decrease mortality and results in better graft survival. It is expensive. It is the only immunosuppressive drug adminis-

Table 72.4 Maintenance Immunosuppressants for Organ Transplant

	Kidney	Liver	Heart	Lungs[b]
Cyclosporine	+	+	+	
Tacrolimus[a]	+	+	+	+
Glucocorticoids	+		+	
Mycophenolate mofetil	+	+	+	
Azathioprine	+			
Sirolimus	+		+	
Everolimus	+	+		
Belatacept	+			

[a]Extended release tacrolimus and LCP- tacrolimus for renal transplant
[b]Many other immunosuppressants are used off label for lung transplant

tered intravenously monthly and is well tolerated. PH 1.50

2. **Rejection regimens** are used in acute rejections, which may be antibody –mediated or T-cell mediated.
   - In case of acute antibody-mediated rejection, plasma exchange followed by IVIG and rituximab can be tried. Plasma cell inhibitor bortezomib or eculizumab can also be used instead of rituximab.
   - If the rejection is T-cell mediated, then IV methylprednisolone (250 to 1000 mg daily) is given for 3 to 5 days. It targets T cells, B cells, and macrophages (Chapter 64). rATG targeting T cell receptors is another alternative, especially for steroid resistant rejection.
   - The dose and the level of the maintenance immunosuppressive drugs should be optimized in all patients.

The transplant patients remain on life-long immunosuppressants and hence are prone to an increased risk of bacterial, viral and fungal infections. The patients may receive long-term prophylactic therapy for infections e.g. cotrimaxazole to prevent Pneumocystis carinii infection. There can be a risk of malignancy such as skin cancer, lymphoma, and cervical cancer. Metabolic derangement is also observed in these patients.

IMMUNOSUPPRESSANTS IN IN HEMATOPOIETIC STEM CELL TRANSPLANTATION PH 1.50

Hematopoietic stem cell transplantation (HSCT) is a curative treatment for many malignant and non-malignant diseases. However the donor cells (in allogenic stem cell transplant) recognize different HLAs of the host cells as foreign and the activated T cells start secreting cytokines such as IL -1, IL-2, TNF and gamma-interferon, which sets in graft versus host disease (GVHD). This can be acute (within 100 days of transplant) or chronic. Immunosuppressants are required to prevent as well as treat GVHD.

Preventive therapy for GVHD includes glucocorticoid (methylprednisolone), methotrexate and CNI. Steroids are used in combination with other immunosuppressants. It helps to reduce their toxicity without altering efficacy.

- In myeloablative conditioning regimens, cyclosporine with short course of methotrexate (intermittently for 4 doses till day 11) is used. Cyclosporine is started a day prior to transplant and continued for 6 months if there is no GVHD. The doses may be tapered after 3 months. Tacrolimus serves as an alternative.
- In reduced intensity conditioning regimens, the preferred combination is cyclosporine and MMF. MMF is given on the day of transplant and continued for 1 month in sibling transplantations, 3 months in unrelated or mismatched donor transplantations.
- ATG is recommended in GVHD prophylaxis of unrelated donor transplantations either in myeloablative or non-myeloablative regimen.

PH 1.50

In acute GVHD, IV methylprednisolone (2 mg/kg/day given in two divided doses) is used for 7 days along with other immunosuppressants. It is tapered based on clinical response. ATG is the second line option.

Chronic GVHD has no standard therapy. **Rituximab and ruxolitinib** are used. Anti TNF agents, extracorporeal photopheresis, and mesenchymal stem cell infusion are some other options. Ruxolitinib is a selective Janus kinase (JAK) 1/2 inhibitor. Janus kinase (JAK) 1/2 is involved at multiple steps in GVHD process. It is effective in both, acute and chronic GVHD.

IMMUNOSTIMULANTS AND IMMUNOMODULATORS PH 1.50

The use of a variety of agents to enhance immunological and nonspecific host defences and thus to modify the defences favourably is an exciting development in immunopharmacology. Such agents may act by:

- **Increasing the humoral antibody responses**
- **Enhancing the phagocytic activity of macrophages**
- **Modifying the cell-mediated immune responses**

No ideal immunostimulant is yet available.

Drugs like **amantadine** and **tilorane** stimulate the humoral immune system. Nonspecific immunostimulation with **BCG** increases the clearing of antigen by macrophages. It activates NK cells and production of haemopoietic stem cells. It has been used along with conventional therapy in the treatment of leukaemias, melanoma and lung and bladder carcinoma with some beneficial results (Chapter 52).

THALIDOMIDE: This drug, chemically related to barbiturates, and introduced as a hypnotic and antiemetic, was found to be teratogenic and hence rejected. It has now staged a comeback in therapeutics as an **immuno-modulator/stimulator.**

Mechanism of action:

1. **Anti-inflammatory:** It inhibits the production of TNF-alpha and interferon, and has stimulatory effects on IGF1, IL-6 and IL-2.
2. **Immunomodulatory:** Its effects vary with different conditions. It decreases circulating TNF-alpha in patients with ENL but increases it in patients who are HIV seropositive. It reduces phagocytosis by neutrophils and enhances CMI. It enhances natural killer (NK) and T cell–mediated cytotoxicity.
3. **Anti-proliferative/pro-apoptotic antitumour effects:**
4. **Antiangiogenic:** It inhibits the induction of COX-2 and the biosynthesis of PGE_2 needed for angiogenesis.

Given orally, it is well absorbed and is metabolised to several metabolites. 5-Hydroxy thalidomide is an active metabolite. It is administered in the dose of 100–300 mg daily at bed time 1 h after dinner.

Adverse reactions: It can cause sedation, dizziness, constipation, tremors, mood changes, increased risk of deep vein thrombosis (DVT), brittle nails and palmer erythema. Peripheral sensory neuropathy and hypothyroidism may occur **after long-term therapy. It is highly teratogenic.**

Indications:

- **Drug of choice in symptomatic treatment of moderate to severe ENL** (Chapter 53)
- **Multiple myeloma and lymphomas, refractory to other treatments**
- **Refractory cutaneous lupus lesions**
- **Crohn disease**
- **To inhibit angiogenesis**
- **Treatment of cachexia and weight loss in HIV and that due to TNF-alpha in cancer patients; it counters nausea, vomiting and anorexia due to TNF-alpha in cancer patients**
- **In advanced prostatic cancer, as an immunomodulatory**

Lenalidomide and **Pomalidomide** are derivatives of thalidomide and are used for multiple myeloma and myeloplastic syndrome. They are teratogenic.

Levamisole, an anthelmintic (Chapter 58), has **immunotropic** properties and may help in restoring the efficiency of host defence mechanisms. It probably acts by modulating CMI responses and enhances it. Like BCG and **clofazimine,** (Chapter 53), its effect is associated with enhanced phagocytic activity of the macrophages. The drug may cause GI disturbances, headache, dizziness, insomnia, thrombocytopenia and agranulocytosis. It is used as an adjuvant therapy for chronic infectious diseases, warts, steroid dependent nephrotic syndrome and cancer.

Interferons are naturally occurring species specific cellular glycoproteins with complex effects on immunity (Chapter 57).

Interferons have been shown to produce some beneficial effect on certain human lymphoreticular and other cancers (Chapter 59), in MS (Chapter 15) and in hepatitis B, C and D (Chapter 57).

HUMAN RECOMBINANT IL-2: See Chapter 25

GLATIRAMER ACETATE: This is a synthetic co-polymer with some immunological similarity to myelin basic protein, one of the major components of myelin. Given subcutaneously, it is claimed to reduce the relapse rate in relapsing–remitting multiple sclerosis. It probably acts as an immunomodulator.

Tinospora cordifolia: This Ayurvedic plant drug (Guduchi) has been studied widely for its immunomodulatory effects. It stimulates nonspecific immune cells, neutrophils and macrophages as well as NK cells. It activates cellular and humoral immunity. It has been shown to release cytokines and GMCSF from the activated immune cells. Clinical studies have revealed its therapeutic application in conditions associated with immunosuppression *viz.* obstructive jaundice, patients taking cancer chemotherapy, tuberculosis and CKD.

For use of **monoclonal antibodies,** see section, Monoclonal antibodies in therapeutics.

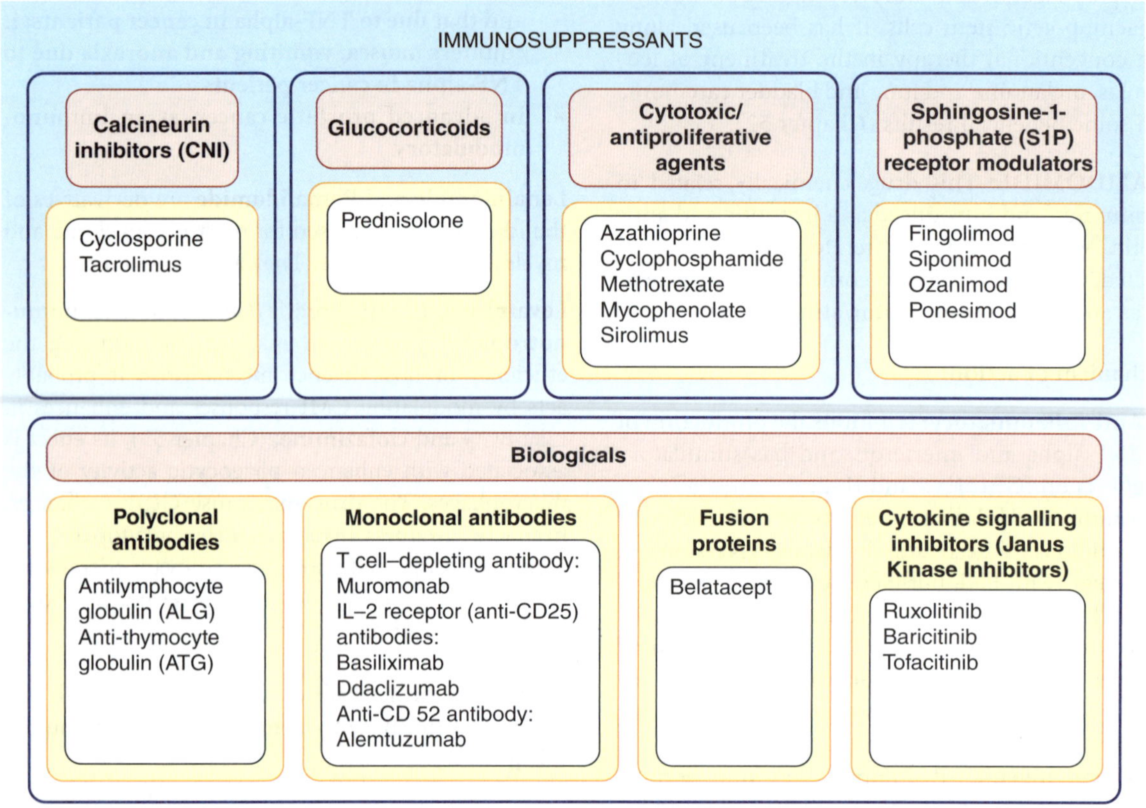

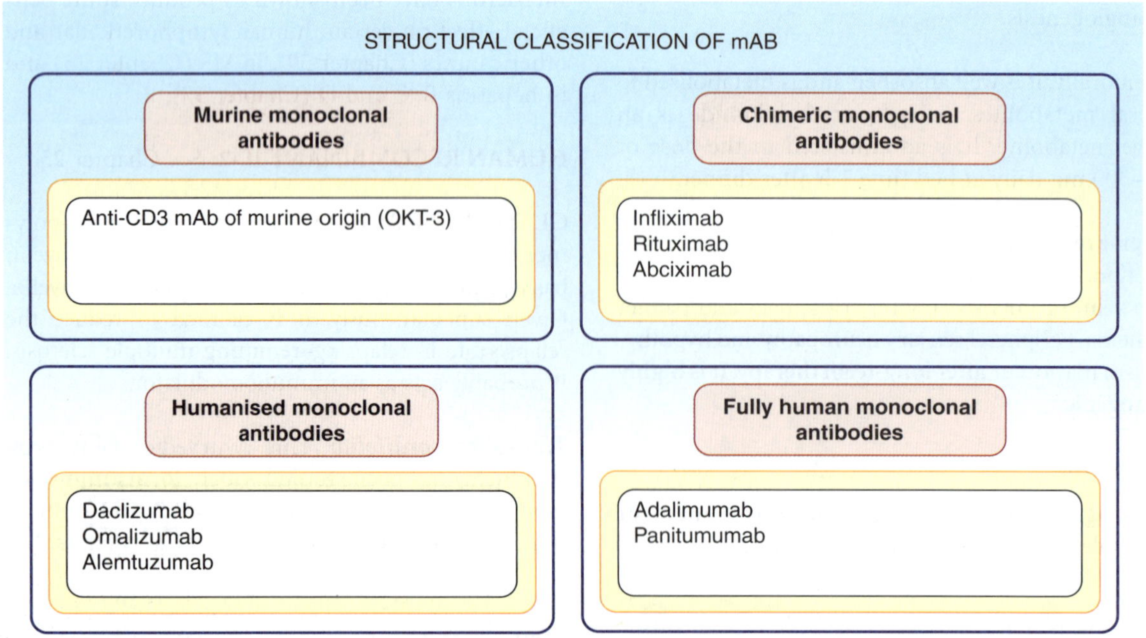

16

SECTION

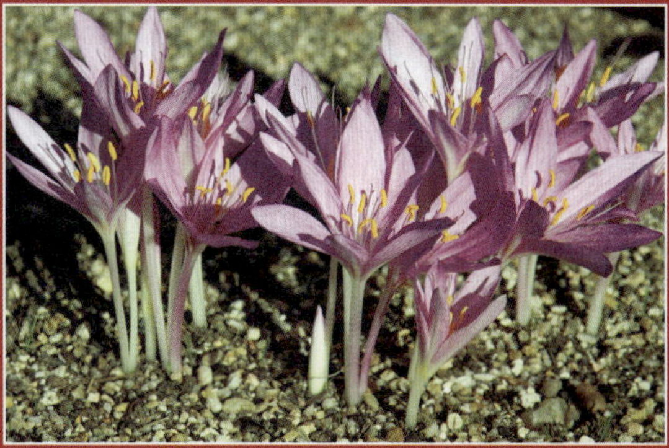

Colchicum autumnale

Miscellaneous

Section Outline

This section consists of the following chapters:

SECTION 16

Miscellaneous

CHAPTER 73

Pharmacotherapy of Gout, Rheumatoid Arthritis and Osteoarthritis

Learning Objectives

This chapter will enable the reader:

1. To be aware of the pathophysiology of gout and its clinical manifestations.
2. To enlist drugs causing hyperuricaemia.
3. To state the dietary principles in prevention and treatment of hyperuricaemia and gout.
4. To explain the mechanism of action, salient pharmacokinetic features, ADR of drugs used in the treatment and prevention of acute attacks of gout and in long-term therapy.
5. To be aware of the pathophysiology of rheumatoid arthritis (RA).
6. To classify drugs used in management of RA.
7. To explain the rationale for anti-inflammatory analgesics and glucocorticoids in the treatment of RA.
8. To state the mechanism of action, salient pharmacokinetic features, ADR and indications for DMARDs in RA.
9. To enumerate various biological agents used in the treatment of RA stating their mechanism of action, indication/s for use and ADR.
10. To outline the management of RA stating the goals and principles of therapy.
11. To outline the management of OA highlighting the role of pharmacotherapy.

KEY TERMS

drug induced hyperuricaemia, p. 1102
colchicine, p. 1103
allopurinol, p. 1104
febuxostat, p. 1105
Rasburicase, p. 1105
probenecid, p. 1105
Azapropazone, p. 1106
disease-modifying antirheumatic drugs, p. 1107
NSAIDs in RA, p. 1107
glucocorticoids in RA, p. 1107
methotrexate, p. 1107
biological agents, p. 1108
TNF-alpha blockers, p. 1108
osteoarthritis, management, p. 1111

OR 3.1

Acute or chronic arthritis or periarthritis can be caused by **monosodium urate (MSU)**, calcium pyrophosphate dihydrate (CPPD), calcium hydroxyapatite (HA) and calcium oxalate (CaOx). In spite of differences in composition, the deposition of crystals in the joints causes clinically indistinguishable arthropathies. *The definitive diagnosis of the type of arthritis can only be made by aspiration analysis of the synovial effusion for the type of microcrystals.*

Gout is a metabolic disorder that results from increase in body pool of urate. It comprises of:

- **Arthritis due to a reaction to the deposition of MSU in the joint.** It is acute, recurrent, monoarticular, at least in the initial years, and usually involves a peripheral joint in the lower limbs.
- **Painless deposition of urate crystals in the soft tissues such as cartilage, bursae and tendons.**
- **Development of 'tophi'** in the latter after many years of recurring gouty arthritis; tophi may not be seen clinically but are often diagnosed radiologically.
- **Renal calculi and nephropathy.**

The first episode of acute MSU gouty arthritis often begins at night with dramatic joint pain and swelling which mimic cellulitis. Less commonly, the arthritis may be less severe and more indolent, and involve more than one joint at one time.

The diagnosis of MSU gout depends upon:

- **A characteristic clinical arthritis**
- **Tophi**
- **The presence of typical urate crystals** in the joint fluid and the tophi

The disease largely affects middle aged to elderly men and only 5%–15% of women.

Box 73.1 Drugs Causing Hyperuricaemia

- Alcohol
- Thiazides, loop diuretics, amiloride
- Cytotoxic drugs
- Isotretinoin
- Ethambutol, pyrazinamide
- Salicylates in low doses
- Cyclosporine
- Levodopa
- Niacin

The incidence of gout rises with the serum uric acid level and the duration of hyperuricaemia; however, *hyperuricaemia per se does not confirm or exclude the diagnosis of gout.* Hyperuricaemia is necessary but not sufficient for the development of gout; only about 5% of patients with hyperuricaemia, in fact, ever develop gout.

Hyperuricaemia is due to either increased urate production or decreased urate excretion. It may be primary; or secondary to:

1. Renal impairment
2. Drugs (Box 73.1)
3. Massive lysis of cells during cancer chemotherapy

Only about 10% of patients with primary gout overproduce urate; majority of patients have diminished fractional renal clearance of urate in spite of normal overall renal function. In humans, who genetically lack uricase, urate which is less soluble circulates as such in the plasma. In MSU gout, the patient has uric acid pool, several times that of normal.

Asymptomatic hyperuricaemia (serum urate >6.8 mg%) does not warrant drug treatment. However, the *correction of reversible* **risk factors** *such as obesity, hyperlipidaemia, excess alcohol consumption, high purine diet (meat and fish) and drugs known to cause hyperuricaemia is wise.* Preference should be given to losartan and fenofibrate in asymptomatic hyperuricaemic patients with hypertension and hyperlipidaemia, respectively.

Box 73.2 outlines the principles of diet in prevention and treatment of hyperuricaemia.

Patients with clinical MSU gout need drug therapy (Box 73.3).

Box 73.2 Diet in Prevention and Treatment of Hyperuricaemia and Gout

- ***Avoid/minimise consumption*** of fatty meats (red meat), sea food and fats.
- ***Consume regularly*** cereals, pulses, fruits, vegetables, nuts in moderation and low-fat milk and milk products.
- ***Purine-rich fruits, beans and legumes have not been shown to be a risk factor in gout.*** Consumption of eggs is not a risk factor but they have high cholesterol content. Tea, coffee and spices pose no risk. Salt and pickles are not a risk factor in gout but an excess salt consumption is a risk factor in hypertension, and in hypercalciuria± renal calculi.
- ***Carbonated beverages may contain added phosphoric acid and their regular consumption may be a risk factor for calcium oxalate renal calculi.***

Box 73.3 Drugs Used in Gout

I. ***To treat acute gouty arthritis:***
   a. **Colchicine:** Specific, slow acting, adverse effects
   b. **NSAID** (short acting such as ibuprofen and indomethacin): nonspecific, rapid, better tolerated
   c. **Corticosteroids:** Effective intra-articularly and systemically; potential for rebound inflammation and adverse effects

II. ***To prevent acute attacks:***
   a. **Colchicine:** Effective in a dose adjusted not to cause diarrhoea
   b. **NSAID:** Less well tolerated for this purpose but may be used if colchicine alone is not sufficient to prevent frequent acute attacks

III. ***To lower serum urate levels:***
   a. **Probenecid:** Well tolerated; interferes with excretion of many drugs; risk of urolithiasis. Uricosuria is reversed by salicylates
   b. **Allopurinol:** Inhibits uric acid synthesis; once a day dosage increases convenience; excretion impaired in renal insufficiency
   c. **Sulphinpyrazone and benzbromarone** are less commonly used drugs

Classification of Anti-Gout Drugs PH 1.16

I. **Drugs Used During Acute Stage**
   - **Anti-inflammatory drugs**
     i. *Synthetic:* NSAID, glucocorticoids
     ii. *Natural:* Colchicine

II. **Drugs Used for Correction of Hyperuricaemia**
   - **Inhibitors of uric acid synthesis**
     i. *Xanthine oxidase inhibitors*

- Purine analogues: Allopurinol
- Non-purine analogues: Febuxostat

ii. *Enzymes:* Rasburicase, pegloticase

- **Promoters of uric acid secretion (uricosuric drugs):** Probenecid, sulphinpyrazone, benzbromarone, azapropazone IM 7.20

DRUGS USED DURING ACUTE STAGE

COLCHICINE, an alkaloid obtained from *Autumn crocus* (colchicum), is highly effective and specific for the treatment and prevention of acute gouty arthritis.

Mechanism of action: Sodium urate crystals in joints are coated by either anti-urate IgG antibody or lipoprotein containing apolipoprotein B and then ingested by granulocytes; the latter then release a glycoprotein which amplifies neutrophil infiltration into the joint. Colchicine by binding to tubulin, damages the microtubules in the granulocytes and inhibits the migration of cells into the inflamed area. It thus prevents the intra-articular release of mediators of inflammation by neutrophils. It also inhibits the release of histamine by mast cells.

Absorption, fate, excretion: Oral absorption of colchicine is variable. It is 50% protein bound and accumulates in the kidney, liver and spleen. It undergoes enterohepatic circulation. It is metabolised in the liver by CYP3A4. Urinary excretion is only 10%–20%. Its plasma t½ is 9 h. The drug is contraindicated in patients with hepatic or renal impairment.

Adverse reactions: It commonly produces GI upset and diarrhoea. Occasionally, it may cause anaemia, leucopenia, agranulocytosis and alopecia. Prolonged therapy may rarely cause myopathy (proximal muscle weakness). Because of the troublesome diarrhoea, indomethacin/NSAID may be preferred to colchicine.

P-glycoprotein inhibitors like cyclosporine can cause fatal toxicity of colchicine. Colchicine is rapidly degraded by exposure to light and loses its therapeutic efficacy.

Indications:

- **Treatment of acute attacks of gouty arthritis:** The drug is administered orally using single dose of 1.2 mg, followed by 0.6 mg 1 h later. It relieves pain in most cases within 24–48 h. If taken early in the attack, it can relieve the attack within a few hours. **Therapy must not be repeated within 4 days to avoid cumulative toxicity.** Unlike indomethacin, colchicine does not cause fluid retention; hence, is valuable in patients with heart failure. Furthermore, it can be given to patients receiving anticoagulants.
- **Prevention of acute attacks of gouty arthritis:** Prophylactically administered in small doses of 0.6 mg twice daily for 6 months, it can reduce the frequency of attacks in patients suffering from three or more attacks in a year. *For chronic use, in small doses it is better tolerated than NSAID.*
- **Prevention of attacks of familial Mediterranean fever** (familial paroxysmal polyserositis.)

INDOMETHACIN: This NSAID, in the dose of 25–50 mg t.i.d. for 5–7 days, can promptly relieve pain. However, the incidence of gastric intolerance is high. The drug can also be given as 100 mg suppositories. **Naproxen** or **ibuprofen** is equally effective and less toxic (see Chapter 11).

GLUCOCORTICOIDS: Glucocorticoids can be used in very severe cases, that are refractory to colchicine and NSAID. Their actions are not specific and the relapse rate is very high following the withdrawal. Prednisolone is given in the dose of 20 mg b.i.d. till the patient is asymptomatic for 1 week and then is progressively reduced by 5–10 mg every day. When a large joint such as the knee joint is affected, aspiration and intra-articular injection of hydrocortisone acetate, methylprednisolone or triamcinolone may give dramatic relief.

In severe cases with excruciating pain, colchicine, an NSAID (in maximum dose) and prednisolone may be combined. An opioid analgesic may be necessary until pain is relieved by other agents.

IM 7.21

DRUGS USED FOR CORRECTION OF HYPERURICAEMIA

These drugs are indicated when any of the following criteria are fulfilled:

- **The cause of hyperuricaemia cannot be corrected** or such correction does not lower the plasma urate to less than 7 mg%.

- **Acute attacks with serum uric acid level of 9 mg% or higher.**
- **The patient has had at least two definite attacks of acute gouty arthritis or has tophi.**
- **The patient agrees to take the medication regularly almost lifelong.**

The drugs act by reducing the plasma urate levels either by:

1. **Preventing uric acid synthesis,** e.g. xanthine oxidase inhibitors or
2. **Excreting uric acid,** e.g. uricosuric drugs

These drugs do not prevent the acute attacks, but decrease the frequency of attacks and may diminish the incidence of complications due to urate deposition. Reduction of plasma urate level to less than 6 mg% is required to prevent acute gouty arthritis and less than 4 mg% for reabsorption of tophi.

The initial treatment is always with uric acid synthesis inhibitors. If it fails, uricosuric drugs are added.

Therapy to reduce plasma urate level should be started only after the subsidence of acute joint inflammation as otherwise it may delay recovery from the acute attack. *However, pre-existing therapy with plasma urate lowering drugs should not be stopped in case of an acute attack.* If started in the interval between acute attacks, it should be preceded by prophylactic treatment with colchicine as rapid lowering of uric acid sometimes precipitates an attack probably due to mobilisation of uric acid from the tophi. Prophylactic colchicine should be continued for one year after the plasma urate level has returned to the target level.

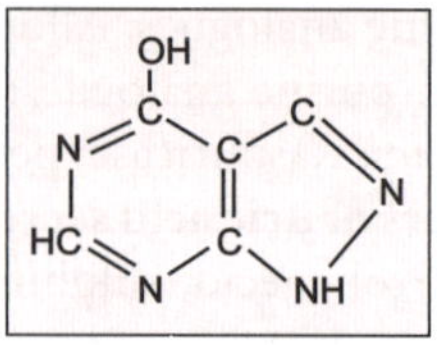

FIG. 73.1 Allopurinol.

XANTHINE OXIDASE INHIBITORS

ALLOPURINOL: It is used for long-term management of gout (Fig. 73.1).

Mechanism of action: During purine metabolism, the purine nucleotides are degraded to hypoxanthine and xanthine, which are then oxidised to uric acid by xanthine oxidase. **Allopurinol and its metabolic product alloxanthine (oxipurinol) inhibit xanthine oxidase** (Fig. 73.2), and hence they:

- **Inhibit the oxidation of hypoxanthine and xanthine to uric acid**
- **Lower serum and urine uric acid**
- **Reduce size of tophi**
- **Increase the excretion of hypoxanthine and xanthine in the urine.** Both these oxypurine compounds are cleared rapidly by the kidney and hence, there is less hazard of their crystallisation in the kidneys and nephrolithiasis. This is an advantage.

Adverse reactions: The incidence of adverse reactions is 15%–20%. The most common are allergic skin rash, nausea, vomiting and diarrhoea. Leucopenia, hepatic damage and vasculitis can occur. Haemosiderosis is a rare but serious complication. The other rare severe ADR are toxic epidermal necrolysis, bone marrow suppression and ototoxicity.

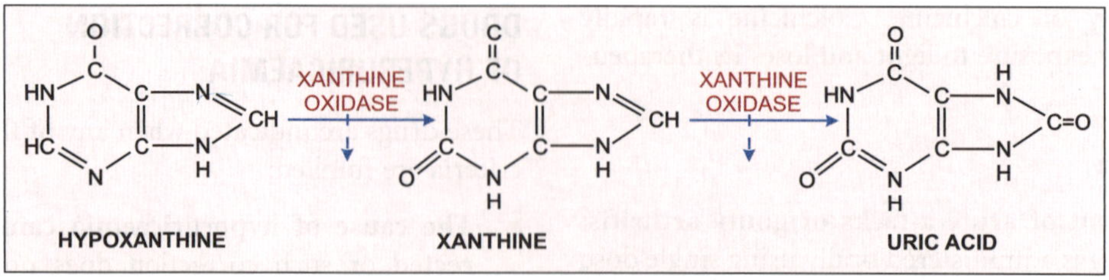

FIG. 73.2 Synthesis of uric acid.

Preparation and dosage: Available as 100 and 300 mg tablets. It is started in a dose of 100 mg per day with monitoring of serum uric acid levels after 2 weeks. The dose is increased gradually every 2 weeks till the serum uric acid falls below 6 mg%. The maximum approved dose is 800 mg/day. A single dose is preferred as the half-life of the active metabolite, oxypurinol, is about 20 h. In chronic renal failure, the dose of allopurinol should be lowered proportional to reduction in GFR.

Indications:

- **Gout:** Allopurinol is used for controlling hyperuricaemia. It is useful in patients with gouty tophi or uric acid calculi and in those with renal failure which renders uricosuric drugs less effective. It may be combined with uricosuric drugs.
- **Secondary hyperuricaemia:** This occurs following the use of cytotoxic drugs in the treatment of leukaemia and lymphoma. Therefore, allopurinol is started before starting chemotherapy. Inhibition of xanthine oxidase, which also metabolises 6-mercaptopurine, prolongs its t½; hence, its dose is reduced to one-third or one-fourth to avoid serious toxicity.

FEBUXOSTAT: This orally active, nonpurine analogue of allopurinol acts as an inhibitor of xanthine oxidase. It is well tolerated and can be used in patients allergic to or intolerant of allopurinol. The maximum daily dose is 80 mg. It is mainly metabolised in the liver. Mild to moderate renal insufficiency does not alter its serum uric acid lowering ability. Its ADR include liver function abnormalities, headache, nausea, and rarely, Stevens–Johnson syndrome.

Rasburicase, a recombinant urate oxidase, **causes enzymatic degradation of uric acid to soluble allantoin.** It is usually used to reduce the elevated uric acid levels in tumour lysis syndrome (TLS) that is seen following cancer chemotherapy. Its ADR include vomiting, fever, headache, GI upset, mucositis, acute renal failure, anaphylaxis and haemolysis in G6PD deficiency patients. **Pegloticase** is pegylated mammalian recombinant uricase produced by genetically modulated strain of *E. coli.* It is used for the treatment of chronic resistant gout. The ADR include infusion reactions, anaphylaxis and development of antipegloticase antibodies, which results in loss of efficacy.

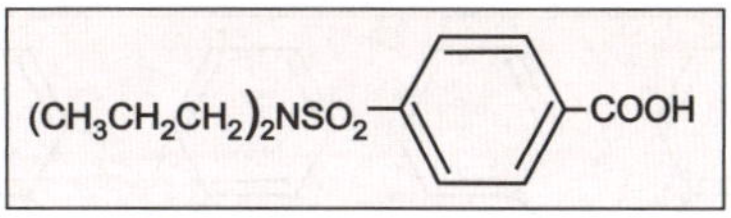

FIG. 73.3 Probenecid.

URICOSURIC DRUGS

Uric acid is freely filtered by the glomerulus, and nearly 90% is reabsorbed by in the proximal tubule. Uricosuric drugs, e.g. probenecid, are organic acids that **inhibit uric acid transporter** in the proximal tubule, which decreases uric acid reabsorption, resulting in an increased urinary excretion.

PROBENECID: This uricosuric agent (Fig. 73.3) *in low doses, causes a decrease in distal tubular secretion of uric acid but in larger therapeutic doses, it increases its excretion, by blocking* proximal *tubular reabsorption.* After treatment for some months, the serum uric acid may return to normal levels together with significant mobilisation of gouty tophi. It is given orally, initially in doses of 0.5 g once daily, gradually increasing to three times daily.

In addition, probenecid also inhibits both the organic anion transporters (OAT) in the basolateral membrane of cells in the proximal tubule. This results in reduced clearance and increased plasma levels of drugs normally secreted by this mechanism (e.g. penicillin).

Adverse reactions: The drug is relatively nontoxic and is well tolerated. Occasionally, it causes dyspepsia, skin rashes and deposition of urate crystals in the renal tubules/pelvis; this risk can be minimised by maintaining a high volume of alkaline urine with 1 g of sodium bicarbonate orally 3–4 times a day. The drug inhibits the renal excretion of drugs such as penicillin, indomethacin, methotrexate and dapsone. It also impairs heparin metabolism thus reducing the dose of heparin necessary for anticoagulation.

SULPHINPYRAZONE: This is a sulphoxide derivative of phenylbutazone (Fig. 73.4) with some anti-inflammatory activity but marked uricosuric property. This effect is dose related. *Like probenecid its smaller dose prevents the tubular secretion of uric acid, whereas higher dose promotes its excretion.* It is

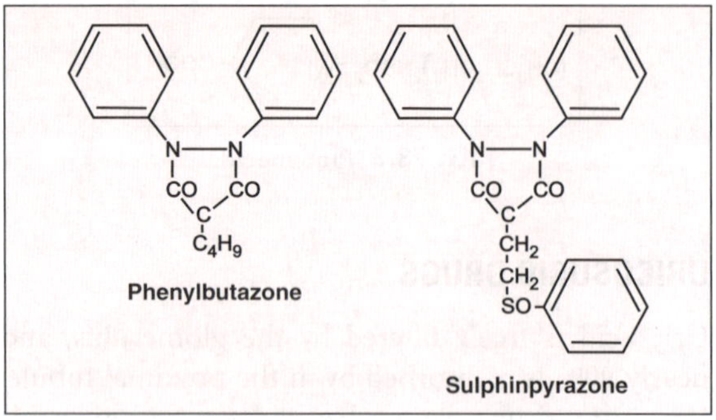

FIG. 73.4 **Phenylbutazone and sulphinpyrazone.**

administered orally in doses of 100–200 mg t.i.d. The daily dose should not exceed 600 mg.

Adverse reactions: These include vomiting, upper abdominal discomfort and skin rashes. Rarely, it can aggravate an existing DU and may cause bone marrow depression. Sulphinpyrazone inhibits platelet aggregation.

Both probenecid and sulphinpyrazone are ineffective in the presence of impaired renal function.

Benzbromarone, a benzofuran compound, is another uricosuric drug. It is potent and is claimed to be effective even when the GFR is reduced to 25%–50 % of normal.

AZAPROPAZONE: This uricosuric agent **has weak analgesic, antipyretic and anti-inflammatory actions.** It is a weak inhibitor of cyclooxygenase. The drug is rapidly and almost completely absorbed from the gut. It is relatively toxic. The common ADR comprise GI effects and headache. It has also been used for the treatment of RA and osteoarthritis (OA).

Uricosuric drugs can be hazardous in:

- **Urate overproducers** (24 h urine urate more than 800 mg)
- **Those with urine flow consistently less than 1 mL/min**
- **Those with creatinine clearance less than 50 mL/min**
- **Those with history of renal calculi**

Aspirin, an analgesic, relieves joint pains (Chapter 11). Although it has a uricosuric action, the dose required for persistent uricosuria is large, which is intolerable.

In smaller doses, it acts as anti-uricosuric and also blocks the uricosuric effect of other drugs. Salicylates, therefore, should be avoided in gout.

Other measures in gout: With the uricosuric drugs, a **fluid intake** sufficient to yield daily urinary output of at least 2 L and the maintenance of a neutral or slightly alkaline urine pH are desirable to prevent renal damage. This is particularly important during hot weather and in the tropics.

IM 7.20

Other crystal-induced arthropathies: Acute CPPD arthritis was formerly known as pseudogout because of its similarities with MSU gout. There is no effective therapy to remove the synovial deposits, and the treatment is symptomatic, i.e. NSAID, colchicine and intra-articular glucocorticoid.

The treatment of HA arthritis and calcium oxalate arthritis is also symptomatic. OR 3.1

PHARMACOTHERAPY OF RHEUMATOID ARTHRITIS (RA)

Rheumatoid arthritis (RA) is a chronic, systemic, inflammatory disease predominantly affecting joints, and periarticular (synovial) tissues and is **autoimmune in origin.**

Of all the rheumatoid disorders, RA remains a formidable disease, being capable of producing severe crippling deformities and functional disabilities. Common clinical signs and symptoms are pain and/or joint swelling, morning stiffness at least for 1 h, fatigue, fever and weight loss. The disorder is more common in women and elderly persons. Its aetiology is unknown.

Autoantibodies such as RA factor (RF), are associated with more severe joint disease with extra-articular manifestations. Other important antibodies are those directed against citrullinated peptide (ACPA) which seems to be more specific and sensitive marker. About 50%–80% of RA patients have RF or ACPA or both. Clinical diagnosis is confirmed by estimating ESR, autoantibody and radiographs. Antibodies can be detected years before onset of disease.

Pathophysiology: It comprises three basic interrelated pathological processes:

- **Inflammation**
- **Synovial proliferation**
- **Joint tissue destruction**

The focus of RA is the synovial lining. RA factor-containing immune complexes found in the joints activate the pathological process.

The earliest lesion is vasculitis, an inflammation of small blood vessels. It is now believed that the monokines *IL-1 and IL-6, and TNF-alpha are the central mediators of active rheumatoid process.*

Joint damage occurs early in the course of RA. Fibroblasts like synoviocytes invade the cartilage. **Osteoclasts activation is considered to be a key event in bone destruction.**

Classification of Drugs Used in RA

PH 1.16, IM 7.22, IM 7.23

I. **Anti-inflammatory analgesic drugs:** Aspirin and other NSAID (Chapter 11)

II. **Anti-inflammatory drugs with indirect analgesic action:** Glucocorticoids (Chapter 64). They also have immunomodulatory activity.
These two groups act rapidly, relieve pain and control inflammation; they thus help to improve and maintain joint function. *However, they do not halt the underlying destructive process.*

III. **Disease-modifying antirheumatic drugs (DMARD),** e.g. methotrexate, sulphasalazine, chloroquine and leflunomide.
They have no analgesic or immediate anti-inflammatory effect and begin to act after 6–12 weeks. They probably modulate immune function. They arrest the basic destructive process in the joints and modify the course of the disease. They may induce remission.

IV. **Biological agents:** This heterogenous group includes complex protein molecules which are developed using molecular biological techniques. Their action is predictable and results from interaction with cytokines or cell surface molecules. These are as follows:
   a. **TNF-alpha blockers:** infliximab, adalimumab and etanercept
   b. **IL-1 receptor antagonist:** anakinra
   c. **IL-6 receptor antagonist:** tocilizumab
   d. **T cell activation inhibitors:** abatacept
   e. **Anti–B-lymphocyte antibody:** rituximab
   f. **Tyrosine kinase inhibitor:** tofacitinib

V. **Immunosuppressants:** Azathioprine and Cyclosporine-A. They can be life saving when severe vasculitis complicates the clinical picture.

I. ANTI-INFLAMMATORY ANALGESICS

NSAIDs act symptomatically, relieve pain, decrease swelling (Chapter 11) and help to improve the joint movements. Aspirin is required to be given in the dose of 3–5 g daily to maintain therapeutic blood levels of 20–30 mg%. Such high doses cause GI adverse reactions. Enteric coated aspirin may cause less gastric irritation. It should be avoided in the elderly. Aspirin and indomethacin can be given as rectal suppositories so as to avoid gastric irritation. Other NSAIDs used are ibuprofen (200–400 mg thrice daily), diclofenac (75–100 mg twice daily), naproxen (250 mg twice daily) and ketoprofen (50 mg thrice daily), given with food. A single dose of naproxen 500 mg taken at bedtime may also be effective. **Ibuprofen is perhaps the best tolerated among the NSAIDs.** Since piroxicam and diclofenac have prolonged action, a single dose at bedtime often may be effective for relieving the night pain and the early morning stiffness (Chapter 11). *The risk of GI bleeding in patients taking NSAID and/or glucocorticoids is very high in RA.* This can be prevented to some extent by prophylactic use of PPI (Chapter 41).

II. GLUCOCORTICOIDS

These potent anti-inflammatory drugs on oral administration produce dramatic symptomatic relief which lasts as long as they are used. They act by inhibiting the synthesis and/or by suppressing the actions of inflammatory mediators (Chapter 64). Prednisolone is started in the dose of 1 mg/kg/day, and then tapered gradually to a maintenance dose of 7.5 mg/day. The small maintenance dose may be continued as needed. *Glucocorticoids are not used as monotherapy.* Low doses of prednisolone (5 mg/day) that do not affect clinical inflammation may have a joint protective effect and can be combined with DMARD. Larger doses are required to control severe systemic manifestations of RA such as pericarditis and vasculitis. Their major drawback is their toxicity (Chapter 64). Furthermore, relapse rate after stoppage is high.

III. DMARDs: IM 7.23

METHOTREXATE (MTX): This folic acid antagonist (Chapter 59), **given intermittently, appears to be highly effective, has acceptable long-term**

toxicity and is cost-effective. The initial dose is usually 5–7.5 mg orally, taken as a single dose once a week. When administered in such low **doses, methotrexate shows anti-inflammatory action but no immunosuppressive or cytotoxic action**. Its action is probably related to inhibition of aminoimidazole carboxamide (AICAR) transformylase and thymidylate synthetase, thereby preventing neutrophil chemotaxis. Clinical response is usually seen in 4–8 weeks. If no response is seen even after 8 weeks of therapy, the dose may be increased by 2.5 mg every other week to a maximum of 15 mg once weekly. After improvement sets in, it is given at the lowest possible effective dose indefinitely, as relapse occurs following its discontinuation.

Its toxicity is dose related. *In the dose recommended (7.5 mg or less per week), the risk of toxicity is* less. Folic acid 5 mg/day may reduce its toxicity. However, long-term use is suspected to cause liver cirrhosis and fibrosing alveolitis. Hence, it is best avoided in patients with pre-existing liver disease and chronic alcoholics. It should also be avoided in patients with significant renal dysfunction.

Methotrexate is teratogenic and it should not be used during pregnancy. Men should not take the drug for 3 months, and women for one menstrual cycle, before a planned pregnancy.

CHLOROQUINE and **HYDROXYCHLOROQUINE:** These antimalarials (Chapter 54) are taken up by macrophages and lymphocytes. **They inhibit phagocytosis, decrease T-cell activation and reduce inflammatory cytokines, i.e. TNF-alpha.** They have mild anti-inflammatory action and probably act as immunomodulators.

Hydroxychloroquine is preferred because of the lower incidence of gastrointestinal adverse reactions compared with chloroquine. The dose of hydroxychloroquine sulphate is 400 mg/day; the maintenance dose is 200–400 mg (maximum of 6.5 mg/kg/day. *After getting good relief, the frequency of the daily dose is progressively reduced to once a week;*

They are perhaps the best tolerated and relatively safe DMARD. Long-term therapy may rarely cause retinopathy and irreversible visual impairment. Hence, periodic ophthalmic examination during therapy is mandatory.

SULPHASALAZINE: This drug, used in the treatment of ulcerative colitis, is discussed in Chapter 43. The mesalamine component of sulphasalazine inhibits pro-inflammatory cytokines, immunoglobulin, COX and lipo-oxygenase and thus exerts anti-inflammatory action. Sulphapyridine, which is absorbed more, reduces IL-8 synthesis and probably inhibits angiogenesis.

It is a useful and reasonably safe drug in the treatment of RA. The dose required (1–2 g/day) is larger than that required to treat ulcerative colitis. With this dosage, adverse reactions are common and include allergy, nausea, vomiting and headache. Rarely, neutropenia, haemolytic anaemia and thrombocytopenia may occur. It interferes with absorption and metabolism of folic acid

LEFLUNOMIDE, a pyrimidine synthesis inhibitor, is as effective as sulphasalazine in decreasing signs and symptoms, and slowing the radiological progression of RA. After absorption, it is converted to active metabolite which inhibits RNA synthesis and cell growth; it also prevents T cell proliferation. It remains in the body for a long time (up to 2 years). The dose is 100 mg daily for three days, followed by maintenance dose of 10–20 mg per day. The adverse effects are diarrhoea, reversible alopecia, skin rash, hypertension and hepatic damage. Anaphylaxis and Stevens–Johnson syndrome have been reported. *The drug is carcinogenic and teratogenic*. Hence, it is advisable for a woman to postpone conception and for a man to postpone fathering a child for at least 2 years after stopping the treatment.

IV. BIOLOGICAL AGENTS IM 7.23

All biological agents are very expensive and need to be given parenterally. Most of them can precipitate opportunistic infections. They are used in combination with DMARD in severe cases or alone in refractory cases.

a. TNF-alpha blockers:

TNF-alpha agents in treatment of RA.

INFLIXIMAB: This is a chimeric, monoclonal anti-TNF antibody. The cytokine TNF-alpha is actively produced at the synovial sites in RA. Infliximab binds to the TNF-alpha with high

affinity, avidity and specificity and inhibits its binding with the TNF-alpha receptors and thus prevents its biological activity. Given by IV infusion once in 2 months, it causes dose-dependent neutralisation of human TNF-alpha. It has t½ of 8–12 days. It can cause consistent and sustained benefit in patients with RA, *even those who are resistant to DMARD, and methotrexate.*
It is well tolerated in the doses used. The most common ADR are headache, nausea, cytopenia, rash and cough. It may precipitate respiratory tract infections including TB. The recipient can develop antibodies to infliximab. It has also been used in the treatment of Crohn disease, psoriasis and ankylosing spondylitis.

ADALIMUMAB: This recombinant, human anti-TNF monoclonal antibody has similar actions as infliximab. It is given subcutaneously every second week and has t½ of 9–14 days. **Certolizumab pegol** and **golimumab** are the newer anti-TNF agents.

ETANERCEPT: This fusion protein unlike infliximab, selectively binds to active trimeric portion of TNF-alpha. In addition, it also binds to *the cytokine lymphotoxin alpha (TNF-beta).*
TNF alpha inhibitors are generally considered safe for use in pregnancy. Individual agents in this class have probable similar efficacy.

b. IL-1 receptor antagonist:

ANAKINRA is recombinant human IL-1 receptor antagonist and is given daily subcutaneously. Evidence for its efficacy as compared to other biological agents is limited.

c. IL-6 receptor antagonist:

TOCILIZUMAB, an anti-IL-6 receptor blocker, is effective in patients not responding to DMARD or anti-TNF agents, or both. It is administered intravenously. Its ADR are similar to anti-TNF agents. In addition, it may increase total and LDL-cholesterol and cause neutropenia.

d. T-cell activation inhibitors:

ABATACEPT: This fusion protein prevents T-cell activation and lowers the serum concentration of inflammatory cytokines in RA. It is given intravenously, slowly, on day one and repeated at 2 and 4 weeks thereafter. It has been used to treat RA not responding to other agents. *Abatacept can be combined with DMARDs but not with TNF-alpha inhibitors.*

e. Anti–B-lymphocytic antibody:

RITUXIMAB is a monoclonal antibody which selectively depletes the CD20 B-lymphocytes which play a role in the auto-immune response and in the chronic synovitis associated with RA. It is claimed to be useful in RA resistant to TNF-alpha blockers.
The major drawbacks of all TNF-alpha inhibitors and other biological agents is increased risk of serious infection. They should be avoided in the presence of infections, particularly tuberculosis and viral hepatitis, as well as in the presence of a demyelinating disease or CHF. Live virus vaccines are contraindicated in patients receiving biological agents.
The patient should be tested for tuberculosis before starting the treatment, and should be watched for any infection.

f. Tyrosine kinase inhibitor

TOFACITINIB is the first oral janus kinase inhibitor (JAKi /JAKinib) approved for RA patients, who had inadequate response or are intolerant to methotrexate. Janus kinases are protein tyrosine kinases that serve as signalling mediator and initiate intracellular signalling cascade in various immune pathways. *Tofacitinib prevents the activation of intracellular mediators involved in immune response and inflammation that lead to joint destruction.* Adverse effects include diarrhoea, hypertension, hypercholesterolaemia, opportunistic infections, leucopenia, anaemia and increased liver enzymes. *It is metabolised by CYP3A4. It should not be used with biological agents.*
Other janus kinase inhibitors include **baricitinib, filgotinib, upadacitinib** and **peficitinib.**

V. **Immunosuppressive agents** (Chapter 72): Various alkylating agents like **azathioprine, cyclosporine-A, cyclophosphamide** have been

PH 1.1

Box 73.4 Principles of Management of RA

- Rest to acutely inflamed joints
- Symptomatic relief of pain and inflammation by use of adequate doses of NSAID which act as bridge drugs. However, they do not cause a change in the cytokine-mediated acute phase reactants.
- Prevention of articular damage by early use of *DMARD (methotrexate, hydroxychloroquine or sulphasalazine)* with rapid escalation
- Use of combination therapy, which reduces joint swelling and delays bone damage
- Short course of low-dose prednisolone (5–10 mg/day) along with DMARD
- In severe cases, short-term glucocorticoid in high doses at the onset, which is to be tapered to a maintenance dose later
- Use of biological agents if DMARD combination fails
- Quick changes in drug combination depending on the response
- Graded exercises and physiotherapy
- Treatment of comorbid conditions such as infections and osteoporosis
- Modification of the diet, using more omega-3 fatty acids in place of omega-9 fatty acids; in this respect, vegetarian diet may be beneficial
- Frequent follow-up and monitoring of the progress is mandatory.

used to induce remission in RA. These drugs act as suppressors of B and T lymphocytes. However, **they are less effective and more toxic.**

The principles of management of RA are outlined in Box 73.4.

The current goals of therapy of RA are as follows:

- **Suppression of disease activity as soon as possible and reduction of symptoms**
- **Arrest of the erosive and functional joint damage**
- **Improvement in laboratory indices**
- **Induction and maintenance of a long-term clinical and radiological remission after cessation of drug therapy.** There is now convincing evidence that *early treatment (preferably within 12 weeks) with DMARD has the potential to improve the quality of life and long-term outcome in patients with RA.*

Choice of drug therapy: Selection of a preferred drug would be guided by drug efficacy, safety and affordability. Although associated inflammation may be reversible, the cytokine-induced damage is not. *Bone loss has been shown to occur rapidly at the onset of the clinical disease.*

The treatment should be started immediately without waiting for results of lab tests if the clinical diagnosis and ESR indicate RA. Weekly methotrexate is currently favoured because of its relatively rapid onset of action, long-term benefit, acceptable toxicity, good compliance and low cost. The maximum improvement usually occurs after 6 months of therapy. **Methotrexate is usually combined with sulphasalazine and low-dose prednisolone.** Some experts advise more aggressive initial treatment with methotrexate, sulphasalazine, glucocorticoid and hydroxychloroquine.

The TNF-alpha inhibitors and other biological agents, though highly effective, are prohibitively expensive and their long-term safety is not clear. They should be used only in RA resistant to DMARDs.

Local intra-articular injection of a glucocorticoid is useful in controlling inflammation. Its indications are as follows:

- **One or two joints that are 'resistant' in the patient, otherwise well controlled on medical therapy**
- **Patients with one active joint in whom oral NSAID are contraindicated**

Usually, hydrocortisone acetate suspension is given in the dose of 25–50 mg for big joints and 5–10 mg for small joints. The number of injections depends upon the response, but it is advisable to avoid them more often than once in 3 months. The drug may also be injected extra-articularly into painful ligaments, tendons and inflamed bursae with beneficial results.

Supportive therapy: RA being a chronic disease, general supportive therapy including good nutrition and attention to psychological aspect is as important as drug therapy. Both physical and mental rest is essential. During the acute stage the rest must be complete, along with proper splinting of affected joints. *Proper exercises and physiotherapy during and after the recovery stage are essential for achieving maximum benefit.*

Use of warm baths and hot packs helps to loosen joints and relieve the stiffness. Exercise following heat helps to maintain the mobility of joints. Other comorbid states such as osteoporosis, CV disorders and depression need to be treated.

In spite of recent advances, 'cure' in RA is still elusive. Majority of patients recover partially and only a few lucky may get long remission.

OSTEOARTHRITIS IM 7.20, OR 3.1

OA is a common disease in the ageing population and results from a complex interplay of genetic, metabolic, biochemical and biomechanical factors with secondary local inflammation. The process involves the interaction of degradation and repair of the articular cartilage, bone and synovium. **The most important cells in the entire disease process are the chondrocytes.**

The initiating event in OA seems to be injury to the chondrocytes from a single macrotrauma or repeated microtrauma to the joint. The chondrocytes react by proliferation and release of enzymes which degrade the articular cartilage. The products of degradation, released into the synovial fluid, evoke the formation and release of mediators of inflammation by the synovial macrophages leading to cartilage destruction and faulty repair process.

Early OA may be clinically silent. The important symptoms, when they occur, are pain, tenderness, movement limitation, disability and deformity. *Muscle wasting is common and contributes to the disease process. Unlike in RA, there are generally no systemic symptoms.* In most patients, the disease stabilises after initial progression.

Management: *No treatment available at present can halt the degradation of the cartilage or stimulate its fresh synthesis and cannot reverse the pathological changes of OA.* The treatment is aimed at

a. pain relief and
b. improvement in joint mobility.

1. **Nonpharmacological treatment:** This includes physical therapy (heat, cold and transcutaneous electrical nerve stimulation) and exercise. Proper posture and weight reduction are important. Intermittent rest during the day, use of a walking stick and properly cushioned shoes are helpful.

2. **Pharmacological treatment:** Local application of **methylsalicylate** ointment or **diclofenac 1% gel** containing additional capsaicin may bring relief in mild cases. When oral therapy is required, preference should be given to **paracetamol** in the dose of 2–3 g/day in divided doses; this relieves the pain in most patients. A mild NSAID such as **ibuprofen** may be added to paracetamol in the presence of joint stiffness or swelling, or pain which interferes with work or sleep. *Stronger NSAID should be avoided.* This is especially important in the elderly who are particularly prone to the adverse effects of NSAID; they should be prescribed in the smallest possible dose for the shortest possible period. COX-2 inhibitors though 'stomach-friendly' can cause cardiovascular adverse effects (Chapter 11). Their routine use is not recommended.

The use of **intra-articular glucocorticoids** at 3 monthly intervals should be limited to patients with severe pain, especially with an effusion. Intra-articular injection of hyaluronic acid has also been claimed to relieve pain. *Systemic glucocorticoids have no place in the treatment of osteoarthritis.*

Glucosamine is derived from marine shells or is synthetic. It is the sulphate or hydrochloride of amino monosaccharide glucosamine, a normal constituent of glycosaminoglycan in the cartilage. Similarly, **chondroitin sulphate,** a component of cartilages and bones is obtained from animal sources, such as shark and cow cartilages. **Both,** given individually or in combination have no clinically relevant effect on joint pain. Their usefulness in OA is still doubtful.

There is no evidence at present that these supplements prevent OA in healthy persons or in patients with knee pain but normal X-rays.

Surgical treatment: Joint replacement helps selective patients with advanced OA and unbearable pain.

ANTI-GOUT DRUGS

Drugs Used During Acute Stage

Anti-inflammatory drugs

Synthetic
- NSAID
- Glucocorticoids

Natural
- Colchicine

Drugs Used for Correction of Hyperuricaemia

Inhibitors of uric acid synthesis

Xanthine oxidase inhibitors
- *Purine analogues*
  - Allopurinol
- *Non-purine analogues*
  - Febuxostat

Enzymes
- Rasburicase
- Pegloticase

Promoters of uric acid secretion (uricosuric drugs)
- Probenecid
- Sulphinpyrazone
- Benzbromarone
- Azapropazone

DRUGS USED IN THE TREATMENT OF RA

Anti-inflammatory analgesic drugs
- Aspirin

Anti-inflammatory drugs with indirect analgesic action
- Glucocorticoids

Disease-modifying antirheumatic drugs (DMARD)
- Methotrexate
- Sulphasalazine
- Chloroquine
- Leflunomide

Biological agents

TNF-alpha blockers
- Infliximab
- Adalimumab
- Etanercept

T cell activation inhibitors
- Abatacept

IL-1 receptor antagonist
- Anakinra

Anti–B-lymphocyte antibody
- Rituximab

IL-6 receptor antagonist
- Tocilizumab

Tyrosine kinase inhibitor
- Tofacitinib

Immunosuppressants
- Azathioprine
- Cyclosporine-A

CHAPTER 74

Metals and Their Antagonists

Learning Objectives

This chapter will enable the reader:

1. To enlist the various heavy metals and their toxic effects.
2. To outline the treatment of common heavy metal poisoning stating the choice of drugs in each poisoning.
3. To explain the term, chelating agents.
4. To explain the mechanism of action, salient pharmacokinetic features, adverse drug reactions and indications for heavy metal antagonists.

KEY TERMS

chelating agents, p. 1116
dimercaprol, p. 1116
succimer, p. 1117
D-Penicillamine, p. 1117
trientine, p. 1118
calcium disodium edetate, p. 1118

Several heavy metals such as lead, arsenic, cadmium, mercury compounds are important environmental pollutants and are also important from the toxicological point of view. Many herbomineral products like *bhasmas* of zinc, copper, mercury, arsenic, lead and gold available over the counter (OTC) may contribute to heavy metal toxicity. Reckless disposal of industrial waste particularly in river water is perhaps the major cause of chronic poisoning. This chapter gives an overview of the toxicity caused by heavy metals and its treatment with chelating agents. PH 1.51, PH 1.53, FM 9.3

Common heavy metals, which are known to cause poisoning, along with their toxic effects are listed in Table 74.1.

Pharmacological actions: The organic and the inorganic salts of heavy metals possess astringent, corrosive and caustic properties on local application. They also act as general protoplasmic poisons, interfering with various enzymes and altering cell membranes, thus impairing cell function. **The heavy metal salts, in very small quantities, are lethal to several Gram-positive and Gram-negative organisms.**

Heavy metals exert their toxic effects by combining with several reacting groups such as the SH groups, essential for normal physiological functions. The heavy metal antagonists (chelating agents) compete with these groups for the metals and spare the former; they prevent or reverse the toxic effects and enhance the excretion of the metals.

Adverse reactions: All the heavy metals are **cumulative and potentially toxic.** They can cause widespread damage to various organs like the liver, kidney, gut and brain. Rapidly proliferating tissues such as the bone marrow, the GI mucosa and other delicate cells such as neurons and renal tubular cells are also affected. Some of them serve as environmental toxins and may be responsible for neuropathy (Box 74.1).

The **major treatment** of metal toxicity is to prevent or terminate exposure to them. Chelating agents are used to bind metals into stable cyclic compounds of low toxicity (see section, heavy metal antagonists). **Activated charcoal does not bind metals** and hence is not useful in acute metal poisoning.

Table 74.1 Common Metals and their Toxicity Profile PH 1.53, FM 9.3

S.No	Metal	Symptoms and Signs
1	**Arsenic**	**Acute poisoning:** GI irritation, vomiting, diarrhoea, circulatory collapse and renal failure. GIT symptoms begin in 1 h. **Chronic poisoning:** *Early symptoms* – Weight loss, anorexia, fatigue and diarrhoea or constipation *Late symptoms* – Edema (particularly of eyelids and ankles), hyperpigmentation (especially on eyelids, neck, nipples and the axillae), dermatitis, hyperkeratosis of palms and soles may undergo malignant change resulting in basal cell carcinoma, inflammatory lesions of the mucous membranes, loss of hair; brittle finger nails, garlic odour breath and organ toxicity as cirrhosis, nephritis, aplastic anaemia, encephalopathy and peripheral neuropathy
2	**Lead**	**Acute poisoning:** Metallic taste, GI irritation, paraesthesiae, muscle cramps and weakness, dark-coloured stools, haemolytic anaemia and haemoglobinuria **Chronic poisoning:** *Gastrointestinal:* Metallic taste, greyish *lead line* along the gingival margin, anorexia, constipation, abdominal pain due to intestinal colic ('lead colic') *Skeletal muscles:* Muscle weakness, fatigue, paralysis ('lead palsy'), unilateral wrist or foot drop *Haemopoietic system:* Punctate basophilic stippling of erythrocytes (exceeding 35,000 per million erythrocytes), microcytic hypochromic anaemia, jaundice, excretion of abnormal products of porphyrin metabolism in urine *Nervous system: Lead encephalopathy* manifested as increased irritability, headache, restlessness and tremors, followed by delirium and convulsions or by lethargy and coma. Visual disturbances and stippling of the retina adjacent to the optic disc, which may be an early diagnostic sign; toxic peripheral neuropathy with motor neuropathy is more common. *Kidney:* Interstitial nephritis, tubular damage, hyperuricaemia and renal failure
3	**Antimony**	**Acute poisoning:** Local irritation, severe vomiting **Chronic poisoning:** Toxic effects of antimonials resemble those of arsenic
4	**Bismuth**	**Acute poisoning:** Nausea, vomiting and abdominal pain, (occur within hours) and precede features of nephrotoxicity and neurotoxicity **Chronic poisoning:** Incoordination, behavioural changes, memory deterioration, psychiatric symptoms and these may lead to encephalopathy. These may be associated with erythematous rashes, renal failure, and thrombocytopenia. Herxheimer reaction, renal failure, a blue gumline, stomatitis, generalised skin eruptions, osteoporosis, spontaneous fractures and jaundice have been reported with parenteral bismuth therapy.
5	**Mercury**	**Acute poisoning:** Metallic taste, excessive salivation, inflammation of gums, severe GI irritation, diarrhoea, electrolyte disturbances, arrhythmias, circulatory collapse and marked renal impairment **Chronic poisoning:** Increased irritability, tremors, headache, easy fatiguability, stomatitis, colitis, increased salivation, dermatitis, electrolyte imbalance, neurotoxicity, hepatotoxicity and renal damage. *Minamata disease,* reported from Japan, was found to be due to consumption of fish from waters contaminated by methyl mercury from the industry. It was characterised by birth defects and neurological toxicity such as dementia, peripheral neuropathy, ataxia and tremulousness. *Pink disease or acrodynia:* An allergic manifestation seen in children, due to systemic absorption of topically applied mercurial antiseptics, manifested by marked swelling and erythema of the extremities with sweating, itching and polyarthritis
6	**Cadmium**	**Acute poisoning:** Severe GI irritation, cough, sore throat, vertigo, dyspnoea, cyanosis, bronchopneumonia and circulatory collapse **Chronic poisoning:** Yellow pigmentation of teeth (the yellow ring of cadmium), anosmia, emphysema, proteinuria and kidney damage

Box 74.1 Environmental Toxic Neuropathy PH 1.51

- Arsenic
- Carbon disulphide
- Dimethylamino propionitrile (DMAPN)
- Lead (polyurethane foam)
- Mercury (inorganic)
- Methylbromide
- Thallium
- Vacor

Table 74.2 Metal-Chelating Agents Used in Therapy

Drug	Used Against
$CaNa_2EDTA$[a]	Lead
Dimercaprol[a]	Arsenic, copper, bismuth
Succimer	Lead, arsenic, mercury
Penicillamine	Copper, mercury, lead
Trientine	Copper
Desferrioxamine[a]	Iron
Deferiprone	Iron

[a]Given by injection. Others are effective orally.

HEAVY METAL ANTAGONISTS PH 1.53, FM 9.3

The toxicity of the heavy metals is attributed to their ability to form complexes with important biological radicals like the sulphhydryl (SH), the hydroxyl, the carboxyl, the amino and the imidazole. Inhibition of various enzymes leads to the toxic effects. Thus, affinity for SH group leads to inhibition of vital SH-containing enzymes. Attempts were, therefore, made to develop organic compounds which would have a high affinity for the metallic ions. Such drugs would combine with the metallic ions to produce relatively nontoxic and easily water-soluble complexes which are subsequently eliminated by the kidneys. The process by which these organic compounds combine with the metals to form relatively stable nonionised ring complexes is called **chelation** (chele = claw), the compounds being designated as **chelating agents** (Table 74.2).

DIMERCAPROL (BAL): Dimercaprol, or British Anti-Lewisite, was synthesised by Stocken and Thompson during the World War II to ensure protection against poisoning by the arsenical war gases such as Lewisite. Chemically, it is a dithiol having two SH groups (Fig. 74.1).

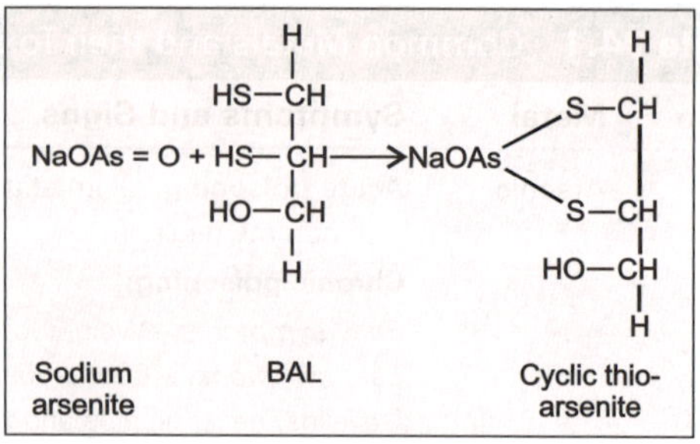

FIG. 74.1 **Mode of action of BAL.**

Pharmacological actions: Dimercaprol forms poorly dissociable complexes with **arsenic, mercury, gold** and **cadmium** ions and thus protects the SH enzymes. In case of mercury and cadmium, the dimercaprol–metal complex further reacts with another molecule of dimercaprol to form a still more stable, inactive complex.

Even though the dimercaprol–metal complexes are poorly dissociable, some amount of dissociation does occur in vivo, causing the release of the toxic metal in the active form. To overcome this drawback, the dosage schedule of dimercaprol is adjusted in such a way that an excess of free drug is always present in the body to bind the free metal released as a result of dissociation. Dimercaprol also reactivates the inhibited enzymes. though to a limited extent, *it fails to protect or reactivate the SH enzymes if administered late or in the presence of overwhelming amounts of the metal.*

Dimercaprol itself inhibits enzymes peroxidase, catalase and carbonic anhydrase in which the heavy metals constitute prosthetic groups.

Absorption, fate and excretion: Following the IM administration, the peak plasma levels are reached in about 2 h and the drug is largely metabolised within 6–24 h. A part is excreted as a glucuronide in urine.

Adverse reactions: Injection of BAL is painful and can cause sterile abscesses and drug fever. Doses of dimercaprol in the range of 4–5 mg/kg body weight produce a variety of ADR in approximately 50% of patients. These include nausea, vomiting, headache, burning sensation in the mouth and eyes, lacrimation, sialorrhoea, paraesthesiae of the extremities, muscle pain and muscle spasm. It can also cause anginal pain, tachycardia and hypertension.

Dimercaprol–metal complex dissociates more readily in an acidic medium. *The urine, therefore, should be made alkaline during dimercaprol therapy to protect the kidneys from the toxic effects of the released free metal.*

The use of dimercaprol is contraindicated in the presence of hepatic damage and in iron poisoning, as it forms a toxic complex with iron. It should be used with caution in hypertensive individuals.

Preparation: Dimercaprol injection 50 mg/mL arachis oil. It has a strong characteristic smell.

Indications:

- **Acute poisoning** due to arsenic, mercury, gold, antimony, bismuth and thallium.
  In severe cases of arsenical and gold poisoning, 3 mg/kg is given deep intramuscularly, at 4 hourly intervals for the first 2 days, at 6 hourly intervals on the third day, and twice daily for the next 10 days or until the recovery is complete.
  Dimercaprol is effective in protecting the eyes from the effects of accidental contamination by arsenical vesicants. Complete recovery is usually achieved if 5%–10% oily solution of dimercaprol is instilled into the conjunctival sac within 5 min of contamination.
  In acute mercurial poisoning, dimercaprol is administered initially in the dose of 5 mg per kg followed by 2 or 3 injections of 2.5 mg per kg during the next 12 h, or until recovery is assured. However, to be maximally effective, it must be injected within the first hour or two after poisoning. It is ineffective if extensive renal damage occurs, for which haemodialysis is indicated. Acetyl penicillamine and succimer have also been used. Supportive treatment with IV fluids, treatment of shock and prophylactic antibiotics to prevent secondary infection are also instituted. Administration of proteins in the form of raw eggs or milk, which form nontoxic proteinates, and of medicinal charcoal in suspension adsorb a mercuric ions from the GIT. This is followed by gastric lavage with sodium formaldehyde sulphoxylate, which reduces the mercuric ion to the less soluble mercurous form.
- **Lead poisoning:** Dimercaprol can be substituted for succimer (See section, Therapeutic uses of calcium disodium edetate).

Both dimercaprol and ethylene diamine tetraacetic acid (EDTA) are not recommended in cadmium poisoning as they may further aggravate the kidney damage caused by cadmium.

SUCCIMER (2,3-Dimercaptosuccinic acid): This water soluble analogue of dimercaprol, is effective orally. After absorption, it is biotransformed to a mixed disulphide with cysteine. It is an effective and better tolerated **chelator of lead, arsenic, cadmium** and **mercury**. Adverse effects are nausea, vomiting, diarrhoea, loss of appetite and skin rash. It is recommended for children with lead poisoning.

D-PENICILLAMINE: This compound, contains one SH group and is a derivative of benzyl penicillin.

Pharmacological actions: Penicillamine forms a water soluble complex with **copper, mercury** and **lead** ions and thus facilitates their excretion in urine. Like dimercaprol, it inhibits a number of enzymes, including transaminase and desulphhydrase which have one of these metals as the prosthetic group.

Penicillamine is well absorbed on oral administration and rapidly excreted in urine.

Adverse reactions: Penicillamine is a toxic drug. It causes:

- **General toxicity** such as headache, sore throat, fever, rash, nausea lymphadenopathy, and ecchymosis; loss or impairment of sense of taste can be very upsetting, neuritis
- **Haematologic toxicity:** Leucopoenia, thrombocytopenia, agranulocytosis and aplastic anaemia
- **Renal toxicity:** Proteinuria, reversible nephrotic syndrome, haematuria
- **Autoimmune syndrome:** Myasthenia like syndrome, diabetes, polymyositis and SLE

Allergic reactions occur occasionally and patients who are sensitive to penicillin may have a similar reaction to penicillamine. Long-term use may cause optic neuritis, myasthenia-like syndrome, iron and pyridoxine deficiency. Hence, pyridoxine 25 mg/day is supplemented.

It is now rarely used because of its toxicity.

ACETYL D-PENICILLAMINE: This drug, a less toxic but weaker chelating agent than D-penicillamine, has been shown to be particularly effective in mercury poisoning. It is administered in the dose of 1 g daily in 3 or 4 divided portions, for 10 days. The course may be repeated after a week's interval.

TRIENTINE (triethylene tetramine): Given in doses of 400–800 mg thrice daily on empty stomach, it is as effective in **reversing the neurological lesions of Wilson disease.** It appears to be less toxic than penicillamine and may cause less iron deficiency.

Wilson's disease is a rare, hereditary disease of **abnormal copper metabolism** characterised by degenerative changes in the basal ganglia and cirrhosis of the liver. The copper content of the liver, brain, kidneys and other tissues is grossly increased, the total serum copper and ceruloplasmin copper content are reduced and the urinary excretion of copper is enhanced. The *Kayser–Fleischer ring*, brownish pigmented ring at the corneal margin, is diagnostic of this condition.

Treatment of Wilson's disease or copper poisoning is directed towards reducing the total body copper. This is achieved by administration of **zinc acetate plus trientine.** As trientine can chelate zinc, they are administered at least 1 h apart. This therapy is given in conjunction with a high protein, low copper diet with potassium disulphide (20 mg thrice daily with meals). The latter precipitates dietary copper and thereby reduces its absorption. Zinc acetate and zinc sulphate 50 mg t.i.d. also reduce copper absorption.

Foods rich in copper (shell fish, nuts, chocolates, mushrooms and organ meats) should be avoided.

PE 14.1

CALCIUM DISODIUM EDETATE AND **DISODIUM EDETATE:** The calcium-disodium and the disodium salts of EDTA form stable and highly water

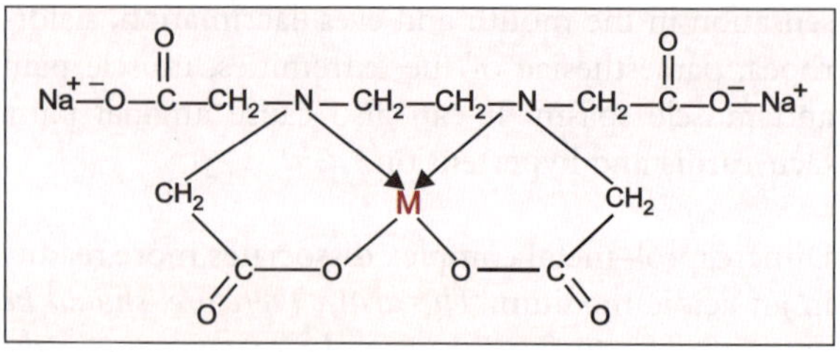

FIG. 74.2 **Mode of action of disodium edetate. 'M' stands for chelated metal.**

soluble complexes with many divalent and trivalent metallic ions and owe their therapeutic application to this chelating property (Fig. 74.2).

The calcium disodium salt has a high affinity for lead, whereas the disodium salt exhibits a high affinity for calcium. The affinity for other metals like sodium, magnesium and potassium is much less and this permits their selective use in the treatment of **lead poisoning** and hypercalcaemia, respectively.

Absorption, fate and excretion: Both the salts are poorly absorbed from the GI tract and are given by IV or IM routes. The latter is very painful. They are excreted almost completely within 24 h, both by glomerular filtration and tubular secretion.

Adverse reactions: Besides thrombophlebitis, these agents cause nausea, diarrhoea and toxic nephrosis. Oliguria and renal failure have been reported but generally, the damage is reversible. Renal damage has been attributed to the free metallic ion released as a result of dissociation of the metal-chelate complex.

A febrile reaction, followed by myalgia, nausea, vomiting, histamine-like reaction with rhinorrhoea, lacrimation and dermatitis are the other adverse effects reported. The disodium salt may also cause hypocalcaemic tetany due to excessive chelation of calcium.

Preparations:

i. Calcium disodium edentate: It can be given IM mixed with a local anaesthetic agent. Same preparation can be given by IV infusion by diluting with normal saline or 5% dextrose.
ii. Disodium edetate injection 20 mL ampoules containing 4 g of the drug

Indications:

- **Lead poisoning:** Disodium calcium edetate is used in the treatment of acute and chronic lead poisoning. It acts by exchanging its calcium for lead in the blood to form a stable, nonionisable, water-soluble lead compound which is rapidly eliminated in urine. This exchange between lead and calcium is selective.

In acute lead poisoning, the agent is given by slow IV infusion in the dose of 40 mg/kg in two divided doses/day, as a 0.5%–3% solution in 0.9% saline or 5% dextrose, for a maximum period of 5 days. The course may then be repeated after an interval of 2–3 days. Smaller doses are recommended in the presence of encephalopathy and increased intracranial pressure. In children, the dose should not be larger than 55 mg/kg. This should be divided into two portions and given by IV drip. It is necessary to monitor urine output as the chelator–lead complex is nephrotoxic.

Disodium calcium edetate has also been used in the treatment of porphyria and in poisoning with iron, cadmium and plutonium.

The drugs of choice in lead poisoning are **calcium disodium edetate** and **succimer**. The latter is more effective for mobilising lead from soft tissue. Hence, a combination of succimer and calcium disodium edetate is preferred. Dimercaprol can be substituted for succimer.

Lead colic can be controlled by the administration of antispasmodics and calcium gluconate 2 g IV Convulsions are best treated with diazepam. Increased intracranial tension can be relieved by mannitol or by lumbar puncture.

DITHIOCARB: This agent, administered orally in the dose of 2 g daily for 7 days, preceded by an initial dose of 200 mg intravenously, has been found useful in the **treatment of nickel carbonyl poisoning** and also to some extent in **acute thallium poisoning** and in **Wilson disease**. The toxicity reported in animals includes visual disturbance and blindness.

DESFERRIOXAMINE and other iron-chelating agents are discussed in Chapter 34.

CHAPTER 75

Gases: Therapeutic and Toxic

Learning Objectives

This chapter will enable the reader:

1. To enumerate therapeutic and toxic gases.
2. To explain the pharmacological effects, methods of administration, ADR and indications for oxygen and hyperbaric oxygen.
3. To state the pharmacological effects, ADR, preparations and indications for carbon dioxide.
4. To mention the indications for helium, nitric oxide and water vapour.
5. To explain the toxic effects of carbon monoxide (CO) inhalation and outline the treatment of CO poisoning.
6. To state the toxic effects of sulphur dioxide, ozone and nitrogen dioxide.
7. To enumerate organic solvents and list their toxic effects.
8. To state the symptoms of cyanide poisoning and outline its treatment.

KEY TERMS

The gases of therapeutic importance are oxygen, carbon dioxide, nitric oxide and inhalational anaesthetic gases for e.g. nitrous oxide, sevoflurane, etc. Helium, an inert gas present in the atmosphere in minute amounts, has also found therapeutic applications.

Some gases and organic solvent vapours exist as environmental pollutants and are of toxicological concern, e.g. carbon monoxide (CO), sulphur dioxide and ozone.

THERAPEUTIC GASES

OXYGEN: Inspired air contains 21% of oxygen. It is carried in the body largely in combination with haemoglobin and a small quantity is transported in non-haeme forms in plasma.

Effects of oxygen administration: Inhalation of 100% oxygen in a normal individual produces the following effects:

- **Ventilation:** Oxygen at atmospheric pressure initially depresses and later mildly stimulates the ventilation; *Oxygen also directly decreases the sensitivity of the respiratory centre to carbon dioxide.* This effect is apparent when the gas is given under more than one atmospheric pressure.
- **Cardiovascular system:** It reduces the heart rate and the cardiac output. The coronary and the cerebral blood flow are probably reduced, whereas the pulmonary vessels are dilated. It does not modify BP significantly.
- **Nitrogen concentration:** Inhalation of oxygen leads to a reduction in the partial pressure of nitrogen within the pulmonary alveoli, with its subsequent diffusion from the body cavities and blood into alveoli from where it is eliminated.

Methods of administration: Equipment available for administering oxygen include those which:

- **provide the highest concentration of oxygen in the inspired air.** These include the oxygen tent and the various types of closely fitting aero-nasal masks with a nonreturn valve and either a reservoir bag or a demand valve on the oxygen supply line. Masks are particularly useful at high altitudes and in the treatment of bronchial asthma, pulmonary oedema and chronic pulmonary diseases. *Because of its irritant effect on the respiratory tract, oxygen in high concentration is humidified by passing it through either a humidifier or a nebuliser.*

- **achieve a steady concentration, < 60% in the inspired air.** These include simple devices such as the nasal cannula and the nasal catheter (*inserted through the nostril into the nasopharynx*) and the more sophisticated equipment like the **Ventimask.** A flow of 1–6 L of oxygen per minute through a cannula or a catheter ensures 24%–44% oxygen concentration in the inspired air. *Larger flow rates of oxygen do not achieve higher concentrations of oxygen and are, therefore, wasteful.*

Adverse reactions:

1. **Due to formation of reactive O_2 species:**
   - **Respiratory tract:** *Inhalation of oxygen in the concentration of 60% or more for 36 h or longer may damage the pulmonary epithelium and inactivate the surfactant* secreted by the alveoli, which helps to keep the alveoli patent by reducing the surface tension within them. Consequently, extensive pulmonary atelectasis may occur. Administration of oxygen at a pressure greater than 1 atmosphere may cause respiratory distress in neonates, particularly in premature ones.
   - **Central nervous system:** Inhalation of pure oxygen at pressures > 2 atmospheres may lead to paraesthesiae, mental disturbances, twitching, loss of consciousness and generalised convulsions. Convulsions may occur within a few minutes or several hours after inhalation of the gas.
   - **Retrolental fibroplasia:** High arterial oxygen tension (over 100 mm Hg) interferes with the retinal blood supply and produces an occlusive proliferative retinal disease termed retrolental fibroplasia. This is observed mainly in premature infants and may either regress or progress to blindness.

2. **Others:**
   - **Hyperoxia** can reduce coronary blood flow.
   - **Carbon dioxide narcosis:** In patients with COPD, status asthmaticus, weakness of the respiratory muscles (from polyneuritis, poliomyelitis or myasthenia gravis), and in those with central respiratory depression (head injury or raised intracranial tension), the alveolar ventilation is inadequate to prevent a rise in the arterial carbon dioxide tension ($PaCO_2$). With increasing hypercapnea (raised $PaCO_2$), the respiratory centre becomes more tolerant of CO_2 and its activity is solely maintained by the stimulus of hypoxaemia (**hypoxaemic drive**) reflexly through the carotid and aortic bodies. A removal of this stimulus by oxygen administration reduces the ventilation still further with a consequent rise in $PaCO_2$. This gives rise to the syndrome of **carbon dioxide narcosis** with raised intracranial tension, clinically manifested by sweating, twitchings, drowsiness, convulsions, papilloedema and coma. It is a potentially lethal condition.
   - **Fire hazard:** Every oxygen appliance is a potential fire hazard and no naked flame, lighted cigarette or electric switch should be brought near a patient receiving oxygen.

Preparations: Oxygen is dispensed in a compressed state in cylinders painted black with a white shoulder. Cylinders of oxygen mixed with carbon dioxide are also painted black but have grey and white quarterings on neck and shoulder.

Indications:

- **Correction of hypoxia:** The primary indication of oxygen therapy is hypoxia (See under the section Hypoxia and hypoxaemia)
- **Reduction in the partial pressure of an inert gas:** Oxygen is used by workers in pressurised spaces to reduce the inhaled nitrogen concentration and thus to prevent the decompression sickness. It is also commonly used during general anaesthesia with the inhalational anaesthetic agents.
- **Oxygen as a diluent:** Oxygen is used as a diluent for anaesthetic gases.

HYPOXIA AND HYPOXAEMIA

Hypoxia may be defined as **inadequate tissue oxygenation.**

The brain is the most sensitive organ to hypoxia, and irreversible damage usually results within 3–4 min of its onset. Hypoxic damage to the kidney, liver and heart (multiple organ failure) is also seen. Types of hypoxia are shown in Box 75.1.

The oxygen in the alveoli equilibrates with the blood in the pulmonary capillaries. It produces in the arterial blood a partial pressure of oxygen dissolved in the plasma (**arterial oxygen tension, PaO_2**) of 80–100 mm Hg and an oxygen saturation (SaO_2) of over 95%. *A reduction in the arterial oxygen tension is called* **hypoxaemia.** This must be distinguished from **hypoxia.** Hypoxaemia generally (but not always) leads to hypoxia; on the other hand, hypoxia can arise from causes other than hypoxaemia.

The carotid and the aortic bodies are the chemoreceptors which sense hypoxaemia and stimulate breathing (mechanical ventilation) and the heart reflexly so that the hypoxaemia tends to be corrected.

Hypoxaemia can arise in several ways and can be detected by measurement of PaO_2.

The carbon dioxide tension in the arterial blood ($PaCO_2$) *faithfully reflects the adequacy of alveolar ventilation.* In any cardio-pulmonary disease where $PaCO_2$ is low or normal, it is safe to administer oxygen in high concentration without special precautions. *In any condition accompanied by elevated $PaCO_2$, oxygen in high concentration tends to precipitate carbon dioxide narcosis.* These patients are, however, badly in need of oxygen which should not be withheld from them. Only, it should be administered in low concentration so that the hypoxaemia is only partly corrected, unless they can also be given mechanical assistance to ventilation.

Box 75.1 Types of Hypoxia

I. ***Hypoxic***, characterised by hypoxaemia
II. ***Anaemic***, due to deficiency of haemoglobin as in anaemia or due to inability of the altered haemoglobin to take up oxygen as in methaemoglobinemia, and carbon monoxide poisoning. In this variety, the oxygen tension in the arterial blood is normal but the 'oxygen content' is reduced
III. ***Stagnant***, due to excessive slowing of blood supply to the peripheral tissues, e.g. in shock
IV. ***Histotoxic***, due to increase in metabolic oxygen demand of the tissues as in thyrotoxicosis, and/or the tissue may be unable to utilise the available oxygen either as a result of paralysis of essential enzyme systems (cyanide poisoning) or due to a mechanical barrier (tissue oedema)

Administration of sedatives, hypnotics and opioids makes patients drowsy and abolishes their voluntary ventilatory drive, leading to CO_2 narcosis.

The clinical recognition of 'hypoxia' is largely inferential. **Hypoxia cannot be measured** but has to be surmised by the presence of:

- **A clinical situation known to produce hypoxia**
- **Hypoxaemia which can be detected by measurement of PaO_2**

The results of oxygen administration are the best in situations where there is a deficiency of oxygen in the inspired air such as at high altitude, where breathing 100% oxygen is beneficial. CT 2.16

In cardiopulmonary disorders, the conditions maximally helped by oxygen therapy are those associated with alveolar hypoventilation due to any cause, venous admixture as in COPD and alveolo-capillary block as in interstitial lung disease. *Those in which $PaCO_2$ is elevated should be treated with* ***oxygen in low concentration*** *and the effect on the patient's clinical condition (and on the $PaCO_2$ if possible) should be watched carefully. Others can be safely treated with* ***high-concentration oxygen therapy.***

Administration of oxygen in high concentration to patients in shock increases the amount of dissolved oxygen in the plasma. Though this may be small, it may be sufficient to tip the scales in patient's favour in this critical condition. Besides, it can relieve the pain of MI, an important cause of shock.

HYPERBARIC OXYGEN: The amount of oxygen dissolved in the plasma can be increased by breathing oxygen at an absolute atmospheric pressure greater than one. The larger amount of oxygen present in the plasma enables better tissue oxygenation.

Hyperbaric oxygen (HBO) therapy is defined as 'a mode of treatment in which the patient is entirely immersed in a pressure chamber and breathes oxygen at a pressure greater than 1 atmosphere absolute (ATA)'. HBO is administered by using a special chamber which is pressurised by either (a) 100% oxygen at 2–3 ATA, which the patient breathes or (b) compressed air, with the patient breathing 100% oxygen at 2–3 ATA through special masks or oxygen hoods. At these pressures, the amount of oxygen dissolved in the plasma rises from 0.3 mL% at 1 ATA to 4.4 mL% at 2 ATA and 6.8 mL% at 3 ATA, respectively (hyperoxygenation).

Pharmacological actions: HBO exerts several beneficial actions in the body.

Mechanical:

- **Reduction in the size of the gas (mainly nitrogen) bubbles** in the circulation and the tissues in patients with decompression sickness and air/gas embolism, leading to amelioration of the symptoms of the former and improvement in the circulation in the latter

Hyperoxygenation:

- **Displacement of CO from carboxyhaemoglobin** in CO poisoning and smoke inhalation
- **Peripheral vasoconstriction in tissues, with, nonetheless, increased oxygen delivery to the tissues.** This helps to restore oxygenation of the ischaemic tissues and to clear oedema surrounding an abscess, especially in the brain and spinal cord. The heart is slowed and the cardiac output is reduced.
- **Increased neovascularisation in hypoxic areas**
- **Direct bactericidal action on anaerobic organisms**
- **Killing of other pathogens by stimulating** phagocytic and killing capacity of the leucocytes
- **Promoting wound healing in radiation-damaged tissues,** e.g. osteonecrosis, cystitis and enteritis

Adverse reactions: Up to 3 ATA, HBO is safe. Yet, adverse effects and accidents can occur:

1. **In the patient**
    - **Claustrophobia**
    - **Damage to the ear drums** (otic barotrauma)
    - **Barotrauma to the lungs** resulting in pneumothorax or air embolism
    - **Pulmonary and neurological toxicity** from oxygen free radicals
    - **Retrolental fibroplasia**
    - **Hypersensitivity to oxygen**
2. **In the attendants** in the multiplace chambers, who may suffer from decompression sickness if the chamber is decompressed rapidly
3. **Fire hazard** is a real but avoidable risk

Indications:

- **Metabolic:** Carbon monoxide poisoning, smoke inhalation and cyanide poisoning blood loss with severe anaemia
- **Mechanical:** Decompression sickness and air/gas embolism
- **Ischaemic conditions:** Acute traumatic ischaemia and crush injuries; retinal artery thrombosis
- **Infective conditions:** Clostridial infections (gas gangrene), severe/refractory infections such as chronic osteomyelitis, diabetic foot ulcers and brain abscess
- **Wound healing problems:** Nonhealing ulcers and wounds; compromised skin grafts, thermal burns
- **Early and late radiation damage** to bone (radio-osteonecrosis) and soft tissues (e.g. cystitis and enteritis)

CARBON DIOXIDE: Normally, it is produced in the body during tissue and food metabolism. The inspired atmospheric air contains 0.04% of carbon dioxide. **Carbon dioxide has marked effects on the CNS, the respiration and circulation.**

Effects of carbon dioxide inhalation:

Respiration: Carbon dioxide stimulates respiration by:

a. Its direct action on the brain stem
b. Its action on the peripheral arterial chemoreceptors to a smaller extent

It increases both the rate and the tidal volume. This effect is seen with inhalation of even 2% carbon dioxide.

Circulation: Carbon dioxide, by a direct action, tends to decrease the heart rate and the myocardiac force of contraction. It also relaxes the vascular smooth muscle, tending to cause vasodilatation.

The direct circulatory effects are antagonised by the sympathetic activation, causing an increase in the peripheral release of the catecholamines. The total circulatory response, therefore, is the outcome of two opposite actions. *Cerebral and coronary vessels, which are devoid of a significant sympathetic control, dilate after carbon dioxide inhalation and so do the splanchnic and the skeletal muscle blood vessels. It is probably the most potent cerebral vasodilator.*

CNS: Inhaled in low concentration, it stimulates the cerebral cortex and reduces seizure threshold. Higher concentrations depress the cortex, while activating the subcortical areas that have cortical projections.

Adverse reactions: Above a concentration of 7% in inhaled air, carbon dioxide gives rise to headache, dizziness, mental confusion, palpitation, dyspnoea and an increase in BP. Concentration > 10% causes loss of consciousness. Withdrawal of carbon dioxide after prolonged inhalation often leads to pallor, hypotension, dizziness, nausea and vomiting. Carbon dioxide narcosis has already been discussed earlier.

Preparations:

i. Carbon dioxide is marketed in steel cylinders painted grey, usually in a liquid form, under a pressure of 58–72 atmospheres
ii. Combinations of oxygen and 5%–10% carbon dioxide are marketed as 'carbogen'.
iii. Solid carbon dioxide is available in two forms: dry ice and carbon dioxide snow.

Indications:

- **Hiccups:** See under the section, Management of hiccups
- **Neuropsychiatry:** Inhalation of 30% of carbon dioxide with 70% oxygen has been employed for the treatment of anxiety neurosis and personality maladjustments. Its therapeutic value is not well established.
- **Local uses:** Carbon dioxide snow, which has a temperature of –80°C is used to destroy warts and naevi by local application. The procedure is almost painless and scarring is minimum. The surrounding tissue should be protected with soft paraffin.
- **Miscellaneous:** Supersaturated solution of carbon dioxide or aerated waters possesses a mild rubefacient action and is believed to increase the secretion of gastric juice particularly hydrochloric acid. They are often used as carminatives and for masking unpleasant taste of saline purgatives.

MANAGEMENT OF HICCUPS

Hiccups are the sudden involuntary contractions of inspiratory muscles terminated by abrupt closure of the glottis, resulting in a peculiar sound. They may occur due to a wide variety of causes including gastric distension, alcohol ingestion, excessive smoking, psychogenic disorders, irritation of the diaphragm and drugs. They serve no useful purpose. They are usually self-limiting and harmless, but sometimes they are indicators of a serious underlying disease.

Inhalation of 10%–25% of carbon dioxide may be used in the treatment of intractable hiccups. Rebreathing into a paper bag is a household method of achieving the same effect.

The other measures tried are:

a. **Nonpharmacological:** Stimulation of the uvula or the nasopharynx (touching the uvula with a spoon; sipping iced water; sucking hard candy; swallowing dry, granulated sugar; breath holding; inhalation of ammonia); Valsalva manoeuvre; sneezing; phrenic nerve block.
b. **Pharmacological:** A variety of drugs such as chlorpromazine; haloperidol; metoclopramide; carbamazepine orally; phenytoin intravenously; magnesium sulphate intramuscularly have been used to treat hiccups with variable results.

Benzodiazepines are not useful in hiccups.

HELIUM: This inert gas, along with oxygen (80:20), has been used by intermittent inhalation for treating prolonged asthmatic attacks resistant to other therapy. Because of its lower density, it minimises the breathing effort. It is also employed prophylactically for prevention of Caisson disease, and in the treatment of oedema and spasm of larynx.

NITRIC OXIDE (NO): (Chapter 29) When inhaled, it has selective vasodilatory effect on the pulmonary circulation. It is used to improve oxygenation in hypoxic respiratory failure with pulmonary hypertension in term and near-term neonates; and in adults with various types of pulmonary hypertension and in adult respiratory distress syndrome (ARDS). It is administered by inhalation in the concentration of 10–80 ppm. Higher concentrations can be toxic because of its metabolic degradation to NO_2 and because of methaemoglobinemia.

Water vapour: Water, administered either as a vapour (from a humidifier) or in particulate form (from a nebuliser), decreases crusting of the respiratory mucosa, liquefies thick secretions, promotes mucociliary drainage (Chapter 26), limits loss of body water and conserves body heat by reducing the evaporation in the airway. It is used in patients with respiratory infection/irritation and also in those with chronic airway intubation. Aerosol is used to deliver drugs such as bronchodilators and mucolytics to the airways. Vaporisation with water containing drops of tincture benzoin or eucalyptus oil is used as a home remedy.

TOXIC GASES PH 1.51, FM 9.6

Due to environmental pollution, people are exposed to various pollutants in the air, which enter the body not only through the lungs but also through skin and eyes, and cause local and systemic toxicity. Several of these are respiratory irritants and can cause chronic bronchitis, emphysema, pulmonary fibrosis and cancer. The major air pollutants are shown in Box 75.2.

CARBON MONOXIDE (CO): This is a colourless, odourless, nonirritating gas which constitutes almost 50% of the air-pollutants. CO is responsible for many accidental deaths every year. The automobile is the largest source of CO. Incomplete combustion of organic matter and smoking also generate CO.

Actions: Carbon monoxide combines with haemoglobin to form carboxyhaemoglobin (COHb) which cannot carry oxygen. This reduces the oxygen delivery to the issues. **The affinity of CO for Hb is more than 200 times that of O_2.** CO interferes with ferroproteins like myoglobin and cytochrome oxidase.

Box 75.2 Major Gaseous Air Pollutants

- Carbon monoxide (CO)
- Sulphur dioxide (SO_2)
- Nitrogen dioxide (NO_2)
- Hydrocarbon vapours
- Glycols (Chapter 6)

The signs and symptoms of acute CO poisoning are those of hypoxia. Acute CO poisoning causes headache, weakness, dizziness, nausea, vomiting, coma and intermittent convulsions. The patient is cyanosed. *Sudden exposure to very high concentrations of CO can cause immediate death without any warning symptoms.* Lack of O_2 causes cardiac and delayed neurological damage. **Cherry-red colour of the blood is highly suggestive of the diagnosis**, which is confirmed by spectroscopy of the blood.

Early symptoms of poisoning are flu-like and may be wrongly diagnosed.

Chronic exposure to low concentrations of CO probably facilitates the development of atherosclerosis, cardiac disease, neurological damage and Parkinsonism.

Treatment of acute CO poisoning: COHb is fully dissociable and CO is rapidly excreted through the lungs. Treatment, therefore, consists of transport to an open space with fresh air, rapid administration of 100% oxygen with a tight fitting mask, and supportive therapy to correct hypotension and acidosis. Recovery is almost complete if the patient is treated early. It can also be treated with HBO (see section on Therapeutic uses of HBO).

SULPHUR DIOXIDE (SO_2): This gas is primarily generated during burning of fossil fuels that contain sulphur. It rarely causes death. Being a **respiratory irritant**, it leads to the production of thick mucus and causes bronchospasm. Chronic exposure results in abnormal pulmonary function. A part of the atmospheric sulphur is converted to sulphuric acid and particulate sulphates. Sulphuric acid in the atmosphere causes further damage to the respiratory passages, increases airway resistance and like sulphur dioxide predisposes to chronic respiratory diseases. Sulphuric acid also dissolves in rain water and returns to the earth as **acid rain** which can cause environmental damage. The treatment is essentially symptomatic.

OZONE (O_3): This gas is formed from a complex reaction of a major atmospheric pollutant NO_2 with UV light. Thus:

$$NO_2 \rightarrow NO + O$$
$$O + O_2 \rightarrow O_3$$

Ozone is a respiratory irritant and can cause pulmonary oedema and death. It is a potent oxidant, and pulmonary injury may be due to the formation of highly reactive free radical intermediates. Chronic exposure to ozone may cause chronic bronchitis, emphysema and pulmonary fibrosis. It increases the sensitivity of the lung to other bronchoconstrictors such as histamine, acetylcholine and to allergens. The treatment of the toxicity is symptomatic. Antioxidants such as vitamins C and E may be useful.

NITROGEN DIOXIDE (NO_2): This pollutant gas is also a pulmonary irritant and, like ozone, can cause pulmonary oedema and changes in pulmonary function.

ORGANIC SOLVENT VAPOURS: In addition to the above pollutant gases, we are constantly exposed to **organic solvent vapours such as petrol, crude oil, aerosol sprays and floor cleaners.** *Some of these solvents and hydrocarbons cause pleasant sensations when inhaled and are frequently abused.* The common hazardous solvents are shown in Box 75.3.

Kerosene and **petroleum** products contain a variety of hydrocarbons. Petroleum vapours, when inhaled, cause sensitisation of the myocardium to noradrenaline and may precipitate ventricular arrhythmias. Ingestion of kerosene causes symptoms similar to ethyl alcohol poisoning and pulmonary oedema.

Many of the hydrocarbons are capable of causing GI disturbances, CNS depression, neurological damage, polyneuropathy and aplastic anaemia. They are also carcinogenic.

CYANIDE: This is one of the deadliest of all poisons causing death within a matter of minutes when inhaled as hydrogen cyanide. If ingested, it may take several hours before serious symptoms develop. **It acts by forming a complex with cytochrome C oxidase, thereby inhibiting cellular O_2 use leading to marked tissue anoxia.** Small amounts of cyanide normally present in the body are biotransformed to the much less toxic thiocyanate; this reaction is catalysed by an intracellular enzyme rhodanase which requires thiosulphate or colloidal sulphur as a substrate. As the availability of this substrate is limited, rhodanase is unable to biotransform large amounts of cyanide. Symptoms of acute poisoning include dizziness, anxiety, perspiration, chest pain and in serious cases acidosis, coma and death. The breath smells of bitter almonds.

Box 75.3 Common Hazardous Organic Solvents

- ***Aliphatic hydrocarbons:*** Methane, ethane, *n*-hexane
- ***Aromatic hydrocarbons:*** Benzene, toluene
- ***Halogenated hydrocarbons:*** Carbon tetrachloride, tetrachlorethylene

Treatment of Cyanide Poisoning: *The treatment must be instituted immediately to prevent the fatal outcome:*

1. **Dicobalt edetate,** a chelating agent, is the treatment of choice in cyanide poisoning. It is given intravenously in the dose of 300 mg (one 20 mL ampoule) over 1 min followed by 50 mL of 50% glucose by IV infusion. Both may be repeated once or twice as necessary. The drug is toxic and can cause severe hypotension.
   Owing to its serious toxicity its use should be limited to a serious patient who is tending to lose, or has lost, consciousness; it should not be used as a precautionary measure.
2. Sequential **sodium nitrite** and **sodium thiosulphate therapy: Sodium nitrite** 300–500 mg in 10–15 mL of water is given intravenously over 3 min. It acts rapidly by converting haemoglobin to methaemoglobin. Methaemoglobin competes with cytochrome C oxidase for cyanide, to form cyanmethaemoglobin and thus protects the enzyme. This is followed by IV **sodium thiosulphate** given slowly in the dose of 25 mL of 5.0% solution (containing 12.5 g of sodium thiosulphate) over a period of 10 min. This results in the formation of relatively nontoxic thiocyanate, which is excreted in the urine. It is slow acting but more safe.
3. **Hydroxocobalamin** in large doses (4–5 g) may also be useful and is safe. It is converted to cyanocobalamin.
4. **Hyperbaric oxygen** and **IV methylene blue** (1%) 1–4 mg/kg are the other measures employed. Methylene blue, a water soluble dye, facilitates the conversion of methaemoglobin to haemoglobin and is used for idiopathic and drug induced methaemoglobinaemia (Chapter 36).

CHAPTER 76

Enzymes in Therapy

Learning Objectives

This chapter will enable the reader:

1. To enlist enzymes that are used in therapeutics.
2. To state the physical properties, contraindications and indications for hyaluronidase.
3. To state the preparations, ADR and indications for streptodornase and trypsin.
4. To mention the source and indications for streptokinase, chymotrypsin, alpha-chymotrypsin, collagenase and deoxyribonuclease.
5. To discuss the rationality of fixed dose combination of NSAID and serratio-peptidase.

KEY TERMS

hyaluronidase, p. 1127
streptokinase, p. 1128
trypsin, p. 1128
collagenase, p. 1129
serratiopeptidase, p. 1129

Enzymes being extremely potent substances, the possibility of their therapeutic application is attractive. However, majority of these substances have to be administered parenterally as they are inactivated within the gastrointestinal tract. In addition, because of their proteinic nature, they are likely to evoke allergic reactions and because of their high potency, their careless use may result in alarming adverse effects. Lastly, because of the complicated method of their preparation, the cost of such therapy is likely to be high.

Enzymes, such as **pancreatin, diastase, pepsin** and **papain,** used in the treatment of certain GI disturbances have been described in Chapter 38. The enzymes **fibrinolysin, thromboplastin, urokinase** and **arvin** involved in the process of blood coagulation and **streptokinase** used as fibrinolytic agent are discussed in Chapter 33. The therapeutic application of **dornase alpha** is discussed in Chapter 26 and the use of **asparaginase** in Chapter 59. Similarly the utility of enzymes **rasburicase** and **pegloticase** in management of gout is discussed in Chapter 73.

The other enzymes used therapeutically are as follows:

HYALURONIDASE: This enzyme, prepared from mammalian testes acts by depolymerising hyaluronic acid, an essential component of the intercellular ground substances which determines the permeability of the tissues. Thus, hyaluronidase, administered subcutaneously, increases the tissue permeability or exhibits 'spreading activity'. Certain snake venoms and bee venoms also contain hyaluronidase. Similarly, certain virulent organisms also liberate hyaluronidase.

Hyaluronidase is an odourless, fluffy powder containing not less than 300 U of activity per mg. It is antigenic and may occasionally produce allergic reactions. Because of the danger of spreading the infection, the enzyme should not be injected into or around an infected area. Malignancy is also considered a contraindication for hyaluronidase for similar reasons.

Indications:

- It is employed to promote the rapid absorption of drugs and fluids given subcutaneously or intramuscularly, especially in infants and young children, in whom IV injection may be difficult. For hypodermoclysis 1500 U are added to each litre of fluid to be administered.

- Substances used in radiography are rapidly absorbed on IM injection with the aid of hyaluronidase, thus providing an alternative to their IV administration.
- It can be used to promote the absorption of blood and fluid in traumatic or postoperative oedema or haematoma.
- Sodium hyaluronate in highly purified form is used in a number of ophthalmic surgical procedures. *It should not be applied directly to the cornea and should not be used to reduce the swelling of bites and stings.*

STREPTODORNASE: This is not a single enzyme but a group of rapidly acting enzymes which promote the depolymerisation of the complex nucleoproteins derived from degenerated leucocytes and injured tissue cells. *They act directly and not through plasminogen activation.* Their action results in a rapid conversion of thick, viscous and purulent material to thin, easy flowing fluid. The enzymes do not attack the nucleoproteins of living cells. Their optimum activity is observed between the pH 7.0 and 8.5 and requires the presence of magnesium ions.

These enzymes are stable for several months in desiccated form but solutions at room temperature deteriorate rapidly.

Adverse reactions: As with other enzymes, the use of streptodornase may occasionally result in allergic reactions like urticaria, rash, fever and anaphylaxis. A febrile reaction may occur. It should not be employed in the presence of acute cellulitis and inflammation, as it may encourage the spread of localised infection. Since these substances are bacterial antigens, therapy with them results in rapid antibody formation rendering further treatment ineffective.

Preparations and dosage: Powder for topical application containing 25,000 U of strepodornase with 1,00,000 U of streptokinase, buffered with sodium phosphate to pH 7.5 is available.

Indications: Streptokinase+streptodornase is used topically, for debridement of chronic ulcers. Streptodornase is no longer used for intracavitary instillation as in empyema of the pleural cavity; some physicians use streptokinase instead, for this purpose.

TRYPSIN: This enzyme is obtained from an extract of the ox pancreas. It is available as a white powder soluble in water. The enzyme is active at a pH range of 5–8 with optimum activity at pH 7. Trypsin directly hydrolyzes natural proteins, including the respiratory mucins.

Adverse reactions: Application of the dry powder to surface lesions may cause a severe burning sensation. Intramuscular injection causes pain and induration at the site of injection and occasionally fever, leucocytosis, angioneurotic oedema and urticaria.

Contraindications and precautions for the use of trypsin are similar to those with streptodornase. The agent should be used cautiously in the presence of renal damage and be avoided in individuals with hepatic insufficiency. *It should never be given intravenously.*

Indications: For infiltration into cavities or for instillation on wound surface, it is used as a solution containing 3–5 mg of the enzyme per millilitre. The dry powder may be applied every 15–30 min to small areas and every 3 h to large areas; wet dressings and irrigations should be repeated 3 hourly. Small gelatin capsules containing the enzyme may be inserted into non-irrigable sinuses and fistulae. An aerosol of trypsin has been used to liquefy excessive bronchial secretions but its irritant nature makes it of doubtful value.

Proteolytic enzymes from ***Carica papaya*** **(papase)** and **concentrated protease (bromelains) obtained from pineapple plant** have the same indications as trypsin. They act by depolymerising the soft fibrin deposits in the inflamed areas and by facilitating the drainage of fluids. Their therapeutic use is not well established.

CHYMOTRYPSIN: This is a proteolytic enzyme obtained from the bovine pancreas. It is available as tablets containing 50,000 U of the enzyme per tablet. Tablets containing trypsin and chymotrypsin are also available.

Chymotrypsin is proposed for use as an adjunct to the conventional treatment of inflammation and oedema of soft tissues especially due to trauma. It is applied locally or given orally. However, its usefulness is doubtful. Its oral toxicity is mild.

ALPHA-CHYMOTRYPSIN: This proteolytic enzyme has been reported to dissolve the suspensory ligament of the lens to facilitate the dissection of the lens during intracapsular extraction of cataract. The procedure is called zonulolysis. It can also be applied locally. The adverse effects include transient glaucoma, wound disruption, loss of vitreous and rarely retinal damage, if it penetrates the vitreous.

COLLAGENASE: This enzyme is derived from fermentation of *Clostridium histolyticum.* It acts on both denatured and undenatured collagen. *Newly formed collagen and healthy tissue collagen are not attacked.* The activity is optimal at pH 6–8. Adverse effects are uncommon. It is used for debridement of dermal ulcers and in severe burns. It is applied in the form of an ointment once daily.

Deoxyribonuclease: DNA released from neutrophils forms long fibrils that contribute to the viscosity of sputum in cystic fibrosis. Inhaled recombinant human deoxyribonuclease which cleaves DNA has been tried in patients with cystic fibrosis who have purulent sputum and airway obstruction.

Serratiopeptidase: This proteolytic enzyme, administered orally, is claimed to be useful for 'digesting' necrotic tissue, cell debris, cellular exudate and coagulated blood. It is promoted in combination with other active agents such as NSAID for the oral treatment of inflammatory oedema and haematoma. Adequate evidence, however, is lacking to substantiate its usefulness.

CHAPTER 77

Vitamins and Antioxidants

Learning Objectives

This chapter will enable the reader:

1. To classify vitamins and state the situations leading to their deficiency.
2. To be aware of the sources, daily requirements, mechanism of action and physiological functions of vitamin A.
3. To enlist vitamin A preparations including synthetic analogues, and state their salient pharmacokinetic features, ADR and indications.
4. To state the physiological functions, symptoms of deficiency, preparations, ADR and indications for commonly used water-soluble vitamins (vitamins B and C)
5. To discuss the advantages and drawbacks of multivitamin combinations.
6. To enlist the sources of oxidants in the body and the host defence mechanisms against them.
7. To enumerate antioxidants giving current recommendation for their use.

KEY TERMS

uses of vitamin A, p. 1133
synthetic analogues of vitamin A, p. 1133
treatment of beriberi, p. 1135
pellagra, p. 1136
uses of pyridoxine, p. 1137
scurvy, p. 1138
multivitamin combinations, p. 1139
antioxidants, p. 1140

Vitamins are organic substances that are essential in minute quantities for the body. They act especially as coenzymes and precursors of coenzymes in the regulation of metabolic processes but do not provide energy or serve as building units. Many are present in natural foodstuffs or sometimes produced within the body e.g. vitamin K, pantothenic acid, folic acid and cyanocobalamin are synthesised by the intestinal bacterial flora. Vitamins form components of important enzyme systems which catalyse the reactions by which the body metabolises carbohydrates, proteins and fats. It is beyond the scope of this book to discuss in detail the physiological aspects of vitamins. The discussion is, therefore, limited to the pharmacological aspects when vitamins are employed as drugs.

A normal individual ingesting a well-balanced diet, containing a wide variety of foods, gets adequate supply of vitamins and needs no supplementation. Vitamin deficiency, however, can arise in various ways:

- **Deficient dietary intake:** Undernutrition from any cause including food fads.
- **Inadequate absorption from the GI tract:** Chronic diarrhoea, malabsorption syndrome, alcoholism, obstructive jaundice, interference with the function of the intestinal flora by oral antibiotics leading to decreased production or decreased absorption by drugs like liquid paraffin.
- **Interference with utilisation** usually by drugs, e.g. pyrimethamine, trimethoprim and methotrexate which interfere with folic acid utilisation; INH prevents the conversion of pyridoxal to pyridoxal phosphate.
- **Increased demand:** During growth, in pregnancy, during lactation, under stress, in fevers and other catabolic conditions such as hyperthyroidism. Groups vulnerable to develop vitamin deficiency are socio-economically disadvantaged persons, institutionalised persons, elderly persons on medications, heavy smokers who often lose interest in eating, women of childbearing age, infants (especially premature infants) and food faddists.

A diet that is deficient in one vitamin is likely to be deficient in others as well. Using food as the source of vitamins is the best safeguard against vitamin toxicity; in general, vitamin supplements should be used only when a dietary solution is not available.

Vitamins are classified as:

a. **Fat-soluble vitamins** such as A, D, E and K
b. **Water-soluble vitamins** such as B complex and C

The former are stored in the body and cannot be excreted easily; hence, excessive administration of these can cause serious toxicity. Water-soluble vitamins, on the other hand, are rapidly excreted in the urine following excessive administration.

FAT-SOLUBLE VITAMINS

VITAMIN A: Vitamin A is available from the diet either:

- **As preformed vitamin, retinol,** which is a complex, primary alcohol or
- **Esters of retinol in the form of carotenoid pigments** (particularly beta carotene) which is considered as provitamin A

Sources: Beta carotene, the major carotenoids in the food, is present in green and yellow vegetables and fruits: carrots, papaya, mango, etc. *Retinol is present in animal foods: eggs, milk, milk products and meat. Animal liver (cod, halibut and mammals) is a rich source of retinol.*

The daily requirements of vitamin A is about 5000 U in adults and older children and about 3000 U in children below 5 years. About 35 g of dark leafy vegetables will supply the daily dietary requirements of children. Small fish, eaten whole (with their livers), are a good supplementary source of vitamin A in diet. Human milk supplies sufficient vitamin A for infants unless the mother's diet is grossly inadequate; in the latter instance, enough vitamin A should be given during the first 6 months after birth to provide about 1500 U daily to normal birthweight infants and 2000–2500 U daily to premature infants.

Vitamin A values are now expressed as the **retinol activity equivalent (RAE)**. One RAE is equal to 3.33 IU (1 mcg) of retinol and 20 IU of beta carotene.

Vitamin A and the carotenes are stable to moderate heat in the absence of oxidising agents. **The ordinary cooking processes do not destroy the vitamin A in vegetables.** Prolonged, high temperature cooking, exposure to light and rancidity of fat hasten vitamin A destruction but *frozen foods retain their vitamin A content for a long time.*

Mechanism of action: Vitamin A binds to steroid family receptors such as retinoic acid receptors (RAR) and retinoid X receptors (RXR) and activates gene transcription. RARs predominantly are involved in cellular differentiation and proliferation, and RXRs are involved in cellular apoptosis.

Physiological functions: Vitamin A is essential for:

- The synthesis of rhodopsin, the photosensitive pigment of rods. Rhodopsin decomposes when light strikes the rod, thus initiating the nerve impulse
- The integrity of epithelial cells
- Maintenance of CMI
- Normal morphogenesis, somatic growth and cell differentiation
- Protection against infection

Deficiency of vitamin A *affects the immune system* at multiple sites. It affects certain subsets of T lymphocytes, natural killer (NK) cells, cytotoxic activity and the antibody response to bacterial polypeptides. *Mortality from infectious diseases, which accompany xerophthalmia, can be reduced by intermittent, massive vitamin A therapy.*

Clinical vitamin A deficiency is characterised by:

- **Night blindness, xerosis of conjunctivae** (manifested as Bitot spots) and **xerophthalmic** or **dry eye**
- **Squamous metaplasia of the mucosal surface of the upper respiratory tract** and the periodontal tissues
- **Follicular hyperkeratosis of the skin** (also termed *toad skin*)
- **Increased incidence of renal calculi**

Similar changes may occur in the intestinal epithelium leading to diarrhoea.

In advanced stages, true **keratomalacia** may occur, leading to blindness. The manifestations of this condition are necrosis, ulceration and finally, perforation of the cornea and panophthalmitis. *Vitamin A deficiency is one of the major preventable causes of blindness in children in* some *developing countries.*

Absorption, fate and excretion: Retinol is readily absorbed from the GI tract but requires the presence of dietary protein. The absorption is reduced in the presence of biliary obstruction or liver disease.

Following absorption, vitamin A is stored in the Kupffer cells of the liver as **retinyl ester**. Almost 90% of vitamin A in the body is in the liver. It is released into the plasma as **free alcohol (retinol)** in combination with specific proteins, retinol binding protein. Liver disease, therefore, may be associated with low plasma retinol levels. In kwashiorkor, plasma retinol levels are low, probably owing to the deficiency of the carrier protein.

As opposed to vitamin A, GI **absorption of carotene is slow and requires the presence of bile and absorbable fat.** Carotene is converted to vitamin A in the intestinal wall and is subsequently stored in the liver. Only about 30% of the dietary carotene is converted to retinol. In the event of large dietary intake of carotene, some of it may escape into the circulation, leading to carotenaemia, which causes a characteristic yellow discolouration of the skin.

Vitamin A is metabolised in the body to:

- **Esters** which are stored in the liver
- **The aldehyde retinal** which is the active element of the visual pigment
- **Retinoic acid,** an intracellular messenger that modulates cell differentiation

Normal human urine does not contain any vitamin A.

Adverse reactions:

- **Acute intoxication:** Consumption of the liver of polar bear (vitamin A content, 10,000–34,000 IU/g) leads to anorexia, nausea, vomiting, abdominal pain, headache, papilloedema, diplopia, convulsions, delirium and coma. Bulging of fontanelles and vomiting have been reported in infants given a single, large dose of 300,000 IU of vitamin A.
- **Chronic intoxication** usually develops following the administration of large doses of vitamin A (over 25,000 IU daily) for prolonged periods. The usual symptoms are anorexia, dry itching skin (hyperkeratosis), loss of weight, increased irritability, low grade fever, alopecia, dependent oedema with erythema and ecchymosis, refractory skin ulcer, anaemia and hepatosplenomegaly. Headache, increased ICT and papilloedema are often encountered. Tenderness over long bones and bony exostoses are other notable features. X-ray studies reveal premature closure of epiphyses and consequent retardation of growth in children. The symptoms usually appear after a latent period of 6–15 months. *The characteristic skin desquamation is a major diagnostic point to hypervitaminosis A.*

Large doses (more than 20,000 IU/day in the form of fish oil) of vitamin A should not be used during pregnancy or in infants; similarly, large amounts of liver in the diet should be avoided. Pharmacological doses of vitamin A are teratogenic. In pregnancy the daily dose must not exceed 6000–8000 IU.

Although beta carotene/vitamin A is claimed to act as antioxidant, it also has pro-oxidant effect *in vivo.* Its excessive intake may in fact, increase the risk of lung cancer and prostatic cancer.

Preparations and dosage:

i. Concentrated vitamin A solution contains not less than 50,000 IU/mL of vitamin A activity. Dose: 0.06–0.6 mL.
ii. Vitamin A tablet: Contains 50,000 IU of vitamin A. Dose: 1–2 tablets daily.
iii. Vitamin A injection: Contains 100,000 IU/mL. Dose: 1 mL IM once or twice a week.

Synthetic and natural preparations containing both vitamin A and vitamin D are as follows:

i. Vitamins A and D capsule or tablet contains 4000 IU of vitamin A and 400 IU of antirachitic activity. Dose: 1–2 capsules daily.

ii. Shark liver oil is obtained from the livers of the shark and allied species. Shark liver oil gelatin capsules in a dose of 500 mg are available. It contains not less than 6000 IU of vitamin A activity in 1 g. Dose: 1-2 capsules orally.

Indications:

- **Prophylactic uses:** Prophylactic use of this vitamin is important in the high risk, malnourished populations to prevent blindness and other disturbances. *Furthermore, even mild degree of vitamin A deficiency is associated with increased morbidity and mortality in children, largely as a result of vulnerability to diarrhoea and repeated infections.* PH 1.55

The prophylactic schedule recommended by WHO is shown in Table 77.1. Vitamin A has been introduced in the national immunisation schedule by the Indian government (Chapter 71). First dose of vitamin A (1 mL, 1 lakh units orally) is given at 9 completed months with measles-rubella vaccine while second dose (2 mL, 2 lakh units orally) is given at 16–18 months and subsequently every 6 months till the age of 5 years (total 9 doses).

- **For treatment:**
  a. **In the treatment of nightblindness and xerophthalmia,** vitamin A is administered in the dose of 100,000 IU by IM injection repeated if necessary. Improvement begins within a week after administration but several months are required for complete healing. A complete response is rare except in early stages. For severe deficiency with corneal changes: dose is 500,000 IU/day for 3 days, followed by 50,000 IU/day for 2 weeks and then 10,000-20,000 IU/day for 2 months as follow-up therapy. For cases without corneal changes: dose is 10,000-25,000 IU/day until clinical improvement occurs (usually 1-2 wk).
  b. **Measles** *can precipitate acute, severe vitamin A deficiency by depleting the hepatic stores of vitamin A.* WHO/UNICEF have recommended, *'High dosage of vitamin A supplementation should be provided to all children diagnosed with measles in communities in which vitamin A deficiency is a recognised problem'.* The recommended dose, to be administered as soon as measles is diagnosed, is 100,000 IU in children under the age of 12 months and 200,000 IU in children over that age. If any ocular sign of vitamin A deficiency is present, the same dose should be repeated the next day and again after 1–4 weeks.
  c. **Deficiency of vitamin A is also seen in coeliac disease, sprue, and with excessive use of liquid paraffin** and responds to the treatment outlined above

Table 77.1 WHO Recommended Prophylactic, Oral Vitamin A Doses (in International Units)

• **At birth (neonate)**	50,000 (single dose)
• **Up to 1 year**	100,000 once in 4–6 months
• **Children older than 1 year**	200,000 once in 4–6 months
• **Immediately after delivery (mother)**	300,000 (single dose)
• **Pregnant and lactating women**	5000 daily

Synthetic Analogues of Vitamin A

Vitamin A has the important **antikeratinising** property. Retinol, to be effective, must be administered in doses that cause hypervitaminosis A. Hence, synthetic analogues of retinol (**retinoids**) are used in a variety of skin disorders in doses that do not cause hypervitaminosis A. The analogues are:

1. **First generation**
   - **Tretinoin** (vitamin A acid, 13-transretinoic acid, retin-A) which is used **locally as a comedolytic in the treatment of acne vulgaris** (Chapter 69). It is also used to treat facial fine wrinkles, mottled pigmentation and promyelocytic leukaemia.
   - **Isotretinoin** (13-cis retinoic acid) which is used locally and orally as a sebostatic in the treatment of **severe acne vulgaris** (Chapter 69).
   - **Alitretinoin** is a topical retinoid used in the treatment of Cutaneous Kaposi sarcoma. It binds to both the types of retinoid receptors, RARs and RXRs.
2. **Second generation**
   - **Etretinate** (a derivative of tretinoin) and

acitretin (a metabolite of etretinate, Neotigason) which are used orally in the treatment of psoriasis (Chapter 69). They have been used to treat mycosis fungoides, basal cell carcinoma of the skin, oral leukoplakia and superficial bladder tumours.

3. **Third generation**
   - **Tazarotene,** and **adapalene** are used in the treatment of **acne** and **bexarotene** for **cutaneous T cell lymphoma.** Tazarotene is also used to treat plaque psoriasis, facial fine wrinkles and mottled pigmentation.
4. **Fourth generation**
   - **Trifarotene** selectively binds to RAR-γ receptors, which are present in the skin. It is used for acne vulgaris on the face and trunk.

VITAMIN D: See Chapter 68.

VITAMIN E: Vitamin E is a family of 4 tocopherols and 4 tocotrienols. Humans acquire vitamin E from plants and plant products like soya bean oil, corn oil, sunflower oil, wheat germ oil, rice germ oil, nuts and lettuce. *Natural vitamin E is gamma tocopherol whereas the synthetic vitamin E is l-alpha tocopherol.* The former is more bioavailable and is retained longer than the latter. *The daily requirement of vitamin E is believed to be 3–15 mg.*

Experimentally vitamin E has been shown to have antioxidant properties. It scavenges free radicals produced during metabolic processes, which damage the PUFA in the cell membrane. PUFA is essential for the maintenance of normal structure and function of the nervous system. Vitamin E deficiency is characterised by low serum levels, and increased fragility of RBCs, haemolytic anaemia and peripheral neuropathy.

Therapeutic usefulness of vitamin E is controversial. Commercial vitamin E supplement is mostly alpha tocopherol, which can block the antioxidant activity of natural vitamin E in diet and may have a pro-oxidant effect *in vivo*. Further higher dose of vitamin E (more than 800 mg) interferes with vitamin K metabolism and reduces platelet aggregation. *A meta-analysis clearly indicated that vitamin E alone or in combination with vitamin A/carotene has no protective effect on cancer or cardiovascular events.* In fact, vitamin E supplements during pregnancy have been reported to increase the gestational hypertension and cause premature rupture of the membrane.

VITAMIN K: See Chapter 33.

WATER-SOLUBLE VITAMINS

Vitamin B complex group includes thiamine, riboflavin, nicotinic acid, pyridoxine, pantothenic acid, inositol, biotin, methionine, folic acid and cyanocobalamin.

THIAMINE (Aneurine, vitamin B_1): This first member of the B complex series *can withstand boiling but is easily destroyed in an alkaline solution.* Peas, beans, oatmeal, the outer germ layer of the cereal grains, peanuts and mammalian organ meat are the rich sources of thiamine. Appreciable amounts are also present in yeast, vegetables and fruits. Tea and coffee contain an enzyme thiaminase which can destroy thiamine.

Physiological functions: The physiologically active form, **thiamine pyrophosphate** constitutes the prosthetic group of the decarboxylases involved in the metabolism of pyruvic and alpha-ketoglutaric acids, amino acids, and thus, it plays an important role in the intermediary carbohydrate metabolism and energy generation. *The daily thiamine requirement is estimated to be between 1 and 2 mg.*

Thiamine deficiency produces a symptom complex with characteristic neuropathy termed beriberi. Beriberi occurs in three main forms:

- **Wet beriberi** characterised by neuritis, oedema and high output cardiac failure
- **Infantile beriberi** which occurs within the first few months of life, with a high output failure, cyanosis, tachycardia, convulsions, anorexia, vomiting, greenish stools and sometimes sudden death as the noteworthy features
- **Dry beriberi,** which is usually seen in adults and in which symmetric **peripheral neuropathy** and muscular atrophy are predominant

Even though neuropathy in some form is common to all the three varieties, it is the most important manifestation in dry beriberi, whereas nervousness, increased irritability and depression may occur in all the types. In addition to beriberi, **Wernicke encephalopathy,** characterised by confusion, ophthalmoplegia, nystagmus, tremors and often peripheral neuropathy, is looked upon as a manifestation of severe thiamine deficiency; **Korsakoff psychosis** encountered in chronic alcoholics may owe some of its symptoms due to the lack of this vitamin and similarly the neuritis encountered in pregnancy and pellagra.

Vague symptoms like epigastric pain, anorexia, flatulence, constipation and lethargy or easy fatigability are also attributed to thiamine deficiency.

Absorption, fate and excretion: Thiamine is incompletely absorbed from the duodenum and the small intestine. It is distributed in all tissues. Thiamine appears in urine only when the minimal requirements are satisfied and the stores (liver, heart, brain, kidney) are saturated.

Adverse reactions: Thiamine administered orally usually does not evoke any adverse effects. Administration of large dose by IM/IV route, however, may rarely result in anaphylactoid shock. **Large doses** may also interfere with the metabolism of other members of B complex group. *Except in the initial treatment of acute wet beriberi, there is no justification for exceeding 100 mg daily, parenterally.*

Preparations and dosage:

i. Thiamine hydrochloride tablet 10, 25, 50 and 100 mg available, also as modified release tablets in a strength of 100 mg. Dose: prophylactic, 10–25 mg daily; therapeutic 25–100 mg daily.
ii. Thiamine hydrochloride injection. Dose: 25–100 mg SC or IM

Indications: Thiamine deficiency can be prevented by improvement in the dietary intake and by preventing overmilling of cereals, particularly rice.

- **Acute wet beriberi** responds to oral or parenteral administration of thiamine. Treatment is initiated with 50–100 mg, given parenterally, for 7 days. A maintenance dose of 5–10 mg is given subsequently orally. Most of the oedema fluid is eliminated within 48–72 h.
- **In dry beriberi,** it is advisable to use thiamine with other members of vitamin B complex.
- **Alcoholic and pregnancy associated neuritis** respond well to the oral administration of 5–10 mg daily. In Wernicke encephalopathy, a dose of 50 mg is usually advocated. In contrast, the neuritis of Korsakoff psychosis may respond slowly.

RIBOFLAVIN (vitamin B_2): Riboflavin occurs as yellow or orange yellow crystals; it is heat stable.

It is present in the yeast, green vegetables, legumes meat, fish, eggs and milk. In plants, it is present as a greenish fluorescent pigment. It is highly sensitive to sunlight and undergoes photodegradation. *The daily riboflavin requirement in an adult is estimated to be 1.5–3 mg and in a child 0.6–2 mg.*

Physiological functions: The physiologically active form of riboflavin is formed by phosphorylation. The two coenzymes flavin mononucleotide (FMN) and flavine adenine dinucleotide (FAD), which contain this active form, play an important role in oxidation of carbohydrates, fats and amino acids. FAD also modulates homocysteine metabolism.

Riboflavin deficiency (ariboflavinosis) is characterised by angular stomatitis, glossitis, a peculiar magenta pigmentation of the tongue and cheilosis (loss of epithelium at the mucocutaneous junction of lips resulting in reddened, shiny and denuded lips). The other features are seborrhoeic follicular keratosis of nose and forehead, and 'burning feet'. Certain ocular manifestations such as conjunctivitis, blepharospasm, photophobia, burning, lacrimation and vascularisation of the cornea are observed in some cases.

Absorption, fate and excretion: Riboflavin is synthesised in the large intestine, but whether it is available for absorption is uncertain.

Riboflavin and FMN are readily absorbed from the gut. It is phosphorylated to the active form in the intestinal wall, liver and erythrocytes. Excess of vitamin B_2 is stored in liver and kidneys. Only 9% of the orally administered dose appears in urine; the metabolic fate of the remainder is not known. Riboflavin does not produce any significant toxic effects. *Excess of riboflavin is readily excreted in the urine to which it imparts yellow colour and fluorescence.*

Preparations and dosage:

i. Riboflavin tablet 2, 10 mg. Dose: prophylactic, 1–2 mg daily; therapeutic, 5–10 mg daily.
ii. Riboflavin injection 10 mg/mL. Dose: 2–5 mg daily SC or IM.

Indications: In the treatment of **ariboflavinosis,** 5–10 mg of the vitamin is given daily in combination with other members of vitamin B group.

NICOTINIC ACID AND NICOTINAMIDE (vitamin B_3): Nicotinic acid and its, nicotinamide are used for in the treatment of pellagra. Nicotinic acid is present in large quantities in polished rice, liver, milk, eggs and lean meat, and to a smaller extent in potatoes and in vegetables. It is also synthesised from tryptophan in the intestines and in the tissues. *The normal daily requirement is 15–20 mg.*

Physiological functions and pharmacological actions: Nicotinic acid as nicotinamide adenine dinucleotide (NAD) and its phosphate (NADP) is the constituent of a number of coenzymes **involved in the metabolism of proteins** necessary for cellular respiration. They also play a possible role in DNA repair.

Pellagra, a symptom complex due to deficiency of nicotinic acid, occurs endemically in individuals consuming mainly a diet of maize. Nonendemic pellagra occurs in chronic alcoholism, malabsorption syndrome, carcinoid syndrome, cirrhosis, poorly controlled diabetes mellitus, and in cachexia secondary to malignancy.

The characteristic features are dermatitis and pigmentation of the skin, especially in regions exposed to sunlight (such as neck; Casal necklace) and at various pressure points, anorexia, stomatitis, glossitis, diarrhoea, irritability and mental confusion (dementia). Hallucinations may occur. Spinal cord degeneration leading to spastic paraplegia has been rarely reported.

Associated folic acid deficiency is responsible for the megaloblastic anaemia.

Serum lipids: Large doses lower the serum cholesterol and triglyceride levels and activate fibrinolysis (Chapter 38).

Vascular smooth muscle relaxation: Nicotinic acid, *in pharmacological doses*, causes peripheral vasodilatation by direct action on the vascular smooth muscle and causes flushing. This may be accompanied by pruritus. Nicotinamide is devoid of these effects.

Absorption, fate and excretion: Both nicotinic acid and nicotinamide are readily absorbed from the GI tract and from parenteral sites. They are distributed to all the tissues. Inactivation occurs mainly by *N*-methylation and to some extent by conjugation; the products are eliminated in the urine. Following large oral doses, the vitamin may appear in urine in the active form.

Adverse reactions: Besides flushing, urticaria and pruritus, *large doses* may cause furunculosis and other skin lesions, malaise, GI disturbances, activation of peptic ulcer, amblyopia, impairment of liver function, decrease in glucose tolerance and hyperuricaemia. Nicotinic acid potentiates the action of vasodilator drugs.

Preparations and dosage:

i. Nicotinic acid tablet 50 mg. Dose: prophylactic 15–30 mg daily; therapeutic, 50–200 mg daily, for Hartnup disease higher doses of 300-500 mg / day are administered.
ii. Nicotinamide tablet 50 mg. Dose: 100-300 mg in divided doses.

Indications:

- **Pellagra:** Nicotinic acid or its amide is used in the treatment of pellagra in the daily dose of 50–500 mg. Usually, nicotinamide is preferred because of its lack of adverse effects. The neuropathy and the lesions of face and lips, may need adjuvant treatment with riboflavin.
- **As a vasodilator:** Nicotinic acid, in the dose of 100–300 mg by subcutaneous or oral route, has been employed as a vasodilator in the treatment

of Meniere disease and in peripheral vascular disorders including chilblains and frostbite.

- **Hyperlipidaemia:** Large doses (3–6 g daily) are used (Chapter 38).

PYRIDOXINE (vitamin B_6): Pyridoxine, pyridoxal and pyridoxamine are collectively called as vitamin B_6. It is present in yeast, cereals, legumes, nuts, milk and meat. All the three forms are converted in the body to **pyridoxal phosphate** which is the physiologically active form. *The daily requirement is estimated at 1–2 mg.*

Physiological functions: Pyridoxal phosphate acts as a coenzyme for amino acid decarboxylases and transaminases. *It is involved in amino acid metabolism and the synthesis and degradation of biogenic amines like the catecholamines, 5-HT and other compounds like GABA, steroids.*

A syndrome in infants secondary to ingestion of proprietary milk preparation deficient in pyridoxine has been described. The characteristic features include irritability, abdominal distension, twitching, failure to gain weight, **hypochromic microcytic anaemia** and convulsions. The anaemia is probably due to inadequate utilisation of iron for erythropoiesis. Pyridoxine deficiency in adults may lead to lesions of the skin and mouth resembling those seen in ariboflavinosis and pellagra, **peripheral neuritis** and mental changes. Its deficiency may cause abnormal GTT.

Absorption, fate and excretion: All the three forms of the vitamin are readily absorbed from the GI tract. The end product of metabolism, 4-pyridoxic acid, is eliminated in urine.

Adverse reactions: Pyridoxine, administered in physiological doses, does not produce any adverse effects. Pyridoxine interferes with therapeutic effect of levodopa (Chapter 15).

Preparations and dosage:

i. Pyridoxine tablet 5, 25, 50 and 100 mg. Dose: 5–150 mg daily.
ii. Pyridoxine injection. Dose: 25–100 mg IM or IV

Indications:

- **Pyridoxine dependent inborn error of metabolism**, e.g. primary hyperoxaluria, homocystinuria
- **Convulsions due to pyridoxine deficiency in infants:** 4 mg/kg/day for short periods
- **Anaemia due to pyridoxine deficiency:** 50–150 mg/day in divided doses
- **Pellagra:** As an adjuvant in the dose of 5–10 mg/day
- **Vomiting of pregnancy, postirradiation vomiting** (Chapter 39)
- **Mental depression during oral contraceptive therapy** (Chapter 66)
- **INH and alcohol-induced peripheral neuropathy** (Chapter 52 and 6)

There is no evidence to suggest that supplementation of vitamin B_6 with or without folate and B_{12} reduces the risk of stroke or cancer.

PANTOTHENIC ACID (vitamin B_7): This is an organic acid which serves its physiological function by being converted into coenzyme A. Yeast, wheat, peanuts, cereals, milk, vegetables and liver contain large amounts of pantothenic acid. *The daily requirement of pantothenic acid is estimated to be 5 mg.*

Physiological actions: Coenzyme A is involved in several fundamental biological reactions such as fatty acid metabolism, synthesis of cholesterol and steroid hormones and acetylation reactions.

Pantothenic acid deficiency in humans under normal circumstances is not known. Artificial deficiency produced in human volunteers is characterised by fatigue, malaise, headache, somnolence, paraesthesiae, nausea, occasional vomiting, abdominal cramps, flatulence and possibly burning feet syndrome.

Absorption, fate and excretion: The vitamin remains stable in foodstuffs for long periods and little is destroyed during cooking. Pantothenic acid is rapidly absorbed from the gut and is concentrated in liver, heart and kidneys. It is mainly excreted in the urine.

Pantothenic acid is almost nontoxic.

Preparations and dosage:

i. Calcium pantothenate: 10 and 50 mg tablets. Dose: 10–50 mg.
ii. Dexpanthenol: *This analogue of pantothenic acid is readily converted to the parent compound on administration.* Dose of 250–500 mg given IM/IV For topical application, 2%–5% cream/ointment.

Indications: Calcium pantothenate has been employed in **postoperative paralytic ileus and as a nutritional supplement** along with other members of the B-complex group. Dexpanthenol has been employed systemically for the prevention and treatment of postoperative intestinal atony and topically for various skin lesions including burns, wounds and ulcers; their utility in these conditions, however, remains doubtful.

BIOTIN: Biotin is an organic acid which functions as a coenzyme for numerous carboxylation reactions. *Biotin deficiency is not encountered naturally in humans* but has been produced in volunteers by administering a diet containing large amounts of raw egg white (albumin), which binds to biotin and reduces its bioavailability. Deficiency is characterised by seborrhoeic dermatitis, lassitude, anorexia and paraesthesiae. The daily human requirement of the vitamin is unknown. The vitamin is synthesised by the intestinal flora. *Clinical deficiency syndrome has not been demonstrated and hence biotin has no therapeutic application.*

Miscellaneous: These include **inositol, choline, methionine** and **para-aminobenzoic acid** *(PABA)*.

Choline plays a role in cholinergic transmission, lipid and cholesterol metabolism, methyl group metabolism and transmembrane signaling. Food items like wheat germ, milk, egg yolk, meat contain lecithin – a choline compound. Choline is also synthesised by the liver.

Choline and methionine, the so-called **'lipotropic factors'**, have been used in the treatment of liver cirrhosis; inositol has been used in the management of diseases associated with fat metabolism. This is based on the observation that their experimental deficiency in animals causes fatty livers. Their efficacy in human conditions is, however, equivocal. *Methionine is used to treat acute paracetamol poisoning* (Chapter 11).

For **folic acid** and **vitamin B_{12}**, see Chapter 35.

ASCORBIC ACID (vitamin C): The dietary sources of ascorbic acid include citrus fruits, tomatoes, plants, potatoes and green vegetables. Lemon juice as a sole source of this vitamin is not reliable. Although cereals and other seeds are devoid of vitamin C, they produce it on germination. Laevo compound is more active. *Vitamin C is unstable and is destroyed by boiling and by alkali.*

The minimum daily requirement of ascorbic acid for an adult is about 30 mg and for infants, 5 mg/kg of body weight.

Physiological actions: Ascorbic acid, along with its oxidation product dehydroascorbic acid, is intimately involved in several physiological functions:

- In biological oxidation–reduction reactions and in cellular respiration
- For the functional integrity of sulfhydryl group of enzymes and also for the formation of collagen and intercellular matrix, and hence, for the development of cartilage, bone and teeth and for healing of wounds
- As a potent antioxidant, in neutralising free radicals (oxidant)
- For absorption of nonhaeme iron, and for conversion of dopamine to NA
- The formation of haemoglobin, erythrocyte maturation, certain immunological reactions of the body and the conversion of folic acid to tetrahydrofolate
- In carbohydrate metabolism and in the oxidation of phenylalanine and tyrosine

Ascorbic acid deficiency leads to the development of **scurvy**. The characteristic features in adults are perifollicular haemorrhages, petechiae, ecchymoses, haemorrhages in subcutaneous tissues, muscles and joints; swollen, inflamed, bleeding and spongy gums and normocytic or microcytic anaemia. In infants, loss of appetite, listlessness and subperiosteal haemorrhages leading to tenderness and restriction of limb movements are the cardinal features. Ecchymoses and gum changes may also be seen. *Infantile scurvy is usually seen in bottle-fed babies; human milk contains appreciable amounts of ascorbic acid.*

Absorption, fate and excretion: Ascorbic acid is almost completely absorbed from GIT when given in smaller doses. However, absorption is only 50% when doses >1 g are used. It is concentrated in the glandular tissues, leucocytes and platelets. It is partly metabolised and excreted in urine as oxalate and a part is eliminated in the free form. Urinary excretion depends upon saturation of body stores and in individuals *with its deficiency, the vitamin may not appear in urine even on administration of large doses.*

In ordinary doses (<1 g), ascorbic acid is essentially nontoxic. Vitamin C in urine gives a false positive test for sugar while using Benedict test and a false negative test while using glucose oxidase test.

Preparations and dosage:

i. Ascorbic acid tablet contains 50 mg. Dose: Prophylactic, 25–75 mg daily; therapeutic 200–500 mg daily.
ii. Ascorbic acid injection: available as 100 mg/ ml; Dose: 0.5–1 g IM/IV

Adverse reactions: Prolonged ingestion of large quantities (>2 g/day) of vitamin C is known to lead to increased urinary excretion of oxalate and possibly stone formation and kidney damage.

Indications:

- **Scurvy prevention and treatment:** In the treatment of scurvy, ascorbic acid is administered in the dose of 100–500 mg per day. As a prophylactic measure, it is important to ensure adequate Vitamin C intake in infancy and old age. *Infantile scurvy can be prevented by adding 5 mg of the vitamin to the feeds of bottle-fed infants.* For prophylaxis, a daily dose of 50–100 mg is advocated in adults.
- **Methaemoglobinaemia:** Because of its ability to function as a reducing agent, ascorbic acid in the daily dose of 300–600 mg is used in the treatment of methaemoglobinaemia; it is, however, less effective than methylene blue.

Table 77.2 Recommended Dietary Allowances (RDA) of Various Vitamins per Day for Adults

Vitamins	Recommended By: ICMR[a] (for Indians)	Recommended By: WHO/FAO Expert Group
Thiamine	1.2–2.0 mg	1.0–1.5 mg
Riboflavin	1.3–2.2 mg	1.3–2.1 mg
Pyridoxine	–	1.5–2.0 mg
Niacin	16–26 mg	–
Vitamin B_{12}	1 mcg	2 mcg
Folate	100 mcg	200 mcg
Vitamin C	50 mg	30 mg
Vitamin A	750 mcg	750 mcg
Vitamin D	5 mcg (200 IU)	2.5 mcg (100 IU)

[a]ICMR, Indian Council of Medical Research.

The vitamin is also used as an antioxidant in emulsions of fats and oils, in certain injections and eye drops, and as a preservative.

High doses of vitamin C fail to reduce the risk of cancer or cardiovascular accidents. It does not have any beneficial effects in common cold. Such doses (>1 g) are poorly absorbed and may cause abdominal pain, diarrhoea, increase in urinary excretion of oxalate and oxalate stones. PH 1.61

Multivitamin combinations: *Prophylactic multivitamin preparations* should contain from one-half to one and one-half times the recommended dietary allowances (Table 77.2) except for vitamin D which should not exceed the daily recommended dietary allowance. Larger doses of ascorbic acid and B-complex in such preparations are wasteful and could be harmful. Multivitamin pills may be useful in old people, who for some reasons cannot get adequate nutrition, malnutrition and during recovery from acute illnesses.

Selective deficiency of a single vitamin B factor occurs less commonly and hence, combined B-complex therapy is commonly employed prophylactically as well as therapeutically.

Commercial multivitamin preparations may contain 4–5 times the recommended dietary allowances.

Table 77.3 Reactive Oxygen Species

Symbol	Name
$^1O_2$	Singlet oxygen
$O^{\bullet -}_2$	Superoxide free radical
$^{\bullet}OH$	Hydroxyl free radical
$R{+}O^-$	Alkoxy free radical
$RO{+}O^{\bullet}$	Peroxyl free radical
H_2O_2	Hydrogen peroxide
LOOH	Lipid peroxide

Box 77.1 Sources of Oxidants in the Body

- ***Cyclooxygenation***
- ***Lipooxygenation***
- ***Lipid peroxidation*** (auto-oxidation on exposure to oxygen)
- ***Neutrophils*** stimulated by exposure to microbes
- ***Re-perfusion of ischemic organs***
- ***Metabolism of xenobiotics*** (foreign chemicals) including alcohol, cigarette smoke and motor car exhaust
- ***Ultraviolet and ionising radiation damage***

Box 77.2 Body Defences Against Oxidants

- ***Intracellular enzymes*** (catalases, superoxide dismutases, glutathione peroxidases) which dispose of the oxidants
- ***Antioxidants obtained along with nutrients***
  Vitamins A, C, E
  Trace elements: selenium
  Flavonoids and polyphenolic substances present in plant foods (fruits, vegetables, *amla*, tea, garlic and others)
  Others present in spices such as coriander, clove and cardamom

They are expensive and should be used only for deficiency states and during periods of increased vitamin requirement. They are not a substitute for a balanced diet. Often, costly multivitamin preparations with several minerals are promoted as general 'tonics' to keep 'good health' and to protect from 'stress' leading to irrational use.

Prolonged use of high doses of vitamin A and vitamin D can cause toxicity.

ANTIOXIDANTS

PH 1.61

Chemically, oxidation is the removal of electrons and reduction is the gain of electrons; oxidation is always coupled with reduction. Many biological oxidations can take place without the participation of molecular oxygen, e.g. dehydrogenations. Furthermore, molecular oxygen has very little capability to oxidise other chemicals. Instead, it must first be converted to an 'active' form called **reactive species of oxygen (an oxidant)**. Many of the reactive oxygen species are free radicals but not all, e.g. singlet oxygen and hydrogen peroxide are not free radicals. **A free radical is an atom or a molecule with one or more unpaired electrons. Its tendency to acquire electron(s) from other substances makes it highly reactive.** Table 77.3 lists the reactive oxygen species.

These oxidants are generated during the normal metabolic reactions in the body. The other sources of free radicals and other oxidants are listed in Box 77.1.

Small amounts of oxidants are continually formed in the cell membrane and close to the cell organelles which can damage cell structures. However, the body has inbuilt mechanisms to mop up the small amounts of oxidants normally formed during metabolic reactions (Box 77.2).

Oxidants formed in controlled amounts by neutrophil leucocytes on exposure to microbes are beneficial to the body in that they participate in destroying the microbes. Excess of oxidants, however, can be harmful to the tissues. However attempts have been made to make a case for supplementation of human diet with antioxidants given as pharmacological agents. *Currently, there is no pharmacological antioxidant agent available which has been convincingly shown to be useful in prevention or treatment of disease in humans.* Hence, the **current recommendation** is to increase the consumption of cereals, pulses, nuts, fruits and vegetables which are good sources of natural antioxidants. Spices used in Indian cooking also contain antioxidants. Evidence indicates that increased fruit and vegetable intake raises plasma concentration of α and β carotene, lycopene, beta cryptoxanthine and ascorbic acid and may decrease both, diastolic and systolic blood pressure. For vitamin E, see earlier. PH 1.61

Coenzyme Q10 (Ubiquinone): This is a **fat-soluble antioxidant,** currently sold as a dietary supplement.

Humans synthesise as well as obtain it from dietary sources. It is present in the mitochondria of human cells, and high concentrations are found in the heart, liver, kidney and skeletal muscle. Tissue concentrations decline with age. Coenzyme Q10 is involved in ATP generation. The usual dose is 100–200 mg/day in divided doses. It has been claimed to be of some benefit in conditions including Parkinson disease and CHF. It is well tolerated and the adverse reactions are mild, comprising nausea, vomiting and abdominal discomfort. Its place in therapeutics needs further substantiation. PH 1.61

Spirulina: This product, obtained from the marine algae, is claimed to contain 70% by weight of protein and many micronutrients. However, the daily recommended dose of 2 tablets (each containing 500 mg of spirulina), contains only 700 mg of protein and minuscule quantities of micronutrients, much below RDA. Hence, the claims are unjustified, and this expensive product cannot be recommended.

SYNTHETIC ANALOGUES OF VITAMIN A

First generation

Tretinoin
Isotretinoin
Alitretinoin

Second generation

Etretinate
Acitretin

Third generation

Tazarotene
Adapalene
Bexarotene

Fourth generation

Trifarotene

CHAPTER 78

Drugs, Pregnancy and the Infant

Learning Objectives

This chapter will enable the reader:

1. To explain the changes in drug pharmacokinetics that occur during pregnancy.
2. To state the factors affecting placental transfer of drugs.
3. To explain the salient features of fetal-neonatal pharmacokinetics and pharmacodynamics.
4. To enumerate the effects of drugs on pregnancy.
5. To enlist the drugs that have teratogenic potential and the effects produced by them.
6. To state the principles followed while prescribing drugs to women in reproductive age.
7. To mention the drugs preferred in pregnant patients for common ailments.
8. To state the factors influencing excretion of drugs in milk.
9. To enumerate drugs to be avoided in women who are breastfeeding.

KEY TERMS

pharmacokinetics during pregnancy, p. 1142
placental transfer of drugs, p. 1143
teratogenic drugs, p. 1146
drug prescribing in pregnancy, p. 1147
drugs avoided during lactation, p. 1150

Drugs are likely to be self-administered or prescribed by the physician during pregnancy. Intelligent use of drugs during pregnancy requires that the physician understands the interaction between drugs and pregnancy so as to avoid indiscriminate use of drugs with disastrous consequences as illustrated by the thalidomide tragedy. At the same time, overcautious timidity on the part of the physician casts the pregnant mother in the role of a therapeutic orphan. It must be remembered that most of the drugs prescribed during pregnancy are given for the benefit of the mother and that one must not deny her adequate treatment for a serious illness.

In addition to drugs, the pregnant woman is likely to be exposed to a variety of environmental, nontherapeutic or illicit agents which can affect the fetal health.

PHARMACOKINETICS DURING PREGNANCY

Most of the available information on **pharmacokinetics** of drugs during pregnancy has been obtained from animal experiments and may not be directly applicable to humans. Although pregnant women do not differ qualitatively from the nonpregnant ones in their response to drugs, certain quantitative differences do occur because of physiological changes during pregnancy, with consequent alterations in pharmacokinetics of drugs. Furthermore, the fetus has its own pharmacokinetic peculiarities.

Drug absorption: High circulating levels of progesterone slow the gastric emptying as well as gut motility, thus increasing the intestinal transit time. As a result, one might expect slower drug absorption during pregnancy. *However, this does not occur except at term when parenteral drug administration is preferred* in order to obtain a quick response. Administration of iron and antacids may also interfere with the absorption of certain drugs. Drug compliance may be poor during pregnancy because of nausea and fear of possible adverse effects.

Drug distribution: Pregnancy is accompanied by an increase in total body water by up to 8 L and a 30%

increase in plasma volume, with consequent decrease in plasma albumin (0.5–1.0 g%) due to haemodilution. Drugs which have low lipid solubility and are also highly plasma protein bound (e.g. warfarin, benzodiazepines) have a low apparent volume of distribution (Vd). **The Vd of such drugs increases markedly during pregnancy.** The protein bound fraction of the drug in the plasma diminishes and so does the concentration of the total drug in the plasma. Although the fraction of unbound drug increases, a greater pharmacodynamic effect is prevented by more rapid elimination of the drug by metabolism and/or excretion (see below). The therapeutic range for drugs whose use is monitored by measurement of total plasma concentration (e.g. phenytoin) must be adjusted downwards to make allowance for the above mentioned changes, if their plasma protein binding changes during pregnancy. There is also likely increase in body fat which acts as a reservoir for lipid-soluble drugs.

Drug metabolism: *Hepatic drug metabolising enzymes are induced during pregnancy, probably by the high concentrations of circulating progesterone.* This can lead to more rapid metabolic degradation, especially of the highly lipid-soluble drugs such as phenytoin and theophylline. However, this is of little clinical consequence because the metabolism of most such drugs is ordinarily so fast that their clearance is limited only by hepatic blood flow, which does not change appreciably during pregnancy, e.g. pethidine. The contribution of the placenta and the fetal liver to the clearance of drugs from the maternal body is thought to be small.

Drug excretion: During pregnancy, the renal plasma flow increases by 100% and the GFR by 70%. Add to this the increase in the unbound fraction of the drug in the plasma. **Hence, drugs which depend for their elimination mainly on the kidney are eliminated more rapidly than in the nonpregnant state.** Examples are ampicillin, aminoglycosides, cephalexin and digoxin.

The conventional dose of ampicillin needs to be doubled during pregnancy if it is used for a systemic infection in the mother, but not if it is used for a urinary tract infection. An increase in the dose of cefuroxime and lithium is needed for similar reasons. In the case of phenytoin (whose unbound plasma level diminishes due to more rapid metabolism, in addition to total plasma level), an increase in the daily dose by 25–100 mg may be required to maintain good seizure control; a similar increase is also required in the dose of carbamazepine. In spite of pharmacokinetic alterations, the doses of benzodiazepines, aspirin, propranolol, sulphafurazole and metronidazole do not require alterations during pregnancy. The pharmacokinetics of furosemide does not alter during pregnancy and no dose adjustment is required.

DRUGS, THE FETUS AND THE NEWBORN

Placental transfer of drugs: The placenta acts as an intravenous portal for entry of drugs into the fetus. As pregnancy progresses and the placenta develops, the surface available for transfer between the maternal and fetal circulations increases; at the same time, the placento-fetal barrier becomes progressively thinner. Transfer across this barrier is governed by the same properties of drugs which regulate the transfer across other biological membranes: *unbound, nonionised, lipid-soluble molecules of low molecular weight cross the barrier more easily than those which do not possess these attributes;* most of the drugs in use fulfil these criteria and are able to cross the placental barrier. However, because of the differences in the plasma protein concentration and the pH between maternal and fetal blood, the concentration of drugs in the two circulations, even at equilibrium, differ considerably. Add to this, the differences in pharamacokinetics between the mother and the fetus. Furthermore, the placenta is capable of metabolising drugs; this is of little relevance to the mother but can protect the fetus from the entry of many drugs. For example, prednisolone and hydrocortisone, which are metabolised by the placenta to inactive compounds are safer for the fetus than dexamethasone and betamethasone, which are not so metabolised.

The method of drug administration to the mother may also decide the fetal concentration. For example, at term, antibiotics given by intermittent intravenous infusion can achieve higher concentrations in the fetal blood and amniotic fluid than when the same total dose is given by continuous infusion; this may be important in the treatment of intrauterine infections.

In spite of above considerations, the fetal: maternal ratio of unbound drug concentration is generally close to unity. Furthermore, the placenta is always available to the fetus as a route of drug elimination.

Compared to adults, both fetus and infants differ in their handling of drugs, as related to pharmacokinetics as well as pharmacodynamics. However, the data available regarding this are far from adequate.

Fetal/neonatal pharmacokinetics: Human growth is not a linear phenomenon. Age-related changes in body composition and organ function are dynamic and can be discordant during the first decade of life. *Hence, the simplified dosage approaches calculated by standard formulae may not be adequate for individualising drug doses across the span of infancy and childhood.*

During the neonatal period, intragastric pH is relatively higher (>7.4). Hence, orally administered drugs such as penicillin G have greater bioavailability in neonates than in adults. On the other hand, weak acids such as phenobarbitone need higher doses in the young children. Generally, the rate at which majority of drugs are absorbed is slower in the neonates than in the older children. Furthermore, developmental differences in the activity of intestinal drug metabolising enzymes and changes in the intestinal microflora may also affect the plasma levels of drugs.

Compared to adults, neonates and infants have relatively larger extracellular and total body water spaces. This, along with the adipose tissue stores that have a higher lipid/water ratio, leads to lower EC concentrations when drugs are given on weight basis. Distribution of highly protein bound drugs is also modified by the amount of circulating plasma albumin and alpha 1-acidglycoprotein.

In infants and young children, the ratio of total body surface area (BSA) to body mass far exceeds that in adults. *Hence, the relative systemic exposure of infants to topically applied drugs such as glucocorticoids may exceed that in adults, leading to adverse systemic effects.*

Delayed maturation of hepatic drug metabolising enzymes in infants can cause increased drug toxicity, e.g. chloramphenicol.

The expression of Phase I metabolising enzymes such as cytochrome P-450 undergoes marked changes during development of neonates. This affects the hepatic clearance of various drugs metabolised by the isoforms of these enzymes. The clearance of carbamazepine is greater in children than in adults. In the case of phenytoin, its $t\frac{1}{2}$ is about 75 h in preterm infants, which decreases to about 20 h during the first week of life and to 8 h after the second week of life. The plasma clearance of morphine is known to quadruple between 27th and 40th weeks of gestational age, thus requiring corresponding increase in the dose of morphine for effective analgesia.

Because of significant developmental changes during the neonatal period, drugs such as methylxanthines, morphine, captopril and third generation cephalosporins need age-appropriate dosage regimens.

Various developmental changes in the kidney function during infancy can alter the plasma clearance of drugs that are primarily excreted by the kidney, e.g. aminoglycosides, famotidine, ceftazidime, digoxin, chlorpropamide, penicillin, salicylic acid, indomethacin and paracetamol. This obviously will need age-appropriate selection of dosage regimen.

In view of the above problems, it is safer to consult worked-out dosage tables for neonates and infants than to use formulae based on body weight and/or BSA.

Fetal–neonatal pharmacodynamics: Age-dependent differences in the interaction of the drugs with specific receptors do probably exist but the data are limited. This may modify the safety and efficacy of drugs in the neonates and infants. For a given plasma concentration, the response of the fetal tissues to most drugs is equal to or less than that of maternal tissues. There are some notable exceptions. Certain drugs given in the second and third trimesters produce either exaggerated effects or effects that are unique to the fetus. For example, tetracyclines get deposited in the fetal teeth and bones and retard their growth; coumarins can cause fetal and neonatal haemorrhages. Salicylates given at term can cause neonatal haemorrhage. PG synthetase inhibitors (NSAIDs) given near term can induce premature closure of ductus arteriosus and pulmonary hypertension in the fetus. Antithyroid drugs can inhibit fetal thyroxine synthesis and can cause goitre formation. Opiates and barbiturates (given to mother) achieve very high concentrations in the fetal brain and can cause respiratory depression at birth. Phenothiazines given to the mother can cause extrapyramidal toxicity in the neonate which may persist for several months (also see Chapter 13).

EFFECTS OF DRUGS ON PREGNANCY

Effective treatment of maternal illness with drugs such as insulin, thyroxine, antibiotics and antihypertensives may be said to have a beneficial effect on the course of pregnancy.

On the other hand, in certain situations drugs can cause harm to the conceptus. These harmful effects depend upon the nature of the drug and its dose and route of administration; the stage of pregnancy at which the drug is used; and the genetic constitution and susceptibility of the fetus, which in turn, depend upon the age, nutritional status and health of the mother. Gestation may be divided into four major stages.

- **Preimplantation stage** (blastocyst formation) which lasts about 16 days from conception to implantation. Exposure to harmful drugs (such as anticancer drugs) can kill the embryo or else the damaged cells are replaced by undifferentiated cells which have the potential to develop normally. This is an all-or-none effect.
- **Period of organogenesis** from 17th to 56th day. Preimplantation stage and the stage of organogenesis together constitute the *first trimester.* Exposure to harmful drugs (and other environmental influences) during the period of organogenesis can cause congenital malformations (**teratogenicity**) or abortion.
- **The second and third trimesters** are periods during which considerable growth and development occur in teeth, bones and in central nervous, endocrine, genital and immune systems. During this period drugs can cause either teratogenesis or a variety of other effects such as retardation of physical or brain growth, behavioural teratogenicity, premature labour, neonatal toxicity and even late post natal effects such as cancer(s).
- **A short labour-delivery stage:** Drug administration during this period is mainly fraught with the danger of toxicity in the neonatal period for reasons already discussed.

TERATOGENICITY

This word was originally used in the sense of congenital malformations grossly visible at birth and caused by exposure to exogenous agents (**teratogens**) in the first trimester. The definition has now been broadened to include any birth defect (morphological, biochemical or behavioural) induced at any stage of pregnancy and detected at birth or later in life. *Birth defects are known to occur in 2%–4% of all births in the population.* Out of all birth defects, the cause is unknown in 65%–70%; 25% can be attributed to genetic defects and 3% to chromosomal aberrations. *Only about 3% can be ascribed to environmental factors* including maternal infection, radiation and drug administration. The overall incidence of congenital malformations does not appear to have increased in the last 30 years in spite of the dramatic increase in the number of drugs available.

Teratogenesis includes restricted growth of the fetus, malformations, carcinogenesis and behavioural teratogenicity (see later). It should be noted that fewer than 30 drugs have been proved to be teratogenic in humans when used in clinically effective doses. Many of the commonly used drugs, once thought to be teratogenic, have been shown by subsequent studies to be safe; they include salicylates, glucocorticoids, diazepam, combination OC pills and spermicides. Much of the information on teratogenicity of drugs has been obtained from animal experiments and mishaps in clinical practice. Because of species variability and the high doses used in these experiments, such data are not directly applicable to humans; but they have a high positive predictive value. Almost every drug that has been found to be teratogenic in humans has caused similar teratogenicity in animals. However, there are drugs that have caused teratogenic effects in animals in large doses that are not teratogenic in humans in clinically effective doses. Individual case reports and limited epidemiological surveys provide the information available about teratogenicity of drugs in humans.

Except in a few instances, congenital malformations produced by drugs are not unique. Most drugs currently suspected of being teratogenic in humans are, in fact, weak teratogens and probably increase the frequency of congenital malformations only 2–3-fold. *In fact, smoking and alcohol are more harmful to the fetus than most drugs. Table 78.1 lists the drugs which are known or suspected to be teratogenic in humans. Absence of a drug from the list should not be interpreted to mean that it is necessarily safe during pregnancy.*

The teratogenic effects of thalidomide have been described in Chapter 1; those of alcohol in Chapter 6; tetracycline in Chapter 47 and retinoic acid derivatives in Chapter 69.

Often, women are advised to delay pregnancy for certain periods of time after completing the course of certain drugs: one month after isotretinoin (Chapter 69); three months after mefloquine (Chapter 54); one year after cytotoxic drugs (methotrexate, cyclophosphamide); and three years after etretinate (Chapter 69) in order to allow the elimination of the drug. However, azathioprine following renal transplantation has not been found to pose an excess risk of congenital malformations in succeeding pregnancies.

Table 78.1 Drug with Proven Teratogenic Effects in Humans

Drug	Teratogenic Effect
Methotrexate	CNS and limb malformations
ACE inhibitors / ARB	Prolonged renal failure in the neonate, renal tubular dysgenesis, decreased skull ossification, IUGR
Aminoglycosides	Hearing defects, vestibular problems
Anticholinergic drugs	Neonatal meconium ileus
Antithyroid drugs	Fetal and neonatal goitre and hypothyroidism, aplasia cutis (with methimazole)
Beta blockers	IUGR, intrauterine deaths, premature deliveries
Carbamazepine	Neural tube defects
Cyclophosphamide	CNS malformations, secondary cancer
Danazol and other androgenic drugs	Masculinisation of female fetus
Diethylstilbestrol	Vaginal carcinoma and other genitourinary defects in female and male offspring
Lithium	Ebstein's anomaly
Methimazole	Premature delivery, scalp defects, esophageal atresia
Misoprostol	Moebius syndrome skull defects, cranial nerve palsies, facial malformations, limb defects
Mycophenolate mofetil	External ear and facial defects; cleft lip and palate; heart, esophagus, kidney and distal limb defects
NSAID	Constriction of the ductus arteriosus, necrotising enterocolitis
Oral hypoglycaemic drugs	Neonatal hypoglycaemia
Phenytoin	Growth retardation, CNS defects
Psychoactive drugs	Neonatal withdrawl syndrome when drug is taken in late pregnancy
Rifaximin	Cleft palate, jaw shortening, incomplete ossification
Statins	Spina bifida
Systemic retinoids (isotretinoin, etretinate)	CNS, craniofacial, cardiovascular and other defects
Tetracycline	Anomalies of teeth and bones
Thalidomide	Limb-shortening, internal organ defects
Trimethadone	Malformed ears, cleft palate, cardiac, urogenital and skeletal defects
Valproic acid	Neural tube defects
Warfarin	Skeletal and CNS defects, Dandy–Walker syndrome

Testosterone and its derivatives, including progestogens derived from 19-nortestosterone, can masculinise the external genitals of a female fetus. Estrogens and progestins, on the other hand, are known to induce defective masculinisation of the external genitals of a male fetus. However, inadvertent continuation of a COC pill during the first month of gestation has not been found to be harmful to the fetus. Diethylstilbestrol administration during pregnancy has been associated with the development of congenital anomalies of external genitals in fetuses of both sexes, and with the development of vaginal adenosis and vaginal adenocarcinoma in girls whose mothers had received the drug.

The use of coumarin anticoagulants is associated with congenital malformations and high incidence of fetal loss from abortion, retroplacental and intracerebral fetal bleeding.

Consumption of even one drink (10 g of alcohol) per day is associated with fetal growth retardation and an increased incidence of abortion. Consumption of large quantities (40 g per day) is associated with 'fetal alcohol syndrome'.

Behavioural teratogenicity: Apart from the structural teratogenicity, drugs can also cause behavioural teratogenicity, i.e. abnormal behaviour in the newborn. So far, behavioural teratogenicity has been observed in human newborns of mothers who were exposed to methylmercury by eating contaminated fish and those who smoked during pregnancy. Animal studies indicate that the developing CNS is highly susceptible to the effects of psychoactive drugs. In humans, the brain development extends into early infancy and hence, the extended vulnerability of the brain in humans to the effects of such drugs.

Box 78.1 lists points to remember while prescribing drugs to women who are of the reproductive age and sexually active.

DRUG-PRESCRIBING DURING PREGNANCY

Box 78.2 summarises the precautions to be taken while prescribing drugs to a pregnant woman.

Nausea and vomiting of pregnancy can be treated without drugs in most women. Reassurance and high carbohydrate diet will help them. If required, an antihistaminic-antiemetic (cyclizine, meclizine, diphenhydramine, dimenhydrinate) may be prescribed. Metoclopramide is safe in the third trimester of pregnancy and may be prescribed in resistant cases.

Box 78.1 Points to Remember While Prescribing Drugs to a Woman of Reproductive Age

- Enquire whether she is pregnant or is likely to become pregnant in near future
- Ask her if she is having unprotected, sexual intercourse. If yes, tell her that if she has an unplanned pregnancy she runs the risk of exposing her fetus to a drug or drugs she may be taking, even before she knows that she is pregnant.
- Advise her to avoid conception for specified periods of time after completing therapy with certain drugs (see text)
- If a known or potentially teratogenic drug must be prescribed, she may be asked to sign a consent form that she agrees to use two effective methods of contraception
- Furthermore, inform her of the availability, efficacy and safety of long acting injectable contraceptives and postcoital contraceptives
- The patient should be encouraged to participate in decision making about whether the drug is necessary and which drug to use

Box 78.2 Precautions While Prescribing Drugs to a Pregnant Woman

- Treat minor ailments without drugs
- If a drug must be prescribed, it should be one which is known to be safe during pregnancy
- Prefer a drug which has been in use for long periods of time to a newly introduced drug as the safety of the latter for the fetus is not likely to be *known* completely
- Adjust the dose of the drug to the pregnant state; with most drugs, it is generally at the lower end of the therapeutic range. However, because of pharmacokinetic factors (increased body weight and more rapid clearance), the dose of certain drugs such as lithium, digoxin and phenytoin is likely to be higher than in the nonpregnant state in some women.
- Discourage the patient from self-administering OTC drugs
- Advise the patient that absolute safety of the fetus cannot be guaranteed even by not prescribing *any* drug to women between the ages of 15 and 45. Therefore, do not sacrifice the mother's interest for the sake of the fetus.

Heartburn is very common in pregnancy and is relieved by a small carbohydrate meal; by avoiding fatty food, smoking and alcohol; and by maintenance of upright posture. Consumption of aerated lemonade 2–3 times a day may also be helpful. Nonsystemic antacids and metoclopramide may be needed in some cases. Anticholinergics usually worsen the heartburn by relaxing the lower oesophageal sphincter.

Peptic ulcer should be treated with dietary modification and nonsystemic antacids. Sucralfate which is not absorbed, H_2-receptor blockers and bismuth subsalicylate are safe during pregnancy. Proton pump inhibitors (except omeprazole) and H_2-receptor blockers can be used to treat GERD.

Constipation generally responds to high fibre diet, plenty of liquids and a mild laxative such as milk of magnesia, docusate sodium, glycerine, mineral oil or bisacodyl.

Infectious diseases: Beta lactam antibiotics (penicillins and most of the cephalosporins) are safe during pregnancy. Ampicillin achieves very high concentrations in the fetal circulation and amniotic fluid and is very suitable for treatment of uterine infections during pregnancy. Erythromycin base is safe but erythromycin estolate should be avoided for fear of hepatotoxicity. Nitrofurantoin and methanamine mandelate are considered to be safe during pregnancy, so are nystatin and miconazole, but ketoconazole and 5-flucytosine should be avoided.

Aminoglycosides are ototoxic to the fetus and should be avoided; if one is needed to treat a serious systemic infection in the mother, gentamicin or tobramycin should be preferred. Tetracyclines damage the fetal teeth and bones and should be avoided. High doses of tetracycline intravenously have been associated with serious hepatotoxicity in the mother. **Chloramphenicol is absolutely contraindicated during pregnancy;** it can cause fetal bone marrow toxicity and 'grey baby syndrome' in the neonate. Cotrimoxazole should be avoided especially in the 1st trimester (because of its trimethoprim content) and the 3rd (because of its sulphonamide content). *Metronidazole is considered to be safe for the treatment of anaerobic infections in pregnancy.* Griseofulvin and nalidixic acid are embryotoxic and should be avoided. The use of sulphonamides at term can cause kernicterus in the neonate by displacing bilirubin from binding with albumin; aspirin, and water-soluble vitamin K analogues can also displace bilirubin from albumin.

Tuberculosis: Isoniazid and ethambutol are safe during pregnancy. Rifampicin should be avoided as far as possible but may be used if a third drug is required. Although using rifampicin, its hepatatoxicity should be kept in mind. *Streptomycin is ototoxic to the fetus and should never be used in pregnant women.*

Parasitic diseases: Amoebiasis is treated with the usual drugs: metronidazole, diodoquin and diloxanide. However, large dose, short-term therapy (e.g. single daily doses of 30 mg/kg with metronidazole) should be avoided.

Primaquine is contraindicated throughout the pregnancy. Pyrimethamine and mefloquine should be avoided in 1st trimester but appear to be safe in 2nd and 3rd trimester. Chronic suppressive use of chloroquine weekly and its use to treat acute attacks of malaria during pregnancy are safe. Quinine may be used to treat acute attacks of chloroquine-resistant falciparum malaria.

Piperazine, bephenium and pyrantel are safe for use during pregnancy. Most people consider mebendazole unsafe during pregnancy. Unless the parasite load is heavy, the treatment of intestinal parasitic infections is best postponed till after delivery.

Pain: Aspirin is not teratogenic but **high dose aspirin treatment** during the last 3 months is associated with increased gestation time, higher incidence of postmaturity and prolonged labour. Furthermore, it can also cause serious postpartum haemorrhage and bleeding in the neonate. NSAID induce premature closure of ductus arteriosus with pulmonary hypertension in the fetus and the newborn. Aspirin and NSAID are, therefore, better be avoided during pregnancy, especially close to term. Paracetamol in the usual doses is safe during pregnancy.

Glucocorticoids: They are administered in pregnancy for the treatment of various conditions such as rheumatoid arthritis, systemic lupus erythematosus, inflammatory bowel disease etc.. The evidence of any risk to the fetus like preterm birth or low birth weight, or to the mother like gestational diabetes or preeclampsia is insufficient. In fact, uncontrolled autoimmune activity is potentially more harmful to both mother and fetus. There may be a small risk of cleft lip with or without cleft palate.

Hypertension: Methyl-dopa is usually safe and preferred. Labetalol intravenously may be used when rapid reduction in BP is desired. However, beta blockers in the second and third trimesters can cause general retardation, whereas ACEI and ARB can cause fetal abnormalities of renal function and skull development. These drugs probably interfere with the maturation of specific organ systems (Chapter 30).

Heart disease: This is treated as in nonpregnant women. Digoxin clearance by the kidney increases during pregnancy. If the dosage remains unchanged by the end of pregnancy, the serum concentration will have fallen to about half the value before pregnancy.

At the therapeutic concentration, quinidine appears to be safe and the drug has only mild oxytocic activity. Quinidine is normally 80% bound to plasma protein. Changes in plasma protein concentration during pregnancy cause total plasma quinidine concentrations to fall and free concentration to be underestimated. After delivery, total concentration of quinidine increases by about half.

Vasopressor agents (noradrenaline, dopamine and dobutamine) all decrease the uterine blood flow and may stimulate uterine contractions. *Their use in pregnancy is justified only if the mother's survival is at stake.*

Anticoagulants: *Warfarin is best avoided in pregnant women, except those who have an artificial heart valve;* in these latter subjects, heparin does not give adequate anticoagulant cover. In other patients, subcutaneous heparin should be used if anticoagulation is required. One dose of heparin should be omitted when labour is imminent, so as to avoid postpartum haemorrhage.

Deep vein thrombosis may be treated with heparin. The use of streptokinase is associated with the risk of bleeding.

Allergic rhinitis: This may be treated either locally (with glucocorticoids or decongestants) or systemically with antihistaminics (diphenhydramine, dimenhydrinate and tripelenamine).

Cough: Diphenhydramine, codeine and dextromethorphan may be used safely to treat dry cough during pregnancy.

Pruritus: This may be treated locally with topical moisturising creams or lotions, e.g. calamine lotion, zinc oxide cream or ointment or glucocorticoids; or systemically with hydroxyzine, diphenhydramine or glucocorticoids.

Bronchial asthma is treated with inhaled beta adrenergic agonists, inhaled glucocorticoids, or with aminophylline. However, intravenously salbutamol used to delay labour is known to cause pulmonary oedema especially (a) in individuals with mitral stenosis and (b) when corticosteroids are administered concurrently to promote fetal lung maturation. The combination may result in fetal death. This therapy should not be used in hypertensive subjects. Furthermore, in diabetic subjects intravenously salbutamol can cause severe hyperglycaemia and ketoacidosis, resistant even to aggressive insulin therapy.

Headache may be treated with paracetamol, codeine and benzodiazepines. Aspirin and NSAID may be used in the first and second but avoided in the third trimester.

Migraine may be treated with analgesics, propranolol, dimenhydrinate and amitryptiline.

Diabetes mellitus should be treated with dietary restriction and insulin, if required; the use of oral hypoglycaemic agents is not recommended. In insulin dependent diabetics who become pregnant, the insulin requirement drops somewhat during the first trimester (owing to nausea and poor food intake), then rises progressively to 2–3 times the prepregnancy level up to 36 weeks, and then drops again up to term. After delivery, insulin requirement dives dramatically to prepregnancy level.

Thyrotoxicosis: Thioamides are the therapy of choice for thyrotoxicosis during pregnancy. The dose should be kept as low as possible. *Stable iodine and radioactive iodine are contraindicated* (Chapter 61).

Epilepsy: Adequate seizure control is important during pregnancy as convulsions themselves are harmful to the fetus. Phenobarbitone, phenytoin and carbamazepine may be used during pregnancy; as discussed earlier, their doses may have to be increased slightly in order to maintain seizure control. *All pregnant women on antiepileptic drugs should be prescribed folic acid 5 mg per day throughout pregnancy.* Vitamin K_1 should be administered to such patients routinely for 3 weeks before delivery and to their newborn babies at birth. *The use of valproic acid is contraindicated during pregnancy.*

Drugs acting on the CNS: Barbiturates, benzodiazepines and antidepressants have not been shown to have any significant teratogenic effects. Lithium has been reported to be teratogenic and also to be deleterious to the fetus in the last trimester.

The use of CNS depressants such as diazepam, antidepressants, phenothiazines and opioids at term and specially during labour, exposes the neonate to the risk of serious CNS depression.

Benzodiazepines are best avoided towards the end of pregnancy.

Phenothiazines, tricyclic antidepressants and SSRI (except paroxetine) can be continued during pregnancy in minimum possible doses. Antiparkinsonian drugs, e.g. benzhexol commonly prescribed together with phenothiazine, should not be used during the first trimester. *MAO inhibitors are contraindicated during pregnancy.* Furthermore, it is desirable to taper and omit tricyclic antidepressants in the last few weeks of pregnancy and to restart them after delivery.

BREASTFEEDING AND DRUGS

Nearly all agents received by the mother are likely to be found in her milk and could theoretically harm the infant. However, the data on excretion of drugs in milk and its possible harmful effects on the newborn are scanty.

Breastfeeding is important not only from nutritional point of view but it also supplies IgA and IgM immunoglobulins which afford protection against gastroenteritis. More and more women are now electing to breastfeed their babies. Although several drugs are known to increase prolactin secretion, no suitable drug is available at present, which could consistently augment the milk production in the human female. Thyrotropin-releasing hormone (TRH) and metoclopramide have been shown to increase milk production in some studies. However, it appears that determination on the mother's part is more important than prolactin-inducing drugs. Lactation will stop if the breast is not suckled. Suckling stimulates the release of prolactin and oxytocin.

Most of the lipid-soluble drugs get into breast milk, though not necessarily in concentrations that can adversely affect the infant. Milk is slightly more acidic (pH 7.0) than plasma and hence, weak bases that become more ionised with decrease in pH will have equal or higher concentrations in milk than in plasma. Nonelectrolytes like alcohol (ethanol) can readily enter into the milk independently of the pH. *Majority of the drugs get into the milk by passive diffusion* although active transport may occur in a few cases, e.g. iodide. Only the unbound drug in the plasma is able to diffuse into the milk. Highly protein bound drugs such as warfarin cannot be detected in breast milk. Even for a lipid-soluble, poorly protein bound, basic drug the milk to plasma ratio does not exceed four. Hence, drug toxicity based on the principal pharmacological action of the drug is considered unlikely in breast-fed infant. However, toxicity based on idiosyncrasy or a particular sensitivity of the infant to very low doses of a drug may occur.

The available data suggest that the net transfer of most drugs in breast milk is too small to produce significant adverse effect in the breast-fed infant. However, in view of such a possibility, drugs, particularly the newer ones, must not be prescribed during parturition unless essential. It must be remembered that the elimination rate for most drugs is slower in neonates than in the adults and this may lead to accumulation of the drug in neonates, particularly when it is taken for long courses by the mother.

Box 78.3 gives a list of the drugs not recommended during breastfeeding. Aspirin and paracetamol have been used extensively in the puerperium without

Box 78.3 Drugs to be Avoided/Not Recommended in Breastfeeding Women

- **Radionuclides and radiopharmaceuticals**
- **Antibacterials:** Sulphonamides, tetracyclines, chloramphenicol, nalidixic acid, isoniazid, fluoroquinolones, erythromycin estolate
- **Analgesics:** Indomethacin, phenylbutazone, aspirin (in large doses for long periods), opioids (regular use of large doses)
- **Psychoactive drugs:** Diazepam, lithium
- **Antihypertensives:** Reserpine, clonidine, atenolol
- **Antineoplastic drugs**
- **Miscellaneous:** Amantadine, lamotrigine, amiodarone, phenindione, cimetidine, anthraquinones, amiodarone, ephedrine, aminophylline, ergotamine, vitamin D (prolonged use of large doses), nitrofurantoin and sulfasalazine (in infants with G6PD deficiency)

apparent ill effects on the infant. Heparin and warfarin are not detected in the milk. There is no contraindication to thyroxine treatment for hypothyroidism during breastfeeding. But, breastfeeding should be discouraged in women taking antithyroid drugs. *Radioiodine is absolutely contraindicated during breastfeeding.* Since most of the antibiotics pass into breast milk, it may be advisable to avoid drugs like chloramphenicol, tetracycline and sulphonamides in breastfeeding women. *Penicillins, erythromycin, lincomycin, quinine and chloroquine appear to be safe for the treatment of nursing mothers.* Aminoglycoside antibiotics, though they appear in breast milk, are not considered dangerous as they are not absorbed from the gut. Metronidazole is considered quite safe during breastfeeding but may make the milk taste bitter. Beta-blockers, thiazide diuretics, captopril and digoxin levels achieved in breast milk are probably too low to have any significant effect on the breast-fed infants. All centrally acting drugs, being lipid soluble, have a high Vd. Hence, the total amount of drug available for concentration in the milk is likely to be small. *Opiate analgesics, phenothiazines, chloral hydrate and antiepileptics may, therefore, be used safely by the mothers, if necessary.* However, lithium has a high milk to plasma ratio and the dose available to breast-fed infant is likely to be similar to that of the mother; it should be avoided during breastfeeding. Regular use of opioids in high doses by the mother may lead to dependence and withdrawal in the neonate. Ergotamine may lead to ergotism and chloroquine in the treatment of rheumatoid arthritis may cause retinal damage in the newborn infant. Amiodarone is present in the milk in significant quantities; it is best avoided because of the possible effects of the released iodine on the neonatal thyroid. The neonate has been reported to become irritable when the breastfeeding mother is taking ephedrine, or 200 mg or more of aminophylline every 6 h; slow release preparations of aminophylline are probably safe. High levels in breast milk have been reported for the H_2 blocker, cimetidine. *Cytotoxic drugs, in general, are absolutely contraindicated in mothers who are breastfeeding.*

It should be noted that certain chemicals like DDT, methyl mercury, acquired environmentally, could appear in milk and cause chronic toxicity in breast-fed babies. *Finally, if a drug is used therapeutically in the neonatal period, one may use it safely in breastfeeding women.*

APPENDIX

Guide to Further Reading

During revision for this edition, we have referred to many reviews and seminars published in journals: The Lancet, New England Journal of Medicine, Medical Letter, BMJ, Clinical Pharmacology and Therapeutics, Drugs, American Family Physician, Australian Prescriber and so on in addition to various books on pharmacology and therapeutics. The National and International Guidelines related to treatment of various diseases published at the web site of the Government agencies or professional societies have been referred to.

A selected list for further referencing and reading is given below. This, obviously, does not detract from the extensive and high-quality references available in the literature on various topics.

Brown M.J. Bennet P.N. Clinical Pharmacology, 12th ed., 2018, New York, UK: Churchill Livingstone, Elsevier.

Brunton L.L., Knollmann B.C. (Ed): Goodman & Gilman's The Pharmacological Basis of Therapeutics. 14th ed., 2023, New York: McGraw-Hill.

Jameson J. L. , Fauci A. S. , Kasper D.L., Hauser S.L., Longo D.L., Loscalzo J. (Ed): Harrison's Manual of Medicine, 20th ed. 2020, New York: McGraw-Hill Education

Guyton A.C., Hall J.E. Textbook of Medical Physiology. 14th ed., 2020, Philadelphia: Elsevier Inc.

Katzung B. G., Vanderah T.W. (Ed): Basic and Clinical Pharmacology; 15e ed., 2021, McGraw Hill.

Meyers M.A. Happy Accidents, 1st ed., 2007, New York: Arcade Publishing.

Ritter J.M., Flower R., Henderson G., Loke Y.K., MacEwan D., Rang H.P.: Rang and Dale's Pharmacology, 9th ed., 2020, Edinburgh: Elsevier Health Sciences.

Seshadri, K.G., Kumar, P. K. M., Sridhar, G.R., Sosale, A (Ed): Clinician's Handbook of Diabetes, 2nd ed., 2015, Gurgaon: Macmillan Medical Communications.

LIST OF NATIONAL HEALTH PROGRAMMES

In addition, we urge the readers to visit the websites that display major National health programmes of India. A list of some such programmes with website links and QR codes is given below.

Programmes related to non-communicable diseases

- National Health Mission
  https://nhm.gov.in/

- National Programme for Prevention and Control of Cancer, Diabetes, Cardiovascular Diseases and Stroke (NPCDCS)
  https://main.mohfw.gov.in/Major-Programmes/non-communicable-diseases-injury-trauma/Non-Communicable-Disease-II/National-Programme-for-Prevention-and-Control-of-Cancer-Diabetes-Cardiovascular-diseases-and-Stroke-NPCDCS

- National Program for Control of Blindness and Visual Impairment
https://npcbvi.mohfw.gov.in/Home

- National Mental Health Programme
https://nhm.gov.in/index1.php?lang=1&level=2&sublinkid=1043&lid=359

- National Iodine Deficiency Disorders Control Programme
https://nhm.gov.in/index1.php?lang=1&level=3&sublinkid=1054&lid=230

- National Programme for prevention and control of Fluorosis
https://nhm.gov.in/index1.php?lang=1&level=3&sublinkid=1055&lid=611

- Anaemia Mukt Bharat
https://anemiamuktbharat.info/

Programmes related to communicable diseases

- National Vector Borne Diseases Control Programme (NVBDCP)
https://ncvbdc.mohfw.gov.in/

- National Tuberculosis Elimination Programme (NTEP)
https://tbcindia.gov.in

- National Leprosy Eradication Programme (NLEP)
https://dghs.gov.in/content/1349_3_National-LeprosyEradicationProgramme.aspx

- National Viral Hepatitis Control Programme (NVHCP)
https://nvhcp.mohfw.gov.in/

- National AIDS Control Organization (NACO)
https://naco.gov.in/

Illustration Credits

IMAGES ON THE COVER

1. Cover Background image: Abstract Cells and DNA Strand.
2. Photo: Kjpargeter/Freepik.
3. Icons: The Noun Project.

IMAGES ON SECTION PAGES

Section I:	From Wikipedia Commons. Available at https://commons.wikimedia.org/wiki/File:Digitalis_purpurea_002.JPG; Retrieved 24 August 2017.
Section II:	From Satoskar R.S., et al. *Pharmacology and Pharmacokinetics*, 24th ed., Elsevier/Popular Prakashan.
Section III:	From Wikipedia. Available at https://en.wikipedia.org/wiki/Coca; Retrieved 24 August 2017.
Section IV:	From *Advanced Medical Life Support: An Assessment-Based Approach*, 2011, Mosby/JEMS.
Section V:	From Wikipedia. Available at https://en.wikipedia.org/wiki/Ginkgo_biloba; Retrieved 24 August 2017.
Section VI:	From Wikipedia. Available at https://en.wikipedia.org/wiki/Justicia_adhatoda; Retrieved 24 August 2017.
Section VII:	From The Jammu and Kashmir Medicinal Plants Introduction Centre 'Ginkgo House', Pampore, J&K.
Section VIII:	From Grodner M., Long Roth S., Walkingshaw B. *Nutritional Foundations and Clinical Applications: A Nursing Approach*, 5th ed., 2011, Mosby (Elsevier).
Section IX:	From *Siegfried Bäumler. Heilpflanzen Praxis heute: Band 1 Arzneipflanzenporträts*, 2012, Urban & Fischer in Elsevier (Verlag).
Section X:	From Wikipedia. Available at https://en.wikipedia.org/wiki/Plantago_ovata#/media/File:Plantago_ovata_form.jpg; Retrieved 24 August 2017.
Section XI:	From Wikipedia. Available at https://en.wikipedia.org/wiki/Willow#/media/File:Salix_alba_Morton.jpg; Retrieved 24 August 2017.
Section XII:	From Bronwen B., Kathleen K. *Pharmacology for Health Professionals*, 3rd ed., 2011, Australia: Mosby (Elsevier).
Section XIII:	From Morrison P. *Natural Standard Herbal Pharmacotherapy: An Evidence-Based Approach*, 2009, Mosby (Elsevier).
Section XIV:	From Bäumler S. *Heilpflanzen Praxis heute: Band 1 Arzneipflanzenporträts*, 2012, Urban & Fischer in Elsevier (Verlag).
Section XV:	From Bronwen B., Kathleen K. *Pharmacology for Health Professionals*, 3rd ed., 2011, Australia: Mosby (Elsevier).

Illustration Credits

IMAGES ON THE COVER

Index

B

E

H

M

N

O

Q

U

V

W

Case Based MCQs

SECTION 1. GENERAL PHARMACOLOGY

CASE 1

A drug is being developed for ischaemic heart disease to be administered if the patient develops acute chest pain and also for its prevention. During the clinical development studies, it was found to have following characteristics:

- Oral bioavailability 25%; intersubject variability :10-90%
- Terminal half-life after oral dosing is 8 h

1.1 The time to reach steady state for this drug (in hours) will be:
- A. 8
- B. 16–20
- C. 32–40
- D. 56–60

1.2 The data on bioavailability indicates that if the drug is to be used for acute chest pain, then there is a need for:
- A. development of sublingual formulation
- B. use of high dose of the drug
- C. therapeutic drug monitoring
- D. detailed study of its metabolism

1.3 The plasma-concentration curve of this new drug will be influenced by all of the following EXCEPT:
- A. absorption
- B. distribution
- C. receptor affinity
- D. elimination

CASE 2

A 65-year-old patient with impaired renal function is prescribed a drug that undergoes elimination by the kidneys.

2.1 How will the pharmacokinetics of the drug get altered in this patient?
- A. Increased absorption
- B. Prolonged half-life
- C. Enhanced metabolism
- D. Decreased volume of distribution

CASE 3

A young adult is prescribed a drug (A) with a narrow therapeutic index. It also exhibits high protein-binding.

3.1 If this patient is administered another drug (B) with high protein binding, then the treating physician must be vigilant as there is a possibility of:

A. increased risk of toxic effects of A
B. lowering of efficacy of A
C. rapid elimination of A
D. increased risk of toxic effects of B

CASE 4

A patient is prescribed a drug that exhibits zero-order kinetics.

4.1 What does this imply about the relationship between drug concentration and elimination? The drug:

A. is eliminated at a constant amount regardless of concentration
B. is eliminated at a rate proportional to its concentration
C. elimination is zero at the highest drug concentration
D. concentration and elimination are not related

4.2 How will changes in the drug dose impact the drug's plasma concentration?

A. Linear increase in plasma concentration
B. Nonlinear increase in plasma concentration
C. No change in plasma concentration
D. Inverse relationship with plasma concentration

CASE 5

A 45-year-old patient is prescribed a new drug. Its pharmacokinetic profile indicates a high hepatic elimination. The patient has a history of liver disease.

5.1 Predict how the impaired liver function can affect the drug's overall bioavailability and elimination.

A. Increased bioavailability and prolonged half-life
B. Decreased bioavailability and prolonged half-life
C. Decreased bioavailability and shortened half-life
D. Unchanged bioavailability and shortened half-life

CASE 6

A 30-year-old patient is prescribed a drug with significantly high protein binding. The patient has a genetic polymorphism associated with slower drug metabolism.

6.1 How will the drug's pharmacokinetics be impacted?

A. Decreased bioavailability
B. Increased risk of toxicity
C. Faster elimination
D. Unchanged distribution

CASE 7

A 55-year-old patient with chronic kidney disease is prescribed a medication that primarily follows renal elimination. The patient is also taking a medication that inhibits a renal transporter responsible for drug excretion.

7.1 **How will the pharmacokinetics of the prescribed drug be potentially influenced?**
A. Increased glomerular filtration
B. Increased protein binding
C. Decreased absorption
D. Prolonged half-life

CASE 8

A patient is prescribed Drug A to manage hypertension. The dose administered is 25 mg once a day on an empty stomach.

8.1 **Which of the following best describes the pharmacodynamics of Drug A?**
A. Food interferes with its absorption
B. Antagonist activity at beta receptors
C. Dose requirement for the patient
D. Frequency of Drug A administration

CASE 9

A patient experiences a severe allergic reaction and is administered an epinephrine injection.

9.1 **The therapeutic effect of epinephrine is mainly due to its:**
A. physiological antagonism
B. chemical antagonism
C. physical antagonism
D. competitive antagonism

CASE 10

A patient is prescribed a medication with a narrow therapeutic window.

10.1 **Which statement accurately reflects the concept of a narrow therapeutic window?**
A. The dose to produce therapeutic effect is small requiring multiple dosing
B. A wide range of doses results in desirable therapeutic effects
C. The drug's effects are highly variable among individuals
D. The difference between the minimum effective and minimum toxic dose is small

CASE 11

A patient is prescribed a drug that is more potent than morphine but acts as a partial agonist of morphine at Mu receptors.

11.1 **What can be expected regarding the pharmacological effects of this partial agonist? It:**
A. has intrinsic activity similar to morphine
B. shows maximal response similar to morphine
C. can display both, agonistic and antagonistic effects
D. potentiates effects of morphine if administered concurrently

CASE 12

A 40-year-old patient is prescribed an analgesic, codeine for postoperative pain relief. The patient complains that there is no pain relief.

12.1 What could be the possible reason?
- A. There is extensive metabolism of codeine
- B. Patient may be poor metaboliser
- C. Patient may have increased expression of metabolising enzymes
- D. Metabolising enzymes may be inhibited

12.2 The mixed function oxidase system responsible for above situation is:
- A. CYP3A4
- B. CYP2C19
- C. CYP2D6
- D. CYP1A2

CASE 13

A 30-year-old patient with epilepsy is on long-term treatment with phenytoin. The patient is prescribed an antibiotic, ciprofloxacin, for a urinary tract infection. The patient presents with symptoms of phenytoin toxicity.

13.1 What is the reason for toxicity?
- A. Ciprofloxacin inhibits the metabolism of phenytoin
- B. Additive adverse effects of Ciprofloxacin potentiating phenytoin toxicity
- C. Worsening of UTI prevents Phenytoin elimination
- D. Ciprofloxacin displays Phenytoin from protein binding site

CASE 14

A 35-year old patient with bipolar disorder is prescribed lithium carbonate for mood stabilization. After several weeks of treatment, the patient reports increased tremors, nausea, and confusion.

14.1 What is the most appropriate action while managing this patient?
- A. Increase the lithium dose
- B. Discontinue lithium therapy
- C. Order a serum lithium level
- D. Add an antipsychotic medication

CASE 15

A pharmaceutical company is conducting a Phase 3 clinical trial to evaluate the efficacy and safety of a new antihypertensive drug. The trial involves a large number of participants, randomized into treatment and control groups.

15.1 What is the primary objective of this clinical trial?
- A. Investigate the mechanism of action of the new drug
- B. Assess the drug's safety profile in a controlled setting
- C. Determine the optimal dosage of the new drug
- D. Evaluate the efficacy of the new drug compared to standard treatment

CASE 16

A company plans a Phase 1 clinical trial to assess the safety and pharmacokinetics of a new anticancer drug.

16.1 What is the key objective of this Phase 1 trial and in which participants should the trial be conducted?

A. Determining the long-term safety of the new anticancer drug in normal volunteers
B. Evaluating the drug's pharmacokinetics in patients suffering from various cancers
C. Investigating potential drug interactions with other medications in normal volunteers
D. Establishing the safety and tolerability in cancer patients

CASE 17

A rural health clinic is planning to establish an essential medicines list for maternal and child health.

17.1 Which factor should be a priority when selecting medicines for this specific list?

A. Availability of medicines in paediatric formulations
B. Selection of generic medicines
C. Incorporating medicines that meet health needs
D. Focusing on medications for communicable diseases

CASE 18

A humanitarian aid organization is establishing a mobile clinic to provide medical care in disaster-stricken areas.

18.1 When selecting essential drugs for the mobile clinic, what factor should be a priority?

A. Long shelf life of medicines
B. Wide range of specialty medicines
C. Cost-effective medicines
D. Ease of transportation and stability

SECTION 2. DRUGS ACTING ON THE CENTRAL NERVOUS SYSTEM

CASE 1

A 8-year-old boy PS, suffering from grand mal epilepsy since the past 1 year is controlled on Tablet Carbamazepine 100 mg three times a day. One morning, PS's mother administers the tablet to PS before he leaves for school. While playing with his friends during the lunch break, PS develops convulsions that last for one minute and he loses consciousness. Within the next 2 minutes, he develops another convulsion without recovery. PS is immediately taken to the school clinic. The doctor at the clinic diagnoses PS to be suffering from generalized convulsive status epilepticus.

1.1 Which drug should be administered to PS immediately to stop the convulsions?

A. Carbamazepine orally
B. Midazolam intranasally
C. Propofol intravenously
D. Glucose intravenously

CASE 2

A 35-year-old man, Mr. JS, known case of grand mal epilepsy is stabilized on phenytoin therapy (200 mg tablet thrice daily) since the past two years. One day he visits his neurologist along with his wife who tells the doctor that that he is lethargic, confused, and dizzy. On examination, the neurologist finds that JS has nystagmus and enquires if JS had taken any concomitant medication/s. JS tells him that he was taking Tab. Cotrimoxazole twice daily for 5 days as prescribed by his general practitioner for fever and cough with expectoration.

2.1 What will be the first action taken by the treating neurologist?

A. Refer JS to an ophthalmologist
B. Refer for phenytoin levels estimation
C. Change the antiepileptic drug to sodium valproate
D. Refer for estimation of folic acid levels

2.2 JS had an adverse drug reaction because cotrimoxazole:

A. increases phenytoin levels by preventing its metabolism
B. being a folate antagonist, decreases folic acid levels
C. causes dizziness and visual adverse effects of its own
D. potentiates the adverse effects of phenytoin

CASE 3

Miss LN, an 18-year-old girl presents with complaints of severe dysmenorrhea. She informs the doctor that initially she usually gets mild to moderate pain during her menstrual cycle, but since the last month the pain is unbearable and she is unable to do her daily activities. The doctor reassures her and informs her that he will prescribe a drug to relieve dysmenorrhea.

3.1 Which of the following drugs should be prescribed?

A. Tramadol
B. Chlorzoxazone
C. Dextroprophoxyphene
D. Mefenamic acid

CASE 4

Ms. XYZ, a 35-year-old woman presents to the OPD with stabbing unilateral right sided facial pain triggered by chewing or touching the affected area on the face. The pain shoots from the right corner of the mouth to the angle of the right jaw. The pain is severe giving a sensation of electric shocks followed by a burning ache which lasts for 1-2 minutes. She gets about 5-6 attacks per day but the attacks do not occur during sleep.

4.1 What medication will you advise her for the pain?

A. Nimesulide
B. Carbamazepine
C. Morphine
D. Glyceryl trinitrate

4.2 Which other drug may also be prescribed for the above condition?

A. Tizanidine
B. Verapamil
C. Lamotrigine
D. Dantrolene

CASE 5

Mr. SR, a 70-year-old man with metastatic lung cancer presents to the emergency medical services with complaints of severe pain in the chest and mid-thoracic spinal region. He tells the physician that he has been prescribed fentanyl transdermal patch, which he takes off and on for relief of his pain. Recently, the pain has been progressively increasing since the last two months and now he is experiencing severe pain which is not getting relieved by the prescribed analgesic. The physician prescribes morphine for his pain relief.

5.1 Which of the following side effects of morphine needs to be treated prophylactically?

A. Sedation
B. Pupillary constriction
C. Vomiting
D. Dependence

CASE 6

Mr. MN aged 34 years is brought to the clinic by his wife with complaints of heroin addiction since the past 4 years. The wife informs the physician that MN spends a lot of time obtaining the drug and has lost his job due to absenteeism. He often steals money from the house to pay for the illegal drugs. He has tried to quit taking the drug on his own in the last 2 years but he relapses. MN tells the doctor that he now wishes to undergo a medically supervised withdrawal from the drug.

6.1 Which of the following opioids will MN be switched on to during the detoxification procedure?

A. Methadone
B. Pethidine
C. Nalbuphine
D. Levorphanol

CASE 7

A 21-year-old male patient, TS is on Triflupromazine therapy for schizophrenia is brought to the emergency department by his parents. He is having prolonged contracture of the facial muscles. While being examined, he experiences opisthotonus. The patient is clinically diagnosed as having acute dystonia.

7.1 Which of the following drug would be most beneficial in reducing these symptoms?

A. Diazepam
B. Bromocriptine
C. Lithium
D. Benztropine

TS is referred back to his treating psychiatrist from the emergency department.

7.2 The most preferred approach for TS will be to:

A. continue Triflupromazine on low dose
B. switch over to Thioridazine
C. switch over to Olanzepine
D. not change the therapy and counsel the patient about adverse effects

CASE 8

VT, a 35-year-old adult male, accompanied by his mother presented to the psychiatric OPD. He complained of hearing voices for the past 8 months and loss of appetite. His mother complained to the doctor that VT roams around the city aimlessly and was sometimes physically abusive to her and his sister. VT further added that he felt unsafe and thought that people wanted to harm him. There was no history of alcohol intake or any other substance abuse. The treating psychiatrist diagnoses VT to have schizophrenia.

8.1 What is the preferred next line of action?

A. Prescribe clozapine
B. Initiate cognitive behaviour therapy
C. Prescribe risperidone
D. Counsel VT

The psychiatrist decides to start on antipsychotic agent and advices to double the dose after 3 days if no adverse effects are seen. VT starts the medication and stops it after 5 days. After a week VT is brought by the relatives to the emergency department as he is now violent, aggressive and has hit her sister who is profusely bleeding.

8.2 To calm VT immediately, the doctor at emergency department must administer:

A. IM haloperidol
B. ECT
C. Oral clozapine
D. IM risperidone

CASE 9

SM, a 40- year-old married lady, working as executive officer in a reputed company visits her family physician along with her husband. She states that she feels lethargic and is disinterested in work since last 2 months. She is finding it difficult to maintain her responsibilities at workplace and home. She also complains of loss of appetite, sleeplessness and feelings of guilt. Her husband adds that there are episodes of uncontrollable crying by SM at home. SM is neither alcoholic nor takes any recreational drugs.

9.1 The family physician diagnoses SM to have depression and decides to prescribe:

A. diazepam
B. fluoxetine
C. tranylcypromine
D. risperidone

SM is started on appropriate antidepressant therapy. Her husband visits the family physician after 1 week saying these medicines are not effective as SM still has crying episodes.

9.2 The most appropriate approach to be followed by the family physician is to:

A. increase the dose of the antidepressant drug
B. change the antidepressant drug
C. counsel that medication effect will start after 2 weeks
D. reconsider the diagnosis

CASE 10

A 45-year-old patient with depression is prescribed a selective serotonin reuptake inhibitor (SSRI). The patient also regularly takes a migraine medication, sumatriptan.

10.1 What potential adverse effect should be monitored in this case?

A. Serotonin syndrome
B. Hypertension
C. Hypoglycemia
D. Gastrointestinal bleeding

10.2 Which type of drug-drug interaction is responsible for this adverse effect?

A. Pharmacokinetic
B. Pharmaceutical
C. Pharmacodynamic
D. Pharmacogenomic

CASE 11

Mr. BK, a 62-year-old man visits the clinic with his son with complaints of tremors at rest, difficulty in walking and rigidity which have slowly worsened since the past 1 year. His wife informs the family physician his father's facial expressions have also changed. After a detailed clinical evaluation, the physician diagnoses that BK is suffering from Parkinson's Disease. He refers BK to a neurologist who prescribes him Tab. Levodopa (100mg) with carbidopa (25 mg). After a week BK presents to family physician with severe nausea since the past 3 days and 2 episodes of vomiting since today morning.

11.1 What is the immediate action the family physician must do?

A. Stop the offending drug levodopa+ carbidopa
B. Counsel to take levodopa on empty stomach
C. Prescribe domperidone 10 mg as antiemetic
D. Stop levodopa and start carbidopa alone three times a day

After 6 months, BK's son visits the neurologist along with his father. He states that his father complains entire day that insects are crawling over his body and all insects are invading him. The neurologist diagnoses these as hallucinations due to levodopa therapy.

11.2 What will be the preferred course of action for BC?

A. Decrease the dose of levodopa
B. Prescribe haloperidol
C. Prescribe oral pimavanserin
D. Counsel patient to tolerate these adverse effects

While on therapy for 3 years, it is noticed that before the next dose is due, there is worsening of BC's tremors, rigidity and bradykinesia. The symptoms improve 15 – 20 minutes after taking the scheduled dose of levodopa. However, there is frequent involuntary twitching of the hands.

11.3 Which effects of levodopa BC is experiencing now?

A. Wear off phenomenon
B. On-off phenomenon
C. Muscular dystrophy
D. Psychosis

SECTION 3. LOCAL ANAESTHETICS

CASE 1

Mr. RS, a 29-year-old male factory worker, gets a deep laceration on his hand while working and is brought to the emergency medical services of a nearby hospital. The attending doctor examines the wound and informs Mr. RS that the wound will require suturing under local infiltration anaesthesia. On hearing this, Mr. RS worriedly tells the doctor that while undergoing a dental procedure a year back, the dentist had applied benzocaine gel to his gums to give local anaesthesia, after which he had developed an allergic reaction.

1.1 **Which of the following local anesthetics should the doctor not use for Mr. RS?**
A. Lignocaine
B. Tetracaine
C. Bupivacaine
D. Ropivacaine

CASE 2

Mrs. AM, a 42-year-old woman suffering from inguinal hernia is taken up for surgery. The anaesthetist gives spinal anaesthesia before the surgery. While monitoring Mrs. AM's BP, the anaesthetist notes that her systolic blood pressure is 75 mm of Hg. He immediately suspects spinal hypotension and decides to treat it.

2.1 **Which of the following drugs should the anaesthetist administer to reverse the hypotension?**
A. Ergotamine
B. Methoxamine
C. Dopamine
D. Atropine

SECTION 4. AUTONOMIC NERVOUS SYSTEM

CASE 1

A 26-year-old man, NK is brought to the emergency department following ingestion of some berries. He is found to have an elevated temperature, flushing, dilated pupils, dry mouth, tachycardia, loss of balance, urinary retention, and delirium.

1.1 **Which one of the following agents present in the berries is most likely to cause these findings?**
A. Nicotine
B. Atropine
C. Strychnine
D. Ephedrine

1.2 **Which drug would you give as an antidote to NK?**
A. Diazepam
B. Labetalol
C. Phenobarbitone
D. Physostigmine

CASE 2

Mrs. PS, a 78-year-old elderly woman presents with complaints of sudden urinary urgency with leakage of urine especially when she coughs or sneezes. She says that she feels embarrassed by this condition and has started to wear diapers. She stays alone, is independent, and has no other complaints other than hypertension for which she is taking enalapril. She tells the doctor that she does pelvic floor exercises and bladder training but this hasn't helped her condition and requests the physician to prescribe medication.

2.1 **Which of the following drugs should the physician prescribe?**
A. Bethanecol
B. Flavoxate
C. Tamsulosin
D. Oxyphenonium

CASE 3

Mr. DM, a 26-year-old man comes with complaints of nasal stuffiness and a runny nose since last three days. He informs the doctor that he also has a mild fever for which he is taking paracetamol tablets as and when needed. However, he is having difficulty in breathing and tells the doctor to prescribe a medicine for the nasal congestion. Mr. DM does not suffer from any other disease.

3.1 Which of the following is a preferred medication to relieve Mr. DM's symptoms?
- A. Pseudoephedrine
- B. Midodrine
- C. Xylometazoline
- D. Isoetharine

CASE 4

Mr. SN, a 72-year-old man complains of increase in frequency of urine, difficulty in passing urine even after straining, inability to empty the bladder completely and dribbling at the end of urination. A digital rectal examination reveals an enlarged prostate. The physician decides to prescribe an alpha blocker.

4.1 Which of the following alpha blockers is preferred for Mr. SN?
- A. Doxazosin
- B. Prazosin
- C. Tamsulosin
- D. Terazosin

CASE 5

Mr. SM, a 35-year-old man, meets with an accident and is brought to emergency medical services. After a proper history, clinical examination, and investigations, the attending surgeon realises that the patient has an abdominal trauma and he informs the patient and his relatives that Mr. SM will have to be taken up for immediate surgical intervention. Mr. SM is prepared for surgery and the anaesthetist on call decides to administer a skeletal muscle relaxant.

5.1 Which of the following skeletal muscle relaxants will be appropriate in this situation?
- A. Vecuronium
- B. Pancuronium
- C. Rocuronium
- D. Doxacurium

CASE 6

Mrs. AL, a 58-year-old woman underwent a cholecystectomy surgery under general anesthesia. The attending anaesthetist used mivacurium as the skeletal muscle relaxant. However, after the surgery, Mrs. AL's postoperative recovery was prolonged.

6.1 What could be the reason for Mrs. AL's prolonged recovery?
- A. Decreased levels of plasma cholinesterase
- B. Decreased renal excretion of mivacurium
- C. Increased binding of mivacurium to the nicotinic receptor
- D. Longer action of the active metabolite

SECTION 5. OTHER BIOGENIC AMINES AND POLYPEPTIDES

CASE 1

Mrs CY, aged 25 years visits the doctor with complaints of severe unilateral headaches which are accompanied by nausea and, vomiting. She mentions that she is unable to tolerate light and sound during this period. She has also noticed that she gets some visual disturbances before the headache. The headaches continue for 2-3 days and during this period though the intensity decreases after rest, there is no pain-free interval. She also informs that these episodes of headache occur once or twice a month, either before menstruation or if she does not eat on time and stays hungry. She has been suffering from these headaches for the past 3 years but recently their frequency and severity have increased. Earlier her headaches would get relieved with a single dose of 500 mg paracetamol orally but nowadays it is not effective. She is worried about taking other drugs as she fears that she may get habituated to their use.

1.1 The physician suspects that this episodic unilateral headache is a migraine attack. What should he advise?

A. Counsel and prescribe paracetamol 1000 mg if the pain becomes intolerable
B. Counsel her to take meals on time and prescribe oral contraceptive pills
C. Counsel and prescribe paracetamol 1000 mg at the onset of headache and repeat 4-6 hourly for a maximum of 4 doses
D. Counsel and prescribe paracetamol 500 mg every 6 hourly till the headache is relieved

Mrs CY comes to the OPD after 3 months and mentions that she did not find much change even after taking the prescribed medicine. During this period she got 5 attacks but the medicine did not work during 3 headaches and had less effect in the other two.

1.2 What the physician should do?

A. Change over to NSAID like aspirin
B. Change over to sumatriptan
C. Administer combination of triptan with NSAID
D. Use selective CGRP antagonist such as ubrogepant

1.3 Mrs CY also needs advice for contraception. Which contraceptive is preferable for her?

A. Combined estrogen-progesterone pills
B. Vaginal contraceptive gel
C. Copper containing IUCD
D. Any post-coital contraceptive

CASE 2

A 45-year-old patient with depression is prescribed a selective serotonin reuptake inhibitor (SSRI). The patient also regularly takes a migraine medication, sumatriptan.

2.1 What potential adverse effect should be monitored in this case?

A. Serotonin syndrome
B. Hypertension
C. Hypoglycemia
D. Gastrointestinal bleeding

2.2 Which type of drug-drug interaction is responsible for this adverse effect?

A. Pharmacokinetic
B. Pharmaceutical
C. Pharmacodynamic
D. Pharmacogenomic

CASE 3

A patient with diabetes was admitted for pneumonia and was prescribed amoxicillin/clavulanic acid to be given as 1 gm 8 hourly as IV infusion in 0.9% sodium chloride. The resident started the drip and within 15 min the caretaker came rushing to inform the resident that the patient is having difficulty in breathing and making some noise while breathing, his voice is changed, and is sweating profusely.

3.1 What immediate action must be executed by the resident?

A. Stop the infusion
B. Administer adrenaline
C. Start oxygen
D. Do venous canulation for drug administration

The event is reported as anaphylaxis. After the first dose of adrenaline, the resident noticed that the BP is still low and urticarial patches persist.

3.2 Which one of the following is not recommended as the drug to be administered at this stage?

A. IV fluids
B. Cetrizine
C. Hydrocortisone hemisuccinate
D. Adrenaline

3.3 This patient is monitored for at least 12 hrs after the treatment of initial attack because:

A. the patient gets exhausted after the treatment of this life-threatening condition
B. adverse reactions to administered drugs may appear and need to be treated
C. his primary disease (pneumonia) may worsen due to bronchospasm
D. anaphylaxis symptoms may recur after resolution of earlier response

CASE 4

Miss PD, a rape victim case, has been diagnosed to be pregnant and the foetus is of 7 weeks. She does not wish to go ahead with the pregnancy. A therapeutic abortion is planned.

4.1 Which of the following prostaglandin can be used?

A. Alprostadil
B. Misoprostol
C. Latanoprost
D. Epoprostenol

4.2 Which of the following adverse effects are common with prostaglandins?

A. Nausea, vomiting and diarrhoea
B. Growth of eyelashes and brown pigmentation of iris
C. Cough and insomnia
D. Bronchoconstriction and apnoea

4.3 From the group of prostaglandin analogues given in the parenthesis, select the most preferred prostaglandin for the treatment of each of the following conditions and write in the space provided.

(Prostaglandin analogues: A. Alprostadil, B. Misoprostol, C. Latanoprost, D. Epoprostenol)

A. Pulmonary artery hypertension

B. Glaucoma

C. NSAID induced gastric ulcer

D. To maintain patency of ductus arteriosus

SECTION 6. DRUGS USED IN RESPIRATORY DISORDERS

CASE 1

Ms. NM, a 24-year-old woman visits her general practitioner with complaints of 8 attacks of wheezing and breathlessness in the last 2 weeks. She informs the attending physician that earlier she used to get these symptoms only on exposure to smoke. But since the past 6 months her symptoms have gradually increased. She has also started getting cough at night and this has affected her sleep. On examination, she is afebrile with a respiratory rate of 20/min, pulse rate is 85/min. On auscultation, the chest is clear. The physician advises her to undergo lung function tests which reveal variable expiratory airflow limitation; her FEV_1:FVC is less than predicted on spirometry, her peak expiratory flow is reduced and she shows positive bronchodilator responsiveness (increased FEV_1 after salbutamol).

1.1 Which one of the following is the preferred inhalation therapy for Ms. NM?

A. Low dose ICS-formoterol as-needed with Montelukast

B. Medium dose ICS plus as needed SABA and ipratropium bromide

C. Medium dose ICS-formoterol plus as needed ICS-SABA

D. Low dose ICS-formoterol for maintenance and reliever therapy

CASE 2

Mr. SP, a 68-year-old man and a chronic smoker, presents with complaints of fever, bodyache, weakness, moderate dyspnoea and cough with mucopurulent sputum production since the last 5 days. He informs the doctor that he is taking paracetamol for the fever and bodyache but he isn't feeling better. History taking reveals that Mr. SP is suffering from occasional dyspnoea and cough with sputum production for the last 8-9 years and he had 2 such exacerbations in the last 6 months. He shows the doctor the inhaler prescribed by his general practitioner a few years back which he takes whenever he feels breathless. The doctor notes that it is a salbutamol inhaler. He also informs the doctor that he suffers from high blood pressure for which he is taking treatment. On auscultation, he is found to have decreased air entry and bilateral rhonchi. His BP is 126/82 mm of Hg and body temperature is 101^0F. Spirometry reveals that his airflow limitation is only partially reversible with bronchodilator and that his post-bronchodilator $FEV_1/FVC < 0.7$. His blood eosinophils are 200 cells/μL.

2.1 Which of the following treatments should be given to Mr. SP along with azithromycin?

A. As needed SABA plus LABA

B. LABA plus ICS

C. LAMA plus LABA

D. LAMA plus LABA plus ICS

SECTION 7. CARDIOVASCULAR DRUGS

CASE 1

A patient on therapy for hypertension was taking Tab. Atenolol since 2 years. He suffered from anginal pain and was brought to the OPD.

1.1 Which is the preferred dosage form of Glyceryl trinitrate to relieve the pain?

- **A.** Sublingual tablet 0.3 mg
- **B.** Sustained release capsule 2.5 mg
- **C.** Transdermal patch 5 mg
- **D.** Intravenous infusion 5mcg/min

The patient was relieved of his pain. After thorough investigations, the treating physician added Tab. Verapamil 120 mg three times a day to his therapy.

1.2 The patient should be carefully monitored for:

- **A.** Cardiac ischaemia
- **B.** Development of syncope
- **C.** AV node suppression
- **D.** Bronchospasm

CASE 2

A 60-yr old patient was brought to the casualty and was diagnosed as a case of myocardial infarction. The attending physician decided to administer IV Morphine for decreasing his anxiety and chest pain. However due to non-availability of morphine, another opioid pentazocine was given intramuscularly.

2.1 Following this, the patient's condition deteriorated because pentazocine:

- **A.** causes respiratory depression
- **B.** is less potent than morphine
- **C.** increases myocardial oxygen consumption
- **D.** induces more vomiting

CASE 3

Mrs. SP, a 55-year-old non-diabetic, non-hypertensive woman is admitted with an acute myocardial infarction. She was started on aspirin and clopidogrel.

3.1 Which other medication should be added for secondary prevention of cardiovascular events?

- **A.** Nitroglycerine
- **B.** Warfarin
- **C.** Atorvastatin
- **D.** Verapamil

3.2 Mrs SP is also prescribed metoprolol 50 mg twice daily to:

- **A.** limit infarct size
- **B.** prevent transient ischaemic attacks
- **C.** regulate blood pressure
- **D.** prevent venous thrombosis

CASE 4

Mr. AD, a 65-year-old diabetic patient with a history of previous myocardial infarction, experiences frequent episodes of angina despite optimal standard medical therapy.

4.1 Which anti-anginal medication may be considered as an add-on therapy in this case?

- **A.** Ranolazine
- **B.** Diltiazem
- **C.** Metoprolol
- **D.** Isosorbide dinitrate

CASE 5

Ms. NR, a 45-year-old woman, presents with unstable angina and is scheduled for percutaneous coronary intervention (PCI).

5.1 Which agent should be added to aspirin before the PCI procedure to prevent stent thrombosis?
A. Dabigatran
B. Rivaroxaban
C. Enoxaparin
D. Ticagrelor

CASE 6

A 30-year-old person was diagnosed to have hypertension on routine check-up done at his office. The investigations revealed no other abnormality. He was prescribed an antihypertensive drug. Two months later he reported for follow-up. His blood pressure was controlled but he complained of tiredness after his day's work. He had disturbed sleep with frequent awakenings. He also mentioned that his sex life is disturbed due to decreased desire and difficulty reaching orgasm.

6.1 Which one of the following agents was likely to have been prescribed to him?
A. Enalapril
B. Metoprolol
C. Losartan
D. Indapamide

CASE 7

A patient with hypertension and Type 2 Diabetes mellitus is being treated with an ACE inhibitor. The physician decides to add spironolactone to the therapy as an agent to offer cardiovascular benefit.

7.1 Which potential side effect should the physician monitor closely in this patient?
A. Hyperkalemia
B. Hypoglycemia
C. Hyponatremia
D. Hypercalcemia

CASE 8

A 55-year-old farmer RT visits the district hospital for a nasal bleed. He mentions that he has been experiencing repeated attacks of severe headache since the last 3 months. He also complains of shortness of breath while working in the field and fatigue at the end of the day, which is worsening daily. His blood pressure reading is 150/96 mm of Hg. On repeat measurements of BP on different days and after investigations he is diagnosed to have essential hypertension. RT also reveals that since last 3 years he has been getting episodes of intense pain and swelling of the right toe once or twice a year. The episodes are sudden and last for a week or more. Occasionally even the other toes are swollen, discoloured and tender even on light touch disturbing his sleep. So far he has tried some medications from the local doctor but despite that these attacks have continued. The physician gets his uric acid report as 6.6 mg%.

8.1 Which of the following drugs should be avoided in RT to prevent exacerbation of inflammatory symptoms?

A. Atenolol
B. Hydrochlorothiazide
C. Amlodipine
D. Prazosin

CASE 9

Mrs. AD, 32-year-old woman suffers from essential hypertension. She is currently controlled on Tab. Enalapril 5 mg once a day. She is planning to get pregnant.

9.1 What should be the advice of the treating physician?

A. Continue enalapril as blood pressure is well controlled
B. Switch over to losartan to have better control of BP
C. Add thiazide to take care of blood pressure fluctuations in pregnancy
D. Change to alpha methyldopa as a safe antihypertensive

CASE 10

Mrs. TR, a 75-year-old patient with heart failure and reduced ejection fraction, is currently on standard therapy with an ACE inhibitor, beta-blocker, and a loop diuretic. Despite optimal treatment, she continues to experience symptoms.

10.1 Which medication would provide additional benefit in reducing morbidity and mortality?

A. Spironolactone
B. Hydralazine
C. Isosorbide dinitrate
D. Nesiritide

CASE 11

Mr. CP, a 60-year-old man suffering from heart failure with preserved ejection fraction (HFpEF), is experiencing persistent symptoms despite being on diuretics and ACE inhibitor for which he has been hospitalised twice in the past 2 months. He also suffers from hypertension.

11.1 Which medication will benefit Mr. CP in reducing hospitalizations?

A. Atenolol
B. Empagliflozin
C. Digoxin
D. Eplerenone

CASE 12

Mr. JP, a 55-year-old patient with heart failure with reduced ejection fraction (HFrEF) with dilated heart is taking an ACE inhibitor. His physician wishes to add ARNI to his current therapy.

12.1 Which of the following adverse effect can potentially occur due to this combination?

A. Renal failure
B. Hypokalemia
C. Angioedema
D. Fluid retention

12.2 Mr. JP should receive all of the following EXCEPT:

A. ARNI
B. Aliskiren
C. Beta blocker
D. Aldosterone antagonist

SECTION 8. DRUGS ACTING ON BLOOD AND BLOOD FORMING ORGANS

CASE 1

Mrs. JR, a 76-year-old overweight woman with varicose veins presents to the emergency medical services with pain and swelling in her right thigh. A venous ultrasound of her legs shows a blood clot below her right hip joint. Her D-dimer is also elevated. The treating physician, admits her and immediately starts her on enoxaparin.

1.1 The physician prescribed enoxaparin instead of heparin because it:

A. mainly acts against thrombin
B. also interacts with platelets
C. has a shorter half-life
D. has more predictable anticoagulant effect

At discharge, Mrs. JR says that she does not wish to take twice daily injections.

1.2 Which of the following drugs can be prescribed to Mrs. JR instead of enoxaparin?

A. Fondaparinux
B. Ticagrelor
C. Desirudin
D. Rivaroxaban

CASE 2

A 50-year- old patient, admitted in the ICU has been prescribed continuous intravenous unfractionated heparin for anticoagulation.

2.1 What is the most appropriate strategy for therapeutic drug monitoring in this case?

A. Monitor activated partial thromboplastin time (APTT)
B. Assess activated coagulation factor X
C. Assess platelet functions
D. Measure serum heparin levels

CASE 3

Mr. KP, a 45-year-old male with a history of chronic gastrointestinal bleeding due to ulcerative colitis presents with weakness and dizziness. His blood work up shows microcytic hypochromic anaemia.

3.1 Which of the following tests is most specific for confirming iron deficiency?

A. Serum ferritin
B. Total iron-binding capacity (TIBC)
C. Serum iron
D. Hemoglobin electrophoresis

3.2 What is the most appropriate form of iron supplementation for this patient?

A. Ferrous sulphate
B. Iron sucrose
C. Ferric hydroxide polymaltose complex
D. Recombinant epoietin

CASE 4

Mrs PK, a 22-year-old vegetarian woman complains of fatigue and weakness. She has a pale complexion, and her diet mainly consists of fruits, vegetables, and grains.

4.1 Which of the following dietary sources is least likely contributing to her iron intake?
- A. Spinach
- B. Lentils
- C. Fortified cereals
- D. Oranges

4.2 How much oral elemental iron (in mg) should she receive weekly as a prophylactic therapy?
- A. 25
- B. 50
- C. 100
- D. 200

4.3 As per National guidelines for Control of Iron Deficiency Anaemia, the prophylactic therapy with oral iron is supplemented with:
- A. Vitamin C
- B. Folic acid
- C. Cobalt
- D. Zinc

Mrs PK now visits an antenatal OPD with complaints of generalized weakness, giddiness and breathlessness. She is in her 8th month of pregnancy. Clinical examination reveals pallor. Laboratory test revealed that her Hb level is 7 gm%.

4.4 Which of the following complications is most commonly associated with maternal iron deficiency anaemia during pregnancy?
- A. Neural tube defects
- B. Preterm delivery
- C. Macrosomia
- D. Gestational diabetes

4.5 As per National guidelines, which iron formulation will you recommend to Mrs PK?
- A. Intramuscular iron sorbitol citrate complex
- B. Intravenous iron sucrose
- C. Subcutaneous iron polymaltose
- D. Transfusion with packed red blood cells

CASE 5

A 45-year-old female with iron deficiency anaemia develops nausea, vomiting, and abdominal pain after receiving intravenous iron therapy.

5.1 What is the most appropriate management for this patient's symptoms?
- A. Discontinue the iron infusion
- B. Administer antiemetics and continue the infusion
- C. Switch to oral iron supplementation
- D. Administer desferrioxamine

SECTION 9. DRUGS AFFECTING RENAL FUNCTIONS

CASE 1

Mr. AB, a 63-year-old man presents with severe dyspnoea, restlessness and anxiety to the emergency medical services. He said that he had noticed that his sputum was blood-tinged. On examination, the attending physician finds his pulse rapid and of a low volume, pulmonary crackles and neck vein distention. Chest X-ray has a ground glass appearance confirming the diagnosis of pulmonary oedema. The patient is admitted and started on 100% oxygen. The physician decides to administer a diuretic for controlling the oedema.

1.1 Which of the following diuretics should be administered to Mr. AB?

A. Furosemide
B. Hydrochlorothiazide
C. Mannitol
D. Spironolactone

CASE 2

Mrs. GN, a 78-year-old woman who lives with an attendant is brought to the emergency medical services in the morning by her son with complaints of altered consciousness since 3 hours. History taking reveals that she had a fall in the bathroom in the late evening two days back. Mrs. GN had not complained about anything except that her head was hurting and had taken a paracetamol and gone to bed. The next morning, she started getting a headache and feeling nauseous. By bedtime she started feeling dizzy and complained of seeing double vision, but said that she would feel better if she slept it off and went to bed. This morning the attendant noted that she was disoriented and confused, her speech was jumbled. MRI shows cerebral oedema.

2.1 Which of the following diuretics should be administered to Mrs. GN?

A. Hydrochlorothiazide
B. Acetazolamide
C. Mannitol
D. Triamterene

2.2 The mechanism of action of the selected diuretic for Mrs. GN is:

A. Na^+–Cl^- transporter inhibition
B. carbonic anhydrase inhibition
C. blockade of renal epithelial Na channels
D. reduction in the medullary tonicity

SECTION 10. DRUGS USED IN DISORDERS OF THE GASTROINTESTINAL TRACT

CASE 1

Mr. NP, a 48-year-old man, working as a senior manager in a multinational company, visits a clinic with a report of laboratory investigations which were carried out as a part of his company's policy. He tells the doctor that he has come for a routine health check up as there is a history of heart disease in his family and he has not suffered from any major illness till date. On examination the doctor notes that he is slightly overweight (weight above normal for age, gender and height). His BP is 150/94 mm of Hg. His CBC, HbA1c, LFT and RFT are in the normal range. The report of his lipid profile is as follows: Total Cholesterol: 270 mg/dL, Triglycerides: 148 mg/dL, High-Density Lipoprotein Cholesterol (HDL-C): 34 mg/dL, Low-Density Lipoprotein Cholesterol (LDL-C): 164 mg/dL.

Mr. NP's doctor counsels him and advises him to lose weight with regular exercise and diet restriction. He prescribes losartan for his hypertension and also decides to prescribe a hypolipidemic drug.

1.1 Which of the following hypolipidemic drugs should be prescribed to Mr. NP?

A. Atorvastatin
B. Fenofibrate
C. Ezetemibe
D. Colestipol

CASE 2

Mrs. MB, a 50-year-old overweight post-menopausal woman suffering from hypertension and diabetes visits her doctor for a routine health check up with a blood report. The doctor notes that her blood pressure and blood sugar is under control with medication. Her LFT and RFT is also within range. However, her lipid profile report is as follows:
Total Cholesterol: 238 mg/dL, Triglycerides: 370 mg/dL, High-Density Lipoprotein Cholesterol (HDL-C): 40 mg/dL, Low-Density Lipoprotein Cholesterol (LDL-C): 122 mg/dL.

2.1 Which of the following hypolipidemic drugs should be prescribed to Mr. NP?

A. Rosuvastatin
B. Gemfibrozil
C. Niacin
D. Cholestyramine

CASE 3

Mr. TL, a 62-year-old man visits his general practitioner with complaints of difficulty in passing stools since one week. During history taking he informs the doctor that he suffers from this problem off and on but his constipation usually resolves in 2-3 days. However, this time it has continued and he is not only getting abdominal pain but he also has severe pain in the anal region. TL also informs the doctor that for the last 2 weeks he is taking a drug for gastric acidity prescribed by his general practitioner. He does not suffer from any other disease.

3.1 Which of the following drugs must have been prescribed to Mr. TL for his dyspepsia?

A. Magnesium trisilicate
B. Aluminium hydroxide
C. Bismuth subcitrate
D. Sodium bicarbonate

On examination the doctor notes that the patient has also developed an anal fissure. He advises the patient to discontinue the previous medication and decides to prescribe a laxative.

3.2 Which of the following laxatives should be prescribed to Mr. TL?

A. Castor oil
B. Liquid paraffin
C. Bisacodyl
D. Senna

CASE 4

Mrs. RM, a 68-year-old woman is presents with weakness and fatigue. There has been no change in her diet and lifestyle in the recent past. Her blood test reveals that she is severely anaemic. The CT scan is suggestive of colon cancer. Mrs. RM is scheduled for a colonoscopy and the doctor decides to prescribe a laxative for the preparation of her colon before the scopy.

4.1 Which of the following laxatives would be most appropriate for Mrs. RM?

A. Lactulose
B. Lubiprostone
C. Dioctyl sodium sulfosuccinate
D. Polyethylene glycol

CASE 5

Mr. AS, a 40-year-old male executive, smoker and social drinker presents with complaints of pain in the epigastric region which decreases after meals, feeling of bloating, nausea, vomiting and weight gain. Suspecting a duodenal ulcer, the physician advises urease test which turns out to be positive for *H. pylori*. The physician prescribes Omeprazole 20 mg twice daily for 8 weeks.

5.1 Which other drugs should be prescribed along with omeprazole?

A. Tetracycline 500mg + Azithromycin 500 mg twice daily for 2 weeks
B. Clarithromycin 500 mg + Amoxicillin 1000 mg twice daily for 2 weeks
C. Metronidazole 400 mg + Doxycycline 100 mg twice daily for 2 weeks
D. Ampicillin 500 mg + Tetracycline 500 mg twice daily for 2 weeks

CASE 6

Mrs. RM, a 52 year old woman meets with a road accident and is admitted with severe injuries and 2 fractures. She undergoes multiple surgeries and is admitted in the critical care unit. The treating physician is worried that Mrs. RM may develop acute erosive gastritis due to the stress.

6.1 Which of the following drugs should be prophylactically administered to Mrs. RM?

A. Pantoprazole
B. Misoprostol
C. Sucralfate
D. Bismuth subcitrate

SECTION 11. OXYTOCICS AND UTERINE RELAXANTS

CASE 1

A 28-year-old pregnant woman, JS presents to the hospital with labour pains. The fetal monitoring shows a healthy, full-term fetus with normal fetal presentation. The obstetrician decides to induce labour with oxytocin.

1.1 Before starting oxytocin infusion the obstetrician must rule out which of the following conditions?

A. Bronchial asthma
B. Complete placenta previa
C. Hypotension
D. Rh incompatibility

CASE 2

A 32-year-old pregnant woman, KT at 37 weeks gestation presents to the hospital with preterm labour. She is a known case of asthma and has been taking budesonide + formoterol inhaler throughout her pregnancy. The obstetrician decides to use a prostaglandin analogue to induce labour.

2.1 **Which prostaglandin analogue can be prescribed to KT?**

A. Dinoprostone endocervically
B. Carboprost IM
C. Misoprostol orally
D. Gemeprost vaginally

2.2 **Which of the following is a absolute contraindication for the use of prostaglandin analogues in this patient?**

A. Asthma
B. Hypertension
C. Uterine surgery
D. Gestational diabetes

SECTION 12. CHEMOTHERAPY

CASE 1

Mrs. KM, a 66-year-old woman presents with history of fever and productive cough since the last 5 days. Since the last 2 days she is having chest pain and dyspnoea. History taking reveals that she is taking paracetamol which she has purchased over the counter, but the fever reappears and has been rising over the last few days. On examination, her temperature is 103°F. Auscultation of the chest reveals rales and there is dullness on percussion on the right side of the chest. A chest radiograph shows an infiltrate in the right lower lobe. A blood sample drawn for smear culture and antibiotic sensitivity reveals Gram-positive cocci in pairs. The physician admits her in the hospital and decides to start drug therapy.

1.1 **Which of the following antibiotics, administered intravenously, is the most appropriate initial therapy?**

A. Ampicillin
B. Vancomycin
C. Ceftazidime
D. Ciprofloxacin

CASE 2

Ms. RN, a 16-year-old girl presents with fever since 2 days followed by pain and feeling of pressure in the right ear. On examination the attending physician notes that her body temperature is 102°F and that she has difficulty in hearing. Examination of the ear drum reveals a bulging and erythematous tympanic membrane. Ms. RN is diagnosed as suffering from acute otitis media.

2.1 **Which of the following antibiotics should be prescribed to the patient?**

A. Cloxacillin
B. Gentamicin
C. Amoxicillin
D. Norfloxacin

CASE 3

A 25-year-old female, working as a maid, presents with a vaginal candidial infection. The physician prescribes an antifungal drug that interferes with the synthesis of fungal cell walls by inhibiting the enzyme (1,3)-beta-D-glucan synthase.

3.1 **Which antifungal drug has been prescribed to her?**

A. Clotrimazole
B. Miconazole
C. Micafungin
D. Griseofulvin

3.2 **If you were the physician, what would have been a rational antifungal drug for this patient?**
- A. Amphotericin B
- B. Fluconazole
- C. Micafungin
- D. Griseofulvin

3.3 **All of the following are appropriate reasons for your selection EXCEPT**
- A. broad spectrum antifungal agent
- B. safe to prescribe
- C. suitable to administer
- D. cost-effective

CASE 4

Mr. SR, a 50-year-old patient with a history of liver disease is diagnosed with invasive aspergillosis.

4.1 **Which antifungal agent should be used with caution due to its potential hepatotoxicity?**
- A. Voriconazole
- B. Posaconazole
- C. Caspofungin
- D. Itraconazole

CASE 5

Mrs. RG, a 45-year-old house wife has developed *Tinea pedis* and *Tinea manus* since last 2 years. She has been treated with topical antifungal agents but the infection persisted. Hence she visits the dermatology OPD again. The treating doctor decides to prescribe systemic antifungal drug.

5.1 **Which one of the following would be the drug of choice?**
- A. Amphotericin B
- B. Griseofulvin
- C. Ketoconazole
- D. Caspofungin

CASE 6

Mr. PK, a patient on warfarin therapy develops candidemia and is admitted in the intensive care unit.

6.1 **Which antifungal medication should be avoided due to its potential to increase the risk of bleeding by inhibiting warfarin metabolism?**
- A. Fluconazole
- B. Micafungin
- C. Flucytosine
- D. Amphotericin B

CASE 7

Mrs BC, a 25-year-old woman has amenorrhoea of 8 weeks. She visited antenatal care unit. Her routine urine showed presence of bacteria, however she had no symptoms. It was decided to treat her.

7.1 **Which of the following antibiotics should be prescribed to Mrs BK?**
- A. Ciprofloxacin
- B. Cotrimoxazole
- C. Amoxicillin
- D. Gentamicin

She took the treatment for 3 days and did not come for the follow up after 7 days as was advised. She then visited the antenatal care unit after 15 days complaining of pain in lower abdomen, frequent urination and burning pain while passing the urine. Urine culture and antibiotic sensitivity testing was done and organisms were found to be *Escherichia coli* but resistant to previously given antibiotic.

7.2 Which antibiotic will be the most rational choice in this condition for her?

A. Azithromycin
B. Aztreonam
C. Meropenem
D. Cefotaxime

7.3 Urinary tract infections of pregnancy needs to be treated with appropriate antibiotic given for adequate duration for all the following reasons EXCEPT to:

A. reduce risk of pyelonephritis
B. avoid premature delivery
C. prevent microcephaly in newborns
D. avoid low-birth weight newborns

CASE 8

A patient with a complicated upper urinary tract infection (pyelonephritis) is admitted to the hospital.

8.1 What is the preferred empirical intravenous antibiotic therapy in this scenario?

A. Ceftriaxone
B. Vancomycin
C. Cotrimoxazole
D. Doxycycline

CASE 9

Mr. NR, a 40 -year-old male patient having symptoms of lower urinary tract infection visits a doctor. His laboratory reports indicate positive urine culture for *Escherichia coli*. The doctor recalls that this is his 4th visit in a year for treatment of lower UTI.

9.1 What should be the line of action of the doctor?

A. Treat the UTI, do urine culture & antibiotic sensitivity testing and start antimicrobial prophylaxis
B. Start antimicrobial prophylaxis immediately and do investigations
C. Treat the UTI, rule out urogenital anomaly and start antimicrobial prophylaxis
D. Rule out urogenital anomaly and start antimicrobial prophylaxis

CASE 10

A 70-year-old male with benign prostatic hyperplasia (BPH) develops a UTI.

10.1 Which antibiotic is preferred for treating this patient?

A. Cefotaxime
B. Cotrimoxazole
C. Ampicillin
D. Nitrofurantoin

CASE 11

Mr. JK, 26-year-old man presents with complaints of burning during micturition, purulent urethral discharge and painful ulcer on the penis which is gradually increasing in size since the past 1 week. While taking history Mr. JK informs the physician that he does not use condoms during sexual intercourse. His urine examination is positive for leukocyte esterase. Gram stain of the urine shows intracellular diplococci within polymorphonuclear neutrophils. The physician diagnoses the patient to be suffering from gonorrhoea.

11.1 Which of the following regimens is the most appropriate for this patient?

A. Vancomycin intramuscularly as a single dose
B. Ceftriaxone intramuscularly as a single dose
C. Doxycycline orally for 7 days
D. Procaine penicillin G intramuscularly as a single dose plus one gram of probenecid

CASE 12

In a newly diagnosed HIV-positive patient, aged 30 years and weighing 50 kg the viral load was found to be 2000 copies/mL and CD4 count as 350 cells/mm^3.

12.1 What is the recommended antiretroviral therapy according to the national (NACO) guidelines?

A. Zidovudine + Lamivudine + Efavirenz
B. Stavudine + Didanosine + Lopinavir/ritonavir
C. Ritonavir-boosted Atazanavir + Lamivudine + Tenofovir disoproxil
D. Tenofovir disoproxil fumarate + Lamivudine + Dolutegravir

12.2 The first indicator of treatment failure is:

A. CD4 count increases only by 50 cells/mm^3 at 6 months of therapy
B. plasma viral load ≥ 1000 copies/mL at 6 months of therapy
C. CD4 count < 350 cells/ mm^3 any time within 3 months of therapy
D. plasma viral load < 1000 copies/mL within 3 months of therapy

If the above patient develops confirmed virologic failure.

12.3 What is the next step in management?

A. Switch to a regimen with at least two alternative drugs
B. Increase the doses of drugs in the current regimen
C. Continue the current regimen and monitor closely
D. Switch to an entirely new antiretroviral regimen

CASE 13

A healthcare worker reports that he has a needlestick injury 2 days back while collecting blood of a patient. He came to know later that the patient was HIV positive patient. A blood drop was noticed at the site of the injury but he applied gauze piece so no further oozing appeared. The healthcare worker is HIV negative.

13.1 As a treating doctor, what will be your advice regarding HIV prophylaxis?

A. No need of prophylaxis as injury is not significant
B. No use of prophylaxis as 48 hrs have passed since injury
C. Three drug regimen should be taken as prophylaxis
D. Prophylaxis should be started and continued till risk evaluation

13.2 In case you decide to initiate prophylaxis, what will be the regimen as per the National guidelines?

A. Tenofovir disoproxil fumarate + Lamivudine + Dolutegravir
B. Zidovudine + Lamivudine + Dolutegravir
C. Abacavir + Didanosine + Lopinavir/ritonavir
D. Zidovudine + Lamivudine + Lopinavir/ritonavir

CASE 14

A HIV positive mother is planning to breastfeed. She has been taking antiretroviral therapy during pregnancy and her viral load done at 34 weeks of pregnancy was found to be <1000 copies/mL.

14.1 As per the National guidelines, which one of the following antiretroviral drugs is recommended for the infant to prevent mother-to-child transmission during breastfeeding?

A. Nevirapine
B. Ritonavir
C. Zidovudine
D. Lamivudine

CASE 15

A patient with HIV is receiving antiretroviral therapy but his CD4 count has dropped to <50mm^3. The doctor wants to initiate prophylaxis against mycobacterium avium complex (MAC) infection.

15.1 Which one of the following drugs should be prescribed to this patient?

A. Isoniazid
B. Rifampicin
C. Rifabutin
D. Pyrizinamide

CASE 16

Mr. KS, a 42-year-old male factory worker visits the medicine OPD of a Government Hospital with complaints of cough with sputum, mild to moderate fever and generalised fatigue since 7 days. KS informs his treating doctor that he has been taking Tablet Paracetamol 500 mg orally whenever he has fever. The doctor enquires whether KS has lost weight or had tuberculosis (TB) infection in the past. KS informs that he was diagnosed with TB 1 year back for which he had taken treatment for 3 months. The physician asks him to do sputum examination. The report of sputum examination is positive for sensitive acid fast tuberculous bacilli.

16.1 KS must be prescribed:

A. HRZE for 2 months followed by HRE for 4 months
B. HRZES for 3 months followed by HR for 5 months
C. levofloxacin + REZ for 6 months
D. shorter oral bedaquiline containing regimen for 11 months

KS starts receiving anti-TB treatment as per NTEP guidelines. After 2 weeks he presents to the OPD stating tingling and numbness in his hands and feet and hence working has become difficult as things drop from his hands.

16.2 The new management strategy for KS will now be:

A. referral to neurologist
B. addition folic acid 5 mg to the regimen
C. addition of pyridoxine 10 mg to the regimen
D. massaging hands and feet with counter-irritant oil

CASE 17

Dr. PR is a 32-year-old, 58 kg junior doctor working in a city tertiary care hospital. While on rounds one day, PR starts feeling feverish. He develops cough with slight sputum intermittently. His symptoms do not resolve for one week. He has history of pulmonary tuberculosis a few years back. He undergoes sputum examination and antibiotic sensitivity tests for TB as advised by the Chest TB Consultant. The test reveals that the TB strain is resistant to R and H with KatG mutation.

17.1 Which regimen will be prescribed to Dr. PR?

A. Levofloxacin + REZ for 6 months
B. Shorter oral bedaquiline containing regimen for 11 months
C. Shorter injectable MDR TB regimen without bedaquiline for 11 months
D. All oral longer MDR TB regimen for 18 months

Dr. PR is started on treatment in accordance with PMDT guidelines.

17.2 Which investigations will have to performed on Day 15 of the treatment in Dr. PR?

A. Liver function tests
B. Renal function tests
C. ECG and Serum electrolytes
D. ECG and complete blood count

CASE 18

A 23-year-old female, NW is brought to the Medicine OPD of a tertiary care hospital in Mumbai with history of 1 episode of giddiness, skin rash, muscle aches and recurring fever with chills since the past two days. There is no history of seizures. On examination, NW is found to be febrile (38.3°C), disoriented with a blood pressure: 100/64 mm of Hg, respiratory rate: 20 / min and a pulse rate: 110/ min. The chest examination is normal. Per abdomen examination shows palpable spleen. The laboratory investigations reports are as follows: Hb= 6.8 g/dL; platelets = 71000/μl; total bilirubin = 2.9 mg/dL, serum creatinine = 1.2 mg/dL. Microscopic slides of thick and thin Giemsa-stained blood smears show the presence of trophozoites and schizonts of *P. falciparum*.

18.1 What antimalarial drugs will you prescribe to NW?

A. Quinine 600 mg orally thrice a day + doxycycline 100 mg once daily
B. Quinine hydrochloride IV infusion 20mg/kg over 4 h; followed by 10 mg/kg every 8 hourly
C. Sodium artesunate 100 mg orally 12 hourly plus sulphadoxine (750 mg) + pyrimethamine (37.5 mg) 2 tabs once
D. Artmether (20 mg) + lumefantrine (120 mg) 4 tabs twice daily

NW receives the antimalarial treatment for 3 days and is now afebrile and asymptomatic. She is discharged on 4th day.

18.2 NW also receives primaquine:

A. (0.75 mg/kg) as a single dose on Day 2 of treatment
B. (0.75 mg/kg) per day for 14 days after completing initial treatment
C. (0.75 mg/kg) as a single dose after completing initial treatment
D. (0.25 mg/kg) per day for 14 days from Day 1 of treatment

18.3 What advice will be given to NW at the time of discharge?

A. Take Primaquine for 14 days
B. Take Folic acid for 3 months
C. Continue artemisinin therapy for 2 more days
D. Not to continue antimalarial treatment

CASE 19

Mr. SM, a traveler from Saudi Arabia plans a jungle safari trip to North- East states of India. He calls his friend Dr. AJ, who is a clinician practicing in Mumbai regarding advice on malarial prophylaxis.

19.1 The advice AJ must give is:
- A. start proguanil tablet 200 mg once a day 2 days before the travel
- B. start chloroquine tablet 300 mg one week before the travel
- C. start mefloquine tablet 250 mg one day before the travel
- D. start atovaquone 250 mg + proguanil 100 mg tablet one day before the travel

CASE 20

Mrs. RK, a diabetic patient aged 56 years started getting pain in the abdominal region in the morning. She ignored it thinking that the pain would go away. However, the next day she felt feverish and the pain became more severe and was accompanied by a rash with a few vesicles. She therefore paid a visit to her physician who diagnosed the lesion as herpes zoster and decided to prescribe a drug for Mrs. RK.

20.1 Which drug should the physician prescribe to Mrs. RK?
- A. Acyclovir
- B. Ganciclovir
- C. Foscarnet
- D. Fomivirsen

Mrs. RK comes after 10 days complaining that there is no resolution of the lesions even after taking acyclovir as prescribed.

20.2 Which drug the physician should prescribe now?
- A. Acyclovir
- B. Ganciclovir
- C. Foscarnet
- D. Fomivirsen

CASE 21

Mr. NR, a 70-year-old male presents to the emergency department of a medical hospital in Srinagar with complaints of fever, sore throat, headache, muscle aches, and fatigue since 2 days. On examination, he has a temperature of 103°F (39.4°C), and his respiratory rate is slightly elevated. Laboratory testing of combined nasopharyngeal and oropharyngeal swabs is indicative of influenza B virus infection. On enquiry he reveals that he has not taken influenza vaccine.

21.1 Which one of the following antiviral drugs would be the first-line treatment for Mr. NR?
- A. Oseltamivir
- B. Acyclovir
- C. Amantadine
- D. Ribavirin

21.2 Which of the following side effect should Mr.NR be warned about while prescribing oseltamivir?
- A. Anaemia
- B. Diarrhoea
- C. Urinary retention
- D. Bronchospasm

21.3 Which one of the following antipyretic is contraindicated in this condition?
- A. Paracetamol
- B. Aspirin
- C. Ibuprofen
- D. Naproxen

SECTION 13. DRUGS USED IN ENDOCRINE DISORDERS

CASE 1

A 26-year-old woman TR suffering from goitre, presents with high grade fever, confusion, agitation and seizures on admission. Examination reveals that her pulse rate is 240/min and is irregular. She is diagnosed to be in thyrotoxic crisis.

1.1 The emergency management for TR will include:
- A. aspirin IV 500 mg
- B. sodium iodide IV infusion 1 g
- C. high dose radioiodine
- D. amiodarone IV 300 mg

1.2 Propylthiouracil is preferred over other other thioamides in thyrotoxic crisis because it:
- A. inhibits prompt iodination of tyrosyl residues
- B. prevents coupling of MIT and DIT
- C. inhibits peripheral conversion of T_4 to T_3
- D. blocks immediate release of T_4

1.3 All of the following drugs can be used as an adjuvant therapy in thyrotoxicosis EXCEPT
- A. propranolol
- B. paracetamol
- C. dexamethasone
- D. aspirin

1.4 In thyroid storm, propranolol does NOT control:
- A. anxiety
- B. tremors
- C. tachycardia
- D. hyperpyrexia

CASE 2

Mr. SB, a 45-year-old male diabetic patient, reports to the Endocrine OPD. His blood sugar is not well controlled due to poor adherence to therapy. He is also taking amlodipine and nitrate combination as maintenance therapy for chronic stable angina. He is now diagnosed to have hyperthyroidism.

2.1 The best treatment option for hyperthyroidism in SB will be:
- A. subtotal thyroidectomy
- B. radioiodine
- C. lifelong carbimazole therapy
- D. Lugol's iodine

CASE 3

Mr. JR, a 68-year-old retired pensioner with newly diagnosed type 2 diabetes, is started on metformin. Despite lifestyle modifications and administering 2 g metformin, his HbA1c remains 8.5% after 3 months.

3.1 The most appropriate next step in his pharmacotherapy will be to add:
- A. sulfonylurea
- B. DPP-4 inhibitor
- C. SGLT-2 inhibitor
- D. insulin

CASE 4

Mrs. PS, a 55-year-old woman with type 2 diabetes, is concerned about her increased risk of cardiovascular disease.

4.1 Which antidiabetic medication has demonstrated cardiovascular benefits and may be considered for her?

A. Metformin
B. Pioglitazone
C. Gliclazide
D. Canagliflozin

CASE 5

Mr. AB, a 60-year-old man with type 2 diabetes, has a history of heart failure.

5.1 Which class of antidiabetic medications should be avoided in Mr. AB?

A. Sulfonylureas
B. Thiazolidinediones
C. GLP-1 receptor agonists
D. SGLT-2 inhibitors

CASE 6

Mrs. RD, a 25-year-old woman with type 1 diabetes is an executive manager in a corporate company. As a part of her job, she has to travel a lot. She has to attend number of meetings, some of which are not pre-scheduled and her day to day work programme varies so her meal timings are not fixed. She is now planning a pregnancy.

6.1 What is the preferred insulin regimen for optimal blood glucose control during pregnancy?

A. Inj. Regular insulin before each major meal
B. Inj. Glargine insulin at bedtime with NPH insulin before breakfast and dinner
C. Inj. Glargine insulin at bed time and Inj. lispro before each major meal
D. Inj. NPH insulin before breakfast and dinner

CASE 7

Mr. KH, a 70-year-old man with Type 2 Diabetes, is concerned about the risk of hypoglycemia due to his erratic eating habits.

7.1 Which antidiabetic medication has a lower risk of causing hypoglycemia in Mr. KH?

A. Glyburide
B. Sitagliptin
C. Glipizide
D. Repaglinide

CASE 8

Mrs. CS, a 65-year-old woman with Type 2 Diabetes, has chronic kidney disease (CKD). The eGFR is < 30 mL/min per 1.73 m^2.

8.1 Which antidiabetic medication should be recommended for Mrs. CS?

A. Metformin
B. Empagliflozin
C. Acarbose
D. Linagliptin

CASE 9

Mrs. GA, a 70-year-old woman with Type 2 Diabetes, has been prescribed glibenclamide and acarbose. She felt giddy while taking her routine walk and started perspiring and trembling and had palpitations. Hence she entered a nearby stall of sugarcane juice and ordered a glass of juice. But her symptoms were not relieved even after drinking the juice. Her dizziness increased and she collapsed. She was rushed to a nearby hospital. Her blood glucose showed a level of 55 mg%. She recovered after administration of IV glucose.

9.1 What food should she carry with her while going for a walk in the event that such an episode occurs again?

A. Starch biscuits
B. Sugar candy
C. Glucose powder
D. Table sugar

CASE 10

An 10-year-old boy MT, weighing 45 kg presents with swelling around the eyes, both legs, since the past one week which has progressed to generalized swelling. MT's parents inform the physician that he had intermittent fever since 2 weeks. On investigations, he is found to have proteinuria, reduced serum albumin (2.0 g/dL) with elevated lipid levels. MT is diagnosed to be suffering from idiopathic nephrotic syndrome based on clinical and laboratory findings. MT needs to be started on oral systemic steroids.

10.1 The dosing approach in MT will be:

A. high dose followed by maintenance dose
B. low dose followed by high maintenance dose
C. high intensive dose for 2 weeks
D. low maintenance dose for 2 months

MT is prescribed Tab prednisolone 25 mg four times a day. MT's mother goes to the pharmacist to buy the medicine where in the pharmacist hands over a strip of prednisone. MT's mother approaches the pediatrician enquiring whether pharmacist gave the correct drug.

10.2 The treating pediatrician states it is appropriate to take prednisone because:

A. both are same drugs
B. prednisone is a prodrug
C. prednisolone is prodrug
D. there was spelling error in the drug name on the strip

After 3 months MT comes for follow up and his mother informs MT has been taking medicines regularly but now MT's weight is 50 kg and he has developed a moon face.

10.3 This indicates that:

A. steroid therapy is not working hence edema has increased
B. fat deposition due to steroids
C. appetite is increased due to steroids
D. MT has developed primary hyperaldosteronism

CASE 11

A 32-year-old woman SP presents with complaints of paresthesia, tingling, increased skin sensitivity all over her body and pain in her fingers of left hand extending to arm and neck. These symptoms have been present on and off since the past 2 weeks. She also complains of blurring of vision in the right eye, vertigo and fatigue since the past 10 days. On examination, Babinski sign is positive. MRI shows acute demyelinating optic neuritis. Her CSF analysis reveals oligoclonal bands. On the basis of the above clinical features and examination, laboratory and radiological tests, provisional diagnosis of right optic neuritis due to multiple sclerosis is made by the neurologist.

11.1 For immediate symptomatic relief the neurologist must administer Injection:

A. methylprednisolone
B. dexamethasone
C. cortisone
D. prednisone

11.2 After injectable steroids SP has to be put on maintenance steroids. The neurologist will now:

A. taper the injectable steroid to start low dose oral steroids
B. switch to oral steroid of an equivalent dose
C. stop the injectable steroid to give 5 days drug-free interval and restart with low dose injectable steroids
D. taper the dose of injectable steroids till the lowest dose is achieved to continue with

11.3 With maintenance steroids prescribed to SP, the other concomitant medication will be:

A. metoclopramide
B. cotrimoxazole
C. omeprazole
D. ferrous sulphate

CASE 12

Mrs. NJ, a 26-year-old lady having a 2-year-old son visits the clinic. She gives a history of unprotected intercourse on the previous night and wants advice for an emergency contraception.

12.1 What should the treating doctor prescribe NJ?

A. Tab Levonorgestrel 0.75 mg 2 tablets stat
B. Inj Medroxyprogesterone acetate IM
C. Tab Norethisterone (1 mg) + Ethinyl Estradiol (30 mcg) 1 tablet stat
D. Etonorgestrel vaginal ring

CASE 13

A 32-year-old newly married lady SW, went to a gynaecologist to seek advice for contraception. The gynaecologist tells her about barrier and hormonal methods and asks her preference. She tells she would prefer hormonal method considering failure rates of other methods. The treating gynaecologist asks her about any other medical illness. SW informs that she has 1-2 migraine attacks per year.

13.1 Which one of the following contraceptives the gynaecologist should prefer for SW?

A. Barrier contraceptive
B. Combination oral contraceptive tablets
C. Medicated IUCD
D. Follow calendar method for contraception

CASE 14

A 50-year-old man came to the casualty with symptoms of angina and was given sublingual nitroglycerine, following which his BP dropped from 120 mm Hg to 60 mm Hg. History revealed that the patient was on medication for some sexual disorder.

14.1 Which drug could have caused this fall in BP?
- A. Testosterone cypionate
- B. Tadalafil
- C. Alprostadil
- D. Flibanserin

CASE 15

Mrs. LM is a 57-year-old lady who presents to the outpatient clinic with left wrist pain and swelling following a fall on an outstretched hand while mopping the floor at home. This patient has a medical history of hypertension and attained menopause at age of 50. She does no exercise and is fully mobile with no disabilities. The patient is currently taking lisinopril for her hypertension. LM weighs 75 kg, her BP is 145/88 mm of Hg and pulse rate is 90/ min. Her left wrist is swollen and hurts on movement. X-ray of the left hand reveals Colles' fracture. The hospital then puts a cast on the patient's hand. Her blood test was normal except for low levels of Vitamin D. Her DEXA scan, reveals a T score of –2.9 (Less than –2.5 is osteoporosis).
Patient LM is advised to start exercising daily and eat a healthy diet and be careful while walking and working at home.

15.1 What is the dose of prescribed calcium and vitamin D for LM?
- A. Daily calcium 1500 mg + vitamin D 800 IU/day
- B. Daily calcium 500 mg + vitamin D 500 IU/ day
- C. Daily calcium 1000 mg + weekly vitamin D 600 IU
- D. Weekly calcium 1200 mg + daily vitamin D 600 IU

15.2 The treating physician also starts LM on antiresorptive agent. What is the preferred drug?
- A. Alendronate tablet 70 mg daily
- B. Calcitonin nasal spray
- C. Inj. Denosumab once a month
- D. Ibandronate tablet 150 mg per month

15.3 After 6 months LM complains of headache and her BP is 160/ 100 mm of Hg in spite of taking lisinopril daily. The preferred anti-hypertensive drug to be additionally prescribed to LM will be:
- A. atenolol 25 mg
- B. hydrochlorothiazide 25 mg
- C. telmisartan 20 mg
- D. clonidine 1 mg

SECTION 14. DRUGS USED IN COMMON SKIN AND EYE DISORDERS

CASE 1

A 26 -year-old married lady, ST comes to the dermatology OPD, with complains of pimples on her face. She gives a history of similar complaints since teenage, and use of over-the-counter medications for the same, but nothing seemed to work. On examination, the treating dermatologist detects small comedones and some large pustules on her cheeks and forehead, with no evidence of scarring. The dermatologist makes a diagnosis of mild Acne vulgaris with inflammation.

1.1 What will be the preferred medication for ST?

A. Clindamycin (1%) gel for 1 month

B. Tab. Doxycycline 100 mg OD with benzoyl peroxide (2.5%) gel for 1 month

C. Oral Isotretinoin 20 mg BD and Clindamycin (1%) gel for 1 month

D. Oral Azithromycin 500 mg OD for 3 days and benzoyl peroxide (2.5%) gel for 15 days

CASE 2

A 35-year-old male VG, presents to the general OPD with complains of itching and peeling of skin of 2nd and 3rd digits of left foot, since the past 2 weeks. On enquiry, he gives a history of wearing tight shoes all day long, and on examination it was observed that there was toe web scaling, fissuring and maceration. The treating doctor makes a diagnosis of Tinea pedis.

2.1 What drug should he prescribe to VG?

A. Benzoic acid (6%) – Salicyclic acid (3%) ointment for 1 month

B. Nystatin powder twice daily application for 2 weeks

C. Tab. Fluconazole 150 mg as a single dose

D. Tab. Terfinafine 250 mg daily for 1 month

CASE 3

A 60-year-old male BT, presents to the dermatology clinic with severe psoriasis involving his scalp, trunk, and extremities. He has a history of congestive heart failure and hypertension. The treating dermatologist decides to start BT on systemic medications.

3.1 Which of the following medications has the least risk of potential cardiovascular side effects in BT?

A. Methotrexate

B. Cyclosporine

C. Adalimumab

D. Ustekinumab

CASE 4

Mr. AG, a 70-year-old man, visits his ophthalmologist with complaints of blind spots in his peripheral vision which have gradually increased over the past one year. There is no other complaint. He also suffers from diabetes and hypertension for the last 20 years for which he is taking treatment. On examination his BP is 126/84 mm of Hg and his last lab investigation indicates that his diabetes is under control. Clinical examination of the eye indicates that the intraocular pressure is 24 mm of Hg.

4.1 Which of the following drugs would you prescribe to Mr. AG?

A. Acetazolamide

B. Brimonidine

C. Latanoprost

D. Pilocarpine

CASE 5

Mrs. GR, a 36-year-old woman, visits the ophthalmologist with complaints of redness in the eye associated with severe pain, blurred vision since the previous evening. Her discomfort increases when exposed to bright light. On examination the ophthalmologist makes the diagnosis of iridocyclitis.

5.1 Which of the following eye drops should the ophthalmologist use in Mrs. GR?

A. Dipivefrine
B. Atropine
C. Cyclopentolate
D. Phenylephrine

CASE 6

A 16-year-old boy, JY visits the ophthalmologist with complaints of severe pain in the right eye. The ophthalmologist notices that the eye is red and watering. The boy informs the doctor that while walking on the road he felt that something had entered his eye and he rubbed his eye to remove it. Suspecting injury to the cornea, ophthalmologist instills a dye in the eye to find out the extent of damage to the cornea.

6.1 Which of the following dyes do you think was instilled by the ophthalmologist?

A. Methylene blue
B. Gentian violet
C. Rose Bengal
D. Indocyanine green

SECTION 15. IMMUNOPHARMACOLOGY

CASE 1

A 35-year-old male patient MS underwent liver transplant for autoimmune hepatitis. He was started on immediate maintenance immunosuppression therapy to prevent graft versus host disease.

1.1 Which immunosuppressants will be included in this therapy?

A. Prednisone + cyclosporine
B. Hydrocortisone + mycophenolate + azathioprine
C. Azathioprine + cyclosporine
D. Tacrolimus + mycophenolate + prednisone

CASE 2

SM, a 25-year-old woman, who had undergone bone marrow transplantation, developed jaundice and vomiting after a month. She also had rash over her hands and face. The treating physician did her LFT. The liver transaminases were found to be elevated more than 20 times the upper limit of normal. A diagnosis of probable graft versus host reaction is made. SM was already on prednisone + cyclosporine + methotrexate regimen.

2.1 In emergency management, the preferred steroid in this setting will be:

A. prednisone
B. methylprednisolone
C. triamcinolone
D. betamethasone

CASE 3

Mrs. AR delivers a baby boy in a private hospital. She enquires about vaccines to be administered to the newborn.

3.1 The attending doctor will advise which of the following vaccines?
- A. DPT, OPV, Hib
- B. BCG, OPV, Hepatitis B
- C. DPT, OPV, Hepatitis B
- D. BCG, OPV, Rotavirus

CASE 4

Mr. SD, a 67-year-old man has completed his course of cancer chemotherapy 2 months back. He visits his GP saying that he wishes to get immunised against a few diseases as he is worried that he may get infected.

4.1 Which of the following vaccines cannot be administered to Mr. SD immediately?
- A. Pneumococcal vaccine
- B. Influenza vaccine
- C. Meningococcal vaccine
- D. Varicella vaccine

CASE 5

Mr. RK, a 55-year-old man is diagnosed to be suffering from metastatic colorectal cancer. After carrying out the required investigations, his physician decides to initiate chemotherapy with folinic acid, 5-fluorouracil, irinotecan (FOLFIRI) along with targeted cancer therapy with a monoclonal antibody.

5.1 Which of the following monoclonal antibodies will be administered to Mr. RK?
- A. Cetuximab
- B. Rituximab
- C. Abciximab
- D. Basiliximab

5.2 Which of the following antigens is likely to be targeted in the above situation?
- A. CTLA4
- B. EGFR
- C. BAFF
- D. HER2

SECTION 16. MISCELLANEOUS

CASE 1

PT, a 58-year-old male, presents to his family physician stating that he has pain in the right great toe since last night. On inquiry PT states that he did not sleep the entire night. The physician enquires about any history of trauma but PT denies. The physician on examination finds that right great toe is red, swollen and tender and even other toes are inflamed. The physician suspects that PT could have suffered an acute attack of gout.

1.1 Which drug should be prescribed to PT orally for immediate pain relief?
- A. Aspirin 500 mg
- B. Naproxen 500 mg
- C. Methylprednisolone 5 mg
- D. Tramadol 50 mg

The physician advises PT to get serum urate levels done and the reports reflect a reading of 10 mg%. PT is hypertensive and on Tab telmisartan 40 mg.

1.2 Which drug will PT receive now as prophylactic therapy?

A. Prednisolone
B. Low dose colchicine
C. Allopurinol
D. Indomethacin

After starting the prophylactic therapy, PT again visits his family physician after 2 weeks with complains of maculopapular rash all over the body. There is no fever or difficulty in breathing. On inquiry PT informs he has no pain in his right foot but the rash is disturbing.

1.3 What should the family physician do now?

A. Continue the prophylactic therapy for gout
B. Start concomitant colchicine therapy
C. Advise PT to drink 2–3 litres of water/day
D. Change to non – purine prophylactic therapy

CASE 2

A 65-year-old female patient, SY was admitted to AVB Hospital with the chief complaint of pain in her shoulder, swelling and pain in joints of both the hands. On enquiry, SY informed the doctor that she had moderate pain and stiffness in fingers since the past 1 year on and off, accompanied by malaise and fatigue. Since the past 2 weeks, SY was prescribed ibuprofen 800 mg 3 times per day by her family doctor. There was temporary relief but the pain and stiffness has been gradually increasing and yesterday the pain was so severe that family doctor referred her to this hospital. The doctor at the hospital sends blood samples of SY for RA factor, HsCRP and ESR.

2.1 What should the doctor prescribe to SY while awaiting the laboratory reports?

A. Continue with higher dose of ibuprofen
B. Change over to indomethacin
C. Start oral prednisolone
D. Administer triamcinolone intra-articularly

Within 3 days all blood reports of SY are available and diagnosis of rheumatoid arthritis is done by the rheumatologist visiting the hospital.

2.2 What will be the preferred therapy for SY now?

A. Stop earlier medication and start methotrexate
B. Continue earlier medication and start methotrexate
C. Continue the earlier medication and prescribe ibuprofen for acute flares
D. Stop earlier medication and start joint physiotherapy

CASE 3

A male child aged 6 years, was brought to the pediatric emergency department with an acute abdominal pain, vomiting and severe constipation. Ultrasonography revealed that there was no intestinal obstruction. The child was weak and irritable. On detailed history, it was revealed that child has a habit of eating paint flakes which probably contained lead.

3.1 Which of the following treatment should be started immediately for the child to prevent lead encephalopathy?

A. Dimercaprol
B. Calcium disodium edetate
C. d-Penicillamine
D. Trientine

3.2 The child is started with appropriate lead chelation therapy. He needs to be monitored for:

A. tetany
B. hepatoxicity
C. hypertension
D. hypoglycemia

KEYS FOR CASE BASED MCQs

Case scenarios for Section 1

Case 1. 1.1: C; 1.2: A; 1.3: C;
Case 2. 2.1: B;
Case 3. 3.1: A;
Case 4. 4.1: A; 4.2: B;
Case 5. 5.1: A;
Case 6. 6.1: B;
Case 7. 7.1: D;
Case 8. 8.1: B;
Case 9. 9.1: A;
Case 10. 10.1: D;
Case 11. 11.1: C;
Case 12. 12.1: B; 12.2: C;
Case 13. 13.1: A;
Case 14. 14.1: C;
Case 15. 15.1: D;
Case 16.16.1: D;
Case 17. 17.1: A;
Case 18. 18.1: D.

Case scenarios for Section 2

Case 1. 1.1: B;
Case 2. 2.1: B; 2.2: A;
Case 3. 3.1: D;
Case 4. 4.1: B; 4.2: C;
Case 5. 5.1: C;
Case 6. 6.1: A;
Case 7. 7.1: D; 7.2: C;
Case 8. 8.1: C; 8.2: A;
Case 9. 9.1: B; 9.2: C;
Case 10. 10.1: A; 10.2: C;
Case 11. 11.1: C; 11.2: C; 11.3: B.

Case scenarios for Section 3

Case 1. 1.1: B;
Case 2. 2.1: B.

Case scenarios for Section 4

Case 1. 1.1: B; 1.2: D;
Case 2. 2.1: B;
Case 3. 3.1: C;
Case 4. 4.1: C;
Case 5. 5.1: C;
Case 6. 6.1: A.

Case scenarios for Section 5

Case 1. 1.1: C; 1.2: B; 1.3: C;
Case 2. 2.1: A; 2.2: C;
Case 3. 3.1: A; 3.2: C; 3.3: D;
Case 4. 4.1: B; 4.2: A; 4.3: A: Epoprostenol, B: Latanoprost, C: Misoprostol, D: Alprostadil.

Case scenarios for Section 6

Case 1. 1.1: D;
Case 2. 2.1: C.

Case scenarios for Section 7

Case 1. 1.1: A; 1.2: C;
Case 2. 2.1: C;
Case 3. 3.1: C; 3.2: A;
Case 4. 4.1: A;
Case 5. 5.1: D;
Case 6. 6.1: B;
Case 7. 7.1: A;
Case 8. 8.1: B;
Case 9. 9.1: D;
Case 10. 10.1: A;
Case 11. 11.1: B;
Case 12. 12.1: C; 12.2: B.

Case scenarios for Section 8

Case 1. 1.1: D; 1.2: D;
Case 2. 2.1: A;
Case 3. 3.1: A; 3.2: B;
Case 4. 4.1: D; 4.2: C; 4.3: B; 4.4: B; 4.5: A;
Case 5. 5.1: A.

Case scenarios for Section 9

Case 1. 1.1: A;
Case 2. 2.1: C; 2.2: D.

Case scenarios for Section 10

Case 1. 1.1: A;
Case 2. 2.1: B;
Case 3. 3.1: B; 3.2: B;
Case 4. 4.1: D;
Case 5. 5.1: B;
Case 6. 6.1: A.

Case scenarios for Section 11

Case 1. 1.1: B;
Case 2. 2.1: A; 2.2: C.

Case scenarios for Section 12

Case 1. 1.1: B;
Case 2. 2.1: C;
Case 3. 3.1: C; 3.2: B; 3.3: A;
Case 4. 4.1: A;
Case 5. 5.1: B;
Case 6. 6.1: A;
Case 7. 7.1: C; 7.2: D; 7.3: C;
Case 8. 8.1: A;
Case 9. 9.1: C;
Case 10. 10.1: B;
Case 11. 11.1: B;
Case 12. 12.1: D; 12.2: B; 12.3: A;
Case 13. 13.1: C; 13.2:A;
Case 14. 14.1: A;
Case 15. 15.1: C;
Case 16. 16.1: A; 16.2: C;
Case 17. 17.1: B; 17.2: D;
Case 18. 18.1: C; 18.2: A; 18.3: D;
Case 19. 19.1: D;
Case 20. 20.1: A; 20.2: C;
Case 21. 21.1: A; 21.2: B; 21.3: B.

Case scenarios for Section 13

Case 1. 1.1: B; 1.2: C; 1.3: D; 1.4: D;
Case 2. 2.1: B;
Case 3. 3.1: A;
Case 4. 4.1: D;
Case 5. 5.1: B;
Case 6. 6.1: C;
Case 7. 7.1: B;
Case 8. 8.1: B;
Case 9. 9.1: C;
Case 10. 10.1: A; 10.2: B; 10.3: B;
Case 11. 11.1: A; 11.2: B; 11.3: C;
Case 12. 12.1: A;
Case 13. 13.1: C;
Case 14. 14.1: B;
Case 15. 15.1: A; 15.2: D; 15.3: B.

Case scenarios for Section 14

Case 1. 1.1: B;
Case 2. 2.1: D;
Case 3. 3.1: A;
Case 4. 4.1: C;
Case 5. 5.1: B;
Case 6. 6.1: C.

Case scenarios for Section 15

Case 1. 1.1: D;
Case 2. 2.1: B;
Case 3. 3.1: B;
Case 4. 4.1: D;
Case 5. 5.1: A; 5.2: B.

Case scenarios for Section 16

Case 1. 1.1: B; 1.2: C; 1.3: D;
Case 2. 2.1: C; 2.2: B;
Case 3. 3.1: B; 3.2: A.